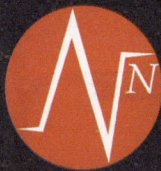

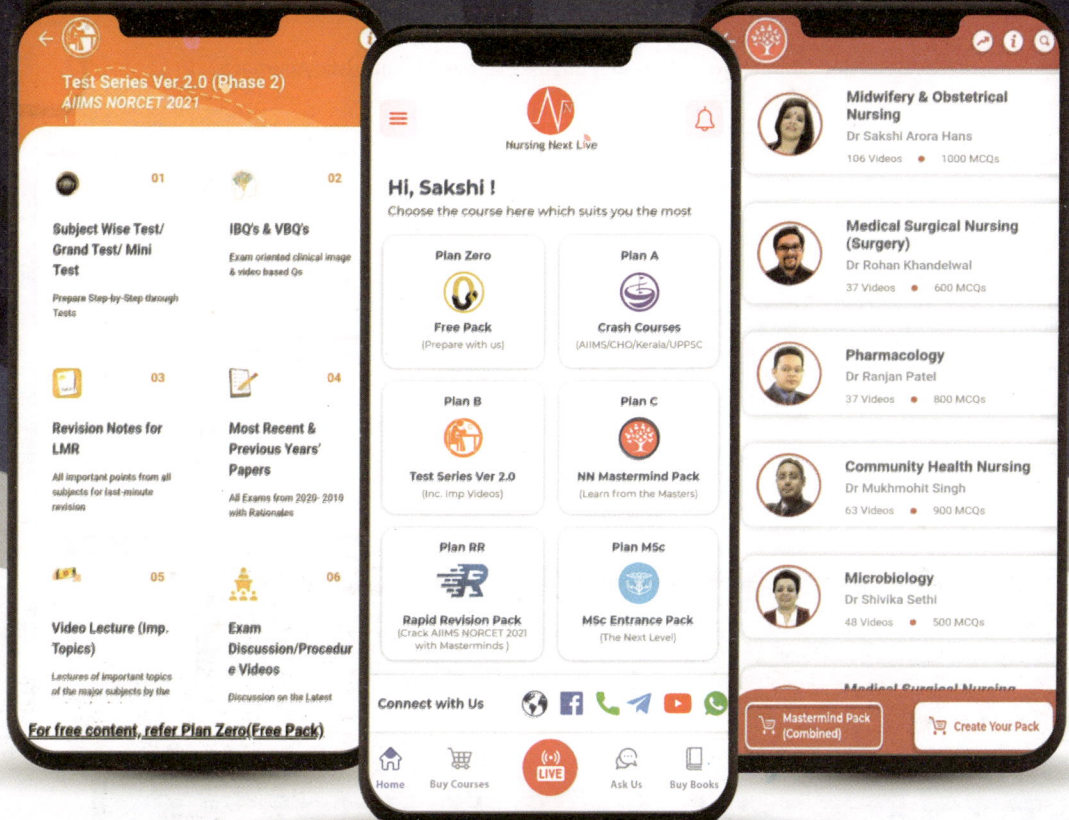

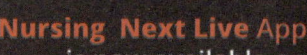
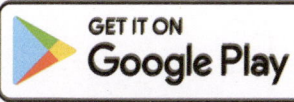
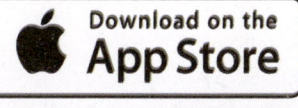
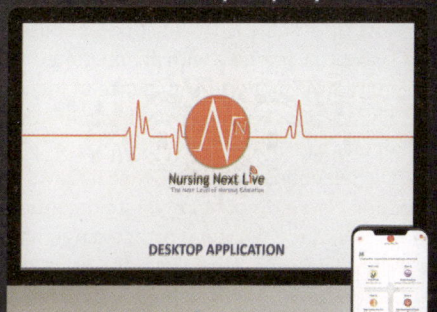

ABOUT US

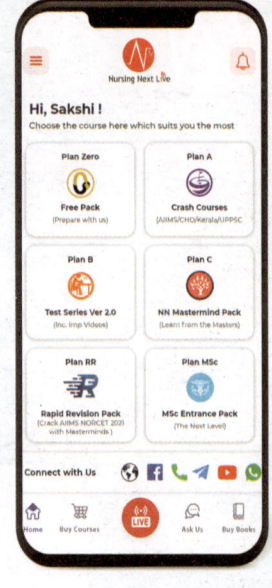

Nursing Next Live has been conceptualized based on the observation that there is a huge gap between the educational services available to the medical graduates and the nursing students. As these two are the strong pillars in providing holistic care to the patients, it is extremely vital that nurses should get equal exposure to access learning. To overcome this issue, we have come forward with the commitment of providing quality education to the nurses in India at their doorstep through Nursing Next Live. And therefore, we say **"We are bringing Learning to the People Instead of People Going for Learning".**

It is India's first and the biggest digital learning platform in the field of Nursing Education. The Nursing Next Live is an interactive self-assessment app, which helps you to build knowledge of nursing specialities any time and anywhere. In a span of one year we have magnified the nursing sector by upscaling it with the strategically designed Quality Content by the Top Medical Faculties of India. We at Nursing Next Live envisage that all students from Kashmir to Kanyakumari should get quality education. We pledge to give the best learning experience to all our students, under one single roof, and that is **"All-in-one and One-in-All platform".**

The Core Values and Principles of Nursing Next Live is:

- First Digital Learning platform for All Nursing Competitive & Undergraduates Exams with Futuristic Approach
- We are bringing Learning to People, Instead of People going for learning!
- Concept Based Teaching by TOP Medical & Nursing Educators (The Masterminds)
- "Quality Content" & "Smart-Study" Approach
- One in All, All in One! Nothing Beyond
- 360 Degree Approach for your complete Preparation
- Most Up to date & updated Content
- Best Guidance & Support at every step
- Best Interface with Unique & Advance Features
- Everything at one Platform ...Buy CBS Nursing Books at Special Discounts/Cashbacks

Nursing Next Live is the fastest-growing Edutech organization in the field of Nursing! With **70k+** downloads, **1200+** total number of selections, **150+** AIIMS NORCET 2020 Selections, and many backend achievements it is the Highest Ranked App on the Play Store. The idea was possible to bring into reality because it was backed by the team of best professionals who did not see time; had One vision and One Goal in Mind of providing the students Nothing but The Best! Their trust towards the vision for the brand and their efforts to continuously make it a success helped Nursing Next to reach to this position

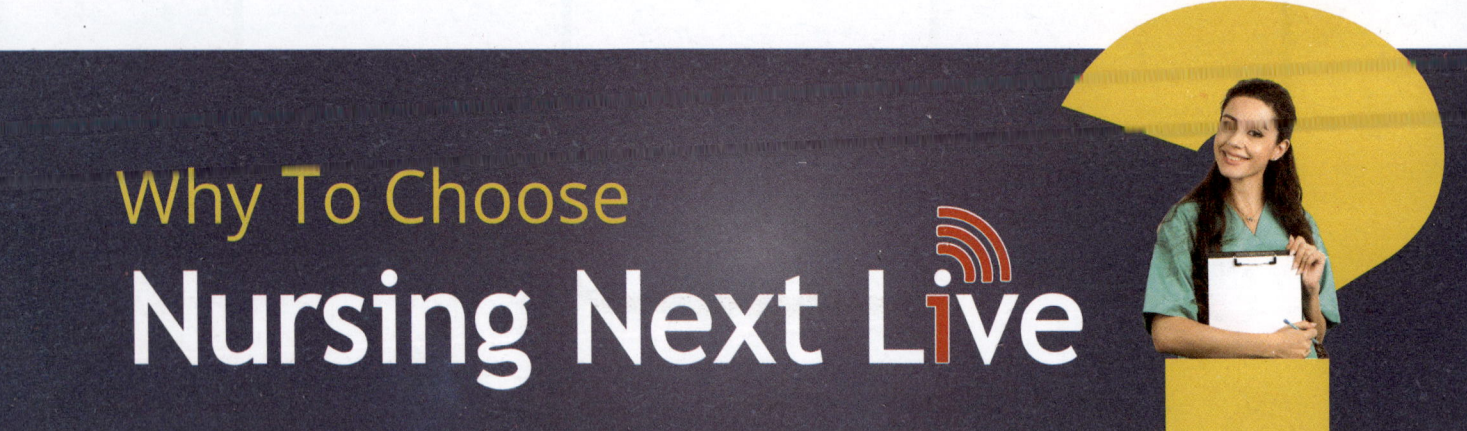

Why To Choose Nursing Next Live

- India's 1st Digital Learning Platform for all nursing competitive, nursing undergraduate and nursing postgraduate exams (One-in-All, All-in-One)
- User friendly interface with unique & advanced features
- Most Up-to-date & Quality Content based on New INC Syllabus
- Conceptual learning with an integrated and futuristic approach
- Smart Study under the guidance of India's Top Educators who are the masterminds of their subjects
- Enhance your learning from Basic To Advance level with a 360-degree approach
- Regular Live Doubt Sessions and Live Tests based on real-time exam pattern
- TOP Selections in AIIMS NORCET, AIIMS MSc, BFUHS, CHO, SGPGI, JIPMER, RRB, DSSSB etc (From Rank 1 to 1000)
- Study Planner that helps you to organize your study
- Faculty-Student Meet (Forthcoming) that provides you an opportunity to meet with faculty and get clarify your doubts
- Printed Booklet: You will get the printed notes of the video lectures that will save your time in notes making and organize your time in a better way
- Customize Study which helps you to create your own pack depending on your needs and wants
- Daily dose of information keeps you updated everyday with new information
- One-in-all all-in-one: You will get exam oriented plan in the app for whatever exams you are targeting. Simulation Videos

THE COMPLETE PACKAGE

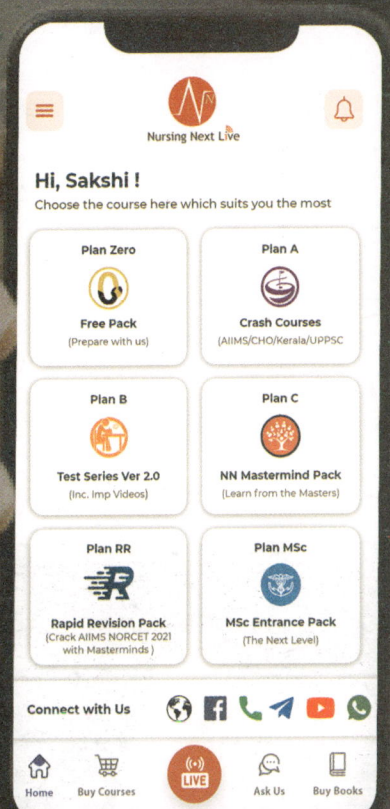

50,000+
MCQs with their Rationale

2000+
Hours of Recorded video lectures (Covering All Subjects/All Topics/ Imp Topics Chanting Videos/Exam Discussions/LMR/IBQ & VBQs Discussions)

150+
Previous years' question papers covering all National & State Level Exams (2021-2010)

Monthly/Weekly/Daily
Live Doubt Sessions & Faculty-Students' Meet (Forthcoming)

1500+
E-Notes/Flash cards of all the subjects for Last-minute Revision

1000+
Image-based Questions with their Rationale

200+
Video-based Questions with their Rationale

Monthly
Special Mega Assessment Tests, National Scholarship Test with up to 100% Scholarship & Reward points

200+
CBS Nursing Books available for purchase

200+
Newly Created Subject-wise cum Topic-wise Test, Mini Test & Grand Tests based on all important National Exams like AIIMS, PGIMER, JIPMER, DSSSB, RRB & ESIC, also State level exams like Kerala PSC

Special Features

Live Classes

Live Doubt Sessions

Mega Assessment Tests

Live Webinars

Faculty-Student Meet on Zoom Sessions

Study Plans

Success Stories

Daily Dose of Knowledge

Blogs

National Scholarship Test with upto 100% scholarship

Any Doubt Ask Us

Exam Notifications

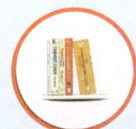
Buy CBS Nursing Books

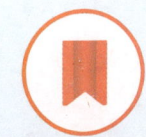
Bookmark Your Imp Topics

Download Videos/ Notes

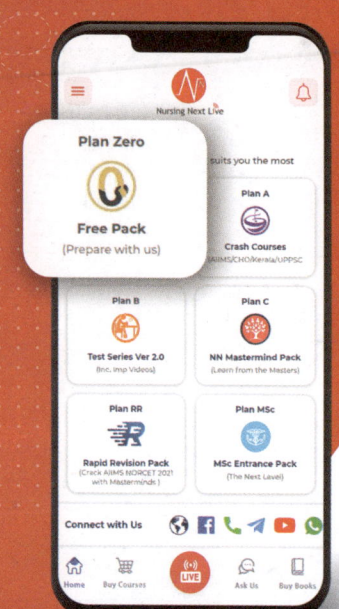

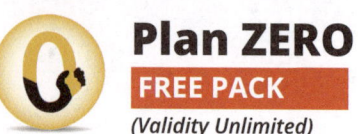

"जांचो, परखो, फिर खरीदो!"

Plan ZERO
FREE PACK
(Validity Unlimited)

Nursing Next Live focuses on providing you the with the best and beyond, nothing less. In Plan ZERO we provide you the glimpse of the content from the various pack that gives you the rights to explore the contents in the App and help in taking the right decisions before selecting the pack.

WHY TO EXPLORE
- Glimpse of the content from the various packs
- TRY-TRUST-OPT. It provides you the rights to first analyze and then go for the best pack
- Enriched content

BEST FOR
- Those who want to explore before selecting the right pack
- Students who have an urge to gain the last momentum by giving a final touch to their preparation.

What all you will get

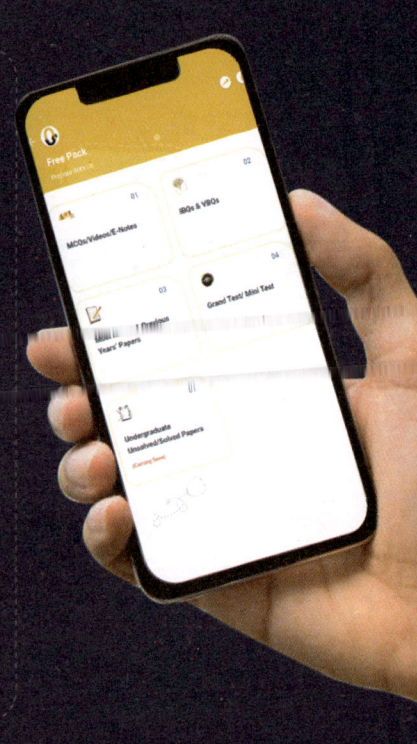

- **2000+** MCQs with Rationale covering All Subjects, Important Topics
- **150+** E-Notes covering All Subjects, Selective important Topics
- **100+** Hours of Lectures covering All Subjects (Topic-wise/Imp Topics/Chanting/Exam Discussions)
- **100+** IBQs & VBQs of All Subjects
- **15** Most Recent/Previous Years Papers with Rationale
- **5+** Grand Test & Bonus Test based on Real Time Exam Pattern
- **5+** National Scholarship test with negaitive marking, National Level Ranking & Cash Rewards
- Daily Dose of Knowledge— Word of the Day, Fact of the Day, Practice Pearls, Question of the Day
- Unsolved & Solved Question Papers of BSc 1st to 4th Year in a consolidated manner covering all Important Universities (Forthcoming)
- Monthly National Scholarship Test with Special Discount for Top Rankers
- How to Prepare for Exams (in the form of Study Planner/Videos)
- Complete Access to Target High Extra Edge Section – which includes additional MCQs & Golden Points in Video Form

Selections in
Various Competitive Nursing Exams

What our glorified achievers say about **Nursing Next Live**

REFURBISHING MY SKILLS WITH THE EXCLUSIVE TESTS!

"MAT and NST helped me in cracking my exams. The regular live sessions by top-notch faculty add to the advantage."

Harjeet Signh
(Rank-1, BFUHS)

CONCEPT BASED LEARNING!

"An effective app in clearing the concepts and doubt of students in very simple terms and the faculty is very professional."

Suresh Kumar
(Rank-1, CHO-MP)

LEARNING MY WAY THROUGH WITH NNLIVE!

"The study content is prepared by the experts, which helped me in polishing my knowledge in all the vital subjects."

Rahul Dahiya
(AIR Rank-3, NORCET'2020)

"लक्ष्य तय है, तो PLAN A सही है!"

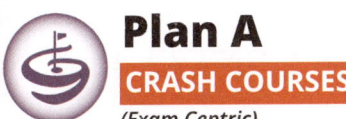

Plan A
CRASH COURSES
(Exam Centric)

If you have a set target and working to achieve it then Plan A is the perfect plan for you. We have come up with this plan to help you prepare for a particular exam that includes exam-centric AIIMS NORCET 2020, SGPGI, CHO & Target Kerala PSC Crash Courses to help you get a hold of every topic in-depth. You get access to in-detailed content of Real-Time Pattern of exams and their latest syllabus. Put your hands on the best!

WHY TO SUBSCRIBE
• Exam specific, it targets the specific exam therefore its pattern syllabus is as per the targeted exam
• Get Acquainted with exam pattern that helps you improve your skills
• Helps in the last minute revision

BEST FOR
• Those who are preparing for specific exams and want to improve their knowledge by practicing
• Those who are working professionals and want to prepare for exams along with their jobs

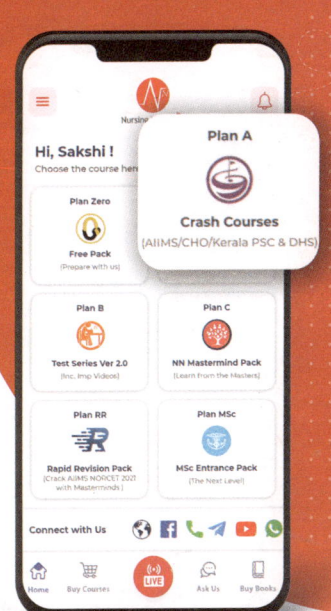

What all you will get

Plan A1
CHO Crash Course

• 35+ Subject-wise Tests & Grand Tests (including Bonus Tests & Previous Years Papers)
• 1500+ Questions with rationale
• 70+ E-notes for last-minute revision covering all the important topics as per the syllabus of CHO
• 30+ (Duration of 30+ Hours) Pre-recorded Videos given by top faculties in Hinglish covering every important topic from exam point of view

MRP ₹689/- | **Validity 2 Months**

Plan A2
AIIMS NORCET 2020 Crash Course

• 60+ Live Tests Subject-wise based on AIIMS Delhi pattern
• 1500+ Qs with Rationale including MCQs, IBQs, VBQs, Clinical skills, Priority setting, and case study
• 15+ Mock Test, Revision Test, and Grand Tests based on Real-time pattern of AIIMS Delhi with Negative Marking and National Level Ranking
• All Subject-wise Tests & Grand Tests are with Detailed Rationale
• 140+ Last-Minute Revision Notes based on Frequently asked Topics of previous Years
• 12+ Videos on Chanting Session by Top Educators/Subject Experts
• 35+ Multiple videos on special tricks for non-nursing subjects, tips on memory retention, strategies to attempt exams, etc.
• Success Guaranteed as we have had 150+ Selections (Rank 3 to 5k) in AIIMS NORCET 2020.

MRP ₹1499/- | **Validity 2 Months**

Plan A3
Target Kerala PSC Crash Course

• 60+ Subject-wise/Grand Tests with Rationale
• 320+ E-Notes in the form of Subject-wisesynopsis
• 50+ Hours of Videos in English (Important Topics Pre-loaded video + Chanting videos)
• In association with our Best-Selling Title- Target High Staff Nurse Entrance Exam

MRP ₹945/- | **Validity 2 Months**

Plan A4
UPPSC Staff Nurse Crash Course

• 40+ subject-wise tests which cover the complete syllabus from basics to advance
• 7 Grand Tests Based on real time exam pattern
• 3 Extra Edge Tests covering Important Positions, Important Nursing Procedures, Drug Calculation, suture techniques & COVID special)
• Previous Year Paper Discussion video helps you how to approach the correct answer
• 25+ Quick Revision videos in one-liner form that covers all the important points from the weightage subject
• 1 **"SUCCESS MANTRA"** video to guide you the right approach for preparation

MRP ₹1499/- | **Validity 3 Months**

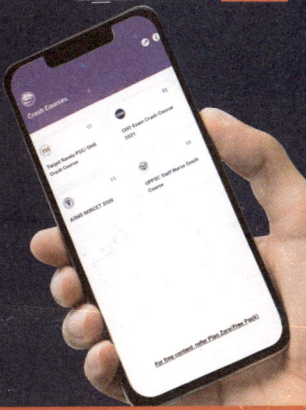

HIGH-END TEST SERIES LEVELS UP THE PROGRESS!
"The Test Series helped me get a quick overall analysis of my progress. "
Nisha Singla
(AIR Rank-12, NORCET'2020)

COMPREHENSIVE AND INFORMATIVE CONTENT!
"You get to be familiar with the Real-Time exam experience. Also, the content provided is very informative and easy to understand. "
Arushi Mittal
(AIR Rank-14, NORCET'2020)

MOVING FORWARD WITH CONFIDENCE!
"This app has helped me boost my confidence, just in my first attempt. The teachers here are superb and deserve a big thumbs up"
Komal Dhull
(AIR Rank-51, NORCET'2020)

BECOME AN ACHIEVER FROM A DREAMER!
"Greatly thankful to the NNL team who have helped me reach my preparation targets of achieving my desired rank. It means a lot to me"
Shivani Bourai
(AIR Rank-72, NORCET'2020)

BEST FOR GAINING THE LAST MINUTE MOMENTUM!
"The Image-Based and overall questions of the Nursing Next Live app are very informative and helpful for last-minute revision"
Nivedita Saini
(AIR Rank-79, NORCET'2020)

NN LIVE IS AS PROMISING AS IT CLAIMS!
"Nursing Next Live has helped me achieve great ranks in all the competitive exams that I have attempted. It does what it has promised and guides you through every step needed to succeed."
Rupali Garg
(AIR Rank-89, NORCET'2020)

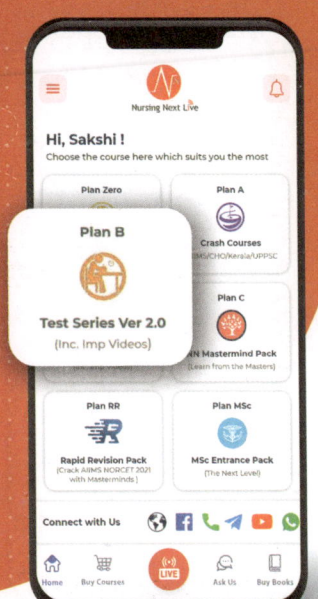

"आज का अभ्यास, आपके कल की सफलता!"

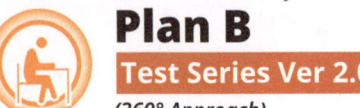

Plan B
Test Series Ver 2.0
(360° Approach)

Test series 2.0, as the name says to excel in any test, you need to base your learnings on two principles 1st is practice, practice, practice, and then 2nd is a 360-degree approach. Variety of subject-wise and topic-wise tests, IBQs, and VBQs that follow the latest exam fashion to help you level up your preparatory work. To give a complete touch to the preparation, we have covered all important national & state level last 15 years papers with important topics/ exam discussion videos.

WHY TO SUBSCRIBE
- Comprehensive test pack with 360 degree approach for those who are targeting any staff nurse examination of National or State level
- Keep track of your progress through test analysis report
- Last-minute revision notes of important topics from all the subjects
- Detailed explanation helps you to enhance your knowledge

BEST FOR
- The students who want to delve into the topic and opt for extensive preparation for any staff nurse entrance exam.
- Who never want to stop learning and always look forward to upgrading their pre-acquired knowledge.
- Working students who don't want to compromise with their preparation and success.

What all you will get

Pre Loaded Content (Phase 1 + Phase 2)

- **190+** Newly Created Subject-wise, Mini Test and Grand Test focusing all important National Exams AIIMS, PGIMER, JIPMER, DSSSB, RRB and ESIC
- **15K+** Qs (MCQs, IBQs, VBQs) with Rationale and updated reference from standard textbooks. All the Tests are designed by the Subject Experts and Topper Students
- **400+** Hours Recorded Video Lectures of Nursing/Non-Nursing Subjects by some of India's best nursing faculties/subject experts. Lectures are in English/Hindi language focusing on concept-based learning.
- **5** Exam Discussion Videos of 2019 Exam papers (Duration 20 Hours)
- **150+** Hours of Recorded Video on Subject-wise Exam Discussion of previous years papers (2017-18) of all nursing exams delivered by subject experts
- **5** Skill Procedure videos demonstrating Nursing Skills in real-time
- **100+** Previous Year Exam Papers of all Nursing Exams from 2020-10 with Rationale (Attempt/View PDF Mode)
- **1500+** Flashcards/E-notes on all the important topics of all the subjects for last minute revision (In 6 months)
- **800+** Image-based Questions with Rationale
- **200+** Video-based Qs with Rationale
- **Complete Access to Plan A-Crash Courses**

New Content (Phase 3) Q Bank Pack

- **8000+** Qs in Q Bank form of all the topics from all the subjects
- **700+** E-Notes covering all subjects/all topics

| MRP ₹3497/- | Validity 4 Months |
| MRP ₹6998/- | Validity 6 Months |

TESTIMONIALS

What our subscribers say about "TEST SERIES PLAN"

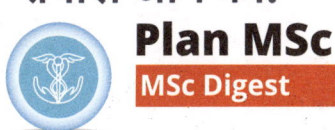

"तैयारी आगे की!"
Plan MSc
MSc Digest

We cant be louder about It, Nursing Next Live is the only growing platform offering MSc preparations to the aspirants. As we say, that your success is our success, so we always look forward to providing the best and beyond study content with a futuristic approach. MSc Digest contains every vital information about the subjects in one place so that it gets easy for all to access the content on one platform.

WHY TO SUBSCRIBE
- Make your preparation easy with your job
- Enriched content helps you to prepare, revise and assess
- Content is prepared by the top Medical & Nursing experts
- Guidance and support

BEST FOR
- Who are always hungry to gain more knowledge from anywhere when they get a chance.
- Who believe in focusing on one topic at a time
- Who want to go further and upgrade their study content to the next level.

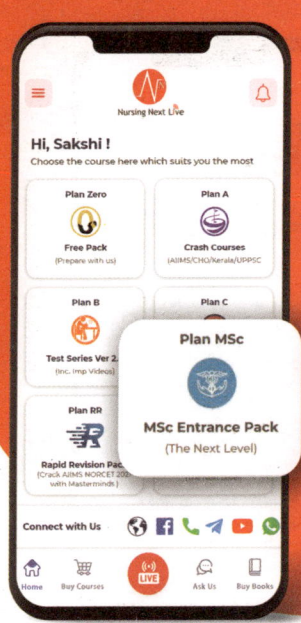

What all you will get

- Subject-wise synopsis covering image base illustrations and interesting Mnemonics to provide an extra edge preparation
- **3500+** MCQs covering the important topics of all subjects
- **800+** IBQs covering all subjects/topics
- **10+** Milestone papers covering more than 1000 MCQs to imbibe the environment of a real examination
- **3** Tests covering 150 IBQs
- **3** Tests covering 75 VBQs
- **10** Previous year papers (2020-2017) covering questions based on important topics/sub-topics from all subjects
- Exam capsules in the form of flashcards & tables
- **400+** LMR flashcards covering all subjects
- Hard copy of notes will be provided

MRP ₹1999/- | **Validity 90 Days**

TESTIMONIALS

What our glorified achievers of MSc Entrance Exam say about Nursing Next Live

ONE APP WITH A COMPLETE GUIDE TO NURSING SUCCESS!
"NNL has helped me a lot in preparing for MSc entrance exam and get a good rank. I will recommend this for every Nursing Aspirant out there."
Sabarni
(AIR Rank-21, AIIMS MSc 2021)

TAKING UNDERSTANDING TO THE NEXT LEVEL!
"It has helped me clear every doubt and that made my understanding of the subjects clearer. Thank you, team!"
Ritika Rajpoot
(AIR Rank-23, AIIMS MSc 2021)

THOROUGHLY RECOMMENDED PLAN 101!
"It was a wonderful experience studying from the top educators and getting counseled by them."
Priti Prajapati
(AIR Rank-39, AIIMS MSc 2021)

NNL FOUND ME WHAT I WAS LOOKING FOR!
"It helped me to polish my subject knowledge and upgraded my preparations. Overall, It is an excellent application for all the Nursing Aspirants."
Pritika Thakur
(AIR Rank-119, AIIMS MSc 2021)

AS EFFICIENT AS THE APP CLAIMS TO BE!
"This app is very helpful if you are looking forward to clearing your doubts in a comprehensive way. The faculty is highly professional and informative."
Aditi Yadav
(AIR Rank-133, AIIMS MSc 2021)

STRESS TURNED INTO THE JOY OF STUDYING!
"NN Live has made me admire the study pattern they follow. The way of teaching of the faculty is very helpful and valuable and filled with enthusiasm."
Shivani Shashni
(AIR Rank-173, AIIMS MSc 2021)

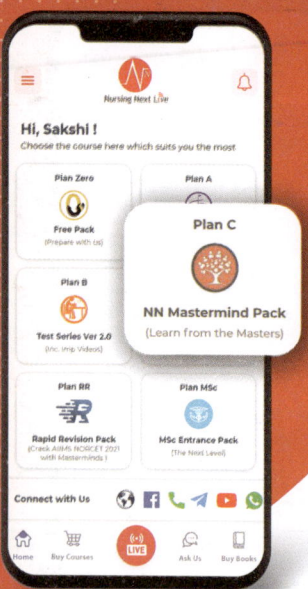

"ज्ञान हो बढ़ाना, तो PLAN C ही लेना!"

Plan C/C Plus
MASTERMIND Pack
(One-in-All, All-in-One)

Nursing Next's One in all, all in one Mastermind pack for complete preparation! Plan C plus is a full package that contains all that you need for your 100% preparation for all the Nursing competitive exams. The content of this package is curated and drafted by the Top-Educators of Nursing Next Live, who are the masterminds of their subjects. NN Mastermind Pack is a gradual phase-wise learning journey with the option of Individual and combined pack and a validity of 12 months!

WHY TO SUBSCRIBE
- Detailed lectures as per the INC syllabus
- Helps you in building the strong foundation
- The MASTERMINDS : India's top medical & nursing faculty is here to guide you
- Sufficient content to cater your undergraduate and entrance exams needs
- Handwritten notes of the lectures that help you to revise the topic
- Question Bank with the topics that help you to assess your understanding in that particular topic

BEST FOR
- Students who are at a good progression level and want to build up their foundation more.
- Those who look forward to studying from the best and beyond educators.
- The students who want to upgrade their knowledge or the one aiming for Staff Nurse Entrance Exam, and also for the Undergraduates.

SPECIAL FEATURES
- Nursing Next's "Mastermind Pack", is a One-Stop solution for all your exam preparation needs for Staff Nurse Entrance Exams & Nursing Undergraduate Exams!
- It is our One-in-All, All-in-One pack for the nursing students of the Digital era!
- NN Mastermind Pack is exactly that 'learning tool' for all the nursing aspirants. It is carefully planned, and strategically designed, under the expertise of TOP Medical/Nursing Educators, just to make learning more authentic and easier for our students.
- Covering All Subjects, All Topics concepts from Basics to Advanced level pattern with the help of Videos/Question Banks & Handwritten Notes
- The Masterminds (TOP EDUCATORS) of NN Live have focused on ALL the upcoming Nursing Exams by giving two convenient options under 'Individual Subject Pack', & 'Combined (NN Mastermind Pack)'
- NN Mastermind Pack is a "road to success" for those who are preparing for any or all staff nurse entrance exams.

What all you will get

Plan C (Including Plan RR)
- **1200+** hours of Video Lectures on All Subject/All Topics
- **11,000+** Questions with Rationale covering All Subject/All Topics
- IBQ/VBQ Video Discussions of All Subjects
- **Monthly Live Doubt Sessions/Live Classes**
- **80+Hours** of Rapid Revision Videos for AIIMS NORCET
- 2021 by Mastermind faculty
- **Handwritten Notes** of videos in PDF format integrated in the App
- Focusing on Quality study over quantity study, using the smart-study approach
- Monthly **Mega Assessment** Tests with National Level Ranking
- All upcoming exam's Important Topics & Exam/Discussions will be covered
- Complete **360-degree approach** for preparation
- Unlimited Watch Time, FREE Download Video option, National Level Ranks, Bookmark the content, Pause & Resume video option
- Best Guidance & Support at every stage
- Monthly Live Doubt Sessions/Live Classes/Live Webinars by Mastermind Faculty

Validity: 12 Months
MRP ₹12974/-

Plan C Plus (Including Plan A+B+C+RR)
- Plan A of NN Live (Complete access to Crash Courses—CHO/AIIMS NORCET 2020/KERALA PSC/UPPSC
  +
- Plan B of NN Live (Complete access to Test Series Pack FOCUSING AIIMS NORCET 2021 & Other Staff Nurse Exams)
  +
- Plan C of NN Live (Complete access to Plan C by the Mastermind Faculty
  +
- Plan RR of NN Live (Complete access to Rapid Revision Pack)

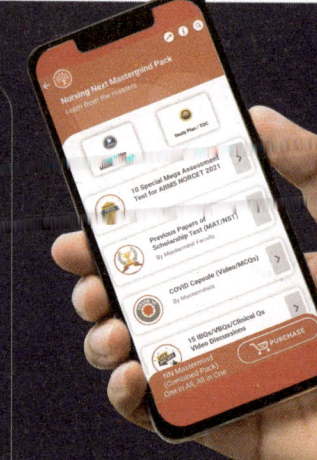

Validity: 6 Months
MRP ₹9995/-

Validity: 12 + 2 Bonus Months
MRP ₹15999/-

Validity: 24 Months
MRP ₹31998/-

Undergraduate Packs (Prof.-wise)

1st Year Students
- ✓ Anatomy
- ✓ Physiology
- ✓ Biochemistry & Nutrition
- ✓ Microbiology
- ✓ Fundamentals of Nursing

2nd Year Students
- ✓ Pharmacology
- ✓ MSN – Medicine
- ✓ MSN – Surgery
- ✓ Community Health Nursing
- ✓ Sociology
- ✓ CET

3rd & 4th Year Students
- ✓ Pediatric Nursing
- ✓ Midwifery & Obstetrical Nursing
- ✓ MSN – Medicine
- ✓ MSN – Surgery
- ✓ Mental Health Nursing
- ✓ Community Health Nursing
- ✓ Nursing Research & Statistics
- ✓ Nursing Management & Administration

Other Mastermind Plans

Mastermind Plan C
For 3rd & 4th Year Students those who are targeting for Staff Nurse Exams

Mastermind Plan C Plus
For Pass out Students those who are targeting for AIIMS NORCET & Staff Nurse Exams

The Masterminds

Learn from the Top Educators of India

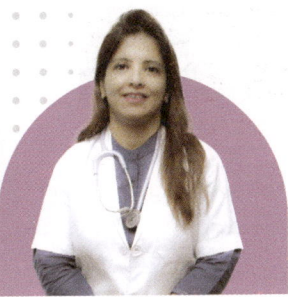

Dr Sakshi Arora Hans

Midwifery & Obstetrical Nursing

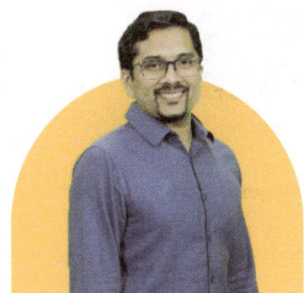

Dr Rohan Khandelwal

MSN - Surgery

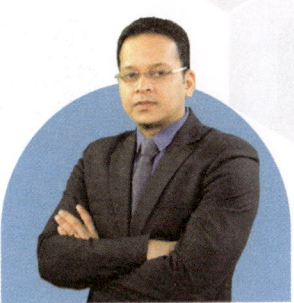

Dr Ranjan Patel

Pharmacology

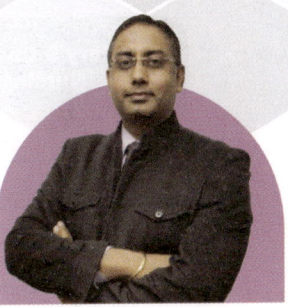

Dr Mukhmohit Singh

Community Health Nursing

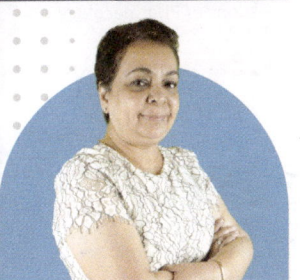

Dr Shivika Sethi

Microbiology

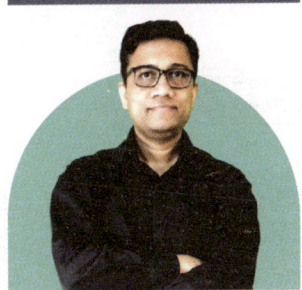

Dr Ashish Kumar

Physiology

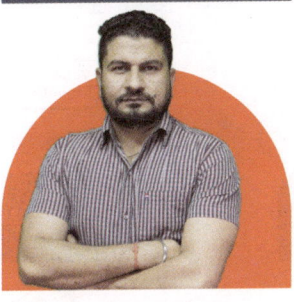

Dr Aman Setiya

MSN - Medicine

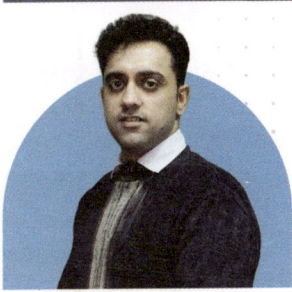

Dr Anand Bhatia

Pediatric Nursing

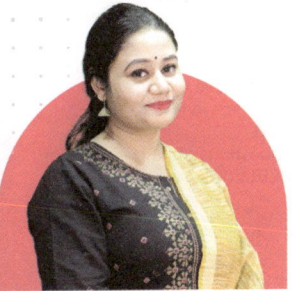

Ms Sabina Ali

Fundamentals of Nursing

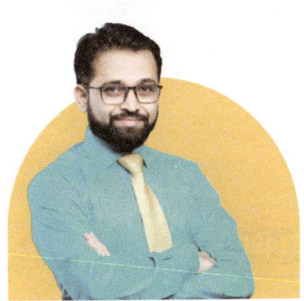

Dr Shrikant Verma

Anatomy

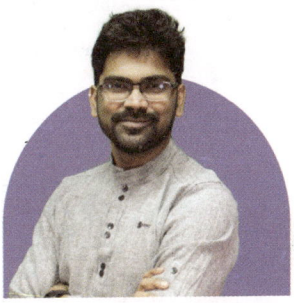

Dr Karthikeyan Pethusamy

Biochemistry & Nutrition

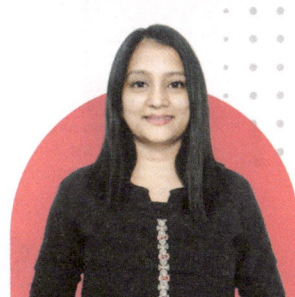

Ms Chetana

Mental Health Nursing

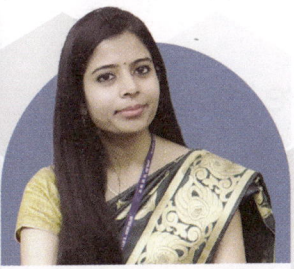

Saumya Srivastava

Nursing Management & Nursing Education

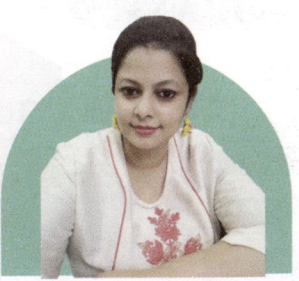

Ms Priyanka Randhir

Sociology & Computers

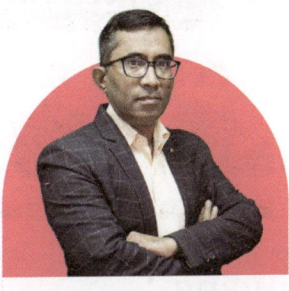

Mr Nitish Dubey

General Arithmetic

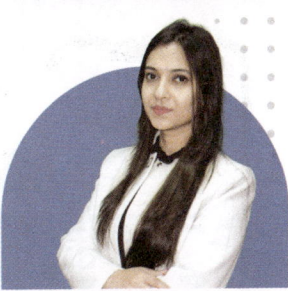

Ms Saloni Sharma

Aptitude & Reasoning

Individual

Midwifery & Obstetrical Nursing
By Dr Sakshi Arora Hans

What all you will get

- **100** hours of Videos on All topics
- IBQs & VBQs Discussion Videos
- **15** hours of Rapid Revision Videos covering Important Topics for AIIMS NORCET 2021
- **1000** Topic-wise MCQs with Rationale
- Live Doubt Sessions/Live Classes
- **88** Hand written Notes in PDF format

Validity: 6 months | **MRP** ₹1994/-

MSN - Surgery
By Dr Rohan Khandelwal

What all you will get

- **50** hours of Videos of All topics
- IBQs & VBQs Video Discussions
- **3** hours of Rapid Revision Videos covering Important Topics for AIIMS NORCET 2021
- **800** Topic-wise Qs with Rationale
- Live Doubt Sessions/Live Classes
- **51** Hand written Notes in PDF format integrated in App

Validity: 6 months | **MRP** ₹1499/-

Pharmacology
By Dr Ranjan Patel

What all you will get

- **50** hours of Videos of All topics
- IBQs & VBQs Video Discussions
- **10** hours of Rapid Revision Videos covering Important Topics for AIIMS NORCET 2021
- **800** Topic-wise Qs with Rationale
- Live Doubt Sessions/Live Classes
- **71** Hand written Notes in PDF format integrated in App
- **100** Probable Questions of Pharmacology for AIIMS NORCET 2021

Validity: 6 months | **MRP** ₹1499/-

Community Health Nursing
By Dr Mukhmohit Singh

What all you will get

- **90** hours of Videos of All topics
- IBQs & VBQs Video Discussions
- **7** hours of Rapid Revision Videos covering Important Topics forAIIMS NORCET 2021
- **900** Topic-wise Qs with Rationale
- Live Doubt Sessions/Live Classes
- **87** Hand written Notes in PDF format integrated in App
- **300** Probable Questions of CHN for AIIMS NORCET 2021

Validity: 6 months | **MRP** ₹1995/-

Microbiology
By Dr Shivika J Sethi

What all you will get

- **54** hours of Videos of All topics
- IBQs & VBQs Video Discussions
- **8** hours of Rapid Revision Videos covering Important Topics for AIIMS NORCET 2021
- **800** Topic-wise Qs with Rationale
- Live Doubt Sessions/Live Classes
- **75** Hand written Notes in PDF format integrated in App
- **100** Probable Questions of Microbiology for AIIMS NORCET 2021

Validity: 6 months | **MRP** ₹1499/-

MSN - Medicine
By Dr Aman Setiya

What all you will get

- **90** hours of Videos of All topics
- IBQs & VBQs Video Discussions
- **5** hours of Rapid Revision Videos covering Important Topics for AIIMS NORCET 2021
- **900** Topic-wise Qs with Rationale
- Live Doubt Sessions/Live Classes
- **90** Hand written Notes in PDF format integrated in App
- **400** Probable Questions of MSN - Medicine for AIIMS NORCET 2021

Validity: 6 months | **MRP** ₹1499/-

" जितनी जरूरत उतना पढ़ो !"

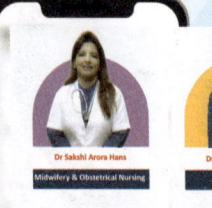
Dr Sakshi Arora Hans
Midwifery & Obstetrical Nursing

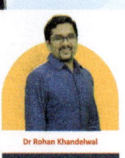
Dr Rohan Khandelwal
MSN - Surgery

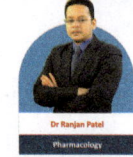
Dr Ranjan Patel
Pharmacology

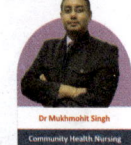
Dr Mukhmohit Singh
Community Health Nursing

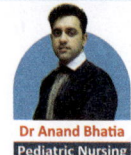
Dr Anand Bhatia
Pediatric Nursing

Now you have
The Freedom to Choose

Introducing
CREATE YOUR PACK

Pack

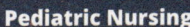

Pediatric Nursing
By Dr Anand Bhatia

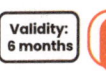 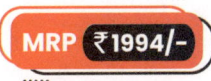

What all you will get

- **80** hours of Videos of All topics
- IBQs & VBQs Video Discussions
- **8** hours of Rapid Revision Videos covering Important Topics for AIIMS NORCET 2021
- **900** Topic-wise Qs with Rationale
- Live Doubt Sessions/Live Classes
- **81** Hand written Notes in PDF format integrated in App
- **300** Probable Questions of Pediatric Nursing for AIIMS NORCET 2021

Validity: 6 months   MRP ₹ **1994/-**

Anatomy
By Dr Shrikant Verma

 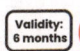 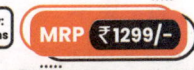

What all you will get

- **60** hours of Videos of All topics
- IBQs & VBQs Video Discussions
- **6** hours of Rapid Revision Videos covering Important Topics forAIIMS NORCET 2021
- **605** Topic-wise Qs with Rationale
- Live Doubt Sessions/Live Classes
- **86** Hand written Notes in PDF format integrated in App
- **100** Probable Questions of Anatomy for AIIMS NORCET 2021

Validity: 6 months   MRP ₹ **1299/-**

Biochemistry & Nutrition
By Dr Karthikeyan Pethusamy

  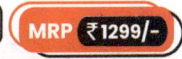

What all you will get

- **50** hours of Videos of All topics
- IBQs & VBQs Video Discussions
- **3** hours of Rapid Revision Videos covering Important Topics for AIIMS NORCET 2021
- **500** Topic-wise Qs with Rationale
- Live Doubt Sessions/Live Classes
- **45** Hand written Notes in PDF format integrated in App
- **100** Probable Questions of Biochemistry & Nutrition for AIIMS NORCET 2021

Validity: 6 months   MRP ₹ **1299/-**

Physiology
By Dr Ashish Kumar

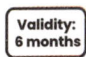 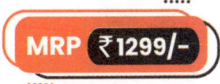

What all you will get

- **60** hours of Videos of All topics
- IBQs & VBQs Video Discussions
- **8** hours of Rapid Revision Videos covering Important Topics for AIIMS NORCET 2021
- **600** Topic-wise Qs with Rationale
- Live Doubt Sessions/Live Classes
- **55** Hand written Notes in PDF format integrated in App

Validity: 6 months   MRP ₹ **1299/-**

Fundamentals of Nursing
By Ms Sabina Ali

  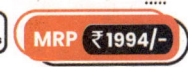

What all you will get

- **200** hours of Videos of All topics
- IBQs & VBQs Video Discussions
- **14** hours of Rapid Revision Videos covering Important Topics for AIIMS NORCET 2021
- **900** Topic-wise Qs with Rationale
- Live Doubt Sessions/Live Classes
- **200** Hand written Notes in PDF format integrated in App
- **300** Probable Questions of FON for AIIMS NORCET 2021

Validity: 6 months   MRP ₹ **1994/-**

Mental Health Nursing
By Dr Dharmendra Singh & Ms Chetana

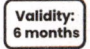 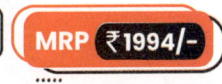

What all you will get

- **90** hours of Videos of All topics
- IBQs & VBQs Video Discussions
- **6** hours of Rapid Revision Videos covering Important Topics for AIIMS NORCET 2021
- **900** Topic-wise Qs with Rationale
- Live Doubt Sessions/Live Classes
- **300** Probable Questions of MHN for AIIMS NORCET 2021

Validity: 6 months   MRP ₹ **1994/-**

 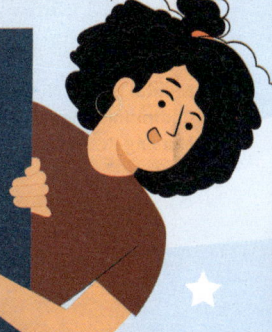

Select any **5 Subjects**
by **The Masterminds** and Create Your Own Pack

MRP ₹ **8450/-**   **Validity: 9 Months**

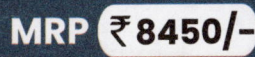

Wondering, HOW? Call us at our helpline number +91-9999117411

Undergraduate Packs

By THE MASTERMINDS

Undergraduate Pack - 1st Year

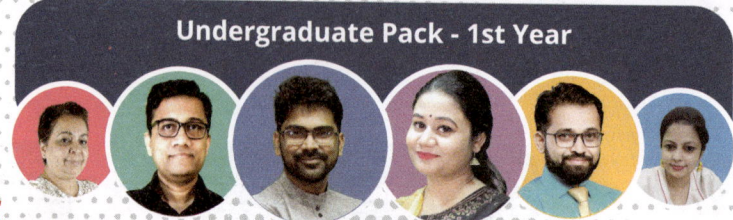

What all you will get

Main Subjects	Video Duration	No. of Questions
Anatomy	60+ Hours	600+ Qs
Physiology	60+ Hours	600+ Qs
Biochemistry & Nutrition	50+ Hours	500+ Qs
Microbiology	50+ Hours	500+ Qs
Fundamentals of Nursing	200+ Hours	400+ Qs

Bonus Subjects:- Computers & Psychology

MRP ₹7997/-

Validity: 18 months

Undergraduate Pack - 2nd Year

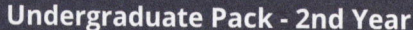

MRP ₹7997/-

Validity: 18 months

What all you will get

Main Subjects	Video Duration	No. of Questions
Pharmacology	50+ Hours	800+ Qs
MSN - Medicine	90+ Hours	900+ Qs
MSN - Surgery	50+ Hours	600+ Qs
Community Health Nursing	90+ Hours	900+ Qs
Sociology	40+ Hours	250+ Qs

Undergraduate Pack - 3rd & 4th Year

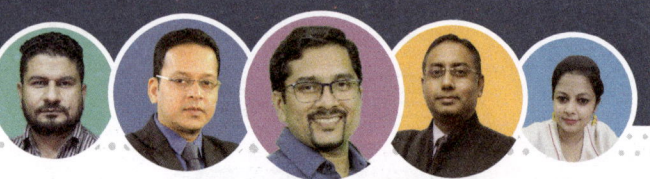

What all you will get

Main Subjects	Video Duration	No. of Questions
Pediatric Nursing	80+ Hours	900+ Qs
Midwifery & Obstetrical Nursing	100+ Hours	1000+ Qs
MSN - Medicine	90+ Hours	900+ Qs
MSN - Surgery	50+ Hours	600+ Qs
Mental Health Nursing	90+ Hours	900+ Qs
Community Health Nursing	90+ Hours	900+ Qs
Nursing Research & Statistics	35+ Hours	400+ Qs

Bonus Subjects:- Nursing Managment & Nursing Education

MRP ₹12992/-

Validity: 24 months

Special Features

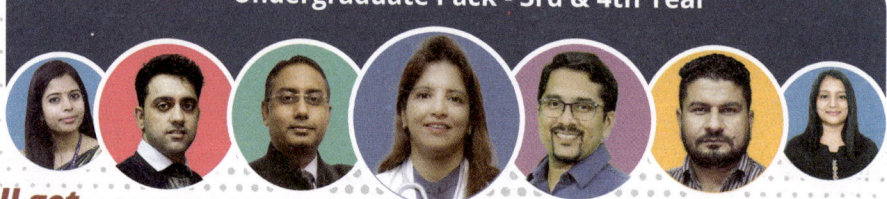

- Handwritten Notes of Videos in PDF Format
- IBQs/VBQs Discussion Videos of above mentioned Subjects
- Monthly Mega Assessment Tests
- Monthly Live Doubt Session/Live Classes/Live Webinar by MM Faculty
- Best Guidance & Support
- Get your query directly resolved by MM faculty

"कम समय में जीत पक्की!"

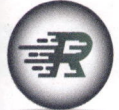

Plan RR
Rapid Revision Pack
(Ready, Steady & Rapid)

We are here to make you a Mastermind for all your Nursing exams, and for that, we believe the last-minute revision works like a wonder. Rapid Revision Pack, as the name says is to make you all ready and rapid for all your Nursing Competetive exams. Learn from basics to advance level and get a hold of every topic. Gain the last-minute momentum with this pack and open the gateway to excellence for yourself.

WHY TO SUBSCRIBE
- Rapid and intense course of study
- Covers important topics in concise yet complete form
- Most probable Qs which have large rate of incidence in exam
- If your foundation is good, then this is good pack to revise before the exam

BEST FOR
- Those who believe in doing extensive preparation for their Nursing competitive exams.
- The students who want to clear all of their last moment doubts.
- Working professionals who never want to compromise with their learnings for the competitive exams.

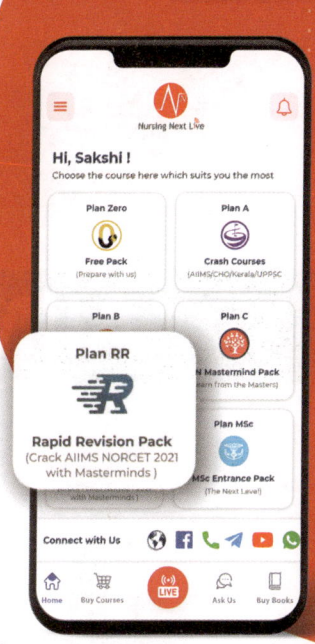

What all you will get

Plan RR

- **80-100 Hours of Rapid Revision Videos** covering Most Imp Topics for NORCET 2021 (Major Subjects including Nursing Management & Nursing Education)
- **2000+** Probable Qs with Rationale (MCQs + NCLEX Pattern)
- IBQ & VBQ Video Discussions by Master Mind Faculties (Relevant Subjects)
- **10 Special Mega Assessment Test** based on AIIMS NORCET Pattern
- Various Imp Tips/Trick & How to Prepare for NORCET 2021 Videos
- **15+** Imp Videos on COVID 19/Test & Discussion covering MCQ & NCLEX Pattern Qs
- COVID-19 Capsule (MCQs & Videos)
- Rapid Revision eBook in PDF format

MRP ₹2777/- Validity: 2.5 Months

Plan RR+Mini TSP

Complete Ccontent of RR Pack + Mini TSP:
- **15k** Questions with Rationale
- **1000+** IBQs/VBQs with Rationale Subject-wise/System-wise approach
- **190+** Tests (Subject-wise/Grand Test)
- **1500** E-notes/Clinical Gems
- **400+** Hours of videos Lectures/Subject-wise Exam discussion/Skill Procedure Videos

MRP ₹7520/- Validity: 3+1 Months

TESTIMONIALS

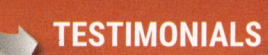

What our Subscribers say about our **Rapid Revision Pack**

SELF-EVALUATION IS THE KEY!
"It has proved the best plan if you look forward to self evaluate before your exams. Great initiative."

Sushma Rani

LESS TIME CONSUMING AND MORE LEARNING!
"Through the Rapid revision pack and test series 2.0, I learned from excellent educators in a time-saving way"

Usha Rani

EXPERIENCE REAL-TIME EXAM VIBE!
"Rapid Revision Pack has helped me clear my doubts by providing real-time exam experience preparation. I gained an overall improvement in my studies."

Akansha Sharma

INNOVATIONS DETERMINES EFFECTIVENESS!
"Excellent pack if you want to do a quick revision effectively. The lectures are in a very comprehensive manner which makes it one of the best initiatives by NNL. "

B. Snegha Varshini

NN LIVE BECAME MY PARTNER-IN-LEARNING!
"Mastermind C Plus Pack became an amazing opportunity for me as I got everything from MCQs to High Standard Questions. Got the RR plan as a bonus too. Also, the faculty is always there to boost you up!"

Rahul Sain

IMPROVING RESULTS AND CHANGING STUDY PERSPECTIVES!
"Even the micro-content helped me to study in a macro way. With NNL, it has become very simple for me to understand the topics in a very comprehensive way. The Live sessions just work as an advantage. Thank you Nursing Next Live!"

Yashpal Vishvakarma

GLORIFIED ACHIEVER

AIIMS NORCET 2020

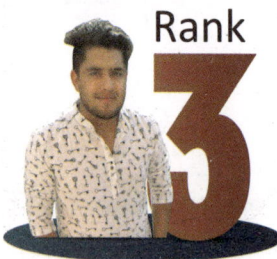

Rank 3

Rahul Dahiya
Roll No. 9016060

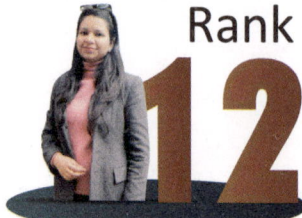

Rank 12

Nisha Singla
Roll No. 9101820

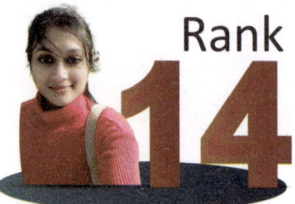

Rank 14

Arushi Mittal
Roll No. 9079646

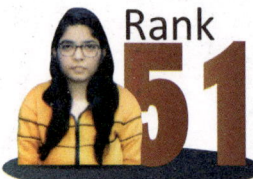

Rank 51

Komal Dhull
Roll No. 9024458

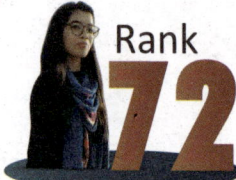

Rank 72

Shivani Bourai
Roll No. 9092877

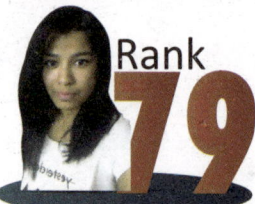

Rank 79

Nivedita Saini
Roll No. 9004587

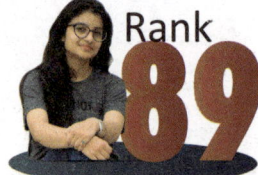

Rank 89

Rupali Garg
Roll No. 9054544

And many more

CHO 2020

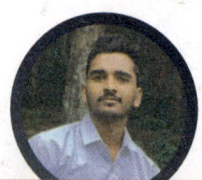

Suresh Kumsr
Rank- 1
Roll No. 12090
MP

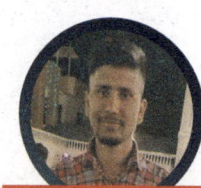

Vikas Kumar Sahu
Rank- 14
Roll No. 10011
MP

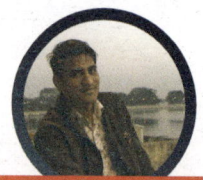

Harish Kumar Lodha
Rank- 18
Roll No. 7930
MP

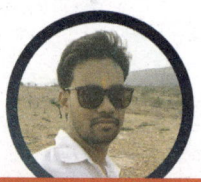

Heeralal Lodha
Rank- 33
Roll No. 10009
MP

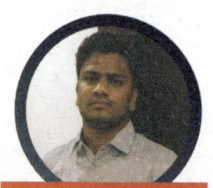

Sandeep Krumar Kumawat
Rank- 44
Roll No. 12585
MP

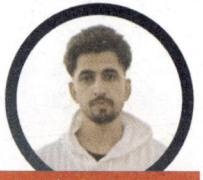

Mahadev Aanjan
Rank- 50
Roll No. 10130
MP

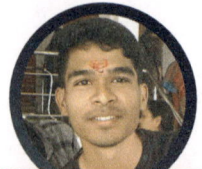

Nilesh
Rank- 81
Roll No. 10572
MP

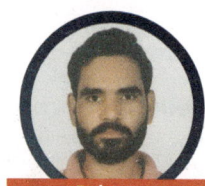

Balveer
Roll No. 619175
RAJASTHAN

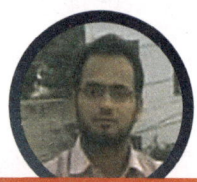

Mahendra Singh Gurjar
Roll No. 626167
RAJASTHAN

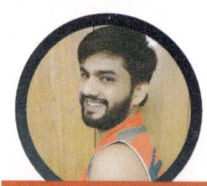

Fateh Singh
Roll No. 108169
RAJASTHAN

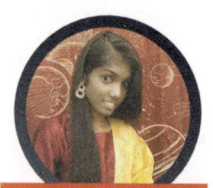

Shivangi
Roll No. 406105
RAJASTHAN

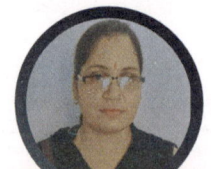

Suneeta Swami
Roll No. 619378
RAJASTHAN

And many more

OF NURSING NEXT LIVE

1200+ STUDENTS who cleared Various National/State Level Nursing Exams

BFUHS 2021

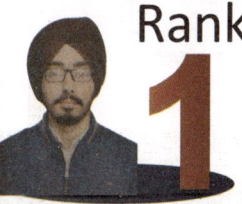 Rank **1**

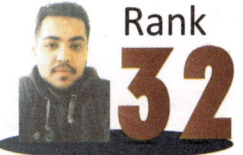 Rank **28**

 Rank **32**

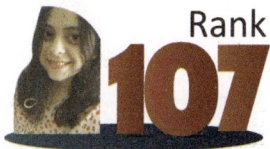 Rank **38**

Rank **107**

Harjeet Singh
Roll No- 472478

Kuljit Kaur
Roll No. 473956

Karan Sharma
Roll No. 469134

Smriti Rana
Roll No. 463342

Harpreet Kaur
Roll No. 474125

And many more

AIIMS MSc ENTRANCE EXAM 2021

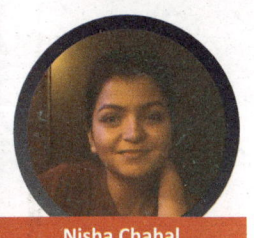
Nisha Chahal
AIIMS AIR-18

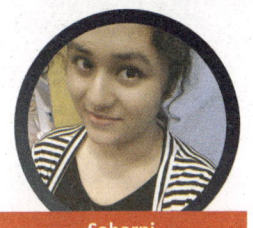
Sabarni
AIIMS AIR-21

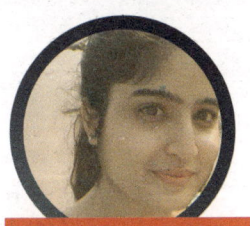
Ritika Rajpoot
AIIMS AIR-23

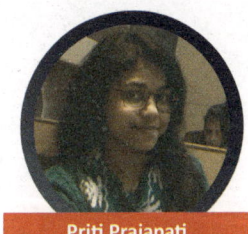
Priti Prajapati
AIIMS AIR-39

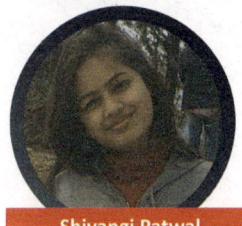
Shivangi Patwal
AIIMS AIR-64

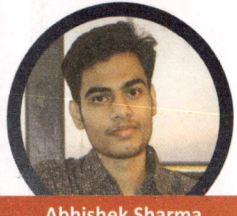
Abhishek Sharma
AIIMS AIR-97

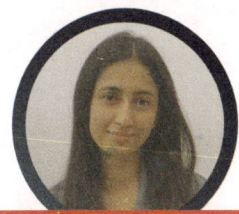
Pritika Thakur
AIIMS AIR-119

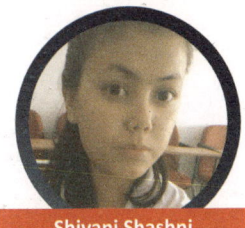
Shivani Shashni
AIIMS AIR-173

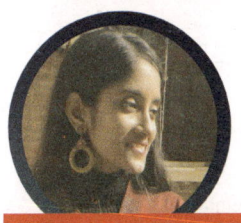
Mahima Paul
AIIMS AIR-175

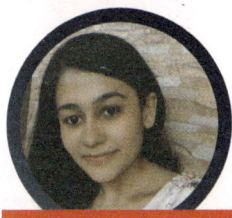
Deeksha Bhatt
AIIMS AIR-281

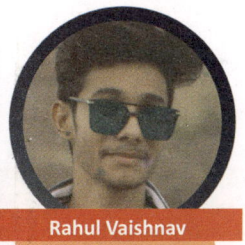
Rahul Vaishnav
AIIMS AIR-301

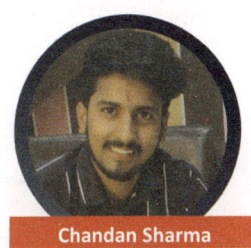
Chandan Sharma
AIIMS AIR-310

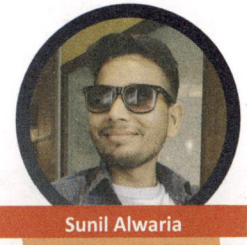
Sunil Alwaria
AIIMS AIR-677

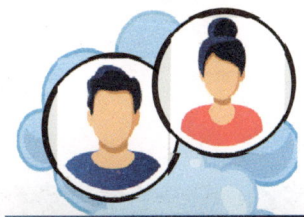
You Will Be The Next...

Scan the QR code to visit to our YouTube Channel to hear their success stories.

ONE PLACE FOR ALL! AN INVITATION FOR ALL THE NURSING FACULTY MEMBERS TO COME.

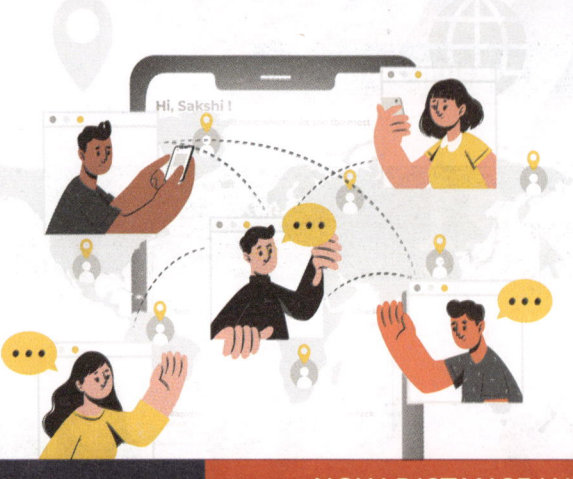

NURSING NEXT S●CIAL

Carrying on the legacy of being the best networking platform for the Nursing Segment!

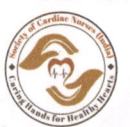 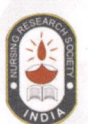 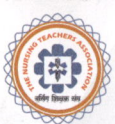 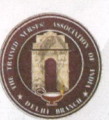

NOW DISTANCE WILL NOT BE A BARRIER

Knowledge is like money: to be of value, it must circulate, and in circulating it, it can increase in quantity!

Nursing Next Live always focuses on providing you with the best and beyond and nothing less than that. We aim to bring all the Nursing Faculties from across the nation closer and together on a single platform.

No social distancing can stop the circulation of learnings from the teachers to students now. With Nursing Next Social, all the faculties from every corner of the country can join at one platform without any barriers.

Nursing Next Social at your service!

ONE PLATFORM TO BECOME THE MENTORS AND MENTEE!

Rewards For You

• Get Acknowledgement & Appreciation Certificates • Get Sponsorships for Educational Programs • Get Credit hours for attending Webinars • Get Free Access to Nursing Next Live Content & CBS Nursing Books • Get Latest Updates related to your subject • Get a chance to become Reviewer, Contributors in Nursing Next Live, Target High & in CBS Nursing Titles

BE THE MENTOR OR MENTEE

SHOWCASE YOUR ACHIEVEMENTS ➡ SHARE YOUR KNOWLEDGE ➡ ENHANCE YOUR KNOWLEDGE

Purposes
• Attend Webinars/ E- Workshops
• Connect with other Faculty Members
• Share Your Knowledge. Be the Mentor or Mentee
• Get Complimentary Books
• Latest Updates on State/National/International Conferences & Webniars

Special Features
• Create your profile
• Add your accomplishments to level up your portfolio
• Earn Reward Points & Redeem through various options
• Set your Professional GOALS with timelines
• Regular Updates on Upcoming Conferences, CNEs & webinars
• Become Mentor or Mentee
• Get a chance to become Reviewer, Contributor or Author
• Get Certificates with credit hours issued by renowned nursing societies

ARE YOU A NURSING FACULTY ?
BE THE PART OF NURSING NEXT LIVE SOCIAL!

PRE-REGISTER FOR NURSING NEXT SOCIAL

& Get 60 Days Free Subscription of **Nursing Next Live App**

Scan the QR Code & Fill the form to Pre-register

Or Use the below link to fill the form

http://nursingnextlive.com/NNSocial/

ONE NATION ONE NURSING COMMUNITY

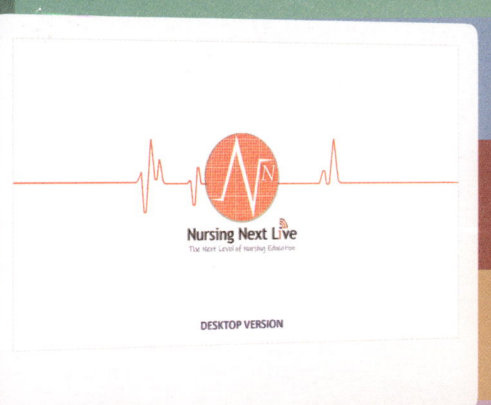

Plan-wise Comparison Chart

Compare and Choose the Best Suited to You

Feature	Plan Zero	Crash Course	Test Series	Rapid Revision	Mastermind Plan C	Mastermind Plan C Plus
Videos						
1. All Subjects /Topics Videos	—	—	—	—	✓	✓
2. Video Lectures of Imp Topics	✓	—	✓	✓	—	✓
3. Exam Discussion Videos	—	—	✓	—	—	✓
4. Procedure Videos	—	—	—	—	—	✓
5. Rapid Revision Videos	—	—	—	✓	—	✓
6. IBQ/VBQ/Clinical Qs Discussion	—	—	—	✓	—	✓
7. Live Doubt Sessions	—	—	—	—	✓	✓
8. Student-faculty Meet	—	—	—	—	✓	✓
9. Zoom Sessions/Webinar	—	—	—	—	✓	✓
10. Youtube Videos	✓	—	✓	—	✓	✓
Tests						
11. Special Mega Assessment Tests	—	—	—	✓	✓	✓
12. Grand Tests	✓	✓	✓	—	—	✓
13. Subject-wise Tests	✓	✓	✓	—	—	✓
14. Mini Tests	✓	✓	✓	—	—	✓
15. IBQs/VBQs	✓	✓	✓	—	✓	✓
16. Most Recent Papers	✓	✓	✓	—	—	✓
17. Previous Years Papers	✓	✓	✓	—	—	✓
18. Kerala Psc Crash Course	✓	✓	✓	—	—	✓
19. CHO Exams Crash Course	—	✓	✓	—	—	✓
20. AIIMS NORCET 2020 Crash Course	—	—	✓	—	—	✓
21. UPPSC Crash Course	—	—	✓	—	—	✓
22. Most Probable Qs	—	—	✓	✓	✓	✓
23. National Scholarship Test	✓	—	✓	✓	✓	✓
24. Subject-wise Qs of All Topics	—	—	—	—	✓	✓
Notes						
25. Handwritten Notes Integrated With Lectures	—	—	—	—	✓	✓
26. Last-minute Revision Notes	✓	—	✓	✓	—	✓
27. Notes Integrated With Rapid Revision Videos	—	—	—	✓	✓	✓
28. Printed Booklets(Forthcoming)	—	—	—	—	✓	—
Features						
29. Desktop Version	—	—	—	✓	✓	✓
30. Any Doubt Ask Us	✓	✓	✓	✓	✓	✓
31. Report A Query	✓	✓	✓	✓	✓	✓
32. National Level Ranking	✓	✓	✓	✓	✓	✓
33. Blogs	✓	✓	✓	✓	✓	✓
34. Daily Dose Of Knowledge	✓	✓	✓	✓	✓	✓
35. Forums Get Latest Info	✓	✓	✓	✓	✓	✓
36. Resume Learning	✓	✓	—	✓	✓	✓
37. Buy Books	✓	✓	—	✓	✓	✓
Supports						
38. Guidance & Counseling	—	—	—	✓	✓	✓
39. Faculty Telegram Channel	—	—	—	✓	✓	✓
40. Faculty Facebook Page	—	—	—	✓	✓	✓

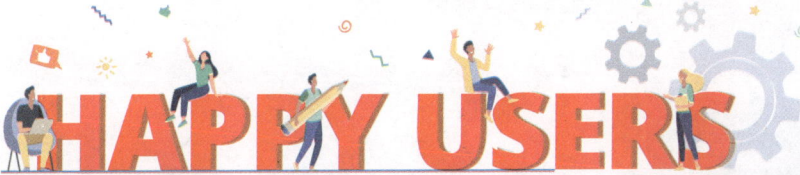

HAPPY USERS

Anisha Manna
★★★★★

DIVERSIFIED SPECIAL FEATURES TO BRACE YOU UP!

"The app is highly recommended for all nursing aspirants. The app has numerous special features with thorough information and is the best Nursing preparation option during these Pandemic times. Used for just 1 year and cleared my M.Sc. with excellent results."

Abhishek Kushwaha
★★★★★

RESULTED TO BE THE BEST NURSING PREPARATION APP!

"Hands down, it is the best Nursing app I have come across. All the tests, study content, CHO Crash Course will not let your expectations down but will prove to be really impressive. If you are a Nursing student/aspirant, then don't think just go for it."

Swatilekha Das
★★★★★

BECOME AN ACHIEVER FROM JUST AN USER WITH NURSING NEXT LIVE

"It has proved to be the best platform for me. If any student is looking for the perfect platform for Nursing Preparations, this is it. To become an achiever from just a dreamer, install this app and study from the plans now."

Nursing Guide Hindi
★★★★★

BEST PLAN FOR THE 1ST YEAR NURSING STUDENT

"The question bank, video lectures are amazing. Extremely helpful for any Nursing Aspirant. It is more preferable if you are in 1st year of Nursing. Do use this app if you want to make your knowledge vaster and achieve all your Nursing goals."

Harshit Upadhyay
★★★★★

IT HAS PROVED TO BE THE BEST NURSING PREPARATION ALLY!

"All the faculties especially Dr Sakshi, Dr Mukhmohit, Dr Rohan, Ms Sabina, all are excellent. The only drawback is that Dr Dharmendra needs to be a bit quick to make the notes and data. Else, it is an excellent prepping platform."

Naga Venkat
★★★★★

GET THE REAL-TIME TEST EXPERIENCE BY USING THE NNLIVE APP

"It is an excellent platform for learning and practicing for Nursing Competitive Exams. It consists of topic-wise explanations and helps us hold command of all. After attempting the real-time tests, I was able to progress gradually."

Sarangi Patel
★★★★★

THE ONE-STOP SOLUTION AS IT SAYS!

"I am grateful to the Nursing Next Live team for making great efforts towards providing us with the best and beyond preparation experience. The video lectures, e-notes, MCQs, and so on will suffice all your preparation needs and take it to the next level. "

Deepak Kumar
★★★★★

10/10 RECOMMENDATION FOR THE NN LIVE APP!

"This app is best for all Nursing students as it has the best quality content to study and learn from."

Shafat Maqbool
★★★★★

CLEAR ALL YOUR DOUBTS-101!

"The video lectures, study content is highly informative and the topics are understood effectively. Clear all your doubts with NNL in no time"

Video Testimonials

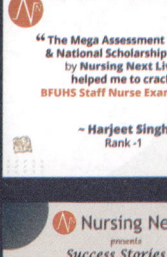

"The Mega Assessment Tests & National Scholarship Tests by Nursing Next Live helped me to crack BFUHS Staff Nurse Exam 2021"
~ Harjeet Singh
Rank -1

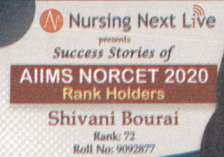
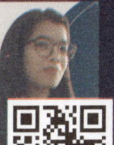

Nursing Next Live presents
Success Stories of
AIIMS NORCET 2020 Rank Holders
Shivani Bourai
Rank: 72
Roll No: 9092877

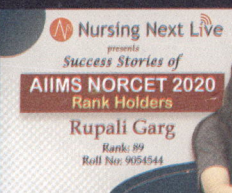
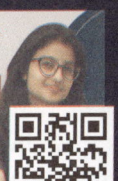

Nursing Next Live presents
Success Stories of
AIIMS NORCET 2020 Rank Holders
Rupali Garg
Rank: 89
Roll No: 9054544

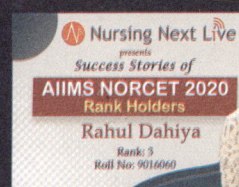

Nursing Next Live presents
Success Stories of
AIIMS NORCET 2020 Rank Holders
Rahul Dahiya
Rank: 5
Roll No: 9016060

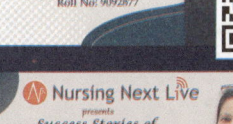

Nursing Next Live presents
Success Stories of
AIIMS NORCET 2020 Rank Holders
Nivedita Saini
Rank: 79
Roll No: 9004587

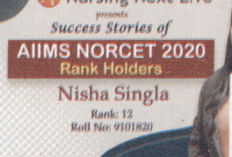

Nursing Next Live presents
Success Stories of
AIIMS NORCET 2020 Rank Holders
Nisha Singla
Rank: 12
Roll No: 9101820

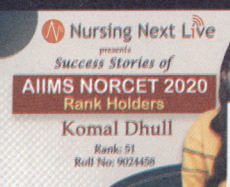
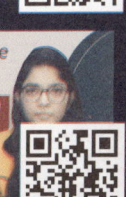

Nursing Next Live presents
Success Stories of
AIIMS NORCET 2020 Rank Holders
Komal Dhull
Rank: 51
Roll No: 9024458

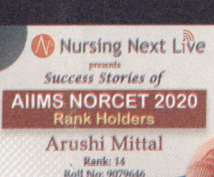
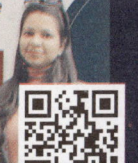

Nursing Next Live presents
Success Stories of
AIIMS NORCET 2020 Rank Holders
Arushi Mittal
Rank: 14
Roll No: 9079646

Scan the QR Codes to watch the videos on our YouTube Channel.

We Are Here 24X7

24×7 Guidance & Support

We provide personalized guidance and counseling to all our Subscribers, to ensure that their preparation is in the right direction, that is, toward success. That's why we have an active support service, handled especially by our:`

Nursing Counselors/Academic Counselors – To suggest you what to refer as per your need and want
Relationship Managers – To guide you throughout your learning journey and help you on every step
Guidance & Counselor – To teach you what to study and how to study
Scientific Team – To clear your Scientific Doubts within 24-48 Hours

How to connect with us?
Any Doubt, Ask Us : (In App Support 24x7)
Helpline and WhatsApp No : 9999117411 (Mon-Sat 9:00 am to 8:00 pm, Sunday 9:00 am to 2:00 pm)
Email : feedback@nursingnextlive.in
Web : www.nursingnextlive.com

Follow Us
(Scan the QR Code to Visit to Our Social Media Pages)

 FACEBOOK
- Latest Updates & Discount Offers
- Read students feedbacks & Testimonials
- Fun & Learn Activities- Participate and win exciting prizes & free subscription

 INSTAGRAM
- Latest updates of upcoming events
- Participate in giveaways, contests, and quizzes
- See what's latest

 YOUTUBE
- Watch Success Stories, Tips & Tricks for easy preparation, from the top rank holders
- Videos of all Subjects/Important Topics by the mastermind faculty
- Various Last-minute revisions, motivational, and chanting videos
- Live Doubt Sessions every month for paid subscribers

 LINKEDIN
- Behind-the-scenes of Nursing Next Live
- Significant days of the staff members
- Get insights into the insides of NNLive

TELEGRAM
- Exclusive content for both paid and free subscribers
- Get Daily MBQs/IBQs, E-Notes, Video Teasers
- Latest updates, Daily dosage of learning, Quiz, Special discounts & Offers

Introducing TARGET HIGH DIGITAL
Now Read & Practice Together

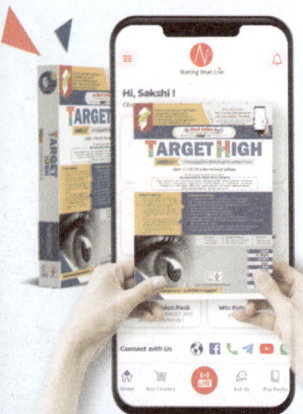

India's No. 1 and the most trusted book with exclusive & complete coverage of all National & State Level Exams is now going digital with no restrictions & additional content.

Explore The Next Level Of Best Preparation, Now!

Buy Best-Selling CBS Nursing Books

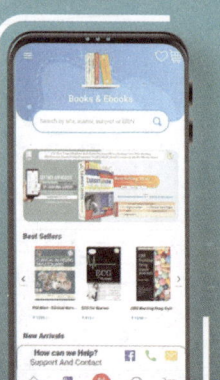

Read, Review & Buy

Now, buying CBS Nursing Books is extra convenient with Nursing Next Live App!

Get a Glimpse of **Sample Pages and TOC** before you proceed to buy the books.

Best Discounts & Special Offers on all the Books.

Textbook of
Nursing Foundations
for BSc Nursing Students

As per the syllabus of Kerala University of Health Sciences

Harindarjeet Goyal PhD, MPhil, MSc (MSN), BSc (Hons.), RN, RM

Former Principal
Rajkumari Amrit Kaur College of Nursing
New Delhi

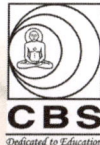

CBS
Dedicated to Education

CBS Publishers & Distributors Pvt Ltd

• New Delhi • Bengaluru • Chennai • Kochi • Kolkata • Lucknow
• Mumbai • Hyderabad • Nagpur • Patna • Pune • Vijayawada

Textbook of
Nursing Foundations
for BSc Nursing Students

As per the syllabus of Kerala University of Health Sciences

ISBN: 978-93-90619-38-2

First Edition: 2022

Published by **Satish Kumar Jain** and produced by **Varun Jain** for

CBS Publishers & Distributors Pvt Ltd

4819/XI Prahlad Street, 24 Ansari Road, Daryaganj, New Delhi 110 002, India.
Ph: +91-11-23289259, 23266861, 23266867   Website: www.cbspd.com
Fax: 011-23243014
e-mail: delhi@cbspd.com; cbspubs@airtelmail.in.

Corporate Office: 204 FIE, Industrial Area, Patparganj, Delhi 110 092
Ph: +91-11-4934 4934   Fax: 4934 4935
e-mail: feedback@cbspd.com; bhupesharora@cbspd.com

Branches

- **Bengaluru:** Seema House 2975, 17th Cross, K.R. Road, Banasankari 2nd Stage, Bengaluru 560 070, Karnataka
  Ph: +91-80-26771678/79   Fax: +91-80-26771680   e-mail: bangalore@cbspd.com

- **Chennai:** 7, Subbaraya Street, Shenoy Nagar, Chennai 600 030, Tamil Nadu
  Ph: +91-44-26680620, 26681266   Fax: +91-44-42032115   e-mail: chennai@cbspd.com

- **Kochi:** 68/1534, 35, 36-Power House Road, Opp. KSEB, Cochin-682018, Kochi, Kerala
  Ph: +91-484-4059061-65   Fax: +91-484-4059065   e-mail: kochi@cbspd.com

- **Kolkata:** 6/B, Ground Floor, Rameswar Shaw Road, Kolkata-700 014, West Bengal
  Ph: +91-33-22891126, 22891127, 22891128   e-mail: kolkata@cbspd.com

- **Lucknow:** Basement, Khushnuma Complex, 7-Meerabai Ma Rg, (Behind Jawahar Bhawan),
  Lucknow-226001, Uttar Pradesh
  Ph: +0522-4000032   e-mail: tiwari.lucknow@cbspd.com

- **Mumbai:** PWD Shed, Gala No. 25/26, Ramchandra Bhatt Marg, Next to J.J. Hospital Gate No. 2, Opp. Union Bank of India,
  Noor Baug, Mumbai-400009
  Ph: +91-22-66661880/89   Fax: +91-22-24902342   e-mail: mumbai@cbspd.com

Representatives

- **Hyderabad**   +91-9885175004
- **Pune**   +91-9623451994
- **Patna**   +91-9334159340
- **Vijayawada**   +91-9000660880

Printed at: Goyal Offset Works Pvt. Ltd.

Textbook of
Nursing Foundations
for BSc Nursing Students

As per the syllabus of Kerala University of Health Sciences

Harindarjeet Goyal PhD, MPhil, MSc (MSN), BSc (Hons.), RN, RM

Former Principal
Rajkumari Amrit Kaur College of Nursing
New Delhi

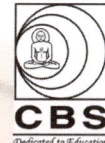

CBS Publishers & Distributors Pvt Ltd

• New Delhi • Bengaluru • Chennai • Kochi • Kolkata • Lucknow
• Mumbai • Hyderabad • Nagpur • Patna • Pune • Vijayawada

Textbook of
Nursing Foundations
for BSc Nursing Students

As per the syllabus of Kerala University of Health Sciences

ISBN: 978-93-90619-38-2

First Edition: 2022

Published by **Satish Kumar Jain** and produced by **Varun Jain** for

CBS Publishers & Distributors Pvt Ltd

4819/XI Prahlad Street, 24 Ansari Road, Daryaganj, New Delhi 110 002, India.
Ph: +91-11-23289259, 23266861, 23266867   Website: www.cbspd.com
Fax: 011-23243014
e-mail: delhi@cbspd.com; cbspubs@airtelmail.in.

Corporate Office: 204 FIE, Industrial Area, Patparganj, Delhi 110 092
Ph: +91-11-4934 4934   Fax: 4934 4935
e-mail: feedback@cbspd.com; bhupesharora@cbspd.com

Branches

- **Bengaluru:** Seema House 2975, 17th Cross, K.R. Road, Banasankari 2nd Stage, Bengaluru 560 070, Karnataka
  Ph: +91-80-26771678/79   Fax: +91-80-26771680   e-mail: bangalore@cbspd.com

- **Chennai:** 7, Subbaraya Street, Shenoy Nagar, Chennai 600 030, Tamil Nadu
  Ph: +91-44-26680620, 26681266   Fax: +91-44-42032115   e-mail: chennai@cbspd.com

- **Kochi:** 68/1534, 35, 36-Power House Road, Opp. KSEB, Cochin-682018, Kochi, Kerala
  Ph: +91-484-4059061-65   Fax: +91-484-4059065   e-mail: kochi@cbspd.com

- **Kolkata:** 6/B, Ground Floor, Rameswar Shaw Road, Kolkata-700 014, West Bengal
  Ph: +91-33-22891126, 22891127, 22891128   e-mail: kolkata@cbspd.com

- **Lucknow:** Basement, Khushnuma Complex, 7-Meerabai Ma Rg, (Behind Jawahar Bhawan), Lucknow-226001, Uttar Pradesh
  Ph: +0522-4000032   e-mail: tiwari.lucknow@cbspd.com

- **Mumbai:** PWD Shed, Gala No. 25/26, Ramchandra Bhatt Marg, Next to J.J. Hospital Gate No. 2, Opp. Union Bank of India, Noor Baug, Mumbai-400009
  Ph: +91-22-66661880/89   Fax: +91-22-24902342   e-mail: mumbai@cbspd.com

Representatives

- **Hyderabad**   +91-9885175004   - **Patna**   +91-9334159340
- **Pune**   +91-9623451994   - **Vijayawada**   +91-9000660880

Printed at: Goyal Offset Works Pvt. Ltd.

Reviewers

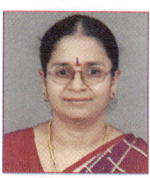

A Tamil Selvi
MSc (N), PhD (N), RN, RM
Principal
Amity College of Nursing, Amity University
Gurugram, Haryana

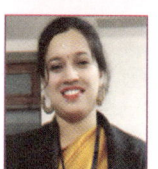

Amandeep Kaur, RN, RM
MSc (Medical Surgical Nursing, Neurosciences)
Assistant Professor
Amity College of Nursing, Amity University
Gurugram, Haryana

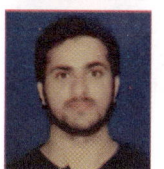

Arshid Nazir Shah
Pursuing PhD (N), MSc (N) Pediatric Nursing,
Diploma in Nursing Administration (DNA)
Government Nursing College, Gandhi Nagar
Jammu, J&K

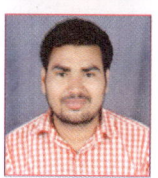

Gaurav Tyagi
MSc (N) Community Health Nursing
Vice Principal
KMC College of Nursing
Meerut, Uttar Pradesh

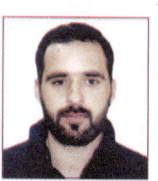

Iqbal Majid Dar
MSc (N) Psychiatry Nursing
Tutor
Government College of Nursing (MA Road)
Srinagar, J&K

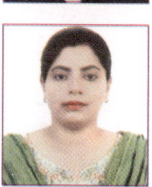

Jamal Fatima
MSc (N) Mental Health & Psychiatric Nursing
Assistant Professor
Rufaida College of Nursing Jamia Hamdard,
New Delhi

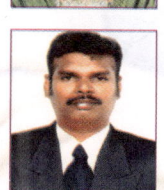

JC Frank
MSc (N) Community Health Nursing
Associate Professor
BEE ENN College of Nursing
Jammu, J&K

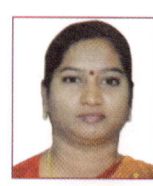

Manohari Sivakumar
MSc (N)
Principal
Saraswathi College of Nursing
Hapur, Uttar Pradesh

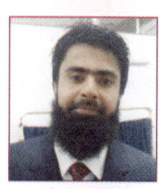

Mohd. Suhail Jogi
MSc (N) Psychiatric & Mental Health Nursing
Nursing Officer
SKIMS (MMINSR)
Srinagar, J&K

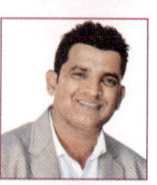

Mukesh Tetarwal
MSc (N) Medical Surgical Nursing
Principal
Government Nursing College
Jodhpur, Rajasthan

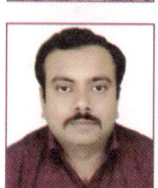

Naveena JH
MSc (N) Community Health Nursing
Associate Professor
NAAC & Outcome Coordinator
Amity College of Nursing, Amity University
Gurugram, Haryana

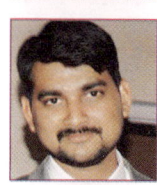

Neeraj Bansal
PhD (N) Medical Surgical Nursing
Associate Professor
Jai Institute of Nursing and Research
Gwalior, Madhya Pradesh

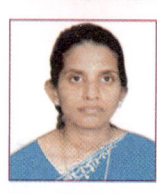

Prathiba Manoharam B
Pursuing PhD, MSc (N) Child Health Nursing
Principal
Keshlata College of Nursing
Bareilly, Uttar Pradesh

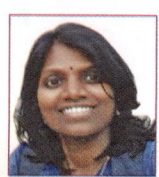

Prema Balusamy
Assistant Professor
Department of Nursing
College of Applied Medical Sciences
University of Hafr-Al-Batin
Kingdom of Saudi Arabia

The names of the reviewers are arranged in alphabetical order

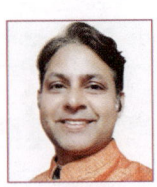

Rajesh Kumar Sharma
MSc (N) Medical Surgical Nursing
Associate Professor & HOD
Himalayan College of Nursing
Swami Rama Himalayan University
Dehradun, Uttarakhand

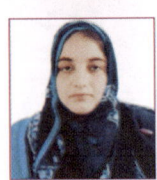

Rehana
MSc (N) Community Health Nursing
Tutor
Government College of Nursing (Shreen Bagh)
Srinagar, J&K

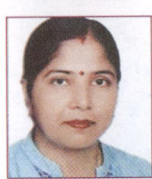

Rekha Anil Kumar
MSc (Mental Health Nursing)
Nursing Tutor
College of Nursing
Dr Ram Manohar Lohia Hospital
New Delhi

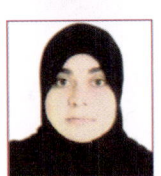

Rohi Jan
MSc (N) Community Health Nursing
Nursing Tutor
Alamdar Memorial College of Nursing &
Medical Technology, Chrar-i-Sharif
Srinagar, J&K

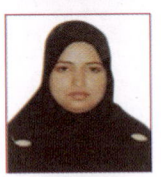

Roohi Jan
MSc (N) Community Health Nursing
Nursing Tutor
Syed Mantaqui Memorial College of Nursing
and Medical Technology
IUST Awantipora, J&K

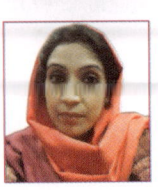

Shazia
MSc (N) OBG Nursing
Nursing Tutor
Bibi Halima College of Nursing &
Medical Technology
Srinagar, J&K

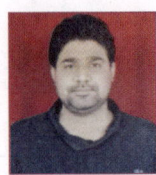

Sheeshpal Chauhan
MSc (N) Psychiatry Nursing
Principal
Florence College of Nursing
Faridabad, Haryana

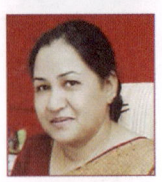

Sunita Lawrence
PhD (N), MSc (OBG Nursing)
(Received National Florence Nightingale
Award–2019)
Principal
Pragyan College of Nursing
Bhopal, Madhya Pradesh

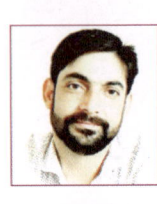

Syed Shahid Siraj
MSc (N) Mental Health Nursing
Nursing Tutor
Alamdar Memorial College of Nursing &
Medical Technology, Chrar-i-Sharif
Srinagar, J&K

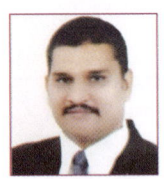

Yogeshwar Puri
Principal
Geetanjali College of Nursing
Udaipur, Rajasthan

The names of the reviewers are arranged in alphabetical order

Preface

Keeping in mind the challenge that today's nurses confront with, it becomes imperative to provide them necessary skills of compassionate nursing care in a variety of health care settings, which they could apply for patients in the various stages of illness. At the same time, there are ample opportunities for health promotion activities for individuals and groups; this is an integral part of providing nursing care.

It gives me immense pleasure and satisfaction to introduce and present this title of **Textbook of Nursing Foundations**. The book is specifically designed for the nursing education in Asia to prepare nurses to think critically and practice collaboratively within today's challenging and complex health care delivery system.

Health care is an exciting and challenging field with opportunities and advancements. The entire health care system reverberates with change. The role of nurses in this system is expanding and extending, hence the process of embracing change inevitably requires adaptation and a constant demand for literary excellence. This textbook has been developed comprehensively with an incredible outlook to help nurses develop their clinical skills which are fundamental aspect of nursing care.

The book is organized into **15 Units having 64 chapters**. The content has been designed for the BSc (N) and MSc (N) students and is based on prescribed curriculum and requirements, which is conforming to Kerala University of Health Sciences (KUHS).

Training is an integral part of the nursing profession. A nurse must possess a strong theoretical base and practical skills. This book will act as a standard prescription for educators and mentors to teach and demonstrate the clinical nursing procedures to budding and practicing nurses. The text has been developed keeping in mind the clinical requirements of a student nurse at all levels of nursing education.

I hope you will enjoy reading the book as much as I enjoyed writing it. Constructive criticism from the readers is always welcome to improve upon in further edition. Happy Reading!

Harindarjeet Goyal

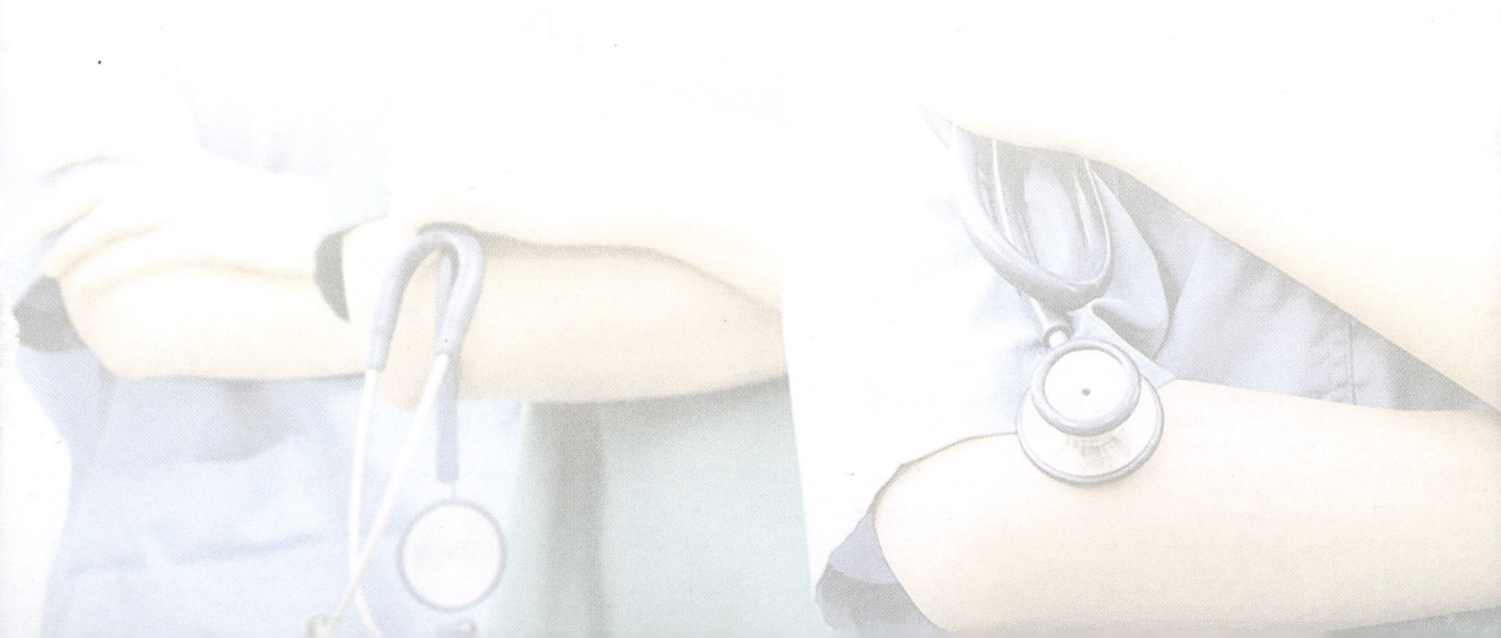

Acknowledgments

Writing a book of this standard demands lots of patience, and focus. I am fortunate enough to have support of many people who helped me in this endeavor.

I want to thank them all who trusted and supported me with their encouragement throughout.

- Fundamentals of Nursing department consisting of Mrs Madhumita Dey, Mrs Usha Phulara, Mrs Rekha Kotnala and Mrs Monika Sharma. They contributed towards many procedures which were carried out in the lab.
- My husband, Mr Ramesh Goyal who had been my source of inspiration to handle the project from beginning till end.
- My daughters: Charu, Khyati and Khushboo for support and patience throughout.

Last but not the least, I extend my special thanks to **Mr Satish Kumar Jain** (Chairman) and **Mr Varun Jain** (Managing Director), M/s CBS Publishers and Distributors Pvt Ltd for their wholehearted support in publication of this book. I have no words to describe the role, efforts, inputs and initiatives undertaken by **Mr Bhupesh Aarora** [Sr. Vice President – Health Science Division (Publishing & Marketing)] for helping and motivating me.

I sincerely thank the entire CBS team for bringing out the book with utmost care and attractive presentation. I would like to thank Ms Nitasha Arora (Publishing Head & Content Strategist – PGMEE & Nursing), and Dr Anju Dhir (Product Manager cum Commissioning Editor – Medical) for their editorial support. I would also extend my thanks to Mr Shivendu Bhushan Pandey (Sr. Manager & Team Lead), Mr Manoj K Yadav (Production Manager), Mr Ashutosh Pathak (Sr. Proofreader cum Team Coordinator) and all the production team members for devoting laborious hours in designing and typesetting the book.

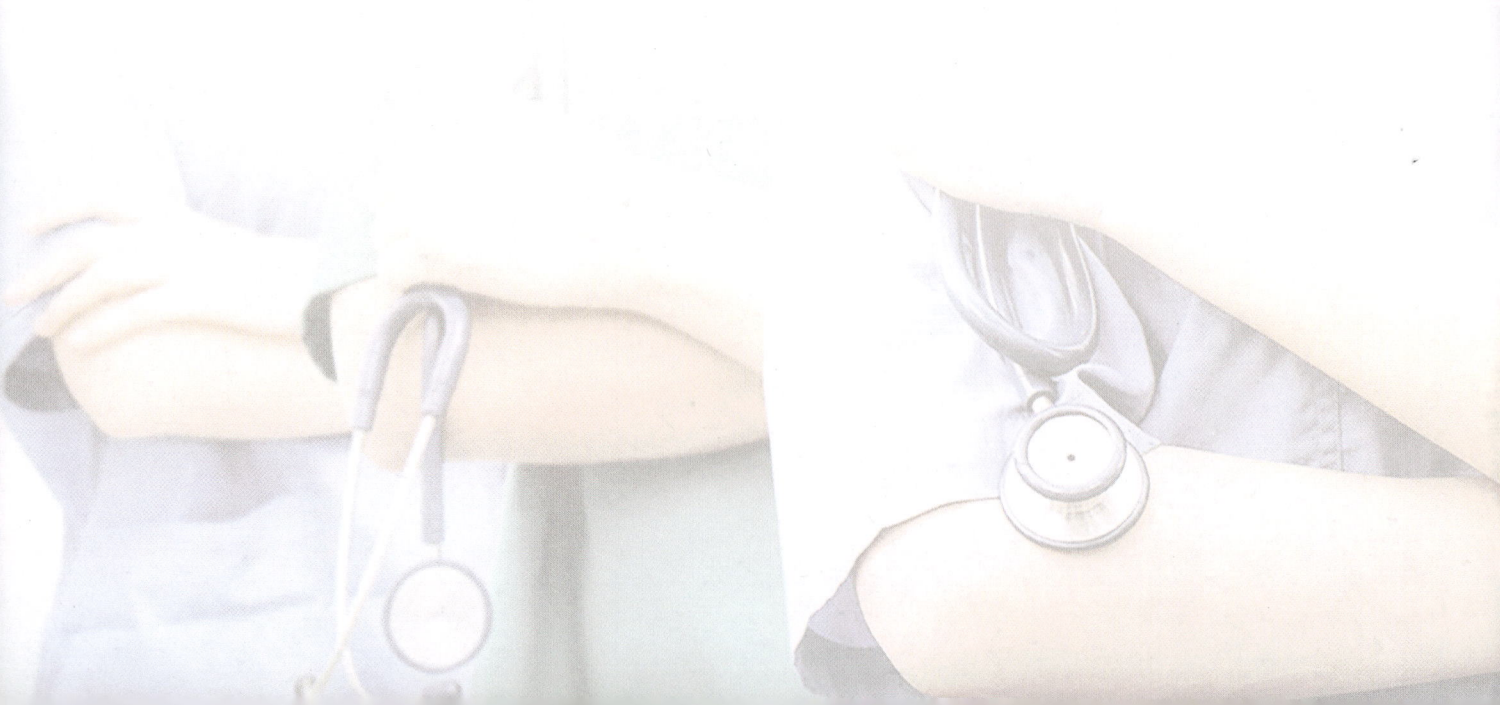

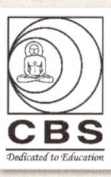

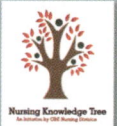

Extends its Tribute to

Florence Nightingale

> *For glorifying the role of women as nurses,*
> *For holding the title of "The Lady with the Lamp,"*
> *For working tirelessly for humanity—*
> *Florence Nightingale will always be*
> *remembered for her*
> *selfless and memorable services to the*
> *human race.*

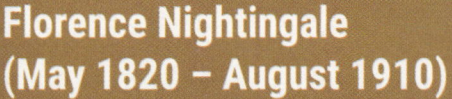

Florence Nightingale
(May 1820 – August 1910)

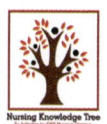

Nursing Knowledge Tree

An Initiative by CBS Nursing Division

"Coming together is a beginning. Keeping together is progress. Working together is success."

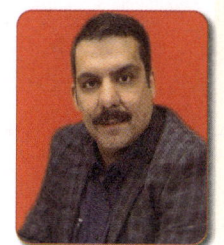

It gives us immense pleasure to share with you that the Nursing Knowledge Tree—An Initiative by CBS Nursing Division, has successfully established itself in the field of nursing as we have been able to stand as a strong contender by sharing approximately 50% of the market share. This growth could not have been possible without your invaluable contribution as our reader, author, reviewer, contributor and recommender, and your outstanding support for the growth of our titles as a whole. You people are the pillars of our series and we are so glad that you all have strengthened our basic foundation.

Nursing Knowledge Tree has been a pioneer and specialist in publishing best quality books for nursing education. Keeping in mind the changing trends in nursing education, we, at Nursing Knowledge Tree, have taken up a mission to bring student-friendly and syllabus-based books written by Subject Experts PAN India.

Our Noteworthy Achievements:

- Our nationally-acclaimed titles
  - *PGIMER NINE Clinical Nursing Procedures*—**Sandhya Ghai**
  - *Target High Staff Nurse Entrance Examination*—**Muthuvenkatachalam S, Ambili M Venugopal**
  - *CBS Nursing Drug Guide*—**Yogesh Gulati/Rakesh Sharma**
  - *Textbook of Nursing Foundations*—**Harindarjeet Goyal**
  - *Essentials of Biochemistry*—**Harbans Lal**
  - *Textbook of Nursing Education*—**Ratna Prakash**
  - *Nursing Research in 21st Century*—**Sukhpal Kaur and Amarjeet Singh**
  - *Essentials of Applied Microbiology*—**D R Arora and Brij Bala Arora**
  - *Textbook of Pediatric Nursing*—**Meharban Singh and Raman Kalia**
- Liaised with the topmost institutes of the country, like **AIIMS, NIMHANS, PGIMER NINE, CMC-Vellore, Manipal University, JIPMER, RAK-Delhi**, etc.
- Published **100+ Quality Nursing Books** and more than **50 New Books** on various subjects for Nursing Undergraduates, Postgraduates and Nursing superspecialty are under process and will be releasing in 2021.
- Increased our social presence by participating in more than **200+ National Conferences, CME's, College Exhibitions & Webinars** in previous years.
- We have come out with **Nursing Next Live**, an EdTech platform, the Next Level of Nursing Education, where we bring learning to people, instead of people going for learning. Through NNL App we are providing various study modules/plans covering All Subjects/All Topics, Video Lectures, Question Banks, E-notes and a Variety of Tests. Students can choose the plan according to their needs and requirements.
- We are excited to announce that we are coming out with our new initiative—**Nursing Next Live Social**, where nursing faculties can share as well as gain knowledge, with the aim to revolutionize the way the nursing segment connects. It's going to be India's first networking platform for Nursing Segment.

Our Journey towards providing Quality Nursing Education is Incomplete without YOU ! Join Us Now !

We specialize in publishing nursing books of superior quality, going ahead we see us publishing more and more quality content and it will only be possible when intellectuals from across the nation come together. Keeping pace with the advancements, we want to strengthen the nursing sector, which was long neglected, and establish a strong foundation when it comes to quality content for the segment.

We are determined to bring about changes in the Nursing Education system and with your support and contributions, we will do it for sure. We will be delighted if you join hands with us in the form of Author, Contributor or Reviewer and take the vision of quality education for nursing students ahead.

Let's join hands together and share our ideas and knowledge. Be the part of this Revolution. We are looking forward to your cooperation in future as well. Share your CVs at **bhupesharora@nursingnextlive.in** or scan the given QR code and fill the form or you can talk to me directly at +9555353330.

With Best Wishes
Mr Bhupesh Aarora
Sr. Vice President – Health Science Division
(Publishing & Marketing)

Special Features of the Book

Learning Objectives → Important learning objectives of every chapter are highlighted in the beginning.

After completing this chapter, you will be able to:
- Define health and its changing concepts
- Describe the health-illness continuum
- Enumerate the various factors influencing health
- Explain the causation of disease with the help of model
- Discuss the impact of illness on patient and family

→ Important key terms used in the chapter are presented to familiarize the readers with the important terminologies.

Key Terms

- Health
- Biomedical concept
- Ecological concept
- Psychosocial concept
- Holistic concept
- Agent
- Host
- Environment

→ Chapter outline is given in the beginning of every chapter to make the reader go through the topics covered in a particular chapter.

Chapter Outline

- Introduction
- Concept of Health and Disease
- Changing Concepts of Health
- Health-illness Continuum
- Factors Influencing Health
- Illness and Illness Behavior

→ Numerous Tables are used to clarify the concept and make the reading enjoyable and informative.

TABLE 1: Clinical observations for nutritional assessment

Parameters/body area	Signs of good nutritional status	Signs of poor nutritional status
Appearance	Alert, responsive	Listless, apathetic
Vitality	Energetic, vigorous, sleeps well	Lacking energy, tired, apathetic
Weight	Normal as per height, age and body build	Overweight or underweight
Hair	Shiny, lustrous, healthy scalp	Dull, dry, brittle, thin
Skin	Smooth, good color, slightly moist, no rashes or swelling	Rough, dry, swollen, pale, pigmented, bruises, petechia
Nails	Pink, firm	Spoon-shaped, pale, brittle

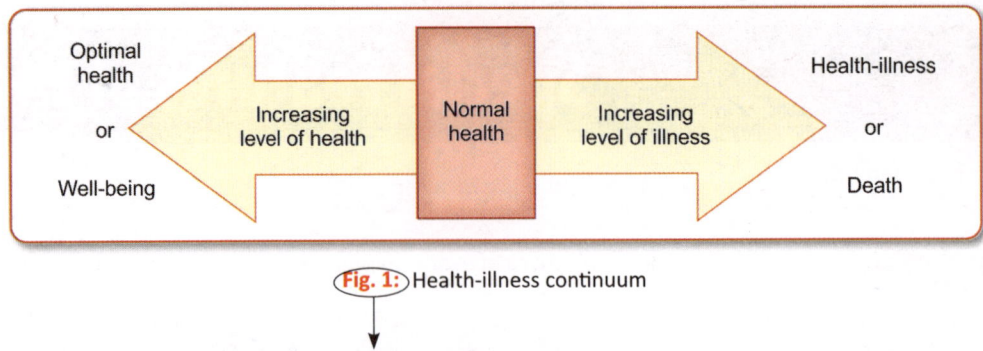

Fig. 1: Health-illness continuum

Studded with 200 + fully colored images and illustrations for easy grasp of the relevant topic.

At the end of every chapter, Bibliography has been added for further reference to enhance knowledge.

Added information boxes have been supplemented throughout the book.

BIBLIOGRAPHY

1. Park K. Park's Textbook of Preventive and Social Medicine, 25th edition: Banarsidas Bhanot. Jabalpur, MP: 2017.
2. Lewis LW. Fundamental Skills in Patient Care, 2nd edition: Lippincott Williams and Wilkins.
3. Christensen K. Fundamentals of Nursing, 8th edition: Mosby Publishing. Maryland Heights Missouri: 2010.
4. Sharma S. Potter and Perry's Fundamentals of Nursing. A South Asian edition: India. Gurugram: Elsevier 2013.

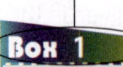

Change of Shift Report

- Bed no. 104- M_2X
- Admitted last night with head injury
- Allergic to penicillin
- I/V Dextrose 5% infusing 100 mL/hour in (L) forearm
- Needs urgent CT scan
- Temp. 102°F Pulse 98/minute, RR 24/minute
- Blood pressure 110/70 mm of Hg
- GCS-11

Nursing Foundations

Placement : *1st Year*

Time (Theory): **465 hours**
Class: 265 hours
Lab: 200 hours

Course description: This course is designed to help the students to develop an understanding of the nursing profession, philosophy, objectives, theories and application of nursing in various clinical settings. It is aimed at helping the students to acquire knowledge, understanding and skills in techniques of nursing and practice them in supervised clinical settings.

Unit	Time (hrs)	Learning objectives	Content	Teaching learning activities	Assessment Methods
I	10	Describe the concept of health, illness and health care agencies	**Introduction** • Health and Illness ▪ Definition ▪ Concept • Health illness continuum • Factors influencing health • Causes and risk factors of illness • Illness behavior • Impact of illness on patient and family • Health care services ▪ Health promotion ▪ Levels of prevention • Health care agencies: ▪ Hospitals—types, organization and functions • Health care team	• Lecture • Discussion • Visit to health care agencies	• Short answers • Very short answers
II	15	• Explain concept and scope of nursing • Describe values, code of ethics and professional conduct for nurses in India	**Nursing as a Profession** • **Nursing:** ▪ Definition ▪ Philosophy ▪ Objectives ▪ Characteristics ▪ Scope of nursing practice • Functions of nurse • Qualities of a nurse • Categories of nursing personnel • Definition and characteristics of profession • Nursing as a profession • Values: Definition, types, values in professional nursing • Ethics: Definition, ethical principles, nursing code of ethics • History of nursing in India	• Lecture • Discussion • Case discussion • Role plays	• Short answers • Very short answers
III	5	Explain the basic concepts of conceptual and theoretical models of nursing	**Conceptual and Theoretical Models in Nursing Practice** • Introduction to models: ▪ Holistic model ▪ Health belief model ▪ Health promotion model • Maslow's hierarchy of needs • Introduction to theories in Nursing: Florence Nightingale environmental theory ▪ Orem's general theory of nursing ▪ Peplau's theory of interpersonal relationship ▪ Henderson's definition of nursing	• Lecture • Discussion	• Short answers • Very short answers

Contd...

Unit	Time (hrs)	Learning objectives	Content	Teaching learning activities	Assessment Methods
IV	10	• Communicate effectively with patient families and team members and maintain effective human relations projecting professional image • Appreciate the importance of patient teaching in nursing	**Communication and Nurse Patient Relationship** • Communication ▪ Definition ▪ Levels ▪ Elements ▪ Types ▪ Factors influencing communication ▪ Methods of effective communication ▪ Attending skills, rapport building skills, empathy skills ▪ Barriers to effective communication • Helping relationships (NPR) ▪ Definition ▪ Goals ▪ Phases of a helping relationship (NPR) • Patient teaching: ▪ Purpose ▪ Principles ▪ Role of nurse	• Lecture • Discussion • Role play • Video film on nurses interacting with the patient • Practice session on patient teaching • Supervised clinical practice	• Essay • Short answers • Very short answers
V	30	• Describe purpose and process of health assessment • Describe the health assessment of each body system • Explain the concept, uses, format and steps of nursing process • Documents nursing process as per the format	**Health Assessment** • Purposes • Process of health assessment: ▪ Health history, physical examination • Methods: Inspection ▪ Palpation ▪ Percussion ▪ Auscultation ▪ Olfaction • Preparation of patient and unit for physical examination • Nursing process • The nursing process: ▪ Overview ▪ Definition ▪ Steps of nursing process • Assessment: ▪ Collection of data—types, sources, methods ▪ Formulating nursing judgment ▪ Data interpretation • Nursing diagnosis: ▪ Identification of client problems ▪ Nursing diagnosis statement ▪ Difference between medical and nursing diagnosis • Planning: ▪ Establishing priorities ▪ Establishing goals and expected outcomes ▪ Selection of interventions ▪ Protocols ▪ Standing orders ▪ Writing nursing care plan • Implementation: ▪ Implementing the plan of care • Evaluation: ▪ Outcome of care ▪ Review and modify • Documentation and reporting	• Lecture • Discussion • Demonstration • Practice on simulators • Supervised clinical practice	• Structured essay • Short answers • Very short answers

Contd...

Unit	Time (hrs)	Learning objectives	Content	Teaching learning activities	Assessment Methods

VI	5	Describe the purposes, types and techniques of recording and reporting	**Documentation and Reporting**
			• Documentation:
			  ▪ Purposes of recording and reporting
			  ▪ General guidelines for recording
			  ▪ Types of documentation system
			  ▪ Computerized documentation
			  ▪ Common record keeping forms
			• Reporting:
			  ▪ Change of shift reports
			  ▪ Transfer reports
			  ▪ Telephone report and
			  ▪ Incident reports
			• Minimizing legal liability through effective record keeping
				• Lecture
				• Discussion
				• Demonstration
				• Practice session
				• Supervised clinical practice
					• Essay
					• Short answers
					• Very short answers

VII	5	• Explain the admission and discharge procedure
		• Performs admission and discharge procedure
			Hospital Admission and Discharge
			• Admission to the hospital:
			  ▪ Purposes
			  ▪ Types
			  ▪ Unit and its preparation
			  ▪ Admission procedure
			  ▪ Medicolegal issues
			• Discharge from the hospital:
			  ▪ DAMA and abscond
			  ▪ Referrals and transfers
			  ▪ Discharge planning
			  ▪ Discharge procedure
			  ▪ Care of the unit after discharge
			  ▪ Medicolegal issues
				• Lecture
				• Discussion
				• Demonstration
				• Lab Practice
				• Supervised clinical practice
					• Essay
					• Short answers
					• Very short answers

VIII	20	Describe principles and techniques for infection control and biomedical waste management in Supervised clinical settings	**Infection Control and Waste Management**
			• Infection control
			  ▪ Nature of infection
			  ▪ Chain of infection
			  ▪ Methods of transmission
			  ▪ Body defenses against infection
			• Types of infection
			  ▪ Nosocomial infection
			• Asepsis: Concepts
			  ▪ Medical and surgical asepsis
			  ▪ Barrier methods
			• Hand washing:
			  ▪ Medical and surgical
			• Isolation: Source and protective
			• Personal protective equipments:
			  ▪ Types, uses
			  ▪ Techniques of wearing and removal
			• Decontamination of equipment and unit
			• Transportation of infected patients
			• Universal safety precautions—standard precautions and transmission-based precautions
			• Biomedical waste management
			  ▪ Importance
			  ▪ Types of hospital waste
			  ▪ Hazards associated with hospital waste
			  ▪ Decontamination of hospital waste
			  ▪ Segregation, transportation and disposal
			  ▪ Hospital infection control committee—Nurse's role
				• Lecture
				• Discussion
				• Demonstration
				• Practice session
				• Supervised clinical practice
					• Essay
					• Short answers
					• Very short answers

Contd...

Unit	Time (hrs)	Learning objectives	Content	Teaching learning activities	Assessment Methods

IX	30	• Describe principles and techniques of monitoring and maintaining vital signs
		• Monitor and maintain vital signs
			Vial signs
			• Guidelines for taking vital signs
			  ▪ Principles
			• Body temperature
			  ▪ Physiology
			  ▪ Regulation and factors affecting body temperature
			  ▪ Sites, equipments, techniques and special consideration
			  ▪ Temperature alterations: Hyperthermia, hypothermia, heat stroke
			  ▪ Care of patients having alterations in body temperature
			• Pulse
			  ▪ Physiology and regulation
			  ▪ Characteristics of pulse
			  ▪ Factors affecting pulse
			  ▪ Assessment of pulse, sites, location, techniques
			  ▪ Alteration in pulse
			• Respiration
			  ▪ Physiology and regulation
			  ▪ Mechanics of breathing
			  ▪ Characteristics of respiration
			  ▪ Factors affecting respiration
			  ▪ Alterations in respiration
			• Blood pressure
			  ▪ Physiology and regulation of BP
			  ▪ Characteristics of BP
			  ▪ Factors affecting BP
			  ▪ Assessment of BP
			  ▪ Sites, equipments and technique
			  ▪ Alterations in blood pressure
			  ▪ Assessment of BP
			• Assessment of TPR
			• Recording of vital signs
				• Lecture
				• Discussion
				• Demonstration
				• Practice session
				• Supervised clinical practice
					• Essay
					• Short answers
					• Very short answers

X	60	• Describe the basic physiological and psychological needs of the patient
		• Describe the principles and techniques for meeting basic, physiological and psychosocial needs of patient
		• Perform nursing assessment, plan, implement and evaluate the care for meeting, basic physiological and psychosocial needs of patient
			Meeting Needs of Patients
			• Basic needs
			• Activities of daily living
			• Provide safe and clean environment: Therapeutic environment
			• Physical environment: Temperature, humidity, noise, ventilation, light, odor, pest control
			• Reduction of physical hazards, fire, accidents
			• Role of a nurse in providing safe and clean environment
			• Patient environment: Room, equipment and linen
			• Making patients' beds:
			  ▪ Types of beds and bed making.
			• Comfort and safety
			• Factors influencing comfort
			• Comfort devices
			• Safety devices—restraints, side rails, airways
			• Hygiene
			• Factors influencing hygienic practices
			• Care of skin:
			  ▪ Bath, perineal care
			• Pressure ulcers
			  ▪ Care of pressure points
			• Care of oral cavity, eyes, ears and nose
			• Care of nail and foot, hair
			• Physiological needs
			  ▪ Sleep and rest
				• Lecture
				• Discussion
				• Demonstration of sponge bath, back care, nail care, foot care and hair care
				• Demonstration of mouth care
				• Practice sessions
				• Supervised clinical practice
					• Essay
					• Short answers
					• Very short answers

Contd...

Unit	Time (hrs)	Learning objectives	Content	Teaching learning activities	Assessment Methods
			• ▪ Physiology of sleep ▪ Factors affecting sleep ▪ Promoting rest and sleep ▪ Sleep disorders • Nutrition ▪ Importance ▪ Factors affecting nutritional needs ▪ Assessment of nutritional needs ▪ Meeting nutritional needs: principles, procedure and special care • Oral, nasogastric and gastrostomy feeding, parenteral feeding • Urinary elimination ▪ Review of physiology of urine elimination ▪ Composition and characteristics of urine ▪ Factors influencing urination • Alteration in urinary elimination: urinary retention and incontinence • Types and collection of urine specimen ▪ Urine testing • Facilitating urine elimination: assessment, types, equipments • Procedures—Providing urinal/bed pan ▪ Condom drainage ▪ Catheterization ▪ Care of urinary drainage ▪ Bladder irrigation • Bowel elimination ▪ Review of physiology of bowel elimination ▪ Composition and characteristics of feces ▪ Factors affecting bowel elimination ▪ Alteration in bowel elimination and its management– ▪ Constipation ▪ Diarrhoea ▪ Fecal impaction • Types and collection of specimen of feces-observation • Facilitating bowel elimination: ▪ Assessment, equipment and procedures ▪ Passing of flatus tube ▪ Enemas ▪ Suppository ▪ Bowel wash • Mobility and immobility • Principles of body mechanics • Maintenance of normal body alignment and mobility • Hazards associated with immobility • Alteration in body alignment and mobility • Nursing intervention for impaired body • Alignment and mobility: assessment, types of devices used, methods and special considerations, rehabilitation aspects • Range of motion exercises • Maintaining body alignment: positions • Moving, lifting, transferring, walking • Restraints ▪ Care of patients having restraints • Alteration of mobility: Assessment of self-care ability and special considerations		

Contd...

Unit	Time (hrs)	Learning objectives	Content	Teaching learning activities	Assessment Methods
			• Oxygenation ▪ Review of cardiovascular and respiratory physiology ▪ Factors affecting oxygenation ▪ Alterations in oxygenation • Nursing interventions in oxygen administration: ▪ Assessment, types ▪ Equipment used, procedure and special consideration • Chest physiotherapy • Fluid, electrolyte, and acid base balances ▪ Review of physiological regulation of fluid, electrolyte and acid base balances ▪ Factors affecting fluid, electrolyte and acid base balance ▪ Alterations in fluid and electrolyte balance ▪ Nursing interventions in fluid, electrolyte and acid base imbalance ▪ Assessment, types, equipment, procedure and special consideration • Measuring fluid intake and output ▪ Correcting fluid and electrolyte–imbalance: replacement of fluids—oral and parenteral, • Venipuncture • Regulating IV flow rates, changing IV solutions and tubing, changing IV • Dressing • Administering blood transfusion • Restriction of fluids • Psychosocial needs: ▪ Concepts of cultural diversity, stress and adaptation, self-concept, sexuality, spiritual health, coping with loss, death and grieving ▪ Assessment of psychosocial needs ▪ Nursing interventions for meeting psychosocial needs: • Recreational and diversional therapies ▪ Nurses role • Meeting the special needs of patients • Care of patients having alterations in sensory functioning: Visual and hearing impairment, Assessment of self-care ability, communication methods and special considerations • Care of patient having altered sensorium—Unconsciousness assessment and nursing management		
XI	5	• Explain the general principles of heat and cold applications • Demonstrate procedures of hot and cold applications	**Therapeutic use of Heat and Cold Applications** • General principles • Effect on the body Hot applications: • Hot water bag • Infrared therapy • Fomentation • Sitz bath Cold applications: • Cold compress • Ice cap • Tepid sponge	• Lecture • Discussion • Demonstration • Practice sessions • Supervised clinical practice	• Essay • Short answers • Very short answers

Contd...

Unit	Time (hrs)	Learning objectives	Content	Teaching learning activities	Assessment Methods
XII	40	• Explain the principles, routes and effects of administration of medications. • Calculate conversions of drugs dosages within and between system of measurements. • Administer drugs by the following routes—oral, intradermal, subcutaneous, intramuscular, intravenous, topical and inhalation	**Administration of Medications** • General principles/considerations • Purposes of medication, principles, rights, special considerations, prescriptions. • Safety in administering medications • Medication errors • Drug forms • Routes of administration • Storage and maintenance of drugs and nurses responsibility • Broad classification of drugs • Therapeutic effect, side effects, toxic effects, idiosyncratic reactions, allergic reactions, drug tolerance, drug interactions • Factors influencing drug actions • Systems of drug measurement: ▪ Metric system, apothecary system ▪ House hold measurements ▪ Solutions • Converting measurement units: Conversion within one system, conversion between systems, dosage calculation • Terminologies and abbreviations used in prescriptions of medications • Oral drug administration: ▪ Oral, sublingual and buccal—Equipment, procedure • Parenteral ▪ General principles, decontamination and disposal of syringes and needles • Types of parenteral therapies • Types of syringes, needles, cannula, and infusion sets • Protection from needle stick injuries • Routes of parenteral therapies: • Intradermal: Purpose, site ▪ Equipment, procedure, special considerations • Subcutaneous: Purpose, site, equipment, procedure, special considerations • Intramuscular: Purpose, site, equipment, procedure, special considerations • Intravenous: Purpose, site equipment, procedure, special considerations • Advanced techniques: ▪ Epidural ▪ Intrathecal ▪ Intraosseous ▪ Intraperitoneal ▪ Intrapleural ▪ Intra-arterial ▪ Role of nurse • Topical administration ▪ Purposes, site, equipment, procedure, • Special considerations for application to skin and mucous membrane • Direct application of liquids • Gargle and swabbing the throat • Insertion of drug into the body cavity • Suppository/medicated pack in rectum/ vagina • Instillations: Eye, ear, nasal, bladder and rectum • Irrigations: Eye, ear, nasal, bladder and rectum.	• Lecture • Discussion • Demonstration • Practice sessions • Supervised clinical practice	• Essay • Short answers • Very short answers

Contd...

Unit	Time (hrs)	Learning objectives	Content	Teaching learning activities	Assessment Methods
			• Spraying—nose and throat • Inhalation: Nasal, oral, endotracheal/tracheal (steam, oxygen and medications): Purpose, types, equipment, procedure, special considerations • Nebulization • Recording and reporting of medications administered		
XIII	5	• Define rehabilitation • Explain the concepts, principles and types of rehabilitation • Discuss the role of nurse in rehabilitation	**Rehabilitation** • Definition of rehabilitation • Concepts of rehabilitation • Types of rehabilitation • Role of nurse in rehabilitation	• Lecture • Discussion	• Short answers • Objective Type
XIV	5	Explain care of terminally ill patient	**Care of Terminally Ill Patient** • Concepts of loss, grief • Signs of clinical death • Care of dying: Special considerations • Advance directives: euthanasia, will, dying declaration, organ donation • Medico-legal issues • Care of body after death—equipment, procedure and care of unit • Autopsy • Embalming	• Lecture • Discussion • Demonstration • Case discussion/role play • Practice session • Supervised clinical practice	• Short answers • Very short answers

XV	20	Explain the principles of first aid and demonstrate application of different types of bandages	**First Aid Nursing**
			• Definition
			• Qualities of a first aider
			• Preparation of equipment
			• Application of bandages and slings
			• Shifting of patients with spine dislocation
			• Padding and splinting fractured limbs
			• First aid measures and antidotes in poisoning: Immediate care of patients with snakebite, rabid dog bite, burns, scalds, frost bite, sunstroke, drowning, electrocution
			• First aid and nursing in simple emergencies
			• Common accidents—preventive measures and emergency care:
			  ▪ Wounds
			  ▪ Food poisoning
			  ▪ Chemical poisoning
			  ▪ Foreign body in the eye, ear, nose and throat
			• Cardiopulmonary
			• Resuscitation—BLS
				• Lecture
				• Discussion
				• Demonstration
				• Case discussion/role play
				• Practice session
					• Short answers
					• Very short answers

Contents

UNIT XI: THERAPEUTIC USE OF HEAT AND COLD APPLICATIONS

UNIT XII: ADMINISTRATION OF MEDICATIONS

UNIT XIII: REHABILITATION

UNIT XIV: CARE OF TERMINALLY ILL PATIENT

UNIT XV: FIRST AID NURSING

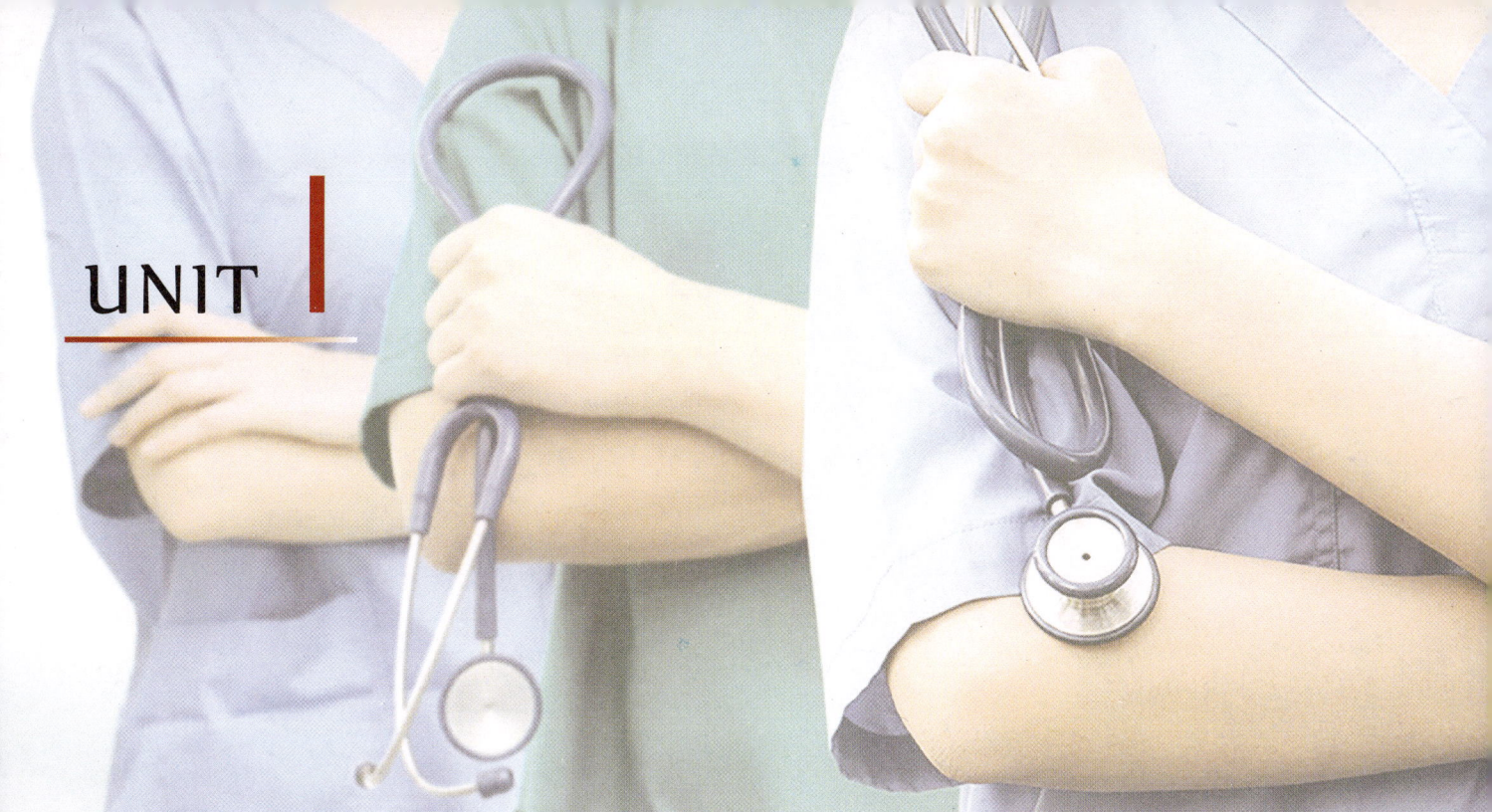

UNIT I

INTRODUCTION

Unit Outline

Concept of Health

INTRODUCTION

In the yesteryears, good health or wellness was viewed as the opposite or absence of disease. We now understand that some conditions of health may lie between disease and good health. Therefore, health should be viewed from a broader perspective. As a nurse, you will use concepts of health, health promotion, wellness and illness to assist your clients in achieving and maintaining an optimum level of health. Models of health and illness can be used to understand and explain these concepts.

The relative presence or absence of disease is both a personal and a social problem. It is a personal problem because a person's ability to work, to be productive, to love, and to play are all related to that individual's mental and physical health. It is a social problem because the illness of one person can adversely affect other people, e.g., family, friends, etc.

People have different attitudes and reactions to illness. The nurse who understands how clients react to illness, can minimize the effects of illness and assist clients and their families in maintaining or returning to the highest level of functioning.

CONCEPT OF HEALTH AND DISEASE

Health and disease are not static conditions. Rather, they are vital concepts that are subject to continuous evaluation and change. It is difficult to derive a universally acceptable definition for the terms 'health' and 'disease' because these concepts are subjective and difficult to measure. People define these terms according to personal value systems that are influenced by culture, socio-economic status, age, knowledge and pre-existing states of health and disease.

Indeed, we all have our own definitions of health and disease based on our individual life experiences.

You will be able to understand better, if you go through the following definitions.

Health is defined as:

- A series of successful and continuous adaptations to a continuously changing environment.
- The condition of being sound in body, mind and spirit and especially free from physical disease or pain *(Webster)*.
- Soundness of body or mind; that condition in which their functions are duly and efficiently performed *(Oxford English Dictionary)*.
- A state of relative equilibrium of body's form and function, which results from its successful dynamic adjustment to forces tending to disturb it. It is not passive interplay between body substance and forces impinging upon it but active response of body forces working towards readjustment *(Perkin)*.
- Health is a relative concept; this may be due to ecological conditions and the fact that standards of health vary among culture: Social classes and age groups.

The above-mentioned definitions give varied views of health. We shall now try to look into the most widely accepted definition of health given by the World Health Organization (WHO) which states:

"Health is a state of complete physical, mental, social and spiritual well-being and not merely an absence of disease or infirmity."

If we look at the above definition, these are four aspects or dimensions emerging from it. These are:

1. Physical health
2. Mental health
3. Social health
4. Spiritual health

Physical health means that an individual has good complexion, a clean skin, bright eyes, good appetite, sound sleep, regular activity of bowel and bladder, and smooth coordinated bodily movements. All the organs of the body function normally. All special senses are intact. The resting pulse rate and blood pressure (BP) are within the range of normality for the individual's age and sex.

Mental health means that an individual has following characteristics:

- He/she feels comfortable about himself/herself. He/she neither overestimates nor underestimates his/her own abilities. He/she accepts his/her shortcomings, is internally adjusted, is self-confident and free from internal conflicts.
- He/she is at peace with others. He/she is able to feel himself/herself as a part of a group and is able to get on well with others.
- A mentally healthy person has good self-control. He/she is not overcome by emotions, not dominated by fear, anger, love, jealousy, guilt or worries. He/she faces problems and tries to solve them intelligently.

Social health means ability of making friendships that are satisfying and lasting, of assuming responsibilities according to one's capabilities, of finding satisfaction, success and happiness in accomplishments of everyday tasks and living happily with others.

Spiritual health is an intangible something that transcends physiology and psychology, i.e., the spirit of man. A spiritually healthy person maintains faith in religion and believes in empathy and goodness for all.

Health as a State of Being

We might describe a person in various terms like energetic, outgoing, enthusiastic, beautiful, caring, loving, intense, etc. Therefore, health involves physical, psychological, spiritual and sociocultural influences that define one's present condition. Even the state of feeling well fluctuates. Some mornings we wake up feeling more energetic and enthusiastic than other mornings. How a person feels varies day by day, even hour by hour; nevertheless, it can be a strong indicator of that person's state of health.

WHO later produced a more specific definition stating:

"Health can be defined as a series of successful and continuous adaptations to a constantly changing environment." This definition of health appears to be a more realistic and complete since health is a dynamic state rather than a static state.

Disease, Sickness and Illness

While all the three terms appear similar, there is a significant difference in the ways they are used and in their meanings. Illness is defined as the ill health, the person identifies himself with, often based on self-reported mental or physical symptoms. Sickness is defined as the state of being sick or of being affected by an illness, infection or disease. Disease is defined as a condition that is diagnosed and identified by a doctor or a medical expert. It is some deviation from the biological norm and have an objectivity about them.

CHANGING CONCEPTS OF HEALTH

In a world of continuous change, new concepts are bound to emerge based on new patterns of thought. The changing concepts of health are mainly of four types discussed as follows.

Biomedical Concept

Traditionally, health has been viewed as "absence of disease." If any person is free from disease, he/she is considered as healthy. This concept is known as biomedical concept and is based on Germ Theory of Disease.

The medical profession viewed the human body as a machine and disease as a consequence of the breakdown of the machine. One of the tasks of a doctor is to repair the machine. This concept was found to be inadequate as it minimizes the role of environmental, social, psychological and cultural determinants of health.

Ecological Concept

Ecologists viewed health as a dynamic equilibrium between man and his environment, and disease as a maladjustment of the human organisms to the environment. Ecological and cultural adaptations determine not only the occurrence of disease, but also the availability of food and the population explosion. This concept supports the need for clean air, safe water, ozone layer in the atmosphere to protect from exposure to unhealthy factors, etc.

Psychosocial Concept

Development in social sciences reveals that disease is both a biological and social phenomenon. There are not only biological factors, but also social, cultural and psychological factors, which must be taken into consideration while defining health and illness.

Holistic Concept

Holistic concept is the synthesis of biomedical, ecological and psychosocial concepts. It recognizes the strength of social, economic, political and environmental influences on health. It has been defined as unified or multidimensional process involving the well-being of an entire person in the context of his environment.

HEALTH-ILLNESS CONTINUUM

Health always involves a continuum; a range of degrees from optimal health at one end to death or total disability at the other (Fig. 1). The health of an individual moves back and forth along this continuum throughout life.

According to health-illness continuum, health is a dynamic state that fluctuates as a person adapts to changes in the internal and external environments to maintain a state of total well-being. Internal environment refers to physiological system, body temperature, blood pressure and external environment refers to atmospheric temperature, humidity, etc.

Health level wellness and severe illness are the opposite ends of the continuum. According to Newman (1990), "Health on a continuum is the degree of client's wellness that exists at any point of time, ranging from an optimal health condition, with available energy at its maximum to death, which represents total energy depletion." A nurse can determine a client's level of health at any point on the health-illness continuum, risk factors are important in identifying level of health. They include genetic and physiological variables such as age, lifestyle and environment.

FACTORS INFLUENCING HEALTH

The factors which influence health are multifactorial, which are both within the individual and externally in the society in which he/she lives. The factors influencing health can be broadly classified into:
- Genetic factors
- Environmental factors.

Genetic Factors/Heredity/Human Biology

The mental and physical traits of every human being are determined by the nature of the genes to some extent. There are a number of diseases that are known to have genetic origin, e.g., diabetes, hemophilia, etc. The state of health, therefore, depends partly on the genetic constitution of man. The steady state of internal environment of the body is called homeostasis.

Environment

Environment has a close relation to the health of an individual. It can be external or internal. The internal environment pertains to each and every component of the body, every tissue, organ and organ system, and their hormones functioning within the system.

The external environment of man is the aggregate of all external conditions, which affect the development of life

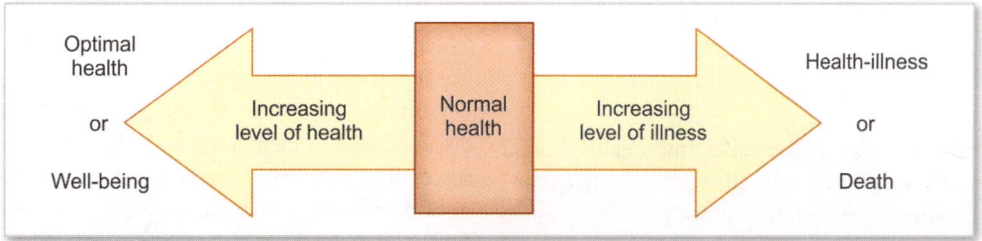

Fig. 1: Health-illness continuum

of an individual. If the environment is favorable, he/she can make full use of physical and mental capacities he/she has inherited. Mostly, ill health results because of poor external environment. External environment comprises three closely related components: physical, biological and social.

Physical environmental factors that affect state of health are water, air, sunlight, climate, season, soil, housing-facilities, waste and excreta disposal, etc.

Biological environmental factors consist of all living things plants, animals, insects and microorganisms.

Social environmental factors consist of people, customs, culture, society, income, occupation, religion, etc.

Lifestyle/Ways of Living

Lifestyle denotes the way people live, reflecting a whole range of social values, attitudes and activities. Lifestyles are learnt through social interactions with parents, peer groups, friends, siblings and through school and mass media. It is composed of cultural and behavioral patterns of life-long personal habits that have developed through process of socialization. Many health problems are associated with lifestyle changes. Risks of illness and death are related with lifestyle such as lack of sanitation, poor nutrition, personal hygiene, habits, systems and cultural patterns. Certain lifestyles like adequate nutrition, enough sleep and sufficient physical activity help in promoting good health. Adoption of healthy lifestyle leads to promoting optimal health.

Resources

The resources which help in maintaining and determining health of an individual are his/her socio-economic conditions. Health status is primarily determined by the level of socio-economic development like per capita income, political system, economy, etc.

The important socio-economic factors of major importance are discussed below.

Economic Status

The per capita income is accepted measure of socio-economic condition. The socio-economic development has a major role in reducing morbidity, increasing life expectancy and improving quality of life. Socio-economic status determines the purchasing power, quality of life, standard of life, family size, pattern of disease, and deviant behavior in the community.

Education

Education is an important factor affecting health. Lack of education closely coincides with ill health, high infant mortality rate, malnutrition, etc. Education compensates the effects of poverty on health irrespective of availability of health facilities.

Occupation

Occupation promotes health while unemployment deteriorates the socio-economic status leading to deterioration in health. Loss of work means loss of income and status resulting in psychological and social changes.

Political System

Health is related to a country's political system as it can affect the implementation of health technologies. Political system is concerned with resource allocation, manpower policy, choice of technology and the degree to which health services are made available and accessible to different segments of society. If health patterns are to be changed, changes must be made in the entire socio-political system.

Health Services

Health services are directed towards treatment of diseases, prevention of illness and promotion of health. Purpose of health services is to improve the health status of the population and make health services available to all sectors of the population. Health services are essential for socio-economic development. To be effective, the health services must reach the social periphery that the community can afford and be socially acceptable.

Causes and Risk Factors for Developing Illness

The concept of disease and health have great impact on health promotion, health protection and health maintenance. The Germ Theory became popular during the end of nineteenth century and early part of twentieth century. According to this theory, there is a single, specific causative agent to every disease (Fig. 2).

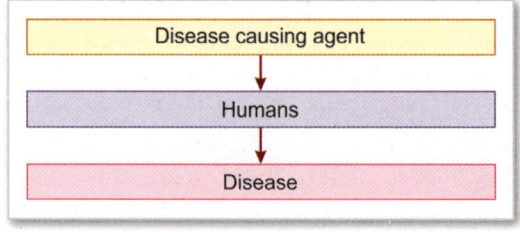

Fig. 2: Germ theory

Tuberculosis is caused by *Mycobacterium tuberculosis*, Cholera is caused by *Vibrio cholerae* and diphtheria is caused by *Corynebacterium diphtheriae*. This theory has many limitations. For example, every one exposed to disease agent does not get the disease. Like in tuberculosis, only those who are malnourished, susceptible and lived in slum get the disease. This means, in addition to specific causative agent, there are many other factors related to host and environment, which contribute to the causation of disease as shown in the model.

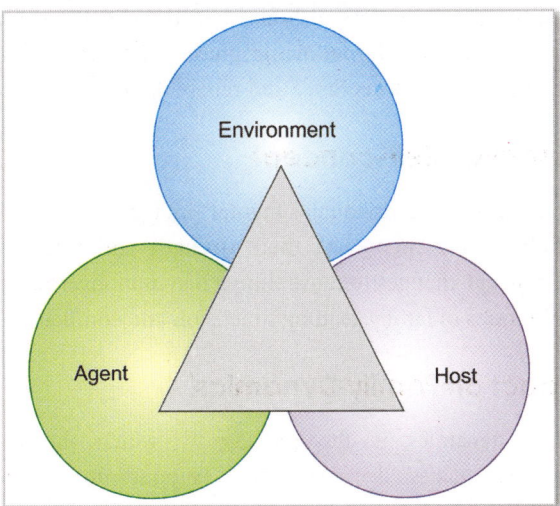

Fig. 3: Epidemiological triad model of causation of disease

The model is known as epidemiological triad (Fig. 3). According to this model, disease is caused by the interaction of agent, host and environment.

This means that disease will occur only when the host is weak, the agent is strong and enters the host through the right channel in sufficient amount and when environmental conditions facilitate the interaction of host and agent. For example, for pulmonary tuberculosis, the organisms must enter through respiratory tract and in sufficient amount; the host should not have specific resistance and should have weak general body resistance; poor, dark and dingy environment is conducive to the prevalence of tuberculosis in patients. This model implies that disease will not occur without the optimal interaction of these factors and remain in balanced state, which is called equilibrium of health.

This model is applicable to infectious diseases and not to new types of chronic and degenerative diseases, which are a result of modern civilization, e.g., cardiac diseases, cancer, diabetes, mental disorders, etc. These diseases are caused due to complex interaction of multiple factors related to lifestyle, human behavior and the environmental conditions.

Risk factors can be modifiable and non-modifiable.

- **Non-modifiable risk factors**
  - Genetic
  - Age
  - Biological characteristics
- **Modifiable risk factors**
  - Personal health habits
  - Lifestyle
  - Environment

Risk factors are key to health promotion. Once identified, risk factors can be individually addressed and a primary prevention program can be initiated.

ILLNESS AND ILLNESS BEHAVIOR

Impact of Illness on Patient and Family

Any illness whether acute (rapid onset) or chronic (slow onset) exhibits certain illness behaviors which are unique to the individual and are influenced by age, gender, family, values, economic status, culture, educational level and mental status (Table 1).

TABLE 1: Stages of illness behavior

Stage 1: Experiencing symptoms
When a person becomes actually ill, certain illness behaviors may occur in identifiable stages. (Suchman, 1965). These behaviors are the way people cope with alterations in function caused by the disease. They are unique to every individual. If the symptoms last for a short time or are relieved by self-care, the person usually takes no further action.
Stage 2: Assuming the sick role
If the symptoms persist, the person may choose to do nothing; may buy over-the-counter medications to relieve symptoms; or may seek out a healthcare provider for diagnosis and treatment.
Stage 3: Assuming a dependent role
During this time person may be dependent on others and seeks assistance in carrying out activities of daily living. If the illness is serious, the patient may have to be hospitalized for treatment or it can be managed at home. To facilitate adherence to the treatment plan, the patient needs effective relationships with caregivers, knowledge about the illness and an individualized plan of care. The patient's responses to care depends on a variety of factors, including the seriousness of illness, the patient's degree of fear about the disease, loss of roles, the supports of others, and personal experiences with illness care.
Stage 4 : Achieving resources and rehabilitation
Recovery and rehabilitation might begin in the hospital and conclude at home. Most patients complete this final stage of illness behavior at home. In this stage, the person gives up the dependent role and resumes normal activities and responsibilities.

Impact of Illness on Family

Whenever any illness occurs, there are role changes for both the patient and the family. For example, a chronic illness creates stress for the patient and family because it might require lifelong alterations in roles or lifestyle frequent hospitalizations, economic problems and decreased social interactions among family members. The responses of family members to an illness are also individualized. Some family members want to be with the patient all the time, while others might avoid visiting.

Behavioral and Emotional Changes

People react differently to illness. Individual, behavioral and emotional reactions depend on the nature of the illness, the client's attitude towards it and the reaction of others to it. Severe illness, particularly one that is life threatening, can lead to more extensive emotional and behavioral changes such as shock, anxiety, denial, anger and withdrawal.

Impact on Family Roles

When an illness occurs, the role of client and family may change. Such change may be simple and short-term or drastic and long-term. The family and individual generally adjust more easily to short-term changes because they know that the role change is only temporary.

Long-term changes require an adjustment process. The client and family often require specific counseling and guidance to assist them in coping with role changes.

Impact on Body Changes

Some illnesses result in changes in physical appearance and family may react differently to these changes. When changes in body occur, e.g., loss of limb, then the client and family may pass through the following phases; shock, withdrawal, acknowledgment, acceptance and rehabilitation.

Impact on Self-concept

Self-concept is individual's mental image of themselves, including how they view their strength and weaknesses. Self-concept changes because illness may no longer meet the expectations of family, leading to tension and conflict.

Impact on Family Dynamics

Family dynamics is the process by which the family functions, makes decisions, gives support to individual members and copes with everyday changes and challenges. If a person in a family becomes ill, family activities and decision making often get delayed because they are reluctant to assume the ill person's roles and responsibilities.

BIBLIOGRAPHY

1. Park K. Park's Textbook of Preventive and Social Medicine, 25th edition: Banarsidas Bhanot. Jabalpur, MP: 2017.

2. Lewis LW. Fundamental Skills in Patient Care, 2nd edition: Lippincott Williams and Wilkins.

3. Christensen K. Fundamentals of Nursing, 8th edition: Mosby Publishing. Maryland Heights Missouri: 2010.

4. Sharma S. Potter and Perry's Fundamentals of Nursing. A South Asian edition: India. Gurugram: Elsevier 2013.

5. Taylor C, Lillis C, LeMone P, Lynn P. Fundamentals of Nursing, 6th edition: Lippincott Williams and Wilkins. Philadelphia: 2008.

6. Gulani KK. Community Health Nursing (Principles and Practices), 3rd edition: Kumar Publishing House. Delhi: 2014.

7. Kadri AM. IAPSM's Textbook of Community Medicine. Jaypee Brothers Medical Publishers. Delhi: 2019.

Body Defenses, Immunity and Immunization

INTRODUCTION

Microorganisms exist everywhere; in water, in soil, and on body surfaces such as skin, intestinal tract and other areas open to outside, e.g., mouth, upper respiratory tract, vagina and lower urinary tract. Most microorganisms are harmless and some are even beneficial in a way that they perform essential functions in the body. Many microorganisms that are normally harmless can cause disease or infection in a healthy individual. Infectious diseases are a major cause of death worldwide. The control of the spread of microorganisms and the protection of people from communicable diseases and infections are carried out on the international, national, state, community and individual level. A susceptible host is any person who is at risk for infection. Impairment of body's natural defenses and a number of other factors can affect the susceptibility to infection.

BODY DEFENSES AND IMMUNITY

Individuals normally have defenses that protect the body from infection. These defenses can be categorized as specific and non-specific.

- **Specific defenses** protect the person against identifiable bacteria, viruses, fungi or other infectious agents.
- **Non-specific** defenses protect the person against all microorganisms regardless of prior exposure.

Non-specific Defenses

Non-specific defenses include anatomic and physiological barriers and the inflammatory response.

Anatomic and Physiological Barriers

Intact skin and mucous membranes are the body's first line of defense against microorganisms. Unless the skin and mucosa become cracked and broken, they are an effective barrier against bacteria. Normal secretions make the skin slightly acidic; acidity also inhibits bacterial growth. The nasal passage filters air and keeps mucous membranes moist because of cilia. The oral cavity has a regular flow of saliva and its partially buffering action helps to prevent infections.

The eye is protected from infection by tears, which continuously wash microorganisms away and contain lysozyme.

The high acidity of gastrointestinal tract prevents microbial growth. Peristalsis tends to remove microbes out of the body.

Vagina also has natural defenses against infection. When a girl reaches puberty, lactobacilli ferment sugars in the vaginal secretions, creating a vaginal pH 3.5 to 4.5. This low pH inhibits the growth of many disease- producing microorganisms. Urine flow has a flushing and bacteriostatic action that keeps the bacteria from ascending the urethra.

Inflammatory Response

Inflammation is a local and non-specific defensive response of the tissues to an injurious or infectious agent. It is an adaptive mechanism that destroys or deletes the injurious agent, prevents further spread of the injury and promotes the repair of damaged tissue. It is characterized by five signs:

1. Pain (Dolor)
2. Swelling (Tumor)
3. Redness (Rubor)
4. Heat (Calor)
5. Impaired functions of the body part.

There are three stages of inflammatory response:

1. **First stage:** Vascular and cellular response
2. **Second stage:** Exudate production
3. **Third stage:** Reparative phase

Vascular and Cellular Responses

During the first stage of inflammation, blood vessels at the site of injury constrict, which is followed by dilation of small blood vessels due to release of histamine released by injured tissues. This increase in blood supply is referred to as hyperemia, which is responsible for signs of redness and heat.

There is also release of chemical mediators (e.g., bradykinin, serotonin and prostaglandin) and of histamine. Fluid proteins and leukocytes leak into the interstitial spaces and the signs of inflammation, swelling and pain appear. Pain is caused by accumulation of fluid on nerve endings and the irritating chemical mediators. In response to the exit of leukocytes, the bone marrow produces a large number of leukocytes and releases them into blood stream. This is called leukocytosis.

Exudate Production

In the second stage of inflammation, exudates that are produced, consist of fluid that is escaped from the blood vessels, dead phagocytic cells and end products of dead tissue cells. The nature and amount of exudate vary according to the tissue involved, and the intensity and duration of the inflammation. The major types of exudates are serous, purulent and hemorrhagic (sanguineous).

Reparative Phase

The third stage of the inflammatory response involves the repair of injured tissues by regeneration or replacement with fibrous tissue (scar) formation.

Specific Defenses

Specific defenses of the body involve the immune system. An antigen is a substance that induces a state of sensitivity or immune response (immunity). The immune response has two components—Antibody-mediated defenses and cell-mediated defenses.

Antibody-Mediated Defenses/Humoral Immunity

Antibody-mediated defenses reside in the B-lymphocytes and are mediated by antibodies produced by B cells. Antibodies, also called immunoglobulins, are part of the body's plasma proteins, which defend against bacterial and viral infections. B cells are activated when they recognize the antigen. They then differentiate into plasma cells, which secrete the antibodies and serum proteins that bind specifically to the foreign substance and initiate a variety of elimination responses. The B cells may produce antibody molecules of five classes of immunoglobulins designated by letters and usually written as IgM, IgG, IgA, IgD and IgE.

Cell-Mediated Defenses/Cellular Immunity

This occurs through the T cell system. On exposure to antigen, the lymphoid tissues release large numbers of activated T cells into the lymph system. These T cells pass into the general circulation. There are three main groups of T cells (i) helper T cells, which help in the functioning of the immune system (ii) cytotoxic T cells, which attack and kill microorganisms and sometimes body's own cells and (iii) suppressor T cells, which can suppress the function of the helper T cells and the cytotoxic T cells.

When cell-mediated immunity is lost, as happens in human immunodeficiency virus (HIV) infection, an individual is defenseless against most viral, bacterial, and fungal diseases.

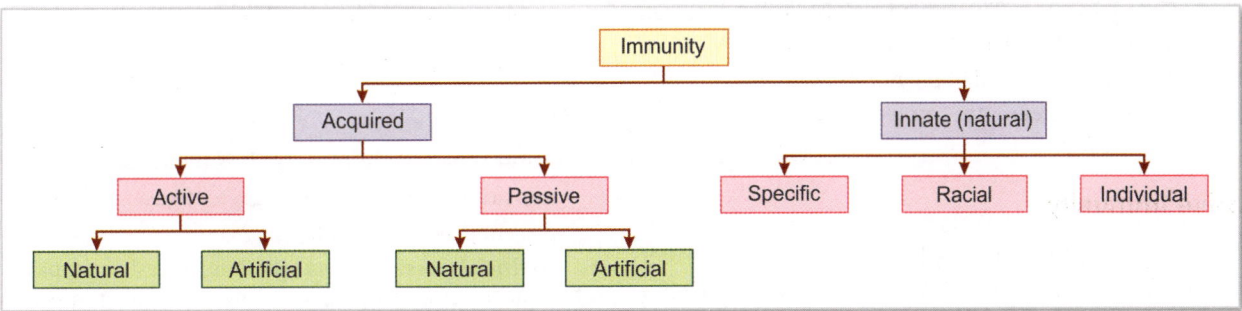

Fig. 1: Types of immunity

Immunity (Fig. 1)

Immunity may be natural (innate) or acquired (Table 1).

Innate Immunity

Innate immunity is the resistance with which an organism is born. It is present throughout the life.

Types

- **Specific immunity**
  - Animals of same species exhibit uniform pattern of susceptibility to infection, e.g., poliomyelitis, measles occur only in humans.
- **Racial immunity**
  - Within a species, races show differences in susceptibility to infection, e.g., Africans are resistant to yellow fever and malaria.
- **Individual immunity**
  - Certain individuals may be found within a highly susceptible population, who cannot be infected by some microorganisms.

Acquired Immunity

Resistance acquired by an individual during illness, infestation, vaccination, etc. is called acquired or specific immunity.

Active Immunity

- Active immunity is the resistance acquired by an individual after effective contact with an antigen.
- It follows either exposure to natural infection or by vaccination.
- Here, the immune system actively participates in producing antibody and often cell-mediated immunity.
- It develops slowly over a period of days or weeks but persists for long time usually for years.

Types

- **Natural active immunity:** It is acquired by natural infection by the organisms predominantly by subclinical infection after repeated exposures to small doses of the infecting organism.
- **Artificial active immunity:** It is the resistance produced by vaccination. The vaccines are prepared of attenuated or killed microorganisms or their antigens or active materials derived from them.
  - **Attenuation:** It is a live vaccine and prepared by culture or cultivation at high temperature passing through animals of different species by continued cultivation in presence of antagonistic substance and by repeated subculture in artificial media.

TABLE 1: Types of immunity

Type	Antigen or antibody source	Duration
Active	Antibodies are produced in response to an antigen.	Long
Natural	Antibodies are formed in the presence of an active infection in the body.	Lifelong
Artificial	Antigens (vaccines or toxoids) are administered to stimulate antibody production	Many years; the immunity must be reinforced by booster
Passive	Antibodies are produced by another source, animal or human	Short
Natural	Antibodies are transferred naturally from an immune mother to her baby through the placenta or in colostrum	6 months to 1 year
Artificial	Immune serum (antibody) from an animal or another human is injected	2–3 weeks

- **Killed vaccine:** The organisms are killed by heat, formalin, phenol, alcohol and ultraviolet (UV) light. These are preserved in phenol and alcohol.
- **Toxoid:** These are preparations of bacterial serotoxins.

Passive Immunity

- The resistance that is induced in the recipient by transfer of preformed (readymade) antibodies against infective agent or toxin in another host is called passive immunity.
- Immune system plays no active role and the protective mechanism comes into force immediately after the transfer of antibodies.

- Passive immunity is short-lasting, i.e. only for few days or weeks.

Types

- **Natural passive immunity:** It is the resistance passively transferred from the mother to fetus and infant, via placenta and breast milk.
- **Artificial passive immunity:** It is the resistance passively transferred to a recipient by the prenatal administration of antibodies.

UNIVERSAL IMMUNIZATION PROGRAMME (UIP) (TABLE 2)

TABLE 2: UIP schedule after introduction of Td vaccine (2019)

Age	Vaccination schedule after Td introduction
At birth	BCG, OPV-zero dose, Hep B-birth dose
6 weeks	OPV-1, Pentavalent-1, Rota-1*, fIPV-1, PCV-1*
10 weeks	OPV-2, Pentavalent-2, Rota-2*
14 weeks	OPV-3, Pentavalent-3, Rota-3*, fIPV-2, PCV-2*
9 months	Measles-1/MR-1, Vit A, JE-1*, PCV-B*
16–24 months	DPT first booster dose, OPV-booster dose, Measles-2/MR-2, JE-2*
5–6 years	DPT second booster dose
10–16 years	Td
For pregnant woman	Td-1 : early in pregnancy Td-2 : 4 weeks after Td-1 Td-B : if pregnancy occurs within 3 years of last pregnancy and 2 Td doses were received

*Td–Tetanus and adult diphtheria

Source: Introduction of Td vaccine in Universal Immunization Programme of India 2019 Replacement of TT with Td vaccine

BIBLIOGRAPHY

1. *Park K. Park's Textbook of Preventive and Social Medicine, 25th edition: Banarsidas Bhanot. Jabalpur, MP: 2017.*
2. *Lewis LW. Fundamental Skills in Patient Care, 2nd edition: Lippincott Williams and Wilkins.*
3. *Christensen K. Fundamentals of Nursing, 8th edition: Mosby Publishing. Maryland Heights Missouri: 2010.*
4. *Sharma S. Potter and Perry's Fundamentals of Nursing. A South Asian edition: India. Gurugram: Elsevier 2013.*
5. *Taylor C, Lillis C, LeMone P, Lynn P. Fundamentals of Nursing, 6th edition: Lippincott Williams and Wilkins. Philadelphia: 2008.*
6. *Gulani KK. Community Health Nursing (Principles and Practices), 3rd edition: Kumar Publishing House. Delhi: 2014.*
7. *Kadri AM. IAPSM's Textbook of Community Medicine. Jaypee Brothers Medical Publishers. Delhi: 2019.*

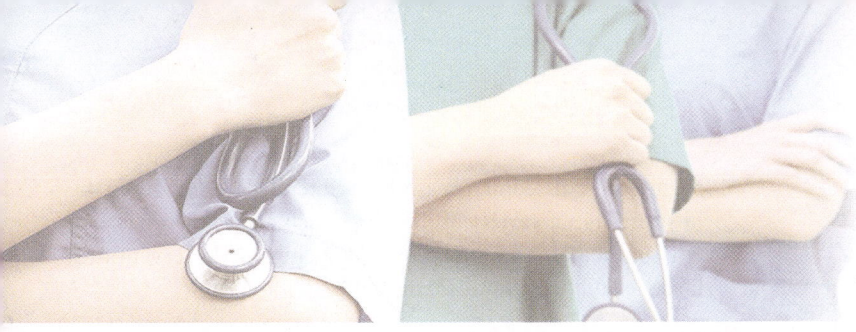

Health Care Services—Health Promotion and Levels of Disease Prevention

HEALTH PROMOTION

Health promotion means a lot more than just preventing illness. It means assisting individuals to enhance their health, well-being and functioning and to maximize their potential. Health promotion focuses on adopting healthy behaviors rather than avoiding illness. The goal is to enable an individual to control and improve his/her health. Pender (1987) describes health promotion as being an activity that is concerned with sustaining or increasing one's level of well-being, self actualization and personal fulfillment.

The concept of self-responsibility is important to health promotion, and it must be accepted and acted upon in order for wellness to become a reality for an individual. No one else can make a person live healthy life; self-responsibility is the only way to make changes. An individual can be given information relating to health and wellness, but only that person can change unhealthy or destructive habits, with an exception of small children. Each individual must take responsibility for behaviors leading to health and wellness. Illness prevention, i.e., hindering, obstructing or thwarting a disease or illness, incorporates both old and new ideas. The taboos, dietary laws and traditions of various cultural, ethnic and religious groups can be initiated for this reason. All stages of life should embody the tenets of preventive health. It must begin before conception with healthy parents and prenatal care and should be continued throughout a person's life span.

Before the full impact of illness prevention can be discovered, major changes are needed in health care delivery, funding and insurance coverage. The health care system must insist on more research relating to prevention and must then apply the results of the research to insurance practices. Preventive practices must be supported and funded by the health care system in order to change from treatment to prevention of illness.

Principles of Health Promotion

- Taking responsibility of oneself is the key to successful health promotion, i.e., to control unhealthy habits, beliefs and practice like smoking, alcohol, risky sexual practices, etc. and to develop healthy practices like balanced diet, regular exercise, etc.
- Understanding the importance of a properly balanced diet that supplies all the essential nutrients.
- Stress, which is a part of the modern way of life, has become inevitable in 'high tech' urban societies. Teaching techniques such as relaxation, yoga, meditation, exercises, etc. are included in health promotion programs to combat stress.
- A regular exercise program can promote health by improving the functions of body lowering body weight, decreasing cholesterol and low density lipoproteins.
- Assertiveness means standing out for one's own rights without violating the rights of others.

LEVELS OF DISEASE PREVENTION

Prevention extends to all stages of health. There are three levels of prevention, primary, secondary and tertiary. Primary prevention has not historically been supported by our health care system, whereas secondary and tertiary prevention have been and still are the main focus. They are also the most expensive. Primordial prevention is a new concept that is becoming popular these days.

Primordial Prevention

Primordial prevention, a new concept, is receiving special attention in the prevention of chronic diseases. In primordial prevention, efforts are directed towards discouraging children from adopting harmful lifestyles. For example, many adult health problems such as obesity, hypertension have their early origins in childhood, because this is the time when lifestyles are formed, e.g., eating habits, exercise, smoking, etc. The main intervention in primordial prevention is through individual and mass education.

Primary Prevention

Primary prevention can be defined as "action taken prior to the onset of disease, which removes the possibility that a disease will ever occur". Primary prevention may be accomplished by measures designed to promote general health and well-being, and quality of life of people or by specific protective measures.

Health Promotion

Health promotion is "the process of enabling people to increase control over, and to improve health". It is not directed against any particular disease, but is intended to strengthen the host through a variety of measures such as health education, environmental modifications, nutritional interventions, lifestyle and behavioral changes (Box 1).

Box 1

Health promotion behaviors
- Wearing seat belts, safety helmets, etc.
- Eating well-balanced diet
- Maintaining ideal body weight
- Refraining from using tobacco, etc.
- Consuming minimal or no alcohol
- Obtaining immunization
- Obtaining sufficient rest and exercise
- Brushing teeth regularly and getting dental check-ups
- Keeping sun exposure to a minimum; using a hat outdoor; applying sunscreen

Specific Protection

There are number of interventions which are aimed at specific protection like immunization, use of specific nutrients, chemoprophylaxis, protection against occupational hazards, protection against accidents, protection from carcinogens, avoidance of allergens, control of specific hazards in the general environment, e.g., air pollution, noise pollution and control of consumer product quality and safety of foods, drugs, etc.

Secondary Prevention

Secondary prevention can be defined as "action which halts the progress of a disease at its incipient stage and prevents complications". The specific interventions are **early diagnosis and adequate treatment**. By this, disease process can be averted and treatment is possible before irreversible pathological changes have taken place (Box 2).

Box 2

Secondary prevention
- Performing monthly breast or testicular examination
- Undergoing regular mammography
- Having regular papanicolaou (pap) or prostate-specific antigen (PSA) tests
- Obtaining bone density studies
- Obtaining regular glaucoma testing
- Undergoing testing for tuberculosis
- If diabetic, regular testing of blood sugar
- Complying with treatment program for chronic disease
- Following cardiac rehabilitation program

Modified from Ignatavicius, D.D., Workman, M.L., and Mishler, M.A. (1999), Medical surgical nursing across the health care continuum, 3rd edn. Philadelphia WB Saunders, P.B.

Tertiary Prevention

Tertiary prevention can be defined as "all measures available to reduce or limit impairments and disabilities, minimize suffering and to promote the patient's adjustment to irreversible conditions." It includes:

- Disability limitation
- Rehabilitation

Rehabilitation has been defined as "the combined and coordinated use of medical, social, educational and vocational measures for training and retraining the individual to the highest possible level of functional ability."

PRIMARY HEALTH CARE

Definition

Primary health care is essential health care made universally accessible to individuals and families in the community, by means acceptable to them, through their full participation and at a cost that community and country can afford.

Characteristics of Primary Health Care

- **Accessibility:** Primary health care permeates uniformly to reach equitably to all segments of population.
- **Acceptability:** Primary health care achieves acceptability through cultural assimilation of its policies and programs.
- **Adaptability:** Primary health system is highly flexible and adaptable to consumer as well as provider.
- **Availability:** Primary health care is always ready to respond to any demand at any time.
- **Appropriateness:** Primary health care system evolves from the socio-economic conditions, social values and health situation of a community, it is quite appropriate from all angles.

- **Closeness:** Primary health care is close to people at their door steps.
- **Continuity:** Primary health care service is a continuous, service which extends from 'womb to tomb' and address the changing needs of an individual in all situations of health and disease.
- **Comprehensiveness:** Primary health care is comprehensive.
- **Coordination:** Primary health care is dependent on intersectoral coordination and community participation.

Elements of Primary Health Care

As per Alma-Ata declaration, primary health care includes:
- Education concerning prevailing health problems and methods of identifying, preventing and controlling them.
- Promotion of food supply and proper nutrition.
- An adequate supply of water and basic sanitation.
- Maternal and child health care including family planning.
- Immunization against the major infectious disease.
- Prevention and control of locally endemic diseases.
- Appropriate treatment of common diseases and injuries.
- Promotion of mental health.
- Provision of essential drugs.

Principles of Primary Health Care

Figure 1 shows the principles of primary health care.
- **Equitable distribution:** Primary health care services must be shared equally by all people irrespective of their ability to pay (rich, poor, urban or rural).
- **Community participation:** Primary health care must be a continuing effort to secure meaningful involvement of the community in the planning, implementation and maintenance of health services.
- **Coverage and accessibility:** Primary health care implies providing health care services to all who require them.

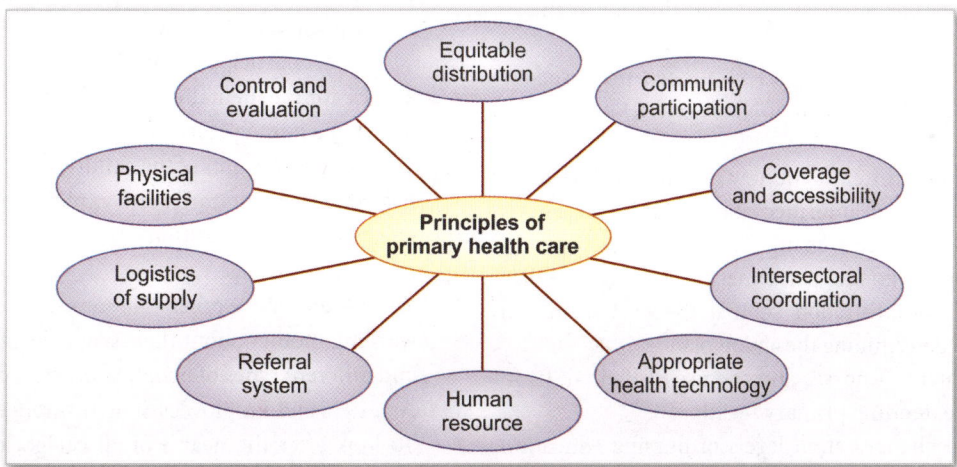

Fig. 1: Principles of primary health care

The care has to be appropriate and adequate to satisfy the essential health needs of the people and has to be provided by methods acceptable to them.

- **Intersectoral coordination:** Primary health care requires joint efforts of other health related sectors such as agriculture, animal husbandry, food, industry, housing, social welfare, communications, etc.
- **Appropriate health technology:** The technology that is scientific, adaptable to local needs and socially acceptable instead of costly methods, equipment and technology.
- **Human resource:** Human resource is very essential to make full use of all the available resources.
- **Referral system:** Referral system should be desirable to develop referring from one level to another with laid down procedures and policies.
- **Logistics of supply:** Include planning and budgeting for the supplies required for procurement or manufacture, storage distribution and control.
- **Physical facilities:** Need to be simple and clean. It should have a spacious waiting area with toilet facility.
- **Control and evaluation:** A process of evaluation has to be built in, to assess the relevance, progress, efficiency, effectiveness and impact of the services.

Role of Nurses in Primary Health Care

- "The nurses are the key persons in the movement of primary care" WHO Director General, Halfdan Mahler (1981).
- "The goal of primary health care cannot be achieved without the participation of nurses "- WHO Division of Manpower, Dr. T Fulap.

Nursing personnel are one of the most valuable assets of any health care system and represent considerable national investment.

In 1981, an informal meeting was convened by WHO to consider the role of nursing in contributing to the achievement of the goal of Health for All (HFA)/2000 through primary health care.

The following **five basic strategies** have been proposed by the WHO-International Council of Nurses (ICN) meeting by nurses:

1. The development of each country depends on the force of nurses that is well informed about health care and is ready to bring necessary changes in the nursing system.
2. The inclusion of nursing personnel at all levels of policy making and administration so that the profession can contribute to determining the action plan.
3. The involvement of nurses and the use of their skills in initiating or extending primary health care.
4. Fundamental changes at all levels of nursing education (basic, post-basic and continuing) to ensure that the priority needs of population are functionally integrated into the education and into nursing practice.
5. Research into nursing administration practice and education, that demonstrate nurse's contribution to primary health care.

Role of Nurse in Various Settings

- To make people realize that health is an asset to them, it is their constitutional right.
- Nurses participate in social activities in the community.
- She serves the self-help group, church group and women's organization.
- She coordinates and cooperates with other personnel who give services to the families and communities directly or indirectly.
- To make concrete efforts to significantly reduce maternal and child mortality and morbidity:
  - Giving high priority to children under six years of age.
  - Pregnant and nursing mothers, premarital counseling, arrangement for safe delivery, post-natal care, care of new born, advises for checking fertility.
- The major nutrition intervention programs:
  - Applied nutrition program
  - Supplementary feeding program
  - Mid-day-meal program for school children
  - National Goiter Control program
  - Vitamin 'A' prophylaxis program
  - Anemia control program
- To facilitate optimum psychosocial development of pre-school children.
  - Universal non-formal education.
  - To assist day care centers and possible preventive, promotive, curative and rehabilitative services.
- To provide special care to the "Save Our Soul Village"
  - Unwanted child in a family set-up.
  - An occupation as a mother for the needy women dedicated to social work.
  - Direct participation in social work.
- To care for the mentally retarded children blind, deaf and dumb taken into priority.
- To secure basic rights of the children and to protect against neglect, cruelty, hazards and exploitation, by promoting effective implementation of existing legislation and enacting new ones.
- To awaken the women laborers and all categories of working mother about their scope, health, safety, welfare and different types of benefits prescribed by the Factories Act, 1976 and Employees State Insurance (ESI) Act, 1984.
- To look after the health of all categories of labor, their living environment and working environment.

- To provide special care of aged people: As these old people are physically, mentally and financially incapable, they always suffer from insecurity.
- To treat minor ailments.
- To provide care to mentally sick persons.
- Nurses should willingly be ready to provide services in interior areas.
- Nurses should be involved in planning for health care programs.
- "Each one teach one": Nurses play an important role in educating the people.
- The nurse plays an important role in organizing appropriate health education program according to needs of the community.

BIBLIOGRAPHY

1. *Park K. Park's Textbook of Preventive and Social Medicine, 25th edition. Banarasidas Bhanot. Jabalpur, MP: 2017.*
2. *Sharma S. Potter and Perry's Fundamentals of Nursing. A South Asian edition. Elsevier India. Gurugram: 2013.*

Chapter
4

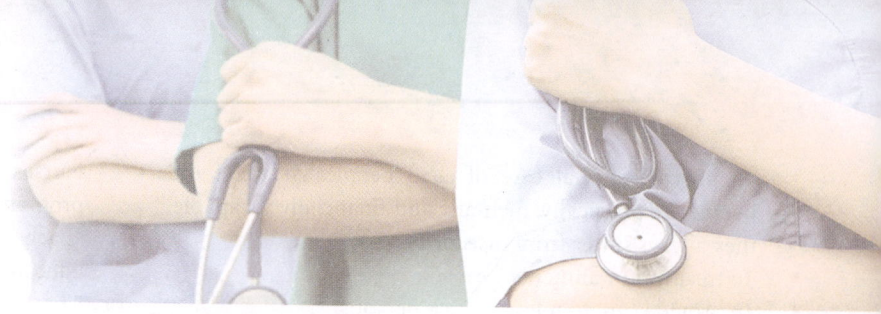

Health Care Agencies

CLASSIFICATION OF HEALTH CARE AGENCIES: HOSPITALS

The health care industry is so large, so diverse, and so complex that it is sometimes difficult to understand. Agencies providing care are classified according to one of the three ways: Length of stay, ownership and type of service. This classification is arbitrary because any agency may be placed in more than one classification with the systemic changes that are occurring. One agency may include multiple lengths of stay and different types of service and may combine many segments with different ownership patterns.

World Health Organization (WHO) defines the hospital as an 'integral part of the social and medical organization, the function of which is to provide for the population, completed health care, both curative and preventive whose outpatient services reach out to families and its environment; the hospital is also a center for the training of health workers and biosocial research. Today, hospital means an institution in which sick or injured persons are treated and healthy persons are helped to promote and maintain an optimum level of well-being.

Classification According to Length of Stay

- **Short-stay hospitals:** Short-stay facilities provide services to patients who are suffering from acute conditions or who have treatment needs that require less than 24 hours of care. Short-stay may take place in separate units in a hospital or even in one section of an emergency department. For example, person having appendectomy or cholecystectomy may stay nowadays for less than 24 hours. Many short-stay procedures or minimal invasive surgeries are carried out these days.
- **Acute-care:** For patients staying more than 24 hours but less than 30 days. However, the length of stay for all acute-care patients regardless of stay and diagnosis has

been declining steadily over the past few years. Length of stay after general surgery is 3–5 days.

- **Long stay hospitals:** Long-term care facilities include those that offer services to patients with major rehabilitation needs and functional losses caused by chronic diseases. The average length of stay extends from 30 days to many years. Some hospitals have a long-term rehabilitation unit. In a long-term care hospital, assisted living facilities for the dependent elderly are designed to make them as permanent residents.

Classification According to Ownership

Agencies may be classified as governmental or public voluntary hospitals, private nursing homes/hospitals, corporate hospitals.

- **Government or public hospitals:** These hospitals are run by the central or state governments or local bodies on noncommercial lines. These may be general hospitals or specialized hospitals or both.
- **Voluntary hospitals:** These hospitals are established and incorporated under the Societies Registration Act 1860; or Public Trust Act, 1882 or any other appropriate act of central or state governments. They are run by public or private funds on a noncommercial basis.
- **Private nursing homes/hospitals:** These are generally owned by an individual doctor or a group of doctors. They run the hospital or nursing home on a commercial basis.
- **Corporate hospitals:** These hospitals are public limited companies formed under Companies Act. They are run on commercial lines. They can be either general or specialized or both.

Classification According to Objectives

- **Teaching cum research hospitals:** A hospital to which a college is attached for medical/nursing/pharmacy/education, e.g., All India Institute of Medical Sciences, (AIIMS), New Delhi, Post-Graduate Institute of Medical Education and Research (PGIMER), Chandigarh, Safdarjung Hospital and Sucheta Kriplani Hospital, New Delhi belong to this category.
- **General hospitals:** These hospitals provide treatment for common diseases and conditions. They provide medical and nursing care for more than one category of medical discipline such as general medicine, general surgery, pediatrics, obstetrics and gynecology, etc. The main objective of these hospitals is to provide medical care to the people, e.g., district hospital, rural hospitals belong to this category.
- **Specialized hospitals:** These hospitals are providing medical and nursing care primarily for only one discipline or a specific disease or condition of one system. For example, tuberculosis, ear, nose and throat (ENT), ophthalmology, orthopedics, pediatrics, oncology, cardiology, psychiatric/mental health, maternity, etc.
- **Isolation hospital:** This is a hospital in which the persons suffering from infectious/communicable diseases requiring isolation from other patients are treated.

Classification According to Size

- **Teaching hospital:** 500 beds, strength to be increased according to the number of students.
- **District hospital:** 200 beds, may be raised up to 300 beds depending upon population.
- **Taluk hospital:** 50 beds, may be raised depending upon population.
- **Community health center:** 30 bedded hospital or more depending upon needs.
- **Primary health centers:** 6 beds may be increased up to 10 depending upon needs.

Classification According to Management

Union Government/Government of India

All hospitals administered by the Government of India, e.g., hospital run by railways, military, defense, public sector undertakings of the central government, etc.

State Governments

All hospitals administered by the state/union territory

- **Local bodies:** All hospitals administered by local bodies; municipal corporation, municipality, zila parishad, panchayat, etc.
- **Autonomous bodies:** Hospitals established under special act of parliament or state legislation funded by the central/state government/union territory e.g., AIIMS, New Delhi, PGIMER, Chandigarh, National Institute of Mental Health and Neurosciences (NIMHANS) Bengaluru, etc.
- **Private:** All private hospitals owned by an individual or by a private organization.
- **Voluntary agencies:** All hospitals operated by a voluntary body/trust/charitable society registered by the appropriate authority under central/state government laws, e.g., Christian Medical College and Hospital (CMC), Vellore.

Classification According to System

- Allopathic hospital
- Ayurveda, Unani, Siddha and Homeopathy (AYUSH)

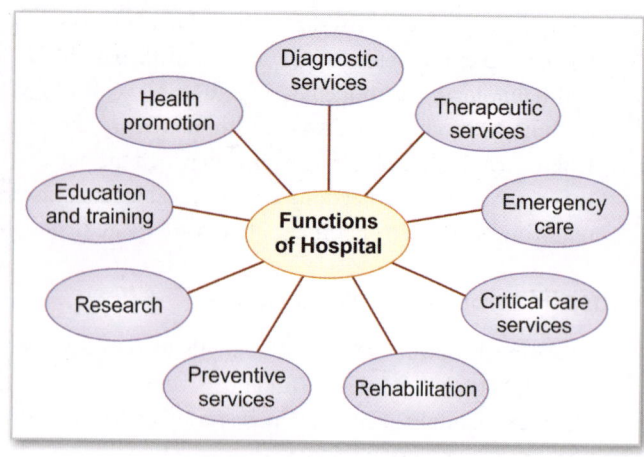

Fig. 1: Functions of hospital

FUNCTIONS OF THE HOSPITAL

Refer to Figure 1 for functions of hospital.

- **Diagnostic services:** Hospitals provide the diagnostic services for the early and prompt diagnosis of illness.
- **Therapeutic services:** Hospitals provide the curative services to the sick people.
- **Emergency care:** Hospital provide the emergency care to patients in acute illness.
- **Critical care services:** Hospitals provide the advanced tertiary care for the patients suffering from life-threatening problems.
- **Rehabilitation:** Hospitals provide facilities for physiotherapy and rehabilitation.
- **Preventive services:** Hospitals provide preventive services such as immunization, well baby clinics, antenatal care, counseling and education, etc.
- **Health promotion:** Hospitals participate in health promotion activities such as health education, family welfare of clients, etc.
- **Education and training:** Hospitals also provide platform for the education for medical, nursing and paramedical students.
- **Research:** Hospitals provide facilities for research for expansion of body of knowledge in the field of health sciences.

HOSPITAL DEPARTMENTS

Outpatient Department

An outpatient department (OPD) is a distinct and important part of the hospital. The OPD is the place of contact between hospital and community. All the patients suffering from minor, acute and chronic diseases are first examined in OPD. OPD is located close to the public entrance and adjacent to the casualty and emergency services. At the entrance to OPD, there should be a reception and inquiry counters, with proper communication facilities like telephone, etc.

The number and type of clinics depend on the needs of the patients that are being served. There are a number of clinics operational in the OPD including services of laboratory and diagnostic facilities for routine tests such as blood examination urine analysis and other facilities like X-ray, electrocardiography (ECG), etc.

Casualty Department

The casualty department provides round the clock immediate diagnosis and treatment for illness of emergency nature and injuries from accident. In casualty department, patients are seen and given immediate treatment, are discharged with instructions to attend OPD for follow-up. Case of serious nature are admitted in casualty and kept for observation for required period and are either discharged or transferred to respective ward.

Department of Medicine

Department of medicine is headed by senior physician with their associates and includes all patients who are admitted to the hospital for treatment other than surgery. The medicine department is further divided into specialties like cardiology, neurology, gastroenterology, nephrology, dermatology, etc. where the patients can be referred and treated depending upon their problems. This department also provides consultation services to other departments of the hospital who require medical services.

Department of Surgery

Patients who require surgery are admitted in the unit. This department also has specialties like, general surgery, orthopedics, urology, gynecology, eye, ear, nose and throat, neurosurgery, vascular surgery, thoracic surgery, etc. depending upon the requirement of the patient.

One of the most important areas of surgical department is operation theater where surgery takes place and attached to that is recovery room for caring patients immediately after surgery. Patients are kept here under observation till the time they are not stable.

Maternity Unit

Maternity unit provides care to pregnant women during and after delivery and provide care to newborns. The department provides antenatal services to mothers in antenatal clinics, which are situated preferably on ground floor, adjoining the maternity wing. There is provision of labor rooms for delivery and those who require surgery, OT provision is for cesarean section. Caring of newborn and providing postpartum services is also the responsibility of this unit.

Pediatric Unit

Pediatric unit is responsible to care for children till 15 years. It provides services to premature infant (Nursery), which is very important area of pediatric unit. In Neonatal intensive care unit, children from their birth to one month of age, who need intensive care, are taken care of. Those children who require surgery are admitted in pediatric surgery department and others who do not require surgery are kept in pediatric medicine department.

Psychiatry Department

General hospital should have psychiatry services which includes OPD services for contacting mental hospitals having day and night treatment facilities in inpatient unit.

Pharmacy Department

The main function of this department includes the stocking of drugs and other medical supplies and equipment, and distribution of drugs to other departments as and when required.

Laundry Department

Laundry department ensures the availability of germ-free washed linen in all the departments of hospital. The linen of different kinds is washed in laundry machines, made germ free and sent accordingly.

Dietary Department

The purpose of the dietary services department in every hospital is the preparation of nutritionally adequate, attractive meals. The services include professional planning of standard and therapeutic diet and distribution from kitchen to various departments of the hospital.

Central Sterile Supply Services Department (CSSD)

The central sterile supply department is supposed to store, sterilize, maintain and issue those instruments materials and garments which are required to be sterilized.

Radiology Department (X-ray Department)

Department of radiology deals with radiodiagnosis and radiotherapy. The department is also known as X-ray department, which provide services for in-patients, outpatients, casualty department, etc. There are number of diagnostic procedures performed in the X-ray department such as barium meal, intravenous pyelography, myelogram, etc.

Radiotherapy is an effective method of treatment in many diseases, e.g., cancer where radiation is used for treatment.

Department of Pathology/Laboratory

The primary function of department of pathology is to assist doctor in the diagnosis and treatment of patients. Blood, bone marrow, cerebrospinal fluid (CSF), tissue biopsy and other body fluids excretions (urine, stool, sputum, etc.) are examined and reported. The laboratory also carries out toxicological, microbiological, biochemical and histopathological investigations.

HEALTH CARE TEAM

Health care team or health professionals also called the providers of health care includes nurses and health personnel from different disciplines who coordinate their skills to assist clients. Their mutual goal is to restore a client's health and promote wellness. The choice of personnel for a particular client depends on the needs of the client. They are:

- Nurse
- Physician
- Dietician/nutritionist
- Physiotherapist
- Occupational therapist
- Dentist
- Paramedics
- Pharmacist
- Respiratory therapist
- Social worker
- Spiritual support personnel
- Unlicensed assistive personnel
- Alternative (complementary) care provider

Nurse

The role of the nurse varies with the needs of the client, the nurse's credentials and the type of employment setting. A registered nurse (RN) assesses a client's health status, identifies health problems and develops and coordinates the care of patient. Nurses can pursue a variety of practice specialties (e.g., critical care, oncology, neonatology). Advance practice nurses provides client care as nurse practitioners, nurse midwives, certified registered nurse anesthetists and clinical nurse specialists.

Physician

The physician is responsible for medical diagnosis and for determining the therapy required by a person who has a disease or injury. Now-a-days many physicians are including health promotion and disease prevention in their practice. Some physicians are general practitioners while others are specialists such as cardiologist, endocrinologist, pediatrician, neurologist, etc.

Dietician/Nutritionist

Dieticians are often concerned with therapeutic diets to meet nutritional needs of individual patients and supervise the preparation of meals to ensure that patients get the proper diet.

Physiotherapist

Physiotherapist assists clients with musculoskeletal problems and treats dysfunctions by means of heat, water, massage, exercise and electric current. The functions of physiotherapists include assessing client's mobility and strength, providing therapeutic measures, e.g., exercises and heat applications to improve mobility and strength, etc.

Occupational Therapist

Occupational therapist assists clients with impaired function to gain the skills to perform activities of daily living. The occupational therapist teaches skills that are therapeutic and at the same time provides some fulfillment, e.g., teaching a person who has arthritis in his arms and hands about how to adjust his/her kitchen utensils so that he/she can contribute to cook.

Dentist

Dentists diagnose and treat dental problems. Dentists are also involved in preventive measures to maintain healthy oral structures (teeth and gums).

Paramedics

They are the technicians in the various departments like radiology, nuclear medicine, laboratory and operation theater.

Pharmacist

A pharmacist prepares and dispenses pharmaceuticals in hospital settings. The role of the pharmacist is monitoring and evaluating the actions and effects of medications on clients.

Respiratory Therapist

The respiratory therapist is skilled in therapeutic measures used in care of clients with respiratory problems. These therapists are knowledgeable about oxygen therapy devices, intermittent positive pressure breathing respirators, artificial mechanical ventilators and accessory devices used in inhalation therapy. Respiratory therapists administer many of the pulmonary function tests.

Social Worker

A social worker counsels clients and their support persons regarding problems such as finances, marital difficulties and adoption of children.

Spiritual Support Personnel

Chaplains, pastors, priests and other religious or spiritual advisors serve as part of the health care team by attending spiritual needs of patients.

Unlicensed Assistive Personnel

Unlicensed assistive personnel (UAP) comprise the health care staff who assume delegated aspects of basic client care. Their tasks include bathing, assisting with feeding and collecting specimens, UAP includes nursing aids, aids/assistants, hospital attendants, nurse technicians and orderlies. Some of these categories of provider may have standardized education and job duties, such as general duty assistants (GDA).

Alternative (Complementary) Care Provider

This category includes herbalists, acupuncturists, massage therapists, chiropractors, reflexologists, holistic health healers, etc.

ISSUES IN HEALTH CARE DELIVERY

The health care today influences both health care professionals and consumers. Nurses who provide patient care need to participate fully and effectively within all aspects of health care. As nursing faces issues how to maintain quality while reducing cost, nurses need to acquire the knowledge, skills and values necessary to practice competently and effectively. It is also becoming important to collaborate with other health care professionals to design new approaches for patient care services.

Shortage of Qualified Nurses

There is an ongoing global shortage of qualified nursing professionals which results from insufficient qualified RNs to fill vacant positions. By 2020, a shortage of nurses will put the nursing work force in critical condition.

This shortage affects all aspects of nursing such as patient care, administration and nursing education but it also represents challenges and opportunities for the profession. There is a direct link between can by registered nurses and positive patient outcomes, reduced complication rates and a more rapid return of the patient to an optimum functional status.

Competency

The health care practitioner competencies are an excellent tool for measuring how well a nurse practices nursing and serves as a guide for the development of a professional nursing career. A consumer of health care expects that the standards of nursing care and practice in any health care setting are appropriate and safe. Health care organizations ensure quality care by establishing policies, procedures, and protocols that are evidence-based and follow accrediting standards. Ongoing competency is a nurse's responsibility and she has to obtain necessary continuing education and follow an established code of ethics in order to provide best services.

In addressing the continued challenge facing the health care system, the Institute of Medicine competencies (IOM), 2001 identified five interrelated competencies that are essential for all health care workers in the 21st century. The IOM also identified 10 important rules of performance for a health care system to meet patient's needs (IOM, 2003)

Institute of Medicine: Competencies for the 21st Century

Provide Patient-centered Care

- Recognize and respect difference in patient's values, preferences and needs
- Relieve pain and suffering
- Coordinate continuous care
- Effectively communicate with and educate patients
- Share decision making and management
- Advocate for disease prevention and health promotion.

Work in Interdisciplinary Teams

- Cooperate, collaborate and communicate
- Integrate care to ensure that care is continuous and reliable.

Use Evidence-based Practice

- Integrate best research with clinical practice and patient values
- Participate in research activities.

Apply Quality Improvement

- Identify errors and hazards in care
- Practice using basic safety design principles
- Measure quality in relation to structure, process, and outcomes
- Design and test interventions to change processes.

Use Informatics

- Use information technology to communicate, manage knowledge, reduce error, and support decision-making.

Adapted from Institute of Medicine (IOM): Crossing the quality chasm: A new health system for the 21st century, Washington DC, 2001, National Academies Press; and Institute of Medicine.

Evidence-based Practice

As professionals, nurses need to be abreast with new information coming from research studies, technological development and practice trends. Evidence-based practice is a research-based practice involving decisions about patient care based on the results of research studies.

Quality and Safety in Health Care

Quality health care is the degree to which the health services for individuals and populations increase the likelihood of desired health outcomes and are consistent with current professional knowledge. Health care providers define the quality of their services by measuring health care outcomes that show how a patient's health status has changed. Examples of outcomes that are monitored are readmission rates of patients after discharge, rate of infection after surgery, etc. Safety is a critical part of quality health care. Examples of safety include, hand hygiene, fall prevention, catheter, associated urinary tract infection prevention, etc.

More and more health care institutions are focused on improving process as a way to improve quality and safety. Six-sigma is a data-driven approach to process improvement that reduces variation in process. It is a measure of quality. For example, a nursing unit collects data on the process of administering the first dose of an ordered chemotherapy. The audit reports delays in getting the drug from the pharmacy to the nursing unit. Using six sigma, the collected data is analyzed, and unnecessary steps in the process are identified. On the basis of this analysis, the process is streamlined to decrease time from ordering to administration.

It is important to know about patient's satisfaction so that measures can be taken to improve the quality of care. Research has shown that hospitals that improved the nursing work environment and lowered nurse-patient ratio had higher patient satisfaction levels and patients were more likely to recommend the hospitals to others.

Nursing Informatics and Technological Advancements

The focus of nursing informatics is not on the technology or the computer; rather its focus is on the organization, analysis, and dissemination of information (ANA 2008).

Advances in technology are constantly evolving and it also influences where and how nurses provide care to patients. Technological advances help nurses improve direct care processes, patient outcomes, and work environments. Sophisticated equipment such as electronic half-infusion devices, cardiac telemetry, computerized medication dispersion system have changed health care. In many ways, technology makes the work of the nurses easier but it cannot replace nursing judgment.

Communication with others also has become challenging tasks due to technology. Personal computers, cell phones, and personal digital assistants (PDAs) allow us to communicate and share information or data with others in a variety of formats around the world. People expect accurate information to be delivered to them. Therefore, it is crucial that nurse helps health care agencies to develop an effective way to manage the collection, interpretation and distribution of information.

Globalization of Health Care

The increasing connectivity of the world's economy, culture, and technology is one of the forces reshaping the health care delivery system. Advances in communication through internet, allow nurses, patients, and other health care providers to talk with others world-wide about health care issues. This has given rise to 'health tourism'. Health tourism is the travel to other nations to seek out health care.

The growth of urbanization is also currently affecting global health. Cities become more densely populated; problems with pollution, noise, over-crowding, inadequate water and improper waste disposal are other environmental hazards becoming more apparent. Children, women, and older adults are vulnerable populations that are most threatened by urbanization.

As a result of globalization, health care providers have to make their services more accessible. The International Council of Nurses (ICN), based in Switzerland, represents nursing world-wide. The purpose of the ICN is to advance the nursing profession world-wide and influence health policies and to bring nursing together.

BIBLIOGRAPHY

1. *Institute of Medicine (IOM). The Future of Nursing: Leading Change, Advancing Health. National Academies Press. Washington (DC): (US); 2011.*

2. *International Council of Nurses (ICN). ICN Mission, Vision and Strategic Plan. [online] Available from www.icn.ch/who-we-are/icn-mission-vision-and-strategic-plan [Accessed November 2019].*

3. *ISIXSIGMA. Statistical sigma definition 2010. [online] Available from www.isixsigma.com/new-to-six-sigma/statistical-six-sigma-definition/ [Accessed November 2019]*

4. *Outon J. Nursing in the International Community. A Broader View of Nursing Issues. St. Louis: Saunders; 2012.*

5. *Bickford CJ. Nursing informatics: scope and standards of practice. Stud Health Technol Inform. 2009;146:855.*

6. *Kutney-Lee A, McHugh MD, Sloane DM, et al. Nursing: A Key to Patient Satisfaction. Health Affairs. 2009;28(4).*

7. *Zuzelo PR, Gettis C, Hansell AW, et al. Describing the influence of technologies on registered nurses work. Clin Nurse Spec. 2008;22(3):132-40.*

8. *Oulton JA. Nursing in the international community A broader view of nursing issues, 6th edition. St. Louis: Saunders; 2012.*

9. *Aiken LH. Economics of nursing. Policy Polit Nurs Pract. 2008 May;9(2):73-9.*

10. *Tanner CA, Bellack JP. Our facility for the future journal of nursing education. 2010:49(3);123.*

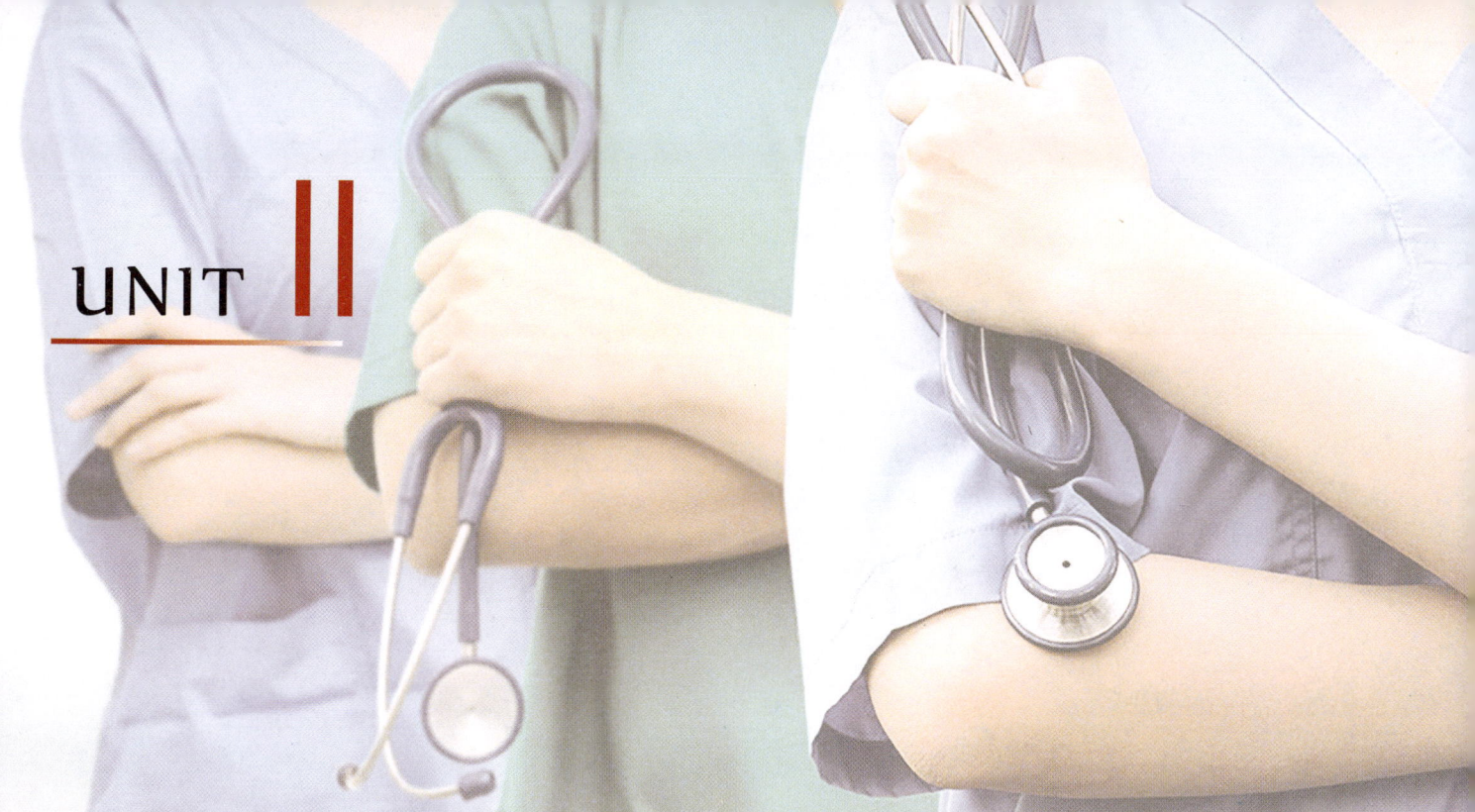

UNIT II

NURSING AS A PROFESSION

Unit Outline

Nursing: A Sacred Profession

INTRODUCTION

The term 'nurse' evolved from the Latin word *nutrix*, which means to nurture of foster someone. The word Nourish means to 'supply which is necessary to life'. Nursing has been called the oldest of the arts and the youngest of the professions. Today, nursing has been merged as a learned profession that is both a science and art.

Science is a body of knowledge based on a large number of carefully collected facts, which have been arranged and classified in such a way so as to establish certain laws and principles. Nursing is a Science, which requires a sound type of education and a thorough knowledge of human behavior.

Art is a skill in doing something that is acquired by study and practice. An art is a body of practical knowledge which tells us how to work to produce certain results.

As an art, nursing requires a sympathetic heart and a willing hand. Nursing today involves many laws and principles not only those of biological and physical nature but also those of social or behavioral science. Nursing, however, is an applied science. Borrowing facts that are needed from pure sciences. The better the scientific background, the safer and more intelligent should be the care, a nurse renders. In addition to scientific knowledge and expert bedside skill, desirable attitudes are necessary in nursing. Therefore, the basic requirements for a nurse are knowledge of nursing science (Head), the desire to nurse, spirit of nursing (Heart), i.e., the attitude and the skill of nursing (Hand) (Fig. 1).

The main core of nursing is prevention of illness, promotion of health, restoration of health and alleviation of suffering for the individual, family and the society.

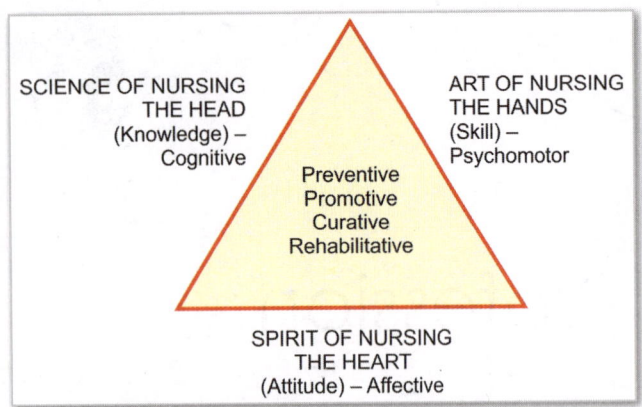

SCIENCE OF NURSING
THE HEAD
(Knowledge) –
Cognitive

ART OF NURSING
THE HANDS
(Skill) –
Psychomotor

Preventive
Promotive
Curative
Rehabilitative

SPIRIT OF NURSING
THE HEART
(Attitude) – Affective

Fig. 1: Basic requirements of a nurse

DEFINITIONS OF NURSING

"The unique function of the nurse is to assist the individual, sick or well, in the performance of those activities contributing to health or its recovery (or to peaceful death) that he would perform unaided if he had the necessary strength, will or knowledge, and to do this in such a way as to help him gain independence as rapidly as possible."

—*Virginia Henderson and adopted by ICN 1972*

Keeping in view of the changes taking place throughout the world, International Council of Nurses (ICN) (2003) defines nursing as:

"Nursing encompasses autonomous and collaborative care of individuals of all ages, families, groups and communities, sick or well and in all settings. Nursing includes the promotion of health, prevention of illness, and the care of ill, disabled and dying people. Advocacy, promotion of safe environment, research, participation in shaping health policy and in-patient and health system management and education are also key nursing roles."

"The protection, promotion and optimization of health and abilities, prevention of illness and injury, alleviation of suffering through the diagnosis and treatment of human responses and advocacy in the care of individuals, families, communities and population.

—*American Nurses Association (ANA), 2004*

Defining nursing is a difficult task since nursing is not static but is always responding to new advances, increased knowledge and consumer needs. However, the expanding roles and functions of a nurse in present days have made every single definition incomplete, therefore, it is better to review the number of definitions of nursing that evolved over the years:

- Florence Nightingale (1860) said that nursing "ought to signify the proper use of fresh air, light, warmth, cleanliness, quietness and the proper selection and administration of diet".

- According to Clara Weeks (1899), nursing includes not only the "execution of the physician order" but also the "administration of food and medicine, and the more personal care of the patient, attention to the condition of the sick room, its warmth, cleanliness, and ventilation, the careful observation and reporting of symptoms and the prevention of contagion".

- Harmer and Henderson (1939) defined nursing as "that service to an individual that helps him to attain or maintain a healthy state of mind or body or where a return to health is not possible, the relief of pain and discomfort".

- Hildegard Peplau (1952) "Nursing is a significant, therapeutic, interpersonal process". This definition tells that effective nursing results from a therapeutic relationship between nurse and patient. Accordingly the goal of nursing in to develop interaction between nurses and client.

- Faye Glen Abdellah (1960) defined nursing as a helping profession. Nursing care is doing something to or for the person or providing information to the person with goal of meeting needs, increasing or restoring self-help ability or alleviating an impairment. Abdellah's concept of 21 problems are the main focus of nursing.

- Dorothea E Orem (1960), described nursing as the giving of direct assistance to a person as required, because of the person's specific inabilities in self-care resulting from a situation of personal health.

So according to this, nursing is doing for a person what he cannot do at particular time due to health-related limitations. The goal of nursing is to care for and help client attain self-care or return to self-care.

- Ida Jean Orlando (1961), said that the function of professional nursing is conceptualized as finding out and meeting the patient's immediate need for help. Orlando viewed three dimensions, i.e., client's behavior, nurse's reactions and nurse's action compared to nursing situation. The goal of nursing is to respond to client's behavior in terms of immediate needs.

- Lydia E Hall (1962) viewed that client is composed of the overlapping parts, i.e., person's pathological stage (core) and treatment (cure) and body (care). Nurse is a caretaker. The goal of nursing is to provide care and comfort to client during disease process.

- Ernestine Weidenbach (1964) said that nursing is a service, helping art and a goal-directed activity. The purpose (goal) of clinical nursing is to facilitate the efforts of the individuals to overcome the obstacles, which currently interfere with his ability to respond to demand made of him by his conditions, environmental situation and time.

- Myra E Strin Levine (1966) said that nursing is a human interaction. Nursing intervention is based on four conservation principles of nursing, i.e., conservation of energy, conservation of structural integrity, conservation of personal integrity and conservation of social integrity. The goal of nursing is to use conservation activities aimed at optimum use of clients resources.

- Dorothy E Johnson (1968) said that nursing is an external force acting to preserve the organization of patient's behavior while the patient is under stress by means of imposing regularity mechanism or by providing resources.

  Nursing is an art and science, it supplies external assistance both before and during system balance disturbances and therefore, requires knowledge of order, disorder and control. The goal of nursing is to reduce stress so that client can move more easily, through recovery process.

- Martha E Rogers (1970) said that nursing is a humanistic science dedicated to compassionate concern for maintaining and promoting health, preventing illness and caring for and rehabilitating the sick and the disabled.

- Imogene King (1971) said that "Nursing is a process of action reaction, interaction and transaction, whereby nurses assist individuals of any age or socioeconomic group to meet their basic needs in performing activities of daily living and to cope with health and illness at one particular point in the life cycle.

- Joyce Travelbee (1971) said, nursing is an interpersonal process whereby the professional nurse assists an individual or family to prevent and cope with experiences of illness and suffering and if necessary, assist the individual or family to find meanings in their experiences.

- Betty Neuman (1972) says 'Nursing' is a unique profession in that it is concerned with all the variables affecting an individual response to stress and believes that nursing is concerned with the whole person. The nursing interventions include primary, secondary and tertiary level of preventions.

- Sister Callista Roy (1979) said, nursing is defined as "theoretical system of knowledge which prescribes a process of analysis and action related to the care of the ill or potentially ill." The goal of nursing is to identify types of demands placed on client, assess adaptation to demands, and help client adapt as nursing is promoting a positive adaptation to changing internal and external environment.

- Madeleine Leininger (1978) said, "Nursing is a learned humanistic art and science that focuses upon personalized core behaviors, functions, and processes directed toward promoting and maintaining health behaviors or recovery from illness which have physical, psychocultural and social significance or meaning for those being assisted generally by a professional nurse or one with similar roles and competencies."

- Kathryn E Barnard (1981) said, "Nursing is a process by which the patient is assisted in maintenance and promotion of his independence. This process may be educational, therapeutic or restorative. It involves facilitation of change, most probably change in the environment."

- Patricia Benner (1982) said that nursing is viewed as caring practice whose science is guided by the moral art and ethics of care and responsibility. Nursing practice is the care and study of the living experience of health, illness and disease and the relationship between these three.

SCOPE OF NURSING

Nurses provide care for three categories of patients: individual, families and communities. Nursing practice involves four areas: promoting health and wellness, preventing illness, restoring health and caring for the dying.

Promoting Health and Wellness

Wellness is a process that engages in activities and behaviors that enhance quality of life and maximize personal potential. Nurses promote wellness in clients who are both healthy and ill. Health promotion is the framework for nursing activities. Through knowledge and skill the nurse facilitates decisions about lifestyle that enhance quality of life and encourage acceptance of responsibility for one's own health. The nurse increases health awareness by assisting in the understanding that health is more than just not being ill. The nurse teaches self-care activities to maximize achievement of goals that are realistic and attainable and encourages health promotion by providing information and referrals.

Preventing Illness

The objective of illness prevention activities is to reduce the risk for illness, to promote good health habits, and to maintain optimal functioning. Nursing activities that prevent illness include educational programs in areas such as prenatal care, immunization, infant care and prevention of sexually transmitted diseases. It also includes literature, television, radio or internet information on healthy diet, regular exercise, and the importance of healthy habits. It also focuses on health assessment in institution, clinics and community settings.

Restoring Health

Activities to restore health focus on the individual with an illness and range from early detection of a disease to rehabilitation and teaching during recovery. Here, the activities include the following:

- Performing assessments that detect illness and providing direct care of the person who is ill.
- Collaborating with other health care providers in providing care and rehabilitation for illness.

Facilitating Coping with Disability and Death

Nurses also facilitate patient and family to cope with altered function, life crises and death. Nurses help patients to achieve optimal level of function through maximizing the person's strength and potentials, through teaching, and referral to community support systems. Nurses provide care to both patients and family during end of life care in hospitals, long term care facilities and homes.

Box 1 provides the different settings where nurses can work.

Box 1

Different settings for nursing care
- Hospitals
- Ambulatory surgery centers
- Clinics
- Homes
- Emergency medical services
- Educational progress
- Public health/community health
- Industry
- Long-term care facilities
- Mobile health care units
- Schools
- Offices
- Hospice
- Market health facilities
- State/National health programs
- Prisons

CONCEPT OF NURSING

Nursing is a call to service. Nursing is a service which includes giving care to sick and care of client's whole environment and provide health education and health services to individual, family and whole community. A nurse is a person who is directly or indirectly helping in constructing the health of the country. The nurse attends the care aspects, curative aspects, protective aspects, teaching aspects, coordinating aspects and the patient advocacy aspects.

Concept of nursing is based on the following factors:

- The delivery of care should be without prejudice, regardless of physical and psychological conditions of individual, their age, gender, race, belief and position in society.

- Respect for the fundamental human rights in delivery of health care to individual.
- Establishment of helping relationship with patient, his family and the society.
- Ability to work independently and in collaboration with multidisciplinary team in order to develop skills and professional knowledge.
- Time-to-time implementation of various health policies and programs.
- Participate in research-based nursing and evaluation of research to propose evidence-based practices.
- Respect the right of patient to accept or refuse care.
- Providing appropriate information to patients and family members about health status, investigations and procedures done, diagnosis, treatment and prognosis of patient.

Nursing is an art, science and a profession. It is an art as all procedures require practice and skills. This directs a nurse to perform work and produce certain results. Nursing care is given to an individual, family and community or in hospital. It is science as it is a body of knowledge based on number of facts to establish certain laws and principles. Nursing is a science because any nursing intervention done for patients is based on knowledge of scientific principles.

Nursing is a helping profession and provides services, which contribute to health and wellbeing of people.

OBJECTIVES OF NURSING

Nursing incorporates both practical and theoretical activities. This is the practice and knowledge that integrates medical, biological, psychological and pedagogical elements. Because of its 'placement', it has always connected with and used the significant care elements of nursing, medical and humanistic knowledge with manual instrumental efficiency.

Nursing is not only an art, which provides skillful care for the sick in appropriate relationship with the patient, family, physician and with others who have related responsibilities.

It is concerned equally with the prevention of illness and conservation of health. Skillful nursing care embraces the whole person, body, mind and soul, i.e., his physical, mental, social and spiritual well-being. In its broadest sense, nursing covers not only the care of the sick, the aged, the helpless and the handicapped, but also cares for the promotion of health and prevention of illness. The main objectives of nursing include:

- Apply principles of philosophy in nursing interventions.
- Apply scientific knowledge from nursing, natural sciences and general education courses as a source for making decisions in nursing.

- Use the nursing process to identify health potential of individuals, groups, families and communities and to meet their health needs.
- Provide comprehensive nursing care to persons without discrimination of race, sex, religion or culture in a variety of settings.
- Use community resources to achieve the goals of nursing.
- Assume individual responsibility for decisions made and actions taken related to nursing intervention.

PHILOSOPHY OF NURSING

The word "philosophy" means love of wisdom. It provides answer to questions such as, of what is this world made? Who made it? Why does this world exist? Who am I? Why do I exist? From where did I come? Where am I going? What is the purpose of what I am doing? These questions are very difficult to answer. The answers to these questions make the philosophy of life, which decides our general behavior and the important choices we make in life. There are many values and beliefs in our philosophy of life and each one guides one behavior. Just as each person has a philosophy of life, each professional nurse has a philosophy of nursing.

An understanding of one's own beliefs, feelings, values, attitudes and culture precedes the development of a philosophy of nursing. Until the nurse has a knowledge of self, it is difficult to state beliefs to guide nursing practice. There are several concepts that must be discussed in any nursing philosophy. These include human beings, health, illness, and nursing. The nurse makes statements of personal beliefs related to each of the identified concepts for example.

The primary function of the nursing department is to provide patient services in a manner conducive to the education of health professionals and supportive of appropriate research activities. The department affirms its commitment to optimal patient outcomes and the highest standards of care possible in the face of increasing technical patient care requirements and the need to make intelligent decisions about the use of resources.

All patients are entitled to excellence in the nursing care they receive. The quality of care given is irrespective of race, sex, religion, political beliefs, socioeconomic status, or ethnic background. Nursing is the primary professional service received during hospitalization. After hospitalization, nurses provide continued care and contribute to effective hospital and community service emphasizing preventive, health maintenance and rehabilitative service.

The department commits to the development of professional nursing through modeling the nursing role in caring for patients, developing new health care providers and expanding nursing knowledge so the belief statements influence the practice of nursing. Each institution has its well laid philosophy which one has to abide to provide highest standard of care.

NURSING PRACTICE

Throughout the 20th century, the definitions of nursing have changed as nurses and nursing as a profession moved towards increasing authority and independence. The need to control the regulatory laws of each state and to define the professional role within the professional nursing organization continued as the social, political and economic world changed. In 1973, in New York State, a definition emerged that described the independent role of the nurse. New York state law defined nursing practice as the "diagnosis and treatment of human responses to actual or potential health problems through such means as case finding, health teaching and counseling."

OBJECTIVES OF NURSING PRACTICE

The purpose of nursing education is to foster high standards of nursing practice, promote the professional and educational advancement of nurses to the end that all people may have better health care services. The objectives of nursing shall include the following:

- To establish and promote implementation of standards of nursing practice, nursing education, and nursing services as defined by statutory bodies.
- To encourage members to adhere to the ethical obligation of nurses as patient's advocates.
- To promote and protect the economic and general welfare of nurses.
- To continually review and clarify the role of the nurse in the delivery of health care services.
- To interpret the aims of various educational programs and career opportunities in nursing.
- To identify the educational needs of practitioners and to work with appropriate groups to provide programs to ensure current nursing practice.
- To initiate legislation and proposals for government regulations and take stand supporting or opposing those which affect the health of the people of the state.
- To speak for the nursing profession in relationships with professional, community and government groups and with the public.
- To provide for representation of nursing interests statewide, nationally and internationally and to present nursing policies and positions on issues that may have statewide, national or international implications.

Concept of Nursing Practice

Nursing is a dynamic and supportive profession, guided by its code of ethics, is rooted in caring a concept evident throughout its four fields of activity, practice, education, administration and research.

In 1965, the ANA's committee on education issued a position paper asserting and elaborated on care, cure and coordination as components of professional nursing practice. The 1965 position paper made the following statement about nursing:

- It is a helping profession and as such, provides services, which contribute to the health and wellbeing of people.
- Nursing is a vital consequence to the individual receiving services; which fulfills the needs, that the person cannot meet by the family or by other persons in the community.
- The essential components of professional nursing are care, cure and coordination. The care aspect is more than "to take care of", it is "caring for" and "caring about" as well. It is dealing with human beings under stress, frequently over long periods of time. It is providing comfort and support in times of anxiety, loneliness and helplessness. It is listening, evaluating and intervening appropriately.
- The promotion of health and healing is the core aspects of professional nursing. It is assisting patients to understand their health problems and helping them to cope. It is the administration of medications and treatments and it is the use of clinical nursing judgment in determining, on the basis of patient's reactions, whether the plan for care needs to be maintained or changed. It is knowing when and how to use existing and potential resources to heal patients towards recovery and adjustment by mobilizing their own resources.

Characteristics of Nursing Practice

- Nursing practice respects the diversity and is individualized to meet the unique needs of the patients, family group or community. All these are health care consumers and the main focus of attention for the registered nurses.
- The nurses establish coordination with in health care team, persons and support systems to address the health needs of the patients and reach the goals of delivering quality health care.
- Professional nursing promotes healing in such a way that builds a relationship between nurse and patient. Caring for individual, families and population is the key focus of nursing. Caring is the center of the nursing practice.
- Nurses use nursing process (cognitive skills and evidence-based practice) to assess, diagnose and identify objectives and plan, and implement and evaluate the care. Critical thinking underlines each step of nursing process.
- Nursing practice is a strong link between the professional work and environment to provide optimal level of health care and to achieve optimal outcomes.

PROFESSION

The dictionary meaning of profession is "vocation, calling, especially one which involves some branch of learning or service as the learned professions of divinity, law, medicine, nursing, etc." One way of defining a profession is to state what it should be. When we state what something should be, we are given the criteria. Criteria are standards of judging something. We have criteria for a nursing profession. These are standards for what a profession should be.

Characteristics of Profession

Many writers have listed the criteria of profession. According to Bixler a profession should be:

- **Intellectual:** The professional person uses specialized knowledge in practice.
- **Scientific:** The education of a professional person is based upon a body of scientific knowledge. A true profession will not only continue research, but will also use the growing body of knowledge and the service of its practitioners.
- **Requires higher education:** The professional person should be educated within an institution of higher education.
- **Essential:** The services of a profession should be vital to human and social welfare. The services are absolutely necessary for survival.
- **Self-governing:** A true profession will be able to provide leadership among its own members. They guide the setting of policies and the control of professional activities.
- **Service-oriented:** The members of a profession should put service first. Their service will be one to which they expect to devote the major proportion of their energies for their rest of their lives.
- **Continuous professional growth:** The profession should provide planned opportunities for its members to continue their professional development.
- **Personal development:** Members of profession should be able to work with a sense of knowing that they are free to make improvements in their work and apply new ideas and methods. They are free to question and evaluate what is being done. Because of this freedom, professional people have great possibilities of improving and developing their practice.
- **Economic security:** Economic security or having enough money to pay for essentials of life is of great importance to every human being. A profession tries to give its

members this security. The profession tries to see that its practitioners are paid adequately so that they will have enough money while working and are able to save for retirement to meet all material needs and the daily expenses of living at that time.

CURRENT TRENDS IN NURSING

Nursing changes continually in response to the needs and resources of society as a whole. It also changes in response to factors such as definition of nursing, the aims of nursing, the educational preparation for nursing and expanded practice roles. The trends are affecting nursing education and practice. As nurses continue to define their own practice, the special and distinctive role of nursing in caring for others has become unceasingly recognized in society.

Shortage of Nursing Professionals

In India there is shortage of nurses in spite of 2000 school of General Nursing and Midwifery (GNM). 1200 Colleges of BSc Nursing and 281 colleges offering MSc Nursing. Annually, they produce 60,000 nurses. Out of this, 20% go to foreign countries due to better pay overseas and job security, competitive environment and better infrastructure. WHO had earlier estimated that India would need 2.4 million nurses by 2012 to achieve the government's aim of a nurse patient ratio of one nurse per 500 population.

Evidence-Based Practice

It is only recently the importance of using scientific evidence to develop guidelines for nursing care has been recognized, by identifying and analyzing the best available scientific evidence, nurses are steadily developing further guidelines for clinical practice that are useful nationally and internationally.

Community-Based Nursing

Health care is unseeingly provided in community-based settings such as clinics, outpatient settings, and homes.

Decreased Length of Hospital Stay

Patients who require in-hospital care are more acutely ill but their length of stay in hospital has decreased. Nurses employed in hospital settings must have the knowledge and skills to provide complex care to very-ill patients. In the home, nurses continue to provide some care, as well as teaching patients and their families how to do self-care.

Aging Population

The older adult population is expanding more rapidly than any other age group. Older population has specific needs, which are to be met. To take care of aging population, there is a need to have specialized nurses to meet specific needs.

Increase in Chronic Health Conditions

Chronic health conditions such as heart disease, cancer, respiratory diseases and acquired immunodeficiency syndrome (AIDS) are major health problems in our society. Meeting the health care needs of so many people will be more different, particularly for those who live in poverty, are homeless or mentally ill, etc.

Independent Nursing Practice

Advanced practice nurses, such as nurse practitioners, and nurse midwives, are increasingly establishing independent practices in which they diagnose and treat illness, promote health and provide care to expectant mothers.

CATEGORIES OF NURSING PERSONNEL

Nursing personnel are among the largest number of health care professionals working in the various fields of health care. They work from the lowest level of care to the highest level.

They work in the varied settings namely:
- Hospital/clinical areas
- Community areas
- Educational settings
- Holistic setting

Nurses Working in the Clinical Settings

The topmost nursing officers are nursing directors, CNO, Nursing Superintendent/Prinicipal matron/Matron in chief.

Nursing Director—Roles and Responsibilities

- Formation of the aims and the objectives, policies
- Staffing based on the nursing requirement
- Planning and directing the nursing care
- Coordinating the interdepartmental activities
- Maintaining the supplies and equipment
- Budgeting
- Keeping records and reports

Chief Nursing Officer (CNO)

- Chief officer for all the staff nurses in hospital. She does planning, coordination, supervision, controlling, reporting to higher medical officer and delegating the work schedules of other nurses.
- Helps to recruit, assign and allocate the required staff at the right place and time.
- Plans the job description, supervise and delegate responsibilities to each staff nurse.

- Conducts rounds in the hospital regularly to check for functioning, cleanliness of the hospital.
- Takes attendance, plans and implement the duty roster for the staff nurses.
- Recruits the staff needed, coordinates the work with the entire department.
- Conducts in-service education, encourages continuing education.
- Conducts nursing audit, does anecdotal reporting to evaluate nursing care.
- Make all staff observe and follow code of ethics and regulations of the hospitals.
- Has authority to terminate any nurse if she misbehaves or violates hospital regulations.
- Encourages and participates in all round development of nurses, especially in nursing research activities.

Nursing Superintendent

- She is responsible for the efficient running of the various nursing departments in the hospital for 24 hours.
- She is accountable to CNO, if there is no CNO, she is responsible to the Medical Superintendent (Director).
- Planning and organizing nursing services.
- Responsible for nursing service administration.

Head Nurse

- To plan the duty roster specific to the ward and allocate ward-in charge to specific wards.
- To control and coordinate the activities of the specific wards.
- To plan all the activities done by ward-in charge in advance, delegates responsibilities and supervise the activities in the wards.
- To supervise the nursing care being rendered for all patients and to take frequent status updates.
- To conduct nursing rounds with ward in charges to assess the problem, plan care, clarify issues, fulfill the requirements and guide the ward-in charge.

Deputy Nursing Superintendent

- Responsible for the efficient running of the various nursing departments in the hospital for 24 hours.
- Responsible to the nursing superintendent and assist in the nursing services, administration of the hospital.
- Officiates in the absence of nursing superintendent.
- Maintains confidential reports and records of the nursing staff.
- Serves on various hospital committees.
- Arranges orientation program for new nursing staff.

Assistant Nursing Superintendent

- Responsible for developing and supervising nursing services of a department specific unit for consisting of two or more wards or units.
- She is responsible to the deputy nursing superintendent/ nursing superintendent, CNO, Director.
- Evaluates the nature and quantum of care required in each unit/ward.
- Plans ward management with the nursing sister of each unit.
- Keeps the DNS/NS officer informed if the needs of the nursing units under her charge if any special problems.
- Arranges classes and clinical teachings of nursing students in the department.
- Acts as a liaison officer between the NS and higher hospital authorities.
- Maintains the enrollment register of all the staff and ward-in charge and ensure that all the staff reported duty on time.
- Allocates the alternative staff in case of absenteeism.
- Conducts meeting with subordinate staff, and provide guidance, and teaching to improve her nursing care.

Ward-in Charges

- Reports to the head nurse for any issue.
- Plans, controls and supervises the activity of the subordinates and also ensures that the staff are allocated at required areas and provide good care to patients.
- Ensures ward cleanliness, safety and security for all the patients in the ward.
- Oversees the patient's condition regularly and to care for the concerns of doctors who take care of the patients.
- Conducts ward rounds with staff nurse and plan her daily activities accordingly.
- Coordinates the shift schedule, day/night off in the coordination with the head nurse.
- Meets the health care needs of all patients in the ward.

Staff Nurse

- Works under the ward-in charge and report to her.
- Provides individual care to patients who are seriously ill and are assisted by the junior nurses.
- Maintains the patient care sheet, record the patient details on the nurse's record.
- Oversees the work of sweepers, attendants and coordinate with student nurses to learn and practice the nursing care.

- Keeps the units neat and tidy, check linen, drugs and other supplies required in ward.
- Identifies the needed supplies with approval form of ward-in charge.

Graduate Nurse

- The nurse directly provides patient care.
- Learns the policies of the hospital and ward and works according to the standards of care.
- Provides health education and directs skilled work.
- She works under the supervision of the senior nurse and holds authority over the nursing assistants and the Aids.

Nurses Working in the Community Areas

- They are also a large part of the health care delivery system.
- They work on various levels and provide care.

Community Health Nurse

There are various community health nurse levels in various states of India. They are classified as:
- DPHNO (District public health nurse officer).
- BPHN (Block public health nurse).
- PHN (Public health nurse).
- ANM (Auxiliary nursing midwifery/female health workers).

Community Health Nurse (CHN)

- Qualified CHN is one who has undergone general training, and basic education in the community health nursing.
- She must have a BSc (Nursing) with a registration to work as a community health nurse.
- Various roles of CHN are: Decision maker, health education, direct care provider, advocate, evaluator, supervisor, research, planner.

ANM/Female Health Workers

- Registers and cares for the prenatal and postnatal mothers at home.
- Registers and follow up all the eligible couples.
- Provides nutritional advice and immunization to mother and children.
- Carries out family planning services, including the distribution of the contraceptives.
- Provides treatment in minor ailments.
- Maintains the records and registers of all the services provided and vital events like birth and death.
- Participates in the various disease control programs.

- Conducts surveys of all sub-center areas and maintains records about every family.
- Coordinates activities with the block level.

Nursing Personnel in Nursing Education

- Director of Nursing Education
- Principal, College of Nursing
- Professor, College of Nursing
- Assistant Professor of College of Nursing
- Nursing tutors/clinical instructors

ROLES AND FUNCTIONS OF THE NURSE

Nurses assume a number of roles when they provide care to clients. The roles required at a specific time depend on the needs of the client (Fig. 2).

- **Caregiver:** This role has traditionally included those activities that assist the client physically and psychologically while preserving the client's dignity. The required nursing actions may involve complete care for the completely dependent client, partial care for the partially dependent client, and supportive, educative care to assist clients in attaining their highest possible level of health and wellness. As a nurse, she provides care directly or delegates it to other caregivers. While performing this role, she utilizes nursing process framework for providing care.
- **Teacher:** As a teacher, the nurse helps clients to learn about their health and health care procedures they need to perform to restore or maintain their health. The nurse assesses the client's learning needs and readiness to learn, sets specific learning goals in conjunction with the client, utilizes various teaching strategies and evaluates learning.
- **Communicator:** Communication is integral to all nursing roles. Nurse communicates with the client and supports persons, other health professionals and people in the

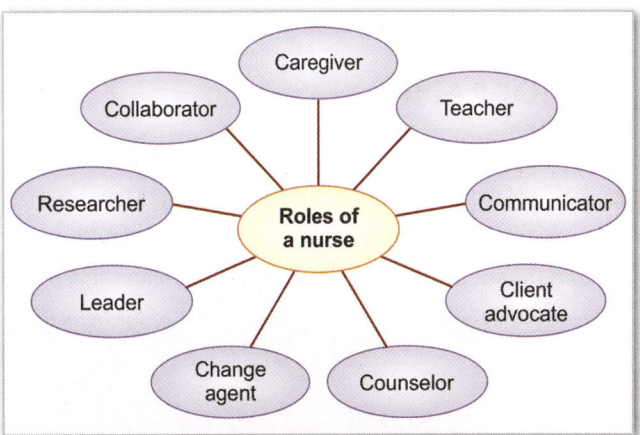

Fig. 2: Roles of a nurse

community. In the role of communicator, nurses identify client's problems and then communicate these verbally or in writing to other members of the health team. The nurse must be able to communicate clearly and accurately in order to meet client's health care needs. The quality of a nurse's communication is an important factor in nursing care.

- **Client advocate:** As a client advocate, a nurse acts to protect the client. Nurses assist clients in exercising their rights and help them speak up for themselves.
- **Counselor:** Counseling is the process of helping a client to recognize and cope with psychological or social problems, to develop interpersonal relationship, and to promote growth. A nurse counsels and helps the person to develop new attitudes, behaviors by encouraging the client to look at alternative behaviors and recognize the choices.
- **Change agent:** The nurse acts as a change agent when assisting clients to make modifications in their behaviors.
- **Leader:** A leader influences others to work together to accomplish a specific goal. A nurse takes up a leader's role, an assertive and self-confident practice of nursing when providing care, effective change, and functioning with groups.
- **Researcher:** A nurse acts as a researcher by participating or conducting research to increase knowledge in nursing and improve patient care.
- **Collaborator:** A nurse acts a collaborator with the effective use of skill in organization, communication, and advocacy to facilitate the functions of all members of the health care team as they provide patient care.

Expanded Educational and Career Roles of Nurses

Clinical Nurse Specialist

A nurse with an advanced degree, education or experience is considered to be an expert in a specialized area of nursing and carries out direct patient care, consultation, teaching of patients, families, staff and research.

Nurse-Practitioner

A nurse who completes a course of study in anesthesia, carries out preoperative assessments, administers and monitors anesthesia during surgery and evaluates post-operative states of patients.

Nurse-Midwife

A nurse who completes a program in midwifery, provides prenatal and postnatal care and delivers babies for women with uncomplicated pregnancies.

Nurse-Educator

A nurse, usually with an advanced degree, who teaches in educational or clinical settings, teaches theoretical knowledge and clinical skills along with conducting research.

Nurse-Administrator

A nurse, who functions at various levels of management in health care settings is responsible for the management and administration of resources and personnel involved in giving patient care.

Nurse-Researcher

A nurse-researcher is the one who has an advanced degree and who conducts research for improvement of nursing practice and education.

Nurse-Entrepreneur

A nurse-entrepreneur is a nurse, usually with an advanced degree, who may manage a clinic or health-related business, conducts research, provides education or serves as an advisor or consultant to institutions, political agencies or business.

BIBLIOGRAPHY

1. *Nursing Services, A report on a WHO Symposium 1978.*
2. *TNAI Nursing Services, Administration and Management, 1st ed. TNAI, New Delhi, 2000; p. 135–67.*
3. *Clement. Management of Nursing Services and Education, 1st ed. Elsevier Publications, New Delhi; p. 247–50.*
4. *The Trained Nurses Association of India. Fundamental of Nursing: Procedure Manual. TNAI Publication.*
5. *Harmer Bertha & Henderson V. Textbook of the Principles and Practice of Nursing. The Macmillan Company, fiftieth ed. 1955.*

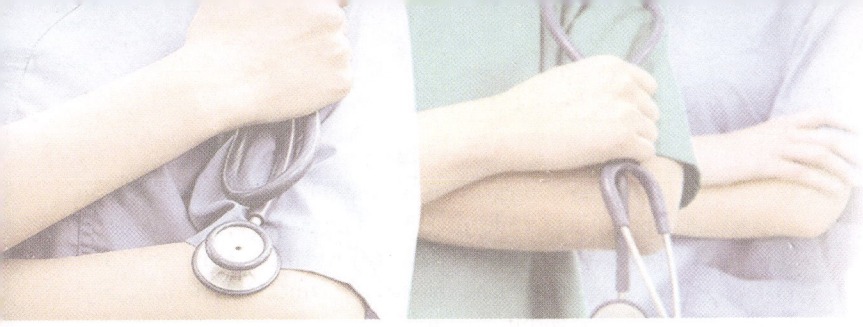

Values and Ethics

VALUES

A value is a belief about the worth of something. It is the importance a person attaches to various endeavors such as amount of time, passion and money you devote to relationships, work study, fitness activities, leisure, etc. A person's values influence beliefs about human needs, health and illness, the practice of health behaviors, and human responses to illness.

Development of Values

Nobody is born with values; rather, values are formed during a lifetime from information available in the environment, family and culture. A child observes the action of others and quickly learns what has high and low value for family members. The common modes of development of values are:

- Modeling
- Moralizing
- Laissez faire
- Rewarding and punishing
- Responsible choice

Children learn through modeling by observing their parents, peers and significant others. It may lead to socially acceptable or unacceptable behavior. Use of moralization by parents or an institution such as school or church allows little opportunity for them to weigh different values, so values are accepted as it is.

Laissez-faire approach helps the children to explore values on their own and develop personal value system.

At times, it leads to confusion and conflict because there is no guidance.

Children are rewarded by demonstrating values held by parents and punished for demonstrating unacceptable values.

Care givers who follow responsible choice as a mode of value transmission, encourage children to explore competing values and to weigh their consequences. Support and guidance are offered as children develop a personal value system.

Values Essential in Professional Nursing

In order to encourage health care professionals to respect and accept the individuality of patients, some educators have advised that professionals be 'value neutral' or 'nonjudgmental' in their professional role. The nurse does not assume that her personal values are right and should not judge the patient's values as right or wrong depending on his/her congruence with the personal values system. This encourages effective care for patients with values different from the nurses.

In 1998, the American Association of Colleges for Nursing identified five values that epitomize the caring. These professional values provide the foundation for nursing practice and guide the nurse's interactions with patients, colleagues and public.

The professional values are:

- **Altruism:** Altruism is a concern for the welfare and well-being of others. In professional practice, altruism is reflected by the nurse's concern for the welfare of patients, other nurses and other health care providers such as:
  - Demonstrating understanding of culture, beliefs of others.
  - Advocates for patients.
  - Takes risk on behalf of patients and colleagues.
  - Mentors other professionals.
- **Autonomy:** Autonomy is the right to self determination. Professional practice reflects autonomy when the nurse respects patient's rights to make decisions about their health care, e.g.,
  - Helps family and patients to make decisions about healthcare.
  - Plans care in partnership with patients.
  - Provides information so that patients can make informed choices.
- **Human dignity:** Human dignity is respect for the inherent worth. In professional practice, human dignity is reflected when the nurse values and respects all patients and colleagues, e.g.,
  - Protect patient's privacy.
  - Preserve the confidentiality of patients and health care providers.
  - Provides culturally competent and sensitive care.
  - Designs care according to patient's needs.

- **Integrity:** Integrity is acting in accordance with an appropriate code of ethics and accepted standards of practice. Integrity is reflected when the nurse is honest and provides care based on ethical framework and accepted within the profession, e.g.,
  - Provides honest information to patients and the public.
  - Documents care accurately and honestly.
  - Seeks to remedy errors made by self or others.
  - Demonstrates accountability for one's own actions.
- **Social justice:** Social justice is upholding moral, legal and humanistic principles. A nurse demonstrates this value in professional practice when she assures equal treatment under the law and equal access to quality health care, e.g.,
  - Supports fairness and non-discrimination in the delivery of health care.
  - Promotes universal access to health care.
  - Encourages legislation and policy consistent with an advancement of nursing care and health care.

Values Clarification

It is a process by which people come to understand their own values and value system. "It is a process of discovery and allows the person to discover through feelings and analysis of behavior, what choices to make when alternatives are presented, and to identify whether these choices are rationally made or are the result of previous conditioning" (Steak & Harmon, 1983, P13).

In nursing, value clarification is beneficial because when nurses understand the values that motivate the decisions and behaviors of patient, they can tap these values when teaching and counseling patients.

The steps involved in valuing process are **Choosing, Prizing and Acting**.

When one values something, one chooses freely from alternatives after careful consideration of the consequences of each alternative. Prizing something one values involves pride, happiness and public affirmation. Finally, the person who values something acts by combining choice into one's behavior with consistency and regularity on the value.

Value clarification is useful in helping individuals or groups to become more aware of their values and how they may influence their actions. By asking patients to agree or disagree with a list of statement or to rank in order of importance a list of beliefs can assist the nurse and client to make the client's values more open so they can be considered in planning the care of patient.

CARING AND ADVOCACY

It is the nurse's responsibility to ensure that patient has access to health care services that meet the health needs. The patients has the right to make decisions and choices. The patient has the right to expect a nurse-patient relationship that is based on shared respect, trust and collaboration in solving problems related to health and health care needs.

When people are ill, they are unable to assert their rights as they would if they were healthy. An advocate is one who expresses and defends the cause of another. If the patient lacks decision-making capacity, is legally incompetent, or is a minor, these rights are exercised on the client's behalf by a designated surrogate, e.g., head of the family or another member of the community. The nurse must ascertain the patient and family's views and honor their traditions regarding decision-making.

Being an effective patient advocate involves being assertive, recognize the rights and values of patients and families, and respecting the patient's right to decide.

Values Basic to Client Advocacy

- The client is holistic, autonomous being, who has the right to make choices and decisions.
- Clients have the right to expect nurse-client relationship in solving problems related to health.
- It is the nurse's responsibility to ensure the client has access to health care services that meet health needs.

TYPES OF VALUES

Nursing is a caring, compassionate profession. Nurses do not just perform tasks or provide services, they develop an empathy for the needs of others and a connection with their patients. Applying nursing care values in all actions ensures the trust of patients in the nurses. The top five nursing care values are:

1. **Compassion:** Compassion encompasses empathy, caring and the promotion of each patient's dignity. Being sensitive to the needs of your patients and your patients families is one of the most fundamental nursing value.
2. **Trust worthiness:** Nurses are among the most trusted groups of people, making trustworthiness one of the most essential nursing values and vital to your integrity and ethical behavior. Patients and fellow medical staff depend on their trust in your confidentiality, faithfulness and responsibility to your patients and their needs.
3. **Humility:** Nursing is one of the most rewarding, fulfilling career paths. With it comes a wealth of medical knowledge and skills that allow you to facilitate healing and alleviate suffering through diagnosis and treatment, but humility should also be your companion. Nurses need to be humble by keeping open mind and heart.
4. **Accountability:** Professional nursing values would not be complete without accountability. There is a need to stress the importance of taking ownership over your practice,

including every mistake, error in judgement or failure to communicate. How can you improve next time? It forces you to take an active role in your life and keeps you from blaming others.

5. **Curiosity:** Nursing knowledge encompasses all the theories, philosophies, research and practice wisdom of the nursing profession. One should never stop learning. Graduation is only the beginning of a nurse's education. Curiosity and an insatiable desire to learn separates mediocre nurses from great ones.

ETHICS

An ethic is a systematic inquiry into principles of right and wrong conduct. It is a branch of philosophy dealing with standard of conduct and moral judgment. They are based on moral reasoning and reflect a set of values

- **Morals** are standards of right and wrong that help people determine the correct or permissible action in a given situation.
- **Values** are ideas or beliefs a person considers important and feels strongly about.

Ethical Principles

The principles offer guidance to action. All things being equal, we ought to act at all times in a manner that respects the autonomy of others, does not harms, benefits others, treats others fairly, and is faithful to the promises we make to others. They are the specific prescriptions for actions.

Autonomy (Self-determination)

It refers to the right to make one's own decisions. Honoring the principle of autonomy means that the nurse respects a client's right to make decisions even, when those choices seem to the nurse not to be in client's best interest. It also means treating others with consideration, provide the information and support patients and families need to make decision that is right for them.

Non-maleficence

Avoid causing harm. Harm can mean intentionally causing any kind of injury or discomfort. In nursing, intentional harm is never acceptable.

Beneficence

Beneficence means "doing good" Nurses are obligated to do good, i.e., to implement actions that benefit clients and their support persons. However, doing good can also pose a risk of doing harm. For example, a nurse may advise a client about a strenuous exercise program to improve general health, but should not do so if the client is at risk of a heart attack.

Justice

Justice is also referred as fairness. Give each his or her due; act fairly. Always seek to distribute the benefits, risk, and costs of nursing care justly.

Fidelity

Fidelity means to be faithful to agreements and promises. Be faithful to the promise you made to the public to be competent and to be willing to use your competence to benefit the patients entrusted to your care. Never abandon a patient entrusted to your care without first providing the patient's needs.

Veracity

Veracity refers to telling the truth. Although this seems straightforward; in practice, choices are not always clear. Should a nurse tell the truth when it is known that it will cause harm? Does a nurse tell a lie when it is known that it will relieve anxiety and fear?

Accountability

Accountability means "answerable to oneself and others for one's own actions".

Responsibility

Responsibility refers to "the specific accountability or liability associated with the performance of duties of a particular role". Thus, the ethical nurse is able to explain the rationale behind every action and recognizes the standards to which he or she will be held responsible.

Nursing Codes of Ethics

A code of ethics is a formal statement of a group's ideals and values that is:

- Shared by members of the group.
- Reflects the moral judgments over time.
- Serves as standard for their professional actions.

Nurses are responsible for being familiar with the code that governs their practice. International, national and state nursing associations have established codes of ethics.

Nursing code of ethics have the following purposes:

- Inform the public about the minimum standards of the profession and help them understand professional nursing conduct.
- Provide a sign of the profession's commitment to the public it serves.
- Outline the major ethical considerations of the profession.
- Provide ethical standards for professional behavior.
- Guide the profession in self-regulation.
- Remind nurses of the special responsibility they assume when caring for the sick.

The ICN Code of Ethics for Nurses

An international code of ethics for nurses was first adopted by the International Council of Nurses (ICN) in 1953. It has been revised and reaffirmed various times since then. Most recently review and revision completed in 2005.

Preamble

Nurses have four fundamental responsibilities: to promote health, to prevent illness, to restore health, and to alleviate suffering. The need for nursing is universal.

Inherent in nursing is respect for human rights, including cultural rights, the right to life and choice, to dignity, and to be treated with respect. Nursing care is respectful and unrestricted by considerations of age, color, creed, culture, disability or illness, gender, sexual orientation, nationality, politics, race, or social status.

Nurses render health services to the individual, the family, and the community and coordinate their services with those of related groups.

The ICN Code

The ICN code of Ethics for nurses has four principal elements that outline the standards of ethical conduct.

Nurses and People

The nurse's primary professional responsibility is for people requiring nursing care. In providing care, the nurse promotes an environment in which the human rights, values, customs, and spiritual beliefs of the individual, family and community are respected.

The nurse ensures that the individual receives sufficient information on which to base consent for care and related treatment.

The nurse holds in confidence personal information and uses judgment in sharing this information.

The nurse shares with society the responsibility for initiating and supporting action to meet the health and social needs of the public, in particular those of vulnerable populations.

The nurse also shares responsibility to sustain and protect the natural environment from depletion, pollution, degradation and destruction.

Nurses and Practice

The nurse carries personal responsibility and accountability for nursing practice and for maintaining competence by continuous learning.

The nurse maintains a standard of personal health such that the ability to provide care is not compromised.

The nurse uses judgment regarding individual competence when accepting and delegating responsibility.

The nurse at all times maintains standards of personal conduct, which reflect well on the profession and enhance public confidence.

The nurse in providing care, ensures that use of technology and scientific advances are compatible with the safety, dignity, and rights of people.

Nurses and the Profession

The nurse assumes the major role in determining and implementing acceptable standard of clinical nursing practice, management, research, and education.

The nurse is active in developing a core of research-based professional knowledge.

The nurse, acting through the professional organization, participates in creating and maintaining safe, equitable social and economic working conditions in nursing.

Nurses and Co-workers

The nurse sustains a cooperative relationship with co-workers in nursing and other fields.

The nurse takes appropriate action to safeguard individual, families, and communities when their health is endangered by a co-worker or any other person.

American Nurses Association Code for Nurses

- The nurse, in all professional relationships, practices with compassion and respect for the inherent dignity, worth, and uniqueness of every individual, unrestricted by considerations of social or economic status, personal attributes, or the nature of health problems.
- The nurse's primary commitment is to the patient, whether as individual, family, group, or community.
- The nurse promotes, advocates for, and strives to protect the health, safety, and rights of the patient.
- The nurse is responsible and accountable for individual nursing practice and determines the appropriate delegation of tasks consistent with the nurse's obligation to provide optimum patient care.
- The nurse owes the same duties to self as to others, including the responsibility to preserve integrity, to maintain competence, and continue personal and professional growth.
- The nurse participates in establishing, maintaining, and improving healthcare environments and conditions of employment conducive to the provision of quality health

care and consistent with the values of the profession through individual and collective action.

- The nurse participates in the advancement of the profession through contributions to practice, education, administration, and knowledge development.
- The nurse collaborates with other health professionals and with the public in promoting community, national, and international efforts to meet health needs.
- The profession of nursing, as represented by associations and their members, is responsible to articulate the nursing values, for maintaining the integrity of the profession and its practice, and for shaping social policy.

From: Code of Ethics for Nurses with Interpretive Statements ©2001 By American Nurses Association.

Canadian Nurses Association: Code of Ethics for Registered Nurses

- Nurses provide safe, compassionate, competent and ethical care.
- Nurses work with people to enable them to attain their highest possible level of health and well-being.
- Nurses recognize, respect, and promote a person's right to be informed and make decisions.
- Nurses recognize and respect the intrinsic worth of each person.
- Nurses recognize the importance of privacy and confidentiality and safeguard personal, family and community information obtained in the context of a professional relationship.
- Nurses uphold principles of justice by safeguarding human rights, equity, and fairness and by promoting the public good.
- Nurses are accountable for their actions and answerable for their practice.

*This represents only one element of the code-values. Nurses in all domains of practice bear the ethical responsibilities identified under each of the seven primary nursing values. These are intended to help nurses apply the code.

From Canadian Nurses Association. (2008). Code of Ethics for Registered Nurses, Ottawa, Ontario.

Code of Ethics for Nurses in India

Indian Nursing Council (INC) has published the code of Ethics for Nurses in India in 2006. The code of ethics for nurses is critical for building professionalism and accountability.

Ethical considerations are vital in any area dealing with human beings including nursing research because they represent values, rights, and relationships. Therefore, same code of ethics may imply for a nurse dealing with human subject during research study.

1. The Nurse Respects the Uniqueness of an Individual in Provision of Care

Nurse

- Provides care for individuals without consideration of cast, creed, religion, culture, ethnicity, gender, socioeconomic and political status, personal attributes, or any other grounds.
- Individualizes the care considering the beliefs, values, and cultural sensitivities.
- Appreciates the place of individual in the family and community and facilitates participation of significant others in the care.
- Develops and promotes trustful relationship with individual(s).
- Recognizes uniqueness of response of individuals to interventions and adapts accordingly.

2. The Nurse Respects the Rights of Individuals as Partners in Care and Help in Making Informed Choices

Nurse

- Respects individuals' rights to make decisions about their care and therefore gives adequate and accurate information for enabling them to make informed choices.
- Respects the decisions made by individual(s) regarding their care.
- Protects public from misinformation and misinterpretations.
- Advocates special provisions to protect vulnerable individuals/groups.

3. The Nurse Respects Individual's Right to Privacy, Maintains Confidentiality and Shares Information Judiciously

Nurse

- Respects the individuals' rights to privacy of their personal information.
- Maintains confidentiality of personal information except in life-threatening situations and uses discretion in sharing information.
- Takes informed consent and maintains anonymity when information is required for quality assurance/academic/legal reasons.
- Limits the access to all personal records written and computerized to authorized persons only.

4. The Nurse Maintains Competence in Order to Render Quality Nursing Care

Nurse

- Nursing care must be provided only by registered nurse.
- Nurse strives to maintain quality nursing care and upholds the standards of care.
- Nurse values continuing education, and initiates and utilizes all opportunities for self-development.
- Nurse values research as a means of development of nursing profession and participate in nursing research adhering to ethical principles.

5. The Nurse is Obliged to Practice within the Framework of Ethical, Professional and Legal Boundaries

Nurse

- Adheres to code of ethics and code of professional conduct for nurses in India developed by INC.
- Familiarizes with relevant laws and practices in accordance with the law of the state.

6. Nurse is Obliged to Work Harmoniously with Members of the Health Care Team

Nurse

- Appreciates the team efforts in rendering care.
- Cooperates, coordinates, and collaborates with members of the health care team to meet the needs of people.

7. Nurse Commits to Reciprocate the Trust Invested in Nursing Profession by Society

Nurse

- Demonstrates personal etiquettes in all dealings.
- Demonstrates professional attributes in all dealings.

SPECIFIC ETHICAL ISSUES

Some of the ethical problems nurses encounter most frequently are issues in the care of human immunodeficiency virus (HIV)/acquired immunodeficiency syndrome (AIDS) clients, abortion, organ transplantation, end of life decisions, cost containment issues and access to health care, and breach of client confidentially.

Acquired Immunodeficiency Syndrome

Nurses will care AIDS victims in every segment of nursing practice. They must utilize standard precautions for control of transmission of HIV virus when caring for all clients. They have the responsibility to safeguard themselves and others from exposure to infectious materials. Issues of disclosure, privacy and confidentiality are important concerns. Testing for HIV client and for the presence of AIDS in health professionals and clients should be done. Questions arise as to whether testing of all providers and clients should be mandatory or voluntary and whether the test results should be released to insurance companies, sexual partners or care givers. As with all ethical dilemmas, there are both positive and negative implications of each possibility for specific individuals.

Abortion

State laws differ as to what type of consents are required. The length of gestation for legal abortion also differs between states. However, nurses have no right to impose their values on a client. Nursing code of ethics support client's rights to information and counseling in making decisions.

Organ Transplantation and Tissue Donation

Ethical issues related to organ transplantation include allocation of organs (either from living donors or from donors who have just died), selling of body parts, involvement of children as potential donors, consent, clear definition of death and conflicts of interest between potential donors and recipients. In some situations, a person's religious beliefs may also present conflict. As per the National Organ Transplant Act, 1984, individuals can be approached for giving consent in the following order:

- Spouse
- Adult son/daughter
- Either parent
- Adult brother/sister
- Grand parent
- Guardian

The law also provides that the physician who certifies death shall not be involved in the removal or transplant of organs or tissues. The law also prohibits selling or purchasing of organs and regulates this area of medical and nursing practice.

End of Life Issues

The most frequent disturbing ethical problems for nurses involve issues that arise around death and dying. These include euthanasia, assisted suicide, termination of life-sustaining treatment and withdrawing or withholding of food and fluids.

Many moral problems relating to end of life can be resolved if client completes *advance directives*. Advance

directives direct the caregivers as to the client's wishes about continuing, withholding or withdrawing treatment. In the event, the person cannot make these decisions for himself or herself. Also advance directive is a legal document in which a person either states choices for medical treatment or names someone to make treatment choices if he or she loses decision-making ability.

Do not resuscitate or DNR orders are written by a doctor when the patient has indicated a desire to be allowed to die if he or she stops breathing or her heart stops. In this situation, no cardiac compressions or assisted breathing (CPR) should be started. It is very important for nursing personnel to know who is to be resuscitated and who is not. A nurse who attempts to resuscitate a patient who has a doctors order for DNR would be acting without the patients consent, and committing a battery.

Euthanasia and Assisted Suicide

Euthanasia, a Greek Word meaning "good death" is popularly known as "mercy killing".

- **Active euthanasia** involves actions to bring about the client's death directly, with or without client's consent, e.g., administration of a lethal medication to end the client's suffering. Regardless of the caregiver's intent, active euthanasia is forbidden by law and can result in criminal charges of murder.
- **Assisted suicide** is a variation of active euthanasia, i.e., giving a client the means to kill themselves if they request it (e.g., providing pills or weapons). Some countries or states have laws permitting assisted suicide for clients who are severely ill, who are near death, and who wish to commit suicide. The question of suicide and assisted suicide are still controversial in our society. The American Nurses Association position statement on assisted suicide states (ANA, 1995) the active euthanasia and assisted suicide are in violation of the code for Nurses.
- **Passive euthanasia,** more commonly referred to now as withdrawing or withholding life-sustaining therapy (WWLST) involves the withdrawal of extraordinary means of life support such as removing a ventilator or withholding special attempts to revive a client. WWLST is both legally and ethically more acceptable to most persons than assisted suicide.

Termination of Life-Sustaining Treatment

Technological advances have helped to prolong life, but not necessarily to restore health. Client may specify in advance directives about their wish to have life-sustaining measures withdrawn or they may appoint surrogate decision maker. However, it is usually more troublesome for health care professionals to withdraw a treatment than to decide initially not to begin it. Nurses must understand that a decision to withdraw treatment is not a decision to withdraw care. As the primary care givers, nurses must ensure that care and comfort measures are given as the client illness progresses. When client is at home, nurses often provides education and supports through hospice services.

Hospice care focuses on support and care of the dying person and family, with the goal of facilitating a peaceful and dignified death. Hospice care improves the quality of life rather than cure, supports the client and family, through the dying process, and supports the family through bereavement.

BIBLIOGRAPHY

1. *Taylor C, Lillis C, LeMone P, Lynn P. Fundamentals of Nursing, 6th edition. Lippincott Williams and Wilkins. Philadelphia: 2008.*

2. *Dewit SC. Fundamental Concepts and Skills for Nursing, 3rd edition. Saunders. 2008. pp. 992.*

3. *Sharma S. Potter and Perry's Fundamentals of Nursing. A South Asian edition. Elsevier India. Gurugram: 2013.*

4. *Berman AT, Snyder S, Kozier BJ, et al. Kozier & Erb's. Fundamentals of Nursing: Concepts, Process and Practice, 8th edition. Pearson Education.*

History of Nursing in India

INTRODUCTION

Nursing like any other discipline or profession, has undergone a lot of changes. The progress in nursing had been relatively slow in the early period of 19th century. During later part of 20th century, there has been definite growth and development in nursing education and nursing practice.

NURSING IN EARLY PERIOD

In the early Judeo- Christian era, women provided nursing services at home as a part of their ethical and humanitarian responsibilities. There was no formal training, rather a woman used her skills as a loving mother to care for the sick on a person-to-person basis. By 500–1500 AD, nursing had become an organized service. Most nurses were part of religions orders, who received training from their practical experience in caring for the sick. Most of them were expected to devote their time outside the home to care for the poor and sick as an expression of Christian love. It was during this period that a rich person like Phoebe of Cenchrea dedicated her life to nursing and was called the first visiting nurse. She founded Deaconess, an order of Christian women who served the sick and poor. Nursing continued in the same fashion for many centuries. The period was referred as the dark-age of nursing when the nurses were treated as a social outcaste. These women worked off jail sentences through nursing duties and had no training or preparation for the care of the sick.

In ancient Egypt, physicians practiced medicine in temples and were assisted by women helpers. Though the records of nursing procedures are available, there is no indication whether these helpers were nurses or not.

Hippocrates, the father of medicine, emphasized on observation of signs and symptoms of illness, but nursing was still not practiced as women remained at home.

NURSING IN MEDIEVAL PERIOD (1000–1450 AD)

During this time, many nursing orders developed in Europe. Clare of Assisi founded 'The Poor clares' which cared for the sick and lepers. Between 1450 and 1800 AD, during Renaissance to the 19th century, there were despair, wars and indifferences to the poor and sick. This was a period of decline for nursing but the field of medicine was growing. During the 17th century, St. Vincent de Paul founded the sisters of charity who cared for the sick. The pattern continued till the Industrial Revolution (1800) until the time of Florence Nightingale of England.

MODERN NURSING

Florence Nightingale (1820–1910) was born in a prominent English family with the benefits of excellent education and knowledge of social conditions and reforms of the time. She believed that nursing should be a separate career, and not part of religious community. Nightingale received the Year Book of the Institution of Deaconesses at Kaiserworth in October, 1846. She went to Kaiserworth in 1847 to work with Deaconesses. She went to Paris in 1853 to study with the Sisters of Charity. She was later appointed as Superintendent of the English General Hospitals in Turkey. During the Crimean war, the major reforms brought in by her were in hygiene, sanitation and nursing practices, which reduced the mortality rate at the Barracks hospital in Scutari, Turkey from 42.7% to 2.2% in 6 months. In 1860, she developed the first organized program of training for nurses, at the Nightingale Training School for nurses at St. Thomas Hospital in London. She elevated nursing to a respectable profession. The civil war stimulated the growth of nursing in the United States. Clara Barton, founder of the American Red Cross, spearheaded the activity followed by Dorothea Lynde Dix, Mary Ann Ball and Harriet Tubman. Between 1872–73, three nursing schools were founded in the United States of America (USA) in New York City, Boston and New Haven. Subsequent to the civil war, nursing schools in the USA and Canada began to create the pattern of their curriculum after the Nightingale School. In Canada, the first training school, St. Catherine's started in Ontario in 1874. In 1884, Mary Agnes Snively became Director of Toronto General Hospital.

HISTORY OF NURSING IN INDIA

The history of nursing in India goes back through the centuries to about 1500 BC. In 700 BC, the practice of medicine was in the hands of Brahmins who were scholars of medical education. Sushruta set standards in surgery. Charaka and Sushruta were authorities in Ayurveda and their samhitas were preserved. They demanded absolute cleanliness and their message was practiced. The emphasis was on prevention. Sushruta was the man who described the technique of cesarean section, plastic surgery, cranial surgery, and cataract operation. Sushruta defined the relation of doctor, patient, nurses and medicine as the four feet on which cure must rest. Ancient people believed more in prevention than in cure.

Doctors were also trained not only in medicine and surgery but also in prevention of diseases Charaka defined a nurse as one who had knowledge of the manner in which drugs should be prepared or compounded for administration. Cleanliness, devotion to the patient, purity of mind and body were the four qualification of the attending nurse. The most advanced period of medicine was from 250 BC to 750 AD.

Army institutions were developed with the arrival of the British. Nurses from Britain arrived to care for British soldiers in hospitals founded in1753. March 25, 1888, is memorable in the medical history, as on this day, ten fully qualified and certified nurses landed in Bombay and Indian Army, Nursing Service was founded. It later developed into one of the finest military nursing services in the world. The first lady superintendent was Ms. Locke.

Though the Indian Military Nursing service (IMNS) was born during the first world war, it developed very slowly until the second world war of 1939. Forty-five nurses were recruited in India for the first time in 1914 and were attached to Queen Alexandria. Military nursing service in India was formed in 1927 and it had 12 matrons, 18 sisters, and 25 staff nurses. They were responsible for the supervision and training of nursing sections of all Indian Hospitals.

It was the Mission Hospitals, which started training of Indians as nurses. Christian girls were mainly attracted towards nursing as Hindus were held back due to caste prejudices and Muslim girls had to follow the purdah system.

In 1908, the Trained Nurses Association of India (TNAI) was established to uphold the unity and honor of the nursing profession, and in 1949, the Indian Nursing council (INC), as per an act of parliament passed in 1947, was established.

Government of India formed a number of committees: Bhore Committee (1946), Shetty Committee (1959), Mudaliar Committee (1961), Mukherjee Committee (1966), Kartar Singh Committee (1973) and Bajaj Committee (1986) which helped in development of nursing. In 1982, National Health Policy was adopted and a high power committee was appointed by the Ministry of Health and Family Welfare in 1987 to review the role, functions, status, preparation of the nursing-personnel, nursing services and other issues related to the development of the profession and to make suitable recommendations.

In August 1988, a national convention of nurses was held, which was a significant development in the field of nursing, who made constructive recommendations for consideration of the high power committee. It had an opportunity to discuss nursing problems with the President and Prime Minster of India. The Central Council of Health, the highest policy making body for health issues recommended improvement in training for nurses in clinical specialties, improving staffing norms, opening more postgraduate courses for nurses, funds for strengthening nursing services and strengthening regulatory mechanism.

DEVELOPMENT OF NURSING EDUCATION IN INDIA

Many changes took place after independence in nursing. Many schools and colleges were opened which gave nursing profession a higher social and economic status. The formation of many commissions and committees, establishment of Indian Nursing Council (INC) and Trained Nurses Association of India (TNAI) brought about changes in nursing education.

CATEGORIES OF NURSING EDUCATION

General Nursing and Midwifery

General Nursing and Midwifery (GNM) is a diploma program offered by schools of nursing under hospital administration. The course is of 3½ years' duration. These schools are recognized by the State Nursing Council and INC. The State Nursing Registration Council conducts examination every year and on completion, certify them as Registered Nurses and Registered Midwife. (RN/RM). GNM diploma nurses are eligible for the post-basic BSc program. The course is likely to be stopped from 2021.

Auxiliary Nurse Midwife

Auxiliary nurse midwife (ANM) course is at present of 2 years' duration (18 months + 6 months internship). The minimum educational requirement is senior secondary school certificate (ANM). (10 + 2). It is recognized by state nursing councils and INC.

Diploma in Nursing Education and Administration

This is the course of 10 months' duration for qualified nurses (GNM) that helps in developing administrative and educational skills.

Diploma Courses in Nursing Specialties

There are various courses ranging from 3 months to 10 months' duration in different specialties, viz. cardio-thoracic nursing, pediatric nursing, oncology nursing, ophthalmic nursing, etc.

University Level Programs

BSc Nursing

The first university program was started by University of Delhi at Rajkumari Amrit Kaur (RAK) College of Nursing in Delhi and Christian Medical College and Hospital (CMC) in Vellore. Gradually, many colleges of Nursing came into existence. This course is of four-year duration conducted by colleges and is duly recognized by state nursing registration council and INC.

Post-Basic BSc Nursing

This course was started in1962 and is of 2 years' duration for qualified registered nurses (GNM). This enables the qualified nurses to augment their professional competence and provides an opportunity for them to advance in their career ladder. There are both regular and distance learning programs available.

Postgraduate Education: MSc Nursing

Course is of 2 years' duration. RAK college of Nursing, Delhi in Delhi and CMC, Vellore in 1969 offered this programme. Specialties such as Medical Surgical Nursing, Pediatric Nursing, Psychiatric Nursing, Community health nursing and Obstetrical Nursing are offered by many colleges.

MPhil in Nursing

It is a one year course for regular candidates and two years for part time candidates. It was started in RAK college of Nursing, Delhi in 1986.

PhD in Nursing

PhD in nursing is offered at RAK College of Nursing, Delhi, College of Nursing, Manipal, PGI Chandigarh and many more institutions.

BIBLIOGRAPHY

1. *The Trained Nurses Association of India. Fundamental of Nursing: Procedure Manual. TNAI Publication.*
2. *Harmer & Henderson V. Fundamentals of Nursing.*

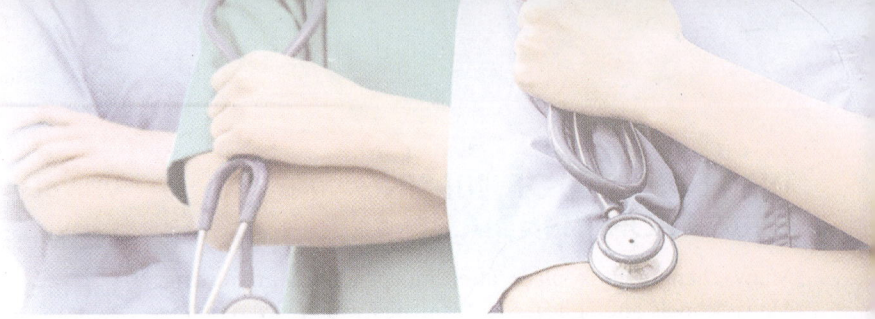

Chapter 8

Legal Implications in Nursing

Learning Objectives

After completing this chapter, you will be able to:
- Describe the laws related to nursing practice
- Explain the difference between malpractice and negligence
- Describe the legal requirements for the practice of nursing

Key Terms

- Accountability
- Accreditation
- Assault
- Crime
- Battery
- Felony
- Liability
- Tort
- Nurse Practice Act
- Negligence
- Consumer Protection Act

INTRODUCTION

Safe nursing practice includes an understanding of the legal boundaries within which nurses must function. Nurses must understand the law to protect themselves from liability and to protect their client's rights. Nurses need not fear the law but, should have knowledge of laws that regulate and affect nursing practice. The laws are needed to ensure that the nurses decisions and actions are consistent with current legal principles and to protect the nurse from liability.

LAW AND ITS FUNCTIONS IN NURSING

Law can be defined as "the sum total of rules and regulations by which a society is governed". The law serves a number of functions in nursing:
- It provides a framework for establishing which nursing actions in the care of clients are legal.
- It differentiates the nurses responsibilities from those of other health professionals.
- It helps in establishing the boundaries of independent nursing action
- It assists in maintaining a standard of nursing practice by making nurses accountable under the law.

LEGAL TERMINOLOGY

Crime

A crime is a wrong committed against a person or property or public good. A crime occurs when there is violation of a law. In a crime, intention to do wrong is also present. Crimes may be
- **Misdemeanor:** It is less serious crime then felony, may result in fines, imprisonment of one year or less, or both.

- **Felony:** It is a serious crime that may result in a prison term of more than one year. Health care workers can be convicted of felonies for offences such as falsification of medical records, insurance fraud, theft of narcotics or practicing without a license.

Liability

It is the responsibility to pay or compensate for a loss or injury that results from one's negligence, e.g., a nurse may be liable if a client receives the wrong medication and is harmed (act of commission) participation in illegal abortion, and participation in euthanasia (mercy killing).

A nurse may be liable if the client did not receive a prescribed medication and was harmed (an act of Omission). Crimes of omission include failure to perform a prescribed treatment, failing to report child or elder abuse and failure to report a specified communicable disease.

Tort

- Tort is violation of a civil law, a wrong against an individual. The injury can be physical, emotional, or financial. It can be (i) intentional or (ii) unintentional (Fig. 1)
  - **Intentional torts:** Include assault, battery, false imprisonment, invasion of privacy and defamation.
    - **Assault:** It is a threat or an attempt to do bodily harm. It includes physical or verbal intimidation. Telling the client that you are going to restrain him in bed, if he tries to get out of bed without assistance is assault.
    - **Battery:** It is physical contact with another person without that person's consent. Touching a person's body, clothing, chair or bed is considered as battery. Giving an injection that the client refuses is battery.

- **False imprisonment:** It is the "unjustifiable detention of a person without legal warrant to confine the person". The client must not be detained against the client will.
- **Invasion of privacy:** It is a direct wrong of a personal nature. It injures the feelings of the person and does not take into account the effect of revealed information or the reputation of the person in the community. The right of privacy is the right of individuals to withhold themselves and their lives from public scrutiny. It can also be described as the right to be left alone.
- **Defamation:** It is communication that is false, or made with a careless disregard for the truth and results in injury to the reputation of a person. **Libel** is defamation by means of print, writing or pictures. **Slander** is defamation by the spoken word, or stating unprivileged or false words by which a reputation is damaged e.g., nurse telling a client that another nurse is incompetent.
- **Unintentional tort:** It is (i) Negligence and (ii) Malpractice
  - **Negligence:** It is defined as harm done to a client as a result of neglecting duties, procedures or ordinary precautions, e.g., performing nursing procedures that have not been taught, failing to follow standard protocols, failure to report defective malfunctioning equipment, failing to meet established standards of safe care, failing to prevent injury to clients and failing to question a physicians order that seems incorrect.
  - **Malpractice:** It is the improper, injurious or faulty treatment of a client that results in illness or injury. Harm that results from a licensed person's actions or lack of actions can be called malpractice.

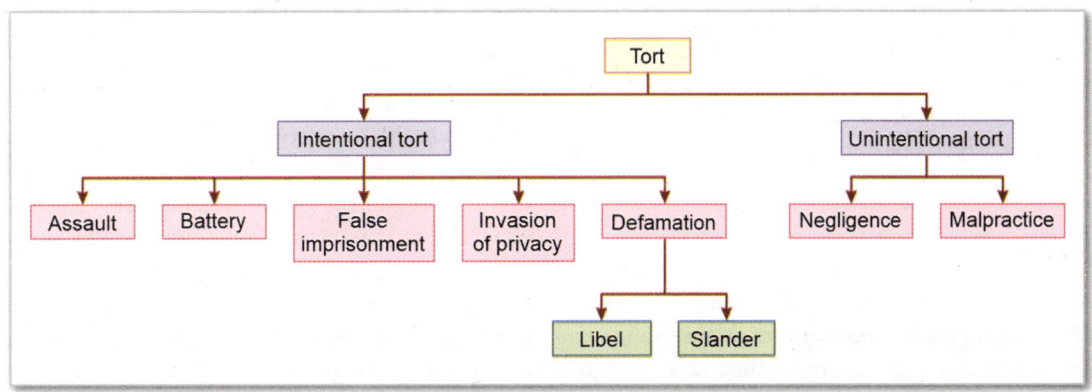

Fig. 1: Classification of tort

LAWS RELATED TO THE PRACTICE OF NURSING AND LICENSURE

Nurse Practice Act (NPA)

State Licensure is required to practice nursing. Each state writes its own laws and regulations regarding licensure, in what is called Nurse Practice Act. This law defines the scope of nursing practice, and provides for the regulation of the profession by a state board of nursing. The nurse practice act in each state sets forth the scope of nursing for the registered professional nurse (RN), advanced practice nurses such as nurse practitioners and nurse anesthetists. NPA also regulate the degree of dependence or independence of a licensed nurse regarding other nurses (LPN), physicians, and other health care providers.

Credentialing

Credentialing is the process of determining and maintaining competence in nursing practice. By this, the nursing profession maintains standard of practice and accountability for the educational preparation of its members. Credentialing includes: licensure, certification and accreditation.

Licensure

Eligibility for licensure is determined by each state's board of nursing, usually involving completion of an approved educational program. In some places like United states, Canada, etc., they have a licensing examination which needs to be passed before they can work as RN. In India presently, the state councils register the nurses who have undergone training from Indian nursing council (INC) approved educational program and this license has to be renewed every five years on completion of 30 CEU. (Continuing Education Units).

Certification

It is the practice of validating that an individual nurse has met minimum standards of nursing competence in specialty areas such as maternal-child health, pediatrics, critical care, mental health, gerontology and school health nursing. These are specialty programs, which one undertakes after basic nursing education.

Accreditation

One of the functions of a state board of nursing is to ensure that schools preparing nurses maintain minimum standards of education. All states require approval/accreditation by the state board of nursing. Some states require that nursing program be both state approved accredited and accredited by a national accrediting/ agency e.g., National League for Nursing Accrediting Commission (NLNAC) and the American Association of Colleges of Nursing (AACN). State accreditation is a legal requirement.

Accountability

Accountability is taking responsibility, for one's actions. Professional accountability is a nurses responsibility to meet the health care needs of the patient in a safe and caring way. Accountability means asking for assistance when unsure, performing nursing tasks in the safe and prescribed manner, reporting and documenting assessments and interventions, evaluating the care given and the patient's response to that care. Accountability also means commitment to continuing education to stay updated and knowledgeable.

Delegation

Delegation is the assignment of duties to another person. An RN may supervise nurse assistants, technicians. When a nurse gives an assignment to another person, the RN is responsible for assuring that the person has the skills and abilities to safely perform the assignment, and that an unlicensed person is not performing acts restricted to nursing under the law.

Standards of Care

Standards of Care are the skills and learning commonly possessed by the members of a profession. Legally, the nurse is responsible for her actions under the nurse practice act and according to the standards of care that are approved by the profession. These standards are defined in nursing procedure books, institutional manuals of procedures or protocols that outline current skills or techniques. These standards provide a way of judging the quality and effectiveness of patient care, and in legal cases determine whether a nurse acted correctly or not.

Occupational Safety and Health Act (OSHA)

The Occupational Safety and Health Act was passed in 1970 to improve the work environment in areas that affect worker's health or safety. It includes regulations for handling infections or toxic material radiation safeguards, and the use of electrical equipment. Health care agencies, as a result of OSHA requirements provide mandatory orientation and continuing education regarding a wide range of topics from isolation procedures and blood borne pathogens exposure, to fire or bomb threats and lifting and evacuation procedures under disaster management.

Safe storage and handling of toxic chemicals and drugs are important part of OSHA. Each facility is required to keep a record of hazardous substances, which includes harmless liquids such as bleach and disinfectants, as well as dangerous chemicals. They must be stored properly in designated areas and maintain manufacturer's safety data sheets (MSDS), which outline the hazard a substance can pose.

Consumer Protection Act (1986)

Consumer Protection Act (CPA) was passed by the Parliament in 1986 (INDIA) to provide better protection in the interest of consumers and focuses on consumer justice through the establishment of consumer councils and other authorities for the settlement of consumer disputes and matters connected therewith. Under this act consumer can complain in redressal forum. It enables the consumer/patient to make a complaint to a redressal forum regarding defective services provided. Right of a consumer/patient are:

- Right of safety
- Right to be informed
- Right to choose
- Right to be heard
- Right to seek redressal
- Right to consumer education

Good Samaritan Laws

Good Samaritan Laws are those that protect a health care professional from liability if he or she stops to provide aid in emergency. In most states there is no legal requirement for a nurse to provide aid in an emergency, but if a nurse provides care in an emergency, liability is limited unless there is evidence of gross negligence, or intentional misconduct.

Patent's Bill of Rights

In 1992, American Hospital Association (AHA) revised the Patient's Bill of Rights; a list of rights the patients could expect and responsibilities that the hospital may not violate. These documents emphasize that patients continue to have rights even if they are helpless and sick. They seek to preserve the dignity, privacy, freedom of movement and information needs of the patient.

Controlled Substances

In 1970, the comprehensive drug abuse prevention and control act was passed in the United States which controls substance such as narcotics, depressants, stimulants, and hallucinogens. As per this act:

- Substances to be kept locked and only authorized personnel should have access to them
- Precise records must be kept
- Criminal penalties are to given in case of misuse of drugs.

LEGAL DOCUMENTS

The Chart or Medical Record

When a person enters the health care system to visit a doctor, clinic, hospital, or emergency room, or to receive home health care, a record is begun that documents the person's health status or problem and the care given. This record is a legal document and include record of all assessments, tests and care provided. The chart, or medical record is confidential which means only people directly associated with the care of that patient have legal access to the information in the chart. The chart is the property of the hospital or agency or physician, not the patient. However, the patient does have the right of access to the chart and copies of information in the chart which may be authorized by the patient to be provided to other agencies, e.g., if the patient transfers from one doctor or health care facility to another. Health care researchers and insurance companies may also gain access to chart information with the patients permission.

Student nurses must protect the confidentiality of their patients while writing care plans, case studies and presentation by not identifying the patient by name.

The chart is used as legal document and used to determine the truth of what happened, what was done or not done, to a patient during a period of time. Therefore, its contents always need to be accurate, pertinent and timely. Charting should be focused on the patient, and the nursing care. Remember that chart is a legal document and may be introduced as evidence in a court case.

Consent and Releases

A consent is a permission given by the patient or his or her legal representative. Consents, or releases, are legal documents that record the patient permission to perform a treatment or surgery, or to give information to insurance companies or other health care providers.

Informed consent indicates the patient's participation in the decision making process. In a consent for surgery or treatment, the patient must be told, in terms he/she can understand the risks and benefits of the proposed treatment, what the consequences may be of not having the procedure done, and the name of health care professional who will perform the procedure. This information is usually provided by the professional performing the procedure. If the patient has any questions, they should be satisfactorily answered before the patient signs the consent. Failure to obtain a valid informed consent may lead to charges of assault and battery or invasion of privacy.

When a person is over the age of 18, and **competent** he or she must sign the consent for treatment. A competent person is legally fit (mentally and emotionally). A person is considered **incompetent** if he or she is unconscious, under the influence of mind altering drugs including alcohol or declared legally incompetent such as in case of chronic dementia etc. In these cases, a next of kin, guardian, or someone who holds a power of attorney has legal authority to give consent. Minors (under the age of 18) may not give legal consent; their parents or guardians have this right.

A **release** is a legal form used to excuse one party from liability (responsibility). A commonly used release is a leave against medical advice (LAMA). This form is used by a hospital or facility when a patient does not accepts the physician's recommendation for hospitalization, and leaves the agency. The form documents that the reasons for continuing hospitalization or treatment, and risks of leaving without treatment have been explained to the patient. If the patient refuses to sign the release, it is noted and witnessed. The term release may also be used for forms used to authorize an agency to send confidential health care information to another agency, school or insurance company.

Witnessing Wills and Other Legal Documents

Many a times, nurses may be asked to witness a will or other legal document. Most hospitals and health care agencies have policies against this. The reason is that wills or legal documents may be contested, and the nurse who witnesses the documents can be called to courts to testify regarding the patient's health or mental condition, or relationship to visitors. To witness the signing of a legal document, one needs to know the content of the document. Legally, it is necessary that the witness confirms that the signature is made under no influence or drug or alcohol and that the person knows what he or she is signing.

LEGAL PROTECTIONS IN NURSING PRACTICE

Maintain Competence

- Learn skills thoroughly
- Know the state law for nursing practice
- Know and follow your employer's institutional policies
- Develop the ability to evaluate your knowledge and performance; identify areas in which you are weak and work to improve those
- Attend continuing education program and keep abreast of changes in health care.
- Keep records of workshops or seminars you attend
- Identify experienced nurses, whose competence you respect, and seek their assistance when you are unfamiliar with some technique or equipment.

Document Fully

- Promptly and accurately, document all assessments and care given. There is an expression in nursing that says "if you did not chart it, it did not get done"
- Use anecdotal records to recollect the incident instead of relying on memory

Establish Rapport

- Develop rapport and treat each patient with respect. Address patient by his/her preferred name.
- Listen to patient's complaints and communicate professionally to attempt to resolve problems.

Communicate Effectively

- Therapeutic communication techniques allow the patient to express feelings.
- Notify your supervisor of any situation in which a patient or family members are dissatisfied with the nursing care received.

BIBLIOGRAPHY

1. Berman AT, Snyder S, Kozier BJ, et al. Kozier & Erb's. Fundamentals of Nursing: Concepts, Process and Practice, 8th edition. Pearson Education. 2008.

2. Dewit SC. Fundamental Concepts and Skills for Nursing. WB Saunders Company; 2001.

3. Taylor CR, Lillis C, LeMone P, et al. Fundamentals of Nursing – The Art and Science of Nursing Care, 7th edition. Wolters Kluwer; 2010.

4. White L. Basic Nursing. Foundations of Nursing Skills and Concepts. Delmar Thomson Learning; 2002. pp. 919.

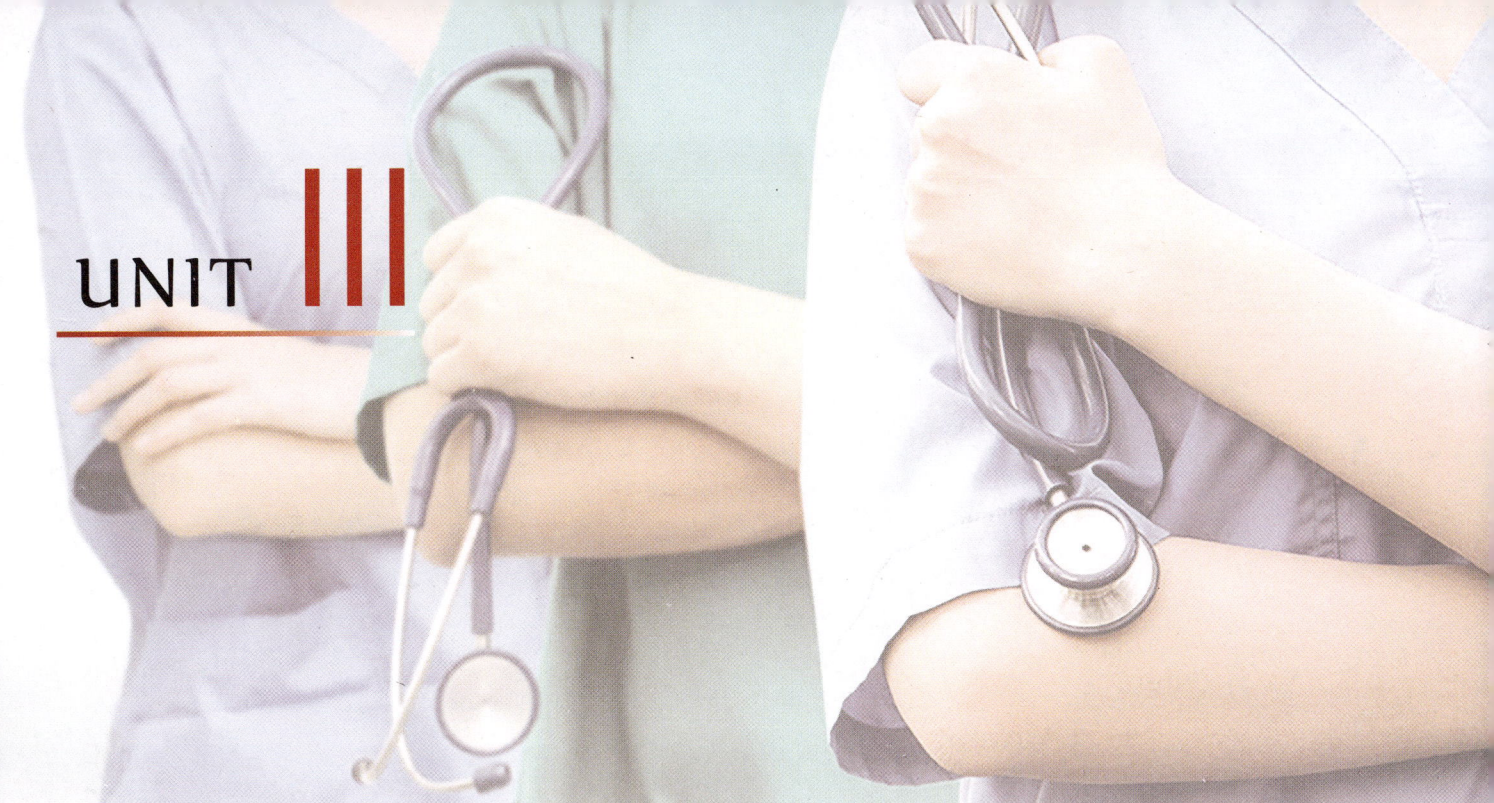

UNIT III

CONCEPTUAL AND THEORETICAL MODELS IN NURSING PRACTICE

Unit Outline

Conceptual and Theoretical Models in Nursing Practice

Learning Objectives

After completing this chapter, you will be able to:
- Explain conceptual and theoretical models of nursing practice
- Define the terminology used in nursing theories
- Describe various theories in nursing and their usefulness in linking with nursing process

Key Terms

- Model
- Holistic health concept
- Conceptual framework
- Theory
- Nursing process

Chapter Outline

- Introduction
- Health Belief Model
- Health Promotion Model
- Holistic Health Concept
- Introduction to Nursing Theories

INTRODUCTION

A model is a theoretical way of understanding concept or idea. Models represent different ways of approaching complex issues. As health and illness are complex concepts, models are used to understand the relationships between these concepts and the patient's attitude towards health and health behavior. Because health behaviors are influenced by health beliefs, they can positively or negatively affect a patient's level of health. Common positive health behaviors include immunizations, proper sleep patterns, adequate exercise, stress management and nutrition. Negative health behaviors include practices, which are potentially harmful to health such as smoking, drug or alcohol abuse, poor diet and refusal to take necessary medications.

The following health models, which are developed, help the nurses to understand patient's attitude and values about health and illness and to provide effective health care. These nursing models help to understand and predict patient's health behavior including how they use health services and adhere to recommended action.

HEALTH BELIEF MODEL

Health Belief Model (Rosenstoch's 1974) and Becker and Maiman's (1975) address the relationship between a person's beliefs and behaviors. This model helps us to understand factors influencing patient's perceptions, beliefs, and behavior to plan care that will most effectively assist patients in maintaining and restoring health and preventing illness (Fig. 1).

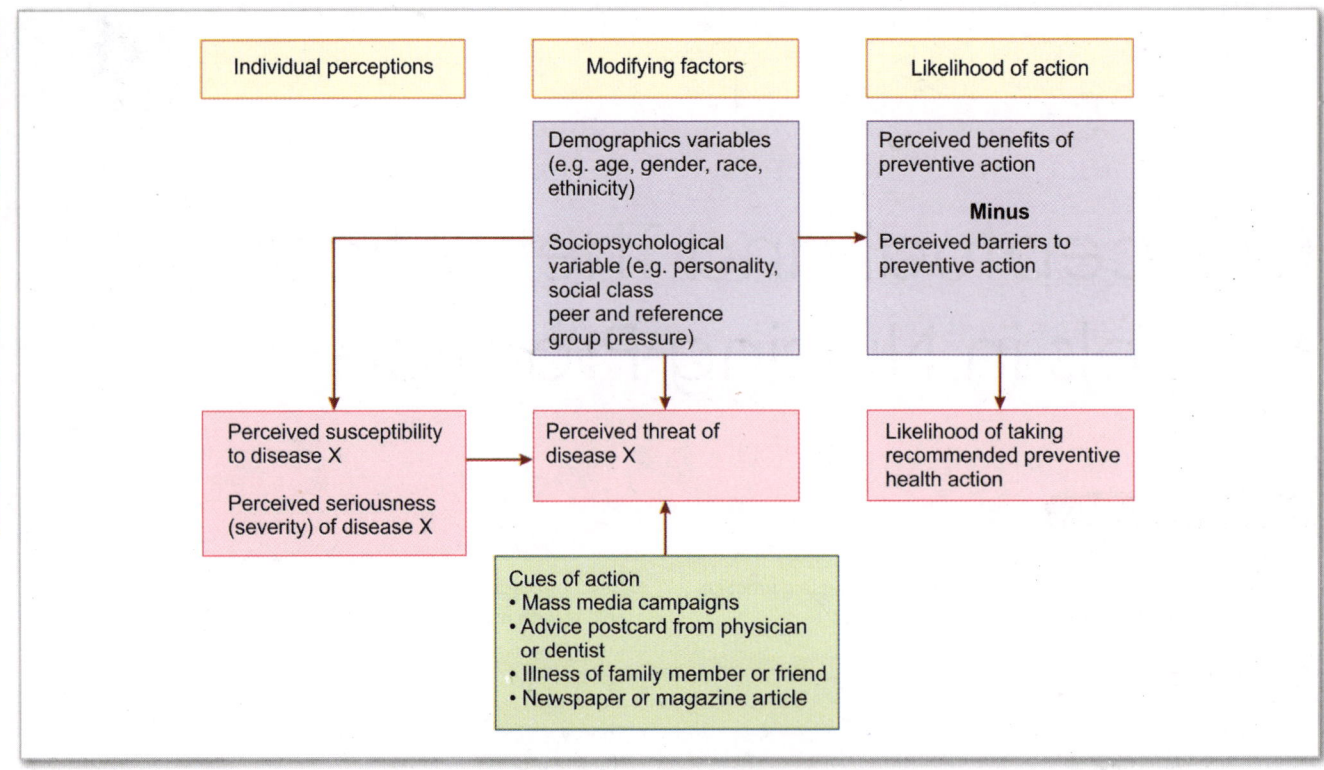

Fig. 1: Health belief model

The **first component** of this model involves an individual's perception of susceptibility to an illness. For example, a patient needs to recognize the familial link for diabetes mellitus. After this link is recognized, particularly when one patient and one sibling have died in their fourth decade from diabetes mellitus, the patient may perceive the personal risk of diabetes mellitus.

The **second component** is an individual's perception of the seriousness of the illness. The perception is influenced and modified by demographic and sociopsychological variables, perceived threat of the illness, and cues to action (e.g., mass media campaigns and advice from family, friends and medical professionals).

The **third component** is the likelihood that a person will take preventive action results from a persons' perception of the benefits of and barriers to take action. Preventive actions include lifestyle changes, increased adherence to medical therapies, or a search for medical advice or treatment, patient's perception of susceptibility to disease and his or her perception of the seriousness of an illness which help to determine the likelihood that the patient will or will not take in healthy behavior.

HEALTH PROMOTION MODEL

The health promotion model proposed by Pender (1982; revised 1996). According to this model, health is defined as a positive, dynamic state, not merely the absence of disease.

Health promotion is directed at increasing a patient's level of well-being. The HPM describes the multidimensional nature of persons as they interact within their environment to pursue health (Fig. 2).

This model focuses on the following three areas:

- Individual characteristics and experiences
- Behavior specific knowledge and effect
- Behavioral outcomes

According to this model, each person has unique personal characteristics and experiences that affect subsequent actions. The set of variables for behavioral-specific knowledge and affect have important motivational significance. These variables can be modified through nursing actions. Health promoting behavior is the desired behavioral outcome and is the end point in the health promotion model. Health promoting behaviors result in improved health, enhanced functional ability, and better quality of life at all stages of development.

HOLISTIC HEALTH CONCEPT

There is no illness which affects only one part of the body or one system alone, but it affects the whole person. Holistic concept emphasizes the care of the 'whole human' not only the cure of disease. This concept is based on the belief that human beings function as a complete unit and cannot be

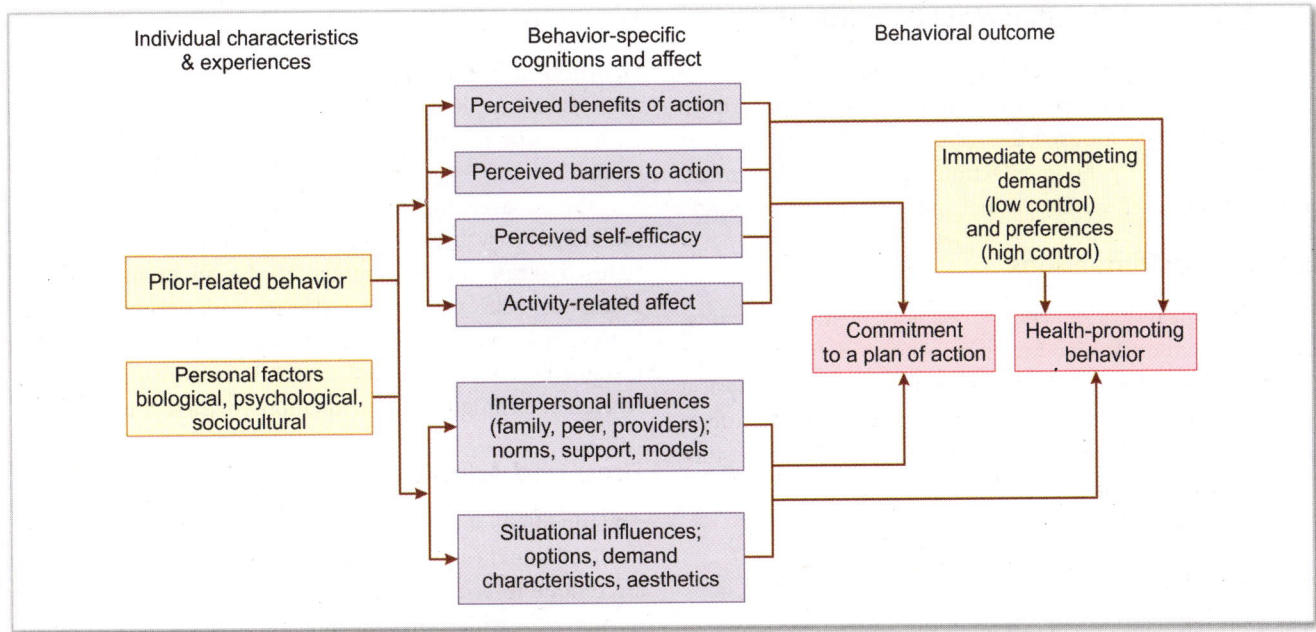

Fig. 2: Health promotion model (revised)

effectively treated as fragmented parts. Holistic nursing recognizes and respects the relationship between physical, mental, emotional, social and spiritual wellbeing and work with the patient on all these dimensions to facilitate healing. The term holistic is an adjective that describes wholeness or integrated system rather than their separate parts, i.e., humans manifest as an essential unity of mind, body and spirit. A holistic health concept recognizes that holism involves identifying the interrelationships of the bio-psycho-social-spiritual dimensions of the persons recognizing the 'whole' is greater than the sum of its parts.

Definition

- Holistic is a term derived from the Greek word "holos" means 'whole' or 'entire'.
- Holistic health care refers to comprehensive and total care of a person by meeting his/her needs in all areas- 'physical, intellectual, psychological, sociocultural and spiritual aspects.
- Holistic nursing is defined as "all nursing practice that has the goal of healing the 'whole person' (American Holistic Nurses Association).
- Holistic nursing is further defined as a practice that draws on nursing knowledge, theories, expertise and intuition to guide nurses in becoming therapeutic partners with clients in strengthening client's response to facilitate the healing process and achieve wholeness.
- Holism is the harmony among all those spheres of body, mind and spirit, and is held to be the highest form of health and the goal of nursing care.

Holistic Health Nursing Concepts

Several concepts are generally accepted as a premise of a holistic orientation to health care. The general concepts are:

- Multidimensionality of the individuals
- Relationship with individual's environment
- Self-responsibility
- Stress and adaptation.

Multidimensionality of an Individual

Each facet of an individual is important and contributes to the quality of life experience. If facets are ignored, the person has difficulty in living in a balanced state.

Physical Dimensions

This involves everything associated with one's body: both internal and external. This includes nutrition, breathing, rest, maintenance of body weight, body image, sleep-wake cycle, etc. The various aspects of the physical dimensions interact constantly with each other. e.g., nutritional status affects energy status, body weight, and other physical process.

Exercise helps to have better eating habits, sleep and helps to control cardiovascular and pulmonary functioning.

The degree to which people experience physical wellness is an indicator of how effectively they are taking care of their complete selves, as well as their interaction with the other dimensions. The physical dimension of an individual affects emotional, intellectual, social functioning and spirituality.

Emotional and Psychological Dimensions

The way a person expresses or ignores feelings and copes up with emotional stress has implications for the whole person. When emotionally aroused, the person undergoes changes that affect every activity thoughts, actions and overall adjustment. It also affects intellectual, spiritual and social dimensions.

Intellectual Dimensions

It involves the individual's receptive ability, memory, learning, cognition and expressive functions. Any thought or message which is communicated to one self can induce physical changes. For example, stressful thinking or relaxation affects heart rate, respiratory rate, skin temperature and other physiological functioning. It also influences the emotional functioning and one's relationship with other people.

Social Dimensions

The social dimension comprises all the aspects of individual that enable him to effectively function in society. It is the interaction and relationship with others. Social interaction helps the people to acquire knowledge, skills and disposition that allows them to function within their society.

Spiritual Dimension

Spiritual dimension includes sensitivity or attachment to religious values. It is the core of individual's existence. Spiritual dimension provides the reassurance that life has meaning and that allows one to experience inner peace and serenity and helps to understand the meaning or reality of existence. Characteristics of spirituality include:

- A sense of wholeness and harmony within oneself.
- A sense of wholeness and harmony with others.
- A sense of wholeness and harmony with God or a supreme power.
- A sense of wholeness and harmony with the ecosystem.

Relationship with the Environment

The environment is an irrevocable aspect of human existence and every living organism is interdependent with the environment. Each individual's environment is composed of many factors that influence his life. One's interaction with the environment contributes to how one lives, what one does and certainly influence one's state of health and illness. Physical, emotional, intellectual and social development of the person greatly depends upon the environmental situations. Therefore, holistic concept considers the ecosystem in relation to the need for health safety and peace of all persons so that healing may take place.

Self-Responsibility

Holistic health philosophy maintains that people are ultimately responsible for their own lives, and health self-awareness is a prerequisite to the genuine acceptance of responsibility to oneself.

When accepting responsibility for personal health, individuals view themselves as active participants in their health status. Holistic nursing emphasizes health promotion, self-awareness, self-exploration, self-care and self-responsibility. For example, management of chronic conditions like diabetes mellitus by diet control and exercise; stress management by relaxation techniques like, meditation, yoga and music therapy.

Stress and Adaptation

An individual's ability to cope with stressors is a primary factor that facilitates health and healing process. Stressful conditions are unique to each person, and are experienced throughout the life cycle, which affect healing of the whole person. People must learn to recognize stressors, and eliminate those that are harmful and learn to choose healthy responses. This includes recognition of needs, strengths and weakness, internal and external factors that affects all dimensions. Holistic nursing provides services that strengthen individuals and enable, them to achieve the wholeness inherent within them.

Holistic Caring Process

Assessment

Each person is assessed holistically using appropriate holistic traditional methods, while the uniqueness of the person is honored.

Problems/Needs

Each person's actual and potential problems, and needs related to health, and disease are identified and prioritized.

Outcome

Each person's actual and potential problems have appropriate outcomes and realistic goals.

Therapeutic Care Plan

Each client engages with the holistic nurses to mutually create an appropriate plan of care that is focused on health promotion, recovery and restoration of health.

Implementation

According to priority. Holistic nursing interventions are applied.

Evaluation

Each persons' response to holistic care is evaluated and recognized and accordingly changes are made in care plan.

Modalities Commonly Used by Holistic Nurses

Holistic nursing incorporates body-mind or behavioral-oriented therapies, to treat the physiological, psychological social and spiritual sequelae of illness.

- Art therapy
- Breathing exercises
- Exercise promotion
- Reiki
- Acupressure
- Therapeutic touch
- Holistic self-assessment
- Music therapy
- Forgiveness facilitation
- Self-care interventions
- Self-reflections
- Smoking cessation
- Weight management
- Guided imagery
- Relaxation training
- Massage
- Meditation
- Yoga
- Hope installation
- Spiritual support
- Emotional support.

Nurse's Responsibilities in Holism

- Attending the physical needs of the patient in detail.
- Care of his immediate environment.
- Carrying out treatment prescribed by the physician.
- Providing emotional support to the patient and relatives by all means.
- Teaching the patients and relatives the essentials of nursing care which they perform.
- Realizing and caring for the spiritual and emotional needs of the patients.
- Honor the individual's subjective experience about health, health beliefs and values.
- Holistic nurses require self-responsibility, spirituality and reflections in their own lives.
- Demonstrates awareness that self-healing is a continuous process.
- Demonstrates awareness that personal presence is as important as technical skills.

- Shares insights with clients without imposing personal values and beliefs.
- Accepts the client's input without judgments.
- Inherent in nursing is the respect for life, dignity and the rights of all persons.

Conclusion

Holistic nursing is the most complete way to conceptualize and practice the professional nursing. It is the focus and heart of nursing practice. The level of nursing care is more comprehensive when it includes physical, psychological, social, spiritual and cultural aspects of clients. "Holistic Nursing takes place wherever healing occurs." It can be done in acute care facilities, outpatient clinics, within the home—any place if you have this kind of direction and philosophy.

INTRODUCTION TO NURSING THEORIES

As a profession, nursing is involved in identifying its own unique body of knowledge essential to nursing practice. To identify this knowledge base, nurses must develop and recognize concepts and theories that are specific to nursing.

Terminology

Concept

Concepts are often called the building blocks of theories.

Concepts are ideas that give meaning to our sense of perceptions, permit generalizations and tend to be stored in our memory for recall and use at later time in new and different situations.

Concepts are said to be "empirical, inferential or abstract depending on their ability to be observed in the real world".

Empirical Concepts

They refer to what we can observe directly in the real world e.g., pen, knife and patient's bed, etc.

Inferential Concepts

They refer to the ones that are indirectly observed, like pain, temperature, blood pressure, etc.

Abstract Concepts

These ideas are difficult to be observed directly or indirectly, such as stress, state of health, etc.

Conceptual Framework

It is a group of related ideas, statements, or concepts. Conceptual framework articulates a broad range of the significant relationships among the concepts of the discipline.

Theory

These are attempts to explain relationships between concepts.

Theory has been defined as a supposition or system of ideas that is proposed to explain a given phenomenon. Theories are also used to describe, predict and control phenomenon.

Model

A model is an idea that explains by using symbolic and physical visualization.

Models are pictorial or diagrammatically representation of a proposition where propositions are explained as the statements that explains relationship between the concept.

Paradigm

It refers to a pattern of shared understandings and assumptions about reality and the world. Paradigm includes our notions of reality that are largely unconscious or taken for granted.

The Metaparadigm for Nursing/Concepts in Nursing Theory

In the late 20th century, most of the theoretical work in nursing is focused on articulating relationships among four major concepts: person, environment, health and nursing. Because these four concepts can be superimposed on almost any work in nursing, they are sometimes collectively referred to as metaparadigm for nursing.

These four concepts are central to nursing.

1. **Person or client:** The recipient of nursing care includes individuals, families, groups and communities.
2. **Environment:** The internal and external surroundings that affect the client. This includes people in the physical environment, such as families, friends and significant others.
3. **Health:** The degree of wellness or well-being that the client experiences.
4. **Nursing:** The attributes, characteristics, and actions of the nurse providing care on behalf of or in conjunction with the client.

According to Kerlinger (1973) "Theory is a set of interrelated concepts, definition and propositions that represent a systematic way of viewing facts or events by specifying relations among variables, with the purpose of explaining and predicting the fact or event".

Importance of Theories in Nursing

- Theory provides nurse with a sound basis to describe, explain and predict factors that influence nursing care. In nursing, caring is the core of nursing practice. As a profession, we need to develop theoretical knowledge based on research findings to form the foundation of nursing practice. Therefore, development and validation of nursing theory will help in strengthening nursing practice.
- Nursing theory is a source of professional autonomy and power.
- It guides nursing education, research and practice and differentiate nursing practice from other disciplines.

Nightingale's Environmental Theory

Florence Nightingale, the first nurse theorist, defined nursing almost 150 years ago as "the act of utilizing the environment of the patient to assist him in his recovery". She linked health with five environmental factors:

- Pure or fresh air
- Pure water
- Efficient drainage
- Cleanliness
- Light-direct sunlight

Deficiencies of these factors produced lack of health or illness.

Nightingale also stressed the importance of keeping the client warm, maintaining a nurse-free environment, and attending to the client's diet in terms of assessing intake, timeliness of the food and its effect on the person.

Nightingale set the stage for further work in the development of nursing theories. Her general concepts about ventilation, cleanliness, noise-free environment, warmth and diet remain integral parts of nursing and health care today.

Handerson's Theory

In 1966, Virginia Handerson's definition of the unique function of nursing was a major stepping stone in the emergence of nursing as a separate discipline separate from medicine.

Handerson describes nursing in relation to the client and the client's environment. Handerson sees the nurse to be concerned with both healthy and ill individuals, acknowledges that nurses interact with clients even when recovery may not be feasible, and mentions the teaching and advocacy roles of the nurse.

Handerson conceptualizes the nurse's role as assisting sick or healthy individuals to gain independence in meeting 14 fundamental needs:

1. Breathing normally
2. Eating and drinking adequately
3. Eliminating body wastes
4. Moving and maintaining a desirable position
5. Sleeping and resting

6. Selecting suitable clothes
7. Maintaining body temperature within normal range by adjusting clothing and modifying the environment
8. Keeping the body clean and well-groomed to protect the integument
9. Avoiding dangers in the environment and avoiding injuring others.
10. Communicating with others in expressing emotions, needs, tears or opinions.
11. Worshipping according to one's faith.
12. Working in such a way that one feels a sense of accomplishment.
13. Playing or participating in various forms of recreation.
14. Learning, discovering, or satisfying the curiosity that leads to normal development and health, and using available health facilities.

Hildegard E Peplau Theory (1909–1999)

Hildegard E Peplau was born in Pennsylvania in 1909. She graduated from a diploma program in Pottstown, Pennsylvania in 1931 after which she received a BA in interpersonal psychology from Bennington College in 1943; an MA in psychiatric nursing from Columbia University New York in 1947 and Ed.D. in curriculum development in 1953. She received honorary doctoral degree from a number of universities like the prestigious professor emeritus from Rutgers University. She started the first post baccalaureate program in nursing. She published her book interpersonal relations in Nursing in 1952. She worked as executive director and president of American Nursing Association (ANA); worked with World Health Organization (WHO), National Institute of Mental Health (NIMH) and nurse corps.

Major Concepts used by Peplau

Peplau's model evolves through the psychodynamic nursing that "psychodynamic nursing is being able to understand ones' own behavior to help others identify felt difficulties and to apply principles of human relations to the problems that arise at all levels of experiences."

Nursing metaparadigm of Peplau's theory includes four concepts, i.e., human being, health, environment and nursing.

Human Being

Peplau defines person in terms of men. Man is an organism that lies in an unstable equilibrium and strives in its own way to reduce tension generated by needs.

Health

Health is defined as "a word symbol that implies forward movement of personality and other ongoing human processes in the direction of creative, constructive, productive, personal and community living.

Environment

Peplau implicitly defined the environment in terms of "Existing forces outside the organism and in the context of culture: from which moral, customs and beliefs are acquired."

Nursing

Nursing is described as "a significant, therapeutic, interpersonal process. It functions cooperatively with other human processes that make health possible for individual in communities.

Major Assumption

Peplau identifies two explicit assumptions

♦ The kind of person the nurses become makes a substantial difference that each patient learns as he or she receives nursing care.
♦ Fostering personality development towards maturity is a function of nursing and nursing education. Nursing uses principles and processes to guide the process towards resolution of interpersonal problems.
♦ One implicit assumption was that the nursing profession has legal responsibility for the effective use of nursing and its consequences to nursing.

Four Phases of Peplau's Theory

Central to Peplau's theory is the use of a therapeutic relationship between the nurse and the client. Peplau identified four sequential steps in interpersonal relationship.

1. Orientation
2. Identification
3. Exploitation
4. Resolution

Each of these phases overlap, interrelate and vary in duration as the process evolves towards a solution. There are some factors which influence the blending of nurse-patient relationship.

Orientation Phase

It is a problem-defining phase and starts when the client meets the nurse as a stranger. During the orientation phase, the individual has a 'felt need'. The nurse help the patient recognize and understand his/her problem and determine his/her need for help. It is the phase that the nurse needs to assist the patient and family to realize what is happening to the patient. It is most important that the nurse works collectively with the patient and family in analyzing the situation, so that together they can recognize, clarify and define the existing problem. It allows the patient to direct energy away from anxiety of unmet needs toward constructive activities. The patient and the nurse work together to understand their reaction to each other, mindful of potential influencing factor such as culture, religion, personal experience and preconceived ideas. To sum up, in this initial phase, the nurse and the patient meet as strangers, but at the end they are concurrently striving to identify problem and are becoming more comfortable with one another and are now ready to progress to the next phase, i.e., identification.

Identification

In this phase, each patient responds differently. The patient identifies with those who can help him or her (relatedness) and might actively seek out the nurse until the nurse approaches (Fig. 3).

The response to the nurse is three fold:
- Participate with and be interdependent with the nurse.
- Be autonomous and independent from the nurse.
- Be passive and dependent on the nurse.

In this identification phase, all the time both the patient and the nurse clarify each other's perceptions and expectations which are more complex than orientation phase. Past experiences of both the patient and the nurse will influence their expectations during this interpersonal process. While working through this phase, the patient begins to have feeling of belongingness and a capacity for dealing with the problem. These positive changes begin to decrease feeling of helplessness and hopelessness and ensue strength. In this phase, patient is prepared to move to the next phase, i.e., exploitation.

Exploitation

During exploitation phase, the patient attempts to derive full value from what is offered to him through the relationship. New goals to be achieved through personal efforts and power shifts from the nurse to the patient.

In exploitation, the nurses use communication tools, such as clarifying, listening, accepting, teaching and interpreting

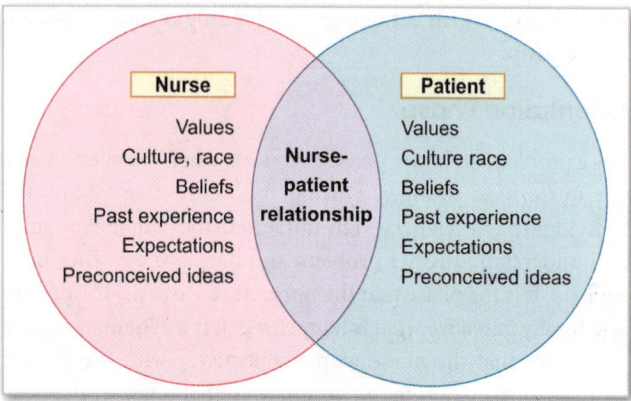

Fig. 3: Identification phase

to offer services to the patient. In the exploitation phase, the patient uses all available services, based on personal interests and needs. The nurse assists the patient in using these services maintaining a therapeutic relationship at all the times. Throughout this phase, the patient works collaboratively with the nurse to meet challenges and work towards maximum health. As the patient develops some of the control in the situation, the patient may become less demanding of the nurse. Thus, in this phase, the nurse aids the patient in using services to help to solve problems. Progress is made towards final step, i.e., the resolution phase.

Resolution

During the resolution phase, after the patient's needs have been met by the collaborative efforts of the nurse and the patient, the therapeutic relationship ends. Resolution is achieved when the patient drifts away from identifying with the nurse and dissolves the nurse-patient bond. Successful resolution results directly from successful completion of the other phases. The patient moves towards new goal during this phase. But dependency needs in a therapeutic relationship often continue psychologically after the physiological needs have been met.

During this phase, patient becomes independent from the nurse as the nurse becomes independent from the patient. Resolution occurs only with the successful completion of the previous phases.

Role of Nurses Based on Peplau's Theory

Peplau describes six different nursing roles that emerge in the various phases of the nurse-patient relationship. They are:
- **Role as a stranger:** Peplau states that because the nurse and the patients are stranger to each other, the patient should be treated with ordinary courtesy. In the initial phase of orientation as they meet as two strangers, the nurse should not prejudge the patient but accept him or her as he/she is.
- **Role as a resource person:** In the role of the resource person, the nurse provides specific answers to questions, especially health information and interprets to the patient the treatment or medical plan of care.
- **Teaching role:** The teaching role is a combination of all roles and always proceeds from what the patient knows and develops around his interest in wanting and ability to use information.
- **Leadership role:** The leadership role involves the democratic process. The nurse helps the patient to meet the task at hand through a relationship of cooperation and active participation.
- **Surrogate role:** Surrogate is one who takes place of another. The patient casts nurse in the surrogate role.

The nurses' function is to assist the patient in recognizing similarities between herself and the person recalled by the patient. She then helps the patient to see the difference in her role and that of the recalled person.

- **Counseling role:** Counseling function is the nurse-patient relationship by the way nurse respond to the patient's demand.

Additional Roles of Nurse

- Teaching experts
- Consultant
- Health teacher
- Tutor
- Socializing agent
- Safety agent
- Manager of environment
- Mediators
- Administrator
- Recorder and observer

Interpersonal Theory and Nursing Process

Peplau's theory of interpersonal relationship can be compared to the nursing process. The nursing process is a deliberate intellectual activity whereby the practice of nursing is approached in an orderly systemic manner.

- Both Peplau's phase and the nursing process are sequential and focus on therapeutic interaction.
- Both stress that the nurse and the patient should use problem solving techniques collaboratively with the end purpose of meeting the patient's need.
- Both emphasize and assist the patient to define general complaints more specifically so that the specific patient's needs can be identified.
- Both use observation, communication and recording as basic tool for nursing practice.

Assessment

Peplau's orientation phase parallels the beginning of assessment phase. In that, both the nurse and the patient come together as strangers. The meeting is initiated by the patient, he/she expresses problems and make the nurse understand. Conjointly, the nurse and patient begin to work through recognizing, Changing and gathering facts are important to this need. Orientation and assessment are not synonymous and must not be confused.

Nursing Diagnosis

The nursing diagnosis identifies the health problem or defects. The nursing diagnosis is a summary of statement of the data collected and analyzed. During the period of orientation, the patient clarifies his first, whole impression of his problem. However, in nursing process, the nurse's judgments form the diagnosis from the data collected.

Planning

In the planning phase, the nurse must specifically formulate how the patient is going to achieve mutually set goals. Planning is still being considered to be within the Peplau's identification phase as the patient responds to people who can meet his or her personal needs.

Implementation

As in Peplau's exploitation phase in implementation phase, the patient is finally reaping benefit from the therapeutic relationship by drawing on the nurse's knowledge and expertise. In both the phases, the individualized plans have already been found, based on patient's interests and needs.

Evaluation

Once needs have been met; resolution and termination are the end result.

Orem's Self-care Deficit Theory

Dorothea Orem's general theory of nursing evolved over a period of four decades from individual work and through collaboration with students, practitioners, researchers, educators, administrators and scholars. She began her work by looking for the uniqueness of nursing. Orem described her work as a general theory of nursing comprising three "articulating" or interrelated theories; **Theory of Self-Care, Theory of Self-Care Deficit** and **Theory of Nursing Systems**. The specific name for Orem's general theory of nursing however is **Self-Care Deficit Theory of Nursing**. She chose the name 'deficit' as it describes and explains a relationship between abilities of individuals to care for themselves and the self-care needs or demands of the individual, their children or the adults for whom they care. The notion of 'deficit' does not refer to a specific type of limitation, but to the relationship between the capabilities of the individual and the need for action.

We need to understand the meaning of some of these forms before describing the details of the theory.

Self-care

Self-care refers to the practice of "activities that individuals initiate and perform on their own behalf in maintaining life, health and well-being" (Orem, 1985, p.84).

Self-care Agency

This refers to the "ability for engaging in self-care" by the client.

Self-care Requisite

Self-care requisites or requirements can be classified as universal (associated with life process, such as air, water), developmental (e.g., adjusting to body changes, adjusting to loss of significant other), and health deviation (e.g., conditions due to illness, injury or disease) (Orem, 1985, p.90-91).

Therapeutic Self-care Demand

Therapeutic self-care demand refers to "totality of self-care actions to be performed to meet the self-care requisites by using valid methods and related actions" (Orem, 1985, p.88).

Self-care Deficit

Self-care deficit is determined by the differences between self-care needs and self-care capabilities, that is when the needs are more than the abilities of the patient to perform self-care activities.

Nursing System Action

Nursing is required when there is self-care deficit, that is, the care abilities are less than those required for meeting the self-care demand (Orem, 1985, p.35). Orem has described three systems; these are (Fig. 4):

1. **Wholly compensatory system:** For example, when individual is unable to perform any form of deliberate action, such as in coma.

2. **Partially compensatory system:** For example, when both nurse and patient perform care because of patient's self-care limitations as in the second postoperative day after surgery.

3. **Supportive-educative system:** For example, when the client is able to perform or can learn to perform required measures for therapeutic self-care as an antenatal mother, requiring information on nutritious diet.

Orem's Conceptual Framework

Orem identified six major concepts in the self-care deficit theory of nursing. **They are self-care, therapeutic self-care demand, self-care agency, self-care deficit, nursing agency and nursing system.** She used these six concepts to express the three constituent theories of the general theory of nursing.

The concept of self-care, self-care agency, therapeutic self-care demand and self-care deficit are related to the patient or the person in need of nursing while the concepts of nursing agency and nursing system are related to the nursing and their actions. Refer Figure 5 to examine the relationship between these concepts ® denotes relationship and the sign < indicates deficit relationship.

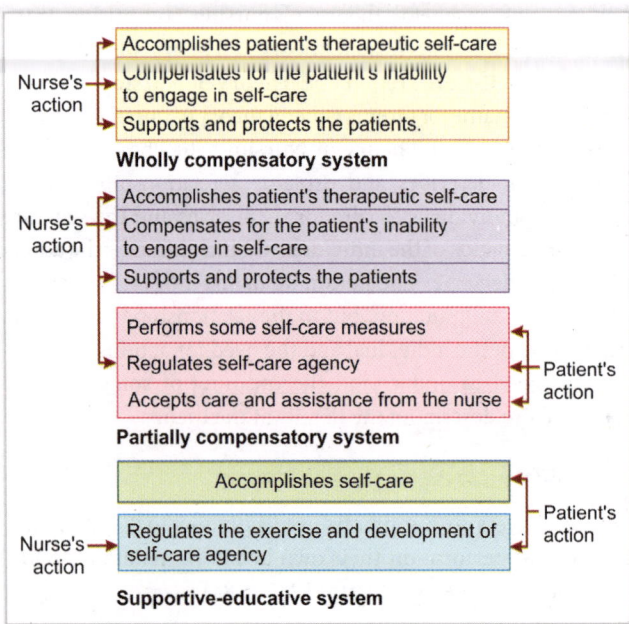

Fig. 4: Basic nursing system

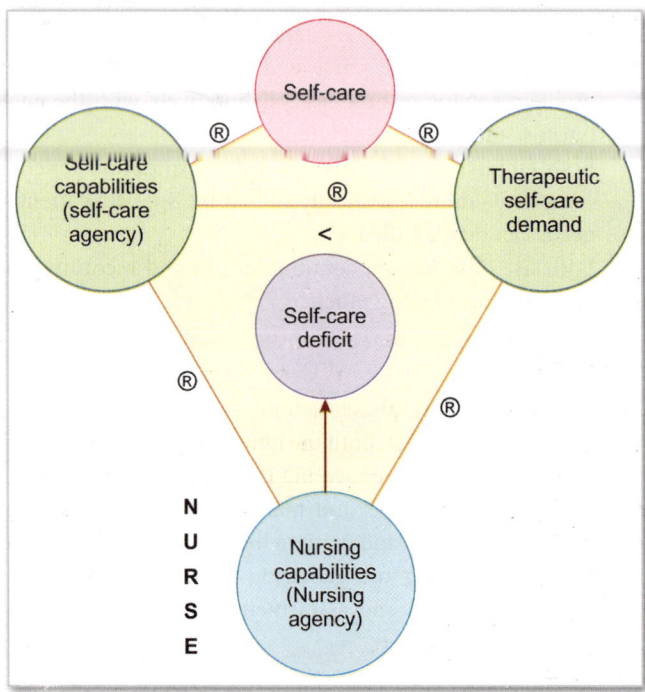

Fig. 5: Conceptual framework for nursing relationship < deficit relationship, current or projected

BIBLIOGRAPHY

1. Paker M. Nursing Theories and Nursing Practice, 2nd edition. Jaypee Brother Medical Publishers, 2007. pp. 51-60.

2. George JB. Nursing Theories: The Base for Professional Nursing Practice, 6th edition. Pearson, 2011, pp. 291-323, 338-65, 114-33.

3. McEven, Melanie, Wills, et al. Theoretical Basis for Nursing, 1st Edition. Lippincott Williams & Wilkins, 2002, pp. 125-144, 182-192.

4. Leahy JM, Kizilay PE. Foundations of Nursing Practice: A Nursing Process Approach, 1st edition. W.B. Sounders Company, 1998, pp. 21-37.

5. Becker MH, Maiman LA. Sociobehavioral determinants of compliance with health and medical care recommendations. Med Care. 1975;13(1):10-24.

6. Pender NJ: Health promotion and nursing practice, Norwalk conn, Appleton century-crofts. 1982.

7. Rosenstock IM. Historical Origins of the Health Belief Model. Health Education Monograph. Sage Journal. 1974;2:334.

8. Roy C. The Roy Adaptation Model and Research, Nurses. 2009;21:209.

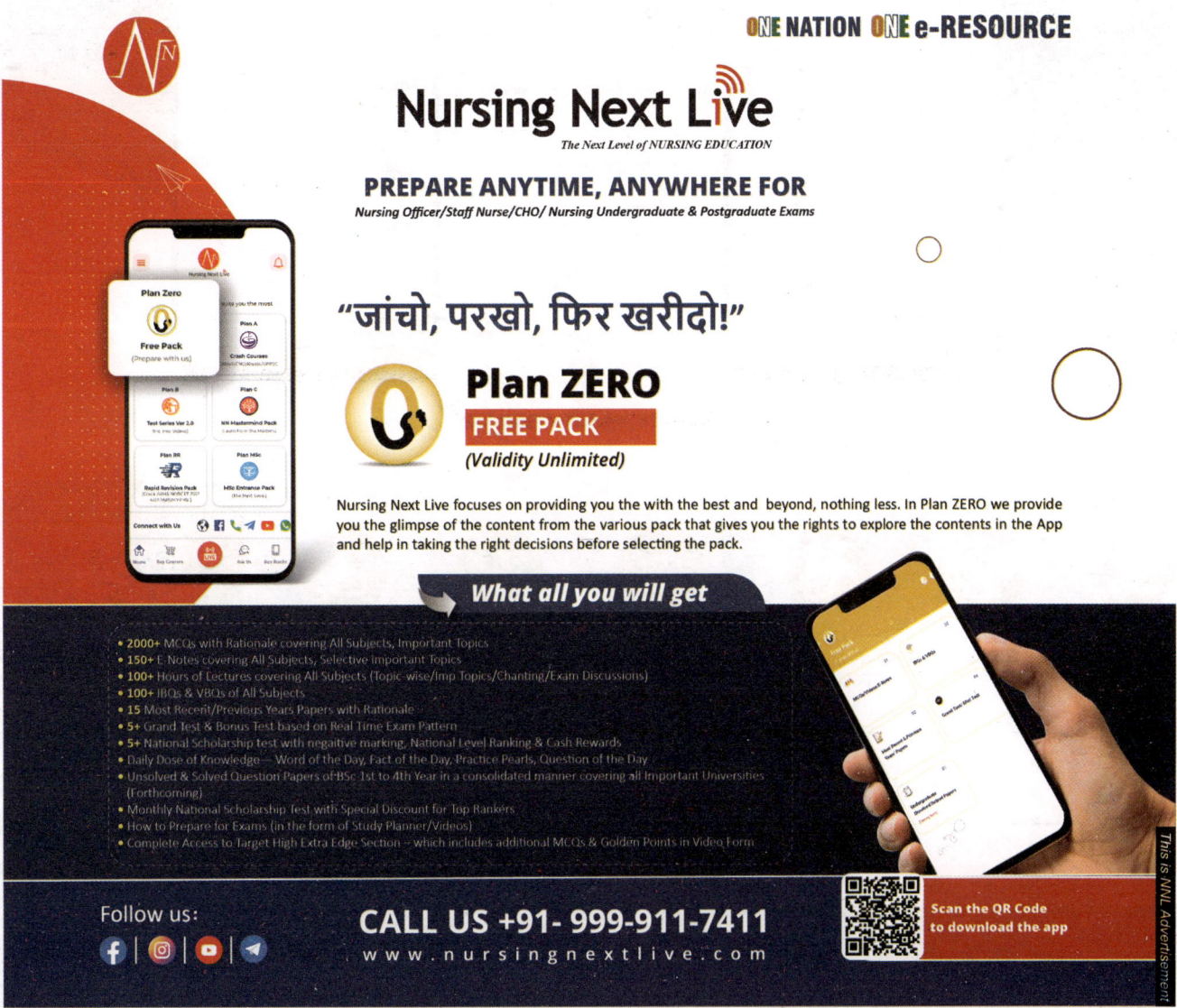

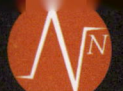
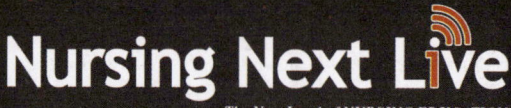
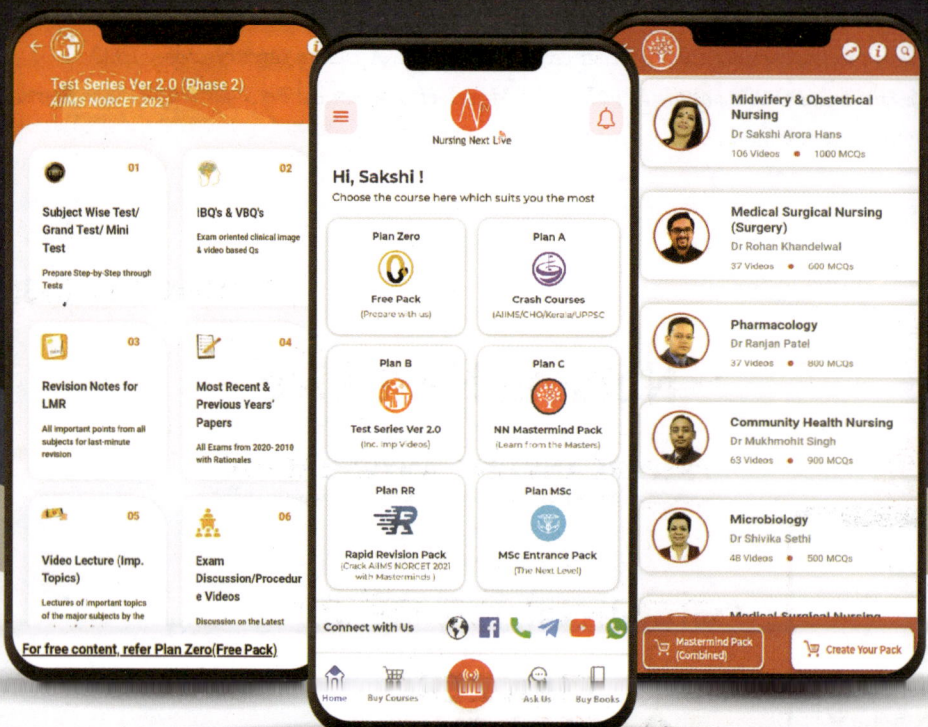

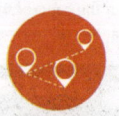

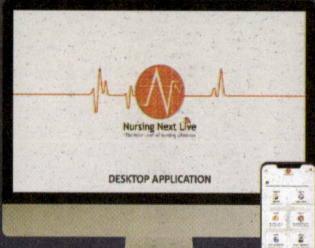
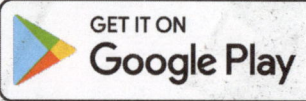
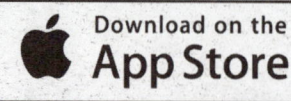

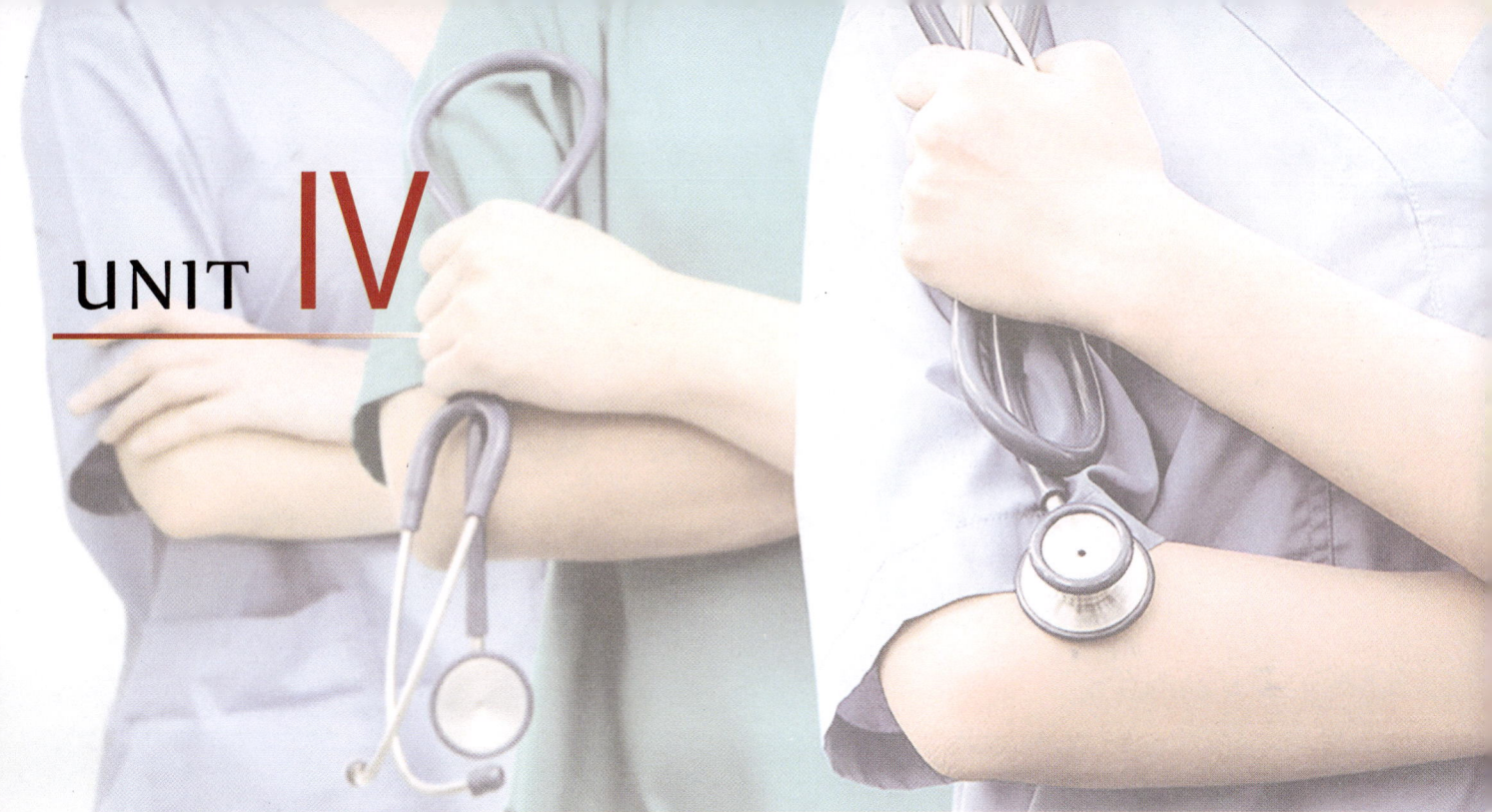

UNIT IV

COMMUNICATION AND NURSE PATIENT RELATIONSHIP

Unit Outline

Communication

INTRODUCTION

Communication is a critical skill for nursing. It is the process by which humans meet their survival needs, build relationships, and experience emotions. In nursing, communication is a dynamic process used to gather assessment data, to teach and persuade, and to express care and comfort. It is an integral part of the helping relationship.

Communication is the process of exchanging information, and generating and transmitting meanings between two or more individuals.

LEVELS OF COMMUNICATION

Throughout our lives and the lives of our patients, communication occurs at various levels. There are four levels of communication in which nurses engage during practice:

- Intrapersonal communication
- Interpersonal communication
- Small-group communication
- Organizational communication

Intrapersonal Communication

It is the communication that happens within the individual or self-talk. It affects the nurse's behavior and has the ability to enhance or downgrade from positive interactions with the patient and family.

Interpersonal Communication

It occurs between two or more people with a goal to exchange messages. The ability to communicate effectively at this level influences sharing, problem solving, goal attainment, team building and effectiveness in critical nursing roles, e.g., roles as a caregiver, teacher, counselor, leader, manager and patient advocate.

Small-Group Communication

It occurs when nurses interact with two or more individuals. It is used in small staff meeting, patient care conferences, teaching sessions or support groups.

Organizational Communication

It occurs when individuals and groups within an organization communicate to achieve established goals, e.g., quality assurance, strategic planning, etc. To determine the effectiveness or ineffectiveness of a group, one studies the group dynamics.

Group dynamics can be described most simply as how individual group members relate to one another during the process of working toward common group goal.

ELEMENTS OF COMMUNICATION/ COMMUNICATION PROCESS

Communication is the process by which information is exchanged between the sender and the receiver.

David K Berlo (1960) gave a classic description of the communication process, which involves a source (encoder), message, channel and receiver (decoder) (Fig. 1).

Source (Encoder, Sender)

The sender is a person or group who wishes to convey a message to another and can be considered the source encoder. Encoding involves the selection of specific signs or symbols (codes) to transmit the message, such as which language and words to use, how to arrange the words, and what tone of voice and gestures to use.

Message

The second component of the communication process is the message itself, which is actually said or written, the body language that accompanies the words, and how the message is transmitted. It might be a speech, interview conversation, chart, gesture, memorandum, or nursing note.

Channel

The medium used to convey the message is the channel. It is important for the channel to be appropriate for the message. The channel might target any of the receiver's senses. The message can be sent to the receiver through the following channels:

- Auditory-spoken words and cues
- Visual sight, observations and perception
- Kinesthetic touch

    Nurses use all three of these channels to communicate with patients.

Receiver (Decoder)

The receiver is the listener, who must listen, observe and attend. The person is the decoder, who must perceive what the sender intended (interpretation). Whether the message is decoded accurately by the receiver, according to the sender's intent, depends largely on their similarities in knowledge and experience. If the meaning of the decoded message matches the intent of the sender, then the communication has been effective. Ineffective communication occurs when the message sent is misinterpreted by the receiver.

Response

It is the message that the receiver returns to the sender. It is also called **feedback** It can be either verbal, nonverbal or both.

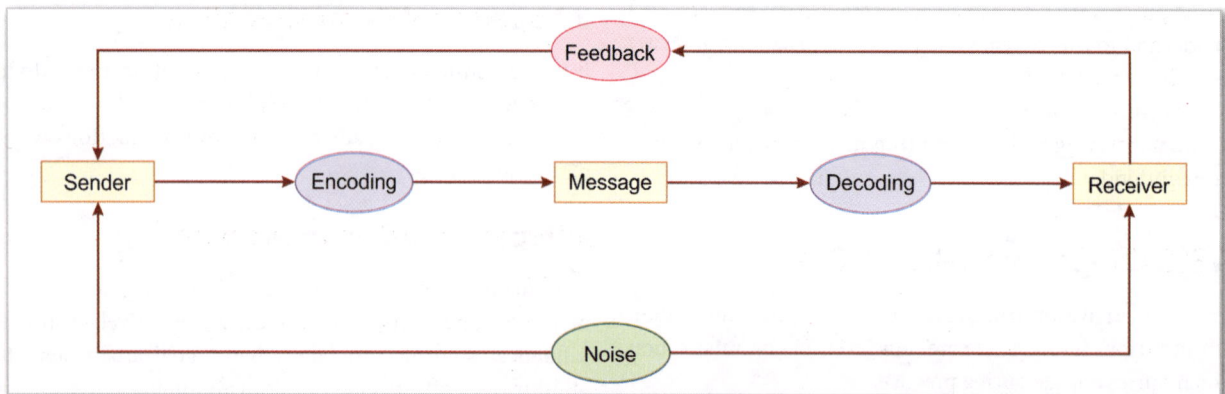

Fig. 1: Communication process

MODES/TYPES OF COMMUNICATION

Communication is generally carried out in two different modes; **verbal** and **nonverbal**.

Verbal communication uses the spoken or written words.

Nonverbal communication uses other forms, such as gestures or facial expressions and touch. Another form of communication has evolved with technology, i.e., **electronic communication**. The most common form of electronic communication is e-mail where an individual can send a message, by computer, to another person or group of people.

Verbal Communication

Verbal communication is an exchange of information using words, including both spoken and written words. Verbal communication depends on language or a prescribed way of using words so that people can share information effectively. The words used vary among individuals according to culture; socio-economic background, age and education.

Criteria for Effective Verbal Communication

- **Pace and intonation:** The manner of speech, the pace or rhythm and intonation, modify the feeling and impact of the message. The pace of speech may indicate interest, anxiety or fear, e.g., speaking slowly and softly to an excited client may help calm the patient. The intonation can express enthusiasm sadness, anger and amusement.
- **Simplicity:** It includes the use of commonly understood words. Nurses need to learn to select appropriate, understandable terms based on the knowledge, culture and education of the client.
- **Clarity and brevity:** Clarity is saying precisely what is meant, and brevity is using the fewest words necessary. One needs to speak slowly and should avoid ambiguity.
- **Timing and relevance:** Nurses need to be aware of both relevance and timing while communicating with clients. They need to be sensitive to the client's needs and concerns.
- **Adaptability:** Spoken messages need to be altered in accordance to behavioral cues from the client.
- **Credibility:** It means worthiness of belief, trustworthiness, and reliability. This is one of the most important criterion of effective communication. Nurses foster credibility by being consistent, dependable, and honest.
- **Humor:** The use of humor can be a positive and powerful tool in the nurse-client relationship, but it must be used with care. It can be used to help clients adjust to different and painful situations.

Nonverbal Communication

The transmission of information without the use of words is termed nonverbal communication, also known as body language. It is generally accepted that nonverbal communication expresses more of the true meaning of a message than verbal communication. Therefore, nurse must be aware of both the nonverbal messages she sends and the nonverbal messages she receives from patients. Nurses working with patients from diverse cultural background should attempt to understand cultural variations to avoid misunderstanding nonverbal communication. The various forms of nonverbal communication are:

- **Touch:** It is viewed as one of the most effective nonverbal way to express feelings of comfort, love, affection, security, anger, frustration, aggression, excitement, etc. Touch is a personal behavior and means different things to different people. Factors such as age, sex, familial, regional, class and cultural influences play a key role in meanings associated with touch.
- **Eye contact:** Communication often begins with eye contact. In many cultures, eye contact suggests respect and a willingness to listen. In some cultures, people are taught to avoid eye contact, out of respect, not to make eye contact with a superior. Eyes carry many nonverbal messages such as eyes fix in a stare during anger, tend to narrow in disgust and wide open in fear. A blank state may indicate inattentiveness.
- **Facial expression:** Face is the most expressive part of the body, e.g., various messages conveyed by facial expressions are anger, joy, suspicion, sadness, fear, and contempt. Some people have extremely expressive faces, whereas others mask their feelings, making it more difficult to determine what the person is really thinking. Nurses need to learn to control their own facial expressions while caring for their clients.
- **Posture and gait:** The way people walk and carry themselves are often reliable indicators of self-concept, current mood, and health. Erect posture and an active, purposeful stride suggest a feeling of well-being. Slouched posture and a slow, shuffling gait suggests depression or physical discomfort. Tense posture and a rapid, determined gait suggests anxiety or anger. The posture of people when they are sitting or lying can also indicate feelings or mood.
- **Gestures:** Gestures using various body parts can carry numerous messages, e.g., thumbs up means victory, kicking an object often expresses anger, wringing the hands or tapping a foot indicates anxiety or anger, and a

waving hand serves to convey someone to come on, or if waved in another way, signify that someone should leave.

- **General physical appearance:** Observing for changes in appearance is an important nursing responsibility for detecting illness or evaluating the effectiveness of care and therapy, e.g., a person with insufficient intake of fluids has dry skin that wrinkles easily, sunken eyes, is dull in appearance and has poor muscle tone.
- **Mode of dress and grooming:** A person's clothing and grooming practices carry significant nonverbal messages, e.g., healthy people who have high self-esteem tend to pay attention to details of dress and grooming, whereas those with low self-esteem often show much less interest to them. People feeling ill often demonstrate little interest in personal appearance and it is often a sign of returning health when interest in their physical appearance and mode of dress returns.

- **Sounds:** Crying, moaning, gasping and sighing are oral but a part of nonverbal forms of communication, e.g., a person might cry because of sadness or joy. Gasping indicates fear, pain or surprise.

Electronic Communication

E-mail is the most common form of electronic communication used in health care facilities for many purposes like schedule and confirms appointments, report normal lab results, conduct client education and follow- up with discharged clients. Many health care agencies are moving toward electronic medical records where nurses document their assessments and nursing care.

BIBLIOGRAPHY

1. Berlo KD. *The Process of Communication: An Introduction to Theory and Practice. Holt: Rinehart and Winston; New York, 1960.*

2. Berman AT, Snyder S, Kozier BJ, et al. Kozier & Erb's. *Fundamentals of Nursing: Concepts, Process and Practice, 8th edition. Pearson Education.*

3. Sharma S. Potter and Perry's *Fundamentals of Nursing. A South Asian edition. Elsevier India. Gurugram: 2013.*

4. Taylor CR, Lillis C, LeMone P, et al. *Fundamentals of Nursing – The Art and Science of Nursing Care, 7th edition. Wolters Kluwer; 2010.*

Factors and Barriers Influencing Communication

FACTORS INFLUENCING COMMUNICATION

Development Level

Knowledge of a client's developmental stage allows the nurse to modify the message accordingly, e.g., a child of 8 years can be explained a procedure in simple language, whereas adolescents who have developed more abstract thinking skills, a more detailed explanation can be given. With aging, there are changes in vision and hearing that may affect nurse-client interactions.

Gender

It is necessary to be sensitive to the fact that men and women might communicate differently, as they possess different communication styles. They might give different interpretations as well to the same conversation.

Values and Perceptions

Values are the standards that influence behavior, and perception is the personal view of an event. As each person has unique personality traits, values, and life experiences, each will perceive and interpret messages and experiences differently.

Personal Space

It is the distance or personal space that people prefer in interactions with others.

- **Intimate distance (1½ feet):** This is an important area to an individual, only those who are emotionally close to the individual are allowed to enter this zone, e.g., spouse, parents, children and close friends. A nurse enters this zone only during certain lines, e.g., cuddling a baby, positioning clients, observing an incision, restraining a toddler for an injection, etc.

- **Personal distance (1½ to 4 feet):** Distance kept in gatherings and social functions, e.g., nurse maintain a distance while taking temperature or giving medications.
- **Social distance (4 to 12 feet):** Individuals keep this distance with strangers. Communication is formal and limited to seeing and hearing, e.g., nursing rounds.
- **Public distance (12 to 15 feet):** This distance is maintained when dealing with large group, e.g., giving health education to group.

Territoriality

It is a concept of the space and things that an individual considers as belonging to self. For a patient, this would be the bed, bed-side locker, bed-side table and chair. Nurses and others need to take permission from clients to enter, remove, rearrange, or borrow objects in their territory.

Roles and Relationship

These roles and the relationships between the sender and receiver affect the communication process. Roles such as nursing student and instructor, client and primary care provider, or parent and child affect the content and responses in the communication process.

Environment

People usually communicate most effectively in a comfortable environment. Extremes of temperature, noise and a poorly ventilated room can all interfere with communication. Lack of privacy, environment distraction can also impair communication.

Interpersonal Attitudes

Attitudes convey beliefs, thoughts and feelings about people and events. Caring and worth convey a feeling of emotional closeness. Respect is an attitude that emphasizes the other person's worth and individuality. It conveys that the person's hopes and feelings are special and unique even though similar to others in many ways.

Acceptance emphasizes neither approval nor disapproval. The nurse receives willingly the honest feelings of a client. An accepting attitude allows clients to express personal feelings freely and nurse needs to restrict acceptance in situations where client's behaviors are harmful to themselves and others.

METHODS OF EFFECTIVE COMMUNICATION

Therapeutic Communication

It is client-and goal-directed communication. It promotes understanding and can help establish a constructive relationship between the nurse and the client. Nurses need to respond not only to the content of the client's verbal message but also to the feelings expressed. It is important to understand how the client views the situation and feels about it before responding.

At times, clients need time to deal with their feelings. Strong emotions are often draining. People usually need to deal with the feelings before they can cope with other matters, such as learning new skills or planning for the future.

Attentive Listening

It is listening actively, using all the senses. It is the most important technique in nursing and is basis to all other techniques. Attentive listening is an active process that requires energy and concentration. It involves paying attention to the total message, both verbal and nonverbal, and noting whether these communications are congruent. Attentive listening means absorbing both the content and the feeling a person is conveying without selectivity. The listener does not select or listen solely to what the listener wants to hear; the nurse focuses not on her own needs but rather on client's needs. Attentive listening conveys an attitude of caring and interest, thereby encouraging the client to talk.

It also involves listening for key themes in the communication. The nurse must be careful not to react quickly to the message. The speaker should not be interrupted and the nurse should take time to think about the message before responding. As a listener, the nurse should also ask questions either to obtain additional information or to clarify. Attentive listening is highly developed skill, which can be learned with practice. A nurse can convey attentiveness in listening to clients in many ways. Common responses are nodding the head, uttering "uhhuh" or repeating the words that the client has used, or saying "I can understand what you mean".

Physical Attending Skills

Egan outlined five specific ways to convey physical attending which he defines as the manner of being present to another or being with another. Listening in his frame of reference, is what a person does while attending. The five actions of physical attending, which convey a "posture of involvement are".

- Face the other person
- Adopt an open posture: in which neither arms nor legs are crossed
- Lean toward the person
- Maintain good eye contact
- Try to be relatively relaxed.

These five attending postures need to be adapted to the specific needs of clients in a given situation.

Rapport Building Skills

Rapport, a feeling of mutual trust experienced by people in a satisfactory relationship, facilitates open communication. Good rapport can be achieved by paying attention to the following:

- **Specific objectives:** Having a purpose for an interaction provides guidance toward achieving a meaningful encounter with the patient.
- **Comfortable environment:** In which both the patient and the nurse are at ease; helps to promote interactions. Suitable furniture, proper lighting and temperature are important.
- **Privacy:** Every effort should be made to provide privacy and to patient conversations from being overheard by others.
- **Confidentiality:** Patient needs to be informed about the information to be shared with whom. The patient's right to privacy needs to be considered.
- **Using nursing observations:** It is the primary source of information and it helps in increasing awareness of patient's nonverbal messages.
- **Optimal pacing:** Let the patient know at the beginning of the interaction if time is limited so that he/she does not feel that you are rushing.
- **Respecting personal space:** It is important to be sensitive to personal space so that patients feel comfortable during interactions.

Empathy Skills

Empathy is identifying with the way another person feels. An empathetic nurse is sensitive to the patient's feelings and problems, but remains objective enough to help the patient attain positive outcomes, e.g., it is helpful to empathize with the family who might be feeling frightened and helpless. "This must be hard time for you … how are you coping?" "Is there any way I can be of help"? When the patient and family sense that you have some idea of what they are experiencing and are committed to helping, the basis is set for a trusting therapeutic relationship.

Interviewing Skills

The purpose of the interview is to obtain accurate and thorough information. In nursing, the interview is a major tool for collecting data during the assessment step of the nursing process. All interviews should begin with an explanation of the purpose of the interview. While interviewing, following techniques are useful:

- **Use of open-ended question:** This allows the patient a wide range of possible responses. It encourages free verbalization. The greatest advantage of this technique is that it prevents the patient from answering with a simple yes or no.
- **Use of closed questions:** It provides the receiver with limited choices of possible responses and might often be answered by one or two words, "yes or no". Closed questions are used to gather specific information from a patient. Closed questions are often a barrier to communication.
- **Validating questions:** This serves to validate what the nurse believes is heard or observed. Overusing validating questions might lead the patient to think that the nurse is not listening.
- **Clarifying questions:** It allows the nurse to gain an understanding of a patient's comment. Overuse of clarifying questions can lead the patient to believe that the nurse is not listening or lacks appropriate knowledge.
- **Reflective questions:** It involves repeating what the person has said or describing person's feelings. It encourages the patient to elaborate on his or her thoughts and feelings.
- **Sequencing questions:** It is used to place events in a chronological order or to investigate a possible cause-effect relationship between events.
- **Summarizing:** Summarizing what has occurred during the interaction is helpful. A summary of alternative solutions to a problem, decisions made, plan for action, or feelings that have been expressed provide closure to the interaction.
- **Assertiveness skill:** While interacting with patients, family members, other health team members, it is important to communicate in a way that demonstrates respect for all parties. Assertive behaviors, which are the hallmark of professional nursing relationships, need to be distinguished from aggressive (harsh, injurious or destructive) behaviors. The key to assertiveness is open, honest and direct communication. The assertive nurse's attitude toward work is characterized by working to capacity with or without supervision, the ability to remain calm under supervision, the freedom to ask for help when needed, the ability to give and accept compliments and honesty in admitting mistakes and taking responsibility for them.

BARRIERS TO EFFECTIVE COMMUNICATION

Nurses need to recognize barriers or non-therapeutic responses to effective communication (Fig. 1).

- **Failure to perceive the patient as a human being:** It is important to focus on whole patient rather than the diagnosis. Patient's report that nothing is more discomforting than to be treated as merely an object of care rather than a patient. It is also of primary importance that the patient is addressed by a formal name.

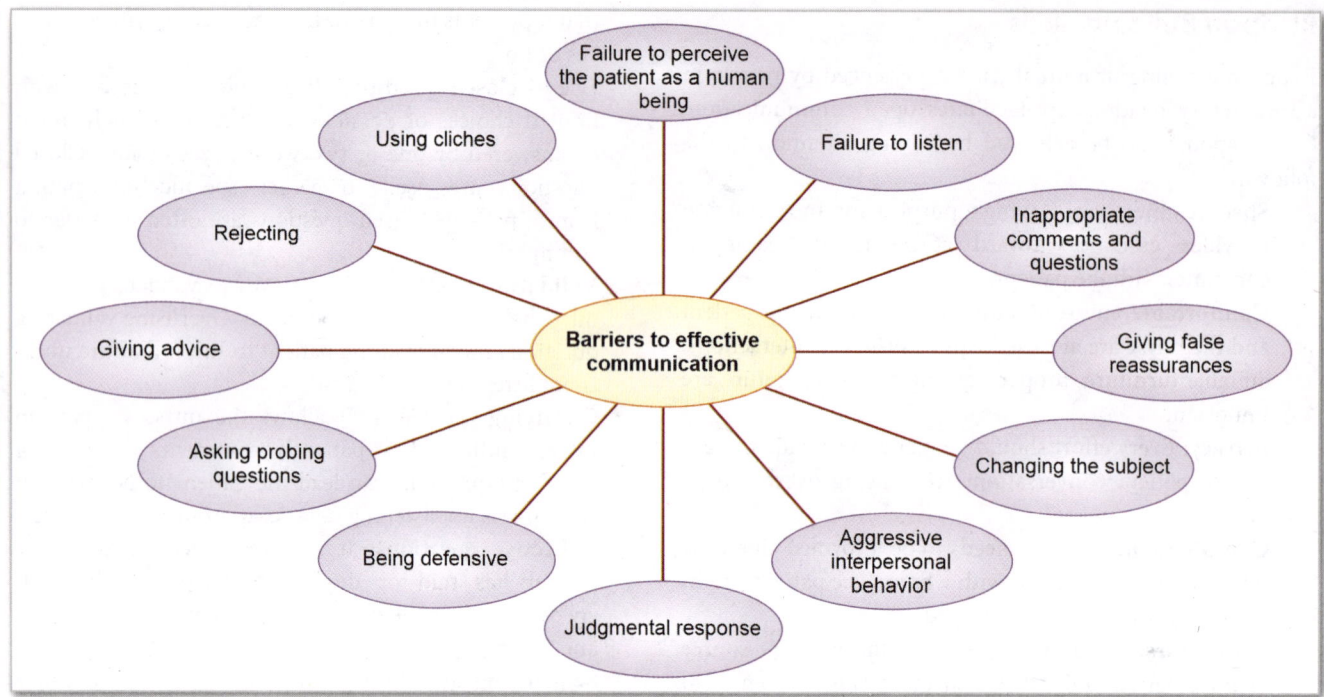

Fig. 1: Barriers to effective communication

- **Failure to listen:** Turning your back when the patient is sharing feelings or pertinent information; showing impatience with body language, i.e., tapping your foot or having your hand on the door to go out; all these indicate that the patient is not important, that the nurse is bored, or that what is being said does not matter. Interrupting or jumping in before the patient has finished speaking also indicates inattentive listening.
- **Inappropriate comments and questions:** Certain types of comments and questions should be avoided in most situations because they tend to impede effective communication.
- **Giving false reassurances:** Giving false hope can destroy trust in the nurse.
- **Changing the subject:** Deprives the patient of the chance to verbalize concerns.
- **Judgmental response:** Giving opinions and approving or disapproving responses or implying one's own values. These responses imply that the client must think as the nurse thinks.
- **Being defensive:** Attempting to protect a person or health care services from negative comments. These responses prevent the client from expressing true concerns. Nurse says "you have no right to blame". Defensive responses protect the nurse from admitting weaknesses in the health care services.
- **Asking probing questions:** Asking for information mainly out of curiosity rather than with the intent to

assist the client. These responses, violate the client's privacy. Asking 'why' is often probing.
- **Giving advice:** Tends to control and diminish patient's responsibility for taking charge of their own health.
- **Rejecting:** Refusing to discuss certain topics with the client. These responses often make clients feel that the nurse is rejecting not only their communication but also the client themselves.
- **Using clichés:** A cliché is an overused expression that may have no real relation to the current situation. Comments such as "you will be fine" "Don't worry, everything will be alright" are clichés. They show a lack of respect for the patient as an individual.
- **Aggressive interpersonal behavior:** Adverse events occur when communication between health care professionals is ineffective, abusive, or negative. Aggressive interpersonal behavior compromises patient's safety, influences satisfaction with care, and contributes to medical errors.

HELPING RELATIONSHIPS

Helping relationship is referred by some as nurse-client relationship or interpersonal relationship. A helping relationship may develop over weeks of working with a client or within minutes. The key to the helping relationship are:
- The development of trust and acceptance between the nurse and the client.

♦ An underlying belief that the nurse cares, and wants to help the client.

Helping relationship is influenced by the personal and professional characteristics of the nurse and the client. Age, sex, appearance, diagnosis, education, values, ethnic and cultural background, personality, expectations, and setting can all affect the development of nurse-client relationship.

Goals of Helping Relationship

♦ Helping relationship is an intellectual and emotional bond between the nurse and the client and is focused on the client.
♦ Respects the client as an individual by:
  ▪ Maximizing the client's abilities to participate in decision making and treatments.
  ▪ Considering ethnic and cultural aspects.
  ▪ Considering family relationships and values.
♦ Respects client's confidentiality.
♦ Focuses on the client's well-being.
♦ Is based on mutual trust, respect and acceptance.

Phases of the Helping Relationship

There are four sequential phases, each phase is characterized by identifiable tasks and skills. The relationship must progress through the phases in succession because each builds on the previous one.

Pre-interaction Phase

This is similar to the planning stage before an interview. In most situations, the nurse has information about the client before the first, face-to-face meeting. The information may include, clients name, age, sex, address, medical history and social history.

Introductory Phase

This phase is also known as the orientation phase or the pre-helping phase, is important because it sets the tone for the rest of the relationship. The three stages of introductory phase are:
1. Opening the relationship.
2. Clarifying the problem.
3. **Structuring and formulating the contract:** In this stage, the nurse and client develop a degree of trust and verbally agree about location, frequency and length of meetings, overall purpose of the relationship, how confidential material will be handled, tasks to be accomplished, duration, and indications for termination of the relationship. The client may develop resistive behaviors which can be overcome by conveying a caring attitude, genuine interest in the client and competence.

Working Phase

During this phase, the nurse and the client begin to view each other as unique individuals. It has two major stages:
1. Exploring and understanding thoughts and feelings.
2. Facilitating and taking action.

For this phase, nurse requires empathetic listening and responding skills, respect, genuineness, concreteness and confrontation skills so that client is willing to pursue self-exploration; the outcome is a beginning to understand on the part of the client behavior.

Termination Phase

This phase is often difficult and filled with ambivalence. Nurse and client accept feelings of loss. The client accepts the end of the relationship without feelings of anxiety and dependence. In some situation, referrals are necessary. Therefore, either meeting or phone call or e-mail are other interventions that ease the client's transition to independence.

BIBLIOGRAPHY

1. *Berlo KD. The Process of Communication: An Introduction to Theory and Practice. Holt: Rinehart and Winston; New York, 1960.*
2. *Berman AT, Snyder S, Kozier BJ, et al. Kozier & Erb's. Fundamentals of Nursing: Concepts, Process and Practice, 8th edition. Pearson Education.*
3. *Sharma S. Potter and Perry's Fundamentals of Nursing. A South Asian edition. Elsevier India. Gurugram, 2013.*
4. *Taylor CR, Lillis C, LeMone P, et al. Fundamentals of Nursing – The Art and Science of Nursing Care, 7th edition. Wolters Kluwer; 2010.*

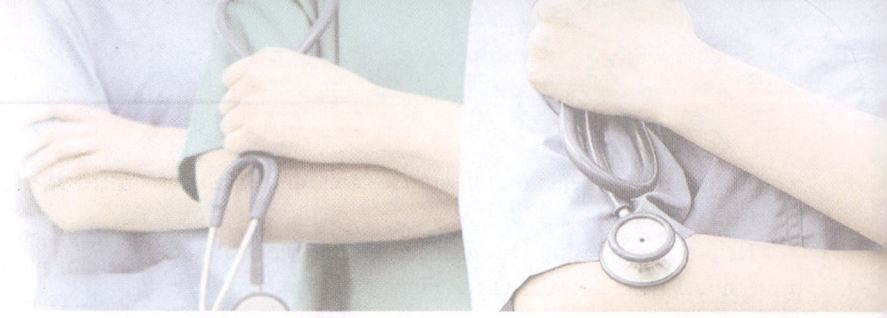

Patient Teaching

INTRODUCTION

Patient education is the process of influencing the patient's behavior to effect changes in knowledge, attitudes and skills needed to maintain health.

PURPOSE OF PATIENT TEACHING

Teaching is done to:

* Assist in prevention of illness or promotion of wellness.
* Care for self at home before discharge.
* Help develop self-care abilities they need.
* Maximize their functioning and quality of life.
* Hasten recovery from trauma or illness with minimal or no complications.
* Enhance ability to adjust to developmental lifestyle changes.
* Acceptance of the lifestyle changes necessitated by illness or disability.

PRINCIPLES OF PATIENT TEACHING

Patients are now expected to learn enough about their own health to be able to participate in health care decisions. Thus, the goal of patient teaching has changed from telling the patient the best actions to take, to now assisting patients in learning about their health care to improve their own health. This newer view of health education is not an easy concept for many patients in our care to grasp and require more intense communication between patients and providers of care.

* To increase knowledge and clarify misconceptions about medical condition.
* Implement new behaviors to adapt to medical conditions and physical limitations.
* Learn strategies to cope up with psychosocial responses to disease and disability.
* Overcome barriers to compliance by articulating.
* To master behavioral changes required to implement and continue with a treatment plan.

ROLES OF NURSE AND INTEGRATING TEACHING IN NURSING PROCESS

Assess Learning Needs and Readiness to Learn

- Use all appropriate sources of information.
- Identify knowledge attitudes, or skills needed by the patient and family member.
- Assess the patient's emotional and experiential readiness to learn.
- Assess factors affecting the patient's ability to learn including age and developmental level, family support network, financial resources, cultural influences, literacy and language barriers, physical problems such as poor hearing, poor vision, literacy, impaired motor function or cognition.
- Identify the patient's strengths.
- Place the identified learning needs on the patient's plan of care.
- Assess the patient's readiness to learn, e.g., motivation, desire to learn, desire to return to independence or to return to comfort of home.

Diagnose the Patient's Learning Needs

- Utilize nursing diagnoses for learning needs, e.g., knowledge deficit related to diet, care, etc.
- Be realistic
- Validate with patient and family through conversation, questionnaires and check list.

Develop Learning Outcomes

- Identify, specific, attainable, measurable, and short term outcomes for patient's learning.
- Prioritize
- Include the patient and family.

Develop a Teaching Plan

- Select contents, content sequencing, and appropriate teaching strategies.
- Relate the teaching content to the patient's learning style, interests, resources and patterns of daily living.
- Pay careful attention to time constraints, scheduling and the physical environment.
- Decide on group versus individual teaching and formal versus informal methodologies.

Implement Teaching Plan and Strategies

- Pay attention to comfort and privacy of patient and prepare the physical environment.
- Gather all audiovisual materials and equipment.
- Communicate effectively with individuals, small groups and large groups.
- Deliver the content in an organized manner using selected teaching strategies.
- Be flexible.
- Keep teaching sessions short.
- Involve the patient in the process. When teaching a procedure, talk about the steps of procedure, demonstrate the procedure and have them write down steps or provide a printed matter for following the steps.
- Review whatever has been learnt and ask for return demonstration of specific skill.

Evaluate Learning

- **Evaluate whether the learner outcomes were met:**
  - Observe return demonstration.
  - Ask patient to restate the instructions.
  - Ask the patient questions to determine whether teaching reinforcement is needed.
  - Use written test or questionnaires.
  - Consult with the patient's family.
  - Consider patient's feedback and comments.
- Revise the plan if the learner outcome is not met.
- Reschedule teaching sessions.
- Document the teaching learning process:
  - Patient and family learning needs and identified barriers to learning.
  - Mechanisms used to overcome barriers.
  - Identification of learning outcomes.
  - Information and skills taught.
  - Teaching methods used.
  - Patient and family response.
  - Evaluation of what patient and family learned and need for follow up.

TEACHING STRATEGIES

The techniques used by a teacher to promote learning are called teaching strategies. These are planned before the actual teaching session so that every content area and learning outcome can be matched with an effective teaching technique. Using a variety of teaching strategies enhances learning. Some methods are better suited for certain learning outcomes as described below.

For cognitive domain (knowledge) teaching strategies are:

- Lecture or discussion.
- Panel discussion.
- Audiovisual materials.
- Printed materials.
- Programed instructions.
- Computer-assisted instruction program like websites.

For affective domain (attitude), teaching strategies are:

- Role modeling.
- Discussion.
- Panel discussion.
- Audiovisual materials.
- Role playing.
- Printed materials.

For psychomotor domains (skill) teaching strategies are:

- Demonstration.
- Discovery-Problem solving and independent thinking.
- Audiovisual materials.
- Printed materials.

BIBLIOGRAPHY

1. *Berlo KD. The Process of Communication: An Introduction to Theory and Practice. New York, Holt Rinehart and Winston; 1960.*

2. *Berman AT, Snyder S, Kozier BJ, et al. Kozier & Erb's. Fundamentals of Nursing: Concepts, Process and Practice, 8th edition. Pearson Education.*

3. *Sharma S. Potter and Perry's Fundamentals of Nursing. A South Asian edition. Elsevier India. Gurugram: 2013.*

4. *Taylor CR, Lillis C, LeMone P, et al. Fundamentals of Nursing – The Art and Science of Nursing Care, 7th edition. Wolters Kluwer; 2010.*

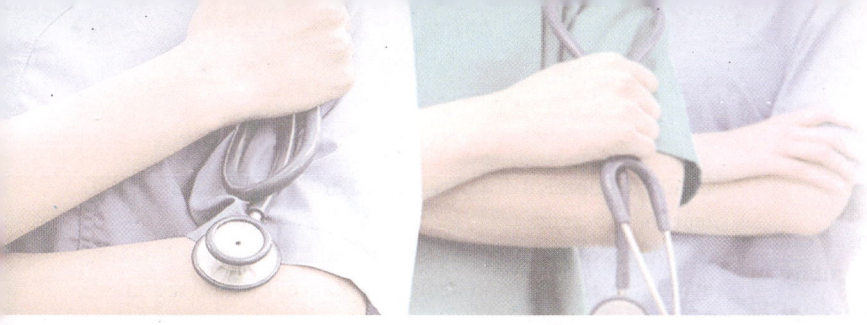

Communication among Health Professionals and Specific Clients

COMMUNICATION AMONG HEALTH PROFESSIONALS

Communication within the health care team occurs through writing and reading nurses notes' physician's orders, dietitian notes and orders of respiratory therapist, physiotherapist, and occupational therapists, and listening to shift report. Filling out a wide variety of forms for the laboratory, radiology, and other departments is another method of communication. Entering information on the computer is an essential tool for communication among hospital departments. The computer is used to transmit requests for laboratory, dietary, radiology, physical therapy, respiratory therapy, and other services. Medication orders are entered into the computer in the pharmacy and the orders are communicated to the nurse. Supplies for patient care are ordered on computer and patient care plans are updated.

End-of-Shift Report

The information can be recorded on audiotape or presented with the members of nursing staff. A full report on each patient should take one to three minutes. Give only essential information. It includes:

- Patient's name, room no., bed no., age, sex, data of admission, medical diagnosis, attending physician's name
- Tests and treatment or therapies performed in the past 24 hours with patient's response
- Significant changes in patient's condition
- Scheduled tests, consultation, or surgery, current intravenous solution, flow rate, amount remaining, oxygen flow rate, current settings, etc.
- Current problems: Dehydration, severe pain, anxiety, depression, insufficient rest, abnormal laboratory values
- Scheduled treatment, medication given, response
- Concerns, need for order charges, teaching emotional status.

Documenting Communication

Assessment of the patient's needs and conditions requires accurate documentation. It helps to promote continuity of care because significant information must be passed on to others through nursing progress notes and care plans.

Hand-off Communication: SBAR Technique

Hand-off communication involves the accurate presentation of all patient-related information to another care giver. **SBAR**, which stands for Situation, Background Assessment and Recommendation, provides a consistent method for hand–off communication that is clear, structured, and easy to use. Details of SBAR are given in Unit VI.

COMMUNICATING WITH ELDERLY

The elderly vary greatly in their communication abilities, interests, and capabilities. Some elders may take more time to think and respond; others may have hearing, sensory, or motor impairments that may interfere with communication. It is best to be certain, to have the person's attention before beginning a purposeful interaction. Eliminate outside distractions. Try to introduce one idea at a time. Do not rush the person because this may cause confusion.

It is important to obtain feedback from an elderly person that the message has been clearly understood. Many elderly person are embarrassed about their hearing deficiency and may just nod their head up and down.

As a nurse you must wait for an answer to one question before asking another. Try not to introduce more than one subject at a time in the conversation, and give only one instruction in one sentence.

COMMUNICATING WITH CHILDREN

The development on language and thought processes must be taken into account to communicate effectively with children. Young children are very responsive to non-verbal messages. Approach the child at eye level and use a calm, quiet and friendly voice when communicating.

When interacting with an infant try to keep the mother within the baby's view. With a toddler, or a preschooler, focus on the child's needs and concerns. Use simple and short sentences.

For school-age child, give simple explanations and demonstrate on how equipment works. Allow the child to

handle equipment if possible. Listen carefully to the child's fears or concerns.

An adolescent needs time to talk. Use active listening, avoid interrupting, and show acceptance. Be honest and talk with the child what to expect.

COMMUNICATING WITH HEARING-IMPAIRED CLIENT

If the patient has hearing aids, see that they are used, that the batteries are functioning and that the device is turned on before trying to communicate. Follow these to promote comprehension for a hearing impaired person.

- Speak very clearly and do not shout
- Speak slowly and keep voice pitch at mid-range
- Get the person's attention, making sure that person is aware of communication taking place.
- The best distance for speaking to a hearing impaired person is $2^{1/2}$ to 4 ft. Face the person at eye level. Never speak directly into the person's ear.
- Be aware of the nonverbal communication. Facial expressions, gestures, lip and body movements all give cues to the meaning of message.
- Use short simple sentences. Rephrase the statement if patient does not understand.
- Give the person time to respond to questions.
- Ask for rephrasing to make sure the patient has understood important information.

COMMUNICATING WITH VISUALLY IMPAIRED CLIENT

- Acknowledge your presence in the patient's room.
- Identify yourself by name.
- Speak in a normal tone and remember that visually impaired person will be unable to pick up most non-verbal cues.
- Explain the reason for touching the patient before doing so.
- Indicate to the patient, when the conversation has ended and when you are leaving the room.
- Keep a call bell within easy reach of patient.
- Orient the patient to room, environment and its furnishings.
- Be sure eyeglasses are clean, intact or contact lenses are in place.

COMMUNICATING WITH THE APHASIC PERSON

Aphasic person has difficulty expressing or understanding language.

- Make the environment relaxed and quiet.
- Assume that the patient can understand what is heard.
- Talk to the patient and do not talk to someone else in the room, about the patient.
- Face the patient, establish eye contact, and speak slowly and distinctly, do not shout.
- Phrase questions so that they can be answered in Yes or No.
- Give the person time to respond to questions.
- Ask only one question at a time, be patient and wait for an answer.
- If there is a need for repetition, use the same words the second time.

- Use body language to enhance the message.
- Allow one person to speak at a time. Be patient.

COMMUNICATING WITH UNCONSCIOUS PERSON

- Be careful of what is said in the patient's presence. Hearing is believed to be the last sense lost; therefore, the unconscious patient is often likely to hear even though there is no response.
- Assume that the patient can hear you. Talk in a normal tone of voice.
- Speak with the patient before touching. Remember that touch can be an effective means of communication with an unconscious person
- Keep environment noises as low as possible. This helps the patient focus on communication.

BIBLIOGRAPHY

1. *Berlo KD. The Process of Communication: An Introduction to Theory and Practice. Holt: Rinehart and Winston; New York, 1960.*
2. *Berman AT, Snyder S, Kozier BJ, et al. Kozier & Erb's. Fundamentals of Nursing: Concepts, Process and Practice, 8th edition. Pearson Education.*
3. *Sharma S. Potter and Perry's Fundamentals of Nursing. A South Asian edition. Elsevier India. Gurugram, 2013.*
4. *Taylor CR, Lillis C, LeMone P, et al. Fundamentals of Nursing – The Art and Science of Nursing Care, 7th edition. Wolters Kluwer; 2010.*

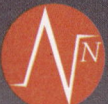   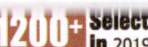

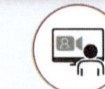
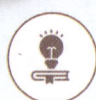

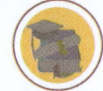

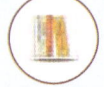

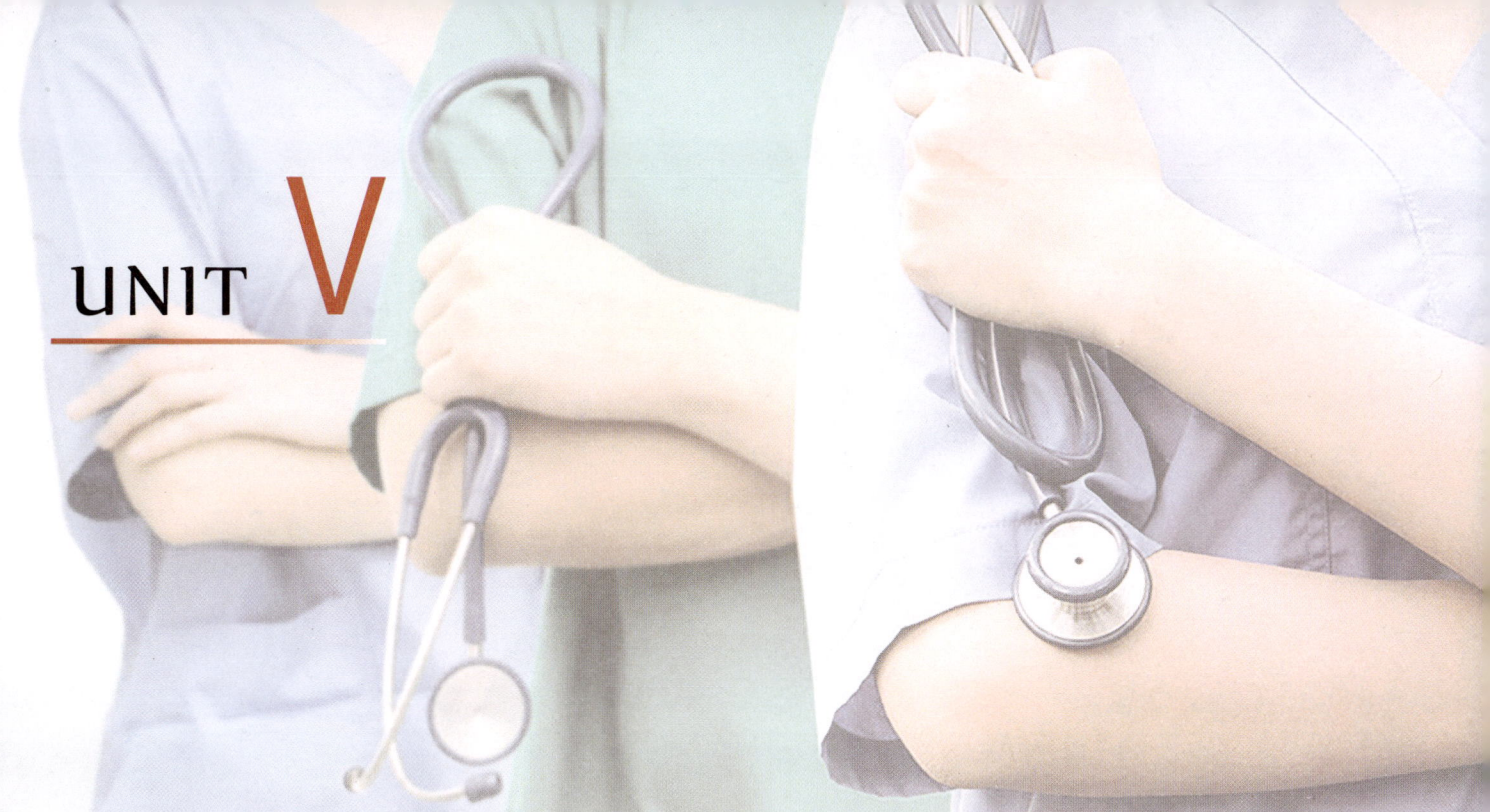

UNIT V

HEALTH ASSESSMENT

Unit Outline

Critical Thinking and Nursing Judgment

INTRODUCTION

Every day all of us utilize critical thinking in our lives, which help us to prepare to face realities. It is necessary to think critically to use nursing process successfully and to develop good clinical judgment in nursing. Critical means requiring careful judgment. Thinking in this context means 'to reason'.

Critical thinking is directed, purposeful, mental activity by which ideas are evaluated, plans are constructed, and desired outcomes are decided.

Critical thinking is necessary to make reliable observations regarding health status and to draw sound conclusions from the data obtained. Critical thinking is needed for creative problem solving and for the production of new ideas and solutions.

SKILLS FOR CRITICAL THINKING

Critical thinking involves a variety of skills

- **Reading skills:** Reading a paragraph and then restating the main ideas yourself is one way to read critically.
- **Writing skills:** Effective writing means writing coherently, concisely, yet clearly. Writing clearly, logically and concisely and evaluating what is written helps improve skill.
- **Attentive listening:** It is consciously focusing on the topic of discussion. Attentive listening takes a lot of practice. Pay attention to each word and the meaning the speaker is trying to convey.
- **Effective communication:** It requires speaking in a disciplined manner about what to say and how to say clearly and concisely in a logical way.

Effective speaking follows attentive listening. Generally, there is a spontaneous response without conscious thought, and misunderstanding often occurs. Taking time to consider your response before beginning to speak is another good way to improve this skill.

Many more skills and attributes found in the critical thinker are the ability to:

- Separate relevant information from irrelevant information
- Recognize inconsistencies in data gathered
- Recognize one's own bias and limitations
- Maintain questioning attitude
- Be persistent in seeking solutions
- Identify missing information
- Consider all possibilities
- Assume an empathetic attitude
- Use an organized and systematic approach to problems
- Consider all possible solutions before making a decision
- Admit what one doesn't know
- Logical reasoning
- Strive for excellence and improvement
- Set priorities and make careful decisions
- Be flexible, realistic, creative, humble, honest, curious and insightful
- Draw valid conclusions from the evidence or data.

LEVELS OF CRITICAL THINKING

The level of critical thinking grows as new knowledge is gained. According to Kataoka-Yahiro and Saylor (1994) critical thinking model has three levels—basic, complex and commitment.

Basic Critical Thinking

Basic critical thinking is an early step in developing reasoning. At this level, the learner trusts that experts have the right answers for every problem. Thinking is concrete and is based on a set of rules or principles. A basic critical thinker learns to accept the diverse opinions and values of experts.

Complex Critical Thinking

As you advance in practice, you adopt complex critical thinking and commitment. Complex critical thinkers begin to separate themselves from experts. They analyze and examine choice more independently. The person's thinking abilities and initiative to look beyond expert opinion begins to change. Thinking becomes more creative and innovative. The complex critical thinker is willing to consider different options whenever situations arise.

Commitment

It is the third level of critical thinking in which a person anticipates when to make choices without assistance from others and accepts accountability for decisions made.

ATTITUDES FOR CRITICAL THINKING

Critical thinking attitude comprises of the guidelines for how to approach a problem or decision-making situations. An important part of critical thinking is interpreting, evaluating and making judgments about the adequacy of various arguments and available data. Knowing when you need more information, knowing when information is misleading and recognizing your own knowledge limits are examples of how critical thinking attitude guides decision-making.

Confidence

When you are confident, you feel certain about accomplishing a task or goal. It grows with experience. When you are not confident in carrying out certain tasks, you become anxious about not knowing what to do. This prevents you from giving attention to the patient. When you show confidence, your patients recognize it and it helps in building trust in your patients.

Thinking Independently

It helps you to challenge the ways others think and look for rational and logical answers to problems. When nurses ask questions and look for the evidence behind clinical problems, they are thinking independently; this is an important step in evidence-based practice. Independent thinking and reasoning are essential to the improvement and expansion of nursing practice.

Fairness

A critical thinker deals with situations without bias or prejudice. Look at the situation objectively and consider all viewpoints to understand the situation completely before making a decision.

Responsibility and Accountability

When caring for patients, you are responsible for correctly performing nursing care activities based on standards of practice. As a nurse, you are answerable or accountable for your decisions and the outcomes of your actions.

Risk-taking

Risk-taking is desirable, particularly when the result is a positive outcome. A critical thinker is willing to take risks in trying different ways to solve problems. The willingness to take risks come from experience with similar problems. Risk-taking often leads to advances in patient care.

Discipline

A disciplined thinker misses few details and follows an orderly or systematic approach when collecting information, making decisions, or taking action. Being disciplined helps the nurse to identify problems more accurately and select the most appropriate interventions.

Perseverance

It means to keep looking for more information/resources, until you find a successful approach. A critical thinker who is not satisfied with minimal effort but works to achieve the highest level of quality care.

Creativity

Creativity involves original thinking. It motivates you to think of options and unique approaches.

Curiosity

A critical thinker's favorite question is "why", Having a sense of curiosity motivates to inquire further and investigate a clinical situation to get all the information you need to make a decision.

Integrity

A person of integrity is honest and willing to admit mistakes or inconsistencies in his or her own behavior, ideas and beliefs.

Your personal integrity as a nurse builds trust from your co-workers.

Humility

Critical thinker admits to any limitations in their knowledge or skill. A nurse may be expert in one area of clinical practice but a novice in another. Therefore, it is important for patient's safety and welfare, if you do not admit your inability to deal with a practical problem.

CRITICAL THINKING IN NURSING

Critical thinking is applied to setting priorities for patient care. Priority setting involves placing nursing diagnoses or nursing interventions in order of importance. Life threatening problems are of a high priority. Problems that threaten health or coping ability are of a medium priority. Low-priority problems are ones that do not have a major effect on the person if not attended on that day or even that week. When all tasks have a rather high priority and there is no way to do them alone. They must be delegated to others.

Priorities constantly change because patient's needs and conditions change frequently. Critical thinking skills help the nurse to skillfully solve problems, make good decisions and develop the clinical judgment necessary for safe nursing practice.

The main purpose of nursing process is to help nurses manage each patient's care scientifically, holistically and creatively. To do this successfully, the nurse needs: **cognitive, technical, interpersonal** and **ethical/legal skills** along with the willingness to use them creatively and critically when working with patients to promote or restore health, to prevent disease or illness, and to facilitate coping with altered functioning. This calls for adequacy of nursing skills for professional practice.

BIBLIOGRAPHY

1. *Berman AT, Snyder S, Kozier BJ, et al. Kozier & Erb's. Fundamentals of Nursing: Concepts, Process and Practice, 8th edition. Pearson Education.*

2. *Shortridge LM, Lal JE. Introduction to Nursing Practice, McGraw Hill Book Company, 1980.*

3. *Christensen BL, Kockrow OE. Foundations of Nursing, Mosby; 2003. p. 764.*

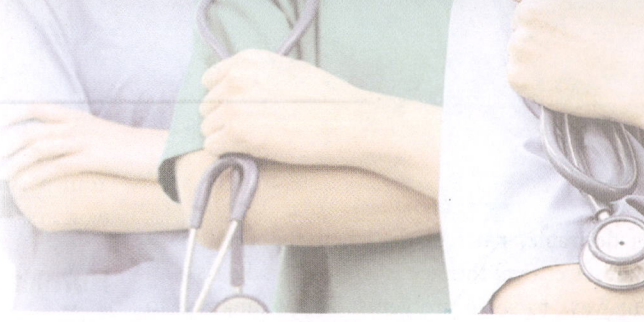

Chapter 15

Assessment of Each Body System

THE INTEGUMENTARY SYSTEM

The Integumentary system includes the skin, hair and nails. Assessing the integumentary structures provide information about the overall health status, as well as clues to local or systemic health problems. It also provides data about self-care activities to maintain health, hygiene and nutrition.

Skin

Inspecting Skin Color

Assessment of skin involves inspection and palpation. The entire skin surface maybe assessed at one time or as each aspect of the body is assessed. In some instances, unusual skin odors in the skinfolds and axillae may be detected related to poor hygiene, hyperhidrosis (excessive perspiration) or bromhidrosis (foul smelling perspiration) changes in skin color include: pallor, cyanosis, jaundice and erythema.

Pallor

It is the result of inadequate circulating blood of less hemoglobin. In black-skinned clients, the skin may appear ashen grey and in brown-skinned clients the pallor may appear as yellowish brown tinge. Pallor in all people is most evident in areas with least pigmentation such as conjunctiva, oral mucous membranes, nail beds, palm of the hand, and soles of the feet.

Cyanosis

It is the bluish discoloration of the skin in response to inadequate oxygenation. It is most evident in the nail beds, lips and buccal mucosa.

Jaundice

It is a yellow color of the skin resulting from liver and gallbladder disease, some times because of anemia, and excessive hemolysis (breakdown of red blood cells). It usually develops first in sclera of the eyes and then in the skin and mucous membranes. Nurses should take care not to confuse jaundice with the normal yellow pigmentation in the sclera of a dark-skinned client. If jaundice is suspected, the posterior part of the hard palate should also be inspected for a yellowish color tone.

Erythema

Redness of the skin is more often seen in the face and the neck. It is associated with sunburn, inflammation, fever, trauma, and allergic reactions.

Inspecting Skin Vascularity and Lesions

The skin is inspected for vascularity, bleeding, or bruising; these signs might relate to a cardiovascular, hematologic, or liver dysfunction.

Ecchymosis

It is a collection of blood in the subcutaneous tissues, causing purplish discoloration.

Petechiae

These are small hemorrhagic spots caused by capillary bleeding, If they are present, assess their location, color, and size.

Lesions are areas of diseased or injured tissue such as bruises, scratches, cuts, burns, insect bites, and wounds. Lesions are categorized as primary or secondary.

Primary Lesions

These lesions may appear from previously normal skin (Table 1).

TABLE 1: Primary skin lesions

Lesion Name	Description	Example	Illustration
Circumscribed, Flat, Nonpalpable Change in Skin Color			
Macule	Lesion ≤ 1 cmww	Petechiae, Freckle	Macule
Patch	Lesion > 1 cm	Vitiligo	Patch

Cotnd...

Lesion Name	Description	Example	Illustration
Palpable, Elevated solid masses			
Papule	Mass < 0.5 cm	Mole	Papule
Plaque	Mass > 0.5 cm	Coalesced papules	Plaque
Nodule	Mass 0.5 cm; Firmer than a papule	Nevus (wart)	Nodule
Palpable, elevated solid masses			
Tumor	Mass > 2 cm	Lipoma	Tumor

Cotnd...

Lesion Name	Description	Example	Illustration
Wheal	Irregular, superficial area of localized skin edema	Hives, mosquito bite	Wheal
Circumscribed, superficial skin elevations formed by free fluid in a cavity within the skin layers			
Vesicle	Filled with serous fluid, $\leq$0.5 cm	Herpes simplex	Vesicle
Bulla	Filled with serous fluid, >0.5 cm	Second-degree burn	Bulla
Pustule	Filled with pus	Acne, impetigo	Pustule

TABLE 2: Secondary and miscellaneous skin lesions

Lesion Name	Description	Example
Secondary Lesions		
Loss of Skin Surface		
Erosion	Loss of superficial epidermis, moist, non-bleeding surface	Moist area after rupture of a vesicle, as in chickenpox
Ulcer	Loss of epidermis and dermis, may bleed and scar	Stasis ulcer
Fissure	Deep linear crack, extends into dermis	Athlete's foot
Material on the Skin Surface		
Crust	Dried residue of serum, pus, or blood	Impetigo
Scale	Thin flake of exfoliated dermis	Dandruff, dry skin
Miscellaneous Lesions		
Lichenification	Thickened and roughened epidermis, with increased visibility of skin furrows	Atrophic dermatitis
Atrophy	Thinning of the skin, loss of skin furrows, shiny appearance	Peripheral vascular disease
Excoriation	Scratch of the skin, loss of skin furrows, shiny appearance	
Scar	Fibrous tissue replaces tissue in the dermis or subcutaneous layer	
Keloid	Hypertrophied scar	
Other Common Skin Lesions, Not Technically Primary or Secondary		
Comedo	Plugged opening of a sebaceous gland, a hallmark of acne	Common blackhead
Telangiectasia	Small, dilated, red or bluish surface vessels; may be a part of basal cells carcinoma or skin injury from radiation	Common mole
Nevus	Flat to slightly elevated, round evenly pigmented	

Secondary Lesions

These result from changes in primary lesions (Table 2)

Assess lesions and wounds for size, shape, depth, locations, and presence of drainage or odor. Scars are healed wounds. Describe rashes (skin eruptions) in terms of their type, size, elevation, coloring and presence of drainage or itching. Document the exact body surface areas involved.

Palpating Skin Temperature, Texture, Moisture and Turgor

The skin is normally warm and dry. An increase in skin temperature and moisture can indicate an elevated body temperature. The texture of the skin varies from smooth and soft to tough and dry. In the dehydrated patient, the texture is dry, loose, and wrinkled, and the mucous membranes are cracked and dry. An excessive amount of perspiration, such as when the entire skin is moist, it is called diaphoresis.

Turgor

It is the fullness or elasticity of the skin. It is usually assessed on the sternum or under the clavicle by lifting a fold of skin

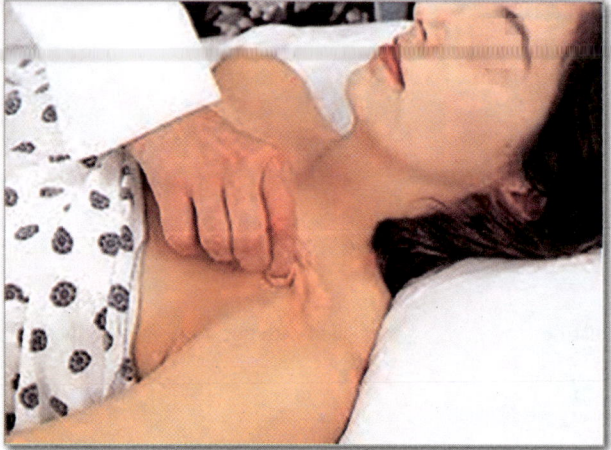

Fig. 1: Assessing skin turgor

with the thumb and first finger (Fig. 1). Skin turgor is normal when the fold returns to its usual shape when released. When the patient is dehydrated, the skin's elasticity is decreased, and the skin fold returns slowly. However this may be a normal finding in older patients.

Edema

Difficulty in lifting a skin fold may indicate edema (excess fluid in the tissues). Edema is characterized by swelling with taut and shiny skin over the edematous area. If the area of edema is palpated with the fingers, an indentation may remain after the pressure is released; if the indentation is very deep, it is called pitting edema. Edema may be graded as 0 (none), +1 (trace, 2 mm), +2 (moderate, 4 mm), +3 (deep, 6 mm) or +4 (very deep, 8 mm). Edema may be the result of overhydration, heart failure, kidney failure, trauma or peripheral vascular disease

Nails

The nails are inspected for shape, angle, texture and color. The nails should be somewhat convex and should follow the natural curve of the finger. The angle between the nail and its base should be about 160 degrees. The nails should be smooth, and the nail base, when palpated, should be firm and non-tender. Abnormal findings include indentations called beau lines (from acute illness), infection, painless separation of the nail plate from the nail bed (onycholysis), due to infection or trauma, (paronychia), increased brittleness or thickness and angulation (from anemia or iron deficiency anemia), and clubbing (from long-term lack of oxygenation) (Fig. 2).

Hair and Scalp

Hair is found on all body surfaces except the palms of the hand and the soles of the feet. Assess the hair for color, texture and distribution. The hair is normally resilient, evenly distributed,

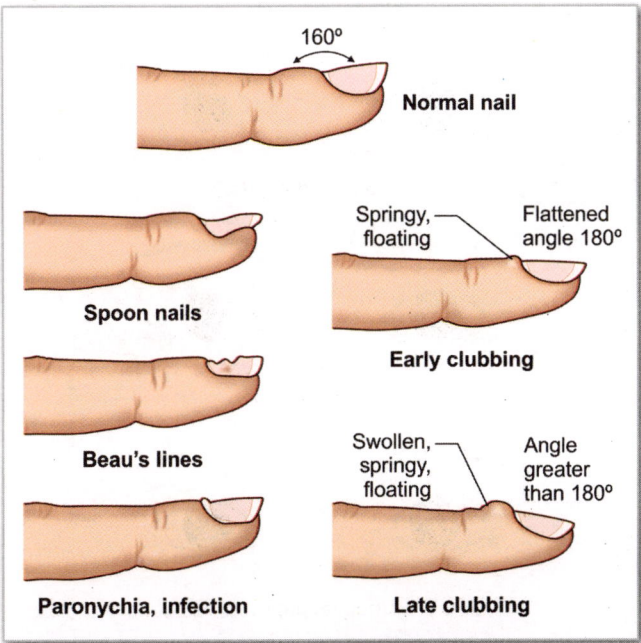

Fig. 2: Examples of nail abnormalities

and neither excessively dry or oily. Abnormal findings include an unusual balding (alopecia) and excessive amounts of hair on the face and body (hirsutism). Hair loss may be normal or may be the result of chemotherapy, radiation therapy, infection, hormonal disorders, or inadequate nutrition. Decreased oxygenation of peripheral tissues, especially of the lower extremities, may cause loss of hair/ excessive hair growth may occur in persons with hormonal disorders.

Inspect the scalp for color, dryness, scaliness, lumps, lesions or lice. Nits, which are the white eggs of lice, can be differentiated from dandruff, because they are attached to the hair shaft. If any lumps or masses are palpated, note their location, size, tenderness and mobility.

Age-Related Variations

Infant/Child

Common/normal variations in newborn and children include:
- Jaundice and milia (whiteheads) in newborn
- Fine downy hair (lanugo) for the first 2 weeks of life
- Smooth, thin skin of birth
- Pubic hair development at the onset of puberty

Old Age-Related Variations

- Wrinkles, dryness, scaling and decreased turgor
- Raised dark areas (senile keratosis)
- Flat brown age spots (senile lentigines)
- Small round red spots (cherry angioma)
- Fine, brittle grey or white hair
- Hair loss
- Coarse facial hair in women, decreased body hair in man and women.
- Thick, yellow toe-nails

INSPECTING HEAD AND NECK

Assessment of the head and neck includes the skull, face, eyes, ear, nose and sinuses, mouth and pharynx, trachea, thyroid gland and lymph nodes. During the health history, note any health problems such as headache or dizziness.

Skull and Face

Inspect and palpate the head for size and shape. The parts of the head and face should be in proportion to each other and symmetric. A normal head size is referred to as normocephalic. Names of areas of the head are derived from names of the underlying bones: frontal, parietal, occipital, mastoid process, temporal, mandible, maxilla and zygomatic bone.

Abnormal findings include lack of symmetry or unusual size or contour of the skull and tenderness. If the skull of a child or an adult appear disproportionately large or small, measure the circumference. Measuring head circumference is a normal part of infant assessment to the age of 2 years, and should be conducted at each visit.

Inspect face for color, symmetry, and distribution of facial hair. Edema of the face, especially around the eye (periorbital edema) and involuntary facial movements (e.g., tics, fasciculation, tremors) are abnormal findings. If abnormalities are noted, document their location, amount, duration and timing.

Inspecting the Eye

Assessment of eyes includes the external and internal eye structures, visual acuity, extraocular movements and peripheral vision

External Eye Structures

The eyes, eyebrows, eyelids, eyelashes, lacrimal glands, pupils and iris are inspected for position and alignment (Fig. 3).

Asymmetry of position and alignment of the eyes may be caused by muscle weakness or a congenital abnormality. The eyebrows should be equally distributed, the eyelashes should curl outward.

Inspect the eyelids for color, edema, and equal coverage of the eyeball. Abnormal findings include drooping of the upper lids (ptosis) which may be due to damage to oculomotor nerve, myasthenia gravis, or a congenital disorder, inward turning of the lower lid and lashes (entropion); outward turning of the lower lid (ectropion); and redness or drainage (from infection of the lid margins, conjunctivae, or hair follicles) Inspect and palpate the lacrimal glands for edema and pain.

Assess the pupils. They are normally black, equal in size, round and smooth. If the patient has cataract (opacity of lens), injury to the eye or glaucoma, the pupil may be cloudy and pale. Certain medications may cause pupil to constrict (miosis), and others may cause pupil to dilate (mydriasis). Pupil may be unequal due to injury or illness of central nervous system. Assess the pupils for reaction to light and accommodation and for convergence (Fig. 4). Decreased or absent puillary response indicates blindness or serious brain damage. Inability of eyes to accommodate or converge is abnormal.

PERRLA is an acronym used to document a common papillary response lest. It is used check the appearance and function of the pupil. It stands for:

- Pupils (P): Pupils are in the center of the iris. They control how much light enters the eye by shrinking or widening.
- Equal (E): Pupils should be of same size.
- Round (R): Pupils should also be perfectly round and need to be further assessed if uneven shapes or borders are found.
- Reactive (R) to: Pupils react to the surroundings by controlling how much light enters the eyes.
- Lights: The pupils should contract when light shines in the eyes.

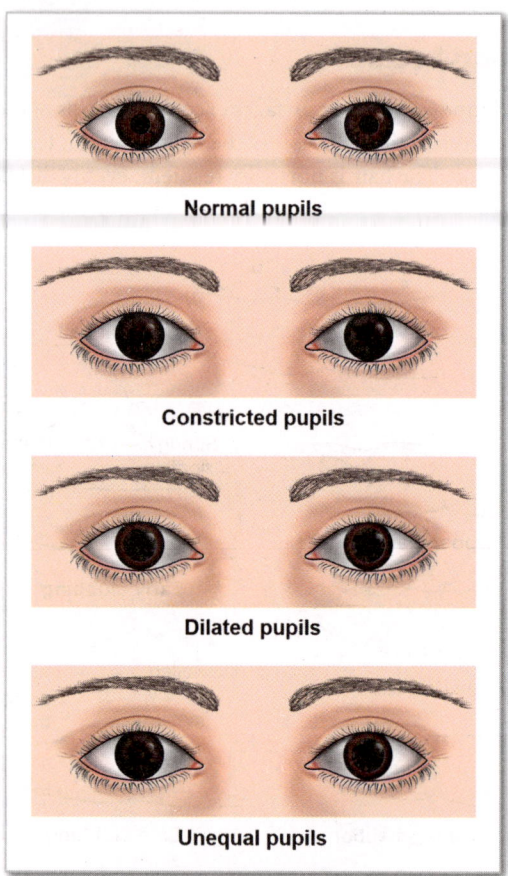

Fig. 4: Assessment of pupil

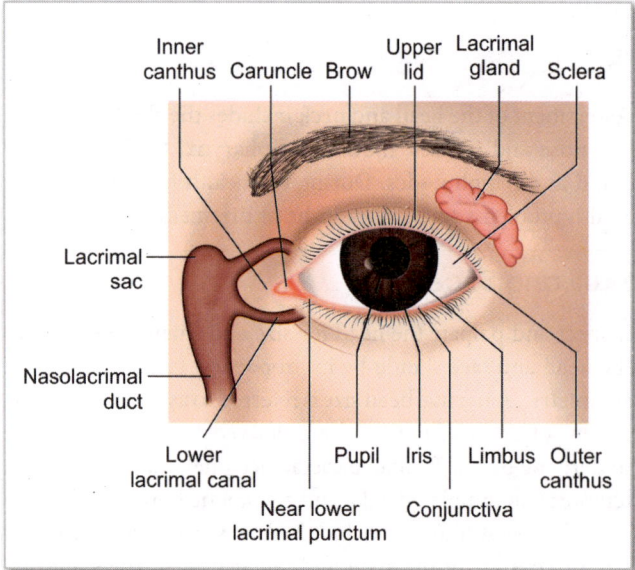

Fig. 3: The eye and surrounding structures

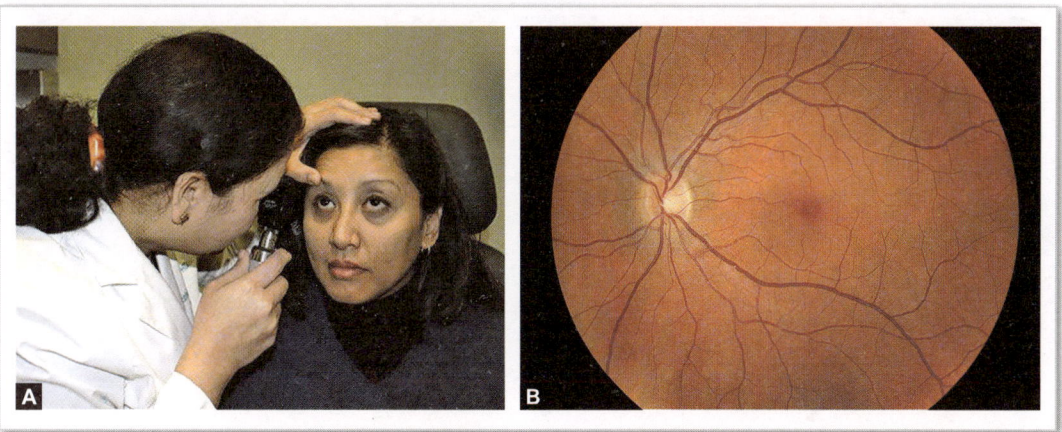

Figs 5A and B: A. Examination of the internal structures of the eye, using an ophthalmoscope; B. The normal fundus as seen through an ophthalmoscope

♦ Accommodation: Accommodation refers to the eyes' ability to see things that are both close and away. The doctor assesses whether the pupils adjust when the focus is shifted.

Internal Eye Structures

The internal eye is examined with the ophthalmoscope to assess the fundus, including the retina, optic nerve disc, macula, fovea centralis and retinal vessels. Normal findings are a uniform red reflex; a clear yellow optic nerve disc; a reddish retina; and light red arteries and dark red veins (Figs 5A and B). Abnormal findings, include cloudiness of the lens (cataract), changes in size and shape of blood vessels (from hypertension or arteriosclerosis), and changes in color and surface characteristics (from diabetes, hypertension, trauma, inflammation and detached retina).

Assessing Visual Acuity, Extraocular Movements, and Peripheral Vision

Visual acuity is checked with the snellen's chart. Have the patient stand 20 feet from the chart and ask the patient to read the smallest line of letters possible, first with both eyes and then with one eye at a time, (with the opposite eye covered). Note whether the patient's vision is being tested with or without corrective lenses.

At the end of each line of the Snellen chart are standardized numbers. The top line is 20/200. The numerator (top number) is always 20, the distance the person stands from the chart. The denominator (bottom number) is the distance from which the normal eye can read the chart. Therefore, a person who has 20/40 vision can see at 20 feet from the chart what a normal sighted person can see at 40 feet from the chart. Thus, the longer the denominator, the poorer the vision.

Test extraocular movements by assessing the cardinal fields of vision for coordination and alignment. Normally both eyes move together, are coordinated and parallel. Test for peripheral vision (vision fields) are used to assess retinal function and optic nerve function. Full peripheral vision is normal.

Testing Extraocular Movements and Peripheral Vision

Extraocular Movements

♦ Ask the patient to sit or stand about 2 feet away, facing you sitting or standing at eye level with the patient.
♦ Ask the patient to hold the head still and follow the movement of your forefinger or a penlight with the eyes.
♦ Keeping your finger or light about one foot from the patient's face, move it slowly through the cardinal positions: up and down, left and right, diagonally up and down to the left diagonally up and down to the right.
♦ Extraocular muscle movements are described in (Fig. 6).

Peripheral Vision

♦ Have the patient stand or sit about 2 feet away, facing you at eye level.
♦ Ask the patient to cover one eye with a hand or an index card.
♦ Ask the patient to look directly at your nose and fix his or her eyes on that spot.
♦ Cover your own eye opposite the patient's closed eye.
♦ Hold one arm outstretched to one side (right or left) equidistant from you and the patient, and move your fingers into the visual fields from various peripheral points.

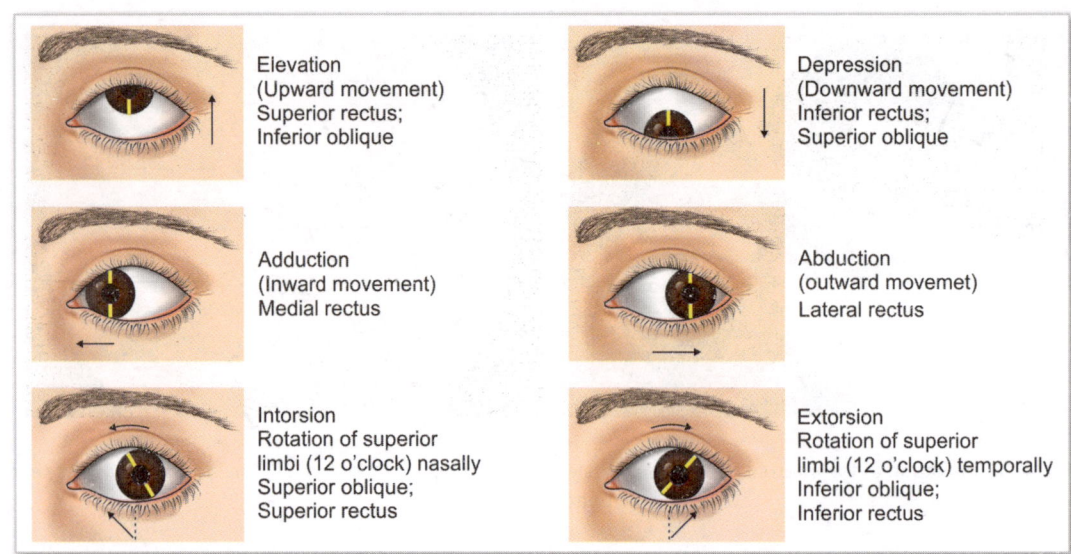

Fig. 6: Actions of extraocular muscles

- Ask the patient to tell you when the fingers are first seen (both you and the patient should see the fingers at the same time).
- Repeat the procedure for the other eye.

INSPECTING AND PALPATING THE EARS

The external ear is assessed by inspection and palpation. The middle ear and tympanic membrane are assessed by inspection. An otoscope with the correct size of ear speculum is used to inspect the ear canal and tympanic membrane. A tuning fork and ticking watch are used to assess hearing acuity.

Inspect the external ear for shape, size and lesions. The external surface of the ear should be smooth, and the size and shape should be symmetric and proportional to the head. Abnormal findings include unequal height and size, uneven color and lesions. Gently palpate the external ear for pain, edema, or presence of lesion. Pain when manipulating pinna is a symptom of an infection of the external ear.

Inspecting the Ear Canal and Tympanic Membrane

Assessment of the ear includes direct inspection and palpation of the external ear and remaining parts of the ear are examined with the help of otoscope. The ear is divided into three parts: external ear, middle ear and inner ear. The external ear includes the auricle or pinna, the external auditory canal, and the tympanic membrane or eardrum. Landmarks of the auricle include the lobule (earlobe), helix (the posterior curve of the auricle's upper aspect), antihelix (the anterior curve of the auricle's upper aspect), tragus (the cartilaginous protrusion of the entrance to the ear canal), **triangular fossa** (a depression of the antihelix), and external auditory meatus (the entrance of the ear canal). Mastoid, although not part of the ear. a bony prominence behind the ear is another important land mark. The external ear is curved, is about 2.5 cm (1 inch) long in the adult and ends at the tympanic membrane. It is covered with skin that has many fine hairs, glands and nerve endings. The glands secrete cerumen (earwax), which lubricates and protects the canal. The curvature of the external ear canal differs with age. In the infant and toddler, the canal has an upward curvature. By age 3, the ear canal assumes the downward curvature of adulthood.

The middle ear is an air-filled cavity that starts at the tympanic membrane and contains three **ossicles** (bones of sound transmission), the **malleus** (hammer), the **incus** (anvil), and the **stapes** (stirrups). The **Eustachian tube,** another part of the middle ear connects the middle ear to the nasopharynx. The tube stabilizes the air pressure between the external atmosphere and the middle ear, thus preventing the rupture of tympanic membrane.

The inner ear **contain** the cochlea, a seashell-shaped structure essential for sound transmission and hearing, the **vestibule** and **semicircular canals**, which contain the organs of equilibrium (Fig. 7).

Sound transmission and hearing are complex processes. Sound can be transmitted by air conduction or bone conduction.

Air-conducted transmission occurs by:
- A sound stimulus enters the external canal and reaches the tympanic membrane
- The sound waves vibrate the tympanic membrane and reach the ossicles

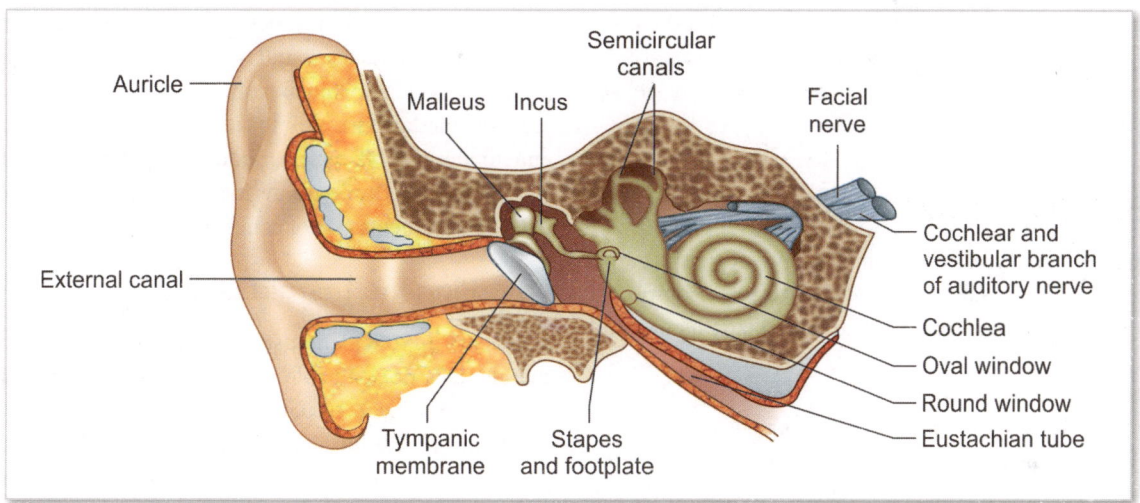

Fig. 7: Internal structures of the ear

- The sound waves travel from the ossicles to the opening in the inner ear (oval window)
- The cochlea receives the sound vibrations
- The stimulus travels to the auditory nerve (the eighth cranial nerve) and the cerebral cortex

Bone-conducted sound transmission occurs when skull bones transport the sound directly to the auditory nerve.

Assessing Hearing and Sound Conduction

Hearing is assessed in one ear at a time by determining whether the patient can hear a whispered voice or ticking watch from a distance of 1–2 feet. Assess hearing acuity out of the patient's line of vision to prevent lip reading with the opposite ear covered.

Tuning fork tests such as the Weber and Rinne tests help assess the type of hearing loss: conductive (the result of a problem with the transmission of sound waves through' the outer and middle ear), sensorineural (from inner ear damage), or a combination of both.

Weber test is used to assess for bone conduction of sound. With this test, the sound is normally heard in both the ears or is localized at the center of the head. Patients with conductive hearing loss hear the sound better in the affected ear. If the sound is heard better in the ear without a problem, it indicates damage to the inner ear or a nerve disorder.

Rinne test is used to compare bone and air conduction of sound With this test, hearing of air-conducted sound is normally greater than bone-conducted sound (documented as AC > BC). If the hearing loss is conductive, sound of bone conduction will be same or greater than air conduction.

The otoscope is used to examine the ear canal and the tympanic membrane. Attach the largest speculum that will fit comfortably into patient's ear to the otoscope. Insert the otoscope speculum as the patient's head is slightly tilted away from the examiner. To achieve better visualization, straighten the ear canal of the adult by pulling gently the pinna up and backward. In children, younger than 3 years of age, straighten the ear canal by pulling the pinna down and back. The ear canal should be smooth and pink. Examine the canal for wax, discharge and foreign bodies. The tympanic membrane should be intact translucent, shiny, and grey. Abnormal findings include redness of the canal, mastoid tenderness, a red and swollen eardrum, a perforated eardrum, wax plugs in the ear canal and drainage from an infection or foreign body in the ear canal.

Inspecting the Nose and Sinuses

Assessment of nose involves examining the external nose, the nares, and palpate the sinuses with the patient sitting with head slightly tilted back. Assess the nose for patency by occluding one nostril at a time and asking the patient to inhale and exhale through the nose. Inspect each nostril using an otoscope or nasal speculum and penlight. Examine the mucous membrane for color and presence of lesions, exudates, or growths. Inspect the nasal septum for intactness and deviation.

Normally, the nasal mucosa is moist and darker red than is the oral mucosa. Abnormal findings are swelling of the mucosa bleeding or discharge, perforation or deviation of the nasal septum and polyps.

The frontal and maxillary sinuses, located in the frontal and maxillary bones, respectively, are palpated for pain and edema. The frontal sinuses are palpated by gently pressing upward on the bony prominences located above each eye. The maxillary sinuses are palpated by gentle pressure on the bony prominences of the upper cheek. Normally, the sinuses are not painful when palpated. Pain may be experienced if the sinuses are infected or obstructed.

INSPECTING THE MOUTH AND PHARYNX

The mouth and pharynx include the lips, tongue, teeth, gums, hard and soft palate, salivary gland and tonsils. Equipment used to assess includes a penlight, tongue blade, gauze and gloves.

Assess the mouth and pharynx by inspecting the lips, gums and teeth, tongue and hard and soft palate. Have the patient sit with head tilted backward and mouth opened wide. Use palpation if any abnormalities are noted during inspection. Wear gloves when assessing patient's mouth and use gauze to hold tongue for palpation.

The lips should be pink, moist and smooth. The tongue and mucous membranes are normally pink, moist and free of swelling and lesions. If the patient wears dentures, ask the patient to remove them for inspection of gums and roof of mouth. The gums should be pink and smooth. With the tongue relaxed on the floor of the mouth, examine the mucous membrane of the oropharynx, while depressing the base of the tongue with a tongue depressor. The uvula is normally centered and freely movable. The tonsils, if present, are small, pink and symmetric in size. The teeth should be regular and free of cavities.

Abnormal findings are pallor, cyanosis, or redness and swelling of the mucous membranes, lesions of the mucosa and lips, swollen red tonsils indicate infection; swollen red, and bleeding gums; poorly aligned, missing or caries teeth; white coating on the tongue (from poor oral hygiene, irritation or smoking); a fissured tongue (due to dehydration); bright red tongue (seen in deficiency of vitamin B_{12} or niacin) or a black hairy tongue (from antibiotic use).

INSPECTING THE NECK

Assessment of the neck includes the trachea, lymph nodes, and thyroid gland. Assess the neck with the patient sitting and the neck slightly hyperextended. Ask the patient to tilt the head backward, forward, and side to side to assess range of motion. The neck should be symmetric, with full range of motion. Also assess the neck for venous distention (indicating heart problems).

Palpating the Trachea and Lymph Nodes

The trachea, normally midline at the suprasternal notch, is palpated for alignment and position. An unusual space between the trachea and sternocleidomastoid muscle on each side is an abnormal finding indicating tracheal displacement.

Palpate the lymph nodes with the pads of the fingers for enlargement, tenderness and mobility. The nodes are generally not palpable, if palpable they should be small, mobile, smooth, and non-tender. Assess for location, size, consistency, mobility, and tenderness. If lymph nodes are palpable and enlarged (lymphadenopathy), it may indicate infection, autoimmune disorders or metastasis of cancer.

Palpating the Thyroid Gland

Assess the thyroid gland using palpation keeping in mind that the gland is not palpable in all patients. Use an anterior or posterior approach to palpate the thyroid gland with sitting position. Palpate for size, shape, symmetry, tenderness, and presence of any nodules. If palpable, the thyroid gland should feel soft but elastic. It should be nontender and should have no enlargement, masses, or nodules (which may indicate infection, or cancer)

ASSESSING THE THORAX AND LUNGS

The thorax comprises the lungs, rib cage, cartilage and intercostal muscles.

Health History

Identify risk factors for altered health during the health history by asking:

- History of trauma to ribs or lung surgery
- Number of pillows used when sleeping
- History of chest pain with deep breathing
- History of persistent cough with or without sputum
- History of allergies
- Environmental exposure to chemicals, asbestos or smoke
- History of smoking (since how long and how many packs/day)
- History of lung disease in family members or self
- History of frequent or chronic respiratory infections

Physical Assessment

Equipment needed are stethoscope and tape measure. The environment should be warm and adequately lit. The techniques for assessment include: inspection, palpation, percussion and auscultation.

Inspecting the Thorax

Inspect the patient's chest for color, shape or contour, breathing patterns and muscle development. The color should be even and consistent with the color of patient's face. The shape or contour should have a downward equal slope at the ribcage. The chest should be symmetric, with the transverse diameter greater than the anteroposterior diameter. An increased anteroposterior diameter, is seen in chronic lung diseases (barrel chest). Respirations should be smooth and ranging from 12 to 20 breaths/min.

Abnormal findings include an increase in chest size and contour, abnormal breathing patterns with use of accessory muscles, unequal chest expansion and abnormal respirations.

Palpating the Thorax

Palpation is used to detect areas of sensitivity, chest expansion during respirations, and vibrations (fremitus). Use the palmar surface of the hands to palpate the anterior and posterior thoracic landmarks in a sequential pattern for temperature moisture, muscular development and any tenderness, or masses. The skin should be warm and dry, with symmetric muscular development and no tenderness, masses or vibrations. Abnormal finding may be cool or excessively dry or moist skin, muscle asymmetry, tenderness, masses and vibrations.

Chest expansion is determined by placing the hands over the posterior chest wall, with the fingers at the level of T9 or T10. Ask the patient to take a deep breath, and observe the movement of your thumbs, The thorax should expand symmetrically.

Auscultating Breath Sounds

Auscultation is used to detect airflow within the respiratory tract. Ask the patient to breathe slowly and deeply through the mouth. Place the diaphragm of the stethoscope over the thoracic landmarks and auscultate breath sounds in the same sequential pattern as used for palpation (Fig. 8).

Normally, breath sounds result from the free movement of air into and out of all parts of the bronchial tree. Listen for the pitch, duration, and intensity of the sounds.

Normal breath sounds vary over different parts of the lungs. **Bronchial sounds** heard over the trachea are harsh sounds, high-pitched, with expiration being longer than inspiration.

Bronchovesicular sounds are heard over the main stem bronchus and are moderate "blowing" sounds, with inspiration equal to expiration. **Vesicular breath sounds** are soft, low-pitched sounds heard best over the base of the lungs and lung periphery during inspiration, which is longer than expiration.

Adventitious breath sounds are not normally heard in lungs but, if present, they may be auscultated. **Stertorous breathing** is a general term used to refer to noisy, strenuous respiration. **Stridor** is harsh, high-pitched sound heard on inspiration, when there is narrowing of the upper airway larynx or trachea. **Crackles** are fine to coarse crackling sounds made as air moves through wet secretion: they are most often heard on inspiration, Crackles are described as "fine" when they are made by air passing through moisture in small air passages and alveoli and as "coarse" when they are made by air passing through moisture in the bronchioles, bronchi and trachea. Coarse crackles can also be documented as **rhonchi. Wheezes** are continuous sounds that originate in small air passages that are narrowed by secretions, swelling, or tumors. A **pleural friction** rub is a grating sound caused by an inflamed pleura rubbing against the chest wall.

ASSESSING THE CARDIOVASCULAR AND PERIPHERAL VASCULAR SYSTEMS

It includes assessment of the heart and the extremities

Health History

Identify risk factors for altered health during the health history by asking:

- History of chest pain, palpitations or dizziness
- Swelling in the ankles and feet
- Number of pillows used to sleep
- Type and amount of medications taken daily
- History of heart defect, rheumatic fever, or chest or heart surgery
- Personal and family history of hypertension, heart attack, coronary artery disease, high cholesterol levels or diabetes mellitus.
- History of smoking (how long, how many packs/day)
- History of alcohol use
- Type and amount of exercise
- Usual dietary pattern each day
- Changes in color or temperature of extremities
- History of pain in the legs when sleeping or pain that is worsened by walking
- History of blood clots or sores on the legs that do not heal.

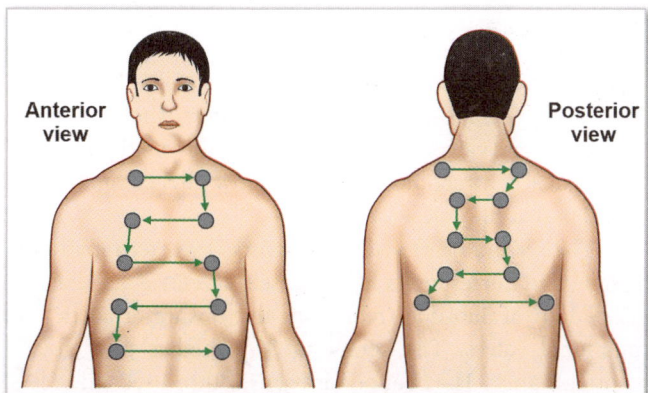

Fig. 8: Auscultating breath sounds

Physical Assessment

The technique used for cardiovascular assessment are inspection, palpation and auscultation. Equipment includes a stethoscope and a sphygmomanometer. The patient may be in sitting position or in supine position with the head raised above 30 degrees. Adequate lighting is essential for inspection of color and for pulsations. A quiet environment is necessary for accurate auscultation of heart sounds.

Peripheral vascular assessment includes measuring the blood pressure and assessing the skin and perfusion of the extremities and the peripheral pulses. Assessments are made by inspection and palpation with the patient in sitting or supine position. Peripheral vascular assessments may be combined with assessment of other body areas.

Inspecting the Neck and Precordium

Inspect the neck for jugular veins distension while the patient is in supine position with the head elevated 30–45 degrees. Normally the veins should be flat. If venous distension is observed, note the level above right atrium. (Fig. 9).

Observe the neck and precordium (the portion of the body over the heart and lower thorax, encompassing the aortic, pulmonic, tricuspid, and apical areas, and erb's point) for visible pulsations. Pulsations usually are absent except for the apical impulse, located at the fourth or fifth intercostal space at the left midclavicular line. Inspect the epigastric area at the tip of the sternum for pulsation of the abdominal aorta. Findings of the neck vein distention (indicating heart disease) or visible pulsations in precordial areas other than the apical impulse (which will result from abnormalities of the ventricles) are considered abnormal.

Palpating the Precordium

Using the palmar surface of the hand with the four fingers held together, palpate the precordium gently for pulsations.

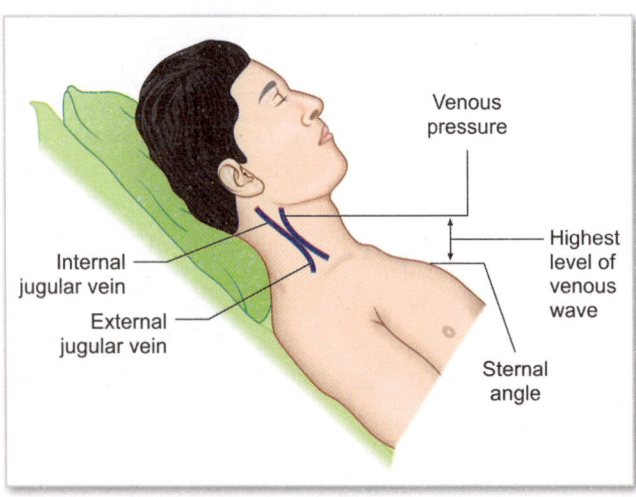

Fig. 9 Inspection of jugular vein

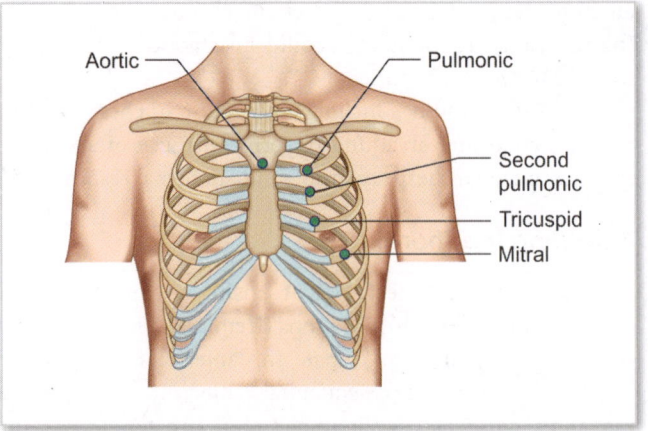

Fig. 10: Anatomical sites for assessment of cardiac function

Keep your hands warm by rubbing together and palpate in a systematic manner, assessing specific cardiac landmarks—the aortic, pulmonic, tricuspid, and mitral areas and Erb's point. Palpate the apical impulse in the mitral area. Note size, duration, force, and location in relationship to the relation line. Normal findings include no pulsation palpable over the aortic and pulmonic areas, with a palpable apical impulse (Fig. 10).

Abnormal findings include precordial thrills, which are fine, palpable, rushing vibrations over the right or left second intercostal space, and lifts or heaves, which involve a rise along the sternal border with each heart beat.

Auscultating Heart Sounds

Auscultation is used to determine the heart sounds caused by closure of the heart valves. Ask the patient to breathe normally. Use systematic auscultation, beginning at the aortic area, moving to the pulmonic area, then to the erb's point, then to the tricuspid area and finally to the mitral area. Use the diaphragm of the stethoscope first to listen high-pitched sounds. Then use the bell to listen to low-pitched **sounds.**

Normal Heart Sounds

During auscultation the first heart sound called S_1, is heard as the "lub" of "lub-dub". This sound occurs when the mitral and tricuspid valves close and corresponds to the onset of ventricular contractions. The sound, low pitched and dull, is heard best at the apical area.

The second heart sound S_2, occurs at the termination of systole and corresponds to the onset of ventricular diastole. The "dub" of 'lub-dub" represents the closure of aortic and pulmonic valves. The sound of S_2 is higher pitched and shorter than S_1. The two sounds occur within 1 second or less, depending on the heart rate. Normal finding includes S_1 that is louder at the tricuspid and apical areas, with S_2 louder at the aortic and pulmonic areas.

Abnormal Heart Sounds

Abnormal findings include extra heart sounds at any of the cardiac landmarks and abnormal rate or rhythm. Extra heart sounds are often heard when the patient has anemia or heart disease. Extra heart sounds may be S_3, S_4, murmurs, or bruits.

- **S_3:** Known as the third heart sound, is often represented by a "lub-dub-dee" pattern ("dee" being S_3); this sound is best heard with the stethoscope bell at the mitral area, with the patient lying on the left side. S_3 is considered normal in children and young adults.
- **S_4:** Is the fourth heart sound, represented by"dee-lub-dub". S_4 is considered normal in older adults but abnormal in children and adults.

Murmurs

Heart murmurs are extra heart sounds caused by some disruption of blood flow through the heart. The characteristics of a murmur depends on the adequacy of valve function, rate of blood flow and size of the valve opening.

Grading of Murmurs (Table 3)

TABLE 3: Grades of murmurs

Grade I	A murmur so faint that can be heard with effort
Grade II	A faint murmur but one that can be easily detected
Grade III	A moderately, loud murmur
Grade IV	A very loud murmur that is usually associated with a thrill sound
Grade V	An extremely loud murmur
Grade VI	An exceptionally loud murmur that can be heard while the stethoscope is lifted off the skin.

Bruits

Bruits are abnormal "swooshing" sounds similar to murmurs and are heard over major blood vessels. The sound indicates a partially blocked artery, causing the blood to swirl, rather than flow normally. Bruits are most commonly heard over carotid arteries, the abdominal aorta, and the femoral arteries.

INSPECTING THE EXTREMITIES

Inspect the skin of the extremities for color, temperature, continuity, lesions, venous patterns, and edema, Normally, venous patterns, varicosities, rashes, ulcers, or edema are absent in the lower extremities. However, if the patient has peripheral vascular disease, the skin of the lower extremities is typically pale and cool, shiny and brown discolorations, and hairless. The toenails are thickened. Phlebitis of the lower extremity is indicated by pain, redness, and swelling of the affected calf or thigh.

Palpating Peripheral Pulses

Palpate peripheral pulses by using pads of the index and middle fingers for amplitude and symmetry. Palpate one at a time: the carotid, brachial, radial, femoral, popliteal, dorsalis pedis, and posterior tibial pulses. These should be strong and equal bilaterally. The amplitude of the pulses may be documented as 0 (absent), 1 + (weak), 2 + (normal), 3 + (increased), or 4 + (bounding)

Abnormal findings include an absent, weak, thready pulse (which may indicate a decreased cardiac output), a forceful or bounding pulse (seen in hypertension and circulatory fluid overload) and an asymmetric pulse (related to impaired circulation).

Assessing Peripheral Circulation

Allen's Test

- Ask the patient to rest hand on the examining table with the palms up and make a fist
- Use your thumbs to occlude the radial and ulnar arteries and ask the patient to open hand (the palm will be pale)
- Release your thumb pressure and observe the return of color to the palm (this should normally take 3–5 seconds)

Buerger's Test

- Ask the patient to assume a supine position and then raise one arm or one arm or one leg about 1 foot (30 cm) above the level of his or her feet.
- Ask the patient to briskly move the leg or arm up and down for 1 minute, then to sit up and dangle the arm or leg downward
- Observe the time it takes for the original color of the patient's skin to return and for the veins to fill. Normally color returns in 10 seconds, and veins fill in 15 seconds.

Capillary Refill

- Using your thumb and forefinger, squeeze the patients fingernail or toenail until it appears white
- Release the pressure and observe the time it takes for normal color to return. Normally, color return immediately,
- Assess capillary refill in children by pressing the skin tightly over the forehead or top of the hand. Release the pressure; observe the time for return of color.

ASSESSING THE BREASTS AND AXILLAE

Physical assessment of the breasts and axillae are primarily conducted to identify any lumps in the breasts or enlargement or pain in axillary lymph nodes; if assessed, the patient should

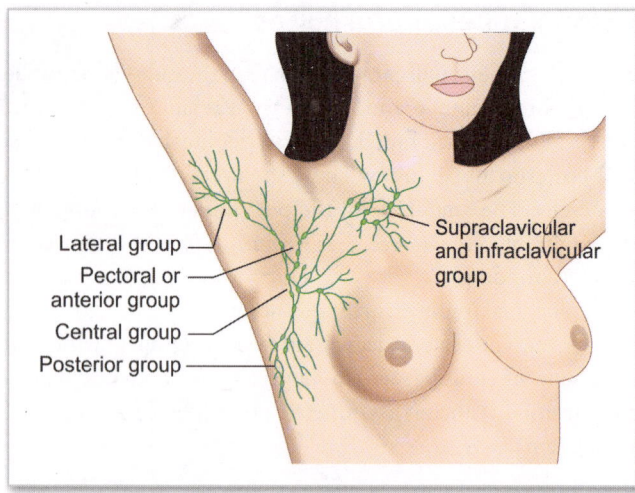

Fig. 11: Location of the cervical, axillary and mammary lymph nodes

have further diagnostic tests. Each breast has a lymphatic network that drains into the underlying axillae (Fig. 11).

Health History

Identify risk factors for altered health during the health history by asking:

* History of pain in one or both breasts, including relationship to menstrual period.
* History of lumps or swelling, redness, change in size, or dimpling of the breasts
* History of discharge from the breast
* Family history of ovarian or breast cancer
* History of breast disease, biopsy, or surgery
* Menstrual and pregnancy history
* Use of hormones and oral contraceptives
* Exposure to radiation, benzene, or asbestos
* Usual dietary intake and alcohol consumption
* Knowledge and practice of breasts self examination
* Most recent clinical breast exam and mammogram.

Physical Assessment

The breasts and axillae are assessed in both men and women using inspection and palpation. The patient can be sitting or lying supine. When sitting, the patient should sit erect, with arms at sides or raised overhead. When supine, the patients hand on the side being examined is placed under the head.

Inspecting the Breasts

Inspect the breasts in size, shape, symmetry, color, texture, and skin lesions. The breasts should be relatively symmetric, although variations are normal. The size varies among individuals. The shape of the breasts is round and smooth, and

there should be no skin depressions (retraction) or puckering (dimpling). The color should be consistent with the rest of the skin and the texture of the skin should be soft.

Inspect the areola and nipples for size and shape and the nipples for discharge, crusting, and inversion. The areolar and nipple areas should be equal in size, round or oval, with a smooth surface. Montgomery's tubercles (sebaceous glands on the areolae of the breasts) are a normal component of the areola. The nipples are normally everted. Discharge from the breast nipples is an abnormal finding except in pregnancy. Other abnormal findings include dimpling, lesions, and asymmetry.

Palpating the Breasts and Axillae

Palpate the breasts in each of the four quadrants (the upper outer quadrant), the lower outer quadrant, the upper inner quadrant and the lower inner quadrant) to detect any abnormality (Fig. 12).

Palpate the nipples and areola and gently compress the nipple between the thumb and forefinger to assess for discharge. The breast tissue should be smooth and firm, with a granular consistency. If a mass is detected, carefully assess its location, size, shape, consistency, and tenderness. The breasts are normally tender during the week before menstruation. An increase in the nodularity and tenderness of the breasts may be associated with the menstrual period or may indicate fibrocystic disease. Discharge, lumps, lesions, dimpling, asymmetry, and palpable lymph nodes may be indicative of breast cancer.

Palpate the axillary areas for lymph nodes which normally are non-palpable and non-tender, If any nodes are palpable, assess their location, size, shape, consistency, tenderness, and mobility. Palpable lymph nodes are an abnormal finding.

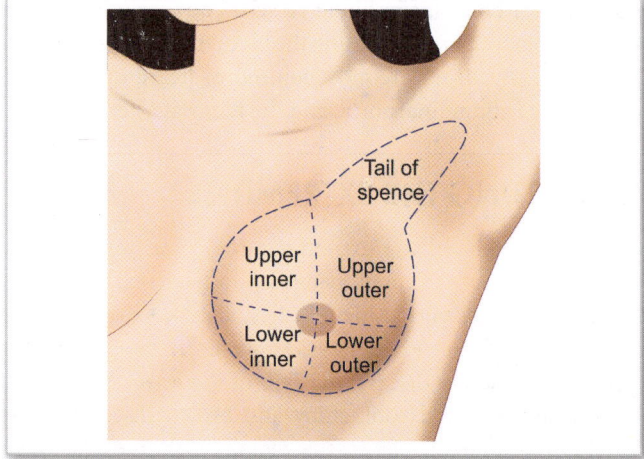

Fig. 12: Location of assessment findings of the breast are identified by quadrant

ASSESSING THE ABDOMEN

The abdominal cavity contains the stomach, the small intestine, the large intestine, the liver, the gallbladder, the pancreas, the spleen, the kidneys, and the urinary bladder. The abdominal cavity also contains the female reproductive organs.

Health history questions are used to identify subjective data, including abdominal pain and nausea and to collect data about the patients elimination patterns, fluid and nutritional intake, and lifestyle. Physical examinations are conducted to further assess problems with pain and to identify abdominal masses. Abdominal assessments are also used to assess the return of bowel sounds after surgery and the retention of urine in the urinary bladder.

Health History

Identify risk factors for altered health during health history by asking:

- History of abdominal pain
- History of indigestion, nausea or vomiting, consti-pation or diarrhea
- History of food allergies or lactose intolerance
- Appetite and usual food and fluid intake
- Usual bowel and bladder elimination pattern
- History of gastrointestinal disorders such as peptic ulcer, bowel disease, gallbladder disease, liver disease and appendicitis
- History of urinary tract disorders such as infections, kidney stones, or kidney disease
- History of abdominal surgery, trauma

- Type and amount of prescribed and over the counter medications used
- Amount and type of alcohol ingestion.
- For women: menstrual history.

Physical Assessment

Equipment needed are stethoscope and proper lighting. When assessing the abdomen, keep your finger nails short and hands warm. Ask the patient to empty the bladder. Position the patient in supine position with the head slightly elevated and arms at the sides. Place small pillows under the head and knees for comfort. Keep the patient warm to prevent contraction of the abdominal muscles, which makes palpation difficult.

To locate organs more easily and to make documentation more specific, the abdomen can be divided into four quadrants: Right upper, right lower, left upper and left lower (Fig. 13).

The sequence of techniques used to assess the abdomen is inspection, auscultation, percussion and palpation. Percussion and palpation are done after auscultation because they stimulate bowel sounds. Ask the patient to breathe slowly and deeply through the mouth during the examination to promote relaxation. Ask the patient to identify painful areas of abdomen and explain you will assess these at the end of the examination.

Inspecting the Abdomen

While sitting at the side of the patient, look across the abdomen tangentially as this enhances shadows and contours. Inspect skin color and surface characteristics, including the

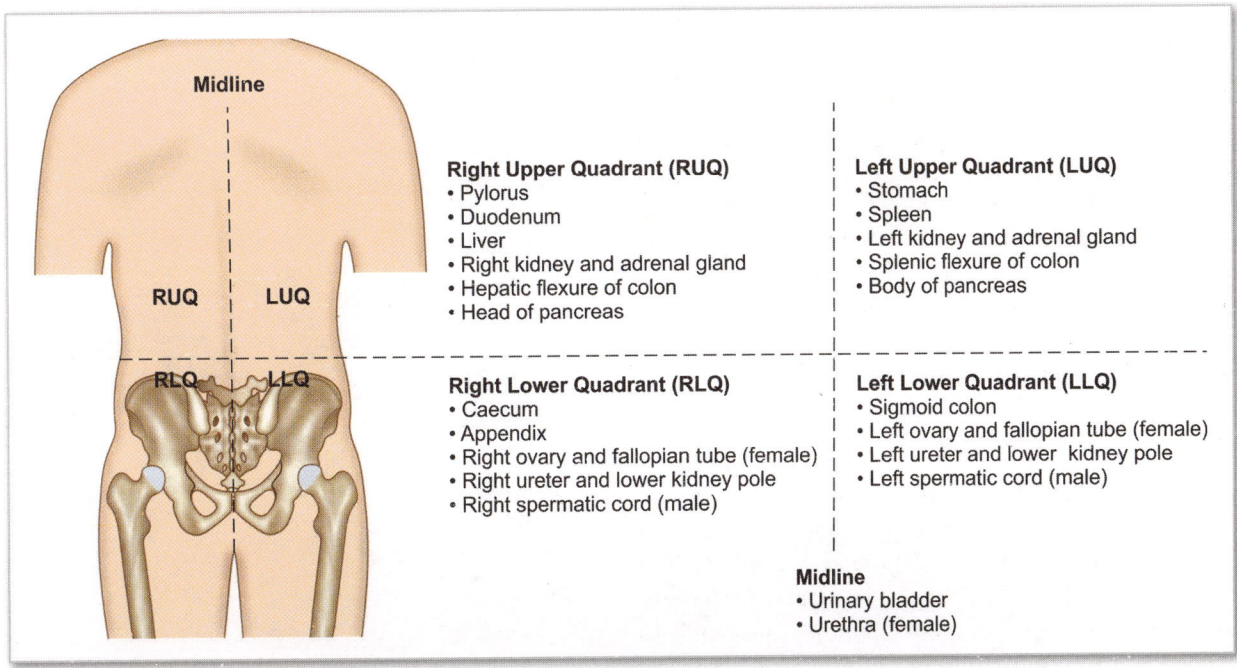

Right Upper Quadrant (RUQ)
- Pylorus
- Duodenum
- Liver
- Right kidney and adrenal gland
- Hepatic flexure of colon
- Head of pancreas

Left Upper Quadrant (LUQ)
- Stomach
- Spleen
- Left kidney and adrenal gland
- Splenic flexure of colon
- Body of pancreas

Right Lower Quadrant (RLQ)
- Caecum
- Appendix
- Right ovary and fallopian tube (female)
- Right ureter and lower kidney pole
- Right spermatic cord (male)

Left Lower Quadrant (LLQ)
- Sigmoid colon
- Left ovary and fallopian tube (female)
- Left ureter and lower kidney pole
- Left spermatic cord (male)

Midline
- Urinary bladder
- Urethra (female)

Fig. 13: Diagram of abdominal quadrants and outline of underlying structures

umbilicus, contour, symmetry, peristalsis, pulsations, and visible masses. The skin color may be slightly lighter than exposed areas. Fine white or silver lines (striae) may be visible, often the result of skin stretching from weight gain or pregnancy. The umbilicus should be centrally located and may be flat, rounded or concave. The abdomen should be evenly rounded or symmetric, without visible peristalsis. In thin people, an upper midline pulsation may normally be visible Abnormal findings include; swelling of the abdomen (ascites), abdominal masses or unusual pulsations and hernias.

Auscultation of Bowel Sounds and Vascular Sounds

By using light pressure, place the warm diaphragm of the stethoscope on the right lower quadrant of the abdomen. Listen bowel sounds carefully and note their frequency and character (usually occur every 5–34 seconds). Before documenting bowel sounds as absent, the nurse must listen for 2 minutes or longer in each abdominal quadrant.

Abnormal findings include increased bowel sounds (often heard with diarrhea or in early bowel obstruction), decreased bowel sounds (heard after abdominal surgery or late bowel obstruction), or absent bowel sounds (indicating peritonitis or paralytic ileus). Bowel sounds of high pitched tinkling. or rushes of high-pitched sounds indicate a bowel obstruction.

Using the bell of the stethoscope, auscultate over the abdominal aorta, femoral arteries, and iliac arteries for bruits (abnormal sounds heard over a blood vessel as blood passes an obstruction). A bruit may be heard if an occlusion or arterial insufficiency is present in an abdominal artery. Report and document changes or absence of bowel and vascular sounds.

Percussing the Abdomen

Percussion is useful in assessing a full bladder or changes in abdominal contents. Percuss the abdomen in all four quadrants in a systematic, clockwise manner to identify fluid, masses, or air. Note the distribution of sounds. Normally tympany, the dominant percussion tone, is heard over the abdomen while dullness is heard over the liver and a full bladder.

Abnormal findings include decreased tympany and increased dullness, possibly caused by fluid or a mass.

Palpating the Abdomen

The pads of the fingers are used to palpate with a light, gentle and dipping motion. Watch the patient's face for nonverbal signs of pain during palpation. Palpate each quadrant in a systematic manner, noting muscular resistance, tenderness, enlargement of the organs, or masses. If the patient complains of abdominal pain, palpate the area of pain in the last. The abdomen should normally be soft, relaxed, and free of tenderness. Abnormal findings include involuntary rigidity, spasm, and pain (which may indicate trauma, peritonitis, infection, tumors, or enlarged or diseased abdominal organs).

Palpating the Liver

The entire liver in not usually palpable, but the lower edge of the liver may be assessed with light palpation. To palpate bimanually, stand at the patients right side and place your left hand under the patients back at the level of 11th to 12th ribs. With your fingertips pointing towards the patient's head, ask the patient to inhale and press up and in with your fingertips. The normal liver edge should feel flrm and smooth and may be mildly tender.

Abnormal findings include a hard and firm liver edge (found in cancer of the liver) nodularity (found with tumor, metastatic cancer, cirrhosis of liver) and pain (from vascular engorgement as in congestive heart failure, hepatitis or abscess). If the liver border is more than 1 – 3 cm below the costal margin, it is considered enlarged. Liver enlargement may result from hepatitis, liver tumors, cirrhosis, and vascular engorgement.

ASSESSING FEMALE GENITALIA

The external female genitalia consists of mons pubis, labia majora and minora, clitoris, vestibular glands, vaginal vestibule, vaginal orifice, and urethral opening. During the physical assessment, the external genitalia may be examined and assessed for lesions, discharge, masses, and enlargement of internal organs (Fig. 14). The rectum and anus may be assessed during part of this examination if a total health assessment is being performed.

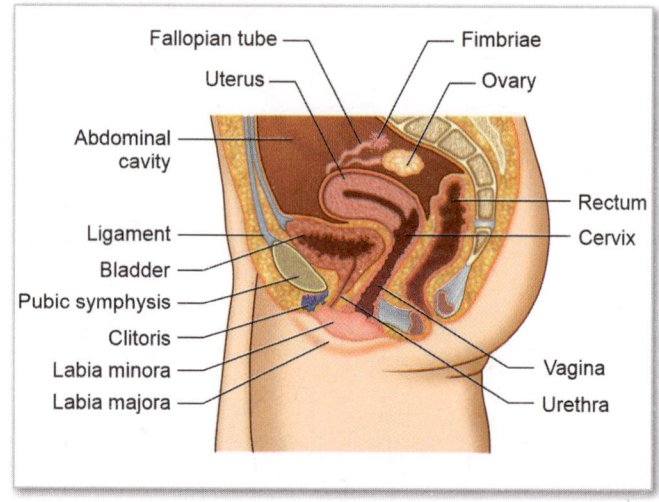

Fig. 14: Female reproductive system

Health History

Identify risk factors for altered female health during the health history by asking:

- Menstrual history (age of first and last period, length of flow, type of flow, pain)
- Sexual history (age at which sexual activity began, number and gender of partners)
- Pain with intercourse, difficulty achieving orgasm
- Number of pregnancies and live births
- History of sexually transmitted infection
- Use of contraceptives
- Frequency of pelvic examination and pap smears
- History of vaginal discharge, itching, or pain on urination
- History of smoking (how long, how many packs/day)
- Family history of reproductive or genital cancer

Physical Assessment

The genitalia are assessed by inspection and palpation. Equipment required include a sterile vaginal speculum, water soluble lubricant and gloves

Inspecting and Palpating the External Genitalia

Ask the patient to empty her bladder before the examination. Place the women in the lithotomy position on the examination table, with the legs in stirrups, and draped so that only the genitalia are exposed. Explain the procedure to her and help her to relax.

Inspect the external genitalia for color, size of the labia majora and vaginal opening, lesions, and discharge, the vulva has more pigmentation normally than other skin areas, and the mucous membranes are dark pink and moist. The skin and mucosa should be smooth, without lesions or swelling. The labia should be symmetric without lesions or swelling. Lesion may be the result of infections, (such as herpes or syphilis). There may be normally clear or whitish vaginal discharge. The vaginal orifice varies in size, depending on the women's age, sexual history, and having vaginal delivery. Palpate the labia for masses and the Bartholin's glands (located slightly below and to the left and right to the opening of the vagina) for swelling, pain, and discharge. Check hymen for its intactness among children, which may be found ruptured due to trauma, intercourse or horse riding.

Inspecting Internal Genitalia (Female)

A speculum is used to examine internal genitalia

- Explain the procedure to the patient
- Apply water soluble lubricant on speculum
- Put on gloves

- Using two fingers placed just inside the vagina, press down gently on the posterior vaginal wall.
- Insert the speculum blades vertically into the vagina, the posterior portion pointed at a 45 degree angle.
- Ensure that no pubic hair is caught in the speculum
- Turn the speculum so that the handle is down and the blades are in a horizontal position
- Open the blades and close the screw that locks the blades open
- Inspect the cervix and os for size, color, shape, lesions, and discharge
- Obtain specimens, if needed
- Withdraw the blades slowly, observing the vaginal walls
- When the speculum blades are clear of the cervix, release the screw, so that the blades close, and withdraw the speculum from the vagina
- Provide the patient with tissues to remove the lubricating jelly

Abnormal findings include redness, swelling of glands, discharge, lesions and pain, which may indicate infection, an abscess, a polyp, or cancer.

ASSESSING MALE GENITALIA

The male genitalia includes the penis, testicles epididymis, scrotum, prostate gland and seminal vesicles. In addition, the inguinal area may be assessed as part of this assessment. The physical examination is focused on detecting abnormal findings so that early diagnosis and treatment can be initiated (Fig. 15).

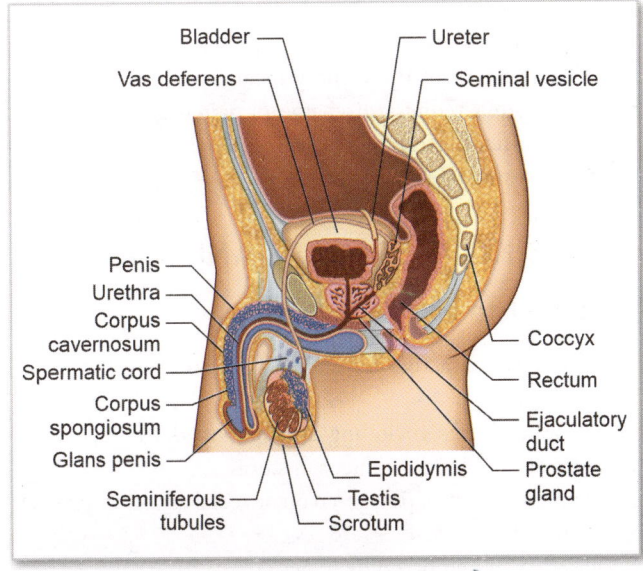

Fig. 15: Male reproductive system

Health History

Identify risk factors for altered male health during health history by asking:

- Frequency of digital rectal examination
- Frequency of testicular self examination
- Use of contraceptives
- Occupational exposure to chemicals
- History of sexually transmitted infection
- History of discharge from the penis
- Difficulty with urination (incontinence, hesitancy, frequency, voiding at night)
- History of erectile dysfunction.

Physical Assessment

The patient may be standing or supine. Gloves are worn during this assessment.

Inspecting and Palpating the External Genitalia

The external genitalia are inspected for size, placement, contour, appearance of the skin, redness, edema, and discharge. If the patient is uncircumcised, retract the foreskin for inspection of the glans penis. Assess the location of the urinary meatus. Inspect the scrotum for symmetry. It is normal that left testicle lies lower in the scrotal sac than the right testicle. The size, shape, and consistency of the scrotal contents (i.e., testis) should be similar bilaterally. Normal findings include skin that is free of lesions, and a foreskin (if present) that is intact, uniform in color, and easily retracted. The urinary meatus is normally located in the center of the glans penis and is free of discharge. The scrotum and testes should be free of masses and non-tender.

Abnormal findings include lesions, redness, edema, pain, discharge, fluid-filled masses in the scrotum (hydrocele), and displacement of the urinary meatus or difficulties with voiding. Edema, redness, discharge, or pain indicate infection. Voiding difficulties may result from scarring caused by infection or prostate enlargement.

ASSESSING THE RECTUM AND ANUS

Health History

Identify the risk factors for altered health during the health history by asking

- Bowel patterns, including constipation, diarrhea, or pain
- History of blood or mucus in stool
- Family history of polyps, colon or rectal cancer or prostate cancer
- History of hemorrhoids
- Frequency of digital rectal examinations
- History of anal intercourse

Physical Assessment

Inspection and palpation are used to assess rectum and anus. Equipment needed are gloves, lubricant and a good light. The patient may be in the Sim's, knee-chest or lithotomy position or may be standing and leaning over the examining table.

Inspection is used to assess the anal area, which normally has increased pigmentation and some hair growth. Palpation is used to assess the rectum, using a well lubricated, gloved finger. Sphincter tone at the anus should be firm and the mucosal lining smooth. Fecal specimens if required may be taken at this time.

Abnormal findings include relaxed sphincter tone; skin cracks, nodules, or hemorrhoids at the anal sphincter, bleeding (which may indicate hemorrhoids or anorectal cancer); and hard or abnormal colored stools.

If a rectal examination is conducted in a women, cervix may be felt as a small, round mass when palpating the anterior rectal wall. Abnormal findings include changes in consistency. The prostate gland in men can be assessed for size, shape, and consistency by palpation through the anterior rectal wall; the gland is normally smooth, firm, and about 4 cm (1¼ inches) in size. Abnormal findings include enlargement or changes in consistency, which occur in benign prostatic enlargement or cancer.

ASSESSING THE MUSCULOSKELETAL SYSTEM

The primary structures of the musculoskeletal system are the bones, muscles, cartilage, ligaments, tendons, and joints. Health history information is used to evaluate the patients ability to carry out activities of daily living and to collect data about areas such as pain, stiffness, and ability to move. Physical examination provides information about posture, gait, bone size and structure, joint, range of motion and muscle strength.

Normally, the joints are bilaterally equal in size, shape and color; are free of swelling, pain, nodules, or crepitus (grating sounds on movement); and can move through full range of motion (ROM).

Abnormal findings include deformity, crepitus, and limited ROM (indicating injury, inflammation and arthritis of the affected joints or bones, muscle pain and weakness caused by injury or disease)

Health History

Identify the risk factors for altered health during the health history by asking:

- History of trauma, arthritis or neurologic disorder
- History of pain or swelling in the muscles and joints
- Frequency and type of usual exercise
- Dietary intake of calcium

- History of any surgery on muscles or joints
- History of smoking (how long, how many packs/day)
- History of alcohol intake

Physical Assessment

The patient assumes variety of positions, including standing, sitting, and supine while assessment of musculoskeletal system is made.

Inspection and Palpating the Muscles

Examine the muscles by inspection and palpation of muscle groups and by testing muscle tone and strength. Muscle groups are observed for bilateral symmetry and palpated for tenderness.

Normally they are symmetric and non-tender. Evaluate muscle tone by putting each joint and extremity through passive range of motion. Assess muscle strength.

Abnormal findings include atrophy (a decrease in size), tremors (involuntary movements) and flaccidity (without tone) of muscles, other abnormal findings are loss of strength and tone, decreased range of motion, uncoordinated movements, swelling and pain, these indicate a musculoskeletal disease, trauma or a neurological disease.

Palpating the Bones

The bones are palpated for normal contour and prominence and for bilateral symmetry. Abnormal findings include pain, enlargement, asymmetry, and changes in contour. These indicate trauma, degenerative joint disease, musculoskeletal disease or neurological disease.

Inspecting and Palpating the Joints

Each joint is put through its full range of motion to assess the degree of movement. Joint movements include flexion, extension, hyperextension, abduction, adduction, supination, and pronation. Normally, each joint has full range of motion is non-tender, and moves smoothly. Palpate joints for the abnormal findings of pain, swelling, nodules, and crepitations (a grating sound heard or felt on movement)

Inspecting Spinal Curves

With the patient standing, inspect the spine from the back and from the side. The spine normally has concave curves at the cervical and lumbar spine and convex curves at the thoracic and sacrococcygeal spine. The lumbar curve may be flattened with a herniated disc. Kyphosis (an increased thoracic spinal curve) is more often seen in older adults. An exaggerated lumbar curve (lordosis) is often seen during pregnancy or in obesity. Scoliosis is a lateral curvature of the spine with increased convexity on the side that is curved.

ASSESSING THE NEUROLOGIC SYSTEM

Neurologic assessment includes cerebral function, cranial nerve function, cerebellar function, motor and sensory function, and reflexes. The health history is useful in obtaining information about activities of daily living and other pertinent data, such as dizziness, loss of sensation, headaches, and ability to see, hear, taste, and detect sensations. Physical examination is conducted to identify mental status and level of consciousness, cranial nerve function, muscle strength and coordination and reflexes. Normally, the patient is alert and responsive, has full sensory function and all muscle groups are bilaterally strong (Fig. 16).

Health History

Identify risk factors for altered health during the health history by asking the following:

- History of numbness, tingling, or tremors
- History of headaches
- History of dizziness
- History of trauma to the head or spine
- History of infections of the brain
- History of stroke
- Changes in the ability to hear, see, taste, smell or feel.
- Loss of ability to control bladder, and bowel
- History of high blood pressure
- History of smoking (how long how many packs/day)
- History of chronic alcohol use
- History of diabetes mellitus or heart disease
- Use of prescription and over the counter drugs
- Family history of high blood pressure, Alzheimer's disease, epilepsy, cancer, or Huntington's chorea.
- Frequency of blood cholesterol tests and results
- Exposure to environmental hazards (lead, insecticide)

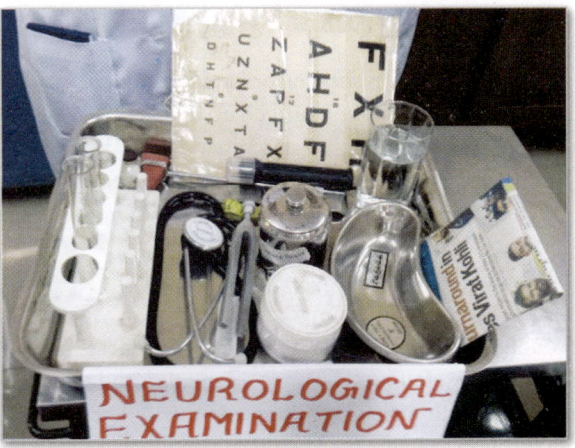

Fig. 16: Tray for neurological examination

Physical Assessment

Evaluate cerebral function by observing the patients behavior throughout the health history interview and physical assessment, Assess the patient's mental status, memory, emotional status, cognitive abilities, and behavior. Evaluate cerebellar function by assisting the motor skills, coordination, and balance. Assess the sensory system by having the patient identify various sensory stimuli, and evaluate the reflexes by contraction of specific muscles.

Equipment for a neurologic assessment includes vials of aromatic substances (for testing smell), a visual acuity chart, a penlight, a sharp object, cotton balls, vials of solution to test taste (sugar, salt), a tuning fork, a tongue depressor, a reflex hammer, and familiar objects, such as coin or key. The patient should be preferably sitting and the environment should be quiet.

Assessing the Mental Status

Mental status assessment includes level of consciousness, behavior and appearance, memory, abstract reasoning, and language. On initial contact, begin to evaluate the patient's orientation to person, place, and time, as well as cognitive abilities and affect (whether the patient knows who he or she is, where he or she is, and time, day or month or year). Observe the patient's appearance, general behavior, ability to speak clearly, and respond to questions. Note any variations in responses.

Assess the patient's overall appearance. The patient should have a clean, neat appearance with erect posture, should be oriented to time, place, person; should have memory recall (both short-term and long-term memory); and should be able to demonstrate coherent and logical thought processes.

Abnormal findings include poor hygiene, inappropriate dress, disorientation, absent memory recall, and incoherent or illogical thought processes. These abnormal findings may indicate a mental health disorder, brain disease, development delay, cerebrovascular disorder, alcohol or drug intoxication, or a tumor.

Assessing Level of Awareness

Assess awareness by evaluating orientation to time, place and person. Following question may be used.

- **Time:** What is today's date? What day of the week is it? What season of the year is this? What was the last holiday?
- **Place:** Where are you now? What is the name of this city? What state are we in?
- **Person:** What is your name? how old are you? Who came to visit you this morning?

Individuals who have impaired awareness lose time orientation first followed by place orientation and then person orientation, although exceptions are there. Therefore, it is often difficult to know the exact date when one is ill.

Assessing Level of Consciousness

Consciousness is the degree of wakefulness or the ability of a person to be aroused. A person may be conscious but may not be oriented. Level of consciousness can be seen:

- **Awake and alert:** Fully awake; oriented to person, place, and time; responds to all stimuli including verbal commands.
- **Lethargic:** Appears drowsy or asleep most of the time but makes spontaneous movements; can be aroused by gentle shaking and saying patients name.
- **Stuporous:** Unconscious most of the time, has no spontaneous movement, must be shaken or shouted at to arouse; can make verbal responses, but these are less likely to be appropriate; responds to painful stimuli with purposeful movements
- **Comatose:** Cannot be aroused, even with use of painful stimuli; may have some reflex activity (gag reflex); if no reflexes present, is in a deep coma.

The Glasgow come scale (Table 4) is a standardized assessment tool that assesses level of consciousness. Three parameters are evaluated; eye opening, motor response, and verbal response. Scores are given in each category, and a total score is recorded, with higher scores indicating a more normal level of functioning. A score of 7 or less defines coma. This is more accurate evaluation of mental status over time.

Assessing Memory

Memory is assessed by asking questions that require answers demonstrating immediate recall and recall for past events. To assess immediate memory, ask the patient to repeat a series of numbers forward or backward (e.g., 4, 8, 12, 16). Start with three or four numbers and gradually increase the digits until the patient can not respond correctly. Most adults can repeat

TABLE 4: Glasgow coma scale

Component	Response	Score
Eye opening	Spontaneous	4
	To verbal command	3
	To pain	2
	No response	1
Motor response	To verbal command	6
	To localize pain	5
	Flexes/with draws	4
	Flexes abnormally	3
	Extends abnormally	2
	No response	1
Verbal response	Oriented/talks	5
	Disoriented/talks	4
	Inappropriate words	3
	Incomprehensible sounds	2
	No response	1

a series of five to eight numbers forward and four to six digits backward. You might ask. "What did you eat in breakfast this morning"? To asses past memory, ask "when is your birthday"? or "when is your wedding anniversary"?

Assessing Abstract Reasoning

Ask the patient to explain a proverb. If intellectual ability is impaired, the patient usually gives a literal explanation or repeats the phrase.

Assessing Language

The cerebral cortex controls the ability to express self through writing, words, or gestures and to understand the spoken and written word. Language can be assessed by asking the patient to name items in the room, To follow simple commands, to read a short sentence.

Injury to the cortex can cause aphasia, which is a disorder of language ability. Aphasia may be expressive, i.e., the individual understands written and spoken words but cannot write or speak to communicate effectively or aphasia maybe receptive, in which individual cannot understand written or spoken words.

ASSESSING CRANIAL NERVE FUNCTION

The function of the 12 cranial nerves in assessed primarily during the neurological assessment (Table 5). Each nerve has a specific function and is evaluated individually.

Assessing Motor and Sensory Function

Motor ability is evaluated by assessing balance, gait, and coordination. Sensory function is assessed by testing sensory discrimination of pain, light touch, and vibrations.

Inspecting Balance and Gait

Evaluate balance and gait by having the patient walk across the room on the toes, on the heels, and heel to toe. Observe posture, balance, and arm and leg movements. The posture should be erect, and the gait even, with simultaneous arm movements.

Abnormal findings include loss of balance, shuffling, wide-based gait, and abnormal patterns of gait. These findings may indicate disorders of the motor, sensory, vestibular and cerebellar lesions.

TABLE 5: Assessing cranial nerves

Nerve (number)	Type	Functions	Methods for examining nerve
Olfactory (I)	Sensory	Sense of smell	Test each nostril for smell reception with various agents and interpretation
Optic (II)	Sensory	Sense of vision	Test vision for acuity and visual fields
Oculomotor (III)	Motor	Pupil constriction, raise eyelids	Test pupillary reaction to light and ability to open and close eyelids
Trochlear (IV)	Motor/proprioceptor	Downward inward eye movement	Test for downward and inward movement of the eye.
Trigeminal (V)	Motor	Jaw movements: chewing and mastication	Ask patient to open and clench jaws while you palpate the jaw muscles.
	Sensory	Sensation on the face and neck	Test face and neck for pain sensations, light touch and temperature.
Abducens (VI)	Motor	Lateral movement of the eyes	Test ocular movement in all directions.
Facial (VII)	Motor	Muscles of the face	Ask the patients to raise eyebrows, smile, show teeth, and puff out cheeks.
	Sensory	Sense of taste on the anterior two-thirds of the tongue	Test for the taste sensation with various agents
Acoustic (VIII)	Sensory	Sense of hearing	Test hearing ability
Glossopharyngeal (IX)	Motor	Pharyngeal movement and swallowing	Ask the patients to say "ah", and have patient yawn to observe upward movement of the soft palate; elicit gag response; note ability to swallow.
	Sensory	Sense of taste on the posterior one third of the tongue	Test for taste with various agents
Vagus (X)	Motor/Sensory	Swallowing and speaking	Ask the patient to swallow and speak; note hoarseness
Accessory (X)	Motor/Sensory	Movement of shoulder muscles	Ask the patient to shrug shoulders against your resistance
Hypoglossal (XII)	Motor	Movement of tongue; strength of tongue	Ask the patient to protrude tongue; ask patient to push tongue against cheek.

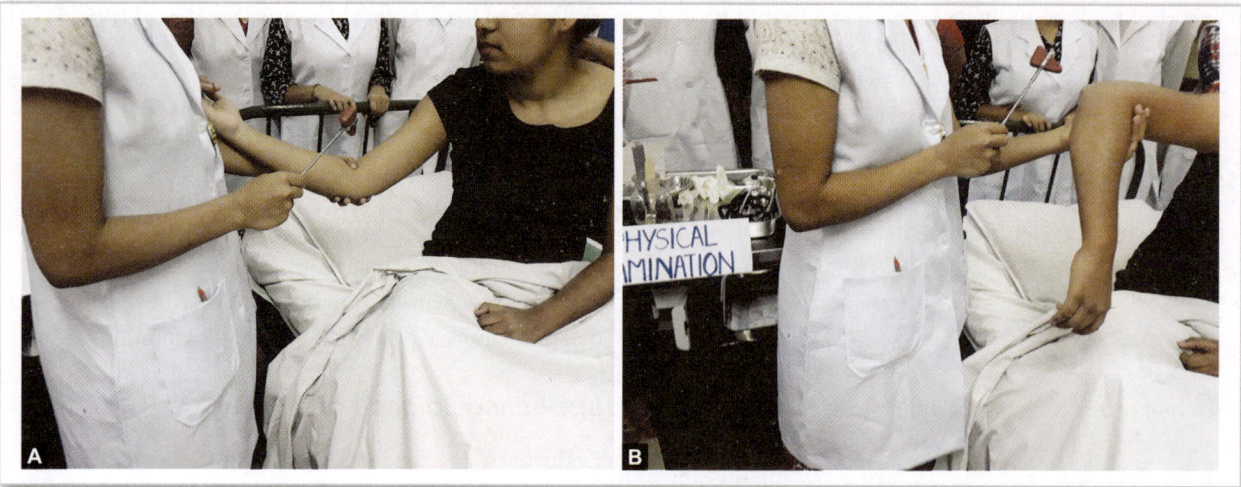

Figs 17A and B: A. Biceps reflex; B. Triceps reflex

Assessing Motor Function and Coordination

Evaluate motor function and coordination by having the patient rapidly touch each finger with the thumb, rapidly pat the hand on the thigh, and tap the foot on the floor. Repeat the sequence on the opposite limb.

Normally, the movements are coordinated. If the patient is unable to perform these movements, it may indicate disease of the upper motor neurons or cerebellum.

Assessing Sensory Perception

Test sensory perception by evaluating the patients response to pain, light touch, normal shapes, and vibration, with the patients eyes closed, randomly touch the skin on the upper and lower extremities and the trunk with a sharp object and soft object. The assessment proceeds from distal (hands, feet, arms) to proximal (the trunk). The patient should be able to distinguish between sharp (painful) and soft or dull touch.

The same process is repeated by using the tuning fork to test for vibratory sensation by placing the activated fork on bony prominences. Sensory perception may also be assessed by asking the patient to close his or her eyes and identify familiar objects (such as coin, button, keys) by touching them.

Abnormal findings includes inability to perceive pain or light touch, inability to identify the location of touch, inability to identify familiar objects, and absence of vibratory sensation.

Assessing Deep Tendon Reflexes

Evaluate deep tendon reflexes to determine the functional ability of specific spinal segment levels. Use the reflex hammer to elicit muscle contraction and reflexes (Figs 17A and B). The patient may be either sitting or supine. Reflex responses are usually graded on a scale of 0 to 4 (Tables 6 and 7).

A grade of 2 is considered normal or active response.

TABLE 6: DTR scale

1.	0–Absent reflex
2.	1 + – Trace or seen only with reinforcement
3.	2 + – Normal
4.	3 + – Brisk
5.	4 + – Non-sustained clonus
6.	5 + – Sustained clonus

TABLE 7: Illustrates the deep tendon reflexes

Deep tendon reflex	Muscle involved	Nerve supply	Root supply
Biceps	Biceps	Musculocultaneous	C5, C6
Triceps	Triceps	Radial	C6, C7, C8
Pectoralis	Pectoralis major	Pectoral	C6, C7, C8
Brachioradialis	Brachioradialis	Radial	C5, C6
Finger flexors	Flexor digitorum	Median and ulnar	C7, C8, T1
Knee	Quadriceps femoris	Femoral	L2, L3, L4
Adductor	Adductors	Obturator	L2, L3, L4
Ankle	Soleus/gastrocneumius	Sciatic/tibial	S1, S2
Plantar	Small foot muscles	Plantar	

DOCUMENTATION OF DATA

After completing the nursing history and assessment, organize, all assessment data to identify actual and potential health problems, make nursing diagnosis, plan appropriate care, and evaluate the patients responses to treatment.

BIBLIOGRAPHY

1. *Beckley LS. Bates' Guide to Physical Examination and History Taking. 8th edition. Wolters Kluwar; 2018.*
2. *Taylor C et al. Fundamentals of Nursing. 1st edition. JB Lippincott Company. 1989.*
3. *White L. Basic Nursing. Foundations of Nursing Skills and Concepts. Delmar Thomson Learning; 2002. p. 919.*
4. *Perry AG, Potter PA. Basic Nursing Essentials for Practice, 5th edition. Elsevier Publications; 2003.*
5. *Craven RF, Hirnle CJ. Fundamentals of Nursing Human Health and Function, 3rd edition. Lippincott Publishers; 2000.*

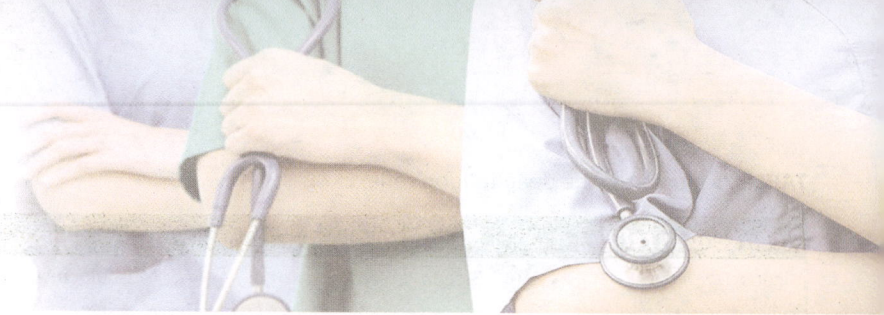

Chapter

16

General Health Assessment

Learning Objectives

After completing this chapter, you will be able to:

- Describe the preparation of patient and the environment for doing health assessment
- Identify the equipment and positions used during a physical assessment
- Use techniques of inspection, palpation, percussion, and auscultation appropriately during physical assessment

Key Terms

- Inspection
- Palpation
- Percussion
- Auscultation
- Olfaction

Chapter Outline

- Introduction
- Physical Health Assessment
- Purposes of Physical Examination
- Role of Nurse in Physical Examination
- Methods of Examination
- General Survey

INTRODUCTION

Health assessment is an integral component of nursing care and is the foundation of the nursing process. The information from the nursing health assessment is used to formulate nursing diagnosis. Assessments are used to plan, implement and evaluate care to promote an optimal level of health through interventions to prevent illness, restore health and facilitate coping with disabilities or death. The information is also used to identify health problems that require interdisciplinary care or immediate referral to other health care providers.

Health assessment has two aspects:

- The nursing health history (discussed in chapter on nursing process).
- The physical examination which can be of three types:
  - Complete assessment when patient is admitted to health care agency.
  - Examination of body systems.
  - Examination of body area.

PHYSICAL HEALTH ASSESSMENT

A physical health assessment is the systematic collection of objective information. It is usually conducted in a head to toe sequence or a system sequence but can be adapted to meet the needs of the patient. It is often necessary to modify the sequence, positions, and specific assessment based on the patient's age, energy level, cognitive and physical state, as well as time constraints. Even when modified, the physical assessment should be conducted in an organized manner.

PURPOSES OF PHYSICAL EXAMINATION

- To obtain baseline data about the client's functional abilities.
- To supplement, confirm or refute data obtained in the nursing history.
- To obtain data that will help establish nursing diagnosis and plans of care.

- To evaluate the physiologic outcomes of health care and thus the progress of a client's health problems.
- To make clinical judgments about a client's health status
- To identify areas for health promotion and disease prevention.

ROLE OF NURSE IN PHYSICAL EXAMINATION

Preparation of the Client

Clients need to be explained about physical examination. The nurse should reassure the client as to where the examination will take place, why it is important, and what will happen. Instruct the client that all information gathered and documented during the assessment is kept confidential and only those health care providers, who have a legitimate need to know the client's information, will have an access to it. Health examinations are generally painless; however it is important to determine in advance about any positions that are contraindicated for a particular client. The nurse assists the client as needed to undress and put on a gown. Clients should empty their bladder before examination. This will help them to feel more relaxed and facilitates palpation of the abdomen and pubic area and if urine analysis is required, urine can be collected for that purpose.

Preparation of the Environment

It is necessary to prepare the environment before starting the assessment. The time for the physical assessment should be convenient to both the client and the nurse. The environment needs to be well lit and the equipment should be organized for efficient use. The room should be warm enough to be comfortable for the client. Providing privacy is important. Most of the people feel embarrassed if their bodies are exposed or if others can overhear or view them during the assessment. Culture, age and gender of both the client and the nurse influence how comfortable the client will be and what special arrangements might be needed. For example, if the client and nurse are of different genders, the client might prefer being examined by same gender person as that of the client.

Positioning

Several positions are frequently required during the physical assessment. It is important to consider the client's ability to assume a position. The client's physical condition, energy level and age should also be taken into consideration. Some positions are embarrassing and uncomfortable and therefore, should not be maintained for long. The assessment is organized so that several body areas can be assessed in one position, thus minimizing the number of position changes needed.

Draping

Drapes should be arranged so that only the area to be assessed is exposed and other body areas are covered. Drapes provide not only privacy but also warmth. Drapes are made of paper, cloth or bed linen.

Instrumentation

All equipment required for the health assessment should be clean, in good working order, and should be readily accessible.

Preparation of Equipment

Refer to Table 1 for purpose of various equipment.

TABLE 1: Purpose of various equipment

Equipment (Fig. 1)	Purposes
Sphygmomanometer	To measure blood pressure
Stethoscope	To listen to the body sounds
Fetoscope	To listen the fetal heart sounds FHS
Temperature, Pulse, Respiration (TPR) tray	To assess the vital signs
Tongue depressor	To examine the mouth and throat
Pharyngeal retractor	To examine the larynx
Tape measure	To measure height, circumference of the head and abdomen
Flash light	To visualize any part
Weight machine	To check the weight
Ophthalmoscope	To examine the inner part of the eye ball
Otoscope	To examine the ear
Tuning fork	To test the hearing
Nasal speculum	To examine the nostrils
Percussion hammer, safety pins, cotton wool, cold and hot water in test tubes	To test reflexes and neurological examination
Vaginal speculum	To examine the genitals in women
Proctoscope	To examine the rectum
Gloves	To examine the pelvis internally
Sterile specimen bottles, slides, cotton applicators	To collect the specimens, if necessary
Thermometer	To check body temperature

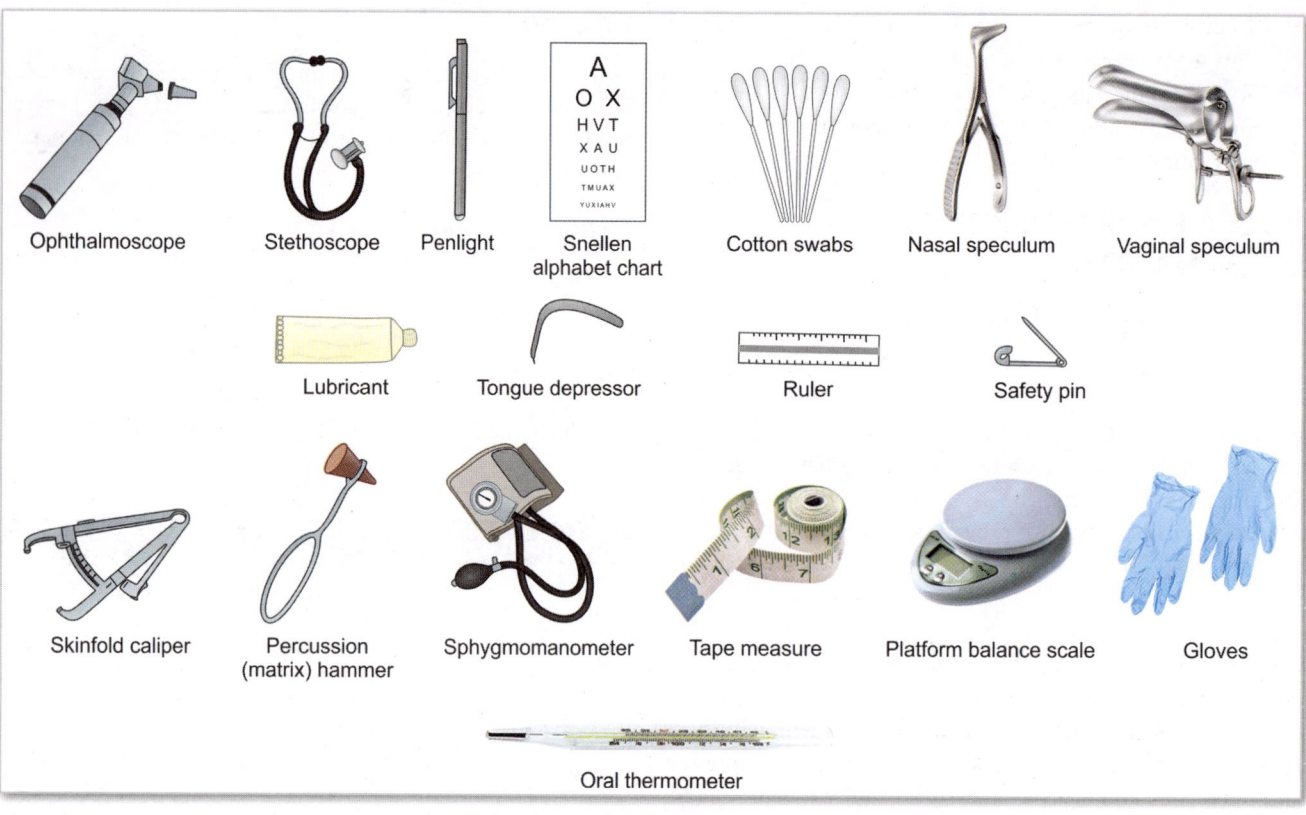

Fig. 1: Equipment used for physical examination

METHODS OF EXAMINATION

There are four methods of examination: Inspection, palpation, percussion and auscultation. Olfaction is another method of examination.

Inspection

Inspection is the visual examination, that is, assessing by using sense of sight. The nurse inspects with the naked eye and with a lighted instrument such as ophthalmoscope (used to view interior of the eye). In addition to visual observations, olfactory (smell) and auditory (hearing) cues are noted. Nurses frequently use visual inspection to assess size, shape, moisture, color, and symmetry of the body. Lighting must be sufficient to see clearly; either natural or artificial. When using the auditory senses, it is important to have a quiet environment for accurate hearing. Observation can be combined with the other assessment techniques.

Palpation

Palpation is the examination of the body using the sense of touch. The pads of fingers are used because the concentration of nerve endings makes them highly sensitive to tactile discrimination. Palpation is used to determine:

- Texture (e.g., of hair).
- Temperature (e.g., of a skin area).
- Vibration (e.g., of a joint).
- Position, size, consistency, and mobility of organs or masses.
- Distention (e.g., of urinary bladder).
- Pulsation.
- Presence of pain upon pressure.

There are two types of palpation, light and deep. Light (superficial) palpation should always precede deep palpation. For light palpation, (Fig. 2) the nurse extends the dominant hand's fingers parallel to the skin surface and presses gently while moving the hand in a circle. With light palpation, the skin is slightly depressed. If it is necessary to determine the details of a mass (Box 1) the nurse presses lightly several times rather than holding the pressure.

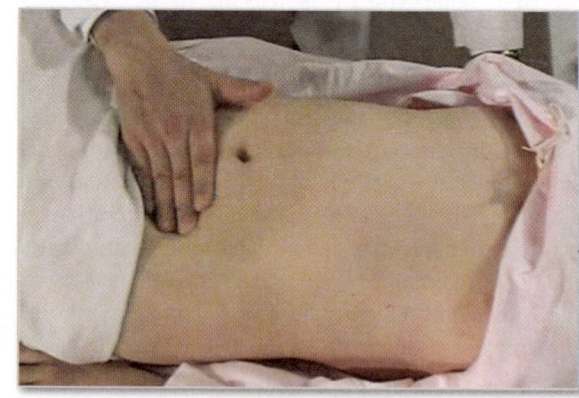

Fig. 2: Light palpation

Characteristics of Masses

➤ **Location:** Site of the body, dorsal/ventral surface
➤ **Size:** Length and width in centimeters
➤ **Shape:** Oval, round, elongated, irregular
➤ **Consistency:** Soft, firm, hard
➤ **Surface:** Smooth, nodular
➤ **Pulsatility:** Present or absent
➤ **Mobility:** Fixed, mobile
➤ **Tenderness:** Degree of tenderness to palpation.

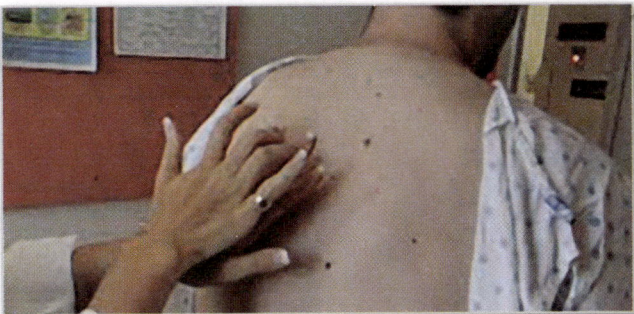

Fig. 4: Percussion

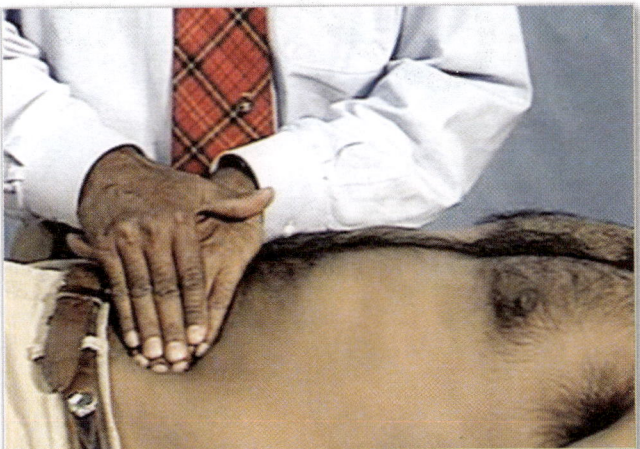

Fig. 3: Deep palpation

Deep palpation is done with two hands (bimanually) (Fig. 3) or one hand. In deep bimanual palpation, the nurse extends the dominant hand as for light palpation, then places the finger pads of the non-dominant hand on the dorsal surface of the distal surface of the distal interphalangeal joint of the middle three fingers of the dominant hand.

The top hand applies pressure while the lower hand remains relaxed to perceive the tactile sensations. For deep palpation using one hand, the finger pads of the dominant hand press over the area to be palpated. Often the other hand is used to support a mass or organ from below.

Deep palpation is usually not done during a routine examination and requires significant skill. It is performed with extreme caution because pressure can damage internal organs. It is usually not indicated in clients, who have acute abdominal pain or pain that is not yet diagnosed.

To test temperature, it is best to use the dorsum or back of the hand and fingers, where the skin is thinnest.

To test for vibration, the nurse should use the palmar surface of the hand.

For doing palpation:
♦ The hands of the nurse should be clean and warm, and the fingernails should be short.

♦ Areas of tenderness should be palpated first.
♦ Deep palpation should be done after superficial palpation. The effectiveness of palpation depends largely on the client's relaxation. Nurses can assist a client to relax by:
  ▪ Gowning or draping the client appropriately.
  ▪ Positioning the client comfortably.
  ▪ Ensuring that their own hands are warm.
♦ During palpation, the nurse should be sensitive to the client's verbal and nonverbal (facial) expressions indicating discomfort.

Percussion

Percussion is the act of striking the body surface to elicit sound that can be heard or vibrations that can be felt. There are two types of percussion: direct and indirect.

In **direct percussion,** the nurse strikes the area to be percussed directly with the pads of two, three or four fingers or with the pad of middle finger. The strikes are rapid, and the movement is from the wrist. It is useful in percussing adult's sinuses (Fig. 4).

Indirect percussion is striking a finger held against the body area to be examined. In this technique, the middle finger of the non-dominant hand, referred to as the pleximeter, is placed firmly on the client's skin. Only the distal phalanx and joint of this finger should be in contact with the skin. Using the tip of the flexed middle finger of the other hand, called the plexor, the nurse strikes the pleximeter, usually at the distal interphalangeal joint. The angle between the plexor and the pleximeter should be 90 degrees, and the blows must be firm, rapid, and short to obtain a clear sound. Percussion is used to determine the size and shape of the internal organs by establishing their borders. It indicates whether tissue is fluid-filled, air-filled or solid. Percussion elicits five types of sound: Dullness, flatness, resonance, hyper-resonance and tympany (Table 2).

TABLE 2: Percussion sounds and location

Sound	Intensity	Quality	Location
Flatness	Soft	Extremely dull	Muscle, bone
Dullness	Medium	Thud-like	Liver, heart
Resonance	Loud	Hallow	Normal lung
Hyper-resonance	Very loud	Booming	Emphysematous lung
Tympany	Loud	Musical	Stomach filled with gas/air

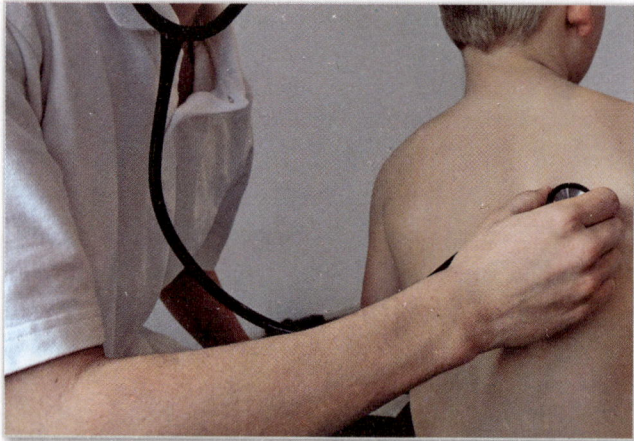

Fig. 5: Auscultation

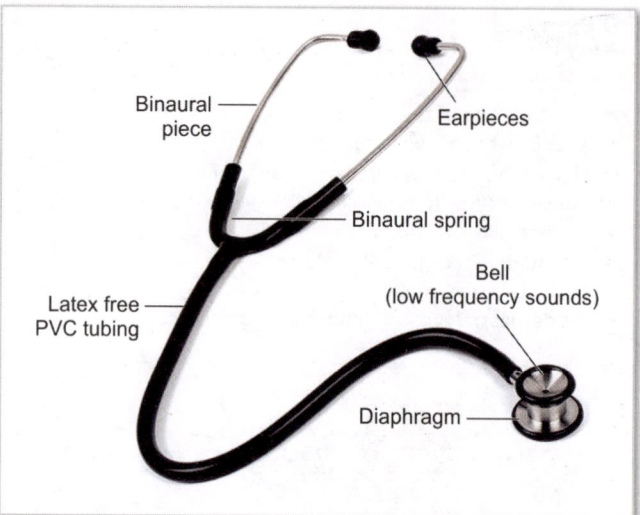

Fig. 6: Stethoscope

Auscultation

Auscultation is the process of listening to sounds produced within the body. It may be direct or indirect. Direct auscultation is use of the unaided ear, for example, to listen to a respiratory wheeze or the grating of a moving joint (Fig. 5).

Indirect auscultation is performed by placing the diaphragm or bell of stethoscope against the body part being assessed. The stethoscope in used primarily to listen to sounds from within the body, such as bowel sounds or valve sounds of the heart and blood pressure (Fig. 6).

The diaphragm best transmits high pitched sounds, e.g., bronchial sounds and the bell best transmits low-pitched sounds such as some heart sounds. If the client has excessive hair, it may be necessary to dampen the hair with a moist cloth so that they will lie flat against the skin and not interfere with clear sound transmission.

Four characteristics of sound are assessed by auscultation

- Pitch (ranging from high to low).
- Intensity, loudness ranging from soft to loud.
- Quality, e.g., gurgling, swishing, whistling.
- Duration as short, medium or long.

For auscultation, the nurse should expose the part to be listened to, use the proper part of the stethoscope and listen in quiet environment.

Olfaction

Olfaction means assessing the patient with the source of body odor. Olfaction helps to detect abnormalities that cannot be recognized by other means. For example, there is fruity smell from oral cavity in a patient with diabetic ketoacidosis or presence of alcohol smell, in which alcohol intoxication can be suspected.

GENERAL SURVEY

Health assessment begins with a general survey that involves observation of the client's general appearance and mental status, measurement of vital signs, height and weight. Many components of the general survey are assessed while taking the client's health history, such as the client's body build, posture, hygiene and mental status.

Note proportion of height and weight, which provides insight into nutritional status. Observe whether the patient has an erect or slumped posture and evaluate movements and gait pattern for coordination. Uncoordinated or spontaneous movements may suggest neurologic problems. Note signs of illness, such as changes in posture, skin color, and respirations, nonverbal communication of pain or distress and short attention span, observe hygiene and grooming and note any deficits, e.g., patients with inappropriate dress (wrong for the season) or dirty/torn clothes, etc. Assess speech content and pattern, orientation to time, place and person and appropriate verbal responses (cognitive processes).

Clues to mood and mental health are provided by speech, facial expressions, ability to relax, eye contact and behavior.

Vital Signs

Vital signs are measured to establish baseline data against which to compare future measurements and to detect actual and potential health problems. Vital signs are discussed in detail in Unit IX (Fig. 7).

Height and Weight

The ratio of height to weight is an assessment of overall health and over nutrition or under nutrition. Height and weight should be measured using accurate scales and measuring devices. If the patient cannot stand erect, weight can be obtained using a chair or bed scale. The patient's actual height and weight can be compared with recommended average weights or from a standardized reference chart (Table 3).

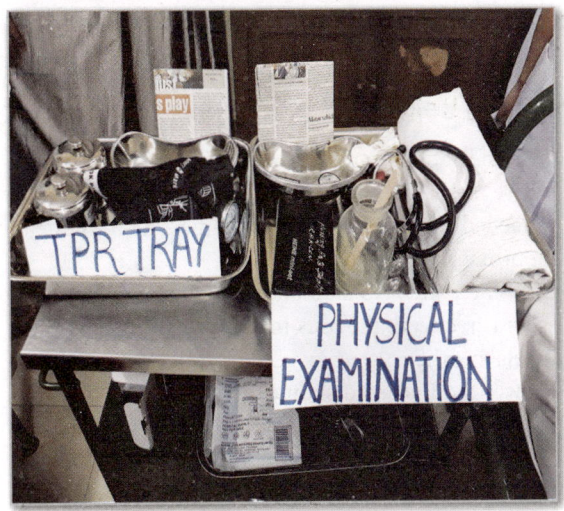

Fig. 7: TPR and physical examination tray

TABLE 3: Height and weight table

Male			Female		
Height in feet	**Height in meter**	**Ideal weight**	**Height in feet**	**Height in meter**	**Ideal weight**
4'6"	1.3524	28–35 kg	4'6"	1.3524	28–35 kg
4'7"	1.3778	30–39 kg	4'7"	1.3778	30–37 kg
4'8"	1.4052	33–40 kg	4'8"	1.4052	32–40 kg
4'9"	1.4286	35–44 kg	4'9"	1.4286	35–42 kg
4'10"	1.454	38–46 kg	4'10"	1.454	36–45 kg
4'11"	1.4794	40–50 kg	4'11"	1.4794	39–47 kg
5'0"	1.5	43–53 kg	5'0"	1.5	40–50 kg
5'1"	1.5254	45–55 kg	5'1"	1.5254	43–52 kg
5'2"	1.5503	48–59 kg	5'2"	1.5503	45–55 kg
5'3"	1.5762	50–61 kg	5'3"	1.5762	47–57 kg
5'4"	1.6016	53–65 kg	5'4"	1.6016	49–60 kg
5'5"	1.627	55–65 kg	5'5"	1.627	51–62 kg
5'6"	1.6524	58–70 kg	5'6"	1.6524	53–65 kg
5'7"	1.6778	60–74 kg	5'7"	1.6778	55–67 kg
5'8"	1.7032	63-70 kg	5'8"	1.7032	57–70 kg
5'9"	1.7286	65–80 kg	5'9"	1.7286	59–72 kg
5'10"	1.754	67–83 kg	5'10"	1.754	61–75 kg
5'11"	1.7794	70–85 kg	5'11"	1.7794	63–77 kg
6'1"	1.8	72–89 kg	6'1"	1.8	65–80 kg

Children up to 2 years of age should have their height measured in the recumbent position with the legs fully extended. Infants should be weighed without clothing.

Obtaining Height and Weight with an Upright Balance Scale

Obtaining Height

- Ask the patient to remove shoes.
- Raise L-shaped sliding arm on the measuring device attached to the scale little higher than the patient's approximate height.
- Ask the patient to step on the platform of the scale and stand erect with the back to the measuring device and the heels together.
- Lower the L-shaped sliding arm till it rests on top of the patient's head.
- Read the height in inches and record.
- Ask the patient to step down from the platform.

Obtaining Weight

- Balance the scale on zero.
- Ask the patient to remove shoes and heavy clothing and step onto the platform.
- Move the sliding indicator to the left until the scale balances.
- Read the weight in kgs and record.
- Ask the patient to step down from the platform.
- Return the scale weight indicator to zero.

Note: Daily weights should be obtained at the same-time each day preferably early morning, with the patient wearing the same clothing, and using the same scale.

BIBLIOGRAPHY

1. Beckley LS. Bates' Guide to Physical Examination and History Taking. 8th edition. Wolters Kluwar; 2018.
2. Taylor C et al. Fundamentals of Nursing. 1st edition. JB Lippincott Company. 1989.
3. White L. Basic Nursing. Foundations of Nursing Skills and Concepts. Delmar Thomson Learning; 2002. p. 919.
4. Perry AG, Potter PA. Basic Nursing Essentials for Practice, 5th edition. Elsevier Publications; 2003.
5. Craven RF, Hirnle CJ. Fundamentals of Nursing Human Health and Function, 3rd edition. Lippincott Publishers; 2000.

Nursing Process

INTRODUCTION

The idea that nursing is a process rather than a set of separate actions, started to emerge in the United States in 1950s.

In 1955, Lydia Hall had presented "Nursing is a Process" to a group of nurses in New Jersey. She defined use of four propositions, nursing at the patient, nursing to the patients, nursing for the patient and nursing with the patient, which described the range in quality of care. In 1960, Orlando first used the term nursing process. She identified nursing situation comprising of three elements:

- Behavior of the patient
- Reaction of the nursing
- Nursing actions designed for the patients benefit. The interaction of these elements is the nursing process.

In 1966, Lois Knowles presented a model of the nursing activities. She suggested that the nurses' success as a practitioner depends on her mastery of 5 Ds. These are:

- **Discover:** She acquires knowledge or information about something that she did not know previously such information should contribute to better patient care.

- **Delve:** She derives information from as many sources as possible to provide data about the client.
- **Decide:** She plans the approach to be used in the client's care.
- **Do:** She administers, and performs activities.
- **Discriminate:** She distinguishes priorities.

In 1967, Yura and Walsh published the first comprehensive book on nursing process, in which they described four steps in the nursing process; assessment, planning, intervention and evaluation. They viewed the element of nursing diagnosis as the logical conclusion of the assessment phase, whereas Gebbie and Lavin (1974) made nursing diagnosis a separate step in the process. This led to the development of the five step nursing process commonly used today, assessment, nursing diagnosis, planning, implementation and evaluation.

In 1973, the steps of nursing process were legitimized, when the American Nurses Association (ANA) Congress of Nursing Practice developed standards of practice to guide nursing performance.

In 1982, the state board examinations for professional nursing practice underwent major revisions and began to use the nursing process as an organizing concept. The revised examinations are structured to test the practitioners' ability to assess patients, to diagnose health problems amenable to nursing therapy, and to plan, implement, and evaluate nursing care.

NURSING PROCESS

Nursing process is a systematic and dynamic method of providing care to client; whether the client is an individual, group, family or community.

"The nursing process is an orderly systematic manner of determining the client's problem, making plan to solve them, initiating the plan or assigning others to implement it and evaluating the extent to which the plan was effective in resolving the problem identified."   —*Yura, Helen and Walsh*

The process provides framework that enables the nurse and patient to accomplish the following:

- Systematically collecting patient data (assessing).
- Clearly identifying patient's strengths and actual and potential problems (diagnosing).
- Developing a holistic plan of individualized care that specifies the desired patient goals and related outcomes and the nursing interventions most likely to assist the patient to meet those expected outcomes (planning).
- Executing the plan of care (implementing).
- Evaluating the effectiveness of the plan of care in terms of patient goal achievement (evaluating).

ELEMENTS/STEPS/PHASES OF NURSING PROCESS

The steps in nursing process are patient-centered and outcome-oriented. Nursing process is dynamic and inter-related. Each of the five steps depend on the accuracy of the preceding step (Fig. 1).

CHARACTERISTICS OF NURSING PROCESS

Systematic

Each nursing activity is part of an ordered sequence of activities. Each activity depends on the accuracy of the activity that precedes it and influences the actions that follow it. The nursing process directs each step of nursing care in a sequential and orderly manner.

Dynamic

There is a great interaction and overlapping among the five steps. No single step in the nursing process is one-time phenomenon; each step flows into the next step. In some nursing situations, all five stages occur almost simultaneously.

Interpersonal

The nursing process encourages nurses to work together to help patients use their strengths to meet all their human needs,

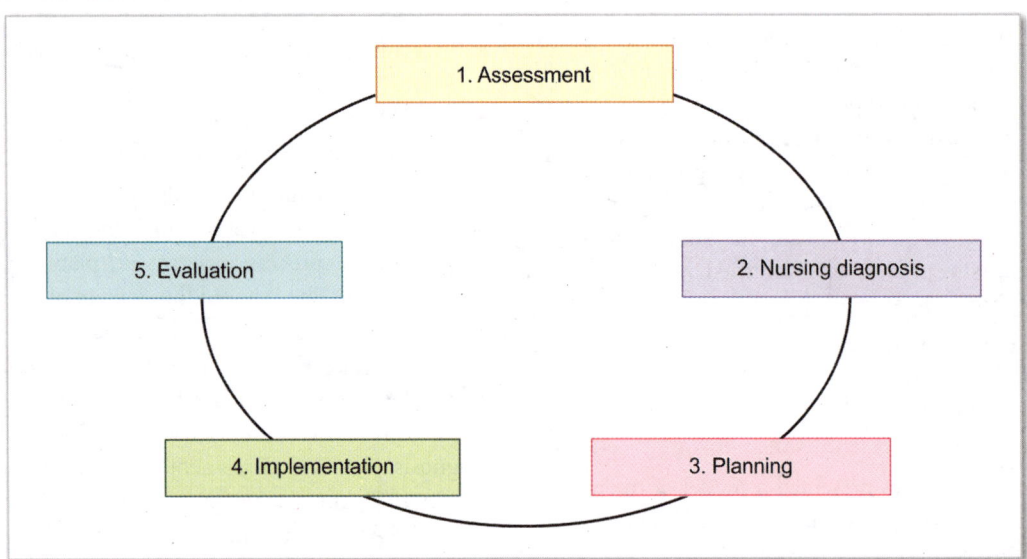

Fig 1: Five-step nursing process

working intimately with patients helps nurses to explore their own strengths and limitations and to develop themselves personally and professionally.

Outcome-Oriented

The nursing process offers means for nurses and patients to work together to identify specific outcomes related to health promotion, disease and illness prevention, health restoration and coping with altered functioning; to determine which outcomes are most important to the patient; and to match them with appropriate nursing actions.

Universally Applicable in Nursing Situations

When nurses have a working knowledge of the nursing process, they find that they can practice nursing with healthy or sick people, young or old or in any type of practice setting.

BENEFITS OF THE NURSING PROCESS

For the Patient

Nursing process achieves individualized care which is scientifically based, holistic, provides continuity of care and works in collaboration with other nurses. It is also cost-effective plan of action.

For the Nurses

The nurses can achieve the best results, have more satisfaction by making 'difference' in the lives of their patients and opportunity to grow professionally as they evaluate the effectiveness of interventions.

BIBLIOGRAPHY

1. Berman AT, Snyder S, Kozier BJ, et al. Kozier & Erb's. Fundamentals of Nursing: Concepts, Process and Practice, 8th edition. Pearson Education.
2. Shortridge LM, Lal JE. Introduction to Nursing Practice, McGraw Hill Book company, 1980.
3. Christensen BL, Kockrow OE. Foundations of Nursing, Mosby; 2003. p. 764.

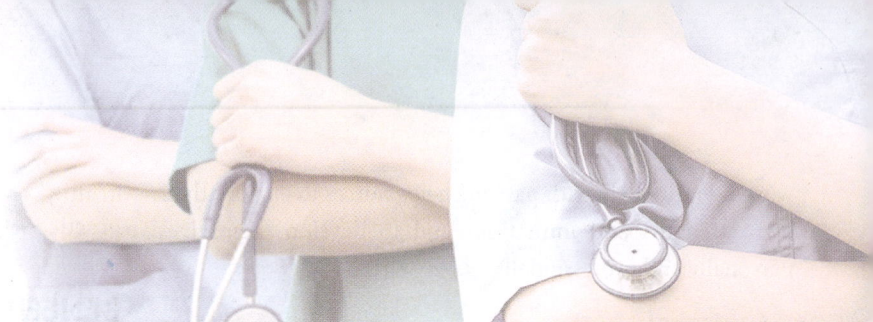

Assessment

INTRODUCTION

Assessment involves data collection and analysis of data. It begins with the nurse's first encounter with the patient. Assessment is the first step of the nursing process. The immediate purpose of assessment is to collect information about the patient's needs or problems, construct a database and identify problems or nursing care needs of the patient.

In collecting data relevant to nursing, subjective and objective data are collected to incorporate patient's perception of his problems and needs, along with observations, findings and results obtained by the nurse.

TYPES OF DATA

- **Subjective data:** It is obtained directly from the patient and elicits information about:
  - How patient feels
  - Difficulties of the patient
  - Problems expressed by the patient
  - Complaints of patient
- **Objective data:** Refers to information based on observation of the nurse and examination of the patient.

SOURCES OF DATA

The data can be collected from patient, family members, records, reports and health team members. Data relevant to nursing is obtained by taking nursing history and by performing a physical assessment.

METHODS OF DATA COLLECTION

The primary methods used to collect data are: Observing, interviewing, and examining.

- **Observation** is the conscious and deliberate use of senses (vision, smell and hearing) to gather data. Observation occurs whenever the nurse is in contact with the client or support persons. Skilled nurses use each nurse–patient interaction to observe and to interpret meaningful stimuli. One can develop such observation skills by training to observe carefully each time you encounter with the patient. For example, what are the patients current responses (physical or emotional) to his/her situation.

Be alert to signs of distress-difficulty in breathing, bleeding, pain, increased anxiety, or sudden eruption of rash or changes in the level of consciousness.

What is the patients current ability to manage his or her care (need for additional information or nursing assistance)?

Consider the immediate environment in terms of safety, functioning of equipment, etc.

- **Interview** is used mainly while taking the nursing health history. It is a planned communication or a communication with a purpose. There are two approaches to interviewing:
  (i) The directive interview—is highly structured and directly ask the questions and the nurse controls the interview.
  (ii) A nondirective interview or rapport building interview and the nurse allows the client to control the interview.

Phases of Interview

- **Preparatory phase:** During this phase, the nurse ensures that the environment in which the interview is to be conducted is private and relaxed. It is best to communicate with patient at eye level, so the sitting arrangement should be such which facilitates an easy exchange of information. The interview should be scheduled when both the nurse and the patient are free of concerns and distractions so that they can concentrate on the task.

- **Introductory phase:** The nurse initates the interview by stating his or her name and status, identifying the purpose of the interview. During the introduction, the nurse should assess the patients comfort and ability to participate in interview. It is also appropriate to assure the client of confidentiality.

- **Working phase:** The nurse gathers all the information needed to form the subjective data base. The accuracy, completeness and relevance of the data base depends on the use of the interviewing and basic communication techniques. Many patient variables such as high anxiety, pain, language difficulty, previous negative experience with nurses and unrealistic expectation can positively or negatively affect the outcome of an interview, unless the nurse responds appropriately.

- **Termination phase:** The successful interview is concluded carefully. The nurse should advise the patient that the interview is coming to an end. It is helpful to recapitulate the interview, highlighting key points.

- **Examining:** This includes physical assessment. The nursing physical assessment involves the examination of all body systems commonly using a head-to-toe format.

  The nursing physical assessment should be performed in an organized, systematic manner in conjunction with the nursing interview. It is accomplished by:

  - **Inspection:** Examination by careful and critical observation.
  - **Auscultation:** Examination by listening with a stethoscope.
  - **Palpation:** Examination by touching and feeling.
  - **Percussion:** Examination by touching, tapping and listening.
  - **Olfaction:** Assessing with the source of body odor, e.g., alcohol smell, fruity smell (diabetic ketoacidosis).

Organization of Data

The nurse uses a format that organizes the assessment data systematically. This is often referred to as nursing health history or nursing assessment form.

Choose a method of organizing your data collection. It the person states, "I can't breathe" assess the respiratory system first. Continue in following order:

- **Respiratory status:** Breath sounds, rate, depth, cough.
- **Cardiac status:** Apical rate, rhythm, heart sounds.
- **Circulatory status:** Rate, rhythm, and quality of pulse (radical, brachial, carotid, femoral).
- **Status of the skin:** Color temperature, turgor, edema, lesions and hair distribution.
- **Neurological status:** Mental status, orientation, pupillary reaction, vision, ability to hear, taste, feel and smell.
- **Musculoskeletal status:** Muscle tone, strength, gait, stability, range of motion, gag reflex, bowel sounds, presence of distention.
- **Gastrointestinal status:** Condition of lips, tongue, gums, teeth, presence of gag reflex, bowel sounds, abdominal distension, tenderness, impaction.
- **Genitourinary status:** Presence of distended bladder, discharge from vagina, urethra.

Validation of Data

The information gathered during the assessment is "double checked" or verified to confirm that it is accurate and complete.

Interpreting Data

Distinguish relevant and irrelevant data. Determine whether and where there are gaps in the data. Identify patterns of cause and effect.

Documentation of Data

To complete the assessment phase, the nurse records client data. Accurate documentation is essential and should include all data collected about the clients health status.

COMPONENTS OF DATABASE

Nursing History

It is a systematic way of collecting relevant nursing information, which is useful for planning nursing care of the patient. It is required to identify both assets and deficits of patient in order to identify problems, which require nursing assistance. Also, identify areas where data is incomplete or needs to be validated.

Purposes

- To collect patient's information in a systematic way.
- To assess patient's needs.
- To make nursing diagnosis.
- To plan and give nursing care depending upon priority of needs.

Methods of Collecting History

- Questionnaire technique, e.g., checklist.
- Interview technique: Structured and semistructured schedule.

Content of Nursing History

- Biographic profile of patient.
- Source of information.
- Chief complaint.
- Medical and post-surgical history.
- Family history of any illness.
- Personal lifestyle, e.g., habit, liking.
- Medication/history of allergy.
- History of alcohol and substance abuse.
- Social history: occupation, income, insurance.
- Pattern of daily living.

Transcultural Issues

- Related to culturally based health beliefs and practices.
- A systematic physical, mental and functional assessment.

ANALYSIS OF DATA

Collected data are analyzed and interpreted utilizing the knowledge of biology and behavioral sciences. Patient's strengths and health problems are analyzed that independent nursing intervention can prevent or resolve. A prioritized list of nursing diagnosis in the form of actual and potential problems is developed. Actual problems are those which the patient is having at present and potential problems are those which the patient is likely to develop in due course of time.

BIBLIOGRAPHY

1. Berman AT, Snyder S, Kozier BJ, et al. Kozier & Erb's. Fundamentals of Nursing: Concepts, Process and Practice, 8th edition. Pearson Education.
2. Shortridge LM, Lal JE. Introduction to Nursing Practice, McGraw Hill Book company, 1980.
3. Christensen BL, Kockrow OE. Foundations of Nursing, Mosby; 2003. p. 764.

Nursing Diagnosis

INTRODUCTION

Nursing diagnosis is a statement of client's health status or problem which can be solved by nursing actions. The process of arriving at a nursing diagnosis involves decision making based on intuitive reasoning, experience and sound theoretical foundation in biological and social sciences.

It is the conclusion reached, based on an analysis of patient's database.

IDENTIFICATION OF CLIENT PROBLEMS

This is most vital step in nursing process, since planning, implementation and evaluation depend on this.

Data Analysis

Data is critically examined for health problem

- Any additional information required to be checked.
- Conflicting information need to be clarified.
- Look for cues which will be significant in decision making.

Data Synthesis

It is the clustering or linking together of cues resulting from the data analysis to determine which cues can be clustered together to form a pattern (Fig. 1).

Nursing Diagnosis

It is a clinical judgment about individual, family or community responses to actual health problems and potential health problems.

A Nursing diagnosis is a statement of a patient problem that is arrived at by making inferences from the collected data.

Nursing diagnosis provides the basic for selection of nursing intervention to achieve outcomes for which the nurse is accountable.

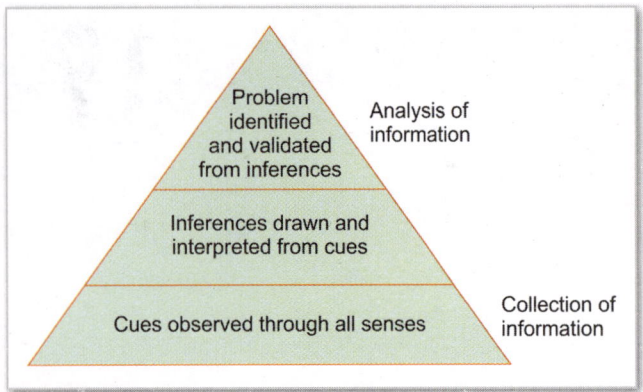

Fig 1: Outline of problem identification based on assessment

Parts of the Diagnostic Statement

A nursing diagnostic statement consists of two parts:
(i) Problem of the client and (ii) the related factor (contributing factor)

♦ **The problem:** The problem is the statement and as identified by the nurse during the assessment phase. The nurse needs to consider two areas while identifying the problem. What is the problem that is inferred by assessment data?

For example:

- Feeling of loneliness.
- Client worried about surgery planned for the next day.
- High glucose level due to lack of knowledge about right selection of food items.
- Pupil dilated with medicine for eye testing.
- Not able to sleep at night.

To what degree is the problem present?

A degree of problem can be explained as:

For example:

- Postoperative patient, a first day require assistance to brush his teeth.
- A malnourished child is at risk for acquiring infection, hypothermia.
- A nurse observes indifferent behavior of mother toward the child.

♦ **The related factor:** The related factors are "Conditions or circumstances that can cause or contribute to the development of a diagnosis."

Examples of related factors:

♦ **Environmental:** Excessive noise, light fumes, pollutants.
♦ **Psychological:** Fear of death, feeling of loneliness, impaired parent–child bonding.
♦ **Socio-cultural:** Inability to procure food, lack of support system, lack of finances, literacy level.
♦ **Physiological:** Breathing difficulty, loss of skin integrity, abnormal fluid/blood loss, sensory deficit.
♦ **Spiritual:** Conflict between religion, beliefs and prescribed health region, inability to practice religious rituals.

Writing the Diagnostic Statement

Nurse can determine the problem by considering the list of NANDA nursing diagnosis. There are several ways to state nursing diagnosis. The widely accepted statement suggests PES of writing the nursing diagnosis.

P Stands for the problems—in clear, concise statement of clients existing or potential health problem or unhealthy response. The statement of problem provides a clear indication of what needs to change.

E Stands for etiology explaining the factors believed to be related to or contributing to the health problem. The related factors are the socioeconomical environmental, physiological, psychological and spiritual factors.

S Refer to the signs and symptoms identified during assessment. These signs and symptoms from the basis for nursing inferences and subsequent nursing diagnosis. They are recorded in the data base.

Example:

♦ First write actual or high risk health problem and not an environmental problem. State environmental factors in the second part, e.g., sensory perceptual alterations (auditory and visual) related to excessive environmental stimuli.

♦ Do not write several unrelated problems in the first part even though the related factor of the problem may be the same, e.g.:
  - Activity intolerance related to frequent episodes of chest pain
  - Anxiety related to frequent episodes of chest pain.

♦ Write the diagnostic statement in a manner that both the problem and related factors refer to different findings, e.g., self-feeding deficit related to muscle weakness

♦ Write the diagnosis in legally advisable terms, e.g., ineffective airway clearance related to effects of sedation.

♦ Write the nursing diagnosis in terms of response rather than the need, e.g., altered nutrition (less than body requirements) related to nausea and vomiting.

♦ Use nonjudgmental language.

♦ Be sure the problem statement indicates what is unhealthy about the patient.

Examples using PES:

♦ Disturbance of self-esteem (problem) related to altered body image (loss of arm) (etiology) manifested by crying and hostility (signs and symptoms).

- Anticipatory grieving (problem) related to husbands terminal illness (etiology) manifested by anorexia and withdrawal behavior (signs and symptoms).
- Altered family processes (problem) related to mothers hospitalization (etiology) manifested by son's unmet physical and emotional needs (signs and symptoms).

Validating Nursing Diagnosis

After a tentative nursing diagnosis is formulated, it should be validated. An affirmative response to each of the following questions validates tentative diagnosis.

- Is my data base sufficient, accurate?
- Does my synthesis of data (significant cues) demonstrate the existence of a pattern?
- Are the subjective and objective data I used to determine the existence of pattern characteristic of the health problem defined?
- Is my tentative nursing diagnosis able to be prevented, reduced, or resolved by independent nursing action?
- Is my degree of confidence above 50% that other qualified practitioners would formulate the same nursing diagnosis on my data?

Remember that you are responsible for validating the diagnosis you write, even when using computer assisted diagnosis. The use of standardized language and electronic health records may make diagnosis writing easier by suggesting possible diagnosis to match your recorded assessment findings. However, computers cannot replace humans and critical thinking, especially when it comes to complex diagnostic reasoning. While the computer can process data faster than you can, it may not be aware of what is happening to your patient at this moment. You need to validate diagnosis. In addition, patients who are able to participate in decision making should be encouraged to validate the diagnosis.

Documenting Nursing Diagnosis

The nurse documents validated nursing diagnosis in the patient record. The statement must also be included on nurses notes or progress notes. Diagnostic statements are reviewed and revised when it is necessary.

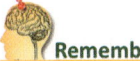

Remember
- The nursing diagnosis must be developed from the data, never the other way round.
- Do not try to fit a client to a nursing diagnosis, rather select the appropriate diagnosis from the data cues presented by the client.

DIFFERENCES BETWEEN MEDICAL AND NURSING DIAGNOSES

Refer to Table 1 for differentiating points between medical and nursing diagnoses.

To facilitate the development of standard nursing language, the groups involved are: North American Nursing Diagnosis Association (NANDA), Nursing Interventions Classification (NIC) and Nursing Sensitive Out-comes Classification (NOC).

TABLE 1: Differentiating points between medical and nursing diagnoses

Medical diagnosis	Nursing diagnosis
• Identifies conditions the physician is licensed and qualified to treat	• Identifies situations the nurse is licensed and qualified to treat
• Focuses on the illness, disease, injury, etc.	• Focuses on the client's responses to actual or potential health problems or life processes
• Remains constant until the cure, e.g., Cancer cervix • Amputation • Diarrhea/ Dysentery • Cerebrovascular accident	• Changes as the clients responds to the health problem changes, e.g., Deficient knowledge, Ineffective coping • Disturbed body image • Fluid volume deficit Electrolyte imbalance • Activity intolerance • Altered nutritional status • Altered skin integrity

TYPES OF NURSING DIAGNOSES

The four types of NANDA nursing diagnoses are Actual (Problem-Focused), Risk, Health promotion, and Syndrome.

1. **A problem-focused diagnosis** (also known as actual diagnosis) is a client problem that is present at the time of the nursing assessment. These diagnoses are based on the presence of associated signs and symptoms. Examples are:
   - Ineffective breathing pattern
   - Anxiety
   - Acute pain

2. **Risk diagnosis** are clinical judgment that a problem does not exist, but the presence of risk factors indicates that a problem is likely to develop unless nurses intervene. The individual (or group) is more susceptible to develop the problem than others in the same or a similar situation because of risk factors. Examples are:
   - Risk for falls
   - Risk for injury

3. **Health promotion diagnosis** (also known as wellness diagnosis) is a clinical judgment about motivation and desire to increase well-being. Health promotion diagnosis is concerned in the individual, family, or community transition from a specific level of wellness to a higher level of wellness. Examples are:
   - Readiness for enhanced spiritual well-being
   - Readiness for enhanced family coping

4. A **syndrome diagnosis** is a clinical judgment concerning with a cluster of problem or risk nursing diagnoses that are predicted to present because of a certain situation or event. Examples are:
   - Chronic pain syndrome
   - Post-trauma syndrome
   - Frail elderly syndrome

NANDA-APPROVED NURSING DIAGNOSES (2018–20)

This list represents the NANDA-approved nursing diagnoses for clinical use and testing.

Domain 1: Health Promotion

Description

The awareness of well-being or normality of function and the strategies used to maintain control of and enhance that well-being or normality of function.

Approved Diagnoses

- Ineffective self-health management.
- Ineffective family therapeutic regimen management.
- In effective health maintenance.
- Impaired home maintenance.
- Readiness for enhanced self-health management.
- Readiness for enhanced nutrition.
- Readiness for enhanced immunization status.
- Self-neglect.

Domain 2: Nutrition

Description

The activities of taking in, assimilating, and using nutrients for the purpose of tissue maintenance, tissue repair, and the production of energy.

Approved Diagnoses

- Ineffective infant feeding pattern.
- Impaired swallowing.
- **Imbalanced nutrition:** Less than body requirements.

- **Imbalanced nutrition:** More than body requirements.
- **Risk for imbalanced nutrition:** More than body requirements.
- Risk for impaired liver function.
- Risk for unstable blood glucose level.
- Neonatal jaundice.
- Deficient fluid volume.
- Risk for deficient fluid volume.
- Excess fluid volume.
- Readiness for enhanced fluid balance.
- Risk for electrolyte imbalance.
- Risk for imbalanced fluid volume.

Domain 3: Elimination and Exchange

Description

Secretion and excretion of waste products from the body.

Approved Diagnoses

- Impaired urinary elimination.
- Urinary retention.
- Functional urinary incontinence.
- Stress urinary incontinence.
- Urge urinary incontinence.
- Reflex urinary incontinence.
- Risk for urge urinary incontinence.
- Readiness for enhanced urinary elimination.
- Overflow urinary incontinence.
- Bowel incontinence.
- Diarrhea.
- Constipation.
- Risk for constipation.
- Perceived constipation.
- Dysfunctional gastrointestinal motility.
- Risk for dysfunctional gastrointestinal motility.
- Impaired gas exchange.
- Ineffective airway clearance.
- Impaired spontaneous ventilation.

Domain 4: Activity/Rest

Description

The production, conservation, expenditure or balance of energy resources.

Approved Diagnoses

- Sleep deprivation.
- Readiness for enhanced sleep.

- Insomnia.
- Disturbed sleep pattern.
- Risk for disuse syndrome.
- Impaired physical mobility.
- Impaired bed mobility.
- Impaired wheelchair mobility.
- Impaired transfer ability.
- Impaired walking.
- Deficient diversional activity.
- Delayed surgical recovery.
- Sedentary lifestyle.
- Disturbed energy field.
- Fatigue.
- Decreased cardiac output.
- Impaired spontaneous ventilation.
- Ineffective breathing pattern.
- Activity intolerance.
- Risk for activity intolerance.
- Dysfunctional ventilator weaning response.
- Risk for decreased cardiac tissue perfusion.
- Risk for ineffective cerebral tissue perfusion.
- Risk for ineffective gastrointestinal perfusion.
- Risk for tissue perfusion.
- Ineffective peripheral tissue perfusion.
- Risk for shock.
- Risk for bleeding.
- Dressing self-care deficit.
- Bathing self-care deficit.
- Feeding self-care deficit.
- Toileting self-care deficit.
- Readiness for enhanced self-care.

Domain 5: Perception/Cognition

Description

The human information-processing system, including attention, orientation, sensation, perception, cognition, and communication.

Approved Diagnoses

- Unilateral neglect.
- Impaired environmental interpretation syndrome.
- Wandering.
- Disturbed sensory perception (specify: visual, auditory, kinesthetic, gustatory, tactile).
- Deficient knowledge.
- Readiness for enhanced knowledge.
- Acute confusion.

- Chronic confusion.
- Impaired memory.
- Disturbed thought process.
- Readiness for enhanced decision-making.
- Risk for acute confusion.
- Ineffective activity planning.
- Impaired verbal communication.
- Readiness for enhanced communication.

Domain 6: Self-perception

Description

Awareness about the self.

Approved Diagnoses

- Disturbed personal identity.
- Powerlessness.
- Risk for powerlessness.
- Hopelessness.
- Risk for loneliness.
- Readiness for enhanced self-concept.
- Readiness for enhanced power.
- Risk for compromised human dignity.
- Readiness for enhanced hope.
- Chronic low self-esteem.
- Situation low self-esteem.
- Risk for situational low self-esteem.
- Disturbed body image.

Domain 7: Role Relationships

Description

The positive and negative connections or associations between persons or groups of persons and the means by which those connections are demonstrated.

Approved Diagnoses

- Caregiver role strain.
- Risk for caregiver role strain.
- Impaired parenting.
- Risk for impaired parenting.
- Readiness for enhanced parenting.
- Interrupted family processes.
- Readiness for enhanced family processes.
- Dysfunctional family process.
- Risk for impaired attachment.
- Effective breastfeeding.
- Ineffective breastfeeding.
- Interrupted breastfeeding.
- Ineffective role performance.

- Parental role conflict.
- Impaired social interaction.
- Readiness for enhanced relationship.

Domain 8: Sexuality

Description

- Sexual identity
- Sexual function
- Reproduction.

Approved Diagnoses

- Sexual dysfunction.
- Ineffective sexuality pattern.
- Readiness for enhanced childbearing process.
- Risk for disturbed maternal/fetal dyad.

Domain 9: Coping/Stress Tolerance

Description

- Contending with life events/life process.

Approved Diagnoses

- Relocation stress syndrome.
- Risk for relocation stress syndrome.
- Rape-trauma syndrome.
- Post-trauma syndrome.
- Risk-for post-trauma syndrome.
- Fear.
- Anxiety.
- Death anxiety.
- Chronic sorrow.
- Ineffective denial.
- Ineffective coping.
- Disabled family coping.
- Compromised family coping.
- Defensive coping.
- Ineffective community coping.
- Readiness for enhanced coping (individual).
- Readiness for enhanced family coping.
- Readiness for enhanced community coping.
- Risk for complicated grieving.
- Stress overload.
- Risk-prone health behavior.
- Grieving.
- Complicated grieving.
- Impaired individual resilience.
- Risk for compromised resilience.
- Readiness for enhanced resilience.
- Autonomic dysreflexia.
- Risk for autonomic dysreflexia.

- Disorganized infant behavior.
- Risk for disorganized infant behavior.
- Readiness for enhanced organized infant behavior.
- Decreased intracranial adaptive capacity.

Domain 10: Life Principles

Description

Principles underlying conduct, thought, and behavior about acts, customs, or institutions as being true or having intrinsic worth.

Approved Diagnoses

- Readiness for enhanced hope.
- Readiness for enhanced spiritual well-being.
- Spiritual distress.
- Risk for spiritual distress.
- Decisional conflict (specify).
- Noncompliance (specify).
- Risk for impaired religiosity.
- Impaired religiosity.
- Readiness for enhanced religiosity.
- Moral distress.
- Readiness for enhanced decision making.

Domain 11: Safety/Protection

Description

Freedom from danger, physical injury, or immune system damage, preservation from loss, and protection of safety and security.

Approved Diagnoses

- Risk for infection.
- Readiness for enhanced immunization status.
- Impaired oral mucous membrane.
- Risk for injury.
- Risk for perioperative positioning injury.
- Risk for falls.
- Risk for trauma.
- Impaired skin integrity.
- Risk for impaired skin integrity.
- Impaired tissue integrity.
- Impaired dentition.
- Risk for suffocation.
- Risk for aspiration.
- Ineffective airway clearance.
- Risk for peripheral neurovascular dysfunction.
- Ineffective protection.
- Risk for sudden infant death syndrome.

- Risk for vascular trauma.
- Risk for self-mutilation.
- Self-mutilation.
- Risk for other-directed violence.
- Risk for self-directed violence.
- Risk for suicide.
- Risk for poisoning.
- Risk for contamination.
- Contamination.
- Latex allergy response.
- Risk for latex allergy response.
- Readiness for enhanced immunization status.
- Risk for imbalanced body temperature.
- Ineffective thermoregulation.
- Hypothermia.
- Hyperthermia.

Domain 12: Comfort

Description

- Sense of mental, physical, or social well-being or ease.

Approved Diagnoses

- Acute pain
- Chronic pain
- Nausea
- Readiness for enhanced comfort
- Impaired comfort
- Social isolation.

Domain 13: Growth/Development

Description

Age-appropriate increase in physical dimension, organ systems, and/or attainment of developmental milestones.

Approved Diagnoses

- Delayed growth and development.
- Risk for disproportionate growth.
- Adult failure to thrive.
- Risk for delayed development.

BIBLIOGRAPHY

1. *Berman AT, Snyder S, Kozier BJ, et al. Kozier & Erb's. Fundamentals of Nursing: Concepts, Process and Practice, 8th edition. Pearson Education.*
2. *Shortridge LM, Lal JE. Introduction to Nursing Practice, McGraw Hill Book company, 1980.*
3. *Christensen BL, Kockrow OE. Foundations of Nursing, Mosby; 2003. p. 764.*

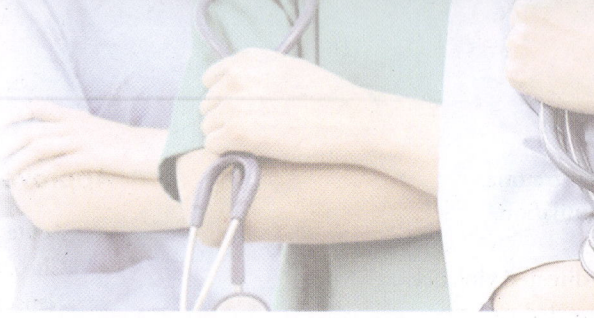
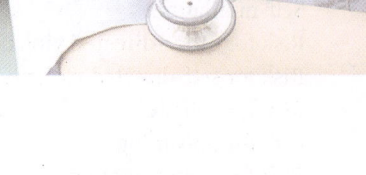

Planning

INTRODUCTION

It is basically a decision-making process mainly to decide appropriate nursing care for the problems of patients and prescribe nursing care in the form of written nursing instructions. The nurse prescribes nursing care which falls within her purview.

NURSING INSTRUCTIONS

These are a list of action which the nurse prescribes for the problem and needs of the patients.

PROTOCOLS

These provide standing guidelines for care to help with management of patients.

PLANNING OF PATIENT CARE

Planning the patient care involve four steps:
1. Establishing priorities.
2. Setting goals/Identify outcomes.
3. Selecting nursing interventions.
4. Writing the plan of care.

ESTABLISHING PRIORITIES

This involves analyzing the problems identified in the assessment stage to decide which problem requires priority of attention. This involves judgments made in relation to the impact of each nursing diagnosis for the clients/ family's immediate and long-term well-being.

- Those problems that involve actual or life-threatening concerns are considered prior to actual or potential health-threatening concerns.

TABLE 1: Prioritizing nursing diagnosis

Nursing diagnosis	Priority
Ineffective airway clearance related to excessive secretions	High
Anxiety related to hospitalization	Moderate
Ineffective coping related to situational crises	Low

- Those diagnosis that the client identifies as important must be given high priority and consideration by the nurse.
- Priority setting is guided by theories, models and principles that provide standard of comparison for evaluating the list of nursing diagnosis, (Table 1).

ESTABLISHING GOALS

A patient goal is desired outcome or change in patient behavior in the direction of health. Goal attainment reflects the resolution of the patients concern or health problem that is specified in the nursing diagnosis. The nursing diagnosis guides the type of goal attainment: goals may reflect health restoration, health maintenance or health promotion (Christensen, 1986).

The purpose of patient goal is to:

- Provide direction for planning nursing interventions that will achieve the anticipated changes in the patient.
- Provide direction for establishing evaluation criteria to measure the effectiveness of the interventions.
  Examples of patient goals:
  The patient/client will
  - Restore fluid volume.
  - Increase actively tolerance.
  - Maintain urinary elimination pattern.
  - Decrease potential for injury.
  - Develop coping abilities.
  - Improve nutritional pattern.
  - Increase parental knowledge.
  - Establish change in family roles.

Establishing Goals from Nursing Diagnosis

Client goals are derived from the first clause of the nursing diagnosis, which the client problems (p) as shown below:

1. Nursing diagnosis	Impaired physical mobility related to pain
Client response or problem	Impaired physical mobility
Client goal	Client will demonstrate increase in physical mobility
2. Nursing diagnosis	Self-care deficit: Inability to feed self related to depression.
Client response or problem	Self-care deficit: Inability to feed self
Client goal	Client will perform self-feeding

Long-term and Short-term Goals/Outcomes

Goals might be either long-term or short-term. Long-term goals require a longer period (usually more than a week) to be achieved than do short-term goals/outcomes. The problem identified in the first part of the nursing diagnoses statement should appear in outcome as an alternative healthful response. The response of client can be classified into the following heading:

Appearance and Functioning of the Body

Within 48 hours after surgery, the client expels flatus, the abdomen is soft, bowel sounds are present. By the time of discharge, client returns to normal elimination pattern.

Specific Symptoms

These refer to symptoms interfering with the client's health status such as nausea, vomiting, burning sensation, pain, frequent urination and so on. The outcome is "verbalises freedom from burning sensation in epigastric region within half an hour of administering antacid."

"Asks for pain medication when needed, expresses relief after initiation of comfort measures."

Knowledge

Refer to client's ability to recall the information taught, e.g., by the end of teaching session, the diabetic client lists common food items to avoid and foods, which are to be added in meal.

Psychomotor Skills

By the time of discharge, the client is able to transfer from bed to wheel chair, test urine for sugar, take insulin injection.

Emotional Status

Prior to discharge the client verbalize feelings about loss of limb, initiate positive interactions with staff, friends, family. Outcome/goals should be determined by the client and nurse together.

DETERMINING OUTCOMES

An outcome is a statement of the behavior or human response that is expected after provision of nursing care. It may involve prevention, modification or correction of behavior stated in the nursing diagnosis.

The identified outcome provides the direction for selecting and evaluating nursing interventions. While determining outcomes, standards determined by legal authorities, professional organizations and the institutions, must be applied. Characteristics of outcome statements are mentioned below:

- Be focused on the client.
- Be concise and explicit.
- Reflect a mutual agreement between nurse and patient.
- Be observable and measurable.
- Be realistic.
- Have a specified time limit. **E.g., Nursing diagnosis:** Risk for altered health maintenance related to lack of knowledge of diabetic self-care.
- **Long-term outcome:** The client will demonstrate knowledge of diabetic self-care by having blood sugar levels over time within expected levels.
- Short-term outcome: The client will demonstrate correct procedure of self-administration of insulin after receiving instructions about the procedure. E.g., Nursing diagnosis: Pain related to rheumatoid arthritis.
- **Short-term goal:** Verbalizes the presence of pain.
  - Identifies factors that influences pain.
  - Client or significant other administers pain medication appropriately.
- **Long-term goal:** Verbalizes comfort.

SELECTING NURSING INTERVENTIONS

Selecting nursing interventions are those actions performed by the nurse that are aimed at the prevention, maintenance and restoration of a client's health.

Guidelines

- Identify possible intervention that are based on scientific rationale.
- Consider a wide variety of possible nursing interventions.
- Determine which interventions are appropriate and related to the identified outcomes and the etiology of nursing diagnosis.
- Standards of nursing practice should serve as a guide for evaluating the appropriateness of selected nursing interventions.

Writing Nursing Orders/Nursing Instructions

Interventions or activities that the nurse identifies as being appropriate in a given situation are termed as nursing orders which include: independent nursing activities and implementation of physician order.

Guidelines for Writing Nursing Order

- There should be separate list of nursing orders for each nursing diagnosis and client outcome.
- There should be sufficient number of nursing order to address each nursing diagnosis.
- Nursing orders should be dated and signed by the nurse to indicate when the orders were written and to verify the accountability of the nurse.
- Nursing orders should be documented in ink.
- Nursing orders should include specific actions that are to be implemented and should indicate the individual who is to carry out the actions.
- Nursing orders should be revised and updated as the client health status changes.
- Nursing orders should incorporate the physician orders and identify all nursing actions related to the implementation of physician's order.
- The nursing plan of care should be a part of client's permanent record to document the process of nursing intervention and achievement of client outcomes.
- All entries on the nursing plan of care should be done using appropriate and acceptable terminologies and abbreviations.

WRITING THE PLAN OF CARE

A written nursing plan is a record, summarizing all information required to carry out appropriate care plan for an individual patient or a family at a given time.

Steps in Planning Nursing Care

Planning the patient's care involves four steps:

1. **Determining priorities:** This involves analyzing the problems identified in the assessment stage, to decide which problem requires priority of attention. This involves judgments made in relation to the impact of each nursing diagnosis for that client's/family's immediate and long-term well-being.
2. **Setting goals:** These state what is to be achieved if the identified problems are to be alleviated.
3. **Selecting nursing actions:** This involves choosing the methods and techniques which will enable us to achieve the stated patient's goal.
4. **Writing the care plan:** The problems, goals and nursing actions are recorded on the nursing care plan.

BIBLIOGRAPHY

1. Berman AT, Snyder S, Kozier BJ, et al. Kozier & Erb's. Fundamentals of Nursing: Concepts, Process and Practice, 8th edition. Pearson Education.

2. Shortridge LM, Lal JE. Introduction to Nursing Practice, McGraw Hill Book company, 1980.

3. Christensen BL, Kockrow OE. Foundations of Nursing, Mosby; 2003. p. 764.

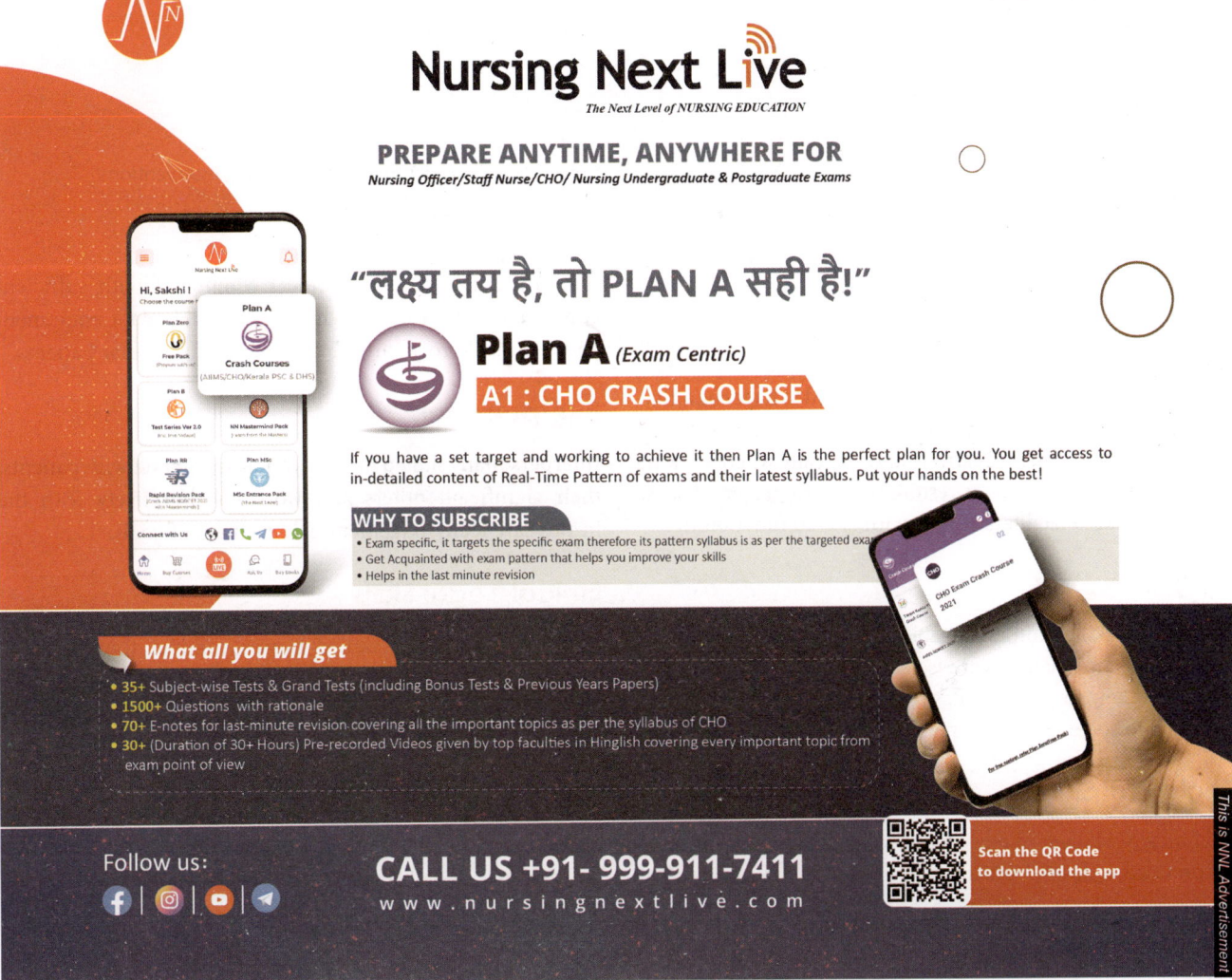

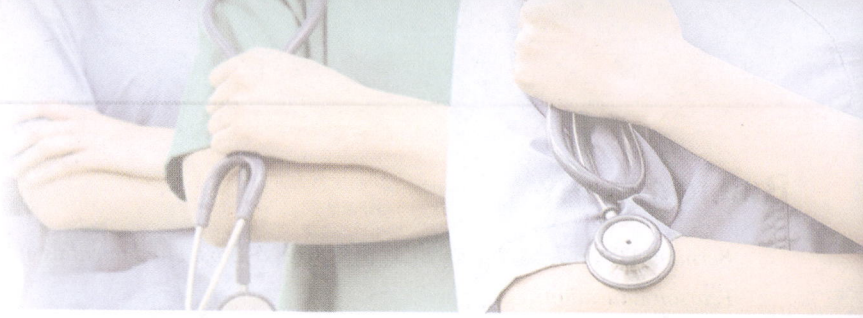

Implementation

INTRODUCTION

It involves actually providing the client with planned care through interventions or orders that are identified in planning phase. To implement the actions, nurses need to have cognitive, technical, interpersonal and ethical/legal skill, along with the willingness to use them creatively and critically when working with patients to promote or restore health, to prevent disease or illness, and to facilitate coping with altered functioning.

Cognitive Skills

Cognitively skilled nurses are able to offer scientific rationale for the patient's plan of care, select those interventions that are most likely to yield the desired outcomes and use critical thinking to solve problems creatively.

Technical Skills

Technically skilled nurses manipulate equipment skillfully to produce a desired outcome or result. Technically skilled nurses are able to use technical equipment with sufficient competence and ease to achieve goals and adapt equipment and technical procedures to the needs of particular patients.

Interpersonal Skills

Interpersonally skilled nurses are able to interact with patients, their significant others and work collaboratively with the health care team to facilitate achievement of goals.

Ethical/Legal Skills

Ethically and legally skilled nurses conduct themselves as effective patient advocates, practice nursing as per code of ethics and appropriate standards of practice, use legal safeguards that reduce the risk of litigation. According to McCloskey "Nursing action is any direct care treatment that a nurse performs on behalf of a client which includes nurse initiated treatments, physician initiated treatment and performance of daily essential functions."

CATEGORIES OF NURSING ACTIONS

Independent Nursing Actions

These actions are initiated by the nurse based on nursing knowledge and skills. These actions are the result of the assessment of client needs and may be initiated without the direction or supervision of another health care professional. These actions are determined by nursing diagnosis and nurses are held legally responsible. Knowing, why, when and how, makes the function an autonomous function.

Dependent Nursing Actions

These actions are carried out according to specific routines, under the supervision of a physician, or as a result of an order by a physician, e.g., medication, injection or any other treatment modalities.

Collaborative and Interdependent Nursing Action

These are performed either as a result of joint decision by a nurse or another health team member, e.g., working with a physical therapist to provide physical exercises to a client who is bedridden, planning a teaching session about a diabetic diet with a dietetics, etc.

FACTORS TO CONSIDER IN SELECTING NURSING INTERVENTIONS

- Desired client outcome.
- Characteristics of nursing diagnosis.
- Research base associated with the intervention.
- Feasibility of implementing the intervention successfully.
- **Acceptability by the client:** Previous response, development stage, psychological and cultural background.
- **The capability of the nurse:** The skills needed, cognitive, interpersonal, technical and ethical/legal skill.
- Ongoing data collection during implementation step is important, this is done by:
  - Interacting with the client.
  - Measuring outcomes.
  - Observing responses.

BIBLIOGRAPHY

1. *Berman AT, Snyder S, Kozier BJ, et al. Kozier & Erb's. Fundamentals of Nursing: Concepts, Process and Practice, 8th edition. Pearson Education.*

2. *Shortridge LM, Lal JE. Introduction to Nursing Practice, McGraw Hill Book company, 1980.*

3. *Christensen BL, Kockrow OE. Foundations of Nursing, Mosby; 2003. p. 764.*

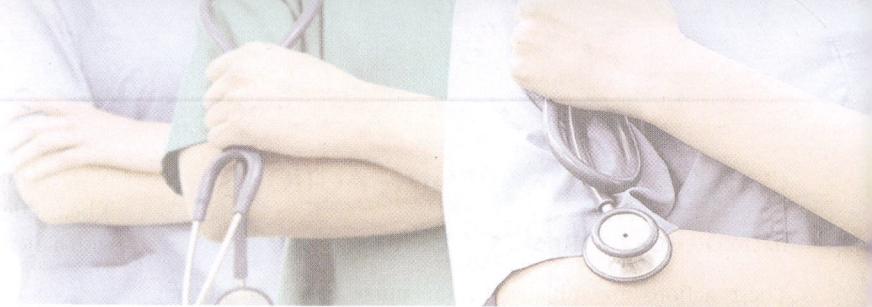

Evaluation

INTRODUCTION

It is an ongoing process which begins when the individual/family/community enters the health care system, provides continuous feedback, and continues until his/her exit from the system. The main purpose of evaluation is to determine the client's progress towards meeting specified outcomes, which will be used as a guide to direct future nurse-patient interactions.

The outcome statements present standards and criteria that are observable and measurable.

Criteria

Kenney (1995) describes criteria as measurable qualities, attributes or characteristics that specify skills, knowledge or attitude that influence a clients' behavior.

* **Skill:** Return demonstration of a dressing change or blood sugar monitoring, etc. The client will be able to perform self-care activities within own capabilities before discharge to home.
* **Knowledge:** Client will verbalize the correct understanding of the discharge instructions. Client verbalizes information about how to determine the amount of insulin to be taken.
* **Attitude:** Clients indifference about taking insulin, which may result in non-compliance.
* **Standards:** These are written rules for clients and nurses that indicate acceptable levels of performance of nursing staff and other health care workers. They are established by custom, authority or general consent.

FACTORS INFLUENCING OUTCOME ATTAINMENT

* **Client variables:** If outcome is to decrease anxiety, a visit by clergymen may have a positive outcome in decreasing client's anxiety, whereas news of a serious illness may result in negative outcome.
* **Nurse variables:** Inadequate assessment by the nurse does not provide enough information and results in negative outcomes, whereas comprehensive assessment increases the likelihood of a positive outcome.
* **Health system variables:** A negative outcome may occur if laboratory results are delayed, resulting in a delay in treatment, whereas timely return of the test results increases positive outcome.

REVIEWING AND MODIFYING THE PLAN OF CARE

When evaluation reveals that the client has made little or no progress towards outcome achievement, the nurse needs to re-evaluate each preceding step of the nursing process to try to identify the contributing factors pointing to problems with the plan of care. New assessment data might need to be collected, diagnosis may be added or altered, outcomes might need to be modified or rewritten, nursing orders may be changed or evaluation may be targeted more frequently.

Review the checklist for helping in evaluating your use of nursing process. Table check list suggests appropriate nursing responses to common problems encountered during evaluation. When the nurse has identified the factors contributing to the outcomes not being achieved, the evaluative statement can be used to suggest the necessary revision in the plan of care.

- Delete or modify the nursing diagnosis.
- Make the outcome statements more realistic.

- Increase the complexity of the outcome statement.
- Adjust time criteria in outcome statement.
- Change the nursing intervention.

Increasing the complexity of an outcome after it has been achieved facilitates optimal function. For example, the initial outcome for a patient with the diagnosis "Impaired physical mobility" might be "patient transfer from the bed to the chair". After this is achieved, however, the outcome needs to be stepped up in complexity to "Patient walks around room with support of a walker".

When it is determined that the care plan needs revising, the nurse follows the above mentioned steps. Reassessment may involve changes in any or all of the previous phases of the nursing process if the nurse determines the extent to which the goals or predetermined outcomes of care have been achieved, partially achieved, or not met.

Checklist for Evaluating Your use of the Nursing Process

Assessing
- The initial database is obtained by means of a nursing history and nursing examination
- Assessment data are documented:
  - **Accurately:** Questionable data are validated.
  - **Completely:** Use of a systematic guide ensures that recorded data describe (1) the patient's functional ability to meet each basic human need, and (2) responses to health and illness.
  - **Concisely:** Irrelevant data and meaningless generalizations are avoided.
  - **Factually:** Patient behaviors are recorded rather than the nurse's interpretation of these behaviors.
  - **Timely:** Current data are recorded for the team.
- The initial database communicates a "real sense" of the patient that makes possible individualized care.
- Focused assessment data are recorded for each patient problem.
- Data collection and documentation are ongoing and responsive to changes in the patient's condition.

Diagnosing
- A prioritized list of nursing diagnoses is on the plan of care.
- Each nursing diagnosis describes an actual or potential patient health problem that independent nursing intervention can prevent or resolve. Each nursing diagnosis:
  - Is derived from an accurate and validated interpretation of a cluster of significant patient data or "cues"
  - Contains a precise problem statement describing what is unhealthy about the patient and what needs to change— suggests patient goals
  - Identifies factors that contribute to the problem (etiology)— these suggest nursing Interventions
  - Uses nonjudgmental language and is written using legal advisable terms
- Old nursing diagnoses are deleted from the plan of care once resolved, and new diagnoses are add as soon as identified.

Outcome identification and planning
- A comprehensive, individualized, and up-to-date plan of care that specifies patient outcomes and nursing orders for each nursing diagnosis is developed with the assistance of the patient and family
- Planning is comprehensive:
  - Initial
  - Ongoing
  - Discharge
- Long-term goals alert the entire nursing team to realistic patient expectations after discharge.
- Short-term outcomes:
  - When achieved, demonstrate a resolution of the problem specified in the nursing diagnosis
  - Describe a single, observable, and measurable patient behavior
  - Are valued by the patient and family
  - Are realistic in terms of the resources of the patient and the nurse
- Nursing orders:
  - Clearly and concisely describe the nursing intervention to be performed (ongoing assessment; nursing treatments and procedures; teaching, counseling, advocacy)
  - Are individualized to the patient
  - Are consistent with standards of care and supportive of other therapies
  - Are effective in accomplishing the desired patient outcomes
- The plan of care encourages patient and family participation.

Implementing
- The patient record contains daily documentation of the nursing measures used to (1) assist the patient to meet basic human needs, (2) resolve health problems, and (3) implement select aspects of the medical plan of care.

Contd...

- The plan of care is implemented:
  - Competently
  - Confidently
  - Caringly
  - Creatively

Evaluating

- Evaluative statements are recorded on the plan of care to document the patient's level of outcome achievement at targeted times.
- Ongoing evaluation of the patient's responses to the plan of care are used to make decisions about terminating, continuing, or modifying nursing care.

EXAMPLE OF NURSING PROCESS

- **Identification date**

Name of the patient	Ms. X	Unit: Medical bed no: 4
Age	32 years	
Sex	Female	
Religion	Hindu	
Address	No. 2X/AA, New Delhi	
Educational Status	B.A. Passed	
Marital status	Married	
Diagnosis	Inflammatory Bowel syndrome	
Assessment:		
Subjective Data:		

- Abdominal pain
- Diarrhea
- Weight loss
- **Objective data**
  - Fever
  - Malnourished

- Pallor present
- Tenderness of abdomen
- Increased bowel sounds on auscultation
- Decreased hematocrit values
- Decreased hemoglobin

Medical Diagnosis–Inflammatory Bowel Disease

Nursing diagnosis	Interventions	Outcomes
Diarrhea related to inflamed intestinal mucosa	• Administer antidiarrheal medications as per order • After every bowel movement, gently clean the skin with warm water and apply a protective moisture barrier cream	• Decrease in diarrhea as evidenced by decrease in frequency and a more solid consistency of stools
Imbalanced nutrition: less than body requirements related to diarrhea and malabsorption	• Monitor the client intake • Encourage intake of fluids and food • Giving small servings to avoid gastrocolic reflex • Foods should be easily digested	• The client will increase the nutritional intake as evidenced by weight gain
Acute pain related to inflamed mucosa	• Assess the client's pain • Administer pain medications as ordered	• Relief of abdominal pain
Risk for ineffective coping related to stress of disease	• Education, counseling and support	• Client will cope effectively with the disease • Improved quality of life

Once these variables are known, the nurse can reinforce the positive factors by using them in future interactions and deal with those variable that are likely to create problems.

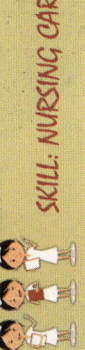

SKILL: NURSING CARE PLAN

45-year-old Mr. Ramesh came to casualty with increased cough, dyspnea and restlessness. On history taking, he is a known case of bronchial asthma.

- **Medical diagnosis:** Bronchial asthma
- **Problem:** Ineffective breathing pattern related to presence of secretions

Assessment	Nursing diagnosis	Scientific explanation	Planning	Interventions	Rationale	Evaluation
Subjective: (none) **Objective:** • Wheezing upon inspiration and expiration • Dyspnea • Coughing, sputum is yellow and sticky • Tachypnea, prolonged expiration • Tachycardia • Chest tightness • Suprasternal retraction • Restlessness • Anxiety • Cyanosis • Loss of consciousness	Ineffective breathing pattern related to presence of secretions, productive cough and dyspnea	Presence of secretion in the bronchi will result into a blockage of air that will enter the body and thus, producing insufficient air needed by the body and inability to maintain clear airway. This obstruction is further heightened by bronchospasm due to the contraction of the smooth muscles in the bronchi. This is caused by parasympathetic stimulation of the muscarinic 2 receptors as well as by chemical mediators released in response to the presence of allergens.	Choose: Patient will demonstrate pursed lip breathing and diaphragmatic breathing. Patient will manifest signs of decreased respiratory effort, absence of dyspnea. Patient will verbalize understanding of causative factors and demonstrate behaviors that would improve breathing pattern.	• Establish rapport. • Assess patient's condition • Monitor vital signs and record • Auscultate breath sound and assess airway pattern • Elevate head of the bed and change position of the patient every 2 hours. • Encourage deep breathing and coughing exercises. • Demonstrate diaphragmatic and pursed-lip breathing. • Encourage increase in fluid intake. • Encourage opportunities for rest and limit physical activities.	• To gain patient's trust. • To obtain baseline data • Serve to track important changes. • To check for the presence of adventitious breath sounds • To minimize difficulty in breathing • To maximize effort for expectoration. • To decrease air trapping and for efficient breathing. • To prevent fatigue. • To prevent situations that will aggravate the condition	Patient will demonstrate pursed lip breathing and diaphragmatic breathing. Patient will manifest signs of decreased respiratory effort, absence of dyspnea Patient will verbalize understanding of causative factors and demonstrate behaviors that would improve breathing pattern

BIBLIOGRAPHY

1. Gebbie K, Lavin MA. Classification of Nursing Diagnosis. Am J Nurs. 1974;74(2):250-3.

2. Herdman TH; North American Nursing Diagnosis Association. NANDA-I nursing diagnoses : definitions & classification, 2009-2011. Oxford: Wiley-Blackwell; 2008.

3. Yura H. & Walsh, BB (1988). The nursing process; Assessing. Planning implementing, evaluating (5th ed.) Norwalk, CT; Appleton- Century- Groups Kratz, Charlotte R. The nursing process. Bailliere Tindall. London; 1979

4. Shortridge LM, Lal JE. Introduction to Nursing Practice, McGraw Hill Book company, 1980.

5. Perry & Potter, Clinical Nursing Skills & Techniques, 5th edition. Mosby; 2002.

6. Hall LE. Quality of Nursing Care. Public Health News (June). New Jersey State Department of Health. New Jersey; 1995.

7. Taylor CR, Lillis C, LeMone P, et al. Fundamentals of Nursing – The Art and Science of Nursing Care, 7th edition. Wolters Kluwer; 2010.

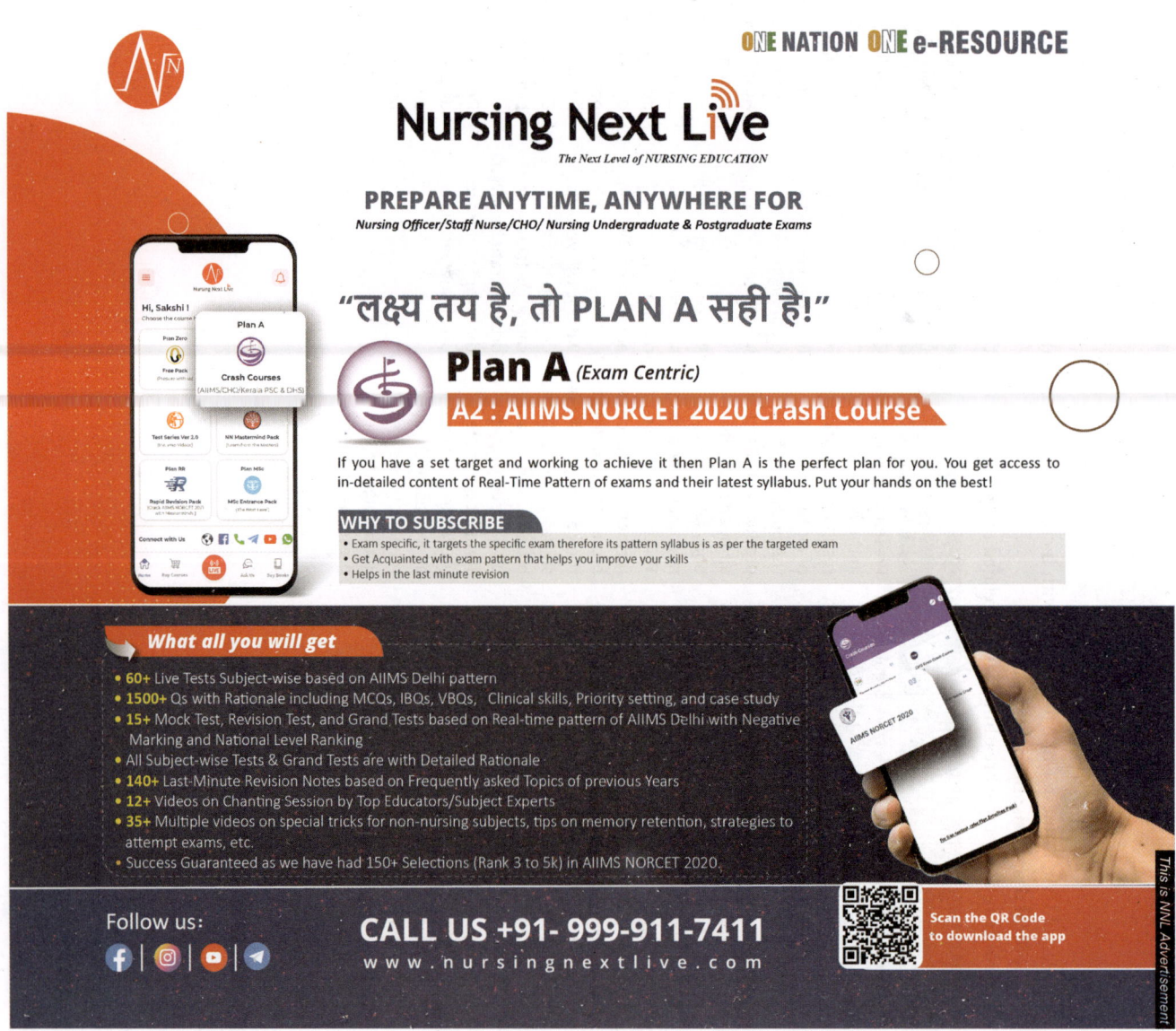

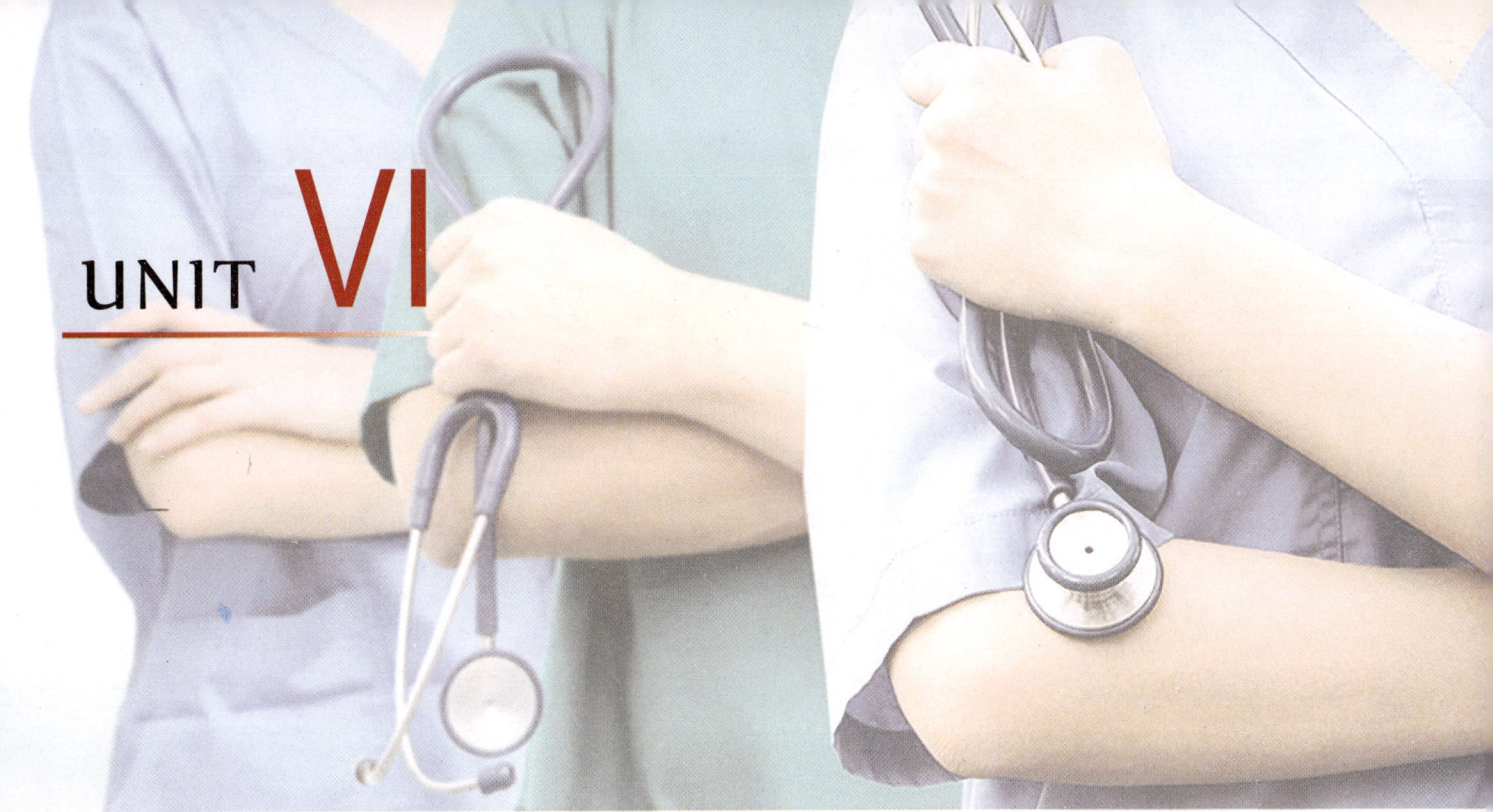

UNIT VI

DOCUMENTATION AND REPORTING

Unit Outline

Documentation

INTRODUCTION

- Communication among health care professionals is essential to the continuation and coordination of care.
- Documentation is the written or typed legal record of all pertinent interactions with the patient: Assessing, diagnosing, planning, implementing and evaluating.

The patient record is a compilation of patient's health information. Each health care institution has policies that specify the nurses' documentation responsibilities.

PURPOSE OF PATIENT'S RECORD

Communication

The primary purpose of the patient's record is to keep health care professionals from different disciplines who communicate with each other to be informed about the patient. It fosters continuity of care, this prevents fragmentation, repetition and delay in client care.

Diagnostic and Therapeutic Orders

Nurses are responsible for entering these orders in the patient's record and getting implemented. These orders must be signed by the professional staff and then only they are executed. Date and time of the order should be documented. Record verbal orders, the name of physician who issued the order and nurse's name and title.

Care Planning

Each health professional uses data from the client's record to plan care for that patient. Nurses use baseline and ongoing data to evaluate the effectiveness of the nursing care plans.

Quality Review

Client records are reviewed for quality assurance. Accrediting agencies such as the Joint Commission on Accreditation of Health Care Organization (JCAHO), National Accreditation Board for Hospital and Health care Providers (NABH) may review client's records to determine if a particular health agency is meeting its stated standards.

Health Care Analysis

Information from records may assist health care planners to identify agency needs, such as overutilized or underutilized hospital services. Records can also be used to establish the cost of various services and those that generate revenue.

Education

Health care professionals and students reading a patient's chart can learn a great deal about the clinical manifestations of particular health problems and their effective treatment modalities.

Legal Documentation

Patient records are legal documents that might be used as evidence in court proceedings; therefore, they play an important role in implicating or absolving health professionals charged with improper care. The record can also be used in accident or injury claims made by the patient.

Reimbursement

Patient's records are used to demonstrate to payers (insurance companies) that patients received the care for which reimbursement is being sought.

Research

The information contained in a record can be a valuable source of data for research. The treatment plans for a number of clients with the same health problems can yield information helpful in treating other clients.

TYPES OF RECORDS

Medical Record

It has following components:
- Patients identification and demographic data
- Present complaints
- Admission history
- Medical history
- Family history
- Physical examination findings
- Tentative diagnosis
- Therapeutic order
- Medical progress notes

- Informed consent for treatment and procedures
- Diagnostic study reports
- Final diagnosis
- Summary of operative procedures
- Discharge plan and summary
- Patient education
- Any other specific instructions.

Nursing Record

- **Admission nursing assessment:** Initial database, nursing history and assessment on admission.
- **Nursing care plans:** Patient's assessment, nursing diagnosis, nursing interventions and patient's outcomes.
- **Kardex:** Concise method of organizing and recording data about a patient, making information quickly accessible to all health care team members. The information in kardexes may be organized into following sections: pertinent information about the patient such as name, room, age, religion, marital status, admission data, diagnosis, etc., list of medication with the date of order and the time of administration, list of intravenous fluids with the data of infusion, list of daily treatment and procedures ordered, e.g., diagnosis tests and a problem list stating goals and list of approaches to meet the goal and relieve the problems. Whether kardex is a written paper or computing, it is important to have a place on it to record data and initials of the person reviewing or revising it.
- **Flow sheets:** It enables nurse to record nursing data quickly and concisely and provides an easy to read and understand format.
- **Graphic record:** Used for recording vital signs of patient—temperature, pulse, respiration and blood pressure.
- **Fluid-balance record:** All routes of fluid intake and all routes of fluid loss or output are measured and recorded on this form.
- **Medication administration form:** Medication flow sheet includes date of medication, order, name, dose, frequency, route and nurses who are taking care of the patient.
- **Skin assessment form:** Skin or wound assessment is often recorded on a flow sheet which includes categories related to: drainage, odor, inflammation and treatment.
- **Progress notes:** Progress notes made by nurses provide information about the progress a patient is making towards achieving desired outcomes.

METHODS OF DOCUMENTATION

Source-oriented Records

A source-oriented record is one in which each health care group keeps data on its own separate form. Sections of the record are designated for nurses, physicians, laboratory, X-ray personnel, etc. The advantage is that each discipline can easily find and chart pertinent data. The main disadvantage is that data is fragmented, making it difficult to track problems chronologically.

Problem-oriented Medical Record

Problem-Oriented Medical Record (POMR) is organized around a patient's problems rather than around sources of information. With POMR, all health care professionals record information on the same form. The advantage of this type of record is that the entire health care team works together in identifying a master list of patient's problems and contributes collaboratively to the plan of care. Progress notes clearly focus on patient's problems. The POMR has four basic components:

1. Database
2. Problem list
3. Plan of care
4. Progress notes

Database

It consists of information about the client when the client first enters the health care agency. It includes the nursing assessment, the physician's history, social and family data, and the results of the physical examination and baseline diagnostic tests. Data is constantly updated as the client's health state changes.

Problem List

The problems list is derived from the database. Problems are listed in the order in which they are identified, and the list in continually updated as new problems are identified and others are resolved. All caregivers may contribute to the problem list. Primary care providers write problems as medical diagnosis, surgical procedures, or symptoms. Nurses write problems as nursing diagnosis.

Plan of Care

Physician writes physician's orders; nurses write nursing orders or nursing care plans. The written plan in the record is listed under each problem in the progress notes.

Progress Notes

A program note in the POMR is made by all health professionals involved in a client's care. Progress notes are numbered to correspond to the problems on the problem list and may be lettered for the type of data. For example, the SOAP format is frequently used. SOAP is an acronym for subjective data, objective data, assessment, and planning.

- **S**: Subjective data consists of information obtained from what the client says. It describes the perception of the client with the problem.
- **O**: Objective data consists of information that is measured or observed by use of senses, e.g., vital signs, laboratory results, etc.
- **A**: Assessment is the interpretation or conclusion drawn about the subjective and objective data. During the initial assessment, the problem is created from the database, so the entry in assessment should be the statement of the problem.
- **P**: The plan is the plan of care to resolve the stated problem. The initial plan is written by the person who enters the problem into the record. All subsequent plans, including revisions are entered into the progress notes.

Over the years, soap format has been modified. The acronyms SOAPIE and SOAPIER refers to the formats that add interventions, evaluation and revision.

- **I**: Interventions refer to the specific interventions that have been actually performed by the care giver.
- **E**: Evaluation includes client's responses to nursing interventions and medical treatments.
- **R**: Revision reflects to care plan modifications suggested by the evaluation.
  Newer versions of this format eliminate the subjective and objective data and start with assessment. The acronym then becomes APIE or APIER.

Focus Charting

The purpose of focus charting is to bring the focus of care back to the patient and his/her concern. Instead of a problem list or list of nursing or medical diagnosis, a focused column is used that incorporates various aspects of a patient and patient care. The focus might be the patient's strengths, problems, or need. The narrative portion of focus charting uses the Data, Action and Response (DAR) format. These three components do not need to be recorded in order, and each note does not need to have all three categories.

Charting by Exception (CBE)

It is a shorthand documentation method that makes use of well-defined standards of practice, only significant findings or 'exceptions' to these standards are documented in narrative notes. Benefits of this approach include:

- Decreased charting time
- Greater emphasis on significant data
- Easy retrieval of significant data
- Timely bedside charting
- Standardized assessment

- Greater interdisciplinary communication
- Better tracking of important patient responses
- Lower costs.

Flow Sheets

These include a graphic record, fluid balance record, daily nursing assessment record and client skin assessment record.

Standards of Nursing Care

Documentation by reference to the agency's printed standard of nursing practice, eliminates repetitive charting of routine care. For example, "the nurse must ensure that the unconscious client has back care at least q4h". Documentation of care according to these specified standards involves only a check mark on the graphic record.

Bed-side Access to Chart Forms

In this system, all flow sheets are kept at the clients' bed-side to allow immediate recording.

Computerized Documentation and Electronic Medical Records (EMR)

Computer systems have revolutionized the nursing documentation as more number of health care institutions have started using EMR. In this, the nurse has a patient database, she develops plan of care using computerized care plans, adds to the patients' data base and modifies care accordingly, receives orders showing treatments, medication procedures necessary for the patient and documents care immediately using the computer terminal at the patient's bedside.

The American Nurses Association (ANA), the American Medical Record Association and the Canadian Nurses Association (CNA) have offered the following guidelines and strategies for safe computer charting.

- Never give your password (personal) to anyone.
- Do not leave computer terminal unattended after you have logged on.
- Follow the correct protocol for correcting errors. If you record information in the wrong chart, write "mistaken entry-wrong chart" and sign off.
- Never change, create, or delete records unless you have specific authority to do so.
- Make sure that stored records have back-up files on important safety check.
- Don't leave information about a patient displayed on a monitor where others may see it.
- Never use e-mail to send protected health information unless it has been encrypted to protect it from an unauthorized access.

- Follow the agency's confidentiality procedures for documenting sensitive material, such as diagnosis of acquired immunodeficiency syndrome (AIDS) or human immunodeficiency virus (HIV) infection.

Personal Health Records (PHRs)

Many individuals today are preparing personal health record on the web to manage their health care via computer. These records contain the individual's medical history, including diagnosis, symptoms, and medications. The chief reason for creating a personal health record is to provide easy access to update complete health information to assist in self-care and communication with providers of healthcare.

FORMATS FOR NURSING DOCUMENTATION

Admission Nursing Assessment

A comprehensive admission assessment, also referred to as an initial database, nursing history, or nursing assessment, is completed when the client is admitted in the nursing unit. These forms can be organized according to health patterns, body systems, functional abilities, health problems and risks, nursing model or type of health care setting, e.g., pediatric intensive care unit. The nurse records ongoing assessments on flow sheets or on nursing progress notes.

Nursing Care Plan

There are two types of nursing care plans *traditional* and *standardized*. The traditional care plan is written for each client. The form varies from agency to agency according to the needs of the client and the department. Most forms have three columns: nursing diagnosis, expected outcomes, and nursing interventions.

Standardized care plans were developed to save documentation time. These plans may be based on an institution's standards of practice, to provide a high quality of nursing care.

Kardexes

The kardex is widely used, concise method of organizing and recording data about a client, making information quickly accessible to all health professionals. The system consists of a series of cards kept in a portable index file or on computer generated forms. The card for a particular patient can be quickly accessed to reveal specific data. The kardex may or may not become a part of the client's permanent record written in pencil for ease in recording frequent changes in client's care.

The information in kardexes may be organized into various sections, e.g.,:

- Pertinent information about the client such as name, room number, age, admission data, physician's name, diagnosis, and type of surgery and date.
- Allergies
- List of medications with the date of order and the times of administration for each.
- List of intravenous fluids with data of infusion.
- List of daily treatments and procedures.
- List of diagnostic procedures ordered.
- Specific data on how the client's physical needs are to be met, such as type of diet, assistance needed with feeding, activity, hygienic needs, and safety precautions.
- A problem list stating goals and a list of nursing approaches to meet the goals and relieve the problems.

It is important to have a place on it to record data and initials of the person reviewing or revising. It is a quick visual guide to ensure that information is current and updated and on a regular basis.

Flow Sheets

A flow sheet enables nurses to record nursing data quickly and concisely and provides an easy-to-read record of the client's condition over time.

Graphic Record

This record typically indicates body temperature, pulse, respiratory rate, blood pressure, weight, and in some agencies, other significant clinical data such as admission or postoperative day bowel movements, appetite, and activity.

Intake and Output Record

Forms are available to document 24-hour intake and output of fluids for patients with special needs. The form includes shift and daily fluid intake and output.

Medication Administration Record

The patient's medication record must include documentation of all the medications administered to the patient (drug, dose, route and time), the nurse administering the drug, and for some medications (e.g., analgesics), the reason the drug was given and its effectiveness.

GUIDELINES FOR EFFECTIVE DOCUMENTATION

The patient's record is the only permanent legal document that details the nurse's interactions with the patient and is the nurse's best defense if a patient alleges nursing negligence. Unfortunately, there are often crucial omissions in the nursing documentation, along with meaningless repetitions or inaccurate entries. Health care personnel must not only maintain the confidentiality of the clients' record but also meet legal standards in the process of recording.

Date and Time

Date and time is essential for each recording for legal reasons and patient's safety. Follow the agency's policy about the frequency of documenting and adjust the frequency as the client's condition indicates. As a rule, documenting should be done as soon as possible after an assessment or intervention. No recording should be done before providing nursing care.

Legibility

All entries must be legible and easy-to-read to prevent errors in interpretation. Hand-written record is permissibly provided it is legible.

Permanence

All entries on the client's record are made in ink so that the record is permanent. Follow agency policies about the type of pen and ink used for recording.

Accepted Terminology

Use only commonly accepted terminology (abbreviations), symbols and terms that are specified by the agency. Many abbreviations are standard and used universally, others are used only in certain geographic areas. Follow the list of approved abbreviations in health care facility where you are working. When in doubt about the use of abbreviation, write the complete form.

Correct Spelling

For accurate recording, correct spelling is essential. If unsure how to spell a word, look it up in a dictionary.

Signature

Each recording on the nurse's notes is signed by the nurse, which includes the name and title with computerized charting, each nurse has her own code through which documentation can be identified.

Accuracy

Before making any entry, check that it is the correct chart. Do not identify charts by room number only, check the client's name. Special care is taken when caring for clients having same name. Notations on records must be accurate and correct. Accurate notations consist of facts or observations rather than opinions or interpretations. When any recording mistake is made, draw a line through it and write the words mistaken entry with your initials or name. Do not erase, or use correcting fluid.

Sequence

Document events in the order in which they occurred, e.g., record assessments, then the nursing interventions and then the client's response. Update or delete problems as needed.

Appropriateness

Record information that pertains to the client's health problem and care only. Recording irrelevant information may be considered an invasion of the client's privacy.

Completeness

Whatever information is recorded needs to be complete and helpful to the client and health care professionals. Nurse's notes need to reflect the nursing process. Record all assessments, dependent and independent nursing interventions, client problems, client comments and responses to interventions and tests, progress towards goals and communication with other members of the health team.

Document what was omitted because of client's condition or refusal of treatment, why it was omitted and who was notified?

Conciseness

Recordings need to be brief as well as complete.

REPORTING

The purpose of reporting is to communicate specific information to a person or group of people. A report, whether oral, written, or computer-based should be concise, including pertinent information. Many methods of reporting are used.

Change of Shift Reports

It is given to all nurses on the next shift. Its purpose is to provide continuity of care for clients by providing the new caregivers a quick summary of client's needs and details of care to be given. Change-of –shift reports may be written or given orally, either in a face-to-face exchange or by audio-tape recording. The face-to-face reports permit the listener to ask questions during the report. Written and tape-recorded reports are often brief and less time- consuming. Reports are given at bed-side sometimes. Box 1 provides a sample change of shift report.

Box 1

Change of Shift Report

- Bed no. 104- M$_2$X
- Admitted last night with head injury
- Allergic to penicillin
- I/V Dextrose 5% infusing 100 mL/hour in (L) forearm
- Needs urgent CT scan
- Temp. 102°F Pulse 98/minute, RR 24/minute
- Blood pressure 110/70 mm of Hg.
- GCS-11

Telephone Reports

Health professionals frequently report about a client by telephone. Nurses inform primary care providers about a change in client's condition, a radiologist reports the result of an X-ray study and a nurse may report to a nurse of another unit about a transferred client.

The nurse receiving a telephone report should document the date and time, the name of the person giving the information, and the subject of the information received, and sign the notation, e.g.,

7/7/15 11:30 Ms Edwina, laboratory technician, reported by telephone that Mr. Deepak's renal function tests were blood urea 35 mg/dl, serum creatinine 1.0 mg/dl_____M.J (RN)

The person receiving the information should repeat it back to the sender for accuracy.

TELEPHONE ORDERS

Most of the agencies have specific policies about telephone orders and they allow only registered nurses to take telephone orders.

Question the primary care provider about any order that is ambiguous, unusual (high dose of medication). Then transcribe the order onto the physician's order sheet, indicating it as a verbal order (VO) or telephone order (TO). Once the order is transcribed on the physician's order sheet, the order must be countersigned by the primary care provider within the time period described by agency policy, e.g., within 24 hours.

CARE PLAN CONFERENCE

It is a meeting of a group of nurses to discuss possible solutions to certain problems of a client. It allows each nurse an opportunity to offer an opinion about possible solutions to the problem. Other health professionals may be invited to attend the conference to offer their expertise.

Care plan conferences are most effective when there is a climate of respect, i.e., non-judgmental acceptance of others even though their values, opinions, and beliefs, may differ. Even when there is disagreement, nurses need to accept and respect each person's contributions and listening with open mind.

NURSING ROUNDS

Nursing rounds are procedures in which two or more nurses visit selected clients at their bed-side to obtain information that will help plan nursing care, provide clients the opportunity to discuss their care and evaluation the nursing care client has received.

During rounds, the nurse assigned to the client provides a brief summary of the client's nursing needs and the interventions being implemented. Nursing rounds offer advantage to both client and nurses. Clients can participate in the discussion and nurses can see the client and the equipment being used. To facilitate client participation in rounds, nurses need to use terms which the client can understand.

SBAR Communication

SBAR communication (Situation, Background, Assessment, Recommendation) is a framework of communication between the members of the health care team about client's condition. It provides a consistent method for handing off communication that is clear, structured, and easy-to-use.

- **Situation:** Communicate why it is occurring and why the patient is being transferred to other department.
- **Background:** Explain what led to the current situation that in context if necessary provides objective data.
- **Assessment:** Give your impression of the problem.
- **Recommendation:** Explain what you would do to correct the problem.

SBAR is an easy-to-remember, concrete mechanism useful for framing any conversation requiring a clinician's immediate attention and action (Fig. 1).

USING NURSING INFORMATICS

Nursing informatics is a specialty that integrates nursing science, computer science, and information science to manage and communicate data, information and knowledge in nursing practice. Nursing information facilitates the integration of data, information, and knowledge to support patients, nurses, and other providers in their decision making in all roles and settings. The main benefits are:

- Increase the accuracy and completeness of nursing documentation.
- Improvement in the work flow and elimination of redundant documentation.

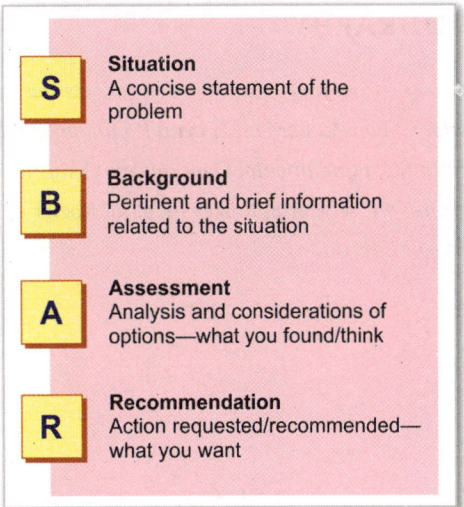

Fig. 1: SBAR communication

- Automation of the collection and reuse of nursing data.
- Facilitation of the analysis of clinical data.

The health care technologies developed and implemented by nurses are: smartphones for perioperative nurses, Accu nurse (a wireless hands free voice recognition documentation and communication system for infusion nurses), bed-side medication system on a PDA (personal digital assistant) device and Vocera B2000 communications badge. These devices allow nurses to answer calls using their voices without breaking sterile-techniques or stopping what they are doing.

MINIMIZING LEGAL LIABILITY

Through effective record keeping, legal problems can be minimized. The nurse has a duty to mention confidentiality of all patient's information. Access to the record is restricted to care givers. The institution or agency is the rightful owner of the client's record.

In documentation of content, the legal problems which can arise are:

- When the content is not in accordance with organizational standards.
- Content is incomplete and does not reflect patient's needs.
- Content does not include description of situation.
- Tampering in documentation.
- Illegibility.
- Dates and times of entries omitted or inconsistently documented.
- Improper nurse initials.
- Transcription errors.

BIBLIOGRAPHY

1. *Spader C. Cool tools. Cutting edge gadgets sharpen nurse's efficiency, Nursing spectrum. Washington DC. 2009;19(11):20-1.*

2. *Taylor C, Lillis C, LeMone P, Lynn P. Fundamentals of Nursing, 6th edition. Lippincott Williams and Wilkins. Philadelphia: 2008.*

3. *DeWit SC. Fundamental Concepts and Skills for Nursing. WB Saunders Company. 2000.*

4. *Berman AT, Snyder S, Kozier BJ, et al. Kozier & Erb's. Fundamentals of Nursing: Concepts, Process and Practice, 8th edition. Pearson Education.*

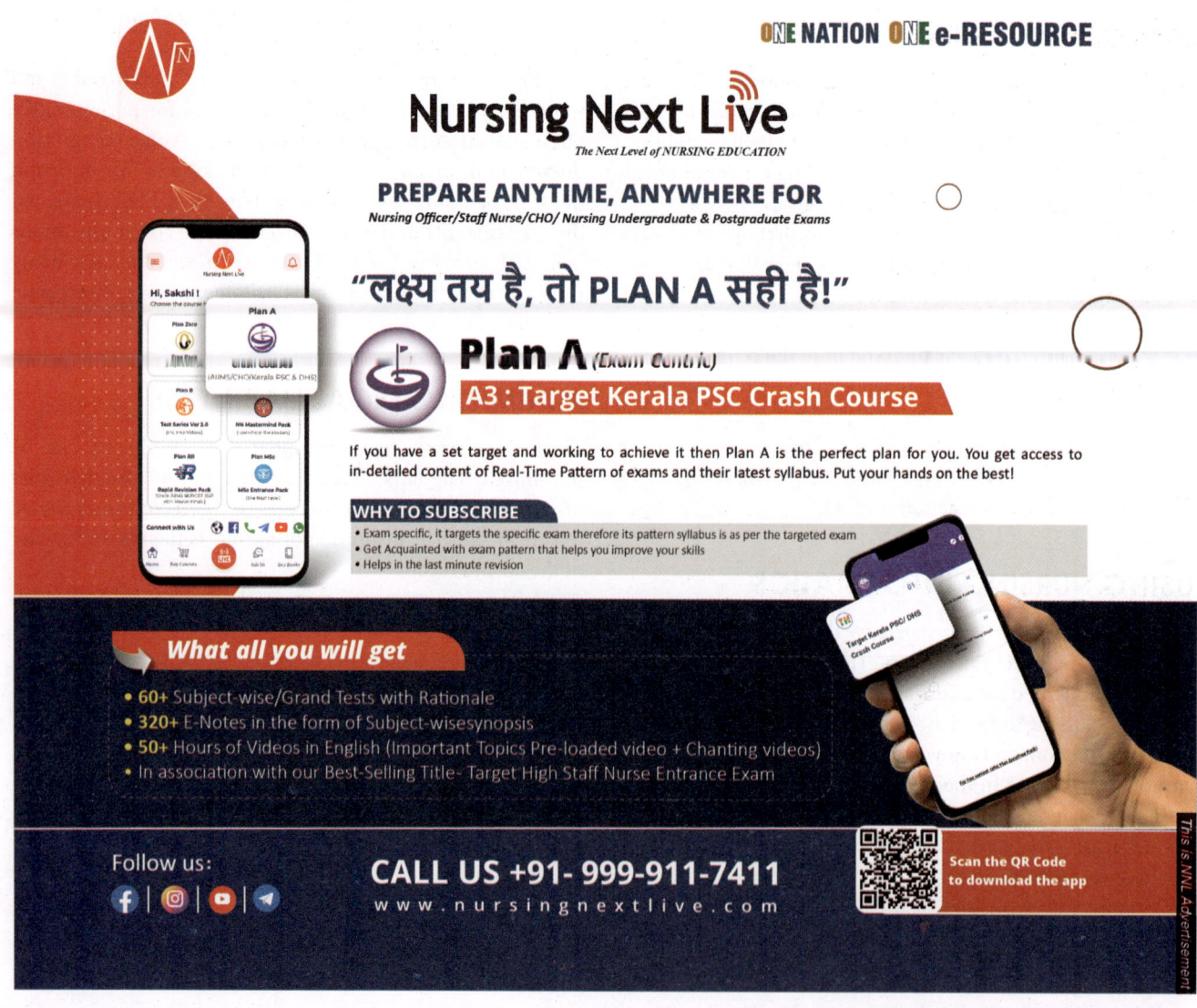

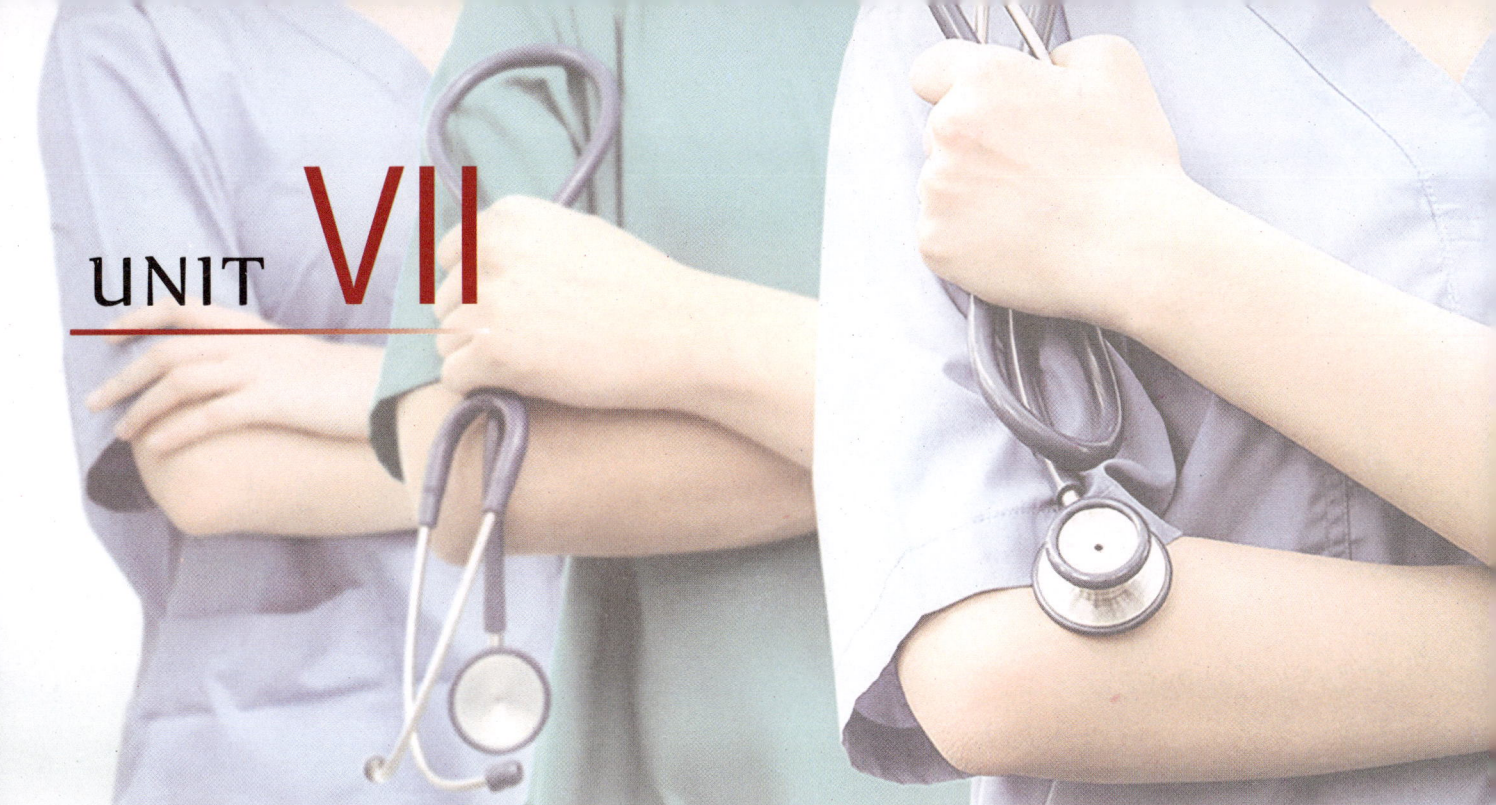

UNIT VII

HOSPITAL ADMISSION, TRANSFER AND DISCHARGE

Unit Outline

Hospital Admission, Transfer and Discharge

ADMISSION TO THE HOSPITAL

Admission refers to the entry of a patient in a health care facility. Admission is an anxious time for patient and their families. Often the patient is having pain or other discomforts. The first contact with nurses and healthcare providers is important, anxiety and fear can be reduced and a positive attitude regarding the care to be received can be initiated. The environment of hospital differs from patient's home in all aspects in relation to new sights, sounds and smell, which may interfere with patient's comforts. Admission routines that the patient perceives as careless or excessively impersonal can heighten anxiety, reduce cooperation, impair response to treatment, and perhaps aggravate symptoms. It is the responsibility of nurses to assist the patient in maintaining dignity and sense of control and in becoming comfortable in the hospital.

Types of Admission

- **Routine admissions** are those that are scheduled in advance. The patient has had at least a short period of time to make plans and arrangements for this interruption in the usual routine.
- **Emergency admissions** are those for which there was no prior planning. Sudden illness, injury or abrupt worsening of an existing condition require immediate admission for treatment. Such admissions are stressful for patient and those closely involved with the patient.

Reaction to Admission

- Fear of the unknown causes insecurity.
- Loss of identity, privacy and autonomy.
- Disorientation.

- Separation-disruption of relationships.
- Loneliness.
- Loss of independence, restrictions on activities.
- Loss of income and its effect on employment.
- Fear of death and pain.

The nurse is the key person to help to reduce the severity of these common reactions to hospitalization with a warm, caring attitude and with courtesy and empathy. Treating each patient with respect, maintaining his/her dignity, involving him/her in the plan of care, and whenever possible, adjusting hospital routine to meet his/her desires will help the patient's adaptation to hospital surroundings.

Preparation of Unit for Admission

Purposes

- To welcome the patient and make him/her feel at home, to adjust to hospital environment.
- To provide comfort and safety to the patient.
- To provide immediate care.
- To make arrangements with patient's family with respect to food, safe water, clothing, valuables, and bringing necessary personal articles.
- To observe and report signs and symptoms.
- To help the doctor obtain the necessary facts from the patient.
- To give necessary information to the family members regarding hospital rules and regulations.
- To relieve anxiety and fear of hospitalization.
- To establish a nurse–patient relationship.

Preparation of Articles

- All articles for an open bed—bottom sheet, draw mackintosh, draw sheet, top sheet, blanket counterpane.
- Full bed-length mackintosh.
- Two bath blankets/bed sheets-one for covering bed-length mackintosh and another to cover the patient.
- Hot water-bags in cold weather.
- Articles for daily care of the patient, e.g., temperature tray, sponge bath tray and set of hospital clothes.
- Special considerations if the patient admitted requires oxygen, suction, intravenous fluids and monitoring equipment.

Admission Procedure

- Prepare the room, equipment and furniture with care and arrange all items in place and adjust height of bed.
- Check the client's identification and greet the client and relatives and introduce self.
- Observe the client's vital signs and symptoms and measure height and weight.

- Check the physicians order for any treatment measures that should be initiated immediately.
- Provide privacy. Give admission bath if needed and change to hospital clothes.
- Orient the client to the nursing unit:
    - Introduce other staff members.
    - Explain visiting hours.
    - Demonstrate use of call-bell, over bed table use, lighting, TV, radio, telephone.
    - Escort the client to the bathroom.
    - Explanation of hospital policies, routines, meal-time, etc.
- Obtain base-line assessment:
    - **Level of consciousness:** Alert, lethargic, drowsy, difficult to arouse, comatose.
    - **Vital signs:** Temperature-route (mention); pulse-rate, quality-bounding, thready irregular; respiratory rate and quality-labored, shallow; blood pressure—systolic and diastolic; height and weight.
    - **Respiratory difficulty:** Dyspnea, wheezing cough (productive or non-productive), shortness of breath, use of accessory muscles, abnormal breath sounds on auscultation.
    - **Ability to communicate:** Language spoken, speech, impediment or impairment, blindness, hearing impairment or deafness.
    - **Condition of skin:** Skin breaks or tears, bruises, abrasions, pressure areas, excessive dryness, birth marks, surgical incisions or wounds.
    - **Prosthetic devices:** Hearing aid glasses contact lenses, dentures, braces, artificial limbs or wigs.
    - **Other health problems and concerns:** Pain or discomfort, loss of function or loss of normal control of function, restricted movement, or alteration in sensation.
- Obtain history of allergies and medication history.
- Give the client a chance to ask questions about procedures and investigations.
- Collect valuables if patient chooses to keep there in the facility (agency policy) and hence, the patient and family member sign it. Place valuables in safe. (color of the metal to be mentioned).
- Complete necessary records according to agency policy.

Medico-legal Issues Related to Admission

- Patient records should be kept confidential.
- The record need to be properly labeled as medico-legal case.
- The chief medical officer and police need to be informed regarding admission of medico-legal case.

TRANSFER OF PATIENTS

Transfer is the movement of a patient from one room to another, within the ward or from one unit to another or from one health care agency to another.

Reasons for Transfer

- For diagnostic procedures.
- Demand for available beds.
- Changes in the patients' condition, e.g., shifting to intensive care unit (ICU) or cardiac care unit (CCU) or transferring to step down unit from these units for observation.
- Surgery has been scheduled.
- Patient requires isolation.
- Transfer to long term rehabilitation unit.
- **Referral** is the transfer of care of a patient from one clinician to another or to a specialist.

Role of Nurse in Transfer

- Make sure there is specific order by the attending physician for the transfer.
- Inform the patient, family or significant others and explain the reasons for transfer.
- Assess whether the patient needs a wheelchair or stretcher.
- Notify the receiving unit of the time, date and the condition of the patient.
- Notify the admission department/business office so that patient's records are updated.
- Record in nurse's notes both by the nurse transferring the patient and the nurse receiving the patient.
- Check the chart for complete recording of vital signs, nursing care, treatment given and assemble the documents, X-rays and medications.
- Inform the dietary department about transfer of patient.
- Assist the relatives to collect their belongings, valuables, glasses, contact lenses, dentures, hearing aids, watch, and jewellery, etc.
- Record the time, mode of transfer, condition of the patient and any ward articles sent with the patient.
- Accompany the patient and transport the patient to receiving unit.
- Introduce the patient to nursing staff of the unit and handover records, medication, etc.
- Collect the ward articles and return them to ward from where the patient was transferred.
- Report to the nurse-in-charge regarding transfer.

DISCHARGE FROM THE HOSPITAL

Discharge or dismissal from the hospital means the departure of the patient from the hospital. It can be the formal discharge of the patient by the attending doctor, when the patient's treatment is over. In Left Against Medical Advice (LAMA), due to personal reasons, the patient may abscond, i.e., leave the hospital without any prior information or the patient may expire during hospitalization.

Purposes of Discharge

- To provide for continuity of care at home.
- To assist the patient to complete hospital formalities before returning home such as medicines, bills, return visit or referral.
- To provide for a safe, efficient return of all the patient's clothing and valuables.
- To assist the patient in managing the change from the hospital environment to the home environment successfully.

Types of Discharge

- **Planned discharge:** Is a process of relieving the patient from the hospital after the completion of the treatment of the patient admitted to hospital.
- **LAMA:** Patient may leave the hospital on his own wish due to the personal reasons, but against the medical advice.
- **Discharge against medical advice (DAMA):** It is a veto power given to a relative of the patient to take discharge if they feel the treatment of their patient is not correct or may be the family is not well to do and cannot afford any further treatment.
- **Referrals and transfer:** Sometimes when patient's condition is not manageable due to any reason, patient is required to be transferred or referred to other health institution. This is known as referrals or transfer.

Other Reasons of Patient Leaving the Hospital

- **Absconding:** If the patient runs away from the ward/hospital, it becomes a major responsibility of the nurse on duty. In such cases, the chief medical officer needs to be informed immediately in writing and record must be kept. The information of absconded patient is made available at the ward so that the nurses in different shifts are aware.
- **Parole:** In mental health hospitals, a patient who has not been discharged from the hospital can be sent home for 2-3 days if requested by the relatives and approved by the attending psychiatrist. If the patient fails to return after

parole, the discharge procedure should be carried as per the hospital policy.

Discharge Planning

It is the systematic process for preparing the patient to leave the hospital for continuity of care. For effective discharge, planning has to start at the time of admission.

Planning for discharge must be individualized to the patient's specific needs. This can be a frightening experience depending on the level of recuperation client has achieved. The amount and type of medications prescribed, dietary needs or restrictions, and other treatment needs to be noted.

Preparation of Patient and Relatives

When the hospitalized patient is ready to be released from health care facility, the physician writes a discharge order. It is the duty of the nurse to make every effort to establish good relations with the patient and the relatives during the discharge process also. The joy of being united with one's family and being restored to a state of good health are after mixed with fear and anxiety about the future. Some may worry about being a burden to their families and their ability to contribute as a member of family and the community. Many of them are anxious about the adjustments they must make in their life situations as a result of physical limitations. Changes in occupation, lifestyles are not easily accepted and are after looked upon with fear. Many a time the patient is sent home with needs that can be met at home, e.g., urine testing, dressing of the wound, injection, etc. Therefore, teaching the family about the care ensures continuity of care. The patient needs to be instructed about diet, medication, activity, rest and follow-up.

The patient and the relatives need to be psychologically prepared and proper arrangement for exit either by wheel chair or stretcher must be made while accompanying the patient at the time of discharge.

Discharge Procedure

- Check the doctor's/written order for discharge.
- Inform the patient and relatives about the discharge.
- Make sure that the family and patient understand the instructions for care, e.g., diet, medication, etc.
- If the patient or relatives decide to leave the hospital against advice of the doctor, have him/her sign LAMA form, so that patient/guardian acknowledges full responsibility and own risk of leaving the hospital care.
- Assist the patient to dress, check and pack belongings.
- Collect the discharge slip and prescriptions that the patient needs to bring for follow-up care. It should include primary and secondary diagnosis, current orders, medications including dosage, route, frequency and time of last dose

given, physician's name and phone number, and brief history of hospital stay.
- Complete the patient's record and discharge summary.
- Send the chart to the billing section with information to pharmacy.
- Once the bill is settled, help the patient to obtain discharge summary, medical certificate and drugs and hand over his/her belongings.
- Accompany the patient up to transport near the exit gate.
- Send the chart (in-patient) to the medical record department within 24 hours.

Special Considerations

- Transfer of the patient from one ward to another ward or hospital must be carefully entered and signed in the ward records as well as to be recorded in patient's file.
- Patient's records or file should not be handed over to police or legal authority without a written permission of the treating physician.
- Name and address of the relative or person should be entered in hospital record with whom the patient has left the hospital.
- On discharge, every patient has full right to see his/her medical records including investigation reports.
- In case of death of the patient in hospital, physician should inform the chief medical officer and ensure that body is appropriately kept in mortuary for the post-mortem examination as per hospital policy.
- Unclaimed dead body must be handed over to police after due permission from the chief medical officer.
- The chief medical officer and police need to be informed regarding discharge of medico-legal case.

Care of Unit after Discharge

Once the patient is discharged, the unit has to be prepared for next patient.

Purposes

- To clean and disinfect the area and equipment.
- To prevent the spread of infection to others.
- To receive a new patient.

Procedure

- Remove the bed linen, mackintosh, mattress, pillows and utensils.
- Wash the bed and locker with soap and water and use antiseptic lotion.
- Clean all the furniture belonging to the unit.
- The mattress, pillow and blanket may be sent to autoclave section or placed in direct sunlight for a day.

- The unit or room is cleaned and aired.
- Rearrange the furniture and the unit.
- Keep the bed ready with clean new sheets for a new patient.

MEDICO-LEGAL ISSUES RELATED TO DISCHARGE

- Patients record is a legal document, should be kept confidential and should not be handed over to the patient or to any other person or even the police without permission from the hospital authorities.
- The signature of the person receiving the records must be obtained if it is indicated.
- The record must be completed and discharge or transfer must be entered with the time, the condition of the patient and details about to whom it was handed over is to be entered and signed by the nurse.
- To safeguard the institution and health care professional, the nurse needs to be careful about legal issues related to patient.
- Any discharge or leaving against medical advice should be recorded and signed by the patient or relative and the nurse.
- Patients have the right to get the discharge summary on discharge and they also have the right to get investigation reports.
- All the patient records have to be handed over to the medical record department and with signatures obtained from those concerned.

BIBLIOGRAPHY

1. *Sharma S. Potter and Perry's Fundamentals of Nursing. A South Asian edition. Elsevier India. Gurugram: 2013.*
2. *Taylor CR, Lillis C, LeMone P, et al. Fundamentals of Nursing – The Art and Science of Nursing Care, 7th edition. Wolters Kluwer; 2010.*
3. *Dewit SC. Fundamental concepts and Skills for Nursing WB Saunders Company; 2001.*
4. *Berman AT, Snyder S, Kozier BJ, et al. Kozier & Erb's. Fundamentals of Nursing: Concepts, Process and Practice, 8th edition. Pearson Education.*

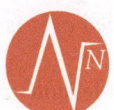 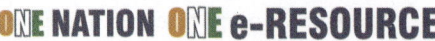
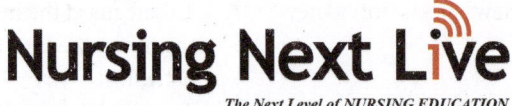
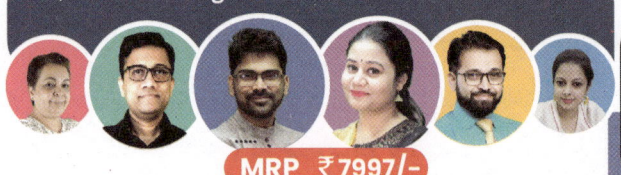
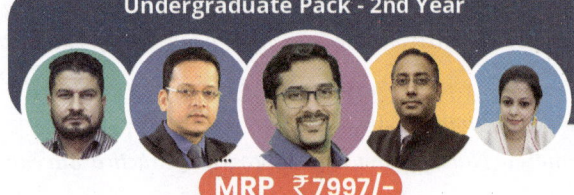
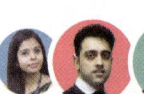 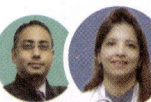 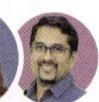 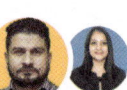

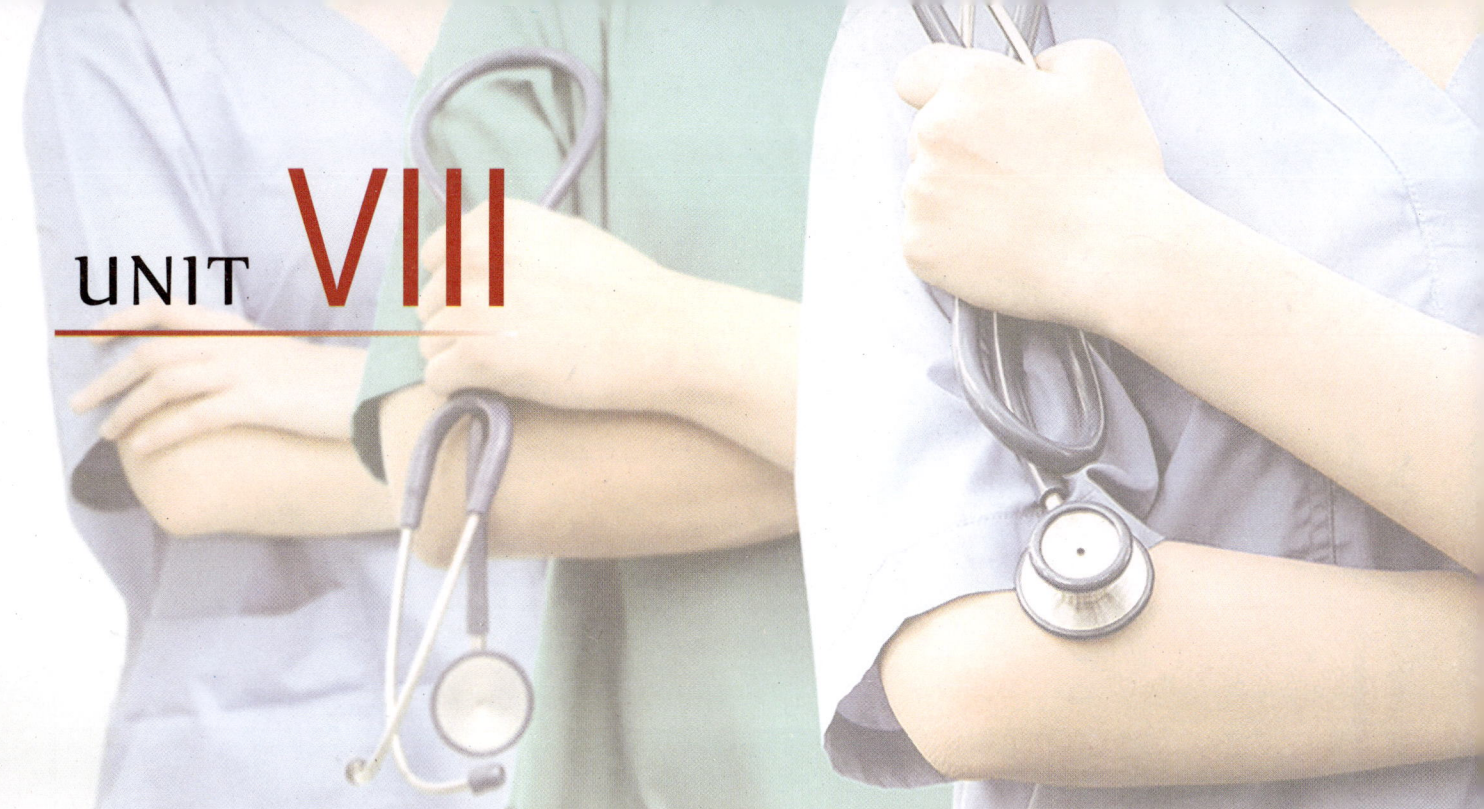

INFECTION CONTROL AND WASTE MANAGEMENT

Unit Outline

Infection Control

INTRODUCTION

Good health depends partly on a safe environment. Practices or techniques that control or prevent transmission of infection help protect clients and health care workers from disease. Clients in all health care settings are at risk of acquiring infections because of lower resistance to infectious microorganism, increased exposure to numbers and types of disease causing microorganisms, and invasive procedures.

Health care workers can protect themselves from contact with infectious material or exposure to a communicable disease by having knowledge of the infectious process and appropriate barrier protection.

DEFINITION

An infection is the entry and multiplication of an infectious agent in the tissues of the host. If the infectious agent (pathogen) fails to cause injury to cells or tissue, then the infection is asymptomatic. If pathogen multiplies and cause clinical signs and symptoms, the infection is then symptomatic. If the infectious disease is transmitted directly from one person to another, it is a communicable or contagious disease.

CHAIN OF INFECTION

The presence of pathogen does not mean that the infection begins. Development of an infection occurs in a cycle that depends on the presence of all of the following elements:

- An infectious agent or pathogen
- Reservoir or source for pathogen growth
- Portal of exit from the reservoir
- A mode of transmission
- A portal of entry to a host
- A susceptible host

An infection develops, if this chain remains intact. Nurses follow infection, prevention and control practices to break the chain so that infection does not develop.

- **Infectious agent:** Microorganism includes bacteria, viruses, fungi and protozoa.
- **Reservoir:** A reservoir is a place where a pathogen can survive but may or may not multiply. For example, Hepatitis A virus survives in shelfish but does not multiply. Pseudomonas organism may survive and multiply in nebulizer reservoir used in the care of clients with respiratory alterations. The most common reservoir is the human body. A variety of microorganism lives on the skin and within the body cavities, fluids and discharges. The presence of microorganism does not always cause illness in a person. Carriers are persons or animals, who show no symptoms of illness but who have pathogens on or in their bodies that can be transferred to others. For example, a person can be a carrier of hepatitis B viruses without having signs or symptoms of infection. Animals, food, water, insects, and inanimate objects can also be reservoir for infectious organisms.

  To thrive, organisms require a proper environment, including food, oxygen, water, appropriate temperature and pH, and light.

  The acidity of an environment determines the viability of microorganism. Most microorganisms prefer an environment within a pH range of 5 to 8. Bacteria in particular thrive in urine with an alkaline pH. Most organisms cannot survive the acid environment of the stomach.

- **Portal of exit:** Once microorganisms find a site to grow and multiply, they must find a portal of exit if they are to enter another host and cause disease. Microorganism can exit through a variety of sites, such as the skin and mucous membranes, respiratory tract, urinary tract, gastrointestinal (GI) tract, reproductive tract, and blood.

- **Mode of transmission:** There are many modes for transmission of microorganism from the reservoir to the host. Four major modes of transmission allow infectious agents to move from portals of exit in reservoir to portals of entry in people. These include contact transmission, common-source transmission, airborne transmission, and vector-borne transmission.

  - **Contact transmission:** It may be direct, indirect contact, or droplet contact.
    - **Direct contact** with infectious agents in most body substances might include touching feces and then putting finger in mouth.
    - **Indirect contact:** It occurs through an intermediate object contaminated with a moist body substance.
    - **Droplet contact:** Droplet contact occurs when infectious agents contained in most respiratory secretions are coughed or sneezed, into environment (usually 3 feet). For example, open sneeze near another person, and moist droplet touch the conjunctiva of the second person's eyes.
  - **Common-source of transmission:** Infectious agents may be transmitted through a common source, e.g., shared food or fluids, through contaminated mediums like water, drugs, blood, food, and improperly handled or stored fruit and vegetables.
  - **Airborne transmission:** Air can carry droplet nuclei. The droplet nuclei can survive suspended in air for long period of time. Very infectious agent can be transmitted this way; however, tuberculosis and chicken pox are examples.
  - **Vector-borne transmission:** Vector-borne transmission includes flies, mosquitoes, rodents, and flies. Transmission of the infectious agents by way of vectors unlikely to occur in modern health care facilities.

- **Portal of entrance:** Portals of entrance are usually the same as portals of exit. For example, agents causing gastrointestinal (GI) infection usually exit from the source or reservoir through the GI tract (i.e., in the stool) and enter in susceptible host through the GI tract.

- **Susceptible host:** Whether a person acquires an infection depends on susceptibility. Depends on the individual degree of resistance to a pathogen. Susceptibility depends upon the individual degree of resistance to an infectious agent.

The stages in course of infection are described in Table 1.

TABLE 1: Course of infection

Stage	Description
Incubation period	Interval between entrance of pathogen into body and appearance of first symptoms, e.g., Chicken pox 2–3 weeks. Common cold-1–2 days.
Prodromal stage	Interval from the onset of non-specific signs and symptoms (malaise, low grade fever, fatigue) to more specific symptoms. Microorganisms grow and multiply and the client is more capable of spreading disease to others during this time.
Illness stage	Interval when the client manifests sign and symptoms specific to the type of infection (e.g., common cold, manifested by sore throat, rhinitis, sinus congestion, etc.)
Convalescence stage	Interval when acute symptoms of an infection disappear, length of recovery depends on severity of infection and the client's general state of health. Recovery may take several days to months.

NOSOCOMIAL INFECTIONS (HOSPITAL-ACQUIRED INFECTIONS)

Nosocomial infections mean infections developed in the patient after admission in hospital, which was neither present nor in the incubation period at the time of hospital.

Types of Nosocomial Infections

- **Iatrogenic infection:** Type of nosocomial infections that result from a diagnostic or therapeutic procedure, e.g., urinary tract infection may result due to catheterization.
- **Exogenous infection:** Arises from microorganisms external to the individual which do not exist as normal flora, e.g., *Clostridium tetani*.
- **Endogenous infection:** Can occur when part of the client's flora becomes altered and an overgrowth results, e.g., infections due to enterococci, yeasts streptococci, etc.

The sites and causes of nosocomial infections are given in Table 2.

TABLE 2: Sites and causes of nosocomial infection

Sites	Causes
Urinary tract	• Insertion of urinary catheter • Closed drainage system becoming open • Catheter and tube getting disconnected • Poor specimen collection technique • Obstruction with urinary drainage • Poor hand washing technique

Contd...

Sites	Causes
Surgical or traumatic wounds	• Skin preparation • Poor hand washing before and after dressing • Use of contaminated antiseptic solutions
Respiratory tract	• Use of contaminated equipment • Improper disposal of mucous secretions
Blood stream	• Contamination of IV fluids by tubing or needle changes • Insertion of drugs to IV fluids • Improper care of needle insertion site • Contaminated needles or catheters • Poor technique during administration of blood products.

PREVENTION AND CONTROL OF NOSOCOMIAL INFECTION

Medical Asepsis

Medical asepsis refers to all practices used to protect the patients and their environment from the transmission of disease-producing organisms that can transmit from one patient to another. It includes all practices intended to confine a specific microorganism to a specific area, limiting the number, growth, and transmission of microorganisms (cross-infection). In medical asepsis, objects are referred to as clean thus, it is also called clean technique.

The nurse follows certain principles and procedures to prevent infection and control its spread. Basic technique is focused on breaking the chain of infection. This can be achieved by the following methods:

Control or Elimination of Infectious Agents Including

- Proper cleaning by water and mechanical action with or without detergents.
- Disinfection
- Sterilization of contaminated objects.
- Handling linens in ways that prevents germs from spreading.

Measures for Control or Elimination of Reservoirs of Infections

- Bathing with soap and water to remove secretion, drainage, perspiration, etc.
- Frequent change of dressings.
- Proper disposal of wastes and contaminated articles.
- Disposal of contaminated needles and syringes.
- Keep the patient's bedside unit clean, dry and biologically safe.

- Bottled solutions should be placed with tight caps as per instructions.
- Keep drainage tubes and collection bags of the patient to prevent accumulation of serous fluid under the skin surface of surgical wounds.
- Drainage suction bottles should be emptied and disposed of as per the agency policy.

Control of Portals of Exit

- Practice aseptic precautions.
- Avoid talking directly into the client's face to prevent droplet infection.
- Wearing of masks is important once the nurse herself has infection or deal with client's suffering from infections.
- Careful handling of wastes like urine, feces, emesis and blood is important.
- Disposable gloves should be worn to prevent direct contact with wastes or infected materials.

Control of Transmission of Infection

- Discourage sharing of bedpans, urinals, basins, eating utensils, etc.
- Use separate thermometers for infectious patients.
- Protect own clothing from direct contact with infected materials.
- Practice hand washing technique.

Control of Portals of Entry

- Maintain integrity of skin and mucous membranes.
- Proper positioning of tubings, etc. may prevent injuries and skin breakdowns.
- Regular skin care is essential with application of lubricants.
- Turning and positioning of debilitated clients help in preventing a skin breakdown.
- Ensure personal hygiene of clients regularly.
- Care should be taken while collecting and handling specimens.

Protection of Susceptible Host

This involves protecting normal defense mechanisms by:

- Proper well-balanced diet.
- Regular oral hygiene.
- Maintaining an adequate fluid intake.
- Encouraging deep breathing and coughing exercises.
- Encouraging proper immunization of children and adult clients.

Cleaning

Cleaning is the removal of all soil (organic and inorganic material) from objects and surfaces. It is the physical removal of visible dirt and debris by washing, dusting or mopping surfaces that are contaminated.

Proper cleaning of items used in health care prior to their being sterilized or disinfected is essential to reduce the number of organisms.

Materials Used in Cleaning

- Mechanical agents: Brushes, dusters or mops.
- Water and soap.
- Absorbent agents.
- Chemical: Solvent, detergents.

Standard Precautions

Treating all patients in the health care facility with the same basic level of "standard" precautions involves work practices that are essential to provide a high level of protection to patients, health care workers and visitors

These include the following:

- Hand washing and hand hygiene.
- Use of personal protective equipment when handling blood, body substances, excretions and secretions.
- Appropriate handling of patient care equipment and soiled linen.
- Prevention of needle stick/sharp injuries.
- Environmental cleaning of spills and appropriate handling of waste.

Universal Precautions

- Use barrier protection to prevent skin and mucus membrane contact with blood or other body fluids.
- Wear gloves to prevent contact with body fluids, infections materials or other potentially contaminated surfaces or items.
- Wear face protection if blood or body fluids one splashed during a procedure.
- Wear protective clothing.
- Wash hands and skin immediately and thoroughly, if contaminated with blood or body fluids.
- Wash hands and skin immediately after gloves are removed.
- Take care while using or handling sharp instruments and needles. Place used sharp in labeled, puncture-resistance containers.
- If you have sustained an exposure or puncture wound, immediately flush the exposed area and notify your supervisor.

- Empty and disposal of drainage suction bottles according to agency policy.

Surgical Asepsis

Surgical asepsis refers to all procedures used to keep objects or areas sterile or completely free from all microorganisms. In the medical asepsis all procedures are directed to the prevention of pathogenic organisms entering into the body; but in the surgical asepsis all practices are directed to elimination of both pathogenic and nonpathogenic microorganisms including spores. In surgical asepsis, a sterile technique is used (Table 3).

Personal Protective Equipment

- **Hair cover:** The surgical head cover or hood should be lint-free and cover all head and facial hair. Hair covers prevent the shedding of hair, squamous cells, and/or dandruff onto the scrub suit.

- **Shoe cover:** Shoe covers protect the footwear and feet from exposure to blood and body fluids. Footwear protects the feet from injury by sharps or heavy equipment and instruments that may accidentally fall on the feet. It also provides a barrier to exposure to blood and body fluids.
- **Wearing mask:** Masks are worn to reduce the risk for transmission of organisms by the droplet contact, air-borne routes, and splatters of body substances.
- **Hand hygiene:** Hand hygiene is the major component of patient and health member's protection. Contaminated hands of health care workers are a primary source of infection transmission in health care setting. Thus, careful washing of hands reduces the numbers of organisms. "Hand hygiene is the act of washing hands with soap and water, followed by rinsing under a stream of water for 15 seconds." [According to, Center for Disease Control and Prevention (CDC)].

TABLE 3: Principles of surgical asepsis

Principles	Rationale
1. Always face the sterile field. Do not turn your back or side on a sterile field.	Sterile objects which are out of vision are considered questionable and their sterility cannot be guaranteed.
2. Keep sterile equipment above your waist level or above table level.	Waist level and table level are considered margins of safety and will promote maximum visibility of the sterile field
3. Do not speak, cough or sneeze over a sterile field. If it is necessary to do so, turn your head away from the sterile field.	To prevent droplet infection
4. Never reach across a sterile field.	When a non-sterile object is held above a sterile object, gravity causes the microorganisms to fall into a sterile field.
5. Prevent excessive air currents around the sterile area. Air currents can be caused by moving fast, flapping the clothes and drapes and by closing doors, etc.	Microorganisms are present in the air and they travel in currents.
6. Keep the unsterile objects away from the sterile field.	Microorganisms may be transferred whenever a non-sterile object touches a sterile field, thus sundering the sterile objects contaminated.
7. Handle liquids cautiously near the sterile field or prevent drapes or wrappers from becoming wet.	When a liquid connects a non-sterile field with a sterile field, the microorganisms may be transferred consequently the sterile area becomes unsterile by capillary action.
8. Keep the sterile field dry.	Microorganisms do not pass easily through a dry surface.
9. The edge of the sterile field is considered unsterile.	Proximity to a contaminated area makes sterility doubtful.
10. Each sterile supply should be clearly labeled as to its contents time and date of sterilization	To ensure sterility.
11. Never assume that an object is sterile. Always check the sterility expiration date.	Sterility of an object wrapped in paper or cloth becomes doubtful after 4 weeks and those sealed in polythene bags becomes doubtful after 1 year.
12. Avoid sweeping and dusting when the sterile objects are opened.	Microorganisms travel in the dust particles.
13. Wash hands and put on gowns, gloves and masks before handling the sterile supplies.	To prevent contamination.

Contd...

Principles	Rationale
14. Open the sterile packages in such a way that the edge of the wrapper is directed away from the worker.	To avoid the possibility of a sterile surface touching the uniform.
Regarding use of transfer forceps	
15. Hold the transfer forceps pointing downward.	To prevent the solution from flowing into the contaminated area (the handle of the forceps) and then back to the sterile area (the tips of the forceps).
16. While removing the forceps from the container, lift it without touching the sides and the rim of the container.	The tip of the forceps becomes contaminated while touching the container that is not in direct contact with the disinfectant solution.
17. Keep the prongs (tip) of the forceps within the vision while using it.	Sterile objects that are out of vision may touch the unsterile objects accidentally.
18. Gently tap the prongs together directly over the container to remove the excess solution.	To prevent the solution dribbling into the sterile field and wet it.
19. Transfer forceps and the container should be sterilized daily.	There is a great possibility of these articles becoming contaminated because of their frequent and varied use.
Regarding use of sterile containers	
20. Remove the cover from the container when necessary and only for a short period of time.	The air currents can contaminate the cover.
21. Lift the cover of the container in such a way that the inside of the lid is pointing down.	The air currents can contaminate the inside of the cover.
22. Invert the cover when it is necessary to place it down.	Contact with the unsterile surface contaminates sterile objects.
23. Consider the rim of the cover and the container to be contaminated.	Proximity to a contaminated area makes sterility doubtful.
24. Do not return the unused sterile objects to the container, once they have been taken out.	It is considered to be contaminated by the air currents.

HAND HYGIENE/HAND WASHING

Hand washing is important in every setting including hospitals. It is an effective infection control measure, as it prevents spread of microorganisms. For routine client care, the Centers for Disease Control and Prevention (CDC) recommends a vigorous hand washing under a stream of water for at least 10–15 seconds using soap.

Hand washing is the single most effective precaution for prevention of infection transmission between patient and staff. When to wash your hand:

- When there are known multiple resistant bacteria.
- Before and after invasive procedures.
- Before and after contact with a patient or caring of wound or the intravenous (IV) line.
- After contact with body fluids and excrete removal.
- After handling contaminated equipment of laundry.
- Before administration of medicines.
- After cleaning spillage after using toilet.
- At the beginning and off duty.
- Before having meals.
- In special units, such as nurseries, intensive care unit (ICUs) and operation theaters (OTs).

- Gloves cannot substitute hand washing, which must be done before putting on gloves and after their removal.

Recent CDC Recommendations on Hand Washing

CDR recently released new recommendation with the intent of improving hand hygiene practices in health care workers.

Effective hand washing requires at least 150 seconds with plain soap or disinfectant and warm water. Hands that are visibly soiled need a longer scrub, if hands are visibly soiled or contaminated with blood or other body fluid:

- Wash hands with either a non-antimicrobial soap and water or an antimicrobial soap and water.
- Wash hands before eating and after using the rest room.
- Use warm, not hot water to prevent further irritation. If hand is not visibly soiled, use an alcohol-based hand rub to decontaminate hands.
- Decontaminate hands before having direct contact with patients, after having direct contact with a patient, before donning sterile gloves for a procedure, and after removing gloves.

- Also decontaminate hands after contact with inanimate objects surrounding the patient, and if moving hands from a contaminated site to a clean site on a patient's body during patient care.
- Perform decontamination also after contact with body fluids or excretions, mucous membranes, non-intact skin and wound dressings.

Purposes

- To remove transient and resident bacteria from fingers, hands and forearms.
- To prevent the risk of transmission of infection to patients.
- To reduce the risk of transmission of infections organisms to oneself.
- To prevent cross-infection among clients.

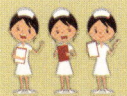 *SKILL: HAND WASHING*

Equipment/Articles

Articles	Rationale
Soap in a soap dish	Soap contains antibacterial agents and has a lasting bacteriostatic effect.
Nail brush	To clean nails
Running water	To rinse soap thoroughly while washing hands
Towel	To dry hands

Steps of Procedure

Action/steps	Rationale
1. File the nails short, ensure that nails are free of nail polish	Short nails are less likely to harbor resident and transient microorganisms.
2. Remove all jewellery and wrist watch	Microorganisms can be inside the settings of jewelry and under rings. Removal facilitates proper cleaning of hands and arms.
3. Turn on the water to adjust the flow so that water is lukewarm.	Warm water removes less of the protective oil of the skin than hot water.
4. Wet the hands thoroughly by holding the hand lower than the elbows so that water flows from arms to finger tips.	It allows water to flow from the least contaminated area (elbow) to the most contaminated area (hands)
5. Apply liberal amounts of soap into hands and lather hands and arms using hand brushes.	Soap emulsifies the oil and lowers the surface tension of water, facilitates the removal of microorganisms, dust and oils, brushes are used to enhance mechanical friction during hand washing.

6. Thoroughly wash hands and rinse using firm rubbing and circular movements to wash the palms, back and wrist of each hand. Interlace the fingers during hand washing:
Follow seven steps of hand washing (Fig. 1):
  i. Palm to Palm: Rub palm together
  ii. Right palm over left dorsum and left palm over right dorsum
  iii. Palm to palm fingers interlaced
  iv. Back of fingers to opposing palms with fingers interlocked
  v. Rotational rubbing of right thumb clasped in left palm and vice versa
  vi. Rotational rubbing backwards and forward with clasped fingers of right hand in left palm and vice versa
  vii. Rotational rubbing of left wrist in with right palm and vice versa
	The circular action helps to remove microorganisms mechanically running water and friction used in cleaning are the mechanical action of cleaning.

Contd...

Action/steps	Rationale
7. Dry arms and hands thoroughly from fingers to wrist and forearms. Discard the towel in a proper container.	Drying helps in removing moisture, prevents chapping and roughening of skin, drying from cleaner to least clean area prevent contamination of washed hands.
8. Turn off the water tap using a paper towel or using an elbow.	Handle is a source of contamination. Use of a paper towel or an elbow prevents contamination of washed hands.

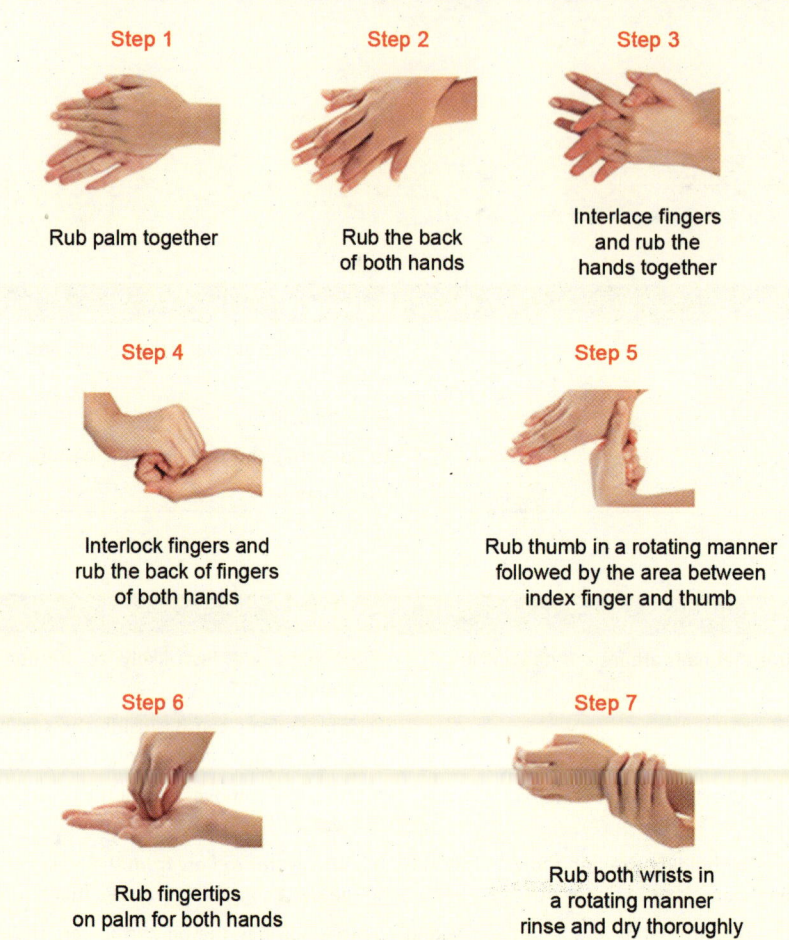

Step 1
Rub palm together

Step 2
Rub the back of both hands

Step 3
Interlace fingers and rub the hands together

Step 4
Interlock fingers and rub the back of fingers of both hands

Step 5
Rub thumb in a rotating manner followed by the area between index finger and thumb

Step 6
Rub fingertips on palm for both hands

Step 7
Rub both wrists in a rotating manner rinse and dry thoroughly

Fig. 1: Seven steps of hand washing

Surgical Scrub

Surgical hand washing is a procedure by which dirt and microorganisms are destroyed and removed from hands and fingers by chemical action and mechanical friction.

Purposes

- To remove dirt and transient microorganisms from hands.
- To reduce the risk of transmission of microorganisms to patients.
- To reduce the risk of cross-infection among the patient.
- To reduce the risk of transmission of infectious agents to oneself.
- To prevent iatrogenic infection.

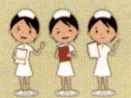

SKILL: SURGICAL SCRUB

Articles

- Soap/antiseptic detergent
- Running warm water
- Nail brush antiseptic lotion
- Towels (sterile)
- Mask and cap

Steps of Procedure

Review and carry out the standard steps as given in Appendix

Action/steps	Rationale
1. Ensure that the nails are short. Remove artificial nail, if any.	Short nails are less likely to harbor organisms, scratch the patient or puncture gloves.
2. Remove nail polish.	Nail polish harbor microorganisms.
3. Inspect hand for abrasion, cuts, or open lesions.	This condition increase likelihood of more microorganisms residing on skin surfaces.
4. Remove jewelry	Microorganisms accumulate in jewelry.
5. After medical hand wash wear cap and mask	
6. Turn on water using knee, foot or elbow	
7. Wet hands and arms under running Lukewarm water and lather with soap/detergent to 5 cm above the elbows. Use firm circular movement to wash palm, back of hand, wrists, forearms and interdigital spaces for 20–25 seconds.	Water flows from finger tip to elbows. Finger tips are considered to be cleaner than elbow.
8. Rinse hands and arms thoroughly under running water (remember to keep hands above elbow)	Rinsing removes transient bacteria from hands.
9. Clean under nails of both hands with nail pick/nail brush.	Removes dirt and microorganisms
10. Scrub nails of each hand with 15 strokes using antimicrobial agent.	
11. Holding the brush perpendicular to scrub palm, each side of thumb and fingers and posterior side of hand with 10 strokes each.	Scrubbing loosens resident bacteria that adhere to skin surfaces.
12. Scrub from wrist to 5 cm above each elbow that is lower arm, upper forearm and antecubital fosse to marginal area above elbows.	Scrubbing is performed from cleanser area to less clean area (upper arms)
13. Entire scrub should last for 5–10 minutes	Scrubbing time can be lengthened according to agency policy/according to the degree of contamination of hands.
14. Discard brush and rinse hands from fingertips to elbows	
15. Take care to not to touch the tap or sides of the sink during the procedure.	Tap and sides of sink are considered to be contaminated.
16. Hold the hands higher than the elbows during the hand wash. Let the water from the fingertips run to the elbows so that the hands become cleaner than the elbows	By this, the water runs the area that now has fewest microorganisms to area with a relatively greater number.
17. Use a sterile towel to dry one hand moving from fingers to elbow. Dry from the cleanest to least clean area. Use new towel to dry the other hand and arm.	Drying facilitates donning of gloves and clean towel prevents the transfer of microorganisms from one elbow to the other.
18. Use one side to dry one hand and reverse side for other hand, if only one towel is available.	

PERSONAL PROTECTIVE EQUIPMENT

Gowning

Clean or disposable gowns or plastic aprons are worn during procedures when the nurse's uniform is likely to become soiled. Sterile gowns may be indicated when the nurse changes the dressings of a client with extensive wounds, burns, etc.

Purposes

- To prevent soiling of clothes during contact with the patient.
- To protect health care personnel from coming in contact with infected material.
- The article tray for personal protective equipment (PPE) is shown in (Fig. 2).

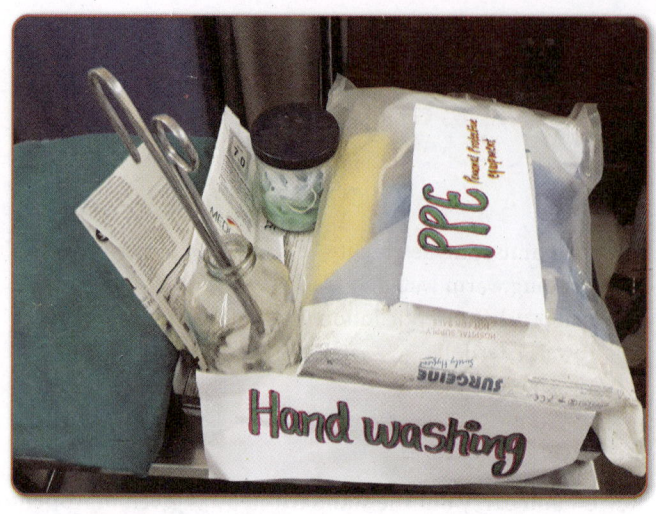

Fig. 2: Article tray for personal protective equipment

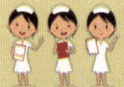

SKILL: GOWNING TECHNIQUE (STERILE)

Action/steps	Rationale
1. Pick up sterile gown and allow it to unfold keeping inside of the gown toward the body without allowing the outside of the gown to touch any area.	To prevent soiling/contamination of the gown.
2. With hands at shoulder level, slip both hands into arm holes simultaneously. Ask the circulating nurse to bring the gown over shoulders (Fig. 3).	It prevents contamination of the sterile gown.
3. The circulating nurse fastens the ties at the neck. Overlap the gown at the back as much as possible and fasten the waist, ties or belt.	It keeps the gown at place and covers the uniform at the back.

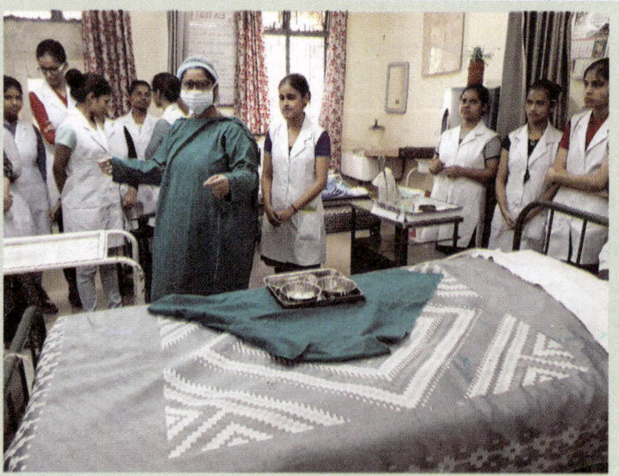

Fig. 3: Gowning

Action/steps	Rationale
4. Prevent the gown from becoming wet.	Moisture allows organisms to pass through the gown to the uniform
5. While removing avoid touching soiled parts on the gown with the soiled part inside and discard in the appropriate container.	It prevents contamination of the uniform, it prevents cross infection.

Wearing Mask

Masks are worn to reduce the transmission of organisms by the droplet contact, air-borne routes, and splatters of body substances. The CDC recommends that masks should be worn:

♦ By personnel who works close to the client if the infection is transmitted by large particle aerosols, e.g., measles, mumps and acute respiratory diseases in children.

♦ By all personnel entering the room, if the infection is transmitted by small particle aerosols (droplet nuclei), e.g., pulmonary tuberculosis.

Purposes

♦ To prevent dispersal of droplets from wearer to environment and patient.

♦ To decrease chances of droplet infection.

♦ During surgical operation to protect wound from staff breathing.

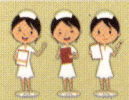 **SKILL: WEARING DISPOSABLE MASK**

Action/steps	Rationale
1. Tie the top two string of the mask, the head above ear	Position of ties at the top of the head provides a tight fix. Ties over ears may cause irritation
2. Tie two lower strings snugly around the neck with the mask well under the chin.	Prevents escape of microorganisms through sides of the mask
3. Ensure that the mask covers the mouth and the nose adequately.	Prevents (inhalation and escape of) microorganisms from and into the air.
4. If glasses are worn, fix the upper edge of the mask under the glasses.	To prevent glasses from clouding
5. Avoid unnecessary talking and, if possible, sneezing or coughing.	To prevent the mask from getting moist.
6. When removing a mask with strings, first untie the lower strings of the mask.	To prevent the top part of the mask from falling into the chest.
7. Discard a disposable mask in the waste container.	To prevent cross infection.
8. Wash the hand if they become contaminated by accidentally touching the soiled part of the mask.	To prevent infection.

*Mask must be of good quality that is properly fixed on mouth and nasal opening.

Eye Wear/Goggles/Face Shields

This protects the mucous membranes of the eyes when conducting procedures that are likely to generate splashes of blood, body fluids.

Gloves

Gloves are worn to protect hands when the nurse is likely to handle any body substances, e.g., blood, urine, feces, sputum, mucous membranes and non-intact skin. Gloves also reduce the likelihood of the nurse's transmitting their own endogenous microorganisms to individuals receiving care. For most activities, disposable clean gloves are used like working with contaminated equipment. Sterile gloves are used when the hands come in contact with an open wound or in invasive procedure, when the hands might introduce microorganisms into a body orifice.

Purposes

♦ To prevent the nurse from pathogenic microorganisms.

♦ To handle sterile articles without contaminating.

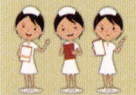

SKILL: WEARING AND REMOVING DISPOSABLE GLOVES

Wearing Gloves

Action/steps	Rationale
1. Thoroughly wash hands.	Removes bacteria from skin surfaces and reduces transmission of infection.
2. Open a sterile glove packet of proper size on a flat surface above waist level.	A sterile object held below waist gets contaminated.
3. If gloves are not powdered take a packet of powder and apply lightly to the hands.	Powder allows gloves to slip on easily.
4. Identify right and left hand. Glove dominant hand first.	Proper Identification of gloves prevents contamination by improper fit.
5. With thumb and first two fingers of the non-dominant hand, grasp an edge of the gloves cuff on dominant hand, touch only the gloves inside surface.	Inner edge of the cuff lies against skin and thus, is not sterile.
6. Carefully pull the glove over the dominant hand. Ensure the thumb and the finger are in proper spaces.	Proper fitting of gloves on fingers.
7. With gloved dominant hand, slip fingers underneath the second glove's cuff.	This prevents gloves contamination.
8. Carefully pull the second glove over the non-dominant hand. Don't allow fingers of the thumb of the gloved dominant hand to touch any part of the exposed non-dominant hand.	Contact of the gloved hand with the exposed hand result in contamination.
9. After the second glove is on, interlock hands together.	Ensure smooth fit over fingers.

Removing Gloves

Action/steps	Rationale
1. Remove the first glove by grasping it on its palmar surface just below the cuff, taking care to touch glove to glove completely off by inverting or rolling the glove inside out.	This keeps the soiled parts of the used gloves from touching the skin of the wrist or hand.
2. Place the first two fingers of the bare hand inside the glove, the second contaminated glove.	To prevent touching the outside of the second soiled glove with the bare hand.
3. Dispose them off in the appropriate glove.	To prevent cross infection.

*Gloves must be of good quality, suitable size, and should never be reused.

Removal of Personal Protective Equipment

What order do you follow to undress PPE? One must think critically as it depends upon the area in which you are working.

As a General Rule

- Gloves are last put on and first taken off.
- If there is a chance of airborne infection, mask must stay on until you are out of the room.
- Consider that outside of your goggles, front of your mask, sleeves, and front of your gown can be contaminated. Remember to wash hand, once all PPE are removed.

- Remove in following order:
  1. Remove gloves
  2. Remove eye wear/goggles
  3. Remove gown (pull of inside out)
  4. Remove mask
  5. Wash hand immediately.

PREPARATION OF ISOLATION ROOM

An isolation room is a specially constructed area in a hospital designed for housing patients with an infectious disease in order to prevent the spread of the disease in the hospital.

Purposes

- To prevent the spread of infections.
- To create a physical barrier that prevents the spread of disease.

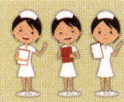 **SKILL: PREPARING ISOLATION ROOM**

Articles Required

- Isolation suite if possible.
- All items required to meet patient's nursing needs during the period of isolation, e.g., instruments to assess vital signs.

Steps of Procedure

Action/steps	Rationale
1. Place a barrier nursing sign outside the door.	Inform the situation to anyone entering the room.
2. List requirements for personnel before entering and after living isolation area.	To decrease entries and exits to the room.
3. Remove all nonessential furniture. The remaining furniture should be easy to clean and should not conceal or retain dirt or moisture either within or around it.	To minimize the risk of furniture harboring microbial spores or growth colonies.
4. Stock the hand basin with a suitable bactericidal soap preparation and paper towels for staff use.	Facilities for hand washing within the infected area are essential for effective barrier nursing.
5. Place yellow clinical waste bag in the room on a foot-operated stand. The bag must be sealed before it is removed from the room.	For contaminated rubbish within the room. Yellow is the recognized color for clinical waste.
6. Place a container for sharp in the room. When the ''sharps'' container is two-thirds full. It must be firmly shut and sent for incineration.	To contain contaminated sharps within the infected area.
7. Keep the patient's personal property to a minimum. Advise him/her to wear hospital clothing. All belongings taken into the room should be washable, cleanable or disposable.	The patient's belongings may become contaminated and cannot be taken home unless they are washable or cleanable. Anything else may have to be destroyed.
8. Provide the patient with his/her own thermometer	Equipment used regularly by the patient should be kept within the infected area to prevent the spread of infection.
9. Keep dressing solution, creams, and lotions, etc. to a minimum and store them within the room.	All partially used material must be discarded when barrier nursing ends, therefore unnecessary waste should be avoided.
10. Setup a trolley outside the door to hold plastic aprons and bactericide alcoholic hand rub. (This is contraindicated, if the trolley causes an obstruction or is a hazard to staff and others.)	Staffs are more likely to use the equipment if it is readily available.

ISOLATION TECHNIQUES

Isolation is the separation of infected persons from the noninfected persons for the period of communicability under conditions which will prevent the transmission of infection to others.

Isolation Practices

Isolation precautions control the transmission of pathogens by prevention of direct contact with the infected client, barrier nursing or isolation technique is intended to confine the microorganism within a given and recognized area.

TABLE 4: Category-specific isolations

Isolation	Purposes
Strict isolation	Prevents transmission of highly contagious or virulent infections that spread by air and contact.
Contact isolation	Prevents transmission of highly transmissible infection, which spread by close or direct contact that does not warrant strict precautions.
Respiratory isolation	Prevents transmission of highly transmissible infections, which spread by close or direct contacts that do not warrant strict precautions.
Enteric isolation	Prevents infection transmitted by direct or indirect contact of feces.
Drainage and secretions precautions (wound and skin isolation)	Prevents infection transmitted by direct or indirect contact with purulent material or drainage from an infected body site.
Universal blood and body fluids precautions (blood isolation)	Prevents contact with pathogens transmitted by direct or indirect contact with infected blood or body fluids containing blood.
Care of severely immune containing blood	Protect the clients with lowered immunity and resistance from acquiring infectious organisms.

There are various isolation techniques, which are broadly classified into two methods for implementation as given by Garner, Simmons, 1987. These are:

- **Disease-specific isolation method:** Certain practices are followed for each infectious disease, e.g., Chicken pox in which the client is placed in a private room with precautions to prevent respiratory spread.
- **Category-specific isolation:** Diseases requiring similar isolation perceptions are grouped as given in Table 4.

USING HAZMAT SPILL KIT

Hazmat spill kits should be used when the spilled chemical poses a risk to health and welfare of those in both the immediate and near vicinity of the spill; depending on the type of chemical that is spilled, certain steps must be taken in order to contain the spill, prevent combustion, and to avoid loss of life or further damage to property.

A quick response to an accident or spill can greatly reduce exposure to a flammable substance. If a spill or accident occurs, first responders must ensure that the contaminated materials are disposed of in the correct hazardous waste bin (ensure stained clothing is removed immediately). A correct spill kit is used on the spill; in the case of a liquid spill, ensure that the spill is cleaned as soon as possible to prevent the formation of aerosols. Managers must have employees tested for exposure to carcinogens, and safety officers must provide medical treatment for specific exposures or dangers. Prepare hazmat spill kits and emergency plans prior to beginning use of the carcinogenic substances, and in the case of a large spill, vacate the area and call for assistance.

Standard containment devices such as fume hoods, glove boxes, use of high efficiency particulate air (HEPA) filters, ventilated containment or weighing, or placing the dangerous substance in a sealed weighed container (Tare Method) are sound preparedness precautions. The employment of these methods and equipment can help reduce the unnecessary exposure to harmful chemicals.

Special care must be taken when using single exposure chemicals, such as polycyclic aromatic hydrocarbons. All surfaces where harmful chemicals are used must be of a suitable material, e.g., stainless steel, plastic trays or absorbent plastic backed paper. Correct signs must be placed outside of the work stating: "No eating, drinking or smoking," "Danger carcinogen in use," and "Authorized personnel Only" are few such signs.

DISINFECTION/DECONTAMINATION AND STERILIZATION

Disinfection of Articles

Disinfection refers to chemical or physical processes used to reduce the numbers of pathogens from the objects surface. These processes do not necessarily remove all potential for infection, because spores may remain present.

Disinfectants are substances that are applied to nonliving objects to destroy microorganisms that are living on the objects. Whereas **antiseptics** are antimicrobial substances that are applied to living tissue/skin.

Classification of Disinfectants (Table 5)

- **Based on consistency**
  - Liquid (e.g., alcohols, phenols).
  - Gaseous (formaldehyde vapor, ethylene oxide).
- **Based on spectrum of activity**
  - High level
  - Intermediate level
  - Low level.

TABLE 5: Disinfectants in use

Name of disinfectants	Methods of dilution	Contact time	Effective time span
Glutaraldehyde 2%, e.g., Cidex	Add activator powder/liquid to the liquid in the 5 Liter jar and use undiluted	Disinfection: 20–30 minutes Sterilization: 10 hours	14–28 days (see hours, manufacturer's instructions) Time span reduces if solution is diluted so utilize in-use test for confirming efficacy
Combination of glutaraldehyde and chemically bound Formaldehyde, e.g., Korsolex, Bacillocid	Korsolex: water 1 part : 9 parts Bacillocid: water 1 part : 49 parts (20 mL : 980 mL)	Disinfection 14 days 15 minutes. Sterilization 5 hours 24 hours 30 minutes	14 days 24 hours
Phenol 5% (Carbolic acid 100%)	Phenol : water 5 mL : 95 mL	10–15 minutes in 5% solution	24 hours
Ethanol Isopropyl alcohol, 70% e.g., Bacillol—25	Do not dilute	2–10 minutes	24 hours
Hydrogen peroxide 6% (available as 30% stabilized solution)	20 mL H_2O_2 - with 80 mL Normal saline = 6% H_2O_2 - (use freshly prepared)	6–8 minutes	Use immediately after preparation
Sodium Hypochlorite solution 1%, e.g., Polar bleach available in 5% and 10% concentrations	5% : 80 mL water + 20 mL bleach solution 10% : 90 mL water + 10 mL bleach solution	20–30 minutes	8 hours
Calcium Hypochlorite, e.g., Bleaching Powder (70% available Cl_2)	14 gm/L dissolved properly for visibly contaminated articles. 1.4 gm per L for clean objects.	20–30 minutes	24 hours
Formaldehyde 40%		30 minutes then open the area after 6 hours	15–30 days

- **Based on mechanism of action**
  - Action on membrane (e.g., Alcohol, detergent).
  - Denaturation of cellular proteins (e.g., Alcohol, Phenol).
  - Oxidation of essential sulfhydryl groups of enzymes (e.g., H_2O_2, Halogens).
  - Alkylation of amino, carboxyl and hydroxyl group (e.g., Ethylene oxide, formaldehyde).
  - Damage to nucleic acids (Ethylene oxide, Formaldehyde).

Types of Disinfection

- **Concurrent disinfection:** It is the immediate disinfection of all contaminated articles and bodily discharges during the course of disease.
  It includes:
  - Cleaning of isolation unit daily
  - Disinfection of all articles
  - Disposal of all wastes by incineration
  - Safe disposal of excreta.
- **Terminal disinfection:** It is the disinfection of the patient's unit with all articles used during discharge, transfer or death of a patient who had been suffering from an infectious disease. It includes: fumigation of room with formalin or sulfur.

Sterilization

Sterilization is the process by which an object becomes free of all microorganisms. By sterilization both the pathogenic and nonpathogenic organisms are destroyed. There are various methods used for sterilization of articles.

Methods of Sterilization

- **Direct sunlight:** It has an effect on acid-fast microorganisms. Place the linen or bed pans in direct sunlight for 6 hours for two consecutive days.
- **Boiling:** Boiling is an effective method of sterilization. Boiling for 5–10 minutes at boiling point kills all the bacteria except spores and viruses. Boiling is the most commonly used method in day-to-day working.
- **Fumigation or gas sterilization:** Total surface exposure to formaldehyde gas under conditions of controlled humidity, temperature and time. This exposure destroys all vegetative forms of bacteria, viruses and most of the spores. The best results can be obtained with high concentration of gas, humidity above 60 and temperature of not less than 18°C. The exposure time varies from 1 hour to 16 hours. The agents commonly used for the fumigation are formalin tablets, ethylene oxide liquids, etc.

- **Ultraviolet light sterilization or radiation:** Ultraviolet light sterilization is effective for disinfecting working surface and air inside rooms.

- **Hot air sterilization:** High temperature and comparatively long exposure time are required. It is not a suitable sterilization agent for fabrics and dresses which are poor and uneven conductors and are mined by excessive heat. It is, however the method of choice for final metal cannula (e.g., lumbar puncture needles) and for glass syringes, since these can be sterilized with a stillet or the piston in position.

- **Autoclaving steam under pressure:** Autoclaving is a method of sterilization by steam under pressure. It is the most widely used, economical and one of the most effective methods of destroying microorganisms, including spore formation. The steam under pressure maintains the necessary high temperature and it allows rapid penetration of articles packed in it.

For effective sterilization autoclaving is done at 15 lbs per square inch pressure and 121°C temperature for at least 20 minutes.

- **Flaming:** Flaming is the method of sterilization by putting the instrument in a flame for a while. This method is used in dire emergency situations.

Differences among various cleaning techniques are enlisted in Table 6.

The level of decontamination should be such that there is no risk for infection when using the equipment. The choice of the method depends on a number of factors, including type of material of object, number and type of organisms involved and risk of infection to patients or staff.

Guidelines for disinfection and sterilization are given in Table 7.

TABLE 6: Differences among various cleaning techniques

Cleaning	Disinfection	Sterilization	Decontamination
Cleaning is a process that removes foreign material (e.g., soil, organic material, microorganisms) from an object.	Disinfection is a process that reduces the number of pathogenic microorganisms, but not necessarily bacterial spores, from inanimate objects or skin, to a level which is not harmful to health.	Sterilization is a process that destroys all microorganisms including bacterial spores. Sterilization cannot be proved except by culturing, so normally an object is said to have been sterilized if it has gone through a controlled process of sterilization.	Use of physical or chemical means to remove, inactivate, or destroy blood borne or other pathogens on a surface or item, to the point where they are no longer capable of transmitting infectious particles, and the surface or item is rendered safe for handling, use, or disposal.

TABLE 7: Guidelines for disinfection and sterilization

Device classification	Devices examples	Types of process	Process examples
High risk (enters sterile tissue or vascular system, includes dental instruments)	Implants, scalpels, needles, other surgical instruments and endoscopic accessories	Sterilisation (cycle time as per manufacturer)	Steam under pressure, Dry heat, Ethylene oxide gas, Chemical gas sterilizers
Intermediate risk (touches mucous membrane or broken skin)	Flexible endoscopes, Laryngoscopes, Endotracheal tubes, Respiratory therapy and Anesthesia equipment, Diaphragm fitting rings, and other similar devices.	High-level disinfection (exposure time 20 minutes)	Glutaraldehyde based formulations (2%) Stabilized hydrogen peroxide (6%) Household bleach (sodium hypochlorite 5.25% 1,000 ppm available chlorine = 1:50 dilution)
	Thermometers (oral or rectal)	Intermediate-level disinfection (exposure time 10 minutes)	Ethyl or Isopropyl alcohol (70% to 90%) (do not mix oral and rectal thermometers)
	Smooth, hard surfaces such as hydrotherapy tanks	Intermediate-level disinfection (exposure time 10 minutes)	Ethyl or isopropyl alcohol (70 to 90%) Phenolic detergent (dilute per label) Iodophor detergent (dilute per label) Household bleach (sodium hypochlorite 5.25% 1,000 ppm available chlorine = 1:50 dilution)

Contd...

Device classification	Devices examples	Types of process	Process examples
Low risk (Touches intact skin)	Stethoscopes, tabletops, floors, bedpans, furniture, etc.	Low level disinfection (exposure time 10 minutes)	Ethyl or isopropyl alcohol (70 to 90%) Phenolic detergent (dilute per label) Iodophor detergent (dilute per label) Household bleach (sodium hypochlorite 5.25% 100 ppm available chlorine = 1:500 dilution)

TRANSPORTATION OF INFECTED PATIENTS

Cover the mouth of the patient with mask and transport the patient out of the room only if necessary. The person moving the patient should also wear a mask and gown. Inform the other health team members about isolation status and the barriers needed to protect themselves and other patients. Take necessary precautions as per disease and in case of serious infections, put the labels, 'isolated' or 'contaminated'.

ROLE OF THE INFECTION CONTROL NURSES

All health care organizations must have multidisciplinary infection control committees. Representatives from the clinical laboratory, housekeeping, maintenance, dietary, and client care areas are included. An important member of this committee is the infection control nurse. This nurse is specially trained to be knowledgeable about the latest research practice in preventing, detecting, and treating infections. All infections are reported to the nurse in a manner that allows for recording and analyzing that can assist in improving infection control practices. She also may be involved in employee education related to infection control practices.

CONCLUSION

The main aim of an aseptic technique is to protect the patients from contamination by microorganisms during nursing and medical procedures from being exposed to potentially infectious blood and body fluids. It is the responsibility of the nurse and health care personnel for providing the patient with a clean and safe environment. The conscientiousness and accuracy of the nurse in performing clean and aseptic procedures increase the effectiveness of infection control.

BIBLIOGRAPHY

1. Taylor FB, Toh CH, Hoots WK, et al. Towards a Definition, Clinical and Laboratory Criteria, and a Scoring System for DIC. Thromb Haemost. 2007;5(3):604-606).

2. Smeltzer SC, Bare BG, Hinkle, et al. Brunner & Suddarth's Textbook of Medical-Surgical Nursing, 11th edition. 2008. pp.1093-1098.

3. Black JM, Hawks JH. Medical Surgical Nursing: Clinical Management for Positive Outcome, 8th edition. Mosby's; St Louise, Missouri; 2009. pp:151-166.

4. Smeltzer SC, Bare BG, Hinkle, et al. Brunner & Suddarth's Textbook of Medical-Surgical Nursing, 12th edition. Lippincott Williams & Wilkins; 2009. pp. 2136-2233.

5. Berman AT, Snyder S, Frandsen G. Kozier & Erb's Fundamentals of Nursing: Concept Process and Practice, 8th edition. Pearson. pp. 668-710.

6. Taylor FB, Toh CH, Hoots WK. Towards definition, clinical and laboratory criteria, and a scoring system for disseminated intravascular coagulation. Thromb Haemost. 2001;86(5):1327-1330.

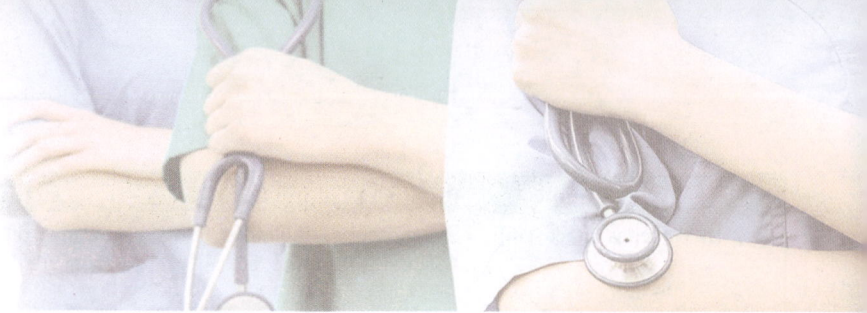

Biomedical Waste Management

INTRODUCTION

The waste produced in the course of health care activities carries a higher potential for infection and injury than any other type of waste. Therefore, it is essential to have safe and reliable methods for its handling.

DEFINITIONS

- **"Authorization"** means permission granted by the prescribed authority for the generation, collection, reception, storage, transportation, treatment, processing, disposal or any other form of handling of biomedical waste in accordance with the rules and guidelines issued by the Central Government or Central Pollution Control Board as the case may be.
- **"Authorized person"** means an occupier or operator authorized by the prescribed authority to generate, collect, receive, store, transport, treat, process, dispose or handle biomedical waste in accordance with the rules and the guidelines issued by the Central Government or the Central Pollution Control Board, as the case may be.
- **"Biological"** means any preparation made from organisms or microorganisms or product of metabolism and biochemical reactions intended for use in the diagnosis, immunization, or the treatment of human beings or animals or in research activities pertaining thereto.
- **"Biomedical waste"** means any waste, which is generated during the diagnosis, treatment or immunization of human beings or animals or research activities pertaining thereto or in the production or testing of biological entities or in health camps.
- **"Biomedical waste treatment and disposal facility"** means any facility wherein treatment, disposal of biomedical waste or processes incidental to such treatment and disposal is carried out, and includes common biomedical waste treatment facilities.

- **"Handling"** in relation to biomedical waste includes the generation, sorting, segregation, collection, use, storage, packaging, loading, transportation, unloading, processing, treatment, destruction, conversion, or offering for sale, transfer, disposal of such waste.
- **"Health care facility"** means a place where diagnosis, treatment or immunization of human beings is provided irrespective of type and site of health treatment system and research activities pertaining thereto. In pretext to these guidelines these health care facilities include— district hospitals, sub divisional hospitals, community health centers, primary health centers and sub centers.
- **"Management"** includes all steps required to ensure that biomedical waste is managed in such a manner as to protect health and environment against any adverse effects due to handling of such waste.
- **"Occupier"** means a person having administrative control over the institution and the premises generating biomedical waste, which includes a hospital, nursing home, clinic. Dispensary, veterinary institution, animal house, pathological laboratory, blood bank, health care facility and clinical establishment, irrespective of their system of medicine and by whatever name they are called.
- **"Operator of a common biomedical waste treatment facility"** means a person who owns or controls a common biomedical waste treatment facility (CBWTF) for the collection, reception, storage, transport, treatment, disposal or any other form of handling of biomedical waste.
- **"Prescribed authority"** means the State Pollution Control Board in respect of State and Pollution Control Committee in respect of Union Territory.
- **"Point of Generation"** means the location where wastes initially generate, accumulate and is under the control of the operator of the waste-generating process.
- **"Storage"** means the holding of biomedical waste for a temporary period at the end of which the biomedical waste is treated or disposed.
- **"Treatment"** means any method, technique, or process, including neutralization, designed to change the physical, chemical, or biological characteristics or composition of any hazardous waste.

CLASSIFICATION OF HEALTH CARE WASTE

Health care facilities (Health care facilities) are primarily responsible for management of the health care waste generated within the facilities, including activities undertaken by them in the community. The Health care facilities, while generating the waste are responsible for segregation, collection,

in-house transportation, pretreatment of waste and storage of waste, before such waste is collected by common biomedical waste treatment facility (CBWTF) operator. Thus, for proper management of the waste in the health care facilities the technical requirements of waste handling are needed to be understood and practiced by each category of the staff in accordance with the Biomedical Waste Management (BMWM) Rules, 2016.

Waste generated from the health care facility is classified shown in (Fig. 1):

- Biomedical waste
- General waste
- Other wastes.

Biomedical Waste

Biomedical waste means any waste, which is generated during the diagnosis, treatment or immunization of human beings or animals or research activities pertaining thereto or in the production or testing of biological or in health camps. Biomedical waste includes all the waste generated from the health care facilities, which can have any adverse effect to the health of a person or to the environment in general, if not disposed properly. All such waste which can adversely harm the environment or health of a person is considered as infectious and such waste has to be managed as per BMWM Rules, 2016 (amendment 2018).

The quantity of such waste is around 10–15% of total waste generated from the health care facility. This waste consists of the materials, which have been in contact with the patient's blood, secretions, infected parts, biological liquids such as chemicals, medical supplies, medicines, lab discharge, sharps metallic and glassware, plastics, etc.

Biomedical waste management rules, 2016 categorize the biomedical waste into four categories based on the segregation pathway and color code. Various types of biomedical waste are further assigned to each one of the categories, as detailed below:

- Yellow category
- Red category
- White category
- Blue category

These categories are further divided as per the type of waste as discussed in Table 1.

General Waste

General waste consists of all the waste other than biomedical waste and which has not been in contact with any hazardous or infectious, chemical or biological secretions and does not include any waste sharps.

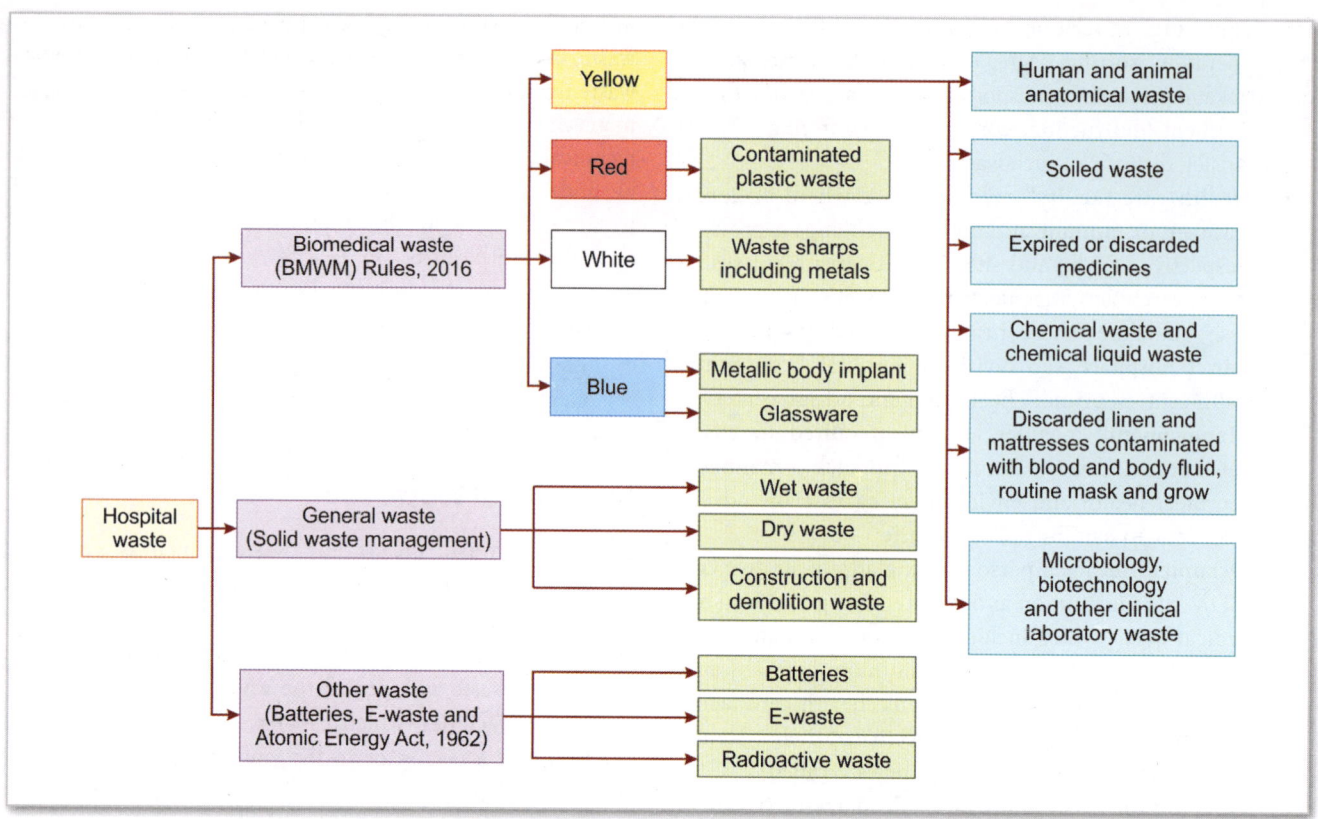

Fig. 1: Classification of health care waste

TABLE 1: Categories of biomedical waste

Category	Types of waste
Yellow	**Human anatomical waste:** Human tissues, organs, body parts and fetus below the viability period (as per the Medical Termination of Pregnancy Act 1971 amended from time to time).
	Animal anatomical waste: Experimental animal carcasses, body parts, organs, tissues, including the waste generated from animals used in experiments or testing in veterinary hospitals or colleges or animal houses.
	Soiled waste: Items contaminated with blood, body fluids like dressings, plaster casts, cotton swabs and bags containing residual or discarded blood and blood components.
	Discarded or expired medicine: Pharmaceutical waste like antibiotics, cytotoxic drugs including all items contaminated with cytotoxic drugs along with glass or plastic ampoules, vials, etc.
	Chemical waste: Chemicals used in production of biological disinfectants and used or discarded disinfectants
	Chemical liquid waste: Liquid waste generated due to use of chemicals in production of biological and used or discarded disinfectants, Silver X-ray film developing liquid, discarded Formalin, infected secretions. aspirated body fluids , liquid from laboratories and floor washings, cleaning, house keeping and disinfecting activities, etc.
	Discarded linen, mattresses, beddings contaminated with blood or body fluid, routine mask and gown.
	Microbiology, Biotechnology and other clinical laboratory waste (Pre-treated): Blood bags, Laboratory cultures, stocks or specimens of microorganisms, live or attenuated vaccines, human and animal cell cultures used in research, industrial laboratories, production of biological, residual toxins, dishes and devices used for cultures.
Red	**Contaminated waste (recyclable):** Wastes generated from disposable items such as tubing, bottles, intravenous tubes and sets, catheters, urine bags, syringes without needles, fixed needle syringes with their needles cut, vaccutainers and gloves.

Contd...

Category	Types of waste
White	**Waste Sharps including metals** Needles, syringes with fixed needles, needles from needle tip cutter or burner, scalpels, blades, or any other contaminated sharp object that may cause puncture and cuts. This includes both used, discarded and contaminated metal sharps
Blue	Broken or discarded and contaminated glass including medicine vials and ampoules except those contaminated with cytotoxic wastes and metallic body implants.

This waste consists of mainly:

- Newspaper, paper and card boxes (dry waste).
- Plastic water bottles (dry waste).
- Aluminum cans of soft drinks (dry waste).
- Packaging materials (dry waste).
- Food containers after emptying residual food (dry waste).
- Organic/Biodegradable waste-mostly food waste (wet waste).
- Construction and demolition wastes.

These general wastes are further classified as dry wastes and wet wastes and should be collected separately.

The quantity of such waste is around 85–90% of total waste generated from the facility. Such waste is required to be handled as per Solid Waste Management Rules, 2016 and Construction and Demolition Waste Management Rules, 2016, as applicable.

Other Wastes

Other wastes consist of used electronic wastes, used batteries, and radioactive wastes which are not covered under biomedical wastes but have to be disposed as and when such wastes are generated as per the provisions laid down under E-Waste (Management) Rules, 2016, Batteries (Management and Handling) Rules, 2001, and Rules/guidelines under Atomic Energy Act, 1962 respectively.

BIOMEDICAL WASTE MANAGEMENT

Steps Involved in Biomedical Waste Management

First five steps (segregation, collection, pretreatment, intramural transportation and storage) are the exclusive responsibility of health care facility. While treatment and disposal is primarily responsibility of CBWTF operator except for lab and highly infectious waste, which is required to be pretreated by the health care facility. Following are the responsibilities of health care facility for management and handling of biomedical waste:

- Biomedical waste should be segregated at the point of generation by the person who is generating the waste in designated color coded bin/container.
- Biomedical waste and general waste shall not be mixed. Storage time of waste should be as less as possible so that waste storage, transportation and disposal is done within 48 hours.
- Phase out use of chlorinated plastic bags (excluding blood bags) and gloves by March 27, 2019.
- No secondary handling or pilferage of waste shall be done at health care facility. If CBWTF facility is available at a distance of 75 km from the health care facility, biomedical waste should be treated and disposed only through such CBWTF operator.
- Only laboratory and highly infectious waste shall be pre-treated onsite before sending for final treatment or disposal through a CBWTF operator.
- Provide barcode labels on all color coded bags or containers containing segregated biomedical waste before such waste goes for final disposal through a CBWTF.

The management of biomedical waste can overall be summarized in the following steps:

- Waste segregation in color coded and barcode labeled bags/containers at source of generation.
- Pre-treat laboratory and highly infectious waste.
- Intramural transportation of segregated waste to central storage area.
- Temporary storage of biomedical waste in central storage area. Treatment and disposal of biomedical waste through CBWTF or captive facility.

Biomedical Waste Segregation

Biomedical waste generated from a health care facility is required to be segregated at the point of generation as per the color coding stipulated under Schedule-I of BMWM Rules, 2016. Following activities to be followed to ensure proper waste segregation:

- Waste must be segregated at the **point of generation** of source and not in later stages. As defined earlier too, **"Point of Generation"** means the location where wastes initially generate, accumulate and is under the control of doctor/nursing staff, etc. who is providing treatment to the patient and in the process of generating biomedical waste.
- Posters/placards for biomedical waste segregation should be provided in all the wards as well as in waste storage area.

- Adequate number of color coded bins/containers and bags should be available at the point of generation of biomedical waste.
- Color coded plastic bags should be in line with the Plastic Waste Management Rules, 2016.
- Provide personnel protective equipment to the biomedical waste handling staff.

Color Coding and Types of Container/Bags to be used for Waste Segregation and Collection

As per Schedule I of the BMWM Rules, 2016 following color coding and type of container/bags is needed to be used by the health care facilities for segregation and collection of generated biomedical waste from the facility (Table 2).

TABLE 2: Storage of biomedical waste

Category	Type of waste	Color and type of container
Yellow category	• Human anatomical waste • Animal anatomical waste • Soiled waste • Discarded or expired medicine • Microbiology, biotechnology and other clinical laboratory waste • Chemical waste (yellow-e) • Chemical liquid waste	Yellow colored non-chlorinated plastic bags **Note:** Chemical waste (yellow-e) comprising unused, residual or date expired liquid chemicals including spent hypo of X-ray, should be stored in yellow container
Red category	Contaminated waste (Recyclable)	Red colored non chlorinated plastic bags (having thickness equal to more than 50 μ) and containers
White category	Waste Sharps including metals	White Colored translucent, puncture proof, leak proof, tamper proof containers
Blue category	• Glassware • Metallic body implants	Puncture proof, leak proof boxes or containers with blue colored marking

Biomedical Waste Collection

Time of Collection

- Biomedical waste should be collected on daily basis from each ward of the hospital at a fixed interval of time. There can be multiple collections from wards during the day.
- Health care facility should ensure collection, transportation, treatment and disposal of biomedical waste as per BMWM Rules, 2016 and health care facility should also ensure disposal of human anatomical waste, animal anatomical waste, soiled waste and biotechnology waste within 48 hours.
- Collection times should be fixed and appropriate to the quantity of waste produced in each area of the health care facility.
- General waste should not be collected at the same time or in the same trolley in which biomedical waste is collected.
- Collection should be daily for most wastes with collection timed to match the pattern of waste generation during the day. For example, in an inpatient department (IPD) ward where the morning routine begins with the changing of dressings, infectious waste could be collected mid-morning to prevent soiled bandages remaining in the area for longer than necessary.
- General waste collection, must be done immediately after the visiting hours of the health care facilities, as visitors coming to facility generate a lot of general waste and in order to avoid accumulation of such general waste in the health care facility. The collection timings must enable the health care facility to minimize or nullify the use of interim storage of waste in the departments.
- Biomedical waste collected by the staff, should be provided with personal protective equipment (PPE).

Packaging

- Biomedical waste bags and sharps containers should be filled to no more than three quarters full. Once this level is reached, they should be sealed ready for collection.
- Plastic bags should never be stapled but may be tied or sealed with a plastic tag or tie.
- Replacement bags or containers should be available at each waste-collection location so that full ones can immediately be replaced.
- Color coded waste bags and containers should be printed with the biohazard symbol, labeled with details such as date, type of waste, waste quantity, senders name and receivers details as well as bar coded label for easy tracking till final disposal.

- Ensure that bar coded stickers are pasted on each bag as per the guidelines of Central Pollution Control Board (CPCB) by March 27, 2019.

Labeling

All the bags/containers/bins used for collection and storage of biomedical waste, must be labeled with the symbol of biohazard or cytotoxic hazard as the case may be as per the type of waste in accordance with the BMWM Rules, 2016 (Fig. 2).

Biomedical waste bags/containers are required to be provided with barcode labels in accordance with CPCB guidelines for "guidelines for barcode system for effective management of biomedical waste".

Interim Storage

- Interim storage of biomedical waste is discouraged in the wards/different-departments of health care facility.
- If waste is needed to be stored on interim basis in the departments it must be stored in the dirty utility/sections.
- No waste should be stored in patient care area and procedure areas such as operation theater. All infectious waste should be immediately removed from such areas.
- In absence of dirty utilities/sections such BMW must be stored in designated place away from patient and visitor traffic or low traffic area (Fig. 3).

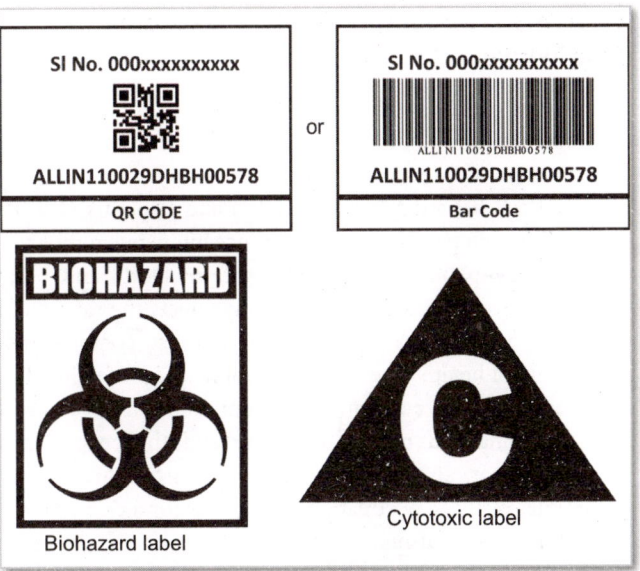

Fig. 2: Correct labeling

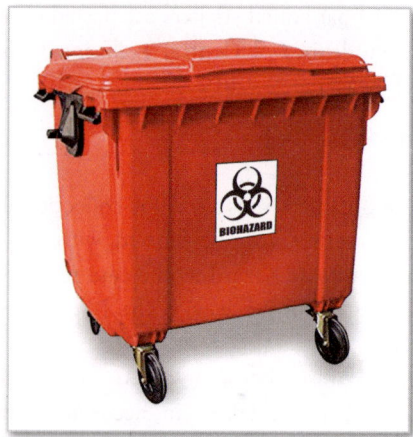

Fig. 3: Typical waste collection trolley for Red category of BMW

In-house Transportation of Biomedical Waste

Transportation Trolleys

In-house transportation of biomedical waste from site of waste generation/interim storage to central waste collection center, within the premises of the hospital must be done in closed trolleys/containers preferably fitted with wheels for easy maneuverability. Such trolleys or carts are designated for the purpose of biomedical waste collection only. Patient trolleys must not be used for biomedical waste transportation. Size of such waste transport trolleys should be as per the volume of waste generated from the Health care facilities.

Biosafety Precautions and Post-exposure Prophylaxis

Health care professionals are at risk of occupational exposure to blood and body fluids, which is a major risk factor in the transmission of infections such as human immunodeficiency virus (HIV), hepatitis B virus (HBV) and hepatitis C virus (HCV) through percutaneous and mucocutaneous routes.

The occupational risk of exposure to blood and body fluids and needlestick injuries not only affects the safety and wellbeing of health care professional, but also compromises the quality of health care delivery. Health care professional in operating, delivery, and emergency rooms and in laboratories have an enhanced risk of exposure and they experience significant fear, anxiety, and emotional distress, which can sometimes result in occupational and behavioral changes.

Thus, it is of utmost importance that all the health care professionals must be aware about the biosafety precautions to be safe from occupational hazards including the regime of post-exposure prophylaxis to prevent the transmission of HIV, HBV and HCV among the care providers.

STANDARD WORK PRECAUTIONS/ UNIVERSAL PRECAUTIONS

"Universal Precautions" as defined by Centers for Disease Control and Prevention (CDCP), are a set of precautions designed to prevent the transmission of HIV, HBV, and other blood-borne pathogens when providing first aid or health care.

Standard safety precautions, if carefully followed, will prevent spread of HIV, hepatitis B, hepatitis C infections in health setting. Thus, all blood and body fluids, substances. secretions, and excretions must be considered to be potentially infectious regardless of the perceived risk of exposure.

Standard work precautions to be followed to control infections are:

- Hand hygiene.
- Disinfection and sterilization of equipment.
- Use of personal protective equipment based on the risk of the procedure.
- Standard precautions against air-borne pathogens.
- Standard precautions against blood-borne pathogens.

Hand Hygiene

Hand washing is one of the simplest, but often overlooked procedure that can be followed to prevent infection from spreading Table 3.

Importance of Hand Hygiene

- Keeping hands clean through improved hand hygiene is one of the most important ways to prevent sickness and spreading germs to others.
- Good hand washing can fight the spread of the common cold, meningitis, bronchitis, influenza, hepatitis A, and most types of infectious diarrhea.

Steps of Hand Washing

- Remove watch and all the jewelry.
- Wet hands up to wrist.
- Apply soap on the palms, back of the hand, between fingers and around the thumb.
- Right palm over left dorsum and left palm over right dorsum.
- Palm to palm fingers interlaced.
- Backs of fingers to opposing palms with fingers interlocked.
- Rotational rubbing of right thumb clasped in left palm and vice-versa.

TABLE 3: Hand hygiene

	When to use	Effect on germs	How to use
Soap and water	Use this technique when hands have visible dirt and whenever you come in contact with a patient.	Removes germs	Apply soap on the palms, back of the hands, between fingers, around the thumb and rub for at least 15 seconds and rinse in running water. The entire handwashing procedure takes 20–30 seconds.
Alcohol rub	If no visible dirt on hands and before procedures needing the aseptic technique.	Kills germs	Place 3–5 mL on dry hands and rub following all the steps of handwashing until dry.
Surgical scrub	Done before surgery or procedure needing sterile technique	Kills germs	• Clean under nails with stick. • Wet up to elbow • Use antiseptic as long for 2–6 minutes with all the steps of handwashing. • Rinse and dry

- Rotational rubbing, backwards and forwards with clasped fingers of right hand in left palm and vice-versa.
- Rinse arms and hands.
- Turn off the tap with elbow or paper towel.

Five Moments of Hand Hygiene

Five Moments of hand hygiene define the key moments when health care workers should perform hand hygiene.

This evidence-based, field-tested, user-centered approach is designed to be easy to learn, logical and applicable in a wide range of settings.

This approach recommends health-care workers to clean their hands.

1. Before touching a patient.
2. Before clean/aseptic procedures.
3. After body fluid exposure/risk.
4. After touching a patient, and
5. After touching patient's surroundings

Differences among various cleaning techniques are enlisted in Table 4.

Disinfection and Sterilization of Equipment

Guidelines for disinfection and sterilization are given in Table 5.

TABLE 4: Differences among various cleaning techniques

Cleaning	Disinfection	Sterilization	Decontamination
Cleaning is the process that remove the foreign material (e.g., soil, organic material, microorganisms) from an object	Disinfection is the process that reduces the number of the pathogenic microorganisms, but not necessarily bacterial spores, from inanimate objects or skin, to a level which is not harmful to health.	Sterilization is a process that destroys all microorganisms including bacterial spores.	Use of physical or chemical means to remove, inactivate or destroy blood borne or other pathogens on a surface or item, to the point where they are no longer capable of transmitting infectious particles, and the surface or item is rendered safe for handling, use or disposal.

TABLE 5: Guidelines for disinfection and sterilization

Device classification	Devices examples	Types of process	Process examples
High risk (enters sterile tissue or vascular system, includes dental instruments)	Implants, scalpels, needles, other surgical instruments and endoscopic accessories.	**Sterilization**	Steam under pressure, dry heat, ethylene oxide gas, chemical gas sterilizers.
Intermediate risk (touches mucous membranes or broken skin)	Flexible endoscopes, laryngoscopes, endotracheal tubes, respiratory therapy and anesthesia equipment, diaphragm fitting rings, and other similar devices.	**High level disinfection (Exposure time 20 minutes)**	2% gluteraldehyde, hydrogen peroxide 6%, Sodium hypochlorite 5.25% in 1:50 dilution
	Thermometers	**Intermediate level disinfection**	Ethyl or Isopropyl alcohol (70% to 90%).

Contd...

Device classification	Devices examples	Types of process	Process examples
	Smooth, hard surfaces such as hydrotherapy tanks	Intermediate level disinfection (Exposure time 10 minutes)	Ethyl or isopropyl alcohol (70% to 90%), sodium hypochlorite 5.25% 1:100 dilution, phenolic detergent, Iodophor detergent.
Low risk (touches intact skin)	Stethoscopes, tabletops, floors, bed, furniture, etc.	Low level disinfection	Ethyl or isopropyl alcohol (70% to 90%), sodium hypochlorite 5.25% in 1:500 dilution, phenolic detergent, Iodophor detergent.

Commonly used Disinfectants

Refer to Table 6 for disinfectants that are commonly used.

TABLE 6: Disinfectants that are commonly used

Name of the disinfectant	Method of dilution	Contact time	Shelf life
Gluteraldehyde 2%, e.g., Cidex	Add activated powder/liquid in the 5L jar and use undiluted.	Disinfection: 20–30 minutes Sterilization: 10 hours	14–28 days
Combination of gluteraldehyde and chemically bound formaldehyde, e.g., Korsolex, bacillocid	Korsolex: Water 1 part: 9 parts Bacillocid: Water 1 part: 49 parts (20 mL: 980 mL)	Disinfection 15 minutes Sterilization 5 hours 30 minutes	14 days 24 hours
Ethanol isopropyl alcohol 70%, e.g., Bacillol-25	Do not dilute	2–10 minutes	24 hours
Hydrogen peroxide 6% (available as 30% stabilized solution)	20 mL H_2O_2-with 80 mL Normal saline = 6% H_2O_2	6–8 minutes	Use immediately after preparation
Sodium hypochlorite solution 1%, e.g., Polar bleach available in 5% and 10% concentrations	5%: 80 mL water + 20 mL bleach solution 10%: 90 mL water+ 10 mL bleach solution	20–30 minutes	8 hours

Preparation of various concentration of sodium hypochlorite solution (household bleach 5.25%):

- **High level disinfection** (approximately 1000 ppm)
  - **Preparing a 1: 50 Household Bleach Solution:**
    - 20 mL (4 teaspoons) household bleach + 1000 mL (4 cups) water.
- Intermediate level disinfection (approximately 500 ppm)
  - Preparing a 1: 100 Household Bleach Solution:
    - 5 mL (1 teaspoons) household bleach + 500 mL (2 cups) water.
- **Low level disinfection** (approximately 100 ppm)
  - Preparing a 1: 500 Household Bleach Solution:
    - 1 mL (1/4 teaspoons) household bleach to 500 mL (2 cups) water.

Note:
- The equipment contaminated by HBV can be sterilized by heating for 60°C for 4 hours.
- The recommended pressure and holding time for autoclaving at 121°C is 15 psi pressure for 20 minutes.
- Blood stained cotton cloth gowns should he disinfected with the help of sodium hypochlorite.

Cleaning up a Blood Spill on the Floor

- Wear appropriate personal protective equipment.
- Put a towel/gauze/cotton over the spill area to cover it completely.
- Pour hypochlorite solution 1% over the covered cloth to soak it completely.
- Leave the solution on the cloth for another 30 minutes without disturbance.
- Carefully lift the cloth from the floor, mopping the whole spill onto the cloth and dispose into the yellow bin.
- Using a routine mop and soap water solution swipe the area and wash the mop and hang it out to dry.
- Remove gloves and dispose into the red bin.
- Wash hands under the running water with soap and dry hands.

Note: The duration of infectivity of the HBV in dried spill of blood is less than 24 hours.

Use of Personal Protective Equipment

Personal protective equipment (PPE) (Table 7) is designed to protect employees from workplace injuries or serious illnesses resulting from contact with chemical, radiological, physical or mechanical or other workplace hazards.

PPE used during common nursing procedures are given in Table 8.

TABLE 7: Personal protective equipment

PPE	When to wear
Gloves	Wear sterile gloves when handling sterile supplies, doing invasive procedures. Wear clean gloves when cleaning or managing waste.
Eye wear (goggles, face shield)	Protect eye when anticipating splash of infectious body fluid
Gowns and aprons	Protect skin when risk of splashing or spraying of blood or blood fluids contact is expected using impervious/plastic gowns. Prevent soiling of clothing during procedures that may involve contact with blood or body fluids.
Masks (Cloth or paper)	Protect mouth and nose from potential splashes from infectious fluid. Use when handling patient with respiratory diseases. Doing any invasive procedures. Conducting delivery.
Caps	Used to keep the hair and scalp covered so that flakes of skin hair are not shed into the wound during surgery.
Footwear	Worn during procedures and patient-care activities when large particle droplet spatter or sprays of blood or body fluids is anticipated.

TABLE 8: Using appropriate PPE during common nursing procedures

Protection required	Common nursing procedures	Types of exposure
Gloves helpful but not necessary	Bed-making, back care, sponge bath, mouth care, minor wound dressing, perineal care, taking temperature, and blood pressure	Low risk (chances of direct contact with infectious body fluids is minimal)
Use gloves with waterproof aprons, for intubation, wear gloves, masks, goggles and apron.	Injections, lumbar puncture, insertion and removal of IV needles, PV examination, dressing large wounds, handling blood spills, intubations, suctioning and collecting blood.	Medium risk
All PPE	Vaginal delivery, uncontrolled bleeding, surgery, endoscopes, dental procedures.	High risk

Note: Special personal protective equipment for protecting against air-borne contagious disease like SARS, anthrax: All PPE including full facepiece air purifying respirator (APR) with P100 or N100 filters, disposable hooded coveralls and shoe coverings, Nitrile or vinyl gloves.

Donning of Personal Protective Equipment

Shoe Cover

Shoe covers are worn to maintain sanitary environment and protect the weaner from accidental spills and body fluids. They need to be picked singly from the box and worn.

Gown

The correct gowning technique includes:

*   Unfold the sterile gown keeping inside of the gown towards the body without allowing outside of the gown to touch any area.
*   With hands at shoulder level, slip both the arms into the armholes simultaneously.
*   Ask the other nurse to fasten the ties at the neck and back.
*   Remove gown avoiding touching of the soiled parts on the outside of the gown.
*   Roll up the gown with the soiled part inside and discard.

Head Cover

Surgical caps or hard covers are worn to minimize the risk of hair falling into the sterile area. If can be simply picked from the box and worn by securing all hair under it.

Mask

The correct way of using mask includes:

*   Hold mask by top two strings and ties two top ties at the top of the back of head.
*   Tie two lower ties snugly around the neck with the mask well under the chin.
*   Ensures the mask covers mouth and nose adequately.
*   When removing a mask, first unties the lower strings of the mask.
*   Discard in appropriate container.

Goggles or Face Shield

Goggles or face shield needs to be worn to recent blood or body fluid spillage into the eyes.

Gloves

The correct gloving technique:

*   Open the sterile glove packet of proper size on flat surface.
*   Identify the right and left hand and glove the dominant hand first.

- With thumb and the first two fingers of the non-dominant hand grasp on the edge of the glove's cuff touching only the inside surface.
- Carefully pull the gloves over the dominant hand.
- With the gloved dominant hand, slip fingers underneath the second glove's cuff.
- Carefully put the second glove over the non-dominant hand.
- After the second glove is on, interlocks the finger together.

The technique of removal of gloves:

- Remove the first glove by grasping it on its palmar surface. Pull the first glove completely rolling the glove inside out.
- Place the first two fingers of the bare hand inside the glove and remove the second contaminated glove.
- Dispose in appropriate container.

Sequence of Doffing Personal Protective Equipment

- Gloves
- Gown
- Goggles
- Mask or respirator
- Head gear
- Shoe cover.

Standard Precautions against Airborne Pathogens

Role of nurse while caring a patient with airborne diseases like tuberculosis.

- Separation of smear of tuberculosis (TB) positive patients.
- Identify procedures that may put a health care provider at risk for TB like suctioning, nebulizer, bronchoscopy, etc.
- Use mask appropriately.
- Ensure good ventilation.
- Educate patient and families to:
  - Report signs and symptoms of TB.
  - Observe cough hygiene.
  - Complete course of treatment.
  - Ensure good ventilation around.

Standard Work Precautions Against Blood-Borne Pathogens

In health care settings, injuries from needles or other sharp instruments are the number-one cause of occupational exposure to blood-borne infections. All staff who come in contact with sharps from doctors and nurses to those who dispose of the trash are at risk of infections.

Sharps

The term sharps refers to any sharp instrument or object used in the delivery of health care services, including hypodermic needles, suture needles, scalpel blades, sharp instruments, IV catheters, and razor blades.

Prevention of Injuries from Sharps

- Handle hypodermic needles and other sharps minimally after use and use extreme care whenever sharps are handled or passed.
- Use the "hands-free" technique when passing sharps during clinical procedures.
- Do not bend, break, or cut hypodermic needles before disposal.
- Do not recap needles.
- Dispose of hypodermic needles and other sharps properly.

Handling Sharps

During a clinical procedure, health care workers can accidentally stick one another or their clients when passing sharps, especially when there is sudden motion by staff members carrying unprotected sharps, when clients move suddenly during injections, or when sharps are left lying in areas where they are unexpected (such as on surgical drapes).

Safe-passing of Sharp Instruments

- Uncapped or otherwise unprotected sharps should never be passed directly from one person to another. In the operating theater or procedure room, pass sharp instruments in such a way that the surgeon and assistant are never touching the item at the same time. This way of passing sharps is known as the "hands-free technique:
  - The assistant places the instrument in a sterile kidney basin or in a designated "safe zone" in the sterile field.
  - The assistant tells the service provider that the instrument is in the kidney basin or safe zone.
  - The service provider picks up the instrument, uses it, and returns it to the basin or safe.

Managing Injuries and Exposure

Studies have shown that cleaning a wound with an antiseptic or squeezing it does not reduce the risk of infection. If you are accidentally exposed to blood or other body fluids, either by a needle stick, an injury from another sharp object, or a splash of fluid:

- Wash the needle stick site or cut with soap and water.
- Flush splashes to the nose, mouth, or skin with water.
- Irrigate splashes to the eyes with water or saline.

Safe Disposal of Sharps

Improper disposal of contaminated sharp objects can cause infections in 'sour health care facility and community. Any delay in the disposal of sharps will increase the occurrence of accidents. To dispose of sharps correctly:

- Do not recap, bend, or break needles before disposal, and do not remove the needle from the syringe by hand.
- Dispose of needles and syringes immediately after use in a puncture-resistant sharps-disposal container.
- Incinerate sharps-disposal containers in an industrial incinerator whenever the containers become three-quarters full.
- To discourage scavenging of discarded sharps, decontaminate needles and syringes that cannot be incinerated and render them harmless before burying them.

Sharps-disposal Containers

Puncture-resistant sharps-disposal containers should be conveniently located in any area where sharp objects are frequently used (such as injection rooms, treatment rooms. operating theaters labor and delivery rooms, and laboratories).

Decontaminating Needles and Syringes

Whenever possible, make hypodermic needles and other sharps unusable by incinerating them. If sharps cannot be incinerated, reduce the risk of infections by decontaminating them before disposal, and bury them in a pit to make it difficult for others to scavenge them.

POST-EXPOSURE PROPHYLAXIS

The term "post-exposure prophylaxis" or PEP refers to the comprehensive management given to minimize the risk of infection following potential exposure to blood-borne pathogens (HIV, HBV, and HCV)

Risk of infection after needle stick from a patient with the infection:

- **HBV: 30% (30 in 100)**
- **HCV: 3% (3 in 100)**
- **HIV: 0.3% (3 in 1000)** Which body fluids have risk for HIV transmission?

How does a Person Becomes Infected?

- Source body fluids, if infected (Table 9).
- Port of exit from infected person (injury, needle stick, etc.)

TABLE 9: Body fluids 'at risk' not at risk of exposure

Body fluids considered "at risk" exposure	Body fluid considered "not at risk" exposure (unless contaminated with visible blood)
Blood	Tears
Semen	Sweat
Breast milk	Urine and feces
Body fluids with blood	Saliva
Vaginal secretions	
Cerebrospinal fluid	
Synovial, pleura, peritoneal, pericardial fluids	
Amniotic fluids	
Other fluids contaminated with visible blood	

- Port of entry into susceptible person (break in the skin, mucus membrane-nose, mouth, eyes).

Factors that Influence Risk for Acquiring HIV

- **Types and extent of exposure**
  - Size and type of needle
  - Depth of injury
  - Amount of blood.
- Types of procedures that carry a higher risk of transmission.
  - Procedures involving a needle placed in artery or vein.
  - Use of invasive devices visibly contaminated with blood.
- Amount of virus present in the contaminated fluid.
- Whether PEP is taken or not within the specified time.

OCCUPATIONAL EXPOSURE PROTOCOL

- Do not put injured part in mouth or squeeze.
- Remain CALM.
- First aid: Wash and irrigate the site.
- Dispose the sharp appropriately.
- Report the appropriate authority.
- Get evaluated for PEP and baseline testing for HIV.
- Post-exposure should be started within 2 hours of exposure, and not later than 72 hours.
- Prophylaxis must be taken for 4 weeks (28 days).
- Follow-up HIV testing (6 weeks, 3 months, 6 months).
- Follow-up counseling and care.

NACO PEP Policy: Procedure to be followed after an Accidental Exposure to HIV Infectious Fluid

Do	Do not
Remove gloves, if appropriate	Do not panic
Wash the exposed site thoroughly with running water.	Do not put pricked finger in mouth.
Irrigate with water or saline if exposure sites is mouth.	Do not squeeze wound to bleed it.
Wash skin with soap and water	Do not use bleach, chlorine, alcohol, Betadine, iodine or other antiseptics/detergents on the wound.

Step 1: Management of Exposure Site-First Aid

For skin: If the skin is broken after a needle-stick or sharp instrument:

- Immediately wash the wound and surrounding skin with soap and water, and rinse. Do not scrub.
- Do not use antiseptics or skin washes (Bleach, Chlorine, Alcohol, Betadine).

After a splash of blood or body fluids:

- **To unbroken skin:**
  - Wash the area immediately.
  - Do not use antiseptics.
- **For the eye:**
  - Irrigate the exposed eye immediately with water or normal saline.
  - If wearing contact lens, leave in the place while irrigating as they form barrier over the eye and will help protect it. Once the eye is cleaned, remove the contact lens and clean them in the normal manner.
  - Do not use soap or disinfectant on the eye.
- **For mouth:**
  - Spit fluid out immediately.
  - Rinse the mouth thoroughly, using water or saline and spit again. Repeat the process several times.
  - Do not use soap or disinfectant in the mouth.

Step 2: Risk Assessment

The evaluation must be done rapidly, so as to start any treatment as soon as possible after the accident (ideally within 2 hours but certainly within 72 hours). This assessment must be made thoroughly because not every accidental exposure to blood (AEB) requires the prophylactic treatment (Table 10).

Step 2a: Assessing the Nature of Exposure and Risk of Transmission

TABLE 10: Categories of exposure

Category	Definition and example
Mild exposure	Mucous membrane/non-intact skin with small volumes, e.g., a superficial wound (erosion of the epidermis) with a plain or low caliber needle, or contact with the eyes or mucous membranes. Subcutaneous injections following small—bore needles
Moderate exposure	Mucous membrane/non intact skin with large volumes or Percutaneous superficial exposure with solid needle, e.g., a cut or needle stick injury penetrating gloves
Severe exposure	• Percutaneous with large volume, e.g., • An accident with a high caliber needle (> = 18G) visibly contaminated with blood • A deep wound (hemorrhagic wound and/or very painful) • Transmission of a significant volume of blood • An accident with material that has previously been used intravenously or intra-arterially

Step 2b: Assessment of the Exposed Individual

The exposed individual must be assessed for pre-existing HIV infection as PEP is intended for people who are HIV negative at the time of their potential exposure to HIV. Exposed individual who are discovered to be HIV positive should not receive PEP. Besides the medical assessment, counseling of the exposed health care worker is essential to allay fear and start PEP at the earliest.

Step 2c: Assessing the HIV Status of the Source of Exposure

Refer to Table 11 for Categories of situations depending on the results of the source.

TABLE 11: Categories of situations depending on the results of the source

Source HIV status	Definition of risk in source
HIV negative	Source is not HIV infected but consider HBV and HCV.
Low risk	HIV positive and clinically asymptomatic
High risk	HIV positive and clinically symptomatic
Unknown	Status of the patient is unknown, and neither the patient nor his/her blood is available for testing (e.g., injury during medical waste management the source patient might be unknown). The risk assessment will be based only upon the exposure.

Step 3: Informed Consent from the Exposed Person

Exposed persons should receive appropriate information about what PEP is about and the risk and benefits of PEP in order to provide informed consent. It should be clear that PEP is not mandatory.

Step 4: Deciding on PEP Medications/Regimen

Determining HIV Source Code

Refer to Figure 4 for determination of HIV source code.

- ◆ **Psychological support:** Every exposed person need to be informed about the risks and measures that can be taken. This helps to relieve part of the anxiety, but some may require further specialized psychological support.
- ◆ Documentation on record is essential.

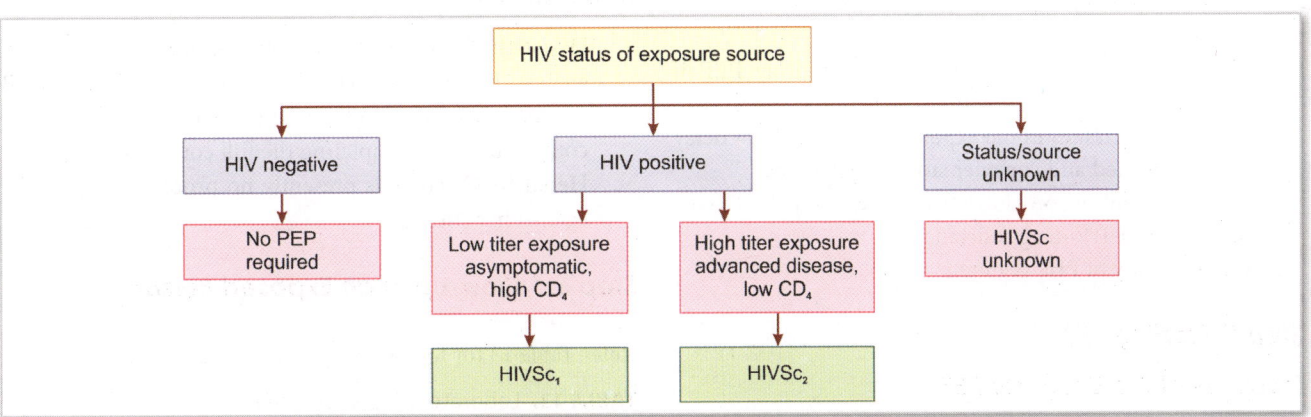

Fig. 4: HIV status of exposure source

Abbreviations: HIVSc, Human immunodeficiency virus source code; PEP, post-exposure prophylaxis

Determining HIV Exposure Code

Refer to Figure 5 for determination of HIV exposure code and Table 12 determining PEP recommendations.

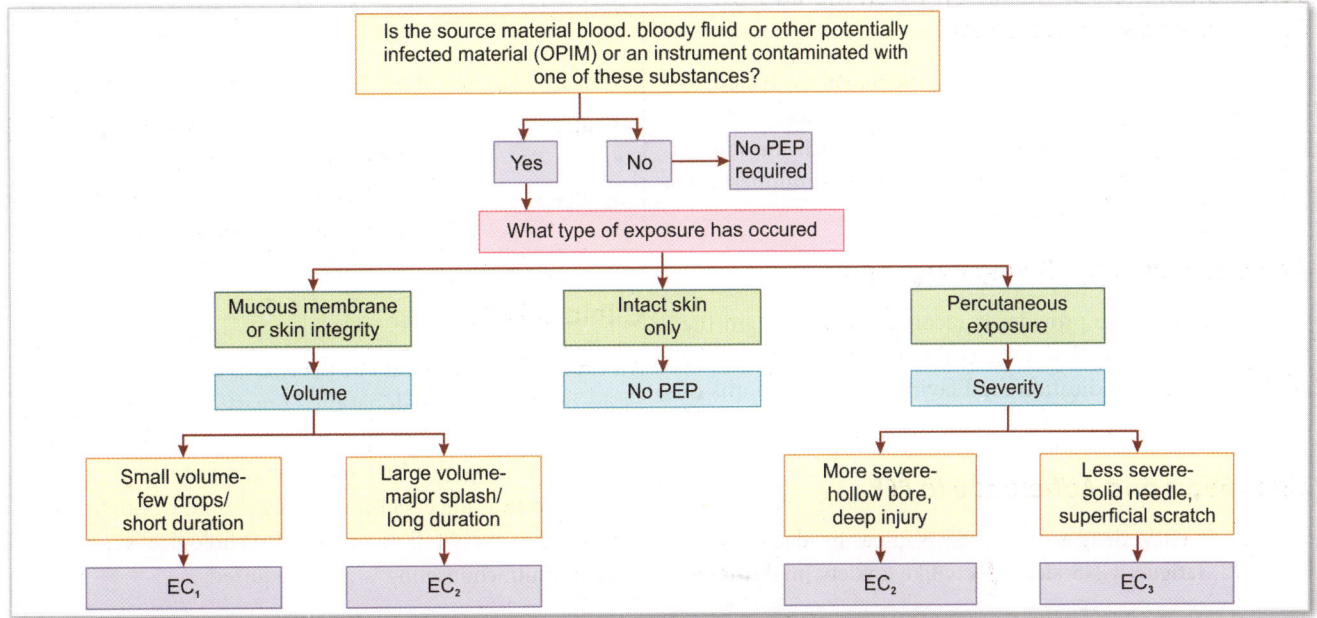

Fig. 5: Determination of HIV exposure code

Abbreviation: EC, exposure code

TABLE 12: Determining PEP recommendations

Exposure code (EC)	Source code (SC)
EC 1	SC 1
EC 1	SC 2
EC 2	SC 1
EC 2	SC 2
EC 3	SC 1 or 2
2/3	Unknown

Expert opinion may be obtained for the following situations:

* Delay in reporting exposure (>72 hours).
* Unknown source.
* Known or suspected pregnancy: Do not delay PEP if indicated.
* Breastfeeding issues in the exposed person: Do not delay PEP if indicated and consider stop breastfeeding.
* Source patient is on antiretroviral therapy (ART) or possibly has I-IIV drug resistance.
* Major toxicity of PEP regimen.

Step 5: Starting PEP

Dosages of the Drugs for PEP

* **Basic regimen (Three-drug regimen):** Tenofovir 300 mg + Lamivudine 300 mg + Efavirenz 600 mg once daily for 28 days.
* **Expanded regimen:** Basic regimen (+ Indinavir - 800 mg/thrice a day, or any other protease Inhibitor).

Selection of the PEP Regimen when the Source Patient is known to be on ART

When the source person's virus is known or suspected to be resistant to one or more of the drugs considered for the PEP regimen, the selection of the drugs to which the source person's virus is unlikely to be resistant is recommended. Refer for the expert opinion.

Antiretroviral Drugs During Pregnancy

Pregnant health care provider is recommended to begin the three drug regimen, Nelfinavir is the drug of choice. There is the clear contraindication for Efavirenz (first 3 months of pregnancy) and Indinavir (pre natal).

Side Effects and Adherence to PEP

* Minor ARV drug side effects: Nausea, headache, diarrhea, fatigue, CNS side effects like anxiety, nightmares.

psychosis. depression (this is mainly due to Efavirenz), blue/black nails, rash, fever, jaundice or abdominal pain, tingling or painful feet/legs.

Amount of Medication to Dispense for PEP

All clients starting on PEP must take 4 weeks of medication. As usage of PEP drugs is not frequent and the shelf life is 1–1.5 years it is proposed that starter packs for 7 days can be put in the emergency department.

Post-exposure Measures Against Hepatitis B and Hepatitis C

* **Hepatitis B:** All the health staff should be vaccinated against hepatitis B. The vaccination for Hepatitis B consists of 3 doses: initial, 1 month and 6 months. Sero conversion after completing the full course is 99%.
* **Hepatitis C:** There is presently no prophylaxis available against hepatitis C.

Step 6: Follow-up of an Exposed Person

Refer Table 13 for follow-up of an exposed person

TABLE 13: Laboratory tests after AEB

Timing	In persons taking PEP	In persons not taking PEP
Baseline	HIV-Ab, anti-HCV, HBsAg, CBC, transaminases	HIV-Ab. anti-HCV, HBsAg
Week 2 and 4	Transaminases, CBC	Clinical monitoring for hepatitis
Week 6	HIV-Ab	HIV-Ab
Month 3	HIV-Ab, anti-HCV, HBsAg, transaminases	HIV-Ab, anti-HCV, HBsAg
Month 6	HIV-Ab, anti-HCV, HBsAg, transaminases	HIV-Ab, anti-HCV, HBsAg

Clinical Follow-up

An exposed person should be advised to use precautions (e.g., avoid blood or tissue donations, breastfeeding, unprotected sex or pregnancy) to prevent secondary transmission, especially during the first 6–12 weeks following exposure. Adherence and side effect counseling should be provided and reinforced in every follow-up visit. Psychological support and mental health counseling is often required.

Refer to Table 14 for HIV vaccination after an accidental exposure of blood (AEB)

TABLE 14: HIV vaccination after an accidental exposure to blood

HBV vaccination status of exposed person	Action after AEB
Anti-HbS level > 10 IU/L	No action
Anti HbS level < 10 IU/L	Hep B vaccine booster
Vaccinated, anti-HbS not known	Hep B vaccine booster
Vaccinated more than 5 years ago	Hep B vaccine booster
Never vaccinated	Give complete hepatitis B vaccine series

SUMMARY

Nurses are in tremendous risk of acquiring occupational exposure to blood, body fluids, needlestick and sharp injuries in day to day work as they are one of the important direct care provider to the patients. Thus, it is of utmost importance for the nurse's to have the knowledge and excellent practice on biosafety precautions and post exposure prophylaxis to safeguard themselves from the blood-borne pathogens. Proper practice of hand hygiene is one of the important maneuver to control the cross infection and use of gowns, gloves, masks and goggles help to safeguard health care providers against exposure to blood and body fluids.

Post-exposure prophylaxis helps to decrease the burden of HIV and HBV among the health care providers who have been exposed to infected blood and body fluids. Fear of side effects is one of the hindrance in the utilization of the prophylaxis for which proper awareness and knowledge regarding the usefulness of the PEP must be incorporated among the health care providers.

BIBLIOGRAPHY

1. Brar NK, Rawat HC. Textbook of advanced nursing practice. 1st edition. The health Sciences Publisher; New Delhi: 2015. pp. 530-53.

2. Gulani KK. Community Health Nursing Principles and Practices, 1st edition. Kumar Publishing House; New Delhi: 2005. pp. 501-2.

3. Park K. Park's Textbook of Preventive and Social Medicine, 22nd edition. M/S Banarsidas Bhanot, 2009. P. 734-9.

4. The Trained Nurses Association of India. Fundamentals of nursing: A procedure manual. 1st edition. TNAI; New Delhi: 2005. pp. 98-100.

5. NACO. HIV/AIDS and ART training for nurses-nurses' manual. 2nd ed. INC; New Delhi: 2011. pp. 58-71, 167-84.

6. Ministry of Health and Family Welfare. Daksh skills lab-training manual for participants. MoHFW. New Delhi: pp. 101-103.

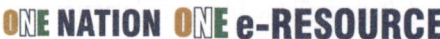
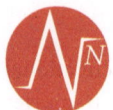
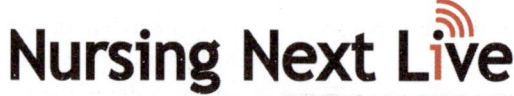
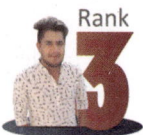
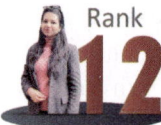
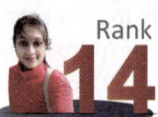
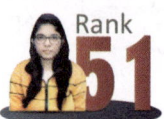
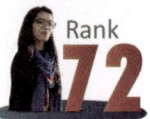
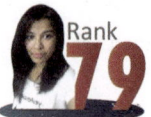
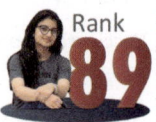
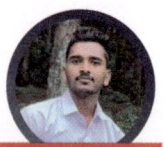
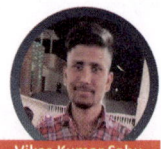
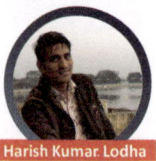
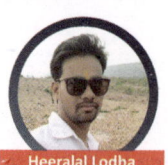
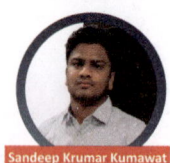
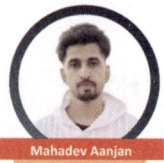
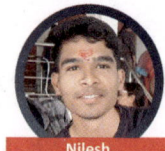
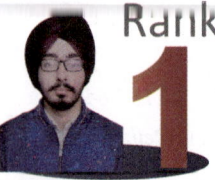
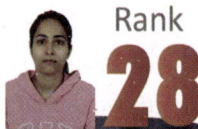

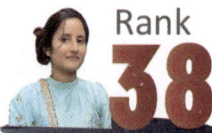
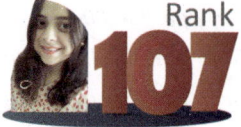
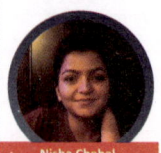
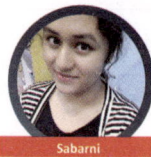
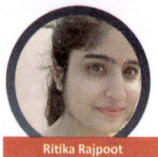
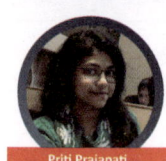
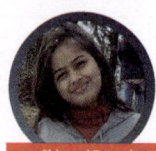
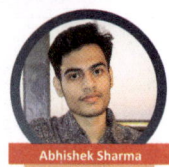
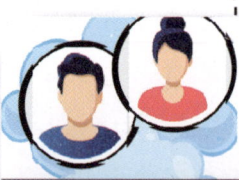

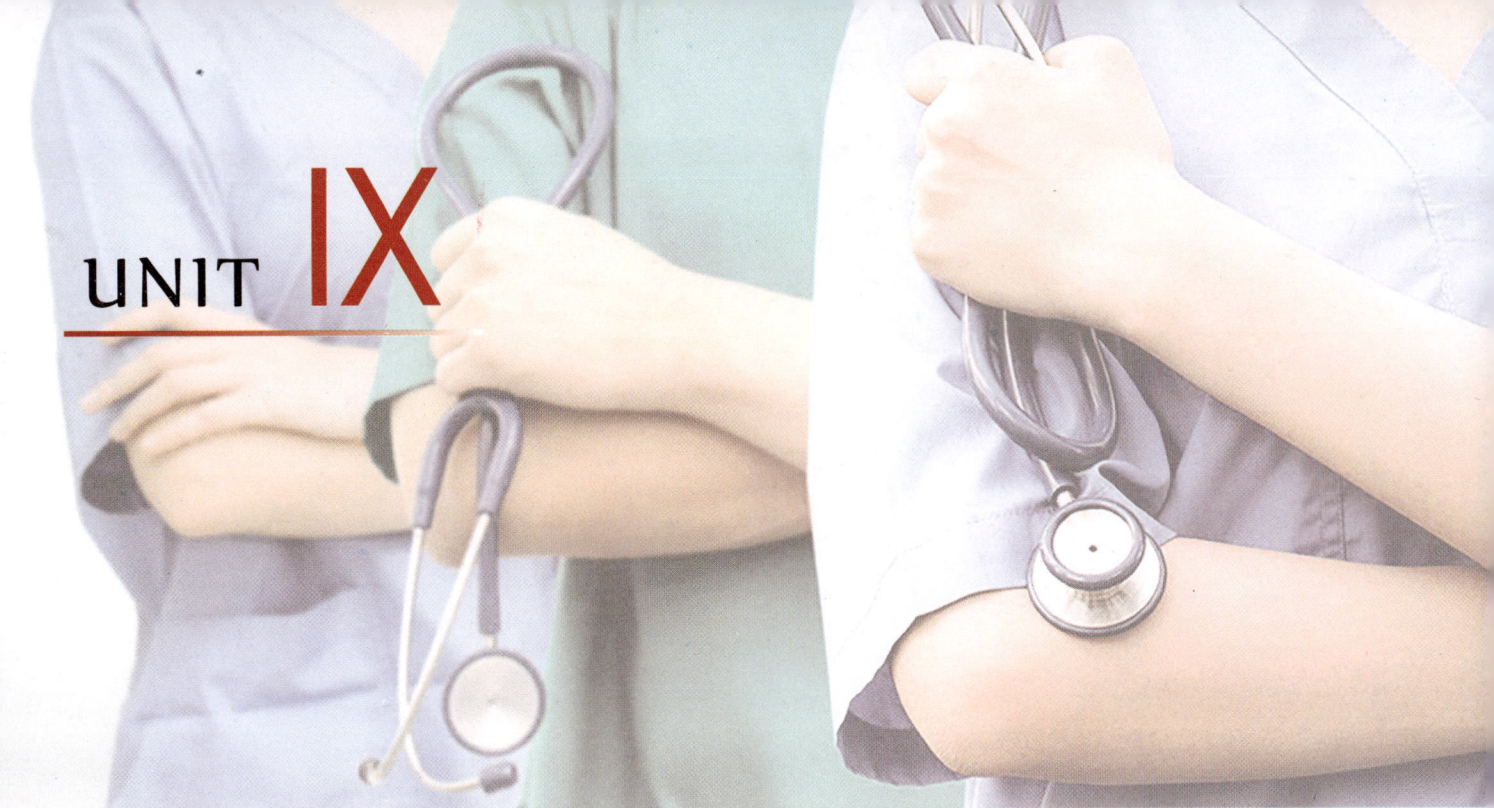

UNIT IX

VITAL SIGNS

Unit Outline

Temperature

After completing this chapter, you will be able to:
- Describe factors that affect the vital signs and their accurate measurement
- Identify the variations in normal body temperature, pulse, respiration and blood pressure that occur from infancy to old age
- Compare methods of measurement of body temperature

Key Terms

- Febrile
- Hypothermia
- Pyrexia

Chapter Outline

- Introduction
- Guidelines for Taking Vital Signs
- Body Temperature
- Factors Affecting Body's Heat Production
- Methods of Heat Loss from Body
- Normal Body Temperature
- Regulation of Body Temperature
- Factors Affecting Body Temperature
- Alterations in Body Temperature
- Common Sites for Assessing Body Temperature
- Measuring Body Temperature

INTRODUCTION

The vital signs are temperature, pulse, respiration and blood pressure. Recently pain has been added as fifth vital sign. All vital signs give some indication of the state of health of an individual.

Vital sign measurement is the initial step in assessment of patients. It is important to understand the physiologic mechanisms that regulate the vital signs and the factors that can affect each one of them.

GUIDELINES FOR TAKING VITAL SIGNS

They are called vital signs because they are important. They include temperature, pulse, respiration and blood pressure. Monitoring vital sings is a basic nursing function in assessing the health status of an individual. It is necessary for the nurse to be able to obtain accurate measurement of vital signs, because they are an indication of basic body functioning. The physiologic status of the body is reflected by these indicators of body functions, which are normally regulated by body through homeostatic mechanism and fall within normal ranges. A change from a person's normal pattern is considered indication of a change in health. Measurement of vital signs provides data that can be used to determine a client's usual state of health as well as the response to physical and psychological stress. An alteration from normal may signal the need for medical and nursing intervention.

The nurse must be able to do all of the following:

- Measure vital signs correctly.
- Understand and interpret the values.
- Vital signs are taken during patient's admission to a health care facility.
- Vitals are taken in a hospital on a routine schedule according to physician's order or hospital policy.
- Vitals are taken before and after an invasive diagnostic procedure.

- Before and after the administration of certain medications that affect cardiovascular, respiratory and temperature control functions.
- When the patients general condition changes.
- In an emergency situation.
- When the patient reports nonspecific symptoms of physical distress, vital signs are taken more frequently.
- The nurse communicate/document findings accurately in graphic flow sheet.
- Begin interventions as needed.
- Any abnormal findings are reported immediately.

BODY TEMPERATURE

Body temperature reflects the balance between the heat production and the heat lost from the body and is measured in heat units called degrees. There are two kinds of body temperature, core temperature and surface temperature.

1. **Core temperature** is the temperature of the deep tissues of the body, such as abdominal cavity and pelvic cavity. It remains relatively constant.
2. **Surface temperature** is the temperature of the skin, the subcutaneous tissue and fat. It rises and falls in response to the environment.

    The body continually produces heat as a by-product of metabolism. When the amount of heat produced by the body equals to the amount of heat lost, the person is in heat balance.

FACTORS AFFECTING BODY'S HEAT PRODUCTION

- **Basal metabolic rate (BMR):** It is the rate of energy utilization in the body required to maintain the essential activities such as breathing. BMR is the rate at which heat is produced when the body is at rest. BMR depends on the body surface area of the person. It deceases with age, i.e., younger the person, higher the BMR.
- **Muscle activity:** Muscle activity including shivering, increases the metabolic rate.
- **Thyroxine output:** Increased thyroxin output increases the rate of cellular metabolism throughout the body which is also called chemical thermo-genesis.
- **Epinephrine, norepinephrine and sympathetic stimulation stress response:** These increase the rate of cellular metabolism in various body tissues.
- **Fever:** Fever increases the cellular metabolic rate and thus, increases the body temperature further.

METHODS OF HEAT LOSS FROM BODY

- **Radiation** is the transfer of heat from the surface of one object to the surface of another without contact between the two objects, e.g., infrared rays.
- **Conduction** is the transfer of heat to another object during direct contact, e.g., body transfers heat to an ice pack causing the ice to melt.
- **Convection** is the dispersion of heat by air currents. The dissemination of heat occurs by motion between areas of unequal density, e.g., an oscillating fan blows current of cool air across the surface of a warm body.
- **Evaporation** is the conversion of liquid to vapor, e.g., body fluid in the form of perspiration and insensible loss is evaporated from the skin.

NORMAL BODY TEMPERATURE

Body temperature varies among individuals, with a range of 0.3°–0.6°C (0.5°–1.0°F) from the average temperature considered to be within normal limits. A person with a normal temperature is referred as afebrile (without fever).

REGULATION OF BODY TEMPERATURE

- The hypothalamus located between the cerebral hemispheres, act as thermostat and controls body temperature by a feedback mechanism. The chemical reactions occur in the body as it fights a pathogen causing the thermostat to reset to a higher level.
- When the body heat rises above normal, the hypothalamus sends out a signal through the nervous system that causes vasodilatation, sweating, and inhibition of heat production.
- If the body temperature drops below normal range, the hypothalamus sends message for vasoconstriction of surface blood vessels to conserve heat and messages to induce shivering to increase heat production.
- Heat loss occurs through the skin's exposure to the environment via radiation, conduction, convection and evaporation.
- Blood flow from the internal organs carries heat to the skin. The heat is radiated to cooler objects in the vicinity of the person.
- When objects in the surroundings are warmer, the body heat is radiated to the body and absorbed.
- When warm skin touches a cool object, heat is lost to the object by conduction.
- Air movement causes heat to be transformed from the skin to the air molecules by convection.
- Sweat glands contribute to loss of heat due to evaporation by secreting sweat in response to a message from the hypothalamus when the body temperature is high.
- As water evaporates from the skin, heat is transferred to the air. There is a loss of 800 mL of water from the skin and lungs due to evaporation.

FACTORS AFFECTING BODY TEMPERATURE

It is necessary for nurses to be aware of the factors that can affect a client's body temperature so that they can recognize normal variations in temperature and understand their significance.

- **Age:** The infant is greatly influenced by the temperature of the environment and must be protected from extreme changes. Children's temperature continues to be more variable than those of adults until puberty. Elderly over 75 years are at risk of hypothermia (temperature below 36°C or 96.8°F) due to loss of subcutaneous fat, lack of activity, inadequate diet and reduced thermoregulatory efficiency. Elders are also sensitive to extremes of environmental temperature.
- **Diurnal variations (circadian rhythm):** Body temperature changes constantly throughout the day, varying 1.0°C (1.8°F) between early morning and the late afternoon. The highest body temperature is reached between 4 pm and 6 pm and the lowest during 4 am and 6 am.
- **Exercise:** Strenuous exercise or hardwork can increase body temperature from 38.3°C to 40°C measured rectally.
- **Hormones:** Women usually experience more hormone fluctuations than men. In women, progesterone secretion at the time of ovulation increases body temperature by 0.3°–0.6°C above basal temperature.
- **Stress:** Stimulation of the sympathetic nervous system can increase the production of epinephrine and nor-epinephrine, thereby increasing metabolic activity and heat production.
- **Environment:** Extremes in environmental temperatures can affect a person's temperature regulatory system. If the temperature is assessed in a very warm room, it will be elevated. Similarly, if the client has been outside in cold weather, the body temperature may be low.
- **Disease conditions:** Bacteria, virus and toxins from some infective agents and the chemical reactions of the inflammatory response may produce fever. Fever is a protective defense mechanism that the body uses to fight pathogens and their toxins.
- **Drugs:** Certain drugs may cause temperature elevation because of the chemical action in the body.

ALTERATIONS IN BODY TEMPERATURE

Two main alterations are: pyrexia and hypothermia.

Pyrexia

A body temperature above the usual range in called pyrexia or fever. A very high fever 41°C (105.8°F) is called hyperpyrexia. The client who has fever is referred as febrile and one who does not have fever is called afebrile.

Types of Fever

- **Intermittent:** The body temperature alternates at regular intervals between periods of fever and periods of normal or subnormal temperatures, e.g., malaria.

- **Remittent:** In this, there is a wide range of temperature fluctuation more than 2°C over 24-hour period above normal, e.g., cold or influenza.
- **Relapsing:** These are short febrile periods of few days and normal temperature of 1–2 days.
- **Constant:** The body temperature fluctuates minimally (less than 2°C) but always remains above normal, e.g., typhoid fever.

Refer to box 1 for crisis and lysis of fever.

Box 1

Terms

➡ **Crisis:** The fever returns to normal suddenly
➡ **Lysis:** The fever returns to normal gradually

Hypothermia

Hypothermia is defined as a core body temperature below the lower limit of normal. The thermal regulatory center in the hypothalamus is greatly impaired when the temperature of the body falls below 94°F (34.4°C). At this level , the activity of the cells is reduced, less heat is produced, and person may go into coma. Those at the risk of hypothermia include postoperative patients who are cooled during surgery, newborn infants whose skin is exposed to cool room temperatures, elderly or debilitated patients and those exposed to cold temperatures for prolonged periods.

Hypothermia may be **induced or accidental**. Induced hypothermia is the deliberate lowering of the body temperature to decrease the need for oxygen by the body tissues such as during surgeries. **Accidental hypothermia** can occur as a result of exposure to cold environment, immersion in cold water, lack of adequate clothing and absence of shelter of heat. In elderly, it can occur due to reduced metabolic rate and use of sedatives.

The skin and underlying tissues are damaged by freezing cold. This results in frost bite in hands, feet, nose and ears.

Management

- Provide warm environment
- Provide dry clothing
- Apply warm blankets (hypothermia blanket-an electronically controled blanket that provides specified temperature)
- Cover the scalp with cap or scarf
- Supply warm oral or intravenous fluids

COMMON SITES FOR ASSESSING BODY TEMPERATURE (TABLE 1)

Oral

This is the most accessible and convenient method. The nurse should make sure that client has not had hot or cold fluid or

TABLE 1: Normal temperature for healthy adults at various sites

	Celsius	Fahrenheit
Oral temperature	37°C	98.6°F
Axillary temperature	36.5°C	97.7°F
Rectal temperature	37.5°C	99.5°F
Tympanic temperature	37.5°C	99.5°F
Forehead temperature	34.4°C	94.0°F

smoked before taking temperature orally. Wait for at least 20 minutes before taking temperature.

Rectal

It is a reliable most accurate measurement of temperature. It is contraindicated for clients with myocardial infarction, as taking rectal temperature can produce vagal stimulation, which might precipitate abnormal heart rhythm. It is also contraindicated in patients who are undergoing rectal surgery, have diarrhea, diseases of the rectum, are immune-suppressed, have a clotting disorder or have hemorrhoids.

Axillary

It is safe, noninvasive and most preferred site for measuring temperature in newborns because it is accessible.

Tympanic Membrane

It is a frequent site for estimating core body temperature.

Temporal Artery

The temperature can be measured on the forehead using a temporal artery thermometer. It is safe, noninvasive and very quick in showing results. Forehead temperature measurements are most useful for infants and children. It requires electronic equipment that may be expensive.

MEASURING BODY TEMPERATURE

Clinical thermometer is used to measure body temperature. There are different types of thermometers available in the market.

Glass Thermometer

They can be hazardous due to exposure to mercury, which is toxic to humans, if it cracks or breaks. Hospitals no longer use mercury glass thermometers, and at several places, it is banned for sale and manufacture. Nowadays plastics have replaced glass and safer chemicals have replaced mercury.

The glass thermometer has a bulb containing mercury and a stem in which the mercury can rise. On the stem, there is a graduated scale representing degrees of temperature from 90°F to 107°F. The range of Celsius thermometer scale is from 32°C to 42°C. The mercury in the bulb expands when the bulb is in contact with body heat and registers on the scale in the stem. The bulb may be long and slender or blunt like the short, fat bulb used for rectal thermometers. Rectal thermometers often have a red tip or color on the stem to signify that they are for rectal use only and should not be used orally. Oral thermometer may also be used to take axillary temperatures. All glass thermometers must have the mercury below the normal range before using, and this is accomplished by shaking down the mercury. This is done by holding the thermometer firmly by the distal glass and flicking the wrist in quick motion several times to bring the mercury down the bulb (Fig. 1).

Reading the Glass Thermometer

The stem of the mercury thermometer contains the scale for measuring the temperature. The scale may be calibrated in either Fahrenheit or Celsius degrees. The Celsius scale has long lines for each one tenth of a degree. In contrast, the Fahrenheit scale has an arrow marking the normal temperature of 98.6°F. Long lines on the scale represent each degree, but only the even numbered degrees are written as 96°F, 98°F, 100°F, and so on. Short lines between the degree lines represent two tenth of a degree. To convert temperature from one scale to another, the formulae are:

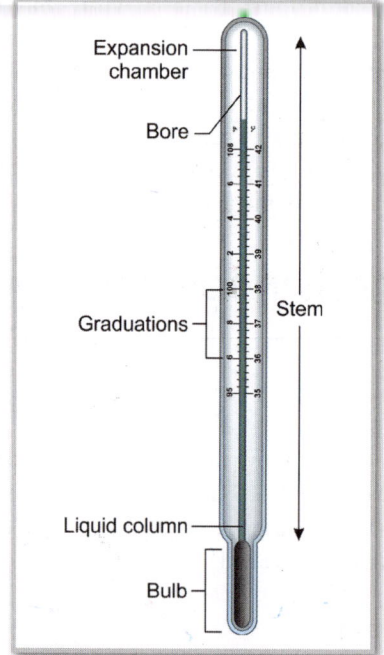

Fig. 1: Glass thermometer

Fahrenheit to Celsius:

(Fahrenheit – 32) × 5/9 = Celsius

Celsius to Fahrenheit:

(Celsius × 9/5) + 32 = Fahrenheit (Table 2)

TABLE 2: Reference table for determining thermometer in Celsius and Fahrenheit scales

Celsius	Fahrenheit
34.0°C	93.2°F
35.0°C	95.2°F
36.0°C	96.8°F
36.8°C	97.7°F
37.0°C	98.6°F
37.5°C	99.5°F
38.0°C	100.4°F
38.5°C	101.3°F
39.0°C	102.2°F
40.0°C	104.0°F
41.0°C	105.5°F
42.0°C	107.2°F
43.0°C	109.4°F
44.0°C	111.2°F

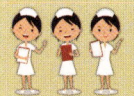

SKILL: MEASURING TEMPERATURE WITH GLASS – MERCURY THERMOMETER

A glass thermometer is used only for patients who are alert, cooperative, able to understand instructions and able to breathe while holding, thermometer in the mouth. Rectal temperatures are contraindicated in patients with rectal bleeding, hemorrhoids, diarrhea, or fecal impaction.

Articles:

♦ Glass thermometer, oral or rectal cotton swabs/tissue
♦ Lubricant for rectal temperature
♦ Gloves
♦ Pencil and paper

♦ Kidney tray
♦ Paper bag to discard tissue/swabs/gloves.
♦ A bottle with disinfectant solution. (Dettol 1:40/Savlon 1:20)
♦ A bottle with water
♦ A wrist watch
♦ Recording sheet.

(**Note:** Review and carry out the standard steps given in Appendix)

Action/steps	Rationale
Assessment	
1. Determine whether the patient can safely use an oral glass thermometer. Ask whether the patient has had any food or drink or smoked in past 15 minutes.	A glass thermometer is never used for uncooperative patient because of risk of biting the thermometer. Eating, drinking and smoking interferes with accurate reading.
Planning	
2. Assemble the equipment and explain to the patient what you are going to do. Hold the stem of thermometer and place it at eye level, rotate it between the fingers to read the mercury level. Shake it down until the reading is below desired level.	Mercury must be below the patient's normal level. Shaking the thermometer returns the mercury to the bulb. Moving away from the objects while shaking prevents breaking of thermometer.

Contd...

Action/steps	Rationale
Implementation	
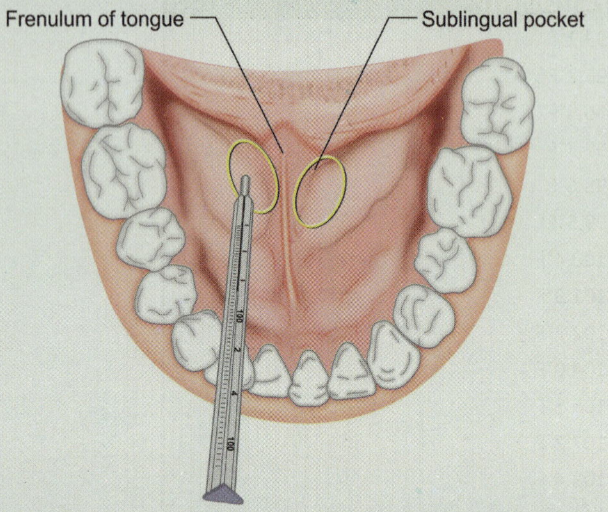 3. Ask the patient to open the mouth and place the thermometer under the tongue. Ask the patient to close mouth with caution not to bite the thermometer (Fig. 2).	Heat from superficial blood vessels below the tongue produces the temperature reading. Keeping mouth closed prevents air from entering the mouth and interfering with the reading.

Frenulum of tongue — Sublingual pocket

Fig. 2: Placement of thermometer while checking oral temperature

4. Leave the thermometer in place for 3–5 minutes	The mercury must warm sufficiently to rise to the correct level.
5. Remove the thermometer from the mouth and wipe with tissue or cotton swab from the stem towards the bulb with a twisting motion to clean off saliva	Prepares the thermometer for proper reading.
Taking rectal temperature	
6. Provide privacy. Ask the patient to turn on side facing away from you with knees slightly flexed and drape the patient.	Draping helps in maintaining privacy so that only anal area is exposed.
7. Don gloves, lubricate the tip of the rectal thermometer and lift the upper buttock slightly so that the anus is clearly seen; insert the bulb into rectum 0.5–1.5 inches.	Gloves protect against fecal microorganisms. Lubricant helps in smooth insertion of the thermometer. Insertion more than 0.5 inches in an infant may cause rectal perforation.
8. Hold the thermometer in place for 3–5 minutes.	Holding the thermometer prevents injury and prevents expulsion.
9. Remove and clean the thermometer by wiping with a tissue/cotton from the stem to the bulb while twisting the thermometer, wipe the buttocks to remove the lubricant and stool and discard tissue in paper bag	Helps to remove feces that might interfere with a visual reading
Taking axillary temperature	
10. Place the thermometer in the center of the patients dry axilla, ask the patient to hold the arm tightly against the chest	A wet axilla will give a false reading of body temperature. If wet due to perspiration, pat dry with a towel. Holding the arm tightly against the chest helps in better contact
11. Leave the thermometer in place for 8–10 minutes	For accurate reading longer contact with thermometer is needed
12. Remove and clean the thermometer as in Step 5.	Removes any moisture that interferes with visual reading.
Common for all Methods	
13. Hold the thermometer horizontally at eye level and rotate it towards you until you can see the column of mercury. Note where the end of mercury is on the lined scale.	Rotating thermometer allows for accurate reading. The end of the mercury column indicates the measured temperature.
14. Record the temperature reading. Tell the patient what the reading was if required.	Putting on the temperature sheet makes it available for all health care providers and patients have a right to their health information.

Contd...

Action/steps	Rationale
15. Cleanse the thermometer according to agency policy and return it to its storage location.	Cleansing reduces the transfer of microorganism storing the thermometer properly prevents breakage.
16. Remove gloves if worn and wash your hands	Prevents transfer of microorganisms
17. Make patient comfortable and tidy the unit	Shows caring and respect
Evaluation	
18. Ask yourself, is the temperature elevated? Is it higher or lower than the previous reading?	Provides data to determine temperature trend
Documentation	
19. Document the time and temperature on the graphic record or enter it in the patients data file on the computer	Notes the temperature taken and the route.

Note: The rectal temperature is usually 1° higher than the oral temperature.

Sample Documentation Form

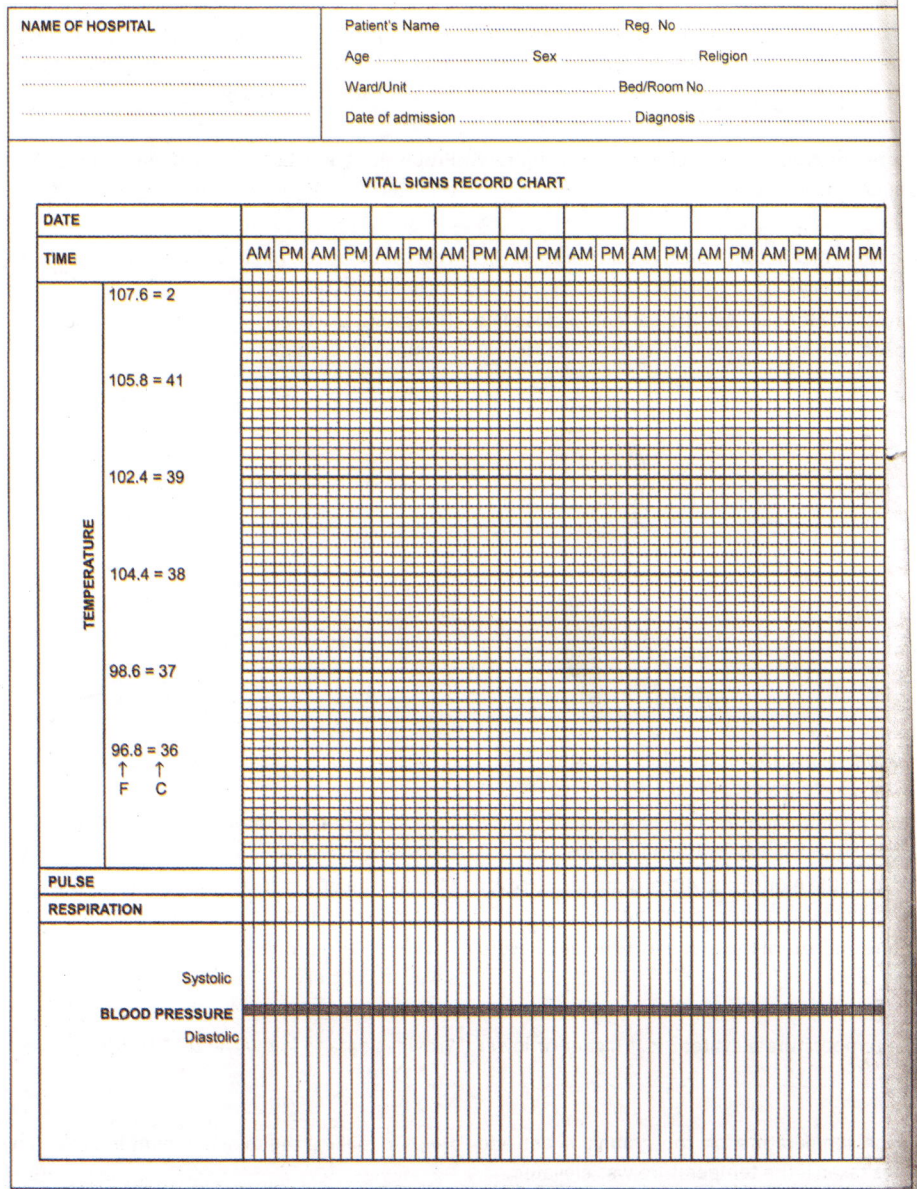

NAME OF HOSPITAL

Patient's Name .... Reg. No ....
Age .... Sex .... Religion ....
Ward/Unit .... Bed/Room No. ....
Date of admission .... Diagnosis ....

VITAL SIGNS RECORD CHART

DATE		AM	PM	AM	PM	AM	PM	AM	PM	AM	PM	AM	PM	AM	PM	AM	PM	AM	PM	AM	PM
TIME																					

TEMPERATURE

107.6 = 2
105.8 = 41
102.4 = 39
104.4 = 38
98.6 = 37
96.8 = 36
↑ F   ↑ C

PULSE

RESPIRATION

Systolic

BLOOD PRESSURE

Diastolic

Digital Thermometer

It is portable, battery-operated electronic thermometer registers body temperature in 5 seconds to 1 minute. There may be on-off button to activate the battery, and a warm-up period may be required. The oral probe is placed in a plastic cover or sheath that is used one time and discarded. The correct disposable probe covers and setting is used when taking oral or rectal temperature. The temperature is displayed digitally on a small screen on the hand-held unit. The reading is in tenth of a degree. A digital thermometer can be used to measure temperature without worry about injury for patients who are at risk for seizure disorders (Fig. 3).

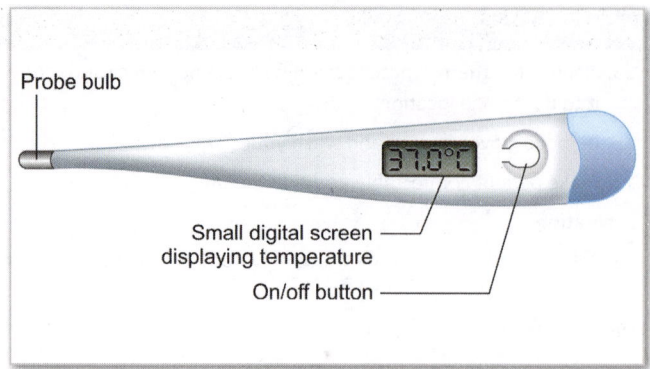

Fig. 3: Digital thermometer

Note: Review and carry out the standard steps in Appendix

Action/steps	Rationale
Assessment	
1. Wash your hands, identify the patient and explain the procedure. Ask whether the patient has had anything to eat or drink in the past 15 minutes.	Reduces transfer of microorganisms. Ensures correct patient and puts the patients at ease. Eating, drinking or smoking alters the temperature of oral cavity.
Planning	
2. Check whether there are probe covers. Check the low battery light to ensure proper functioning of the thermometer.	Probe must not be used without a cover. A low battery must be replaced to obtain accurate reading.
Implementation	
3. Remove the probe from the unit and push it down into probe cover until slight click is heard.	The probe cover must be firmly in place for the unit to operate correctly.
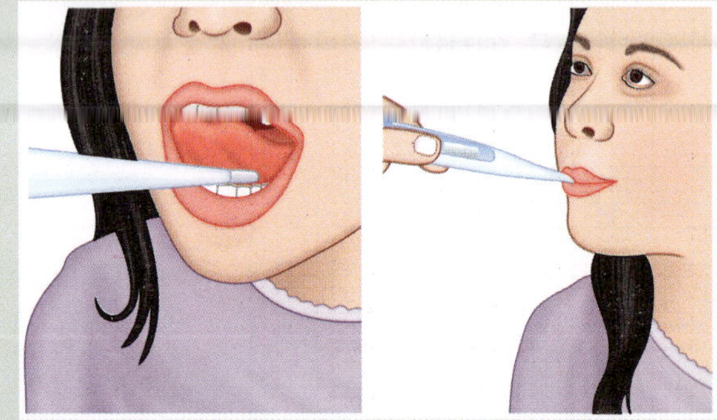 4. Place the probe under the tongue. Ask the patient to close lips and keep them closed (Fig. 4).	The probe must be in contact with tissue rich in blood supply to obtain correct reading

Fig. 4: Placement of digital thermometer while checking oral temperature

5. Allow the patient to hold it, and read the temperature on the screen when the light stops flashing or the unit beeps	If probe is not positioned correctly. It will not beep and refuse to register temperature
6. Remove the probe from the mouth and discard the probe cover into waste container by pressing the ejector button	Ejecting the probe cover directly into waste can prevent handling its contaminated surface.
7. Note the temperature and return the probe to its holder. Record the patient's temperature	Returning the probe to its holder turns off the thermometer and saves the battery
Evaluation	
8. Ask yourself: Is the temperature elevated? Is it higher or lower than last readings	Provides data to know the trend of the temperature
Documentation	
9. Record the time and temperature on the graphic sheet and record the measures taken if the temperature was elevated.	Helps in making the measurement data available.

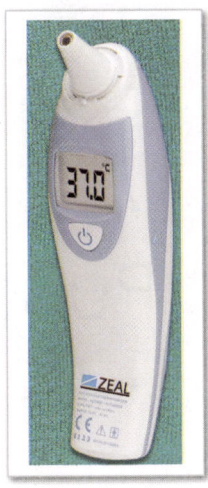

Fig. 5: Tympanic
thermometer

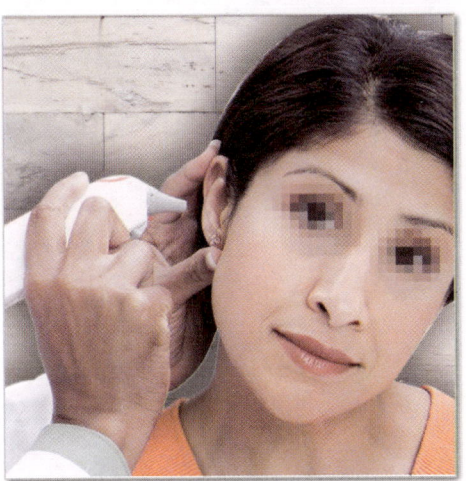

Fig. 6: Measuring tympanic temperature

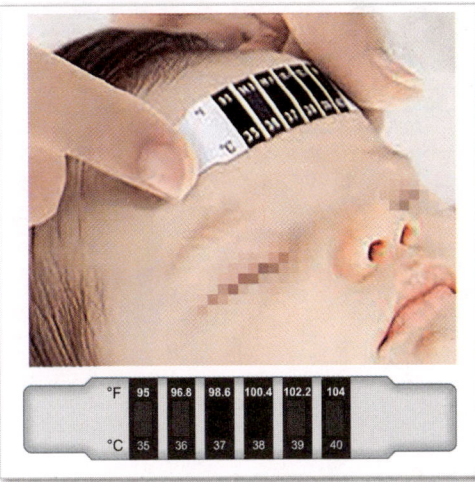

Fig. 7: Disposable thermometer
(temperature-sensitive tapes)

Tympanic Thermometers

It is portable, battery-operated electronic thermometer that registers temperature in 1–2 seconds, when placed in the auditory canal. This thermometer produces a reading of core temperature. It is specifically useful for measuring temperature in children. The auditory canal probe is placed in a plastic cover that is used one time and then discarded. While inserting the probe, gently pull the pinna up and back in adults to straighten the ear canal whereas in children under the age of 2 years pull the pinna of ear down and back. The auditory canal must be inspected for redness, swelling, discharge, or a presence of foreign body before insertion of the probe (Figs 5 and 6).

Disposable Thermometers

Various types of single use disposable thermometers are available. Among them there are temperature-sensitive tapes that are placed on forehead or abdomen to record the heat of the body (Fig. 7).

BIBLIOGRAPHY

1. *Perry & Potter, Clinical Nursing Skills & Techniques, 5th edition. Mosby; 2002.*
2. *Taylor CR, Lillis C, LeMone P, et al. Fundamentals of Nursing – The Art and Science of Nursing Care, 7th edition. Wolters Kluwer; 2010*
3. *Christensen BL, Kockrow EO. Foundation of Nursing. Mosby; 2003.*
4. *Bickley LS, Szilagyi PG. Bates Guide to Physical Examination and History Taking. Lippincott Williams & Wilkins; 2003. p. 862.*

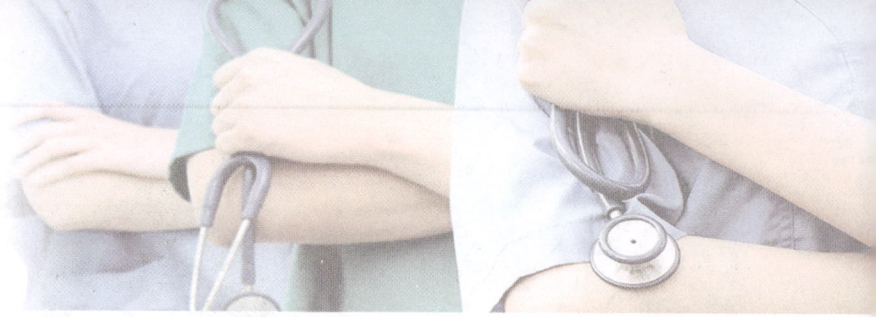

Pulse

INTRODUCTION

The pulse is a wave of blood created by contraction of the left ventricle of the heart. Each time the heart contracts to force blood into the aorta, the arterial walls in the vascular system must expand to accept the increase in pressure. The pressure wave causing this expansion is called the pulse. By counting each pulsation of the arterial wall, we can determine pulse rate.

FACTORS AFFECTING THE PULSE

The pulse rate is expressed in beats per minute (BPM). It varies according to a number of factors and nurse should consider each of the following factors when assessing the pulse rate.

Age

As age increases, the pulse rate gradually decreases. (Table 1)

TABLE 1: Variation in pulse by age

Age	Pulse rate per minute
Newborn	120–160
1-year	110–120
5–8 years	95–100
Adult male	72–80
Adult female	76–80
Athletes	45–60

Gender

After puberty, the average male's pulse rate is slightly lower than the female.

Exercise

The pulse rate usually increases with activity.

Fever

The pulse rate increases due to increased metabolic rate and in response to lowered blood pressure that results from peripheral vasodilation associated with elevated body temperature.

Medication

Some medications decrease the pulse rate and others increase it, e.g., cardiotonics such as digitalis preparations decrease the heart rate, whereas epinephrine increases it.

Hypovolemia

Loss of blood from the vascular system normally increases pulse rate due to the adjustment of the heart rate to increase blood pressure as the body compensates for the lost blood volume.

Stress

Stress increases pulse rate as well as force of the heart beat in response to the sympathetic nervous stimulation.

Position Change

When a person is sitting or standing, there are variations in pulse rate.

Pathology

Certain diseases such as some heart conditions and those that impair oxygenation can alter the resting pulse rate.

Pain

Pain increases the pulse rate.

Body Built and Size

Tall slender persons may have a slower pulse rate than short and stout persons.

SITES OF ASSESSMENT

Common peripheral sites for measuring pulse is described in Figure 1.

Radial

It is noted where the radial artery runs along the radial bone on the thumb side of the inner aspect of the wrist.

Brachial

It is noted at the inner aspect of the biceps muscle of the arm or medially in the antecubital space.

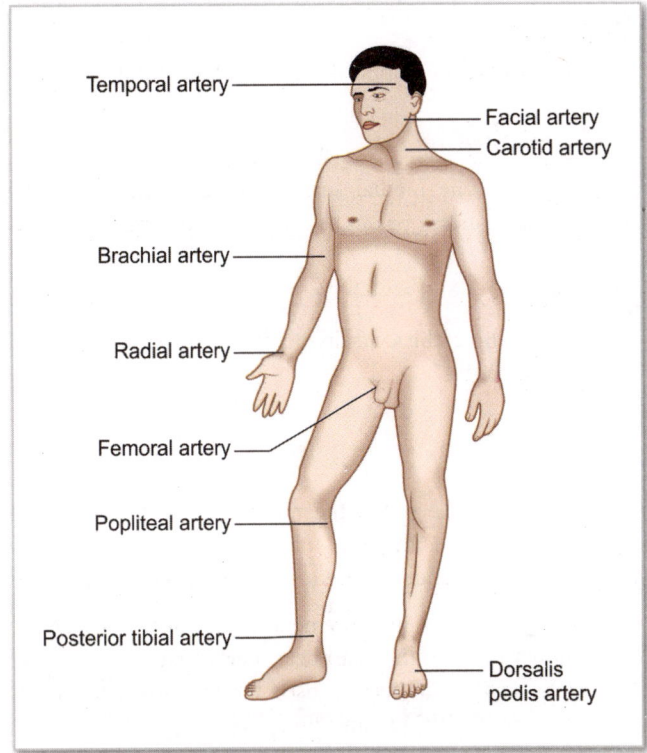

Fig. 1: Common peripheral sites for measuring pulse

Temporal

It is noted where the temporal artery passes over the temporal bone of the head. The site is superior (above) and lateral to (away from the midline of) the eye.

Carotid

It is noted at the side of neck where the carotid artery runs between the trachea and the sternocleidomastoid muscle.

Alert: Never press both carotids at the same time because this can cause a reflex drop in blood pressure or pulse rate.

Apical

It is noted at the apex of the heart. In an adult this is located on the left side of the chest, about 8 cm (3 inches) to the left of the sternum and at 4th, 5th or 6th intercostal space area.

Femoral

It is noted where the femoral artery passes alongside the inguinal ligament.

Popliteal

It is noted where the popliteal artery passes behind the knee.

Posterial Tibial

It is noted on the medial surface of the ankle where the posterior tibial artery passes behind the medial malleolus.

Dorsalis Pedis (Pedal)

It is noted where the dorsalis pedis artery passes over the bones of the foot.

ASSESSMENT OF PULSE

When assessing the pulse, the nurse collects the following data: the pulse rate, rhythm, volume, arterial wall elasticity (tension) and presence or absence of bilateral equality.

- **Pulse rate:** It is measurement of the heart rate at the number of times the heart beats per minute.
- **Tachycardia:** The term is used for excessively fast heart rate over 100 BPM in an adult.
- **Bradycardia:** When the heart rate is less than 60 BPM
- **Pulse rhythm:** It is the pattern of the beats and the intervals between the beats. Equal time elapses between beats of a normal pulse is called pulse having a regular rhythm.

If the pulse has irregular rhythm, it is referred to as dysrhythmia or arrhythmia. If dysrhythmia is detected, the apical pulse is assessed and electrocardiogram (ECG) is necessary for further action.

- **Pulse volume:** Also called the pulse strength or amplitude, refers to the force of blood with each beat. Usually, the pulse volume is the same with each beat. It can range from absent to bounding. A normal pulse can be felt with moderate pressure of the fingers and can be obliterated with greater pressure. A forceful or full blood volume that is obliterated only with difficulty is called a **full bounding pulse.** The pulse that is readily obliterated with pressure from the fingers is referred to as **weak, feeble, or thready.**
- **Tension:** The elasticity of the arterial wall reflects the expansibility. A healthy, normal artery feels straight, smooth, soft and pliable. Elders often have inelastic arteries that feel twisted (tortuous) and irregular upon palpation.
- **Absent:** When pulse is palpable or heard on auscultation. The radial pulse is taken whenever vital signs are measured, the pulse quality and character should be noted while the pulse is being counted. When the radial pulse is irregular, the apical pulse should also be taken.

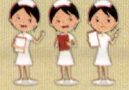 **SKILL: MEASURING THE RADIAL PULSE**

Articles

- Digital watch or watch with second hand
- Pencil
- Paper

Note: Review and carry out the standard steps as given in Appendix.

Action/steps	Rationale
Assessment	
1. Identify the person	Ensures that the pulse is recorded for the right person
Planning	
2. Explain the procedure	Explaining keeps the patient at ease.
Implementation	
3. Wash your hands	Reduces transfer of microorganisms

Contd...

Action/steps	Rationale
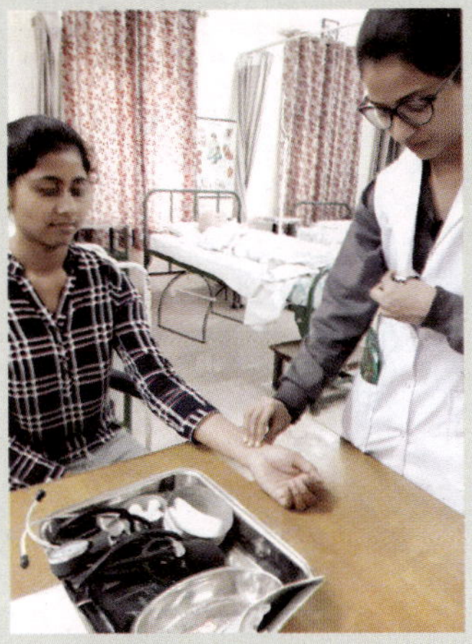 4. Place the pads of two or three fingers lightly over the radial artery with the patient's hand, palm down (Fig. 2).	Fingers are used rather than the thumb because the thumb has a strong pulse that could be confused with that of the patient

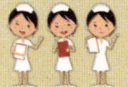

Fig. 2: Checking pulse of a patient

Action/steps	Rationale
5. Count the pulsations for 1 minute and note the regularity, rate, strength and character of the pulse.	Counting for full one minute provides a more accurate measurement of the pulse
Evaluation	
6. Jot down the count	Prevents forgetting the result
7. Wash your hands	Reduces transfer of microorganisms
8. Ask yourself: Is the result within the normal range? Is the pulse slower or faster than previous readings?	Provides data regarding alteration from normal for the patient
Documentation	
9. Record the time and pulse rate on the graphic sheet. Note any abnormalities in quality or rhythm in the nurse's notes and report	Note pulse measurements and any abnormality

Note: There may be a need to take radial pulse and apical pulse when the radial pulse is very irregular, skips beats or is difficult to count. This requires two people to count the radial and apical pulses at the same time to determine whether there is pulse deficit (difference between the apical and radial pulse).

SKILL: MEASURING AN APICAL PULSE

Articles
- Stethoscope
- Digital watch or watch with second hand

Note: Review and carry out the standard steps as given in Appendix.

Action/steps	Rationale
Assessment	
1. Determine if the patient has a known arrhythmia	Provides a baseline against which to compare the apical pulse
Planning	
2. Wash your hands, provide privacy and explain the procedure. Eliminate noise	Reduces transfer of microorganisms. Protects the patient's right to privacy and puts the patient at ease.

Contd...

Action/steps	Rationale
Implementation	
3. Expose the left chest. Warm the diaphragm of the stethoscope in the palm of your hand for a minute or two	Sounds are transmitted through stethoscope best placed on bare skin. A cold stethoscope is unpleasant for patient.
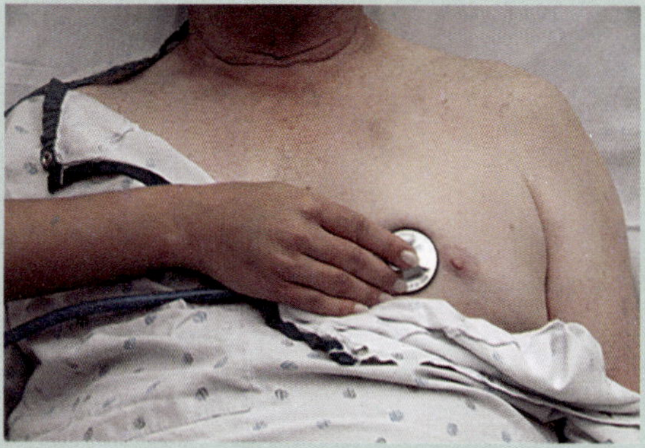 4. Locate the apex of the heart by palpating the fifth intercostal space at the midclavicular line (Fig. 3)	The apex of the healthy heart is located at the fifth intercostal space on the midclavicular line

Fig. 3: Measuring apical pulse

5. Listen to the heart sounds with the diaphragm of the stethoscope	The high pitched heart sounds are heard best with the diaphragm
6. Count the beats for full one minute	While counting, note the rhythm and strength of the beat
7. Cover the chest, make the patient comfortable and jot down the apical pulse	Prevents chilling and protects privacy
8. Wash your hands	Reduces transfer of microorganisms
Evaluation	
9. Ask yourself: Was the apical pulse irregular? Has it been irregular before?	Answer to questions which provide further data regarding heart status of patient.
Documentation	
10. Note down the graphic record of the patient that pulse was taken apically. If irregular, note the finding in nurse's notes	Identifies the method by which pulse was taken. Any abnormality should be documented in the nurse's notes

BIBLIOGRAPHY

1. *Perry & Potter, Clinical Nursing Skills & Techniques, 5th edition. Mosby; 2002.*
2. *Taylor CR, Lillis C, LeMone P, et al. Fundamentals of Nursing – The Art and Science of Nursing Care, 7th edition. Wolters Kluwer; 2010*
3. *Christensen BL, Kockrow EO. Foundation of Nursing. Mosby; 2003.*
4. *Bickley LS, Szilagyi PG. Bates Guide to Physical Examination and History Taking. Lippincott Williams & Wilkins; 2003. p. 862.*

Respiration

INTRODUCTION

Respiration is the exchange of oxygen and carbon dioxide in the lungs and tissues and is initiated by the act of breathing.

It is a combination of two processes: external respiration and internal respiration.

1. **External respiration: It occurs in four ways:**
   - i   Ventilation, which is the mechanical movement of air in and out of the lungs.
   - ii Dispersion of air throughout the bronchial tree of the lungs.
   - iii Diffusion of oxygen and carbon dioxide molecules across the alveolar membrane.
   - iv Perfusion, the movement of blood through the lungs and tissues.
2. **Internal respiration:** It happens at the cellular level, oxygen is released from hemoglobin to the cell and the cell in turn releases carbon dioxide to the blood.

There are basically two types of breathing: Costal (thoracic) breathing and diaphragmatic (abdominal) breathing.

1. **Costal breathing:** Involves the external intercostal muscles and other accessory muscles, such as the sternocleidomastoid muscles. It can be observed by the movements of chest upward and outward.
2. **Diaphragmatic breathing:** Involves the contraction and relaxation of diaphragm, and it is observed by the movement of the abdomen, which occurs as a result of the diaphragm contraction and downward movement.

Normally, breathing is carried out automatically and effortlessly. A normal adult respiration lasts 1–1.5 seconds, and an expiration lasts 2–3 seconds.

CONTROL OF RESPIRATION

Respiratory centers in the medulla oblongata and the pons of the brain and chemoreceptors located centrally in the medulla and peripherally in the carotid and aortic bodies help in the control of respiration. These receptors and centers respond to changes in the concentrations of oxygen, carbon dioxide and hydrogen in the arterial blood.

FACTORS AFFECTING RESPIRATION

Several factors influence respiratory rate. The ones that **increase** the respiratory rate include exercise, stress, increased environmental temperature and lowered oxygen concentration in increased altitudes. Factors that **decrease** the respiratory rate include decreased environmental temperature and certain medications, e.g., narcotics and increased intracranial pressure.

Depth of a person's respiration can be established by watching the movement of the chest. Respiratory depth is generally described as normal, deep or shallow. During normal inspiration and expiration, an adult takes in about 500 mL of air. This is called tidal volume. Deep respirations are those in which a large volume of air is inhaled and exhaled inflating most of the lungs. Shallow respirations involve the exchange of small volume of air and often the minimal use of lung tissue.

ASSESSING RESPIRATION

Respiration is assessed every time the full set of vital signs is assessed. The change in respiratory rate may indicate a change in patient's condition, but is always considered along with the other vital signs and assessment data. The respiration should be counted for full minute. Normal range of respiration is given in Table 1.

As respiration is being assessed, observe for variations in the pattern of breathing. Breathing that is normal in rate and depth in called eupnea. Dyspnea (difficult or labored breathing) is often accompanied by flared nostrils, anxious appearance, and statements such as 'I can't get enough air'. It is important to know, how much activity causes the dyspnea.

TABLE 1: Normal range of respiration

Age group	Respiration per minute
New born	30–80
Infant (age 1 year)	20–40
Child (3 years to 12 years)	20–30
Adolescent	16–20
Healthy adult	12–20
Elderly	16–20

RESPIRATORY RHYTHM

It refers to the regularity of the expiration and inspiration, Normally, respiration is evenly spaced.

RESPIRATORY QUALITY

Character refers to those aspects of breathing that are different from normal, effortless breathing. So, effort required to breathe is referred as **labored breathing** and sound of breathing such as wheeze, stridor, etc. are altered breathe sounds. Normal breathing is silent.

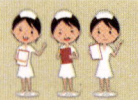

SKILL: MEASURING RESPIRATIONS

Articles

- Digital watch or watch with second hand
- Pencil and paper

Note: Review and carry out the standard steps as given in Appendix.

Action/steps	Rationale
Assessment	
1. Look for the way to distract the patient while you count respiration	Respiration measurement is more accurate when obtained with the patient unaware of the procedure
Planning	
2. Plan to count the respirations after measuring the radial pulse as if you were still counting the pulse	It may make the patient unaware that you are counting respirations
Implementation	
3. Wash your hands and tell the patient you are going to take the vital signs	Reduces transfer of microorganisms and puts the patient at ease

Contd...

Action/steps	Rationale
4. After taking the radial pulse with the wrist lying on the chest, continue holding the wrist while counting respirations. Position the watch so that you can see both its dial and the rise and fall of the chest (Fig. 1). 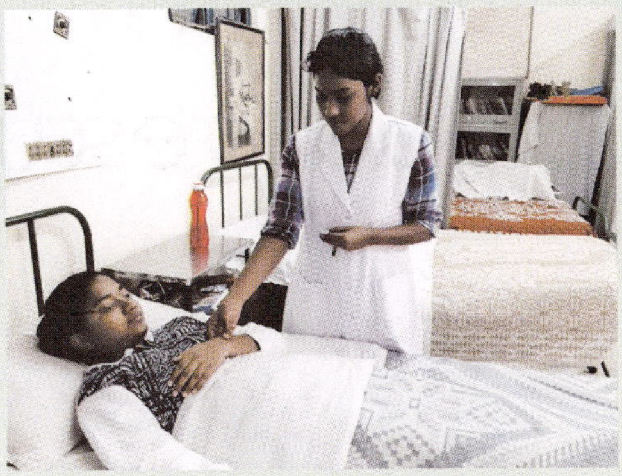	Having your hand on the patient's chest allows for the feeling of the rise and fall of the chest so that you can count the respirations

Fig. 1: Assessing respiration

Action/steps	Rationale
5. Count the respirations, noting rate, depth, pattern, and sounds count for 1 minute.	• While counting recall that a respiration includes both inspiration and expiration
6. Jot down the measurement along with the pulse rate	Prevents forgetting the count.
7. Wash your hands	Reduces transfer of microorganisms
Evaluation	
8. **Ask yourself:** Is the respiratory rate normal? Has it altered since the last measurement?	Provides data to determine whether an alteration from normal is occurring
Documentation	
9. Record the time and respiratory rate on the graphic record, on the patient's chart, or in the computer. If the character of respiration is abnormal or if the rate is irregular, document the findings in the nurse's notes.	Notes respiratory rate and any abnormalities, e.g., respiration: 36 shallow breaths.

BIBLIOGRAPHY

1. *Perry & Potter, Clinical Nursing Skills & Techniques, 5th edition. Mosby; 2002.*

2. *Taylor CR, Lillis C, LeMone P, et al. Fundamentals of Nursing – The Art and Science of Nursing Care, 7th edition. Wolters Kluwer; 2010*

3. *Christensen BL, Kockrow EO. Foundation of Nursing. Mosby; 2003.*

4. *Bickley LS, Szilagyi PG. Bates Guide to Physical Examination and History Taking. Lippincott Williams & Wilkins; 2003. p. 862.*

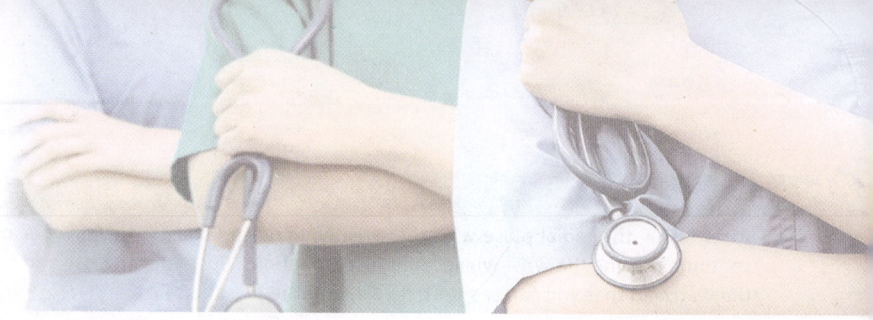

Chapter 30

Blood Pressure

INTRODUCTION

Arterial blood pressure is a measure of the pressure exerted by the blood as it flows through the arteries. Because the blood moves in waves, there are two blood pressure measures. The **systolic pressure** is the pressure of the blood as a result of contraction of the ventricles. The **diastolic pressure** is the pressure when the ventricles are at rest. It is the lower pressure present at all times within the arteries. The difference between the systolic pressure and diastolic pressure is called pulse pressure. A normal pulse pressure is about 40 mm of Hg but can go up to 100 mm of Hg during exercise. A consistently elevated pulse pressure occurs in arteriosclerosis. A low pulse pressure less than 25 mm Hg occurs in conditions such as heart failure.

Blood pressure is measured in millimeters of mercury (mm of Hg) and is recorded as a fraction of systolic pressure over the diastolic pressure. For a healthy adult, blood pressure is 120/80 mm Hg (pulse pressure of 40).

DETERMINANTS OF BLOOD PRESSURE

Pumping Action of the Heart

When pumping action of the heart is weak, less blood is pumped into arteries (lower cardiac output) and the blood pressure decreases. When the heart's pumping action is strong and the volume of blood pumped into the circulation increases (higher cardiac output), the blood pressure increases.

Peripheral Vascular Resistance

Peripheral resistance can increase blood pressure. The diastolic pressure especially is affected. The internal diameter or capacity of the arterioles and the capillaries determines the peripheral resistance to the blood in the body. The smaller the space within a vessel, the greater the resistance. Normally, the arterioles are in a state of partial constriction. Increased vasoconstriction raises the blood pressure, whereas decreased vasoconstriction lowers the blood pressure.

If the elastic and muscular tissue of the arteries are replaced with fibrous tissue, the arteries lose most of their ability to constrict and dilate. This condition is known as **arteriosclerosis**.

Blood Volume

When the blood volume decreases, e.g., in dehydration or hemorrhage, the blood pressure decreases because of decreased blood volume. Conversely, when the volume increases, e.g., rapid infusion of intravenous fluids, the blood pressure increases because of the greater blood volume within the circulatory system.

Blood Viscosity

Blood pressure is higher when the blood is highly viscous (thick), that is, when the proportion of red blood cells to the blood plasma is high. This proportion is referred to as the **hematocrit**. The viscosity increases markedly when the hematocrit is more than 60–65%.

FACTORS AFFECTING BLOOD PRESSURE

Age

The blood pressure rises with age, reaching a peak at the onset of puberty and then tends to decline. In elders, elasticity of the arteries is deceased and the arteries are more rigid. This produces an elevated systolic pressure and diastolic pressure.

Exercise

Physical activity increases the cardiac output and hence, the blood pressure. Thus, 20–30 minutes of rest following exercise is indicated before the resting blood pressure can be reliably assessed.

Stress

Stimulation of the sympathetic nervous system increases cardiac output and vasoconstriction of the arterioles, thus increasing the blood pressure reading; however severe pain can decrease blood pressure greatly by inhibiting the vasomotor center and producing vasodilatation.

Race

African-American males over 35 years have higher blood pressure than European-American males of the same age.

Gender

After puberty, females usually have lower blood pressure than males of the same age; this difference is due to hormonal variations. After menopause, women generally have higher blood pressures than before.

Medications

Medicines like caffeine may increase or decrease the blood pressure.

Obesity

Both childhood and adult obesity predispose to hypertension

Diurnal Variations

Pressure is usually lowest during early morning, when the metabolic rate is lowest, then it rises throughout the day and peaks in the late afternoon or late evening.

Disease Process

Any condition affecting the cardiac output, blood volume, blood viscosity and/or compliance of the arteries has a direct effect on the blood pressure.

ALTERATIONS IN BLOOD PRESSURE

Hypertension

A blood pressure that is persistently above normal is called hypertension. A systolic pressure above 140 mm Hg and a diastolic pressure above 90 mm Hg are regarded as being outside the normal range. A single elevated blood pressure reading indicates the need for reassessment. Hypertension cannot be diagnosed unless an elevated blood pressure is found when measured twice at different times.

Hypotension

A blood pressure that is below normal, i.e., 90/60 mm Hg is called hypotension. Some people have a blood pressure that is low, but they are healthy with no other symptoms. If hypotension is associated with symptoms of shock, i.e., increase in pulse rate, cold and clammy skin, dizziness, blurred vision, it is a dangerous condition that can rapidly progress to death. Unless treated, shock can be caused by hemorrhage, diarrhea, vomiting, burns and myocardial infarction.

Orthostatic hypotension is blood pressure that falls when the client sits or stands. It is usually due to peripheral vasodilatation, in which blood leaves the central body organs, especially the brain, and moves to the periphery causing the person to faint.

EQUIPMENT USED FOR MEASURING BLOOD PRESSURE

The sphygmomanometer (Fig. 1) with an occlusive cuff and the stethoscope are the most commonly used equipment for measuring blood pressure. Two types of manometers are generally used in clinical settings: mercury gauge sphygmomanometer; when greater accuracy is needed, and the aneroid gauge, which is a smaller unit and easy to carry but less accurate. Sphygmomanometer consists of a gauge for measuring blood pressure; tubing from the gauge to a cuff, which is wrapped around the arm or leg; and a control bulb that inflates and deflates the cuff. The cuff must be of correct size to obtain an accurate blood pressure reading. A narrow cuff is used for small children and a wider cuff is needed for muscular or obese persons. This device has a mercury filled manometer.

An **electronic sphygmomanometer** takes the blood pressure automatically. The cuff is placed on the arm and pumped up. As the air is released, the systolic and diastolic pressures are displayed on a screen in the unit. This unit does not require the use of stethoscope for listening to pressure sounds, but it is expensive.

KOROTKOFF SOUNDS

While measuring blood pressure, certain sounds may be heard that relate to the effect of the blood pressure cuff on the arterial wall. These sounds called Korotkoff sounds (Fig. 2) are numbered as follows:

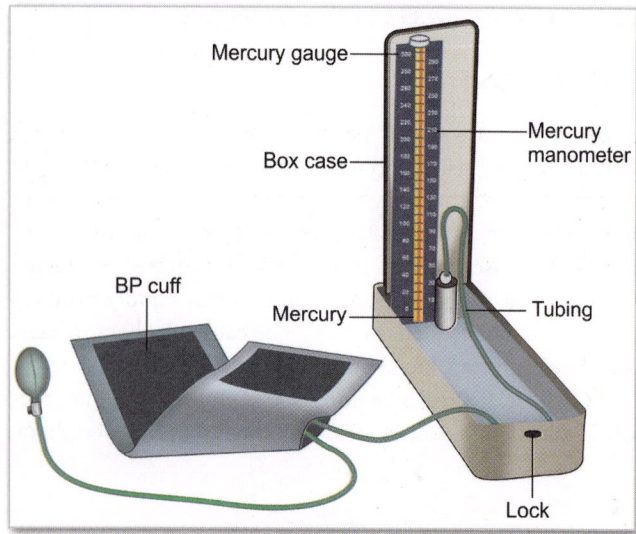

Fig. 1: Mercury sphygmomanometer

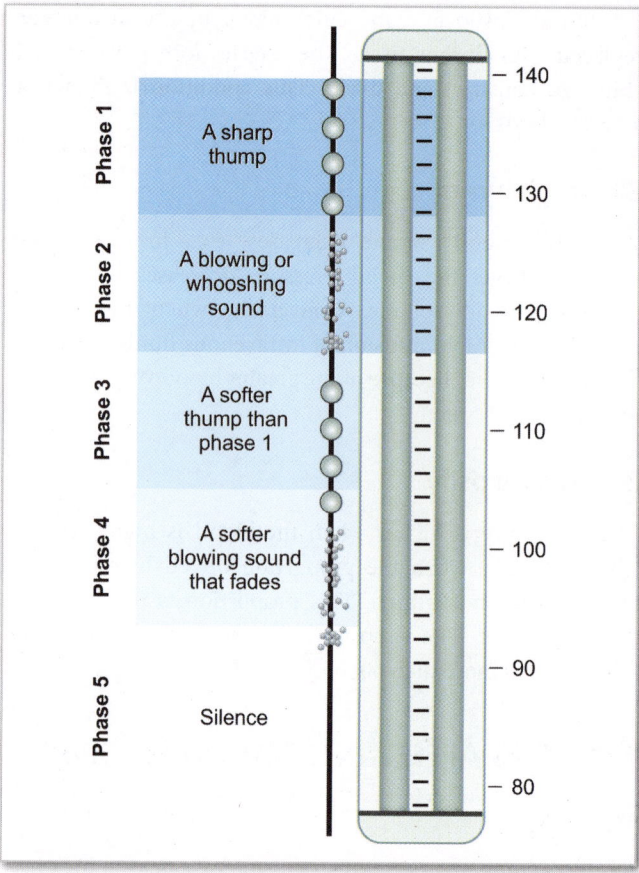

Fig. 2: The sound auscultated during blood pressure measurement can be differentiated into five Korotkoff's phases. For example, blood pressure is 140/90 mm Hg

Phase 1

- **Tapping:** Systolic pressure indicated by faint, clear tapping sounds that gradually grow louder.

Phase 2

- **Swishing:** Murmur of swishing sounds that increase as the cuff is deflated.

Phase 3

- **Knocking:** Louder knocking sound that occurs with each heartbeat.

Phase 4

- **Muffling:** A sudden change or muffling of the sound indicates diastolic pressure in children.

Phase 5

- **Silence:** Disappearance of sound marks diastolic pressure in adults.

GUIDELINES FOR MEASURING BLOOD PRESSURE

- Have the patient lie down or sit for at least 5 minutes.
- Use the brachial artery in the elbow joint of either arm.
- Check the condition of equipment and position of the manometer gauge, so that it can be seen at eye level from a distance of two to three feet. The gauge indicator should be at zero when the cuff is deflated. Use the correct cuff size.
- Inflate the cuff to 30 mm Hg above where the pulse disappeared upon palpation with inflation to prevent missing the auscultatory gap (period where no sound is heard).
- Once the cuff is starting to deflate, while obtaining systolic and diastolic readings, deflate all the way to zero.

Do not stop midway and begin to inflate again, because this gives a false reading.

- Listen for the different sounds while steadily deflating the cuff, and identify the systolic and diastolic blood pressure. The phase 1 sound is systolic pressure; The disappearance of phase 5 sound is the diastolic pressure and record both the readings.

If blood pressure cannot be determined by auscultation, the **palpation method** is used to estimate systolic pressure. Diastolic pressure cannot be measured this way. With the blood pressure cuff in place on the upper arm, palpate the radial artery. Inflate the cuff 30 mm Hg above the point at which the radial pulse disappears. Release the valve and allow mercury to fall 2 mm Hg per second, noting the point on the manometer when the radial pulse is again felt.

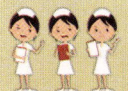

SKILL: MEASURING BLOOD PRESSURE

Articles

- Stethoscope
- Sphygmomanometer with cuff
- Pencil and paper

Note: Review and carry out the standard steps as given in Appendix.

Action/steps	Rationale
Assessment	
1. Identify the patient. Check to see what is the patient's blood pressure (BP).	• Ensure that the BP is recorded for the correct person. Knowing the usual pressure assists in knowing how high to inflate the cuff.
2. Assess the size of the patient's arm to determine the size of cuff needed.	The bladder of the cuff should cover 2/3rd of the circumference of upper arm.
3. Assess if there is a contraindication to taking the blood pressure on either arm.	If a patient has had a mastectomy, serious injury, or a lymph node dissection on the side of the arm chosen, use the other arm. If both arms are contraindicated, use a thigh cuff on a leg.
Planning	
4. Provide privacy and reduce environmental noise. Explain the procedure and wash your hands.	Allows you to hear the blood pressure sounds more accurately. Put the patient at ease. Reduces transfer of microorganisms.
5. Place the patient in comfortable position, sitting down or lying down and allow the blood pressure to stabilize for 5 minutes before measuring it.	• Change of position alter hemodynamics within the body; blood pressure will stabilize within 5 minutes.
Implementation	
6. Apply the cuff smoothly to arm, positioning the center of the bladder over the brachial artery and placing the cuff 1 to 2 inches above the antecubital space. Wrap the cuff firmly and smoothly around the arm and fasten it.	The center of the bladder of the cuff must be over the brachial artery for an accurate measurement to be taken.
7. Position the gauge so that it can be easily visualized.	For accurate reading.
8. Position and support the patient's arm at the level of the heart.	An arm positioned above or below the level of the heart may cause inaccurate reading.

Contd...

Action/steps	Rationale
9. Close the valve of the air pump by turning the screw valve clockwise until it is closed, but not so tightly that it cannot be easily released.	Closing the valve directs air flow into the cuff when the bulb is squeezed.
10. Palpate the radial artery/brachial artery. Pump up the cuff until the artery is occluded, then release the valve and let the air out of cuff.	Locating the pulse before pumping up the cuff is essential to determine the approximate level of systolic pressure. Locating brachial pulse where pulse is strongest, allows placement of stethoscope to hear the sounds.
11. Direct the ear pieces of the stethoscope slightly forward, and place them in your ears. Place the diaphragm or bell of the stethoscope over the brachial pulse.	The bell is smaller and fits more closely over the skin than the diaphragm. If bell is used, it should be only lightly applied to the skin. The diaphragm must be held firmly in contact with the skin to hear sounds clearly.
12. When 30 seconds have passed, reinflate the cuff quickly, while watching the gauge, to at least 30 points higher than the point at which you no longer could feel the pulse (Fig. 3). 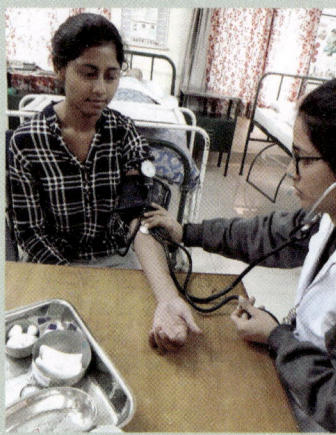 **Fig. 3:** Measuring blood pressure	Ensure that the cuff is inflated to a point above the patient's systolic BP and prevent missing an auscultatory gap (period where sound disappears). Keeping the mercury column at eye level for accurate reading (in sphygmomanometer). The aneroid gauge should be read with the eyes directly over or in line with it.
13. Deflate the cuff at a constant rate of 2 mm Hg per second by unscrewing the valve on the bulb pump counter-clockwise.	Deflating too rapidly or too slowly gives false readings. Avoiding contact of the stethoscope tubing with the clothing, cuff or tubing of the sphygmomanometer will decrease the possibility of extraneous noise.
14. Listen for the first Korotkoff sound, and note this as the systolic BP. Continue to listen and steadily deflate the cuff until muffling is heard; note this point. Continue deflating until the last Korotkoff sound is heard; note this point. Replace the patient's clothing if needed.	The point of muffling of Korotkoff sounds is considered the most accurate measurement of blood pressure in children, the point at which the last Korotkoff sound is heard; note the point; it is most accurate for adults. If sleeve was pushed up, replacing it shows courtesy to the patient.
15. Deflate the cuff completely and note down the reading of blood pressure.	Prepares the cuff for next use. Jotting the BP reading makes it readily available when recording on the patients chart.
16. Wash your hands.	Reduces the transfer of microorganisms
Evaluation	
17. Ask yourself, is the blood pressure within normal range? Is it elevated? Is it dangerously low? Is there a difference between this reading and previous reading?	Answers provide data regarding further plans that may need to be made. Excessively high or low blood pressure should be reported to the physician.
18. Document the time and pressure on graphics sheet; record in nurses notes with systolic BP as the top number and diastolic pressure as the bottom number, e.g., 128/80 mm Hg	Demonstrate trend of blood pressure and communicates any abnormality.

ELECTRONIC SPHYGMOMANOMETER

Electronic sphygmomanometer eliminates the need to listen or the sounds of the client's systolic and diastolic blood pressures through a stethoscope. It should be calibrated periodically to check accuracy.

DOPPLER ULTRASOUND STETHOSCOPES

Doppler ultrasound stethoscopes (DUS) are also used to assess blood pressure. These are used when blood pressure sounds are difficult to hear, such as in infants, obese clients, and when clients are in shock. Systolic pressure may be the only blood pressure obtainable with this method.

AUTOMATED VITAL SIGN MONITORS

Lightweight, portable, automated units are available that measure all vital signs simultaneously. Measurements can be obtained in 20–45 seconds. It is also possible to program most units to measure these vital signs at specified intervals. The vital signs are displayed digitally and may be retrieved using the stored date.

BIBLIOGRAPHY

1. *Perry & Potter, Clinical Nursing Skills & Techniques, 5th edition. Mosby; 2002.*
2. *Taylor CR, Lillis C, LeMone P, et al. Fundamentals of Nursing – The Art and Science of Nursing Care, 7th edition. Wolters Kluwer; 2010*
3. *Christensen BL, Kockrow EO. Foundation of Nursing. Mosby; 2003.*
4. *Bickley LS, Szilagyi PG. Bates Guide to Physical Examination and History Taking. Lippincott Williams & Wilkins; 2003. p. 862.*

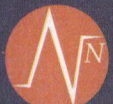
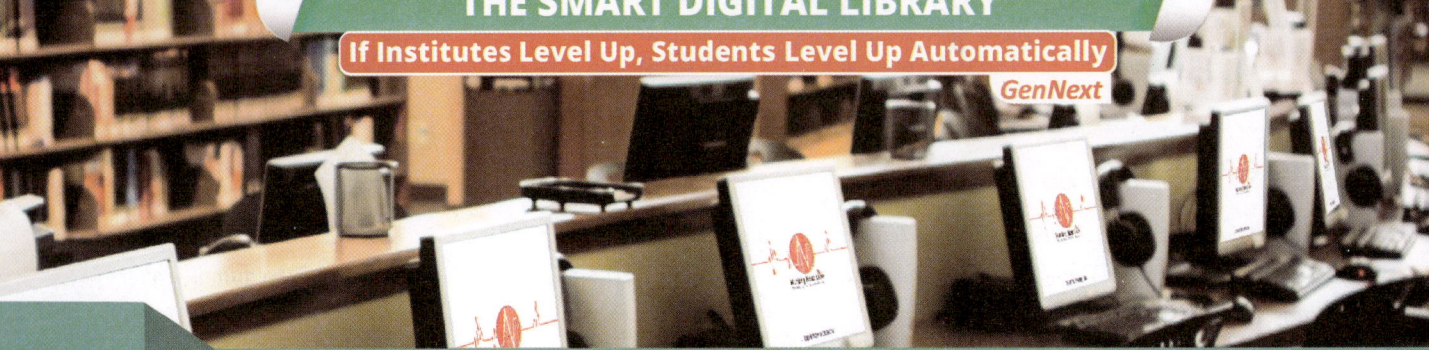
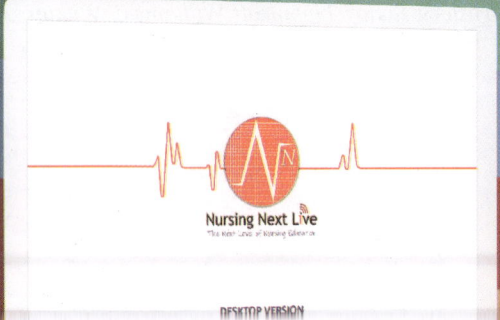

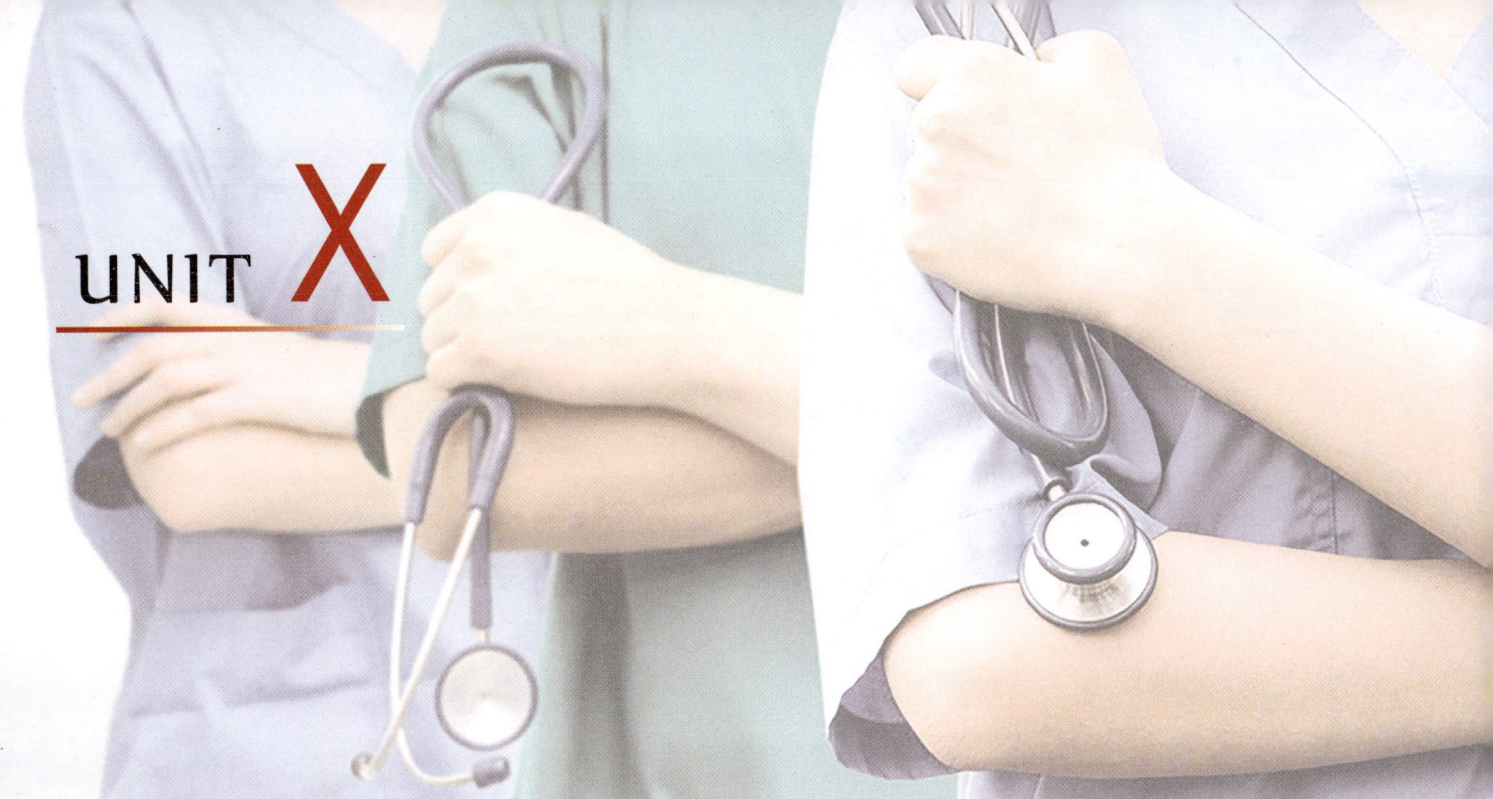

UNIT X

MEETING NEEDS OF PATIENTS

Unit Outline

Providing Safe and Clean Environment

INTRODUCTION

Environment is the total of all elements and conditions that surround us and influence our development. Caring for the patient's environment is important in providing holistic care. The goal is to provide safety while making the patient as comfortable as possible.

FACTORS AFFECTING THE ENVIRONMENT

Temperature

As individuals differ in their reaction to atmospheric conditions, there is a set indoor temperature, which can be ideal for everyone. Infants and older adults may need their rooms warmer than usual due to their poor temperature regulation. For every individual, the most suitable indoor temperature is that which is warm enough to prevent feeling chilly, yet not warm enough to cause perspiration. Keep the temperature between 68°F and 74°F or 20°C and 23°C. Operating rooms and critical care areas are kept slightly cooler to reduce the body's metabolic demands.

Ventilation

Ventilation is the process or act of supplying a building or room continuously with fresh air. Most health care facilities have air-conditioning units that regulate temperature, humidity and air exchange. Fans are discouraged because air currents spread microorganisms. Air in motion increases the evaporation of perspiration and radiation of heat from the skin.

Humidity

Humidity is the amount of moisture in the air. A range from 30% to 50% is normally comfortable. Very low humidity will dry respiratory passages and a person's skin. Most hospitals maintain a low humidity setting to discourage the growth of microorganisms. Vaporizers or humidifiers may be ordered for a patient with a respiratory condition, who requires more humidity.

Lighting

The amount of light is an important factor in comfort and is provided by natural or artificial light. A cheerful and sunny room can improve patients' spirits. Areas must have adequate lighting for tasks and to prevent accidents and injury. The light should be bright enough to see without glare, to avoid eye strain and be soft and diffuse, to prevent sharp shadows.

Odor Control

Illness changes sensory perceptions. Odors that ordinarily are present may make the patient feel nauseated. Health care facilities may have unpleasant odors from bedpans, urinals, wounds, etc. Good ventilation and cleanliness will effectively control odors. Various odor control measures can be taken such as:

- By emptying and rinsing bedpan, bedside commode, urinal and emesis basin promptly.
- Change soiled linens as soon as possible.
- Dispose of used dressings, catheters, urine bags, tubing, intravenous bags, and other disposable equipment by placing in a closed plastic bag according to standard precautions.
- Avoiding being the source of odors yourself. By wearing clean clothes and bathing. Deodorants, perfumes, scented lotions or scented cosmetics should not be worn in a patient care setting.
- Removing old flowers from the unit.
- Use room deodorizer or spray after consulting with your patient as he/she may be allergic or sensitive to deodorizer itself.

Noise Control

Noise is inevitable in health care facilities. The hospital should be a place for rest and should have a quiet atmosphere, yet a patient may experience sensory overload from all of the noise. Moving equipment, visitors and health care personnel are the sources of noise. To avoid noise, use sound absorbing flooring and ceiling materials, carpeting, and plastic equipment to reduce the noise. Encourage staff to limit conversations in the hospital unit and to speak in low volume. Soft, pleasant background music may be played to mask other sounds and promote relaxation.

Interior Design

Patient's rooms and public areas often look more like a hotel now. Rooms have draperies and colorful bedspreads. These changes are to promote comfort by providing a home-like environment for the patient.

Neatness

It is important to provide a neat and tidy atmosphere for your patient. Keep the unit clean in order to be safe. Straighten the patient's unit after making the bed and removing the old dishes and unused equipment. The over-bed table should be cleaned and wiped off if needed, before meals are served. Obtain the patient's permission before disposing off newspapers or magazines.

Privacy

Privacy is essential for a patient's well-being. Always knock gently and identify yourself before entering the room. Close the curtain around the patient for personal tasks such as using a bedpan and bathing. Post a sign on the door when such tasks are being done so as to discourage anyone from entering the room.

Pest Control

Hospital unit should be free from vermin, rodents and other vectors of disease. Keep a fly swatter within easy reach and destroy flies when seen. Keep food well-covered or in a fly-proof net cupboard. Remove soiled dishes immediately after the patient has eaten. Place soiled dressings in covered bins and make sure they are removed twice daily. Cover and remove bedpans at once after use. Make sure that toilets are kept clean.

Encourage the use of mosquito nets when available. Keep screen doors tightly closed and teach patients and attendants to close them properly.

Cockroaches and ants can be prevented by keeping the area clean. Use of gammexane and dichlorodiphenyltrichloroethane (DDT) spray should be done around areas where they appear.

Cleaning beds with a disinfectant can prevent the bed-bugs. Rats and mice can be prevented by reporting holes and cementing and leave no food around to attract them.

REDUCTION OF PHYSICAL HAZARDS

Safety is a primary concern when caring for patients. Safety is needed to prevent accidents and possible injuries to patients, visitors, and health care personnel. The most common accidents among patients are falls, burns, cuts, and bruises.

Fights with others, loss of personal possessions, choking and electric shock also occur.

Role of a Nurse in Promoting Safety

In a Health Care Facility

- Orient the patient and family when admitted to health care facility regarding call bell system, bed and television. Check that the patient can operate the controls.
- Assess the patient's gait and risk for falling on admission. If needed, tell the patient to call for help to get up.
- Evaluate the patient's drug regimen for side effects that may increase the risk of falling.
- Keep the bed in a low position.
- Help the patient to go to toilet on a regular schedule to decrease the chances of patient getting out of bed unassisted.
- Lock the bed wheels to prevent the bed from rolling when the patient attempts to get in or out.
- Provide a night light to aid patients while going to the bathroom at night.
- Encourage the use of firm, non-skid slippers to prevent slipping while walking.
- Answer call lights quickly so that patients learn to trust you and do not feel the need to get up without help.
- Be sure patient is comfortable and all desired items and call bell are within easy reach.
- Encourage the use of grab bars for the toilet, tub and shower.
- Place the high risk or restless patient in a room close to the nurses' station for easy observation.
- Stay with the patient who is confused, agitated, or unsteady whenever the patient gets up and uses side rails.
- Restrict fluids after 6.00 pm so that patient does not have to get up frequently at night.
- Make sure for wheel chair brakes are locked before transferring a patient into or out of it.

In the Home

- Place a non-skid bath mat in the tub and shower
- Use of night light
- Installation of grab bars for bathroom/toilet
- Install door buzzers or bed alarms that sound when the patient leaves the bed
- Encourage removal of extension cords because these may cause a fall.

Hazards

Falls

Falls are a safety hazard. The three most common factors that predispose a person to falls are impaired physical mobility, altered mental status and sensory and/or motor deficits.

Burns

Prevention of burns includes protecting the patient from accidental thermal injury and the threat of fire. Thermal injuries may be caused by either hot or cold materials. A person with diabetes or impaired circulation, or who is paralyzed or on drugs that alter mental awareness, is more easily burned than a person in good health. To prevent these injuries, use a barrier between the patient's skin and the thermal application. Check the temperature of liquids before giving them to the patient. Warn the patient if a food or drink is hot. Caution the patient to avoid lying on, or sleeping with, heating pads or ice packs. Inspect electrical cords that may cause sparks or fires. All electrical appliances brought into the hospital from home must be checked to ensure safety.

Smoking

Smoking is banned in most of the health care facilities, however, some long-term care agencies allow smoking in designated areas. Carefully supervise the patient who smokes and is sedated, confused or irrational. Warn your patient not to smoke in bed. Smoking is never allowed when oxygen is in use because a spark could cause a fire.

Fire

Fire is a possibility in any setting. You must know and be familiar with your institution's fire regulations. This includes knowing the location of the fire extinguishers, fire alarms, escape routes, and how to communicate in case of fire. Most of the health care agencies use the RACE acronym to respond to a fire because it is easy to remember. In case of fire:

- Rescue any patient in immediate danger by removing them from the area
- Activate the fire alarm system
- Contain the fire alarm system
- Extinguish the flames with an appropriate extinguisher.
  One must maintain proper body mechanics to evacuate patients to prevent injury. Protect against possible smoke inhalation by placing wet towels across the bottom of closed doors and have people hold wet washcloths over their nose and mouth. This helps in trapping the smoke.

Fire Safety Measures

- Install smoke detectors on each level.
- Make sure there are two exits to escape in case of fire.
- Never smoke in bed and where the oxygen is administered to patients.
- Store inflammable substances away from heat, sparks, and flame.
- Keep cooking areas free of combustible materials.
- Never overload electrical circuits.

Hazardous Materials: Poison

A poison is a substance that when ingested, inhaled, absorbed, applied, injected, or developed within the body may cause functional or structural disturbances. When reporting a known or suspected poisoning, have the label handy. Report: name of the product, patient's age, amount you believe is involved and any symptoms/complaints you observe.

Caution

- Store all medicines in child-proof containers
- Keep toxic substances in a locked cabinet out of reach of children. Label with poison stickers
- Always keep toxic substances in their original labeled container. Never put toxic substances in beverage or food containers.
- Never induce vomiting unless instructed by professional.

Safety/Protective Devices

Protective devices, formerly called restraints, are used to restrict movement but at present it is an illegal and totally unacceptable practice that constitutes malpractice. It is your responsibility to be aware of and follow the regulations in your health care facility.

Presently health care workers are encouraged to make frequent observations of the patient, which helps to decrease the use of devices. Family and friends of a patient who are confused, can be encouraged to sit with the patient to promote safety. A patient who is confused may try to pull out a nasogastric tube. In order to continue medical treatment, it may be decided to place the patient's hand in a hand mitten (restraint). If this does not prevent the patient from pulling out the nasogastric tube, then a wrist or extremity device may be ordered.

The order must be written before applying a device. When the protective device is no longer needed, obtain an order to discontinue it. The usual time limit is 24–48 hours.

When applying the protective device make sure that patient's movements will not impair circulation or nerve function. Padding the device with a soft washcloth or gauze pads will prevent skin irritation. The device should fit snugly when applied, but should not compromise the patient's neurovascular status. You should be able to easily fit your index and middle fingers between the patient and the device. A device that is secured too tightly may cause injury. Active and passive exercises are performed for immobilized joints and muscles and remove the device at least every 2 hours. Check the area distal to the device every 15–30 minutes. Observe the signs of adequate circulation including pulse, distal to the device. Signs that the circulation or nerve function has been impaired include coolness of the skin, change in color, particularly pallor or a bluish hue, numbness,

pain, edema, and loss of sensation or movement. Remove the device immediately and contact the physician if any of these signs occur.

Selecting a Restraint

Before selecting a restraint, the nurse needs to understand its purpose clearly and measure it against the following five criteria:

1. It restricts the client's movements as little as possible. If a client needs to have one arm restrained, do not restrain the entire body.
2. It does not interfere with the client's treatment or health problem. If a client has poor blood circulation to the hands, apply a restraint that will not aggravate that circulatory problem.
3. It is readily changeable, especially if they become soiled. Changing restraint should be done with minimal disturbance to the client.
4. It is safe for the particular client. Choose a restraint with which the client cannot self-inflict injury, e.g., physically restrained person could be injured trying to climb out of bed if one wrist is tied to the bed frame. A jacket restraint would restrain the person more safely.
5. It is least obvious to others. The less obvious the restraint, the more comfortable people feel.

Types of Restraints

There are several kinds of restraints. The most common for adults are jacket restraint, belt restraint, a mitten or hand restraints (Fig. 1) and limb restraint; use of bed rails is also a restraint. Restraints for infants and children include mummy restraint, elbow restraint and crib knots.

Documentation of the use of protective device must be done. Document the time and from whom the order for device was obtained, the type of device applied, the time of application, the name of the person applying the device, and the location of the device on the patient's body. Include the teaching done for the patient and family prior to the placement of the device. Obtain an informed consent as necessary. Document the periodic observations you make of the patient including skin color and distal pulses. Lastly, record the time when the device was discontinued with the name of the person who discontinued.

FACTORS AFFECTING SAFETY

The ability of people to protect themselves from injury is affected by a number of factors. Nurses need to assess each of these factors when they plan care to provide safety.

Learning about the environment is very essential from the childhood. Thorough knowledge and accurate assessment of the

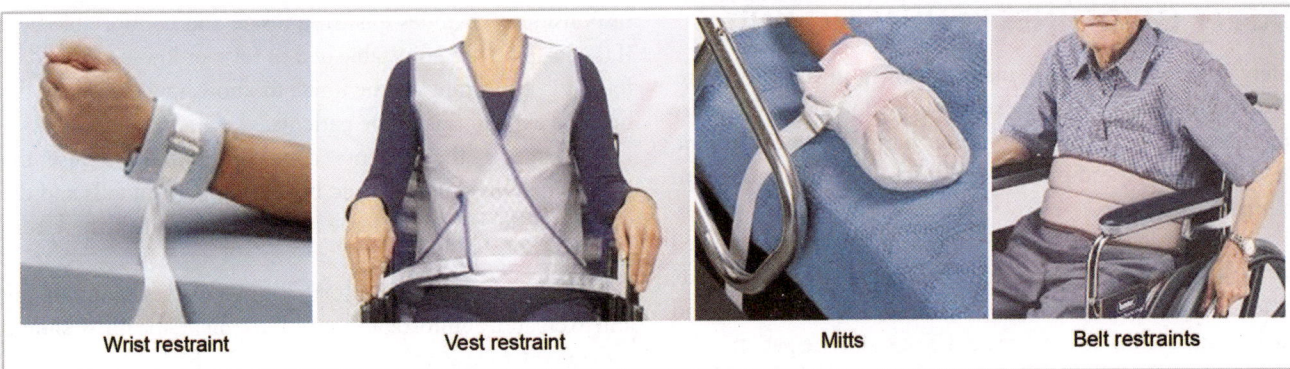

| Wrist restraint | Vest restraint | Mitts | Belt restraints |

Fig. 1: Types of restraints

environment helps people to learn to protect themselves from many injuries. Usually, elderly people have special concerns in protecting themselves from injuries. Often the balance of elderly people is impaired by their flexed posture. Slowness of movement and diminished sensual acuity also contribute to the likelihood of injury.

Lifestyle

Lifestyle factors that place people at risk are unsafe work environment, where workers are in danger from machinery and chemicals; residence in neighborhoods with high crime rates; access to illicit drugs, etc. Risk taking behavior is a factor in accident.

Sensory/Perceptual Alterations

Accurate sensory perception of environmental stimuli is vital to safety.

People with impaired touch perception, hearing, taste, smell and vision are highly susceptible to injury.

Paralysis and other neurologic impairments diminish perceptions.

Some neurologic diseases cause changes in kinesthetic (movement) sense and tactile (touch) perceptions. For example, disease of the inner ear can cause loss of kinesthetic sense and tactile perceptions.

Spinal cord injuries can cause paralysis and loss of tactile perceptions.

Level of Awareness

Awareness is the ability to perceive environmental stimuli and body reactions and to respond appropriately through action. The normal alert person assimilates various types of information at one time, perceives reality accurately, and acts on those perceptions.

Occasionally, people exhibit abnormalities of thoughts; they become absent minded or lose their sense of direction.

Patients with impaired awareness include persons lacking in sleep, unconscious or semiconscious persons, disoriented persons and persons whose judgment is altered by medications, such as narcotics and sedatives.

Mobility Status

Persons who have impaired mobility are obviously prone to injury.

Patient weakened by illness or surgery are not always fully aware of their conditions. It is not uncommon for patients to fall while trying to get up and walk.

Emotional State

Extreme emotional state can alter the ability to perceive environmental hazards.

The acutely anxious or angry person has reduced perceptual awareness. Depressed persons may think and react to environmental stimuli more slowly than usual.

Ability to Communicate

People with diminished ability to communicate are also at risk for injury. Patients who are unable to speak, people with language barriers and those unable to read fall in this category. For example, the person who is unable to interpret the sign "No smoking—Oxygen in use", is at risk.

Previous Accidents

It has been recognized that some people are prone to accidents.

Safety Knowledge

Information is crucial for safety. Patients in hospital and other unfamiliar environments frequently need specific information. Lack of knowledge about physical, (use of equipment), chemical (drugs/disinfectants) and biological (infections) safety is a potential hazard.

SAFETY GUIDELINES IN NURSING UNIT

Safety and security is a main concern in nursing care. The responsibility of nurse is to provide safe and secure environment, and identify the harmful environment. Promoting safety and preventing injury are primary concern in nursing.

Many patients experience fall especially when they need to attend toilet. Any limitation in mobility is dangerous like, an elderly patient with unsteady gait is prone to falling and the hospital setting may increase the risk and the patient with paralysis or spinal cord injury need, support such as walkers, wheel chairs, etc. and they need careful guidance. Nurse must assess the risk for injury to support and to boost self-esteem of the patients.

Environmental Safety

Safe environment contributes to patient's sense of wellbeing.

It is important for the nurse to ensure that bedside environment is clean, safe, and pleasant. The prime nursing responsibility is ensuring that necessary equipment and items are in their proper place and function properly.

On admission, the patient and the visitors should be oriented to the hospital environment, the equipment including the beds, call light, and the layout of the room and unit.

Arrange the equipment in the patient's room so that he or she is able to reach articles on his bedside locker.

The nurse is responsible to allocate the type of bed/crib needed according to patient's age, needs, mental status and capabilities.

Safe bedside unit includes the following:

- Patient's call light should be functioning and always within reach
- Bed should be positioned properly
- Side rails and restraints are safely used
- Provide uncluttered walk space
- Attention to ventilation, odors, room temperature, lighting and noise
- Odors may be decreased by promptly emptying bedpans, urinals and emesis basins, not to dispose of soiled dressing in client's room or near the bed.

Lighting

Many patients find it difficult to sleep in the hospital as they are frequently disturbed for assessment or for treatment purpose, the nurse should be careful to reduce harsh lighting and noises, whenever possible.

Beds

Patients spend most of their time on bed. The bed is an important part of the client's environment. Nursing responsibility includes ensuring a safe and comfortable bed. If the hospital has adjustable bed to raise or lower the head or foot, it is important for the nurse to know how to operate the bed and explain this to the patients.

Whenever the patient's condition indicates, raise the lower side rails. These should be used to prevent falls and the wheels on the beds should be locked to prevent the bed from slipping away.

Ensuring patient's comfort is always a priority in nursing and to create a comfortable bed environment, the nurse should provide the following:

- Linens clean and wrinkle free
- Comfort to the patient
- Pressure points of patient are protected from rough sheet.

Sleep

Providing comfortable bed promotes proper rest and sleep. The bottom linens should be tight and clean while the upper linen should allow freedom of movement and should not exert pressure. A quiet and darkened room with privacy is essential for relaxing. In a strange environment with unfamiliar noises, such as people walking, entering or leaving the room and closing the windows or doors is disturbing. Effort should be made to reduce disturbances. The nurses should be aware of the patient's rituals and should make every effort to meet them.

One of the main problems for sleep is pain. Depending on the cause, severity and the discomfort, appropriate measures have to be taken. Comfort and care should be considered when patient is sleeping.

When care cannot be taken, nurses should explain that checking vital signs or specific nursing measures are more important than sleep.

Noises

- Unfamiliar noises should be explained to the patient on an ongoing basis.
- Nurse helps to keep noises to a minimum range by wearing shoes, which do not cause excessive noise while walking, closing doors quietly, handling the equipment smoothly, avoiding dropping of any objects, and talking and laughing loudly.

Exposure to Microorganisms

- Nurses work in liaison with housekeeping for the patient's room, bathroom, and nursing units to keep them clean and tidy.
- Washing and drying of hands should be practiced before and after contact with each patient.
- Isolation procedure should be utilized and explained to the patients and visitors. For the patients suffering from

communicable diseases or for protective isolation, all policies and procedures on "isolation" should be followed.

- Visitors of isolated patients are taught hand-washing, the use of mask, gowns and gloves, and other precautions as necessary.
- Disposable dishes should be used for isolated patients.
- All patients discharged with continued isolation will be taught the techniques that the patient and the family needs to follow at home.

Electrical Safety
Prevention of Electrical Hazards

- As new machines and equipment are introduced into the hospital, nurses will have to learn the potential dangers before using.
- Inspection on all the equipment, plugs, and outlets should be done daily and the suspected defects should be reported to the maintenance immediately and be repaired. A sign should be placed on the defective items until repaired.
- Water and electricity should not come in contact. Prevent dampness near switches, wiring and appliance items until repaired.
- Protect electrical cord from heat or oil, to prevent the damage in the electrical insulation.
- Electrical cord should always be placed high enough so as to prevent the tripping hazards.
- Nurses should make rounds with maintenance personnel to inspect cords, plugs, switches, socket, etc. for damage. Problems should be alleviated immediately by maintenance.
- Defibrillation paddles should be checked in each shift when the crash carts are checked.

Oxygen Safety

When oxygen is administered, the following precautions should be followed:

- Smoking is strictly prohibited in health institution. "No smoking—Oxygen in use", signs should be placed on the door of the patient's room.
- Flammable or combustible or vapors such as alcohol, oil or grease materials should not be used while oxygen is being administered.
- Nylon, silk, rayon and woolen clothing should not be used by patients, when oxygen is being administered.
- Ether or any other explosive anesthetics should not be used.
- Oxygen administered should be humidified.
- Nurse should understand and be constantly educated on the use of oxygen cylinders, regulators, humidifiers, catheters, inhalers, face masks, tents and ventilators.

- Any new respiratory equipment should be explained to the nursing staff. In-service education on new equipment will include the use and the safety precautions as needed.
- Oxygen cylinders should be stored in a cool temperature away from the inflammable materials and where they are not likely to be knocked over.
- Any problems or questions about respiratory equipment should be immediately reported for inspection and repairs.

Incidents Involving Patient's Visitors and Employees

- All nurses should be aware of correct procedure to follow if a patient is injured in the hospital. The patient's attending physician should be called immediately to examine the patient. The incident should be relayed to the nursing officer/supervisor and an incident report form should be filled out immediately and submitted to the appropriate authority.
- All nurses should be aware of the correct procedure to follow if a visitor is injured in the hospital. The nurse should immediately take him/her to the accident and emergency department and an incident report form should be filled out immediately after examination and submitted to the appropriate authority.
- All nurses should be aware of the correct procedure to follow. If he/she is injured while on duty, he/she should be examined by the appropriate person and incident report should be produced to the higher authority for needful action.

Safety in Moving Equipment

When moving heavy equipment always have sufficient help to:
- Prevent injury to persons and equipment
- Push but do not pull heavy equipment to prevent injury to feet, legs and back
- Open and secure swinging doors before proceeding
- Keep hands and fingers away from the edge of equipment to prevent injury
- When lifting patients and equipment, seek help as and when needed.

Observe the following precautions:
- Keep spine vertical and straight, use leg muscles not back muscles.
- Stand close to the person/object being lifted with feet apart. For balance, bend at knees to use leg muscles to lift.
- Use a safe firm pressure when lifting, do not jerk.
- When lifting as a team, maintain constant level of the object by doing it gradually and gently.

Safety in Transporting Patients

When transporting with stretchers, bed carts and other wheeled equipment, safety precautions must be followed as listed below:

- When assisting patients on to stretchers, beds or wheel chairs, be sure that the equipment is properly secured and brakes are set on the wheels
- Any patient being transferred through stretcher must have side rails in position and safety straps fastened.
- First transport patient on a stretcher.
- Push the vehicle from the end to avoid hand injury
- Move slowly and always have clearance
- When patients are being transported from one room to another by stretcher, they should be secured to a restraining belt and keep their feet, arms and hands covered by blanket and on the stretcher. At doorways, stretchers and carts should be pulled through rather than pushed in blindly.

Safety From Insects

- Flies, mosquitoes and cockroaches should be kept away by spraying
- Make use of insecticides available or supplied from the institute.

Preventing Patient's Fall in the Hospital

Falls may be caused while shifting patients. It can be prevented by keeping floor dry to prevent slipping and securely holding stretchers and wheel chairs while transporting the patient.

Tips to Prevent Fall in the Hospital

- Orient the patient on admission to their surroundings and explain the call system.
- Encourage the patient to use call bell and ensure call bell is within reach.
- Place bed side tables and over bed tables near the bed or chairs so that patient does not lose his/her balance.
- Assess the patient's ability to ambulate and provide assistance as required.
- Instruct the patient to be careful while using toilet.
- Encourage the patient to wear non-skid footwear.
- Keep the environment tidy.
- Maintain clutter free area.
- Ensure adequate lighting.
- Attach side rails to the beds of confused, sedated, restless and unconscious clients.

Safety for Preventing Cross Infection in the Hospital

- Wash hands before and after each procedure.
- Ventilate the patient's room.
- Use damp dusting to prevent the rise of dust in the environment.
- Provide disinfectants for cleaning the floor.
- Keep the environment clean, e.g., bed locker, bed linen, over bed table, floor, etc.
- Cover the mattress and pillow with plastic cover so that it is easy to disinfect after a patient is discharged.
- Wear disposable gloves while handling body fluids and secretions, e.g., urine, stool, vomitus, pus, etc.
- Complete all the cleaning activities, e.g., bed making, dusting, etc. at least one hour prior to commencement of aseptic procedures, e.g., wound dressing, intravenous (IV) infusions injections, etc.
- Wash hands before handling foods.
- Serve the food hot in a covered container.
- Protect the kitchen and pantry from flies, insects and cockroaches.
- Clean and disinfect bedpans, urinals and sputum cups.
- Dispose of all waste materials properly following the hospital protocol.
- Immunize all nurses, who are taking care of patients with infectious diseases.
- Cover all used sharp instruments and discard in an appropriate container.
- Regular health check-ups for all health personnel.
- Keep the toilets clean.
- Instruct people to cover the nose and mouth while sneezing and coughing to prevent droplet infection

Safety Precautions in the Hospital

- Read the bulletin board in order to keep up with change and improvement in the hospital policies and procedures.
- It is the responsibility of each employee to report unsafe conditions to his supervisor.
- All safety measures for disoriented or emotionally disturbed patients should be utilized. Safety measures both for patients and employees shall be put forth into practice while caring.
- Hospital personnel, visitors and patients should be warned when floors are wet, and movable object has been kept in the passage
- Always read warning signs such as "Radiation Precaution", "Isolation", etc.

STRATEGIC OBJECTIVES FOR IMPLEMENTING PATIENT SAFETY

Implementing patient safety framework would require a holistic and pragmatic approach. Patient safety concepts should be interlaced with building blocks of health system. Therefore, safety culture becomes integral part of health care delivery. Six strategic objectives have been identified for this purpose after due consultation with stakeholders and reviewing global and regional frameworks for patients, safety (Fig. 2). Each strategic objective has been further explained in terms of key priorities and specific interventions.

♦ **Strategic objective 1:** To improve structural systems to support quality and efficiency of health care and place patient safety at the core at national, subnational and health care facility levels

♦ **Strategic objective 2:** To assess the nature and scale of adverse events in health care and establish a system of reporting and learning

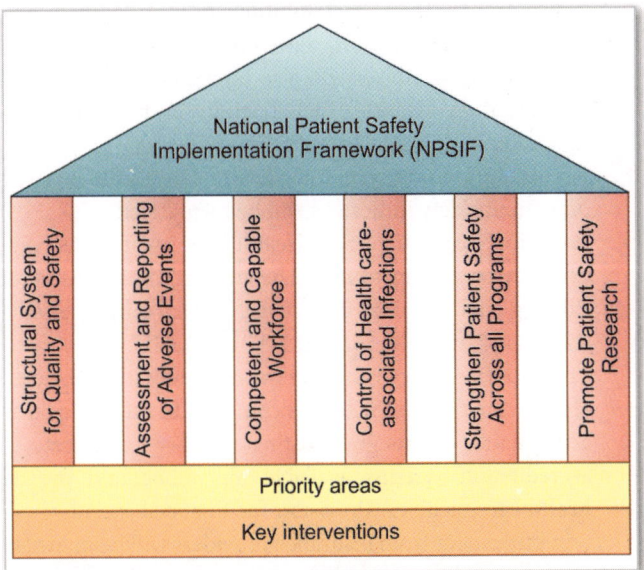

Fig. 2: National patient safety implementation framework

♦ **Strategic objective 3:** To ensure a competent and capable workforce that is aware and sensitive to patient safety

♦ **Strategic objective 4:** To prevent and control health care-associated infections

♦ **Strategic objective 5:** To implement global patient safety campaigns and strengthening patient safety across all programs

♦ **Strategic objective 6:** To strengthen capacity for and promote patient safety research

Strategic Objective 1

To improve structural systems to support quality and efficiency of health care and place patient safety at the core at national, subnational and health care facility levels.

Developing quality and safety culture is a long-term endeavor and requires enabling environment friendly policy, administrative and service provision levels. This requires investments for creating structures for quality and safety and having credible quality accreditation system and regulatory mechanism to ensure compliance to minimum safety standards. India has a vibrant and growing health sector with mix of public and private providers. Further, health is a subject of a state and each state government sets its own legislative, administrative, financing and health care delivery models as per priorities and context. This makes developing a pan-India institutional structure a challenging task. A rational approach would be to have an overarching national framework under which states are given flexibility to design their own institutional mechanism and modalities for quality & safety in public and private sector.

Framework should provide options of quality assurance and accreditation system that private and public health care providers can adapt as per requirements and preference. The institutional framework should be more of a facilitator than regulator so as to let flourish a self-sustainable quality and safety culture. There is also a need for developing culture for safe health care communication and involving patients in their treatment and welfare. Following are key priority areas for improving structural systems for quality and safety.

Key Priority 1.1

Institutionalize patient safety and strengthen legislative and regulatory framework

Patient's safety should become integral part of health care delivery system through institutionalization within the existing policy, regulatory and program management framework. Following is the proposed institutional framework for patient safety in India.

♦ **National level:** National Patient Safety Steering Committee will be constituted under aegis of Ministry of Health & Family Welfare (MoHFW). This committee will have representation from all relevant governmental and non-governmental stakeholders. Quality Assurance mechanisms under National Health Mission (NHM) will also be utilized. This committee will work to implement a robust patient safety framework in the country and coordinate with different stakeholders. Committee will be supported by a dedicated patient safety secretariat in Directorate General of Health Services (DGHS) MoHFW.

This secretariat will provide technical support for implementing patient safety including drafting technical guidelines and developing training material.

- **State level:** At the state level there will be a designated nodal officer for implementing patient safety framework. State quality assurance committees have been constituted in all the states chaired by Principal Secretary (Health). As quality and patient safety are related concepts, it is therefore natural to use existing quality assurance committees for monitoring and implementation of patient safety framework too. A sub-committee on patient safety will be constituted under the state quality assurance committee. If required, large states may engage a dedicated technical staff to support patient safety activities though National Health Mission. Though designated state nodal officers for quality assurance should be over all responsible for patient safety activities also. Terms of references (TORs) and functions of quality assurance committees and officers can be revised to include the patient safety components explicitly. Similarly, district quality assurance committees will be responsible for implementing the patient safety framework at district level through their existing mechanism.

- **Integration of patient safety programs and schemes:** Patients safety concepts should also be strengthened in all vertical disease control program considering safety of both provider and patients/beneficiaries. Some important aspects are injection safety and reporting of adverse event following immunization (AEFI) in immunization programs, infection control in designated microscopy centers (DMCs) under Revised National Tuberculosis Control Program (RNTCP) program, blood safety under National Acquired Immunodeficiency Syndrome (AIDS) Control Program, etc.

- Clinical Establishment Act includes patient safety requirements for registration of clinical establishment. Patient safety concept should also be incorporated in draft of Public Health Act or any such legislation which will contribute regulatory framework in health sector.

- Publicly funded health insurance schemes should incorporate provision for payments based on patient safety performance/safety indicators such as hospital acquired infection rates, medication errors and use of safe surgery checklist.

Key Priority 1.2

Strengthen quality assurance mechanisms, including accreditation system

Quality assurance and accreditation mechanism for public and private health care facilities need to strengthen so patient safety can be assured at the point of delivery. While efforts will be made to increase the coverage of quality certification/accreditation, there is also a need to strengthen the existing quality standards by incorporating the patient safety requirements more adequately in their assessment criteria. Following are the proposed measures:

- At national level, a set of minimum patient safety indicator will be defined by. These MoHFW indicators will be reported by all health care facilities both in public and private sector. Framework recommends leveraging the reporting mechanism instituted under existing quality assurance programs and accreditation systems.

- MoHFW will also define minimum patient safety standards to be incorporated by accreditation agencies in their respective assessment criteria for quality accreditation.

- National Quality Assurance Program for public health facilities has defined set key performance indicators (KPIs) for each level of facilities to be reported on monthly basis. These KPIs will be revised to include minimum patient safety indicators defined at national level.

- For private sector National Accreditation Board for Hospitals and Healthcare Providers (NABH) will be required to include the minimum patient safety indicators in their accreditation programs including entry level certification. Selected indicators applicable to clinical laboratories will also be included in National Accreditation Board for Testing and Calibration Laboratories (NABL) accreditation program.

- A ranking/grading system for health care facilities based on patient safety indicators will be introduced.

- Provision for "Patient Safe Health care Institutions" certification will be instituted. The criteria will be based on existing quality standards such as National Quality Assurance Standards (NQAS) and NABH. MoHFW may institute a special body for issuing patient safety certification.

- Health care facilities will be encouraged to achieve quality accreditation through existing quality certification/accreditation systems available for public and private health care facilities. Provision for financial incentives in reimbursement from insurance providers will be made for certified/accredited hospitals.

- To ensure that quality standards measure patient safety issues adequately, patient safety concerns such as fire safety, seismic safety, medical device safety and structural safety will be included in existing quality standards and norms.

Key Priority 1.3

Establishing a culture of safety and improving communication, patient identification, handing over transfer protocols in health care facilities

Patient safety concepts need to be incorporated in the work culture of health care providers and the way they communicate to each other while delivering the care.

Apart from service providers, patients and community at large also need to be sensitized on patient safety related issues. For this purpose, following activities are suggested:

♦ A comprehensive communication strategy for patient safety will be developed involving all stakeholders. The communication strategy will be developed targeting both patient/community as well as care providers.

♦ For ensuring safe communication amongst care providers for delivery of health care services, standard operating procedures and checklist will be developed for error prone processes such as handover, verbal orders and transfer of patients.

Key Priority 1.4

Establishing patient-centered care and involving patients as partners in their own care

The objective of patient safety framework cannot be achieved without considering perspective of patients. In fact, patient is the most important stakeholder and should be at the center of health care design and delivery process. Following activities are suggested for achieving patient involvement for safe care:

♦ Developing educational and information material on patient safety such as audio-visual material, posters, brochures and IT based aids. Information on patient safety will be disseminated to both patient as well as care providers using communication channels such mass media, print media and social media.

♦ Integrated web based grievance redressal system and toll-free helplines on patient safety within the existing information and communication technology (ICT) system of MoHFW (including toll free number and IT based solutions). This system will also enable anonymous reporting of incidents and practices compromising the safety of patients. The incidents reported will be examined by an independent agency.

♦ Promoting establishment of patient's rights groups and facilitating their involvement in policy discourse and monitoring of patient safety outcome.

Strategic Objective 2

To assess the nature and scale of adverse events in health care and establish a system of reporting and learning

A universal error and adverse events reporting system is crucial to know the extent of harm caused by unsafe care. Although just having reporting system does not mitigate the risk of getting harm. It does serves as the catalyst for improvement, regardless of the level of care. Following actions are proposed for establishing a credible system for reporting of adverse events.

Key Priority 2.1

Generating evidence for policy making

Since limited information is available about overall burden of unsafe care in India, it would be prudent to estimate the baseline quantum of unsafe care in Indian health care system. For this purpose, following activities are proposed:

♦ Scope of errors and adverse events will be defined for Indian context based on internationally agreed benchmarks and best practices.

♦ A baseline assessment of public and private health care facilities will be conducted for estimating the extent of errors and adverse events for defined scope. The survey can be conducted by a designated autonomous national level institution.

Key Priority 2.2

Establishing robust surveillance systems for monitoring patient safety

A universal reporting and feedback system for reporting of errors and adverse events needs to established for the country. This system should be non-punitive, confidential, independent, timely, system-oriented and responsive in nature. Following are the specific activities:

♦ Developing system of reporting of errors, nearly missed and adverse events from facilities to state and national level. This will include standardization of adverse event definitions, reporting formats and establishing a web-based reporting system across public and private health care facilities.

♦ Public health programs such as immunization and National AIDS Control Program (NACP) already have some system of reporting of adverse event specific to their activities. Accreditation programs such as NQAS and NABH also mandate for reporting adverse events. There are national programs for pharmacovigilance and materiovigilance. All these reporting systems will be streamlined and integrated to establish a comprehensive patient safety surveillance system.

♦ Guidelines for errors and adverse events reporting will be developed by MoHFW. This will include definitions, categorization and directory for errors, nearly missed and adverse events as well as process, codes and protocols to be followed by public and private health care institutions for patient safety reporting.

♦ Annual reports on quality of care and patient safety will be released by MoHFW based on the data available from patient safety surveillance system and quality assurance program/accreditation system. A national level Resource Center/Technical Institute will be designated to analyze patient safety data and prepare report on behalf of MoHFW.

- Patient safety risk assessment checklists will be developed for primary, secondary and tertiary care facilities for identifying and mitigating risks through internal assessment and quality improvement approach.
- Health Workers' safety is as important as patient's safety. Minimum health care workers' safety requirements will be issued by MoHFW, which needs to be incorporated in all licensing and accreditation programs.

Key Priority 2.3

Ensuring supportive legislative mechanisms for effective functioning of patient safety surveillance systems

Adequate legal and policy level provisions will be required to create an enabling environment for non-punitive and system-oriented surveillance system.

- A system for analyzing the patient safety reports and feedback mechanism for taking corrective actions will be established with support of National Health Systems Resource Center (NHSRC) and Patient Safety Secretariat.
- The proposed Public Health Act will make provisions for mandatory reporting of adverse events by health care facilities.
- Adequate legal provisions will be made to keep sensitive patient safety reporting confidential and exempted from public access and litigation.

Strategic Objective 3

To ensure a competent and capable workforce that is aware and sensitive to patient safety

To sustain patient safety efforts, it would need to be made part of the work culture at health care facilities. This would require a workforce that is sensitive, well-trained and competent on patient safety issues. Though adverse events can be mainly attributed to failure of the system rather an individual; however, trained and sensitized care providers can prevent the harm and help in building an error-free work environment. The Patient safety framework emphasises a "catch them young" approach, whereby patient safety principles are incorporated in medical and nursing education, and then sustain the accumulated skills through continual medical/nursing education and on the job trainings. Following are the priorities:

Key Priority 3.1

Strengthening education, training and professional performance inclusive of skills, competence, and ethics of health-care personnel

To ensure health worker's competence on patient safety, multipronged approach is recommended which includes making it a part of professional licensing requirements as well creating institutional capacity for trainings. Following are the specific actions:

- Knowledge of basic patient safety concepts will be incorporated as part of evaluation criteria for medical, nursing and paramedical licensing exams. Certain credit hours of attending the online-courses/continued medical education courses on patient safety will be made mandatory as criteria for renewal of professional licenses.
- Academic and technical support intuitions at national and state level will be identified to develop training courses and deliver onsite/online trainings on patient safety.
- An institutional framework will be prepared for developing and updating evidence based standard treatment guidelines in Indian context.
- National Standard Treatment Guidelines for all disease conditions will be developed in phase manner and will be made available for health care providers through user-friendly applications and implementation tools.

Key Priority 3.2

Improving the understanding and application of patient safety and risk management in health care

The understanding of patient's safety should start from the medical and nursing education and should be extended to health care facilities through safe work culture and positive learning environment that enables care providers to apply their learning and strengthen their skills. Following specific actions are planned to achieve this objective:

- Medical, nursing and paramedical educational curricula will be mapped for existing components of patient safety. The syllabus for undergraduate and postgraduate level courses will be revised to incorporate adequate learning objectives for patient safety based on WHO patient safety curriculum guide.
- Patient safety principles will also be incorporated into in-service education programs and on job trainings organized by employers in public and private health sectors.
- Practical guidelines for implanting patient safety at health care facilities will be developed. These guidelines will guide hospital administrators and care providers for implementing patient safety program at facility level.
- Patients safety components will also be incorporated in job description of different cadres of workforces and their performance appraisal criteria. Financial and non-financial incentives such as awards can enhance adherence to safe care practices.
- A National Patient Safety day/week will be observed across the country. Notification on desirable activities for this occasion will be issued by MoHFW.
- Further to facilitate learning on patient safety, a web-based/mobile-based learning platform will be developed.

Strategic Objective 4

To prevent and control health care-associated infections

Health care-associated infections are a major challenge in ensuring patient safety. This situation is further aggravated in public hospitals due to patient overload and inadequate workforce. There is no credible data on burden of health care-associated infection (HCAI) in India. HCAI is a multidisciplinary challenge and requires multipronged approach to contain it. Following are key priorities.

Key Priority 4.1

Strengthening infection prevention and control structure and programs across all health care services and all levels of care

The risk of HCAIs can be mitigated through establishing a sustainable infection control program at health care facilities. A system improvization to this practice would be to connect these facility level programs and committees with policy level objectives and interventions. Following key actions are proposed:

- A national level strategic plan for infection prevention and control will be prepared by MoHFW. This will have close linkage with related programs such as Antimicrobial Resistance Program and National Action Plan on Viral Hepatitis.
- Institutions which have successfully implemented infection prevention and control programs, will be identified and their best practices will be disseminated for evidence-based learning and scaling up.
- Functioning of infection control committees at facility level will be strengthened and development of standard operating procedures are to be undertaken along with regular reporting of indicators.
- Infection control activities in various national health programs will be integrated.
- A system for surveillance of HCAIs will be established in phase manner. Data of HCAI will be collected and analyzed by the agencies responsible for patient safety reporting.

Key Priority 4.2

Providing appropriately cleaned, disinfected or sterilized equipment for patient care as required

Adequate financial resources will be made available to ensure availability of equipment and consumables for disinfection and sterilization of equipment. This will be taken under the overall umbrella of NHM for public health systems and through specific hospital levels budgets for other hospitals.

Key Priority 4.3

Providing a safe and clean environment by improving the general hygiene sanitation and management of health care waste in health care facilities

Hygiene, sanitation and waste management are closely linked with infection control outcomes. Swachh Bharat Abhiyan has given an impetus for improving cleanliness in hospitals and surroundings. Following actions are suggested to further promote sanitation and hygiene in health care facilities:

- Hand hygiene program will be further reinforced in medical and nursing curriculum and in-service training at health care facilities.
- Implementation of Kayakalp (clean hospital scheme) will be further reinforced by disseminating good practices and replicating role models across countries.

Strategic Objective 5

To implement global patient safety campaigns and strengthening patient safety across all programs

Key Priority 5.1

Safe surgical care

- Safe surgery checklist will be adopted for secondary and tertiary care level hospitals to make sure that all elective and emergency surgeries are performed using safe surgery checklist.
- World Health Organization (WHO) 24 × 7 Emergency and essential surgical norms will be adopted in all health care facilities providing surgical care.
- Appropriate sterilization practices will be adopted within National Trauma Care and National Burns program.
- Guidelines for surveillance and prevention on venous thromboembolism will be developed and implemented.

Key Priority 5.2

Safe childbirth

- Quality Assurance standards for maternal health care and assessment tools for labor rooms and maternity operation theater will be reviewed and updated based on latest evidences including respectful maternal care and natural birthing process.
- Quality standards for labor room and operation theater will be expanded and reinforced at private health care facilities to ensure quality of intrapartum and post-partum care.

Key Priority 5.3

Safe injections

- Vaccination of all health care providers against Hepatitis B in addition to waste handlers against tetanus to ensure occupational safety concerns among health care providers

- Strengthen the post-exposure prophylaxis (PEP) for needle stick injuries at all causalities/operation theaters and other intervention sites.

Key Priority 5.4

Medication safety

- Standard operating procedures for disposal of discarded/expired drugs as per biomedical waste management rules 2016 will be developed.
- Adverse drug reaction surveillance will be strengthened and implemented across all public and private health care facilities with close coordination between state health departments, pharmacovigilance agencies, professional associations drug manufacturers and national vertical programs.

Key Priority 5.5

Blood safety

- Voluntary non remunerated blood donation will be promoted though improved donor selection, recruitment, retention and referral through an effective communication strategy and capacity building.
- Adverse donor and transfusion reactions surveillance will be implemented at all levels of care.
- Hospital transfusion committee will be constituted with standard composition and terms of reference and rational use of blood and blood products will be promoted.

Key Priority 5.6

Medical device safety

- Usage of non-mercury devices and equipment will be promoted.
- Availability of biomedical engineers will be ensured at health care facilities.
- Standard operating procedures (SOPs) for utility; breakdown; monitoring of medical devices, restricting reuse of single-use purpose devices, clear policy on condemnation of equipment and SOPs of calibration for electronically operated medical devices will be developed and made available to health care facilities.

Key Priority 5.7

Safe organ, tissue and cell transplantation and donation

- Deceased donor programme will be reinforced and modified as necessary.
- Scale-up Information, education and communication (IEC) for organ donation, training of personnel in addition to registration of organ retrieval centers.
- Dissemination of relevant information and ensure uniform implementation across region/state/institutions/hospital/tissue banks on legislation, National Organ Transplant Programme (NOTP), National Organ and Tissue Transplant Organization (NOTTO), different SOPs, including for selection and safety of donors; allocation policies, and national registries.

Strategic Objective 6

To strengthen capacity for and improve patient safety research.

Key Priority 6.1

Consolidation of patient safety research and utilization for decision-making

A repository of good quality research on patient safety and allied themes will be created at national level. This will be pursued through Indian Council of Medical research (ICMR), which is the nodal medical agency for research in the country.

Key Priority 6.2

Reinforcing research for patient safety

- Studies will be conducted for estimation of the overall burden of unsafe care including point prevalent survey of hospital acquired infections.
- Research on different aspects of patient safety at country and state level will be prioritized.

  Source: National patient safety implementation framework (2018–2015) INDIA.

CONCLUSION

Safety and security is a main concern in nursing care. The responsibility of the nurse is to provide safe, secure environment and identify the harmful environment. Promoting safety and preventing injury are primary concern in nursing.

BIBLIOGRAPHY

1. Trained Nurses Association of India. Fundamentals of Nursing-A Procedure Manual, 1st edition, New Delhi; 2005. p 147-9.
2. Kozier Barbara B, Du Gas Beverly W. Fundamentals of Nursing Patient Care. WB Saunders Company, Philadelphia; 1967. p. 83-9.
3. Alexander MF, Fawcett JN, Phyllis J. Runciman JP. Nursing Practice-Hospital and Home, 1st edition, Longman Group UK Limited; London; 1994. p. 747-50.
4. Leahy JM, Patricia EK. Foundation of Nursing Practice, 1st edition, WB Saunders Company; Philadelphia; 1998. p. 670-6.
5. Craven RF, Hirnel CJ, Henshaw CM. Fundamentals of Nursing-Human Health and Function. Lippincott Williams and Wilkins; Philadelphia; 2000. p. 762-5.
6. Price AL. The Art, Science and Spirit of Nursing, 3rd edition, WB Saunders Company, Philadelphia; 1968. p. 84-94.
7. Thresyamma CP. Fundamentals of Nursing, 1st edition, Jaypee Brother Publication; New Delhi; 2002. p. 154-8.

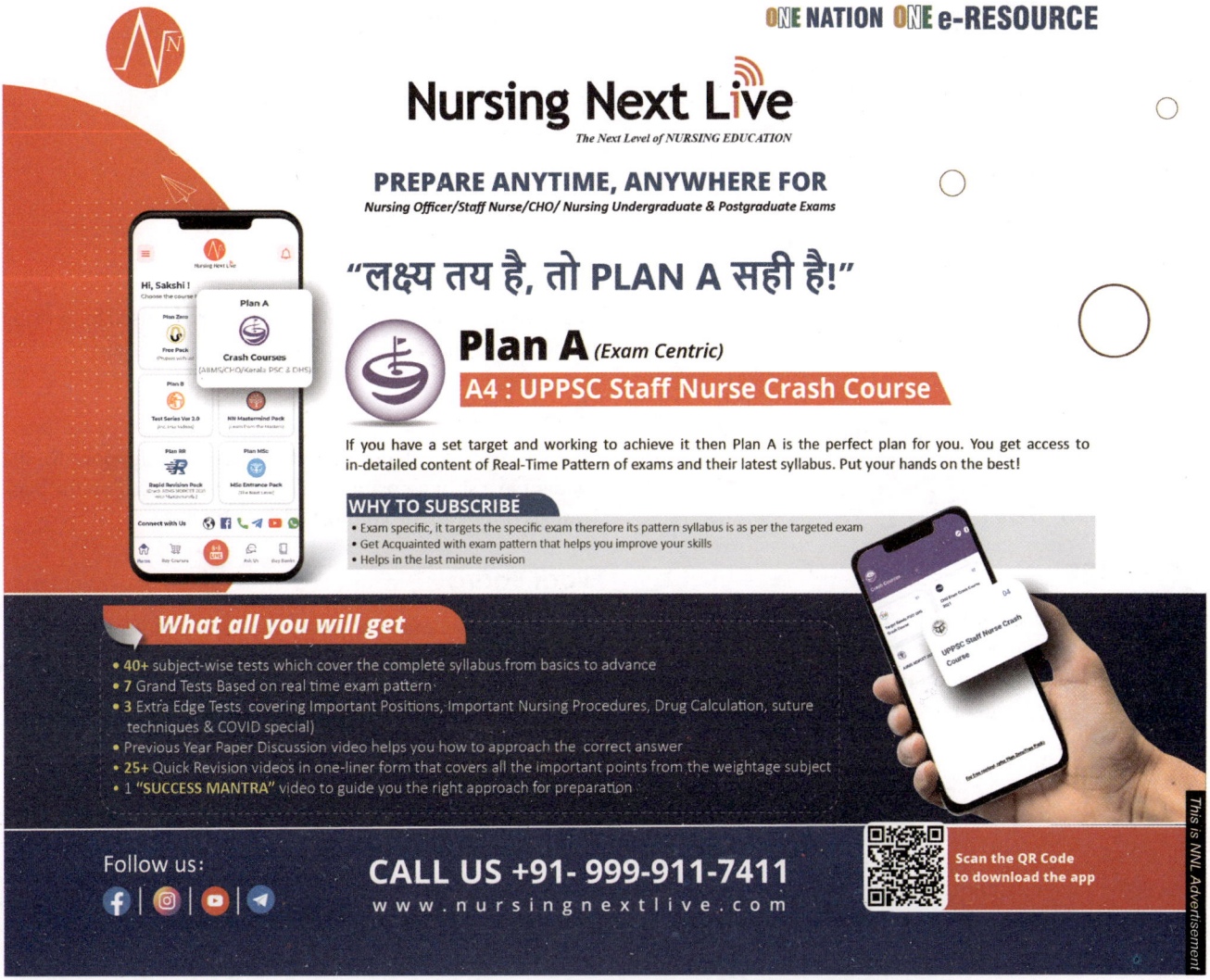

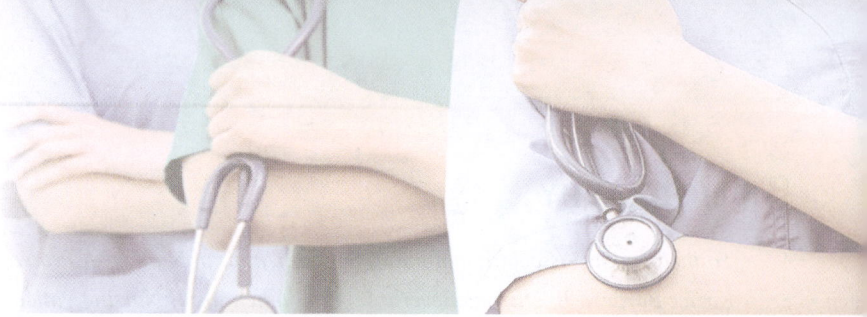

Chapter 32

Providing Comfort

INTRODUCTION

Nursing care meets all client needs. The client's most important basic need is comfort which can be provided by using various comfort devices, positions and a comfortable bed.

COMFORT DEVICES

Mattresses

Most beds have firm and even surface for patients' comfort. A rubber or plastic surface permits easy cleaning. Special mattresses provide extra comfort and support for clients and relieve the pressure on bony prominences, e.g., air-water mattress.

Cardiac Table

It is a device designed as an overbed table and is placed in front of the patients while they are in Fowler's position. It is so called because normally this is used for cardiac patients, who can lean forward on a pillow. This can also be used for writing purpose, serving food and other self-care activities.

Back Rest

It is a mechanical device, which provides support to the patient in a sitting position. Pillows can be placed on the back rest according to the comfort of the patient.

Foot Board

It is a flat panel made of wood or plastic and is placed at the foot end of the bed. It provides support to the patient's feet, keeps the top bed covers off the patient's feet and make the foot comfortable. It helps in preventing foot drop.

Foot Blocks

These are made up of wood, or metal and are used to raise the foot-end or head-end of the bed. They are used to prevent shock, to arrest hemorrhage, to retain enema and after spinal anesthesia.

Air Cushion

These are made of rubber and can be inflated with air. They are used to take the weight of the body off the sacral region. They prevent bed sores at the buttocks and should be always used with cover.

Cotton Rings

These are made of cotton. They are used to relieve pressure on certain parts of the body like elbows, heels, occiput, etc.

Hot Water Bottles

These are rubber bags, which can be filled with hot water, and are used to provide warmth and to make the patient and environment comfortable.

Bed Cradle

It is a comfort device, designed to keep the top bed-clothes off the feet, legs and abdomen of a patient. It is used in cases of burns, or to apply heat for drying plaster casts. It is also used in observing patients with lower limb amputation.

Rubber Ring

They are inflated with air and placed under the patient. Make sure that valve does not come in contact with any part of the body.

Sand Bags

These are used to immobilize a part of the body

BEDS AND BED MAKING

The bed is the equipment used most by a patient, therefore, it should be designed for comfort, safety and adaptability for changing positions.

The typical hospital bed consists of a firm mattress on a metal frame that can be raised and lowered horizontally. The frame is divided into three sections so that the operator can raise and lower the head and foot end of the bed. Most beds are powered by electric motors, but some beds are operated manually. Hospital beds come in two different lengths. Standard length is approximately 6 feet. Longer bed is available for taller patients. Each bed sits on four rollers or casters that allow the nurse to move the bed easily. A hospital bed is usually 65–70 cm (26–28 inches) above the floor. The greater height of a hospital bed prevents undue musculoskeletal strain on the nurse and the client. The position of a bed is usually changed by electric controls on the side of the bed, at the foot of the bed or on a bedside table. Patients can thus, raise or lower sections of the bed without expending much energy. It is important for nurses to instruct clients on the proper use of controls and to caution them against raising the bed to a position that might cause harm.

Beds contain a number of safety measures. Locks located on the wheels, casters at the center of the bed frame should be used whenever the bed is stationery to prevent accidental movement during the performance of a procedure. Side-rails, located on both sides of a bed, protect patients from accidental falls, helps patients position themselves and provide upper extremity support as patient gets out of bed. Side rails are adjustable metal frames that raise and lower the bed by pushing or pulling a knob.

General Rules to be Observed in Bed Making

- Have all equipment on hand and arrange conveniently in the order of use
- Wash hands before and after the procedure
- Do not expose the patient unnecessarily
- Protect the patient from draught of air
- Do not cover the patient's face while placing the linen
- Do not mix clean linen with soiled linen
- Never place the woolen blanket directly on the patient's body and never allow the mackintosh to touch the patient
- Fold dirty linen away from your uniform and body
- Avoid placing dirty linen on the floor
- Start work from head to foot, near to far, and from clean to unclean area
- Make the bed smooth, unwrinkled and firm
- Avoid using torn linen
- Periodical airing and sunning of mattresses to be done
- Maintain body mechanics
- Keep reasonable distance from the face of the patient to prevent cross-infection.

Types of Beds

- Open bed (Fig. 1)
- Closed bed (Fig. 2)
- Occupied bed (Fig. 3)
- Admission bed (Fig. 4)
- Postoperative bed (Fig. 5)
- Cardiac bed (Fig. 6)
- Amputation/divided bed (Figs 7A and B)
- Fracture bed
- Therapeutic bed, e.g., renal bed, rheumatism bed, etc.

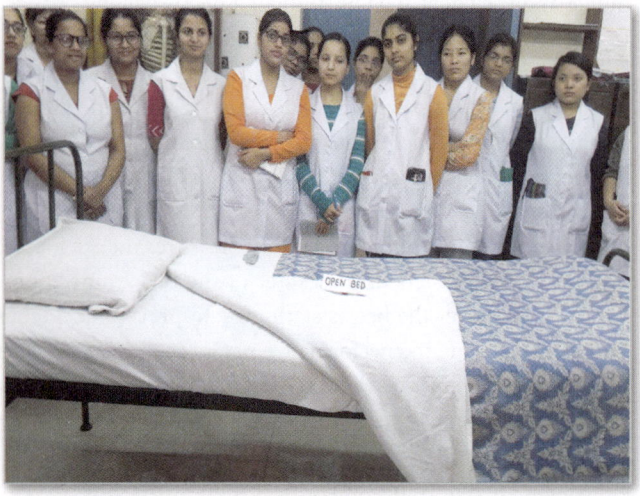

Fig. 1: Open bed

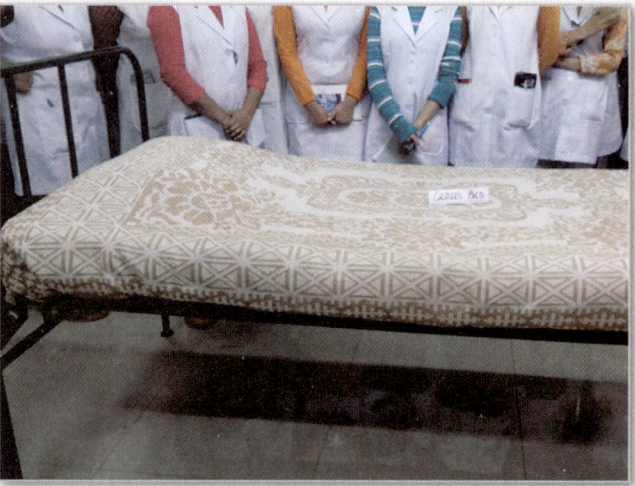

Fig. 2: Closed bed

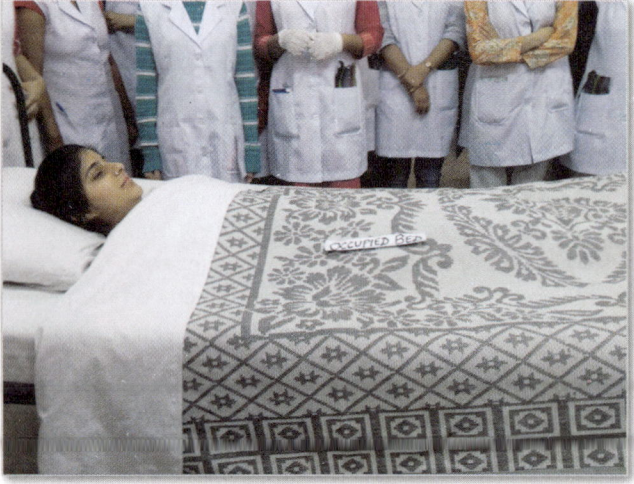

Fig. 3: Occupied bed

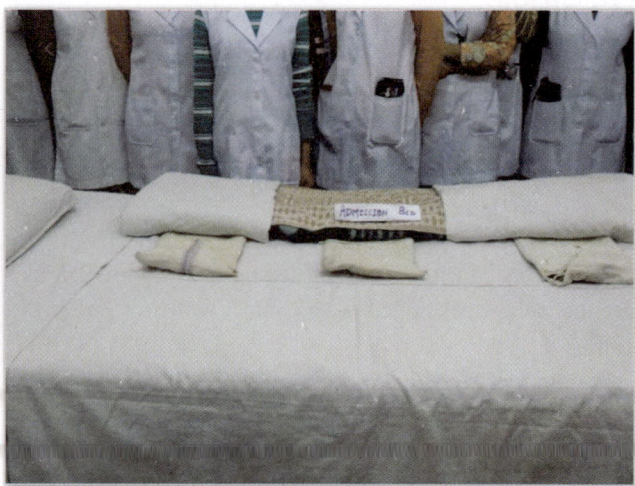

Fig. 4: Admission bed

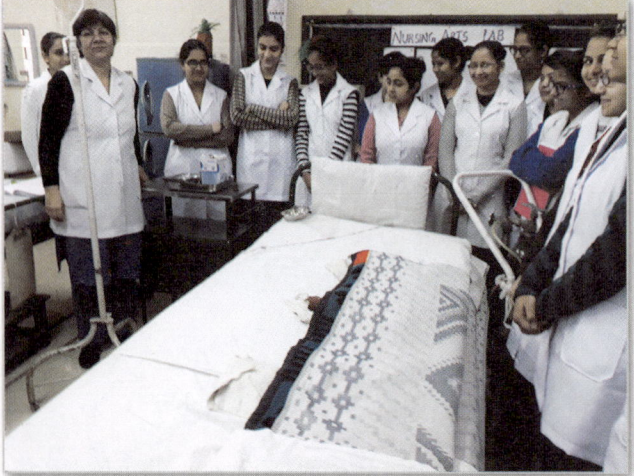

Fig. 5: Postoperative bed

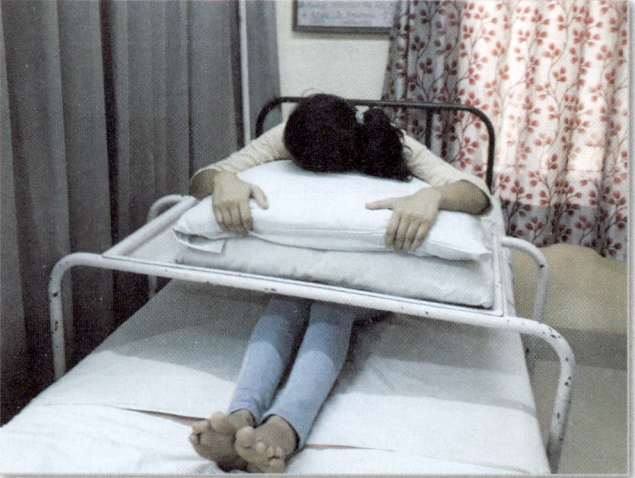

Fig. 6: Cardiac bed

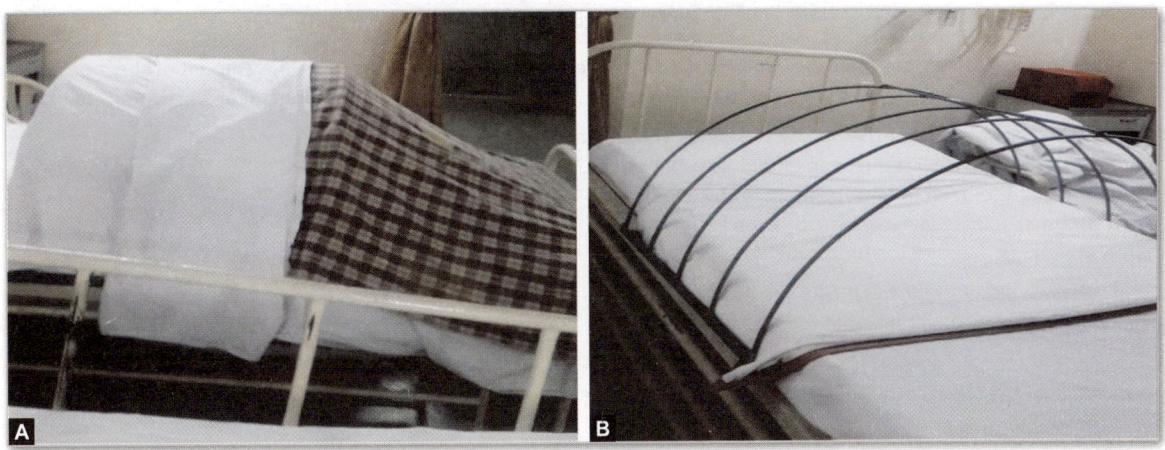

Figs 7A and B: Amputation/divided bed

Skill—Making an Open Bed (Unoccupied Bed)

It is a bed, when it is about to be occupied by either a new patient or an ambulatory patient. Most beds are made when they are unoccupied.

Many patients may be out of bed at that time to reduce the work for both the nurse and the patient.

Purposes

* To provide a comfortable bed for the patient.
* To make the bed, as neat and attractive as possible.

Supplies

Bottom sheet, top sheet, bed spread/blanket, rubber drawsheet (waterproof), drawsheet, pillow cases, linen bag or hamper.

Steps of Procedure

Review and carry out the standard steps as given in Appendix

Steps	Rationale
Assessment	
1. Check patient's ability to be out of bed; obtain help if necessary	Promotes safety for the patient
Planning	
2. Arrange the linens in the order in which they will be used	Saves time if linens are in correct order for use
3. Lower the side rail on your side of the bed. Raise bed to an appropriate working height for you	Provides easy access to materials. Prevents back strain and injury
Implementation	
4. Wash hands and put on clean gloves if there is a chance of contact with blood or body fluids while removing used linen	Prevents spread of microorganisms
5. Loosen all linen on your side of the bed. Go to other side, lower that rail, and loosen the linens from the head to the foot of the bed. Fold bedspread if not soiled, place over the back of patient's chair. Remove sheets and pillow cases. Place pillows on a clean surface. Roll linens together and put them into linen bag or hamper. Avoid shaking or fanning the linen	Permits linens to be removed. Bed spread and pillows are ready to be replaced. Placing soiled linen in linen bag prevents spread of microorganisms
6. Check the mattress; clean if soiled. Move mattress to the head of bed if needed	Mattress cleaned before making the bed. Mattresses tend to move to the foot of bed when the head of the bed is raised
7. Make the bed on one side at a time. Place all center folds in the linens at the center of the bed	Decreases the number of steps for the nurse

Contd...

Steps	Rationale
8. Place the bottom sheet on the mattress. Unfold the right side and tuck about 12 inches of the sheet smoothly over the top of the mattress	Puts the same amount of sheet on both sides of bed. Secures sheet snugly to head of bed
9. Miter the corner at the head of the bed by picking up the side edge of the sheet so that it forms a triangle with the head of bed with the side edge perpendicular to the bed. Using the palm of your hand, hold the sheet against the side of the mattress and tuck excess under mattress. Drop the sheet over your hand; then withdraw your hand and tuck the flap of the sheet under the mattress	Holds the corners in place
10. Position the draw sheet or lift sheet over the middle of the bed. Unfold and tuck both sheets in, on this side, from head to foot. If a lift sheet is used do not tuck it under mattress	Protects the bottom linens from soiling by placing the draw sheet from the patient's shoulders to below the hips.
11. Place top edge of the sheet at the top of the mattress, seam side up, and unfold it towards the foot of the bed	Avoids irritation from the seam
12. Position the blanket or spread 4 inches from the top of the mattress, and unfold it toward the foot	Allows sheet to be cuffed over top covers
13. Tuck the sheet, blankets, and spread under the bottom of the mattress as one unit. Miter the corner by lifting the top linens out from the mattress and up onto the bed about 18 inches from the bottom of the bed. A triangle should be formed. Tuck excess linens hanging below mattress level under it, bring down the upper portion of the linens, and smooth them into a neat diagonal line	Secures the linen under mattress. Top covers are not tucked down the sides of the mattress to allow the patient to get in and out of bed easily
14. Fan fold the top linen back towards the center of the bed while tucking in the bottom sheet and drawsheet	Allows you to see any wrinkles and remedy them. Holds sheet in place
15. Grasp the edges of the bottom sheet tightly in both hands with the knuckles on top. Pull tightly down over the side; tuck under the mattress working down the side from head to foot. Pull the sheet diagonally at the bottom corner of the mattress to remove wrinkles	Provides a smooth bottom sheet without wrinkles that may cause pressure areas
16. Grasp drawsheet if used. Pull tightly and tuck it in over the side of the mattress. If this is used as a lift sheet, do not tuck it under mattress	Saves time because a lift sheet is used often
17. Smooth top linens from the head to the foot of the bed. Fold excess sheet, blanket, and spread under the mattress of the foot of the bed. If a toe pleat is not needed, miter the corner of the top linens at one unit.	Provides patient with a wrinkle-free bed
18. Make the pleats. At the center of the top-linens, at the foot of the bed, make a 6 inch lengthwise pleat in the sheet before tucking the covers under the mattress	Allow room for the patient's feet to move and prevents formation of pressure ulcers from the weight of the linens on the toes
19. Move to the head of bed and fold back the top sheet, forming, a cuff 4–6 inches over the edge of the blanket and spread	Provides a smooth edge under patient's chin and prevents soiling of blanket and spread
20. Grasp the closed end of the pillow case, and with the other hand, gather one side of the open pillow case up over the hand at the closed end. Grasp the pillow with the covered hand while holding it away from your body. With the other hand on an open edge, pull the open edges down over the pillow. Do this until the pillow is completely covered. Adjust the pillow inside the case, keeping it from being contaminated by your uniform	Provides a method for placing a pillow smoothly in the case without contaminating it
21. Place the pillows at the head of the bed with the open ends away from the door	Provides a neater appearance
22. Place the bed in the lowest position, lock the brakes of the bed. Remove the soiled linen. Follow agency policy, or open the bed by folding the top back	Promotes safety in getting in and out of bed. Allows patient to enter bed easily
Evaluation	
23. Assess the patient's area. Is the bed neat, smooth, and wrinkle-free? Is everything within easy reach of patient?	Promotes safety
Documentation	
24. Document linen change if required by agency policy	Records the procedure

Closed Bed

It is an unoccupied bed made to receive the patient and is fully covered with bed spread to protect it from dust and dirt. On admission of the patient, the closed bed is converted into an open bed.

Purposes

- To keep the bed ready for occupancy
- To provide a neat and tidy appearance to the unit

Articles

Same as for open bed

Skill—Making an Occupied Bed

Linens are changed with the patient in bed if bed rest has been ordered.

Supplies

One bath blanket, rest same as unoccupied bed.

Purposes

- To provide a clean and comfortable bed for patient.
- To provide for the neat appearance of the ward.

Steps of Procedures

Review and carry out the standard steps as given in Appendix

Action/steps	Rationale
Assessment	
1. Check patient's orders to ensure patient is not allowed out of bed. Obtain help if necessary.	Promotes safety and assures medical plan to be followed
Planning	
2. Arrange the linens in the order in which they will be used.	Saves time and energy
3. Make sure the bed is locked and lower the side rail on your side. The other side rail should be raised. Raise the bed to an appropriate height.	Prevents back strain and injury
Implementation	
4. Wash hands and put on clean gloves if there is a chance to come in contact with blood or body fluids during procedure.	Prevents spread of microorganisms
5. Loosen the blanket and spread from the foot of the bed and remove each piece separately. If unsoiled, fold and place them over the back of patient's chair. Place any soiled linen in the hamper bag.	Saves time by readying linens to be replaced
Action	
6. Place a bath blanket over the patient and the top sheet, unfold it, and ask the patient to hold the top, or tuck under the patient's shoulders. Remove the top sheet from beneath the bath blanket, and place in linen hamper or bag.	Provides warmth and privacy
7. Move the patient into a side lying position at the far side of the bed, facing away from you. Assist the patient into proper alignment. Place a pillow under the head and at the patient's back to keep the patient in place, if needed.	Provides safety, allow near side of bed to be made
8. Loosen the bottom linens from the top and side of the bed; roll each piece of linen as close to the patient as possible. ▪ Put the bottom sheet on the bed with the center fold at the center of the mattress. Fanfold the sheet that is for the other side of the bed with the center fold at the center of the mattress ▪ Push the folded linen under the rolled, soiled bottom sheets that are being removed. Tuck the near side of the bottom sheet under the mattress and miter the corner. Tuck the sheet under the mattress from the head to the foot of the bed.	Allows soiled linens to be removed and clean linens to be placed when the patient rolls to the other side of the bed
Action	
9. Place the drawsheet on the bed, centering it on the mattress, so that it reaches from the patient's shoulders to below the hips. Fan fold the far side of the sheet, and push it under the rolled bottom sheets. Tuck the near side under the mattress. Raise the side rail.	Allows removal of a soiled drawsheet when the patient is turned

Contd...

Action/steps	Rationale
10. Go to the other side of the bed, lower the rail, and move the patient to the far side of the bed. If the patient can turn easily, ask the patient to roll to the opposite side. Adjust the patient's alignment, and reposition the bath blanket. Ask the patient to grab the raised side rail for support.	Allows removal of soiled linens and placement of clean linens. Raised rail provides safety
11. Loosen the bottom linens and roll them up. Place in the linen hamper bag.	Prevents spread of microorganisms
12. Pull the bottom sheet across the mattress, fold over the top of the mattress and smooth, tighten and tuck the excess sheet under the mattress, and miter the corner	Prevents wrinkles that may cause pressure ulcers
13. Pull the drawsheet from the center of the bed, to pull tightly. Place your knee against the mattress while pulling. Tighten, smooth and tuck sheets under the side of the mattress from head to foot	Protects the bottom sheet from soiling
14. Allow the patients to roll onto back. Place the top sheet over the patient with the top edge folded down a few inches beneath the chin. Have the patients hold the top sheet and remove the bath blanket. Position the blanket if used and spread in the same manner. Smooth the top linens and tuck the excess at the foot under the bottom of the mattress. Miter the corner on the near side, then far side, fold the top edge of the sheet over the blanket, and spread to form a cuff	Keeps the patient warm and protects privacy while the top linens are placed
15. Make a toe pleat in to top sheet and blanket as given in previous skill	Provides extra room for the feet
16. Remove the used pillow case and place it in the linen hamper or bag. Apply the clean pillow case and place beneath the patient's head with the open ends away from the door.	Provides a neat appearance
17. Lower the bed, replace call light and restore the unit. Remove the linen hamper and place at appropriate area	Provides safety for the patient and prevents spread of microorganisms
Evaluation	
18. Assess the patient's area. Are the linens neat, smooth and wrinkle free? Is the unit restored?	Promotes safety because the patient does not have to reach for items
Documentation	
19. Document linen change on the notes, depending on the agency's policy	Documents the completion of the procedure

Admission Bed

This is the bed which is prepared to receive a newly admitted patient.

Steps of Admission Bed

A long mackintosh and a bath blanket are put over the open bed, until a thorough bath is given to patient at the time of admission. After the bath, the mackintosh and bath blankets are removed.

Purposes

- To welcome the patient
- To provide immediate care, safety and comfort,
- To protect the bed linen while giving bath on admission

Articles

A long mackintosh and a bath blanket and articles for bed bath.

Postoperative Bed

It is a bed prepared for a patient who is recovering from the effects of anesthesia following surgery.

Purposes

- To receive the patient after operation
- To provide warmth and comfort
- To prevent shock
- To prevent injury
- To prevent soiling of bed
- To meet any emergency

Articles

Same as open bed with additional articles like.
- Small mackintosh and towel to protect head end of bed
- Temperature tray
- Blood pressure (BP) apparatus to record vital signs
- Intravenous (IV) stand and IV tray: To administer IV fluid to patient

- Hot water bottles 2–3: To keep bed warm
- Oxygen cylinder with tubing and catheter: to meet any emergency
- Suction apparatus: To remove secretions
- **Bed block:** To raise foot end
- **A tray containing:**
  - **Gauze pieces:** To clean mouth off secretion.
  - **Artery forceps:** To prevent falling back of tongue.
  - **Tongue depressor:** To keep the air passage clear.
  - **Airway:** To keep airway open.
  - **Kidney tray and paper bag:** To discard the waste.

Procedure

- Foundation of the bed is the same as that of on open bed
- An extra mackintosh and a towel is placed at head end
- The foot end of the top linen is left untucked and folded back
- Fan fold the top linen lengthwise covering two-thirds of the bed on the right side
- Place the hot water bottles under the top linen
- Place the pillow upright of the head end to protect the patient from injury by hitting against the bars

Cardiac Bed

It is a bed prepared for patients with cardiac diseases.

Purpose

To prepare the bed for the cardiac patient to relieve dyspnea.

Articles

Same as open bed with additional articles back rest/Fowler's bed—to support the patient while sitting
- **Cardiac table:** To provide support and comfort.
- **Extra pillows:** To provide support and comfort.
- **Air cushion:** To relieve pressure from sacral area.
- **Knee Pillow:** To provide support and comfort.
- **Foot rest:** To prevent slipping down.

Procedure

- Make the bed as in the open bed
- Place the back rest and arrange pillows
- Place the air cushion and knee pillow
- Adjust the cardiac table and keep the pillows as needed for the patient to lean on it
- Support the feet on foot rest
- Make the patient comfortable

Amputation/Divided/Cradle Bed

It is a bed in which top linen is divided into two parts to visualize the amputated part of the lower limbs without disturbing the patient.

Purposes

- To watch the stump for hemorrhage and apply tourniquet instantly.
- To keep the weight of bed clothes off the patient.
- To keep the stump in position.

Articles

Same as any open bed with additional articles extra set of top linen—to make a divided bed

- **Bed cradle:** To take weight of top clothes off the patient.
- **Two sand bags:** To keep stump in position.
- **Tourniquet and dressing tray:** To control hemorrhage.
- **Pillow with water proof cover:** To elevate the stump and protect pillow.
- **Hot water bottles:** To keep the bed warm.

Procedure

The foundation and head end of bed is made as in open bed.

- The foot end side of top linen is folded back toward the head end at the level of part/stump to be observed.
- Spread the second set of top linen starting from the level of the stump.
- The second set of top linen should overlap the first by 8–12″.
- Receive the patient and elevate the stump on a small pillow and place the sand bags on either side to support the stump.
- Place the bed cradle in position.
- Cover the patient.

Fracture Bed

It is a bed which is prepared for patients with fracture, bone diseases and deformity.

Purposes

- To prevent undue sagging of mattress.
- To immobilize the fractured part.
- To restrict sudden jerky movements.
- To keep the traction in position.

Articles

Same as an open bed with additional articles. Fracture board to provide firm support to the patient.

Procedure

Arrange the fracture board on the cot. The bed is made as an open bed.

Therapeutic Beds: Renal/Rheumatism Bed

It is a bed made for patients suffering from rheumatism or renal diseases.

Purposes

- To carry the weight of the bed clothes off the painful joints.
- To keep the patient warm.
- To induce sweating.

Articles

Same as in open bed with additional articles:

- **Narrow mackintosh and drawsheet:** To protect the bed linen.
- **Two woolen blankets or bath blankets:** To keep under and over the patient to induce sweating.
- **Bed cradle:** To keep the weight of linen off the patient.
- **Sand bags:** To immobilize the painful joint.
- **Hot water bottles if required:** To provide warmth

Note: In a renal bed, the cradle and sand bags are not required.

Procedure

Bed is made as in open bed. Place a narrow mackintosh and a draw sheet under the patient's buttocks. Place the extra blankets, one over and one under the patient, keeping in mind the principles of body mechanics.

BIBLIOGRAPHY

1. Trained Nurses Association of India. Fundamentals of Nursing-A Procedure Manual, 1st edition, New Delhi; 2005. p 147-9.

2. Kozier Barbara B, Du Gas Beverly W. Fundamentals of Nursing Patient Care. WB Saunders Company, Philadelphia; 1967. p. 83-9.

3. Alexander MF, Fawcett JN, Phyllis J. Runciman JP. Nursing Practice-Hospital and Home, 1st edition, Longman Group UK Limited; London; 1994. p. 747-50.

4. Leahy JM, Patricia EK. Foundation of Nursing Practice, 1st edition, WB Saunders Company; Philadelphia;1998. p. 670-6.

5. Craven RF, Hirnel OJ, Henshaw OM. Fundamentals of Nursing Human Health and Function. Lippincott Williams and Wilkins; Philadelphia; 2000. p. 762-5.

6. Price AL. The Art, Science and Spirit of Nursing, 3rd edition, WB Saunders Company. Philadelphia; 1968. p. 84-94.

7. Thresyamma CP. Fundamentals of Nursing, 1st edition, Jaypee Brother Publication; New Delhi; 2002. p. 154-8.

Hygiene

INTRODUCTION

Hygiene is the practice of cleanliness that is conducive to the preservation of health. Assisting the patient with hygiene and personal care activities is an essential nursing function. Proper care of the skin, hair, teeth and nails promotes good health by protecting the body from infection and disease. In turn, this promotes a sense of well-being for your patient.

FACTORS AFFECTING HYGIENIC PRACTICES

Sociocultural Background

A person's socioeconomic class and financial resources are one of the most basic factors. In some cultures, people do not use deodorant products or bathe daily. Other cultures consider the use of deodorant products and daily bath essential. The economic status of the patient may affect the patient's hygiene because the money or supplies may or may not be available.

Spiritual Practices

Spiritual practices include religious beliefs like purification as a prelude to prayer or eating. Tradition of ritual baths after childbirth and menstruation are considered essential in many cultures.

Developmental Level

Children learn hygiene practices while growing up. Family practices often dictate hygienic habits, such as morning or evening baths; the frequency of shampooing, tooth brushing, and clothing changes and so on. As adolescents become more concerned about their personal appearance, they may adapt new hygiene measures such as taking shower more frequently and wearing deodorant. Bathing frequency commonly decreases as a person ages, possibly due to limitations in mobility and the natural tendency toward dry skin with age.

Health State

Disease, surgery, or injury may reduce a person's ability to perform hygiene measures. Weakness, dizziness and fear of falling may prevent an individual from entering a tub or shower or from bending to wash the lower extremities. Illness may also create a demand for new or modified hygienic measures.

Personal Preferences

People have different preferences regarding hygiene practices such as taking a shower versus tub bath, using bar soap versus liquid soap, having bath in the morning or taking bath to relax before going to bed. A person's self-concept and sexuality also influences personal hygiene practices. Older adults, in an effort to promote a positive self-image, may use skin care products to prevent wrinkles and diminish signs of aging.

Self-care Abilities

Assess ability for self-care, ability to perceive, think and remember. Assess for factors, such as poor vision, decreased sense of touch and limitations in range of motion that interfere with self-care. Assess for coordination, muscle strength, and balance. A patient with these limitations may need additional help with hygiene.

ORAL CARE/ORAL HYGIENE

Oral care is care of mouth and teeth of a patient.

Purpose

The purpose of oral care is:
- To create a sense of well-being.
- To enable the patient to have a clean mouth as an aid to good digestion and better general health.
- To teach the patient to develop good habits of oral hygiene.

Importance of Oral Hygiene

- Mouth is an ideal place for multiplication of germs as there is warmth, moisture and food. Therefore, to prevent infection, it should be kept clean.

- A clean mouth gives a good appearance.
- It prevents bad odor.
- It improves appetite and digestion.
- Gives comfort to the patient.
- Prevents sores and ulceration. Brown crusts are usually seen on the lips and teeth of patients having fever.
- Prevents many diseases because bacteria can enter the mouth and lungs through the mouth.

Complications due to Neglected Oral Care

- Bad odor or halitosis: Foul breath.
- Cracked lips.
- Indigestion along with loss of appetite.
- Discomfort: Patient feels sick.

Common Mouth Infections

- **Glossitis:** Inflammation of the tongue.
- **Stomatitis:** Inflammation of the mouth, mucous membrane and gums.
- **Pyorrhea or periodontitis:** Inflammation of the deeper tissues surrounding the roots of teeth.
- **Gingivitis:** Inflammation of gums.
- **Dental caries:** A substance in saliva converts carbohydrate to lactic acid. The acid dissolves tooth enamel, leading to dental caries.
- **Trench mouth or Vincent's infection:** Gingivitis that progresses to a necrotic state.
- **Plaque:** Invisible soft film that adheres to the enamel surface of the teeth.
- **Tartar:** Visible hard deposits of plaque and dead bacteria formed at the gum lines.
- **Halitosis:** A strong mouth odor.

Care of Mouth during Illness

- Mouth care should be given every four hours or more often.
- Mouth should be rinsed after every drink or feeding.

Mouth Care for the Conscious Patient

- **Equipment:** A toothbrush, glass, toothpaste/powder, water, towel
Note: Encourage patients to go to bathroom to brush their teeth whenever possible. For patients who can take care of themselves, assemble all articles within reach.

Assisting with Mouth Care

- Raise the head of the bed from 45° to 90°.
- Wear gloves when providing or assisting with mouth care.

- If patient is unable to sit up, turn the patient to the side facing you.
- Place a towel under chin.
- Moisten the tooth brush with water or mouth wash and spread toothpaste.
- Brush from the gumline to the edge of teeth.
- All surfaces of each tooth should be brushed.
- Have the patient rinse the mouth and spit the solution onto the kidney tray.
- Repeat as desired.
- Provide the patient with a cloth/towel or tissue to wipe the mouth.

Assisting the Patient to Floss the Teeth

- Obtain 12–15 inches of floss.

- Loosely wrap the floss around a finger on each hand and work the floss between each tooth
- Slide the floss gently down to the gum line, pulling the floss back and forth
- Rinse and wipe the mouth again
- Report any excessive bleeding of the gums after flossing.

Mouth Care for the Unconscious Patient

An unconscious patient should be provided full mouth care at least once every 8 hours. If the patient is mouth breathing, care should be done every 4 hours. Mouth breathing causes the tongue to dry and become crusty. The dry secretions need to be removed because they cause halitosis and may obstruct air flow. Mouth swabbing is done every 2 hours or as needed to maintain the integrity of the oral cavity.

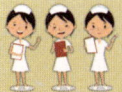 **SKILL: ADMINISTERING ORAL CARE TO UNCONSCIOUS PATIENT**

Equipment

The equipment used for oral care are shown in Figure. 1.

- Artery forceps
- Tongue blade
- Kidney basin
- Feeding cup
- Small bowl
- Towel
- Mouth suction device
- A syringe
- Small rubber sheet
- Swab sticks
- Boroglycerine and gauze pieces
- A glass of water
- Solution for mouthwash: Any of these solutions:
  - Hydrogen peroxide 1:20 mL: Oxidizing agent.
  - Condy's solution 1:5000: Oxidizing agent
  - Soda bicarbonate: Dissolve the mucus

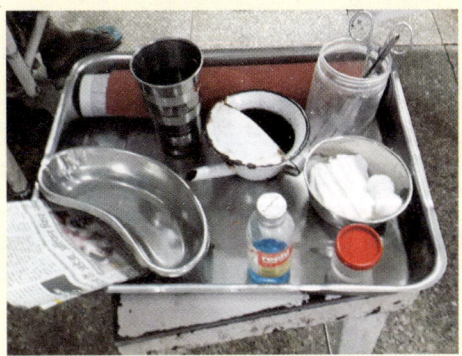

Fig. 1: Mouth care tray

Steps of Procedure

Review and carry out the standard steps as given in Appendix

Action/steps	Rationale
Assessment	
1. Assess gag reflex	Identifies risk of aspiration
Planning	
2. Gather equipment at bedside	Provides easy access to equipment
3. Explain the procedure to the patient	Provides stimulation as unconscious patients may be able to hear
4. Close door or pull curtains	Provides privacy

Contd...

Action/steps	Rationale
Implementation	
5. Raise bed level to comfortable working height. Turn patient laterally on side of bed near to you and lower side rail	Promotes good body mechanics and reduces risk or aspiration
6. Turn on the suction and place the suction device near you. Put a towel under the patient's head and emesis basin beneath patient's mouth and chin	Provides immediate use of suction, towel and emesis basin, keeps linen clean
7. Put on gloves and wrap artery forceps with gauze so that tips are protected	Prevents injury
8. Dip gauze into solution that has been poured into a small bowl	Hydrogen peroxide and water are good cleansing agents
9. Gently sponge the mouth and teeth, paying special attention to tongue (Fig. 2)	Removes crusts and debris

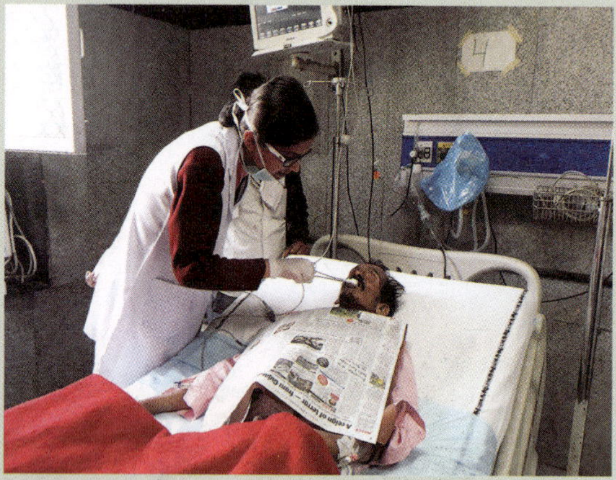

Fig. 2: Performing oral care in an unconscious patient

Action/steps	Rationale
10. Change gauze in the forceps as often as necessary. Discard used one into kidney basin, taking it off the forceps	
11. Rinse mouth by gently squirting water with syringe and use of suction	Reduces risk of aspiration
12. Apply boro glycerine or vaseline on lips with a swab stick	Prevents drying of lips and cracking
13. Explain the patient that you have finished the procedure	Provides stimulation because unconscious patients may be able to hear
14. Remove gloves and dispose them properly. Reposition patient, raise side rails and lower bed	Prevents spread of microorganisms and promotes safety and comfort
15. Clean supplies and tidy unit and leave the patient comfortable	Helps in keeping the equipment ready for next use
Evaluation	
16. Put on gloves and inspect mouth to check effectiveness of procedure	Determines if other actions are needed
Documentation	
17. Note the time when special mouth care was given and the solution used. Mention any cracks, ulcerations or other breaks in the mucous membranes	Notes any abnormalities

Care of Dentures

Patients with dentures who are confined to bed, comatose, weak, or have trouble with hand and finger dexterity may need assistance to provide care for their dentures. Dentures should be cleaned to prevent irritation to the gums and infection. When not in mouth, dentures should be kept in a labeled denture container containing water or normal saline.

- If the patient prefers to clean his own dentures, offer all needed articles.
- Provide privacy.
- If patient does not want to keep them in his mouth, cleanse them thoroughly, place them in a clean gauze and mark the patient's name on adhesive and keep in a safe place or keep in a labeled denture container.
- Encourage patients to use dentures whenever possible.
- Remove dentures before operation.
- Be sure dentures are replaced at once after cleaning.

CARE OF SKIN-BATHING

The type of cleansing bath a nurse provides depends on the patient's physical capabilities and the degree of hygiene required. The nurse is responsible for assessing what type of bath is most appropriate for the patient's need.

Types of Cleansing Baths

- **Complete bed-bath:** This is administered to patients who are totally dependent. The nurse gives the bath with the patient in bed and the entire body is cleaned.
- **Partial bed-bath:** Consists of bathing only those body parts that would cause discomfort if left unbathed such as hands, face, axillae and perineal care. Dependent patients in need of partial hygiene or bed-ridden patients who are unable to reach all body parts receive partial bed bath.
- **Tub bath:** The patient is immersed in a tub of water. The tub bath allows thorough washing and rinsing than a bed-bath. The patient may still require the nurse's assistance.
- **Shower:** Here, the patient sits or stands under a continuous stream of water. The shower provides thorough cleansing than a bed bath.

- **Therapeutic baths:** Therapeutic means having healing or medicinal qualities. A whirlpool bath is done in a bath tub or special whirlpool tub that has a device that agitates the water. The heat of the water and agitation gently massage the skin. Whirlpools are used to cleanse, stimulate peripheral circulation and provide comfort. Starch or oatmeal baths are used for patients with dermatitis. The skin is patted dry after the bath so the nerve endings are not stimulated by rubbing. Sitz baths are used to apply moist heat and clean the perineal or anal area. The bath promotes healing and relieves pain and discomfort. It is commonly used after delivery and vaginal or rectal surgery.

Purposes for Bathing

- To cleanse the skin
- To promote comfort
- To stimulate circulation to all areas of body
- To remove waste products secreted through the skin
- To promote rest and sleep and aid in quick recovery
- To observe the condition of the patient's skin and any abnormalities
- To promote a sense of well-being
- To prevent bed sores

Key Points for Bathing a Patient

- **Maintain safety:** Safety must be maintained. Water should be warm but should not burn the patient (105°F or 40.5°C or according to tolerance). Bed rails must be up when away from that side of the bed. Place the bed in the lowest position if you leave the bed-side.
- **Provide privacy:** Fully draw curtains around the bed to maintain privacy. Appropriately drape the patient, only the part of the body being bathed should be exposed at any one time.
- **Prevent chills:** Draping prevents chills and promotes warmth and comfort. Closing the patient's door and windows provides warmth by decreasing drafts of air.
- **Encourage independence:** Encourage the patient to be independent, but offer assistance as needed. Depending on the patient's activity and ability level, you may plan to give either partial or complete bath.

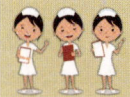

SKILL: PROVIDING A TUB BATH OR SHOWER

If a patient can safely bathe on his own, the area is prepared and then the patient is made ready for the bath or shower. Patients must be checked frequently while in the tub or shower.

Action/steps	Rationale
1. Schedule use of tub or shower room. Clean according to institution's policy. Place towel on floor outside of tub/shower and non-skid mat in tub/shower	Assures area is available when patient is ready. Prevents spread of microorganisms Towel provides a dry warm area and mat decreases chance of falls
2. Gather supplies and assist patient to reach the area. Completely drape patient	Promotes safety, decreases chance of chills and provides privacy
3. Place "occupied" sign on door and demonstrate use of call bell system	Maintains privacy and promotes safety
4. Fill tub half way with warm water; check the temperature. If using the shower, turn water on and adjust as needed. A hand-held sprayer controls water flow and prevents you from becoming soaked. Place toiletry items within patient's reach. Assist patient as and when needed	Prevents burns and decreases chance of falls. Promotes hygiene through helping patient with hard to reach areas
5. Instruct patient not to stay in the tub or shower longer than 20 minutes. Check on the patient every 5 minutes. Knock on the door before entering. Remain within calling distance if the patient has a history of syncope, dizziness or taking shower for the first time.	Decreases chance of light headedness or dizziness from vasodilatation from the warm water. Provides privacy and promotes safety.
6. Assist patient out of tub/shower. Encourage the use of safety bars during transfer. Assist with drying and dressing. Transport back to room	Promotes safety and maintains warmth by preventing chills
7. Clean tub/shower as per instructions or institution's policy	Prevents transfer of microorganisms
8. Document type of bath taken, tolerance of procedure, condition of skin and amount of assistance needed by patient	Promotes continuity of care

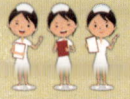

SKILL: ADMINISTERING A BED BATH AND PERINEAL CARE

A complete bed bath is given when the patient is dependent and unable to provide self-hygiene care.

Equipment

- Basin of warm water, soap, towels and washclothes, bath blanket, clean linen for bed, clean gown/clothes, body lotion, toilet articles, bag for soiled linen, bedpan, urinal, toilet paper.
- For perineal care–underpad, gauze pads or wash clothes water and ordered solution

Steps of Procedure

Review and carry out steps as given in Appendix

Action/steps	Rationale
Assessment	
1. Assess patients preferences including cultural factors	Demonstrates respect for patient's preference and encourages participation in care
Planning	
2. Gather supplies	Easy access to equipment needed for hygiene/bathing
3. Explain the procedure to the patient	Decreases the fear of unknown and prepares patient

Contd...

Action/steps	Rationale
4. Prepare environment for bathing–close doors, windows, adjust room temperature, if necessary, pull curtains around bed and place a sign 'Bath in progress' on door	Promotes comfort by warming room and decreasing chance of drafts. Provides privacy
5. Offer bedpan or urinal	Provides comfort and decreases interruption during bath

Implementation

Action/steps	Rationale
6. Wash your hands. Wear gloves if you or patient has broken skin. Gloves must be worn while cleansing perineal area	Reduces transfer of microorganisms
7. Raise level of bed to a comfortable working height. Lower rails on side closest to you and position patient in a comfortable position close to you	Promotes proper body alignment because work is at the center of gravity. Provides comfort for patient
8. If a bath blanket is available, fanfold the blanket horizontally and place it across patient's chest. Ask the patient to hold the top edge of the bath blanket. Pull the blanket and the covers to the foot of the bed from underneath the bath blanket. Use the top sheet if a bath blanket is not available for a drape.	Drapes patient, protecting privacy
9. Remove patient's gown, being careful to keep patient draped. If the patient has an intravenous line in place, remove the gown by gently pulling the gown off the patient's arm over the IV line without pulling on the line. Lift the IV bag and tubing and pass through the sleeve from the outside toward the inside of the gown to free the gown	Prepares patient for bathing. Careful removal of gown protects the IV site
10. Raise the side rail while preparing the bath water. Water should be warm and checked with either bath thermometer or inside of your wrist. Do not leave the soap in the water. Change water when it cools or becomes soiled	Provides safety. Warm water is soothing and maintaining warm clean water is comforting
11. Lower rail and remove the pillow under the patient's head or place a towel over the pillow. Make a bath mitt by grasping the washcloth at an edge and fold it one-third over the palm of your hand. Bring the opposite edge across the palm of your hand and hold it with your thumb. Bring the extreme end of the cloth up to your palm and tuck that edge under upper edge	Provides better control of the wash cloth, loose ends do not drag across patient
12. Fold drape to expose only the area being cleaned. Spread a towel across the patient's chest	Protects patient's privacy and prevents chills
13. Wash the patient's face and neck (soap optional). Moisten the bath mitt with water and wash one eye from the nose to the outer edge near the ear; use a separate part of the mitt to wash the other eye. Do not use soap near eyes. Dry well. Rinse cloth and wash forehead from the center to each side; wash the rest of face using a circular motion around the mouth. Rinse and dry the face well. Wash, rinse, and dry each ear and the neck. Patient may wash face himself if he/she is able to.	Prevents moving bacteria from one eye to the other by using different parts of the cloth. Rinsing will prevent soap from drying the skin.
14. Place a towel under the forearm, make a bath mitt, use soap, and wash the entire arm with long, sweeping strokes from distal to proximal (toward the axilla). Give special care to the axilla with extra soaping. Rinse and pat dry well. Wash the hands and fingers, rinse and dry. Move the towel, wash and dry the near arm and hand in the same manner	Promotes circulation by washing distal to proximal. Towel protects the mattress from getting wet and is available for drying. Bacteria collects in the sweat gland areas, and extra cleansing is needed to remove secretions and decrease body odor
15. Keep the towel in place over the patient's chest and pull the drape down to the waistline. Make a bath mitt and wash under the towel over the entire chest; wash breasts with a circular movement. Wash skin folds under the female patient's breasts by lifting each breast. Rinse and dry well, paying special attention to skin fold areas. Fold the drape to the top of the pubic bone and wash the lower abdomen, rinse and dry well	Provides privacy and protects the patient from chills
16. Expose the leg that is away from you, and tuck the bath blanket around the patient to prevent chilling. Flex the leg and place a towel length-wise on the bed. Wash from the foot to the knee with long sweeping strokes and then from the knee to the hip in the same manner. Rinse and dry the leg well. Place the bath basin on the towel and lift the foot, placing your hand under the heel, and place it into the water. Wash the foot and dry it. Dry each toe separately, and place the leg and foot under the drape. Wash the near leg in the same manner.	Keeps the patient warm. Stroking from distal to proximal encourages venous return. Placing the foot into warm water is soothing and comforting to the patient

Contd...

Action/steps	Rationale
17. Change the bath water after washing the legs and feet	Prevents using water that has been used on the feet or other parts of the body
18. Turn the patient to the side, place a towel lengthwise along the back, and wash the back with long, sweeping motions. Rinse and dry well. Then wash the folds of the buttocks and anus well	Protects mattress from moisture. Offer back rub at this time
19. Change water and washcloth. Provide privacy to the patient to wash the genital area. If patient is unable to do so, put on gloves, place on underpad beneath the perineum to protect the mattress and wash the area thoroughly, rinse well, and pat dry carefully. For the female patient, wash from the front to the back. For the uncircumcised male patient, retract the foreskin and clean the head of penis, rinse, and replace the foreskin. Lift the scrotum and clean the area well. If the catheter is in place, carefully wash around it with soap and water, and rinse the area. Dry the penis and scrotum. Remove the underpad.	Promotes privacy because many patients wish to wash their own perineum. Cleans those areas patient cannot manage. Washing around a catheter removes body secretions
For specially ordered female perineal care	
20. Place the patient in the dorsal recumbent position in bed. Drape with a bath blanket diagonally. Take the point of the bath blanket by the patient's feet and fold it up to the pubic area. Place the lower sides of the bath blanket over the patient's knees and wrap the corners around each foot	Provides privacy and prevents chills
21. With gloves in place, remove any peripad or dressings and observe characteristics of the drainage. Discard soiled items in a waste receptacle	Standard precautions must be used when handling items soiled with body discharges
22. Slip underpad under the patient's hips and position on the bedpan. Raise the head of bed slightly or use pillows to support patient's head	Prevents soiling the linens and mattress. Prevents back stress by supporting the head and shoulders.
23. Carefully pour warm water or the prescribed solution over the perineal area to rinse off urine, feces or vaginal discharge	Cleanses outer perineum
24. Use nondominant hand to separate the labia majora, and with downward strokes from the pubic area to rectum, cleanse the skinfolds with either cotton balls, gauze pads, or a washcloth. Use only one downward stroke with each gauze pad, cotton ball, or portion of the washcloth. Rinse and pat area dry with clean towel or fresh gauze pads. Replace peripad or redress as needed. Remove the underpad	Prevents carrying bacteria from the dirty rectal area up to vaginal and urinary meatus. Provides collection of secretions
Completing care	
25. Put a clean gown on the patient. If the patient has an IV in place, lift the IV bag and line and put it through the sleeve of the gown from the inside of the gown to the outside, just as the arm goes through the sleeve. Then, carefully place the patient's arm through the sleeve of the gown. If a patient has a weak or paralyzed side, dress this extremity first	Maintains IV site and prevents the IV cannula and tubing from coming apart. Dressing is more comfortable and easier for the patient and you
26. Complete personal care by combing the patient's hair, caring for finger nails and toe nails, and permitting the male patient to either shave himself or perform the shaving	Increases patient's sense of well-being and self esteem
27. Lower the bed, raise the rail, and restore the unit. Empty, rinse, and wipe out the basin before returning to storage	Makes patient comfortable and safe. Prepares basin for next use
28. Make an occupied bed	The patient who needs a bed-bath may not be able to get out of bed
Evaluation	
29. Observe the newly bathed patient. Is the patient comfortable? Did the bath tire the patient? Are there any modifications you would make in providing future hygiene care for this patient?	Determines if any changes are needed
Documentation	
30. Document the type of bath given; the patient's tolerance of the procedure, any teaching done, and any abnormalities found during the bath, e.g., reddened area on pressure points, rashes, etc.	Documents effectiveness of nursing care and notes any teaching provided

NAIL CARE

Most of the patients can take care of their nails themselves but those who are unconscious, blind, confused or in cast or traction need to be attended for nail care. Nail care includes regular trimming. Cleaning under the nails, and cuticle care, and is usually done with the bath. Soak the nails in warm soapy water for 5–10 minutes. Push cuticles back gently and use nail clippers to cut the toe nails straight across to prevent them from growing into the skin along the sides.

Observe the color of the nail beds to monitor circulation to the extremities. Nail polish needs to be removed to allow monitoring.

EYE CARE

Assess eyes of patients for drainage, crusting or redness. If crusting is noted, soak the eye with a warm, damp washcloth for 2–3 minutes to soften the crust and ease its removal. Unconscious patients may need more frequent eye care.

EAR CARE

Hearing acuity may be affected if cerumen or foreign material collects in the external ear canal. Remove these materials by gently washing the external ear canal with a warm washcloth. If wax is dried or excessive, there is a need to irrigate the ear after notifying the physician.

PRESSURE ULCERS

Pressure ulcers, also known as decubitus ulcers or bedsores, occur from pressure on the skin. The pressure causes a local area of tissue necrosis (local death of tissue from disease or injury). Most often the area of pressure occurs between a bony prominence and an external surface. Besides pressure, the other main factor in the development of pressure ulcers is a **shearing force**. Shearing is an applied force that causes a downward and forward pressure on the tissues beneath the skin. Examples of shearing force is when a patient slides down in a chair or if bed clothes are pulled from beneath the patient.

The interference with circulation causes the skin to **blanch** (turn white or on darker skin become pale). If the pressure is relieved at this point, the skin will be red or of darker color because of vasodilatation. This process is called **reactive hyperemia** as the blood rushes to where there was a decrease in circulation.

Risk factors for pressure ulcers are given in Table 1.

If the patient is confined to bed or chair, the same areas of the body sustain pressure. This happens if a patient cannot independently change position such as a patient who is paralyzed, unconscious, or has had an orthopedic procedure.

TABLE 1: Risk factors for pressure ulcers

Major factors
◆ Bed or chair confinement
◆ Inability to move
◆ Loss of bowel and bladder control
◆ Poor nutrition
◆ Lowered mental awareness

Contributing factors
◆ Dehydration
◆ Obesity
◆ Excessive diaphoresis
◆ Extreme age due to fragile skin
◆ Edema

Incontinence (loss of bowel and bladder control) puts the patient at risk for ulcer development. Skin that is frequently wet leads to **maceration** (the softening of tissue that increases the chance of trauma or infection). Diaphoresis (perspiration), or a patient who is not dried properly after a bath, also places him/her at risk due to moisture.

A balanced diet is necessary to prevent ulcer development. Without proper nourishment, the body's cells, capillaries, and tissues are easily damaged.

Lowered mental awareness may predispose a patient to pressure ulcers. Patients with impaired cognition may not realize they have been in the same position for a prolonged period. Lowered mental awareness may be caused by medication, anesthesia, or health problems.

Assessment for Pressure Ulcers

Patients at Risk

- Patients with paralysis
- Patients with reduced level of awareness, e.g., unconscious or heavily sedated patients
- Patients who are malnourished and whose diet is insufficient in protein and vitamin C
- Those who are over 85 years of age
- Those who are confined to the bed and wheel chair

Assessing Patients with Pressure Sores

Perform a skin assessment for pressure ulcer risk upon admission. A commonly used tool is the Braden scale for predicting pressure sore risk (Table 2). The cut–off score for onset of pressure ulcer risk with the Braden Scale in the general adult population is 18.

This can be done while you are bathing your patient. Pay attention to the skin over bony prominences.

Check the areas that had pressure when turning and repositioning your patient. If the patient has been in supine position for an hour and is now turned to a right side-lying position (Figs 3A to D), you may notice a 1 inch diameter area of redness on the sacrum. If there has been no damage, then you may expect the redness to subside in 30–45 minutes. If the redness persists, then the pressure will damage the skin and the underlying tissues because they have not received an adequate supply of oxygen, blood, and nutrients. If unrelieved, the damage eventually leads to tissue necrosis and a pressure ulcer.

TABLE 2: Braden scale for predicting pressure sore risk

Patient's Name: _____

Evaluator's Name: _____

Date of Assessment: _____

SENSORY PERCEPTION Ability to respond meaningfully to pressure-related discomfort	1. **Completely Limited:** Unresponsive (does not moan, flinch, or grasp) to painful stimuli, due to diminished level of consciousness or sedation. OR limited ability to feel pain over most of the body surface.	2. **Very Limited:** Responds only to painful stimuli. Cannot communicate discomfort except by moaning or restlessness, OR has a sensory impairment which limits the ability to feel pain or discomfort over half of the body.	3. **Slightly Limited:** Responds to verbal commands but cannot always communicate discomfort or need to be turned. OR has some sensory impairment which limits ability to feel pain or discomfort in 1 or 2 extremities.	4. **No Impairment:** Responds to verbal commands. Has no sensory deficit which would limit ability to feel or voice pain or discomfort.
MOISTURE Degree to which skin is exposed to moisture	1. **Constantly Moist:** Skin is kept moist almost constantly by perspiration, urine, etc. Dampness is detected every time patient is moved or turned.	2. **Moist:** Skin is often but not always moist. Linen must be changed at least once a shift.	3. **Occasionally Moist:** Skin is occasionally moist, requiring an extra linen change approximately once a day.	4. **Rarely Moist:** Skin is usually dry; linen requires changing only at routine intervals.
ACTIVITY Degree of physical activity	1. **Bedfast:** Confined to bed.	2. **Chairfast:** Ability to walk severely limited or nonexistent. Cannot bear own weight and/or must be assisted into chair or wheelchair.	3. **Walks Occasionally:** Walks occasionally during day but for very short distances, with or without assistance. Spends majority of each shift in bed or chair	4. **Walks Frequently:** Walks outside the room at least twice a day and inside room at least once every 2 hours during waking hours.
MOBILITY Ability to change and control body position	1. **Completely Immobile:** Does not make even slight changes in body or extremity position without assistance	2. **Very Limited:** Makes occasional slight changes in body or extremity position but unable to make frequent or significant changes independently.	3. **Slightly Limited:** Makes frequent though slight changes in body or extremity position independently.	4. **No Limitations:** Makes major and frequent changes in position without assistance.
NUTRITION Usual food intake pattern	1. **Very Poor:** Never eats a complete meal. Rarely eats more than one-third of any food offered. Eats 2 servings or less of protein (meat or dairy products) per day. Takes fluids poorly. Does not take a liquid/dietary supplement, OR Is nil per os and/or maintained on clear liquids or IVs for more than 5 days.	2. **Probably Inadequate:** Rarely eats a complete meal and generally eats only about half of any food offered. Protein intake includes only 3 servings of meat or dairy products per day. Occasionally will take a dietary supplement, OR Receives less than optimum amount of liquid diet or tube feeding.	3. **Adequate:** Eats over half of most meals. Eats a total of 4 servings of protein (meat, dairy products) each day. Occasionally will refuse a meal, but will usually take a supplement if offered, OR is on a tube feeding or total parenteral nutrition regimen, which probably meets most of nutritional needs.	4. **Excellent:** Eats most of every meal. Never refuses a meal. Usually eats a total of 4 or more servings of meat and dairy products. Occasionally eats between meals. Does not require supplementation.

Contd...

FRICTION AND SHEAR	1. **Problem:** Requires moderate to maximum assistance in moving. Complete lifting without sliding against sheets is impossible. Frequently slides down in bed or chair, requiring frequent repositioning with maximum assistance. Spasticity, contractures, or agitation leads to almost constant friction.	2. **Potential Problem:** Moves feebly or requires minimum assistance. During a move, skin probably slides to some extent against sheets, chair, restraints or other devices. Maintains relatively good position in chair or bed most of the time but occasionally slides down.	3. **No Apparent Problem:** Moves in bed and in chair independently and has sufficient muscle strength to lift up completely during move. Maintains good position in bed or chair at all times	

Total Score: 23   **Score 3 or 4 = Moderate or low impairment**
Risk predicting score: 16 or less
Risk level
19–23 Not at risk
15–18 Low risk
13–14 Moderate risk
10–12 High risk
≤ 9 Very high risk

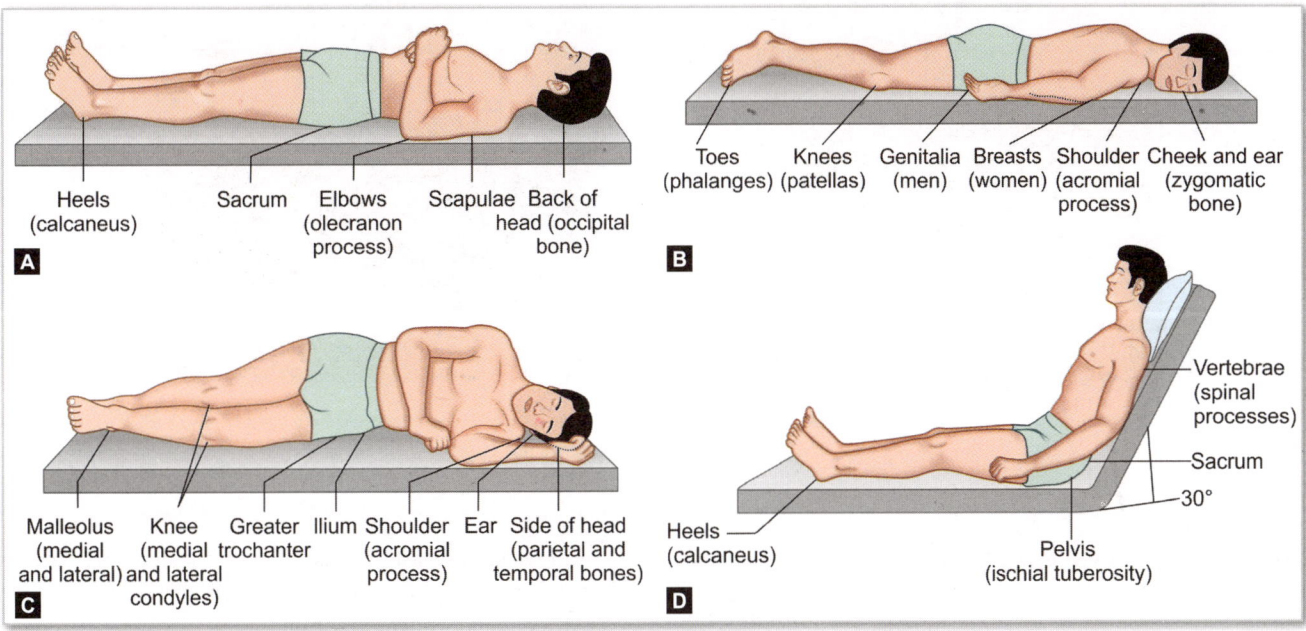

Figs 3A and D: Body pressure areas in A. Supine position, B. Prone position, C. Lateral position; D. Fowler's position

Pressure ulcers have been graded according to depth. There are four stages of pressure ulcers (Fig. 4).

- **Stage I:** If the redness remains, and the skin does not blanch to fingertip pressure, then the patient has a stage I pressure ulcer. In people with dark skin, discoloration of the skin, warmth, edema, or induration (area feels hard) may be a sign of stage I pressure ulcer.
- **Stage II:** Partial thickness skin loss involving epidermis and/or dermis. It may look like an abrasion or blister. The area surrounding the damaged skin may feel warmer.

- **Stage III:** Full thickness skin loss that looks like a deep crater and may extend to the fascia. Subcutaneous tissue is damaged or necrotic. Bacterial infection of the ulcer is common and causes drainage from the ulcer. There may be a damage to the surrounding tissue.
- **Stage IV:** Full thickness skin loss with extensive tissue necrosis or damage to muscle, bone, or supporting structures, sinus tracts may be present. Infection is usually wide spread. The ulcer may appear dry, black in color, with a build-up of tough necrotic tissue (eschar), or it appears wet and oozing. Document the location of any abnormality, its color, and size, and reaction to blanch test.

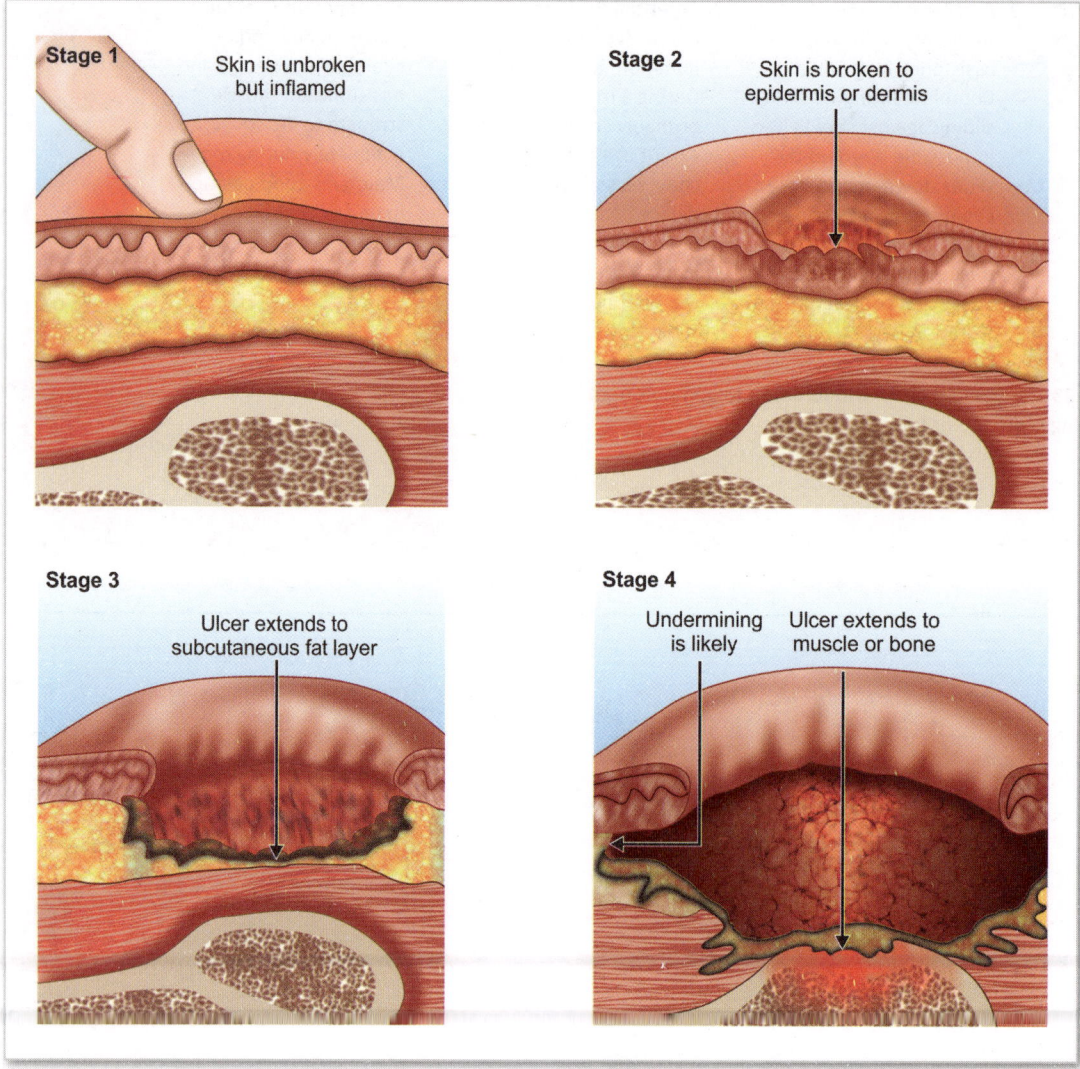

Fig. 4: Stages of pressure ulcer

Prevention of Pressure Ulcers

Excellent nursing care is the main factor in the prevention of pressure ulcers.

- Observe the color of skin carefully and frequently. Skin that is red, blue, or mottled indicates impaired circulation.
- Change the patient's position at least every 2 hours.
- Keep the heels of the totally immobile patient off the bed. Use positioning devices.
- Avoid positioning the patient directly on the trochanter.
- Use of trapeze or lift sheet to move rather than drag patients during transfer and position changes.
- Use pressure reducing devices such as pressure reducing mattress and (air bed mattress) air cushion when in bed.

- Shift weight at least once an hour and restore circulation to a deprived area by rubbing around a reddened area. Use a circular outward motion.
- Do not massage reddened skin as it has already suffered temporary damage. Do not massage directly over bony prominences.
- Wash and dry the incontinent patient quickly and thoroughly to avoid irritation.
- Avoid mechanical and physical injury from improperly fitting splints, braces, casts, prosthesis
- Minimize skin injury by friction and shear forces by using proper positioning, transferring and turning techniques.
- Provide adequate nutrition and fluid intake
- Back rub should be performed with morning care and bed time.

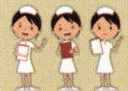

SKILL: CARE OF THE BACK OF BEDRIDDEN PERSON

This involves caring for the skin of the back of a bed-ridden patient

Purposes

- To improve circulation
- To prevent bed sores (pressure sores)
- To keep patient comfortable

Equipment

- Tray containing—Basin with hot water to fill two-thirds and temperature of 110°F–115°F, wash cloth, bath towel, soap in soap dish, dusting powder (spirit oil, lotion), screen for privacy.

Action/steps	Rationale
Assessment	
1. Assess need for back care	To provide back care and to prevent pressure sores
Planning	
2. Gather supplies	Easy access to articles
3. Explain the procedure to the patient	Helps in preparing the patient.
4. Prepare environment for giving back care. Close door and pull the curtain	Promotes comfort and privacy
Implementation	
5. Turn the patient to one side and expose the back, right from the shoulders up to the buttocks	To care for the pressure areas and for proper visualization of the back
6. Protect the bed with bath towel	To prevent sheet getting wet
7. Wash the back with soap and water in circular movements with wash cloth	To cleanse the back and improve circulation
8. Dry the back with patient's towel	To prevent moisture
9. Pour spirit (for moist skin) and lotion/oil (for dry skin) with the palm of the hand and rub the back. Use more pressure on the up strokes toward the head and less pressure on downward strokes. The pressure should be firm but should not cause tension or discomfort for the patient. After few minutes, rub the remainder lotion using short circular strokes	Spirit helps to keep skin tough and dry and oil/lotion helps to keep skin from cracks. Upstrokes, down- strokes and circular strokes help in improving circulation. Rubbing produces heat and causes dilatation of superficial blood vessels and improves circulation.
10. Sprinkle powder on to the back and rub the back (only if spirit is used)	
11. Remove the towel and leave patient comfortable by arranging top linen and leave the unit tidy	Makes patient comfortable
Evaluation	
12. Observe for any reddened areas at the back	To act immediately so that pressure sores do not develop
Documentation	
13. Document in the nurse's notes about back care and if any abnormalities found during back care	Document effectiveness of nursing care

Care for Pressure Ulcers

The most effective method of pressure ulcer treatment is through a team approach. The team should consist of the patient, the family or caregivers, and health care providers. The plan needs to be consistent with the individual patient and family preferences, goals, and abilities. Include education of how pressure ulcers develop and how to prevent additional ulcers.

The initial care of a pressure ulcer involves debridement, wound cleansing and the application of dressings. In most cases, the ulcer is infected and antibiotic therapy is used. Surgery is needed to repair some pressure ulcers.

For cleaning ulcers, use only normal saline and apply light mechanical force with sponges or irrigation fluid to prevent damage to granulation tissue. Use 250–500 mL of solution and irrigate using a syringe with a small catheter to reach undermined areas and tunnels. Cover the wound with a dressing. Thin film dressings are used on stage I ulcers to protect them from shearing forces and to keep them moist. For stage II ulcers that are non-infected, use a hydrocolloid dressing that can be left on for up to a week. For stage III ulcer that is draining, use a dressing that will absorb exudate and maintain a moist environment. For infected ulcers, a non-occlusive dressing is always used. Chemical enzyme formulas may be used in the wound to help debride eschar in stage IV ulcers. A wet to dry dressing may also be applied to help the sloughing of necrotic tissue.

Most pressure ulcers require dressings. The type of dressing is usually based on the stage of the pressure ulcer, the type of tissue in the wound and the function of the dressing. Before placing a dressing on a pressure ulcer, it is important to know the stage of the pressure ulcer. Gauze sponges are the oldest and most common dressing. They are absorbent and are available in different textures and various lengths and sizes. Gauze can be saturated with solutions and used to clean and peck a wound. For pecking, gauze is saturated with the solution usually normal saline. The purpose of this type of dressing is to provide moisture to the wound.

Other type of dressing is non-adherent gauze dressing such as telfa over clean wounds with little or no drainage. Telfa gauze has a shiny, non-adherent surface that does not stick to incisions. Use of self adhesive-transparent film dressing traps moisture over the wound, providing a dry environment. This dressing is ideal for small superficial wounds, such as partial thickness or to protect high-risk skin. It has several advantages:

- Serves as a barrier to external fluid but still allows the wound surface to breathe because oxygen passes through the transparent dressing
- Adheres to undamaged skin

- Provides a moist environment which promotes epithelialization
- Can be removed easily
- Permits viewing a wound
- Does not require a secondary dressing

Hydrocolloid dressings are dressings with complex formulations of colloids, elastomer and adhesive components. The wound contact layer of this dressing forms a gel as fluid is absorbed and maintaining a moist healing environment. These dressing support healing in clean granulating wounds and automatically debride necrotic wounds. It serves the following functionalities:

- Maintains wound moisture
- Absorbs drainage through the use of absorbers in the dressing
- Slowly liquefies necrotic debris
- Is impermeable to bacteria
- Is self adhesive
- Acts as a preventive dressing for friction areas
- May be left in place for 3–5 days
- Useful for shallow to moderately deep dermal ulcers

Hydrogel dressings are impregnated with water or glycerin-based amorphous gel. This type of dressing hydrates wounds and absorbs smaller amounts of exudate. They are useful for partial thickness and full thickness wounds, deep wounds with some exudate, necrotic wounds, burns and radiation damaged skin. They are useful in painful wounds because they are very soothing to the patient and do not adhere to the wound bed and cause little trauma during removal. The only disadvantage is that some hydrogels require a secondary dressing. Other types of dressing are foam and alginate dressings for wounds with large amounts of exudate and those that require packing. Do not use these in dry wounds as they require a secondary dressing. The change of dressing requires the same skill by the health care provider as for taking care of any wound.

CARE OF THE HAIR

The appearance of the hair often reflects a person's feelings of self-concept and well-being. People who feel ill may not groom their hair as before. The hair also reflects the state of health, for example, excessive coarseness and dryness may be associated with endocrine disorders such as hypothyroidism. In elderly, the hair is generally thinner, grows more slowly, and has diminished circulation. Men often lose their scalp hair and may become completely bald.

Each person has a particular ways of caring for hair. Some shampoo hair daily, others shampoo once a week or twice a week. Oil prevents the hair from breaking and the scalp from drying.

Assessment

Normal hair is resilient and evenly distributed. Problems include dandruff, hair loss, ticks, pediculosis, scabies and hirsuitism.

Dandruff

Dandruff appears as a diffuse scaling of the scalp, accompanied by itching. In severe cases, it involves the auditory canals and the eyebrows. Dandruff can be treated with medicinal shampoo.

Hair Loss

Some permanent thinning of hair normally occurs with aging. Baldness, common in males, is thought to be hereditary problem for which there is no known remedy other than wearing a cap or going in for hair transplant.

Ticks

Ticks are small gray-brown parasites that bite into tissue and suck blood. Ticks transmit several diseases to people, e.g., lyme disease, and tularemia. To prevent ticks, place a drop of oil on the tick or cover with petroleum. This will suffocate the ticks and kill them.

Pediculosis (Lice)

Lice are parasitic insects that infest mammals. Infestation with lice is called pediculosis. Three kinds of lice infest humans. They are *Pediculus pubis* (the crab louse), *Pediculus corporis* (the body louse), and *Pediculus capitis* (the head louse).

Pediculus capitis is found on the scalp and tends to stay hidden in the hairs; similarly, pediculus pubis stays in pubic hair. Pediculus corporis tends to cling to clothing, so that when a client undresses, the lice may not be evident on the body; these lice suck blood from the person and lay their eggs on the clothing. The nurse can suspect their presence in the clothing if the person habitually scratches. These are scratches on the skin and there are hemorrhagic spots on the skin where the lice have sucked blood.

Head and pubic lice lay their eggs on the hairs, the eggs look like particles, similar to dandruff, clinging to the hair.

Scabies

Scabies is a contagious skin infection by the itch mite. The characteristic lesion is the burrow produced by the female mite as it penetrates into the upper layers of the skin. The mites cause intense itching that is pronounced at night because the increased warmth of the skin has a stimulating effect on the parasites. Treatment includes application of scabicide lotion and washing of all clothes and bed linen in hot or boiling water.

Hirsutism

The growth of excessive body hair is called hirsutism. It may be due to action of the endocrine system.

Diagnosis

Nursing diagnosis related to hair hygiene and hair and scalp problems include:
- Self-care deficit is related to
  - Activity intolerance
  - Imposed immobility (bed rest)
  - Pain in upper extremities
  - Altered level of consciousness
  - Lack of motivation associated with depression
- Impaired skin integrity related to
  - Scalp laceration
  - Insect bite
- Risk for infection related to
  - Scalp laceration
  - Insect bite
- Disturbed body image related to alopecia

Planning

In planning care, the nurse sets outcomes for each nursing diagnosis. The nurse then performs nursing interventions and activities to achieve the client outcomes.

Implementation

Hair needs to be brushed and combed daily and washed, as needed, to keep it clean. Nurses may need to provide hair care for clients who cannot meet their own self care needs.

Brushing and Combing

Using a clean brush or comb, brush from the scalp toward the hair ends. Separate the hair into smaller sections as it is easier and more comfortable for the patient. Be sure to be gentle when providing hair care. A patient may have tangled or matted hair. To decrease pain, hold the hair between the scalp and the area you are brushing or combing. Braiding the hair helps to reduce tangles but seek patient's permission before braiding. Do not cut the hair to remove tangles.

Shampooing

Shampooing patient's hair removes dirt, blood, or solutions from the hair, stimulates circulation of the scalp, and eases brushing and combing. If the patient is able to be out of bed or in the chair, the shampoo maybe done in front of the sink. If the patient is bedridden, shampoo a patient's hair in bed.

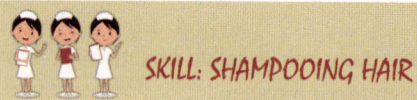

SKILL: SHAMPOOING HAIR

Equipment

Shampoo, comb and brush, bucket for waste, basin for water (hot and cold), waterproof pad (mackintosh with towel) washcloth, bath blanket, bath towel, and cotton plugs for ear.

Steps of Procedure

Review and carry out the standard steps as given in Appendix

Action/steps	Rationale
Assessment	
1. Assess need for shampoo and any special order in case of dandruff or pediculi	Medicated shampoos may be ordered if there are any abnormalities
Planning	
2. Explain the procedure to patient	Decreases fears and anxiety over procedure
3. Gather supplies	Provides easy access to equipment
Implementation action	
4. Wear gloves if patient's scalp has lesions, cuts, infestation or dried blood in the hair	Prevents spread of microorganisms
5. Raise the bed, lower the near side-rail, remove the pillow, and move the patient to the near side of the bed. Place the water-proof pad under the patient's shoulders and head. Drape patient with bath blanket. Place a towel around patients shoulders	Promotes proper body alignment and mechanics. Waterproof pad keeps linens dry. Drape prevents chills and towel helps to keep patient dry
6. Brush or comb a patient's hair	Removes tangles
7. Place bucket at the head of the bed to collect waste water. Lower bed and obtain water at proper temperature	To receive waste water in bucket and protect bed
8. Offer a patient a folded washcloth to cover the eyes. Plug the ear with cotton balls. Pour a small amount of water through patient's hair. Start at the front and move to the back of the head. Wet entire hair surface completely. Apply shampoo and lather. Use your fingertips to massage all parts of the scalp. Again start from the front and work to the back. Lift the head slightly to fully massage and wash the back of the head. Add water as needed to maintain lather	Promotes comfort by using warm water. Promotes proper body alignment. Protects the eyes from soap and water. Ears are protected from entry of water. Friction aids in making the lather, which will cleanse the hair
9. Rinse thoroughly by pouring warm water through the hair. Rinse until the soap is completely out of the hair. Apply soap again, if hair appears still dirty.	No soap should be left and hair appears clean
10. Wrap head in towel, dry face and shoulder and remove articles (basin, bucket) Dry hair and scalp. Comb hair	Decreases chills and prevents spills. Promotes the hair to dry and removes tangles
11. Position patient comfortably and finish arranging the hair as desired by patient	Promotes comfort and demonstrates respect for patient's wishes.
12. Clean equipment and restore the unit. Lower the bed and raise the rail	Makes equipment ready for next use. Promotes safety

Contd...

Action/steps	Rationale
Evaluation	
13. Assess condition of hair and scalp and how does the patient feel.	Promotes a sense of well-being and cleanliness as hair is left clean and groomed.
Documentation	
14. Document the patient's response and tolerance of the procedure. Note any abnormalities of the hair or scalp found during the procedure	Documents effectiveness and measures taken in case of any abnormalities

Pediculosis Treatment

Dangers of Pediculi

- Causes itching and discomfort
- Sucks blood and causes anemia
- Spreads diseases like typhus fever
- Spreads easily to others

Prevention

- Maintaining personal cleanliness
- Use of fine tooth comb
- Keeping comb separate.

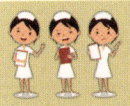 **SKILL: PEDICULOSIS TREATMENT**

Equipment

Water proof sheet, bath towel, cotton balls, kidney basin, cap, ounceglass, spoon, disinfectant (7% lysol), vaseline, medications, e.g., equal parts of kerosene oil and coconut oil.

Action/steps	Rationale
Assessment	
1. Assess the need for pediculosis treatment	To prevent spread to others
Planning	
2. Explain the procedure to patient	Gain cooperation of patient and decreases fear and anxiety
3. Gather supplies	Provides easy access to equipment and saves time
Implementation	
4. Prepare the patient and provide privacy	To prevent embarrassment
5. Protect the patient's bed and your uniform (wear gown) from lice	To prevent spread of lice
6. Apply vaseline to the skin on the forehead at the hairline	Lice will not fall on face
7. If the head is badly infested with pediculi, do not comb the hair, before the treatment is given. If not badly infested, loosen the hair and comb out the tangles. Discard any lice into 7% Lysol in the kidney basin	Lice may drop on the clothes and bed linen
8. Part the hair into small sections and apply the medicine on the hair and scalp by using cotton or gauze pieces, rubbing gently. For long hair, the medicine should be applied along the whole length of hair	So that the medicine can be applied all over the hair and scalp
9. Roll up the hair to the top of the head and cover the head with cap or sling (triangular bandage)	Treatment is done preferably in evening and left overnight. Commercial preparation can be applied any time and requires only 3 minutes (see instructions for use)

Contd...

Action/steps	Rationale
10. Remove all equipment and tidy the unit and replace the articles	Make equipment ready for next use
11. Wash hands	To prevent infection
Evaluation	
12. Assess hair and scalp and repeat after one week if nits are present	If the nits remain after the second treatment, shampoo using vinegar (6% acetic acid)
Documentation	
13. Document when the pediculosis treatment is given and what pediculocide is used	For further reference and action

CARE OF THE HANDS AND FEET

Special attention is often required to prevent infection, odor and injury of the patient's hands and feet. Problems often arise from abuse or poor care of hands and feet, such as biting the nails and wearing ill-fitted shoes.

Assessment of the feet involves a thorough examination of all skin surfaces. Areas between toes should be carefully checked. Patients with diabetes mellitus or peripheral vascular disease should be observed for adequate circulation of the feet. Because of poor vision and decreased mobility, the elderly people are at risk for foot disorders. Care of hands and feet can be provided during the morning bath or at any other convenient time.

Care of the Feet

- Inspect the feet daily including the top and soles and the area between the toes
- Wash and soak the feet daily using lukewarm water (37°C)
- If the feet perspire, apply a foot powder.
- If dryness is noted along the feet, apply soft oil and rub gently into the skin.
- File the toe nails straight across and square.
- Avoid wearing elastic stockings.
- Wear clean socks daily.
- Do not walk barefoot.
- Wear properly fitted shoes.
- Exercise regularly to improve circulation to the lower extremities
- Immediately wash minor cuts and dry them thoroughly. Mild antiseptics may be applied to the skin.

Common Foot and Nail Problems

- Callus is a thickened portion of epidermis caused by local friction or pressure.
- Corns are caused by friction and pressure from shoes. They are seen mainly on toes and over bony prominence.
- Plantar warts are fungating lesions, appearing on sole of foot and are caused by Papilloma virus.
- Athlete's foot (Tinea pedis) is the fungal infection of foot mainly induced by wearing of constricting footwear.
- Ingrown nails: Toe nails or finger nails grow inward into soft tissue during nail trimming.
- Paronychia is the inflammation of tissue surrounding nails following an injury. It is common among diabetic patients.
- Foot odor is the result of excessive perspiration promoting microorganisms growth.

Purpose of Care of Hands and Feet

- To keep the feet clean and dry.
- To trim nails and keep them short to prevent injury.
- To teach the patient in a proper way to inspect the feet and hands for any dryness and signs of infection.

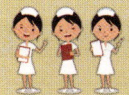

SKILL: CARE FOR HAND AND FEET

Articles

A tray containing:

- A pair of scissors or nail clipper
- A jug with water for washing hands
- Soft nail brush
- A towel
- Wash cloth
- Mackintosh and drawsheet

- Wet swabs in a small bowl
- A kidney tray with Dettol 1 in 40 solution
- A paper bag
- Wash basin
- Mat

Steps of Procedure

Review and carry out the standard steps as given in Appendix

Actions/steps	Rationale
Assessment	
1. Check the client's identification and doctor's order	To assess needs
2. Explain the client about the purpose and the procedure	Providing explanation fosters cooperation
Planning	
3. Gather all the required articles	To prevent interruption during procedure
4. Perform hand-hygiene and put all the required articles to the bed-side	To prevent spread of infection and to promote effective care
5. Provide privacy and assist the client to a comfortable upright position	To provide comfort
Implementation	

6. **Soaking the hands**
  ▪ Put a mackintosh with covering towel on the bed
  ▪ Put the basin with warm water over the mackintosh
  ▪ Soak the client's hands in the basin and apply mild soap (Fig. 5)
  ▪ Scrub and wash them up
  ▪ Dry the client's hands thoroughly by using the towel
	Mackintosh can prevent the sheet from getting wet
	To make nails soft, thereby you can cut nails easily and safely

Fig. 5: Soaking the hands	

7. **Cutting the nails**
  ▪ Trim the client's nails with nail clippers
  ▪ Wipe all fingernails from thumb to 5th nail side by side by wet cotton ball. One cotton ball is used for one nail finger
  ▪ Shape the fingernails with a filer, rounding the corners and wipe both hands by a sponge towel
	Special orders are required before cutting the nails on cuticles of a client with diabetes to avoid accidental injury to soft tissues.

8. Apply lotion or cream to hands	To prevent dryness

Contd...

Actions/steps	Rationale
9. Position patient on chair, place disposable mat under patient's feet if possible and provide patient with privacy	To provide for comfort
10. Fill the basin with water at 100°F–110°F (38°C–44°C) place the basin on a disposable mat and help the patient to place feet into basin, soak feet for 15–20 minutes (Fig. 6) 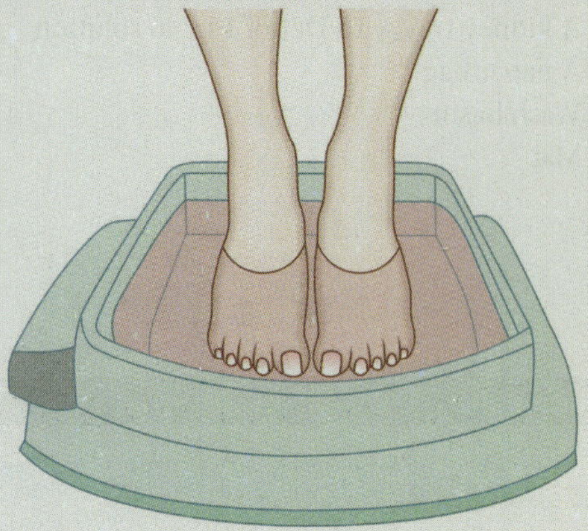	To make nails soft, thereby you can cut nails easily and safely

Fig. 6: Care of feet

Actions/steps	Rationale
11. Cut toe nails straight across and do not round off the corners	If the nails are found to grow inward at the corners, place a wisp of cotton under the nail to prevent toe pressure. A notch in the center will pull in edges and corners. Sometimes, very thick, hard toe nails require surgical removal.
12. Apply lotion or cream to feet	To prevent dryness
13. Make the client comfortable. Replace equipment and discard the water and swabs	To prepare equipment for the next procedure
14. Perform hand hygiene	To prevent the spread of infection
Documentation	
15. Document on chart the condition of hands and feet and report any deviations	Provides the data that care has been given and nails have been cut.

BACK MASSAGE OR BACK CARE

Back care means, "cleaning and massaging, individual's back as therapeutic and comfort measure."

Purposes

- Decreases muscle tension and promotes relaxation
- Increases circulation to the area
- Aids in the development of the therapeutic nurse-patient relationship
- Prevents pressure ulcers
- Keeps the skin clean and dry
- Helps to detect early signs of pressure sores
- Increases elimination through the skin
- Induces sleep
- Provides comfort to the patient
- Regulates body temperature
- Aids in observation of patient

Contraindications

- Burns
- Rib fracture
- Spinal injuries
- Surgeries on back

Basic Principles of Back Massage

- The psychological benefits of back massage cannot be overstressed for the hospitalized patients.
- Agents used for back massage:
  - Lotions or emollients:
    - Lotions or emollients reduces friction and lubricate the skin

- They are appropriate for most patients especially those with a tendency towards dry skin; that is elderly patients
  - **Rubbing alcohol:**
    - Alcohol evaporates quickly, so it has a cooling but very drying effect
    - A certain amount of alcohol is absorbed by the skin so it should not be used on infants, elderly patients or patients with liver disease.
  - **Powder:**
    - Powder reduces friction but also has a drying effect on the skin
    - It may be appropriate for those patients who perspire freely and/or confined to bed.

General Guidelines

- A back massage should take about 5–10 minutes and can be given with the patient's bath before bed time or at any other time during the day.
- Determine if any allergies or skin sensitivities exist before applying lotion to the patient's skin.
- The greatest relaxation effect of a massage occurs when the rhythm of the massage is coordinated with the patient's breathing
- Give special attention to bony prominences
- Avoid using powder and lotion together because this may lead to skin maceration
- Develop a training schedule and give back care at each position change.

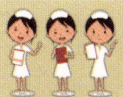 **SKILL: BACK MASSAGE**

Articles

A tray containing:

- Basin 1 with warm water
- Sponge cloth: 1
- Small bowl: 1
- Soap with soap dish
- Towel: 1
- A kidney tray with paper bag
- Spirit
- Talcum powder/lotion/oil
- Mackintosh with cover
- A set of patient's clothes

Steps of Procedure

Review and carry out the standard steps as given in Appendix

Actions/steps	Rationales
Assessment	
1. Check the client's identification and condition	To assess the condition of the client
2. Explain the client about the purpose and the procedure	Helps in promoting relaxation and cooperation
Planning	
3. Put all required articles to the bedside and set-up	Appropriate setting can make the time of the procedure minimum and effective
Implementation	
4. Close all windows and apply screen	To ensure that the room is warm and maintain the privacy
5. Perform hand hygiene with warm water	Cold water causes muscle tension
6. Place the client in an appropriate position 　■ Move the client toward your side 　■ Turn the client to her/his side and put the mackintosh covered by big towel under the client's body	To make him/her more comfortable and provide the care easily. Mackintosh prevents the linens from soiling

Contd...

Actions/steps	Rationales
7. Expose the client's back fully and observe it whether there is any abnormality	To find any abnormality to prevent further complications and to provide proper medication as soon as possible If you find some redness, heat or sores, you cannot give any massage to that place. If the client has some red sore already or broken down area, you need to report to the senior staff or doctor.
8. Wipe back with wet wash cloth. Lather soap on hands. Apply soap from down to upward direction in circular motion giving special attention to the pressure areas and rinse with plain warm water. Dry the area thoroughly.	To clean the back before we give massage with oil/lotion powder.
9. Put some lotion or oil into your palm. Apply the oil or the lotion and massage at least 3 – 5 minutes by placing the palms: ■ From sacral region to neck, use firm smooth strokes to massage over scapular area ■ From upper shoulder to the lowest parts of buttocks gently but firmly knead skin by grasping area between thumb and fingers work across each shoulder and around nape of neck. Continue downward along each side to sacrum	Oil or lotion keep the skin dry by absorbing the moisture and protects the skin from friction

Steps for back massage

10. **Effleurage:** Using your palm, stroke from the buttocks up to the shoulders, over the upper arms and back to the buttocks. Use slightly less pressure on the downwards strokes (Fig. 7).

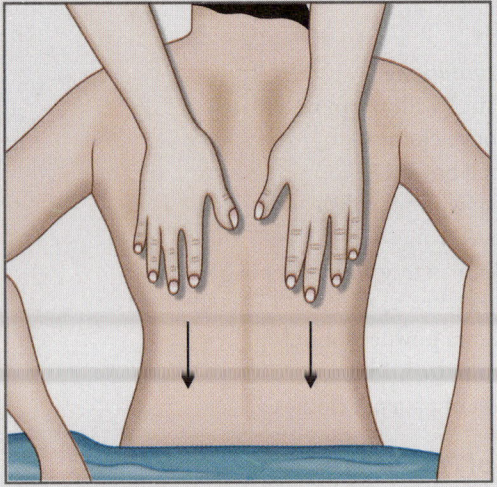

Fig. 7: Effleurage

11. **Petrissage:** Using your thumb to oppose your fingers, knead and stroke half the back and upper arms, starting at the buttocks and moving towards the shoulder. Then knead and stroke the other half of the back, rhythmically alternating your hands (Fig. 8)

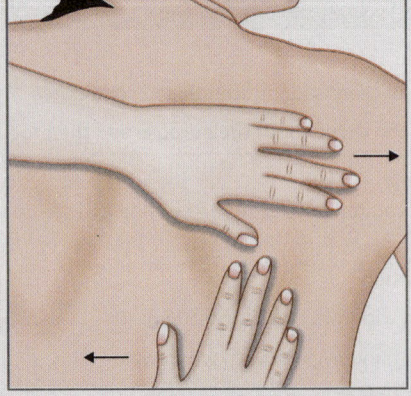

Fig. 8: Petrissage

Contd...

Actions/steps	Rationales
12. **Friction:** Use circular thumb strokes to move from buttocks to shoulders; then, using a smooth stroke, return to the buttocks (Fig. 9)	 **Fig. 9:** Friction
13. **Hand over Hand:** Massage the back with short quick strokes using alternate hands	
14. **Brush Strokes:** Lightly stroke the back with finger tips while massage finger tips while massage	
15. **Kneading:** Stroke the back with both hands together	
16. **Tapping:** Tap the back with both hands	
17. Help the client to put the clothes and return the client to comfortable position	To provide warmth and comfort
18. Replace all articles in proper place	To prepare for the next procedure
19. Perform hand hygiene	To prevent the spread of infection
Documentation	
20. Document on the chart with your signature, including date, time and skin condition. Report any findings to senior staff	Documentation provides coordination of care. Giving signature maintains professional accountability.

BIBLIOGRAPHY

1. *Trained Nurses Association of India. Fundamentals of Nursing-A Procedure Manual, 1st edition, New Delhi; 2005. p 147-9.*
2. *Kozier Barbara B, Du Gas Beverly W. Fundamentals of Nursing Patient Care. WB Saunders Company, Philadelphia;1967. p. 83-9.*
3. *Alexander MF, Fawcett JN, Phyllis J. Runciman JP. Nursing Practice-Hospital and Home, 1st edition, Longman Group UK Limited; London; 1994. p. 747-50.*
4. *Leahy JM, Patricia EK. Foundation of Nursing Practice, 1st edition, WB Saunders Company; Philadelphia; 1998. p. 670-6.*
5. *Craven RF, Hirnel CJ, Henshaw CM. Fundamentals of Nursing-Human Health and Function. Lippincott Williams and Wilkins; Philadelphia; 2000. p. 762-5.*
6. *Price AL. The Art, Science and Spirit of Nursing, 3rd edition, WB Saunders Company. Philadelphia; 1968. p. 84-94.*
7. *Thresyamma CP. Fundamentals of Nursing, 1st edition, Jaypee Brother Publication; New Delhi; 2002. p. 154-8.*

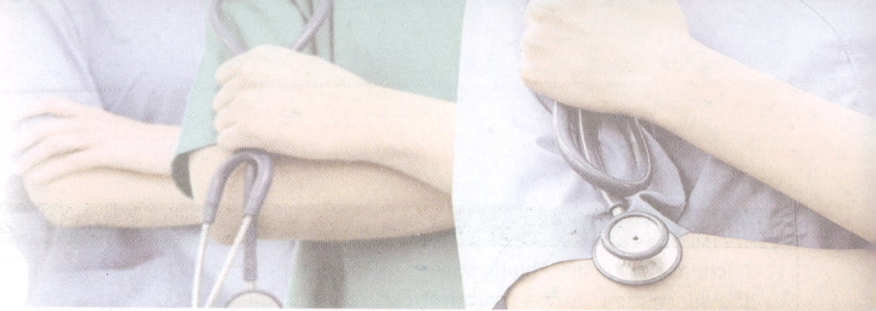

Chapter 34

Rest and Sleep

Learning Objectives

After completing this chapter, you will be able to:

- Explain the function and physiology of sleep
- Identify the stages of sleep: NREM and REM sleep
- Describe variations in sleep patterns throughout the life span
- Identify factors that affect normal sleep
- Describe common sleep disorders
- Identify the components of a sleep pattern assessment
- Plan, implement and evaluate nursing care related to selected nursing diagnosis involving sleep problems

Key Terms

- Circadian rhythm
- Dyssomnia
- Hypersomnia
- Insomnia
- Melatonin
- Narcolepsy
- Non-rapid eye movement (NREM) sleep
- Rapid eye movement (REM) sleep
- Sleep cycle
- Sleep apnea
- Sleep hygiene
- Somnambulism

INTRODUCTION

Rest connotes a condition in which the body is in a decreased state of activity, with the consequent feeling of relaxation physically and emotionally and free from anxiety. Even when rest is possible, one's environment is not always conducive for physical and mental relaxation.

Sleep is a state of rest accompanied by altered consciousness and relative inactivity. It is a complex rhythmic state involving a progression of repeated cycles, each representing different phases of body and brain activity.

Sleep is a basic human need. It is a universal biological process common to all people. Humans spend about one third of their lives asleep. We require sleep for many reasons:

- To cope with daily stresses
- To prevent fatigue
- To conserve energy
- To restore the mind and body
- To enjoy life fully.

Sleep enhances day time functioning. It is vital for not only optimal psychological functioning but also physiological functioning; sleep is an important factor in a person's quality of life.

PHYSIOLOGY OF SLEEP

Two systems in the brainstem, the reticular activating system (RAS) and the bulbar synchronizing region, are believed to work together to control the cyclic nature of sleep. The RAS comprises many nerve cells and fibers. The fibers have connections that relay impulses into the cerebral cortex and spinal cord. During sleep, the RAS experiences few stimuli from the cerebral cortex and the periphery of the body. Wakefulness occurs when this system is activated with stimuli from the cerebral cortex and from periphery sensory organs and cells. For example, an alarm clock makes us wake up from sleep to a state of consciousness, in which we prepare for the day. Sensations such as pain, pressure and noise produce wakefulness by means of peripheral organs and cells.

The hypothalamus has control centers for several involuntary activities of the body, one of which concerns sleeping and waking. Injury to the hypothalamus may cause a person to sleep for abnormally long periods.

Various neurotransmitters are involved with the sleeping process. Norepinephrine and acetylcholine, in addition to dopamine, serotonin, and histamine, are involved in excitation; gamma aminobutyric acid (GABA) appears to shut off the activity in the neurons of the RAS. Another key factor to sleep is exposure to darkness. Darkness and preparing for sleep causes a decrease in stimulation of the RAS. During this time, the pineal gland in the brain begins to actively secrete the natural hormone melatonin, and the person feels less alert. During sleep, the growth hormone is secreted and cortisol is inhibited.

CIRCADIAN RHYTHMS

Biological rhythms exist in plants, animals, and humans. In humans, these are controlled from within the body and synchronized with environmental factors, such as light and darkness. The most familiar, biological rhythm is the circadian rhythm. The term circadian is from the Latin word circa-diem, meaning "about a day." Although, sleep and waking cycles are best known for the circadian rhythms; body temperature, blood pressure, and many other physiologic functions also follow a circadian pattern.

Sleep is a complex biological rhythm. When a person's biological clock coincides with the sleep wake cycles, the person is said to be in circadian synchronization; that is, the person is awake, when the body temperature is the highest, and asleep when the body temperature is the lowest.

STAGES OF SLEEP

There are two stages of sleep: NREM (nonrapid eye movement) sleep and REM (rapid eye movement) sleep. These stages have been studied and analyzed with the help of the electroencephalograph (EEG), which records electrical currents from the brain; the electrooculogram (EOG), which records eye movements; and the electromyography (EMG), which records muscle tone.

NREM Sleep

NREM sleep comprising 75% of total sleep consists of four stages. Stages I and II, constituting about 5% and 50% of a person's sleep time, respectively, are light sleep from which the person can be aroused easily. Stage III and IV, each representing about 10% of total sleep time, are deep sleep states, termed delta sleep or slow wave sleep. The arousal threshold (intensity of stimulus required to awaken) is usually greatest in stage IV NREM. Throughout the stages of NREM sleep, the parasympathetic nervous system dominates, and decrease in pulse, respiratory rate, blood pressure, metabolic rate, and body temperature are observed.

REM Sleep

It is more difficult to arouse a person during REM sleep. In normal adults, the REM stage consumes 20–25% of a person's sleep time. People who are awakened during the REM state almost always report that they have been dreaming. During REM sleep, the pulse, respiratory rate, blood pressure, metabolic rate, and body temperature increase, whereas skeletal muscle tone and deep tendon reflexes are depressed. REM sleep is believed to be essential to mental and emotional equilibrium and plays a role in learning, memory and adaptation.

SLEEP CYCLE

Normally during sleep cycle, a person passes consequently through the four stages of NREM sleep (Fig. 1). This pattern is then reversed, and the person returns from stage IV to stage

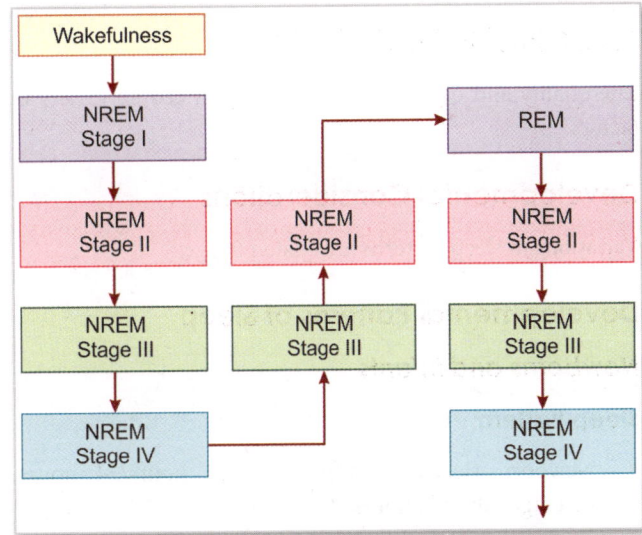

Fig. 1: A single normal sleep cycle. In the normal nocturnal pattern, the shaded cycle is repeated four or five times. Periods of REM sleep generally in duration, and periods of deep sleep (stage IV) progressively decrease as morning approaches.

III to stage II. Instead of reentering stage I and awakening, the person enters into REM stage of sleep, after which the person reenters NREM sleep at stage II and returns to stage III and IV. If a person is awakened from sleep at any time, person return to sleep. Most people go through four or five cycles of sleep each night. Each cycle lasts about 90 to 100 minutes. The cycles tend to become longer as morning approaches (Fig. 1).

Sleep Requirements and Patterns

It is important that each person follows a pattern of rest, i.e., 8 hours of sleep a night which has been accepted as standard for adults. The recommended amount of sleep for adults is 7–9 hours. Those who are able to relax and rest easily, even while awake, often find that less sleep is needed, whereas, others may find that more sleep is required to overcome fatigue. Fatigue can be considered a normal, protective body mechanism and nature's warning that sleep is necessary. Chronic fatigue, is abnormal and is a symptom of illness.

Sleep patterns may vary in old adults. Old people often need more time to fall asleep, wake earlier and more frequently during the nights. Many older individuals nap during the day, which often results in sleeping fewer hours at night. Illnesses in older adults may also affect their sleep patterns.

Pattern of sleep periodicity appears to be learned. For example, most people learn to sleep at night and to be awake and work during the day. However, many night workers learn to sleep equally well during the day.

On an average, infants require 14–20 hours each day. Growing children require from 10 hours to 14 hours of sleep.

FACTORS AFFECTING SLEEP

The quality and quantity of sleep is influenced by variety of factors.

Developmental Considerations

Variations in sleep patterns are related to age.

Developmental Patterns of Sleep

Newborns and Infants

Sleep Pattern

- Newborn sleeps an average of 16 hours/24 hours, (averages about 4 hours at a time).
- Each infant's sleep pattern is unique. On an average, infants sleep 10–12 hours at night with possibly several naps during the day.
- Usually by 8–16 weeks of age, an infant sleeps through the night.

- REM sleep constitutes most of the sleep cycle of a young infant.

Nursing Implications

- Teach parents to position infant on the back. Sleeping in the prone position increases the risk for sudden infant death syndrome (SIDS).
- Advise parents that eye movements, groaning, grimacing, and moving are normal activities at this age.
- Encourage parents to have the infant sleep in a separate area rather than their bed.
- Caution parents about placing pillows, crib bumpers, quilts, stuffed animals, and so on in the crib because this may pose a suffocation risk.

Toddlers

Sleep Pattern

- Need for sleep declines as this stage progresses. They may initially sleep 12 hours at night with two naps during the day and end this stage sleeping 8–10 hours at night and napping once during the day.
- Toddlers may begin to resist naps and going to bed at night.
- They may move from crib to youth bed or regular bed around 2 years.

Nursing Implications

- Advise parents to establish a regular bedtime routine (e.g., reading a story, singing a lullaby, saying prayers, etc.)
- Advise parents regarding the value of a routine sleeping pattern with minimal variation.
- Encourage attention to safety once child moves from crib to bed. If child attempts to wander out of room, a folding gate may be necessary across the door of the room.

Preschoolers

Sleep Pattern

- Children in this stage generally sleep 9–16 hours at night, with 12 hours being the average.
- The REM sleep pattern is similar to that of an adult.
- Daytime napping decreases during this period, and by the age of 5 years, most children no longer nap.
- This age group may continue to resist going to bed at night.

Nursing Implications

- Encourage parents to continue bedtime routines.
- Advise parents that waking from nightmares or night terrors (awakening, screaming about 20 minutes after falling asleep) are common during this stage.

Waking the child and comforting him or her generally helps. Sometimes use of a night light is soothing.

School-aged Children

Sleep Pattern

- Younger school-aged children may require 10–12 hours at night, whereas older children in this stage may average 8–10 hours
- Sleep needs usually increase when physical growth peaks.

Nursing Implications

- Discuss the fact that the stress of beginning school may interrupt normal sleep patterns.
- Advise that a relaxed bedtime routine is most helpful at this stage.
- Inform parents about child's awareness of the concept of death possibly occurring at this stage. Encourage parental presence and support to help alleviate some of the child's concerns.

Adolescents

Sleep Pattern

- Sleep needs of teenagers vary widely. The growth spurt that normally occurs at this stage may necessitate the need for more sleep, however, the stresses of school, activities, and part-time employment may cause adolescents to have a restless sleep
- Many adolescents do not get enough sleep

Nursing Implications

- Advise parents that complaints of fatigue or inability to do well in school may be related to not enough sleep.
- Excessive daytime sleepiness (EDS) may also make the teenager more vulnerable to accidents and behavioral problems.

Young Adults

Sleep Pattern

- The average amount of sleep required is 8 hours, but in fact, many young adults require less sleep.
- Sleep is affected by many factors: physical health, type of occupation, exercise. Lifestyle demands may interfere with sleep patterns.
- REM sleep averages about 20% of sleep.

Nursing Implications

- Reinforce that developing good sleep habits has a positive effect on health, particularly as an individual ages.

- If loss of sleep is a problem, explore lifestyle demands and stress as possible causes.
- Suggest use of relaxation techniques and stress-reduction exercises rather than resorting to medication to induce sleep. Sleep medications decrease REM sleep, may be habit forming, and frequently lose their effectiveness over time.

Middle-aged Adults

Sleep Pattern

- Total sleep time decreases during these years with a decrease in stage IV sleep.
- The percentage of time spent awake in bed begins to increase.
- Individuals become more aware of sleep disturbances during this period.

Nursing Implications

- Encourage adults to investigate consistent sleep difficulties to exclude pathology or anxiety and depression as causes.
- Encourage adults to avoid use of sleep-inducing medication on a regular basis.

Older Adults

Sleep Pattern

- An average of 5–7 hours of sleep is usually adequate for this age group.
- Sleep is less sound, and stage IV sleep is absent or considerably decreased. Periods of REM sleep shorten.
- Elderly people frequently have great difficulty falling asleep and have more complaints of problems in sleeping.

Insufficient sleep may affect normal growth and development and may be a contributing factor in performance deficits and behavioral problems.

Motivation

A desire to be wakeful and alert helps overcome sleepiness and sleep. When there is minimal motivation to be awake, sleep generally follows.

Culture

An individual's cultural beliefs and practices can influence rest and sleep. Children's bedtime rituals, sleeping position and place, and pattern of sleep may vary based on culture. Methods to enhance sleep may also be culturally influenced. Sensitivity to a patient's culture must be included in the plan of care for preparing the patient for sleep.

Lifestyle and Habits

People working in shift other than the day shift must reorganize their priorities, or sleep difficulties may occur. Based on the circadian rhythm, the body prepares for sleep at night by decreasing the body temperature and releasing melatonin (a natural chemical produced at night that decreases wakefulness and promotes sleep). Working in night shift disrupts this natural process and can result in loss of sleep and other adverse effects, such as anxiety, personal conflicts, loneliness, depression, gastrointestinal symptoms and substance abuse.

Nurses who work long hours and varying shifts have difficulty finding time to exercise and this can promote weight gain. Sleep can be affected by watching some types of television shows and participating in stimulating outside activities.

Physical Activity and Exercise

Activity and exercise increase fatigue, and promote sleep. Moderate exercise is a healthy way to promote sleep. The fatigue that results from normal work activities or exercise is believed to contribute to a restful sleep, whereas excessive exercise or exhaustion can decrease the quality of sleep.

Dietary Habits

It is believed that the dietary amino acid L-tryptophan acts to promote sleep. Protein increases alertness and concentration, whereas carbohydrates appear to affect brain serotonin levels and promote calmness and relaxation. Therefore, a small protein and carbohydrate containing snack may be effective for patients with insomnia.

Alcohol Intake

Alcoholic beverages, when used in moderation, induce sleep; however large quantities have been found to limit REM and delta sleep. Most studies recommend that alcohol and products containing alcohol should not be used within 6 hours of sleep.

Caffeine Containing Beverages

Caffeine is nervous stimulant. Beverages containing caffeine include coffee, tea, and most cola drinks should not be consumed before sleep.

Smoking

Nicotine has a stimulating effect, and smokers usually have a more difficult time falling asleep. Eliminating cigarette smoking after the evening meal appears to improve the smoker's ability to fall asleep. Total withdrawal from smoking may be associated with temporary sleep disturbances.

Environmental Factors

Home environment is considered best for sleep by most people. Sleeping in strange environment tend to influence both REM and NREM sleep. A person who is accustomed to sleep in a quiet environment may find it difficult to sleep in noisy environment.

Psychological Stress

Psychological stress affects sleep in two ways: the person experiencing stress may find it difficult to obtain the amount of sleep he or she needs and REM sleep decreases in amount, which tends to add to anxiety and stress.

Illness

Illness, a physiologic as well as a psychological stressor, induces sleep. Certain illnesses are more closely related to sleep disturbances, such as, gastric secretions increase during REM sleep. Many people with peptic ulcers awaken at night with pain and eating snack or using antacids to neutralize stomach acidity relieves discomfort and promotes sleep.

The pain associated with coronary artery disease and myocardial infarction is more likely with REM sleep. Epilepsy seizures are most likely to occur during NREM sleep and appear to be depressed by REM sleep.

Medications

Sleep quality is influenced by certain drugs. Drugs that decrease REM sleep include barbiturates, amphetamines and antidepressants.

COMMON SLEEP DISORDERS

The international classification of sleep disorders includes four major categories of sleep disturbances:
- Dyssomnia
- Parasomnia
- Sleep disorders associated with medical or psychiatric disorders
- Other proposed disorders

The most common sleep disorders are the dyssomnia and parasomnia. **Dyssomnia** are sleep disorders characterized by insomnia or excessive sleepiness.

Parasomnia are patterns of waking behaviors that appear during sleep.

Dyssomnia

Insomnia

Insomnia is characterized by difficulty in falling asleep, intermittent sleep, or early awakening from sleep. It is the most common of all sleep disorders. People older than 60 years of age, women after menopause and persons with history of depression are more likely to experience insomnia. This sleep disorder can also occur during periods of stress, after traveling across time zones (jet lag) and as a result of the side effects of medications. A person with insomnia often reports feeling tired, lethargic, and irritable during the day.

Treatment

Treatment is usually unnecessary because most episodes last for only a short period.

Nonpharmacological approaches should be attempted initially to resolve insomnia. Cognitive behavioral therapy (CBT) is a safe, effective means of managing chronic insomnia and may include sleep hygiene measures. It may also include biofeedback and relaxation techniques. Pharmacologic options include the use of sedatives and hypnotics.

Sleep hygiene include

- Avoiding intake of caffeine, nicotine, and alcohol especially later in the day
- Avoiding activities after 5 pm that are stimulating
- Avoiding naps
- Eating a light meal before bedtime
- Sleeping in a cool, dark room
- Taking a warm bath before bedtime

Hypersomnias

Hypersomnia is a condition characterized by excessive sleep, particularly during the day. A person may fall asleep for intervals during work, while eating or even during conversations. When they awake, they are often disoriented, irritated, restless, and have slower speech and thinking processes. The causes are:

- Drug or alcohol abuse
- Head trauma or other injury to CNS
- Depression
- Obesity
- Other medical conditions-epilepsy, multiple sclerosis

Treatment

Treatment includes stimulant drugs and antidepressants. Attention to diet includes avoidance of alcohol and caffeine. These people should not drive.

Narcolepsy

Narcolepsy is a condition characterized by an uncontrollable desire to sleep. A person with narcolepsy can literally fall asleep standing up, while driving a car, in the middle of the conversation, or while swimming. It is considered as a neurologic disorder. The common features of narcolepsy are:

- Sleep attacks or irresistible urge to sleep
- During a sleep attack the person moves directly into REM sleep

Treatment

Including CNS stimulant that causes wakefulness may be used to control narcolepsy. A person with narcolepsy is not permitted to drive vehicle.

Sleep Apnea

Sleep Apnea is a condition in which person experiences the absence of breathing (apnea) or diminished breathing efforts (hypopnea) during sleep between snoring intervals. Breathing may cease for 10 – 20 seconds and may be as long as 2 minutes. During long periods of apnea, the oxygen level in the blood drops, the pulse usually becomes irregular, and the blood pressure often increases.

Obstructive sleep apnea (OSA) can result when the airway is occluded because of the collapse of the hypopharynx or from structural abnormalities such as enlarged tonsils and adenoids, a deviated nasal septum and thyroid enlargement.

Clinical information and polysomnography can confirm the diagnosis of sleep apnea. It consists of an overnight sleep study which includes EEG recording of the stages of sleep and any episodes of apnea, an electrooculogram (EOG) that detects eye movements and electromyographic (EMG) recording of muscle movement.

Treatment

Moderate obstructive sleep apnea consists of removal of tonsils. If this is ineffective, continuous positive airway pressure (CPAP) is recommended, which delivers positive air pressure and holds the airway open. CPAP is noninvasive and consists of a mask connected to an air pump that is worn during sleep.

Sleep Deprivation

Sleep Deprivation refers to a decrease in the amount, or quality of sleep. It may result from decreased REM sleep or NREM sleep. Deprivation produces changes in physical and mental functioning. The strange environment of the hospital, physical discomfort and pain, the effects of medications, and the need for 24-hour nursing care may contribute to sleep deprivation in hospitalized patients.

Parasomnias

Parasomnias are patterns of waking behavior that appear during REM or NREM stages of sleep. Common example is somnambulism (sleep walking). Another type of parasomnia is sleep related eating disorder, in which the person eats but does not remember. So people with sleep-related eating disorder can gain weight and experience injury either from cooking in their sleep or eating potentially dangerous raw food.

NURSING MANAGEMENT

Promoting Rest and Sleep

Assessment

A complete assessment of a client's sleep difficulty includes a sleep history, health history, physical examination, a sleep diary if available and diagnostic studies.

Sleep History

A brief sleep history should be obtained from all clients entering health care facility. Key questions to ask include the following:

- When do you usually go to sleep? And when do you wake up? Do you nap?
- Do you have any problems with your sleep? Has anyone told you that you snore loudly?
- Do you take any prescribed medications, over the counter medications
- Any preferred room temperature, lighting and preferred bedtime routine.

Health History

A health history is obtained to rule out medical or psychiatric causes of the client's difficult sleeping, e.g., depression, Parkinson's disease, Alzheimer's disease, arthritis. Information should be obtained about all and the prescribed and nonprescription medications.

Physical Examination

Client who has obstructed sleep apnea may have enlarged tonsils and adenoids, obesity and neck size greater than 17.5 inches. Deviated nasal septum may also be noted.

Sleep Diary

A sleep specialist may ask clients to keep a sleep diary for 1–2 weeks in order to get complete picture of their sleep complaints. Sleep diary include selected aspects of the following information:

- Time of going to bed, trying to fall asleep, falling asleep (approximate time) any instances of waking up and duration of these periods, and waking up in the morning
- Activities performed 2–3 hours before bedtime
- Consumption of caffeinated beverages and alcohol

- Any prescribed medications taken during the day
- Bedtime ritual before sleep
- Any difficulties remaining awake during the day

Diagnostic Studies

Polysomnography, Electroencephalogram (EEG), Electromyogram (EMG) and electrooculogram (EOG)

Nursing Diagnosis

Sleep pattern disturbances include the following:

- Risk for injury related to somnambulism
- Ineffective coping related to insufficient quality and quantity of sleep
- Fatigue related to insufficient sleep
- Risk for impaired gas exchange related to sleep apnea
- Anxiety related to sleep apnea
- Activity intolerance related to sleep deprivation

Planning

The major goal for clients with sleep disturbances is to maintain a sleeping pattern that provides sufficient energy for daily activities. Other goals are related to improving the quality and quantity of the client's sleep. The nurse plans specific nursing interventions to reach the goal which include reducing environmental distractions, promoting bedtime rituals, providing comfort measures, scheduling nursing care to provide for uninterrupted sleep periods, and teaching stress reduction, relaxation techniques, or good sleep hygiene.

Implementation

Sleep hygiene refers to interventions used to promote sleep mainly non pharmacologic measures and includes:

- Client teaching: Teaching importance of sleep and conditions that promote sleep and those that interfere with sleep; safe use of sleep medications
- Supporting bedtime rituals: Listening to music, reading, taking a soothing bath and praying, washing hands, brushing teeth and voiding
- Creating a restful environment: All people need a sleeping environment with minimal noise, a comfortable room temperature, appropriate ventilation and appropriate lighting.
- Promoting comfort and relaxation
- Providing loose–fitting nightwear
- Assisting clients with hygienic routines
- Making sure that the bed linen is smooth, clean and dry
- Assisting or encouraging the client to void before bedtime
- Offering to provide back massage before sleep

- For clients who have pain, giving them analgesics
- Encouraging relaxation techniques such as deep breathing, yoga and meditation
- Enhancing sleep with medications: When parenteral medication is prescribed, the nurses and clients need to be aware of the actions, effects and risks of the specific medications prescribed.

Evaluation

To know whether client's goals and outcomes have been achieved. Collect data about the duration of the client's sleep, how the client feels on awakening and observation of the clients' alertness during the day. If the desired outcomes are not achieved, the nurse should explore the reasons and modify the plan of care.

BIBLIOGRAPHY

1. *Goldsmith C. Insomnia: Sleepless in America. Nursing Spectrum. 2007;16(5):16-9.*
2. *Taylor CR, Lillis C, LeMone P, et al. Fundamentals of Nursing - The Art and Science of Nursing Care, 7th edition. Wolters Kluwer; 2010.*
3. *Schaller J. Myths and Facts about Obstructive Sleep Apnea. Nursing. 2008;38(1):27.*
4. *Goldberg R. Obstructive Sleep Apnea. Advance for Nurses. Pennsylvania, New Jersey, Delaware. 2007.*

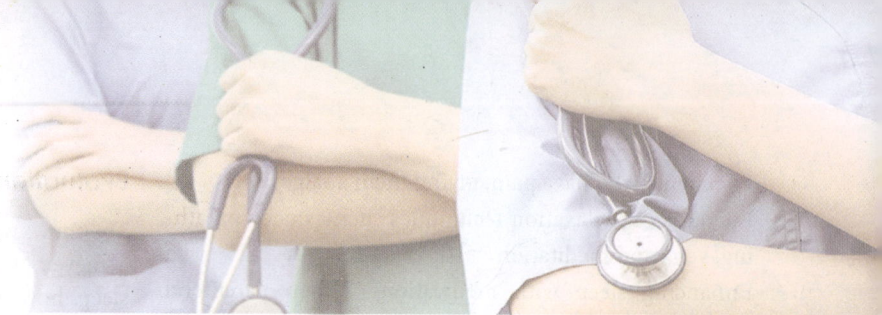

Nutrition

INTRODUCTION

Nutrition is vital for life and health, and poor nutrition can seriously decrease one's level of wellness, which makes it a vital component of nursing.

PRINCIPLES OF NUTRITION

The science of nutrition is the study of how food nourishes the body. It includes the study of nutrients and how they are handled by the body. **Nutrients** are specific biochemical substances used by the body for growth, development, activity, reproduction, lactation, health maintenance, and recovery from illness or injury. Need for nutrients changes throughout the life cycle in response to changes in body size, activity, growth, development and state of health.

Some nutrients are considered **essential** because either they are not synthesized in the body or are made in insufficient amounts. Essential nutrients must be provided in the diet or through supplements. Essential nutrients that supply energy and build tissue such as proteins, carbohydrates and fats are referred to as **Macronutrients. Micronutrients**, such as vitamins and minerals, are required in much smaller amounts to regulate and control body processes.

Out of six classes of nutrients, three nutrients supply energy, i.e., carbohydrates, proteins and fats, and three nutrients are needed to regulate body processes—vitamins, minerals and water.

The body needs energy to function. Energy is derived from foods consumed. Energy is measured in the form of kilocalories, commonly called as calories, or cal. Only carbohydrates, proteins, and fat provide energy. Vitamins and minerals needed for the metabolism of energy, do not provide calories.

One gram of carbohydrate provides four calories, one gram of protein provides four calories and one gram of fat consumed provides nine calories. If a person's daily energy intake is equal to total daily energy expenditure, the person's weight will remain stable. However, if the energy intake is less than the energy expenditure, the person's weight will decrease and if the energy intake exceeds energy consumption, weight will increase.

FACTORS AFFECTING NUTRITIONAL NEEDS

Developmental Stage

Nutritional needs change in relation to growth, development, activity, and age-related changes in metabolism and body composition. Periods of intense growth and development, such as during infancy, adolescence, pregnancy, and lactation, cause an increase in nutritional needs. Nutritional needs stabilize during adulthood. Age influences not only nutrient requirements, but also food intake. The consistency of food consumed, eating patterns and the significance of food change with physical and psychosocial development.

Gender

Males require more nutrition due to differences in body composition and their longer muscle mass.

State of Health

Illness, trauma and stress change the needs for nutrition due to indigestion, loss of appetite and hormonal changes which affect the body's use of nutrients.

Alcohol Abuse

Alcohol Abuse alters the body's use of nutrients and their requirements. The toxic effects of alcohol on the intestinal mucosa interfere with normal nutrient absorption. Need for vitamin B increases because it is used to metabolize alcohol.

Medicines

Many medicines have the potential to influence nutrient requirements. Nutrient absorption may be altered by drugs that:
♦ Change the pH of the gastrointestinal tract
♦ Increase the gastrointestinal motility
♦ Damage the intestinal mucosa
  ▪ Bind with nutrients, rendering them unavailable to the body

Nutrient metabolism can be altered by drugs that:
♦ Act as nutrient antagonists
♦ Alter the enzyme systems that metabolize nutrients
♦ Alter nutrient degradation

Factors that Influence Food Choices

Dietary choices are influenced by economic, culture, religion and personal feelings and meanings associated with food. The financial income can directly influence the ability to purchase sufficient food/or food of high nutritional value. Diverse lifestyles and eating habits directly impact the person's nutritional health. Religious belief restrictions, and cultural practices may affect the patient's acceptance with dietary therapies.

Sociocultural Factors

Sociocultural factors are as follows:
♦ Illiteracy
♦ Language barriers
♦ Knowledge of nutrition
♦ Lack of caregiver or social support
♦ Social isolation
♦ Limited ability to obtain or purchase food
♦ Lack of or inadequate cooking preparation.

Combination of factors can affect an individual's nutritional intake. They can result in decreased food intake, leading to anorexia, underweight or increased food intake, leading to obesity.

ASSESSMENT

Nutritional assessment is a systematic approach used to identify the patient's actual or potential needs, formulate a plan to meet those needs, initiate the plan or assign others to implement it and evaluate the effectiveness of the plan. For healthy persons, good nutritional status can help to maintain health, promote normal growth and development, and protect against disease. For sick persons, good nutritional status can help to reduce risk for complications and speed up the recovery time. Conversely, poor nutritional status can increase the risk for illness or death.

Nutritional assessment involves

- Obtaining a dietary history
- Collecting anthropometric measurements
- Clinical data
- Biochemical data.

Obtaining Diet History

Diet History includes data about eating patterns and habits, food preferences and restrictions, daily fluid intake, use of vitamin or mineral supplements, any dietary problems such as problem in swallowing and chewing. It also covers data on food allergies or intolerances, concerns related to buying food, preparation, storage and type of diet.

The nurse elicits a 24-hour diet history which enables her to compare the data listed with recommended daily allowances or to determine whether the patient is receiving a nutritionally balanced diet. It is also important to ask about patient's medications as some medicines are to be taken before meals, after lunch or at bedtime.

Collecting Anthropometric Measurements

Anthropometric measurements are used to determine body dimensions. In children, these measurements are used to assess growth rate; in adults, they can give indirect measurements of body protein and fat stores. For the data to be accurate and reliable, standardized equipment and procedures must be used, and the data must be compared with the appropriate reference standards for the patient's age and sex. Anthropometric measurements include height, weight, triceps, skin-fold measurements, a measure of subcutaneous fat stores, mid-arm circumference, a measure of skeletal muscle mass and fat store. Height and weight should be determined when the patient is admitted to the health care facility. A patient should be weighed on the same scale each time and at the same time of day, preferably before breakfast. Body weight should be compared with BMI Standards. Body mass index (BMI) is the most preferred method to establish ideal body weight measurement. BMI can be calculated in the following manner:

$$BMI = \frac{\text{Weight in kilograms}}{\text{Height in meters} \times \text{Height in meters}}$$

$$BMI = \frac{\text{Weight in pounds}}{\text{Height in inches} \times \text{Height in inches}} \times 703$$

BMI also provides an estimation of relative risk for diseases such as heart disease, diabetes, and hypertension.

Normal BMI ranges from 18.5 to 24.9. Less than this is considered as underweight and more than this is overweight.

Waist circumference is measured by placing a measuring tape around the patient's waist at the level of umbilicus. This is a good indicator of abdominal fat, where excess of body fat is deposited, and is important indicator of risk for disease such as type 2 diabetes, dyslipidemia, hypertension and cardiovascular disease. The risk increases with a waist circumference over 40 inches in men and 35 inches in women.

Clinical Data

Since nutrition affects most body systems, an assessment of these systems can reveal nutritional problems. It is important to determine whether abnormal findings are actually caused by a nutritional deficiency. Assess for barriers to eating. Dysphagia (difficulty in swallowing) can be the result of poor dental health, cancer, neurologic state such as stroke. Dental problems are associated with impaired chewing. Table 1 lists some of the data that can be collected to assist nursing personnel in determining a patient's nutritional status.

Biochemical Data

Biochemical measurements can be used to detect nutritional problems in the early stages. Blood and urine levels of nutrients measure protein status, measures of body vitamin and minerals and trace element status. Hemoglobin, the oxygen carrying protein of the red blood cells, and hematocrit are measures of plasma proteins that also reflect a person's iron status. Protein status can be measured by measuring serum albumin and transferrin levels and by a total lymphocyte count. Serum albumin levels are a good indicator of a patient's nutritional status. The albumin level does not change with increasing age, but malnutrition and various disease states cause its levels to decrease. Serum albumin levels can also be affected by the patient's hydration status. Over hydration can cause low albumin levels and dehydration may cause a very high level. The total lymphocyte count reflects immune status and is directly affected by impaired nutritional status.

Blood glucose, cholesterol and triglycerides are additional laboratory tests relative to nutritional status. Twenty-four hour urine tests used to measure protein metabolism include urine creatinine excretion and urine urea nitrogen. Creatinine levels are directly proportional to the body muscle mass, and a reduction in this value reflects malnutrition. Table 2 indicates laboratory tests with nutritional implications.

TABLE 1: Clinical observations for nutritional assessment

Parameters/ body area	Signs of good nutritional status	Signs of poor nutritional status
Appearance	Alert, responsive	Listless, apathetic
Vitality	Energetic, vigorous, sleeps well	Lacking energy, tired, apathetic
Weight	Normal as per height, age and body build	Overweight or underweight
Hair	Shiny, lustrous, healthy scalp	Dull, dry, brittle, thin
Skin	Smooth, good color, slightly moist, no rashes or swelling	Rough, dry, swollen, pale, pigmented, bruises, petechia
Nails	Pink, firm	Spoon-shaped, pale, brittle
Eyes	Bright, clear, no sores at corners of eyelids, moist	Pale, dry eyes, bitot's spots, increased vascularity
Lips	Smooth, good color, no swelling, moist	Swollen and puffy, lesion at corners of mouth
Gums	Firm, good, pink color, no swelling or bleeding	Spongy, bleed easily, marginal redness, swollen
Glands	No enlargement of thyroid, lymph glands	Enlargement of thyroid, parotid, lymph glands
Muscles	Firm, well developed	Poor tone, soft, underdeveloped
Gastrointestinal system	Good appetite, normal and regular elimination	Anorexia, indigestion, diarrhea, constipation
Cardiovascular	Heart rate and blood pressure in normal range, rhythm regular	Rapid heart rate and blood pressure elevated, irregular heart rhythm
Neurologic system	Reflexes normal, alert, good attention span, emotionally stable	Deceased reflexes, irritable, confused, emotionally labile

TABLE 2: Biochemical data with nutritional implications

Test	Normal	Abnormal
Hemoglobin	12–18 g/dL	Decreased in anemia
Hematocrit	40–50%	Decreased in anemia, Increased in dehydration
Serum albumin	3.5–5.5 g/dL	Decreased in malnutrition, malabsorption
Prealbumin	23–43 mg/dL	Decreased in protein depletion, malnutrition
Transferrin	240–480 mg/dL	Decreased in anemia, protein deficiency
Blood urea nitrogen	7–20 mg/dL	Increased in starvation, high protein intake, severe dehydration. Decreased in malnutrition and overhydration
Creatinine	0.4–1.5 mg/dL	Increased in dehydration. Decreased in reduction in total muscle mass and severe malnutrition

DIAGNOSIS

Assessment data may reveal actual or potential nutritional problems such as:

- **Altered nutrition:** Less than body requirements (insufficient intake)
- **Altered nutrition:** More than body requirements (excessive intake)
- **Altered nutrition:** Potential for more body requirements related to inappropriate eating, metabolic and endocrine disorders, and inappropriate use of supplements.

There are several nursing diagnoses where nutritional problem is the cause of another problem. They are:

- Activity intolerance related to inadequate calorie intake, iron deficiency anemia
- Impaired dentition related to nutritional deficits
- Anxiety related to obesity
- Ineffective health maintenance related to lack of knowledge about adequate nutrition
- Constipation related to inadequate fluid or fiber intake
- Diarrhea related to overeating and excessive fiber intake
- Deficient fluid volume related to inadequate fluid intake
- Risk for infection related to inadequate calorie and inadequate protein intake
- Inadequate home maintenance management related to inability to purchase, store, or food for family
- Impaired skin integrity related to protein malnutrition, and vitamin A deficiency
- Noncompliance to a particular diet order related to lack of motivation

♦ Disturbed sleep pattern related to excessive caffeine intake.

PLANNING

The goal is to maintain or restore optimal nutritional status using foods the patients like and tolerate. It also includes alleviating the symptoms or side effects of disease or treatment and to prevent complications. Actual patient outcomes should list specific behaviors and criteria such as, the patient will:

♦ Attain and maintain ideal body weight, as indicated by BMI and waist circumference
♦ Eat a diet adequate but not excessive in all nutrients
♦ Follow the appropriate modified diet
♦ Eat variety of food each of three or more meals
♦ Choose healthy foods within their financial means

IMPLEMENTATION

Providing proper and adequate nutrition to the patient is a team effort. Diet is ordered by the doctor in the in-patient setting, sent to the dietician, and explained to the patient by the nurse. The nurse is also responsible for screening patients at home who are at nutritional risk, observing intake and appetite, evaluating the patient's tolerance, assisting the patient with eating, administering enteral and parenteral feeding, monitoring food and participating in nutrition education. Providing special diets like liquid diet, soft diet, clear liquid diet, full liquid diet, salt free or salt restricted diet, high protein diet, low calorie diet, diabetic diet, high fiber diet and, bland diet, cholesterol-control diet.

ASSISTING WITH SPECIAL DIETS

Special diets are needed to treat a disease process such as diabetes mellitus, to prepare for a special examination or surgery, to increase or decrease weight, to restore nutritional deficits, or to allow an organ to rest and promote healing. Diets are modified in one or more of the following aspects: texture, kilocalories, specific nutrients or consistency.

A variation of the regular diet is the light diet, designed for postoperative and other clients who are not ready for the regular diet. Foods in the light diet are plainly cooked and fat is usually minimized, as the bran and foods containing a great deal of fiber.

Diets that are modified in consistency are often given to clients before and after surgery or to promote healing in clients with gastrointestinal problems. These diets include clear liquid, full liquid, soft diet and diet as tolerated.

Clear Liquid Diet

Clear Liquid Diet is limited to water, tea, coffee, clear broths, ginger ale, or other carbonated beverages, strained and clear juices. This diet provides the client with fluid carbohydrate (in the form of sugar) but does not supply adequate protein, fat, vitamins, minerals, or calories. It is a short-term diet (24–36 hours) provided for clients after certain surgeries or in the acute stages of infection, particularly of the gastrointestinal tract. The major objectives of this diet are to relieve thirst, prevent dehydration, and minimize stimulation of the gastrointestinal tract.

Full Liquid Diet

Full Liquid diet contains only liquids or foods that turn to liquid at body temperature, such as ice cream. Full liquid diets are often eaten by clients who have gastrointestinal disturbances or are otherwise unable to tolerate solid or semisolid foods. This diet is not recommended for long-term use because it is low in iron, protein and calories. In addition, its cholesterol content is high because of the amount of milk offered. Examples of foods are shown in Table 3.

TABLE 3: Examples of foods given in various diets

Clear liquid	Full liquid	Soft
♦ Coffee, regular and decaffeinated ♦ Tea ♦ Carbonated beverages ♦ Bouillon, fat-free broth ♦ Clear fruit juices (apple, cranberry, grape) ♦ Other fruit juices, strained ♦ Popsicles ♦ Gelatin ♦ Sugar, honey ♦ Hard candy	All foods on clear liquid diet plus ♦ Milk and milk drinks ♦ Puddings, custards ♦ Ice cream, sherbet ♦ Vegetable juices ♦ Refined or strained cereals (e.g., cream of rice) ♦ Cream, butter, margarine ♦ Eggs (in custard and pudding) ♦ Smooth peanut butter ♦ Yogurt	All foods on full and clear liquid diets, plus: **Meat:** All lean, tender meat, fish, or poultry (chopped, shredded); spaghetti sauce with ground meat over pasta **Meat alternatives:** Scrambled eggs, omelet, poached eggs, cottage cheese and other mild cheese **Vegetable:** Mashed potatoes, sweet potatoes, or squash; vegetables in cream or cheese sauce; other cooked vegetables as tolerated (e.g., spinach, cauliflower, asparagus tips), chopped and mashed as needed; avocado **Fruits:** Cooked and canned fruits; bananas, grapefruit and orange sections without membranes, apple sauce **Breads and cereals:** Enriched rice, barley, pasta; all breads; cooked cereals (e.g., oatmeal) **Desserts:** Soft cake, bread pudding.

Soft Diet

The soft diet is easily chewed and digested. It is often ordered for clients who have difficulty in chewing and swallowing. It is a low-residue (low-fiber) diet containing very few uncooked foods. The puréed diet is a modification of the soft diet.

Modification for Disease

Many special diets may be prescribed to meet requirements for disease process or altered metabolism. For example, a client with diabetes mellitus may need a diet, which is calorie restricted, a cardiac client may need sodium and cholesterol restrictions and a client with allergies will need a hypoallergenic diet.

ASSISTING CLIENTS WITH MEALS

Because clients in health care agencies are frequently confined to their beds, meals are brought to the client. The client receives a tray that has been assembled in a central kitchen. It is the duty of the dietician and nurse to give meals to the respective clients (Fig. 1). There are some groups of people who require help with their meals: Elders who are weakened, and persons with disabilities such as blind clients, those who remain in a back-lying position, or those who cannot use their hands.

The nurse must be sensitive to client's feelings of embarrassment, resentment, and loss of autonomy. Whenever possible, the nurse should help incapacitated clients feed themselves rather than feed them. Some clients are depressed because they require help and because they believe they are burdensome to busy nursing personnel. Although feeding a client is time consuming, nurses should try to appear unhurried and convey that they have ample time.

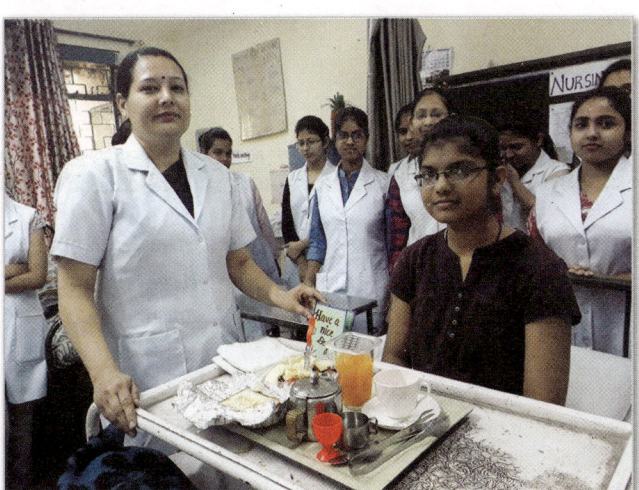

Fig. 1: Serving meal to the patient

When feeding a client, ask in which order the client would like to eat the food. If the client cannot see, tell the client which food is being given. Always allow ample time for the client to chew and swallow the food before offering more. Also, provide fluids as requested, or if the client is not able to communicate, offer fluids after every three or four mouthfuls of solid food. Although normal utensils should be used whenever possible, special utensils may be needed to assist a client to eat. For clients who have difficulty drinking from a cup or glass, a straw often permits them to obtain liquids with less effort and less spillage. Special drinking cups are also made available which has a spout.

NOTHING BY MOUTH

Sometimes, before surgery to prevent aspiration related to anesthesia and after surgery until bowel sounds return, patients are ordered nil per os (NPO) or nothing by mouth. NPO may also be necessary for patients undergoing certain medical tests, for patients experiencing severe nausea and vomiting, or inability to chew or swallow, those who are comatose and women during labor and delivery. The following measures provide comfort to patients who are ordered NPO:

- Encourage or provide good oral hygiene
- Give sips of water or ice chips to keep mouth moist.

If patients are NPO for a short period, they can withstand the stress of NPO if they are well nourished but being NPO for an extended period of time may require nutritional support from **enteral nutrition**, and mustering nutrients directly into the stomach, or **parenteral nutrition** providing nutrition via intravenous (IV) therapy.

ENTERAL NUTRITION

An alternative feeding method to ensure adequate nutrition includes enteral (through the gastrointestinal system) methods. Enteral nutrition (EN) also referred to as total enteral nutrition (TEN), is provided when the client is unable to ingest food or the upper gastrointestinal tract is impaired and the transport of foods to the small intestine is interrupted. Enteral feedings are administered through nasogastric and small bore feeding tubes, or through gastrostomy or jejunostomy tubes.

Nasogastric Tube

Nagogastric (NG) tube is inserted through one of the nostrils, down the nasopharynx, and into the alimentary tract (Fig. 2). For example, Levin tube 12 Fr in diameter is a flexible rubber or plastic single lumen tube with holes near the tip and a double lumen tube is Salem sump tube. The longer lumen of the tube allows delivery of liquids to the stomach or removal of gastric contents, the smaller vent lumen allows for

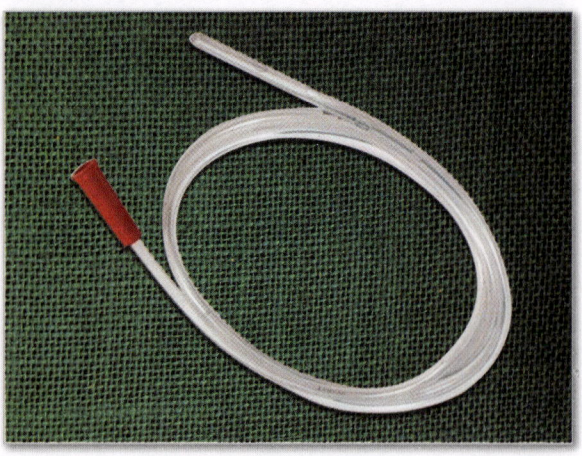

Fig. 2: Nasogastric tube

an inflow of atmospheric air. When these tubes are used for feeding purpose it is called gastric gavage.

Indications for Insertion of Nasogastric Tube

- To prevent nausea, vomiting, and gastric distention following surgery
- To remove gastric contents for laboratory analysis
- Clients who are at risk for aspiration such as:
  - Clients with altered level of consciousness
  - Poor gag or cough reflex
  - Endotracheal intubation
  - Recent extubation
  - Fracture jaw, cleft palate which makes chewing and swallowing impossible
  - Operation on mouth, throat to keep operation site clean
- For gastric lavage (washing out) for patients with gastrointestinal bleeding or for removal of ingested toxins and poisons.
- For administration of medications

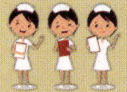 **SKILL: INSERTING A NASOGASTRIC TUBE**

Articles

- Stethoscope
- Gloves
- Drape or towel
- Tongue blade
- NG tube
- Glass of water
- Tape
- Water soluble lubricant
- Plug for tube
- Irrigation syringe
- Tissues/gauze pieces
- Suction machine
- Emesis basin.

Review and carry out standard steps as given in Appendix.

Action/steps	Rationale
Assessment	
1. Assess the patient's understanding of the procedure by explaining the steps	Patients are more cooperative when they understand what is happening to them
2. Position the patient with the head of the bed elevated to 30–90 degree	Elevating the bed enable the tube to move by gravity down the digestive tract
3. Place the emesis basin beside the patients face and tissues near the pillow	To catch emesis if the patient vomits
4. Put on gloves	Barrier protection is needed in case the patient vomits or there is spillage

Contd...

Action/steps	Rationale
Planning	
5. Measure the length of tube to be inserted by measuring from tip of the nose to the tip of the ear lobe and then to the xiphoid process. Mark it (Fig. 3) 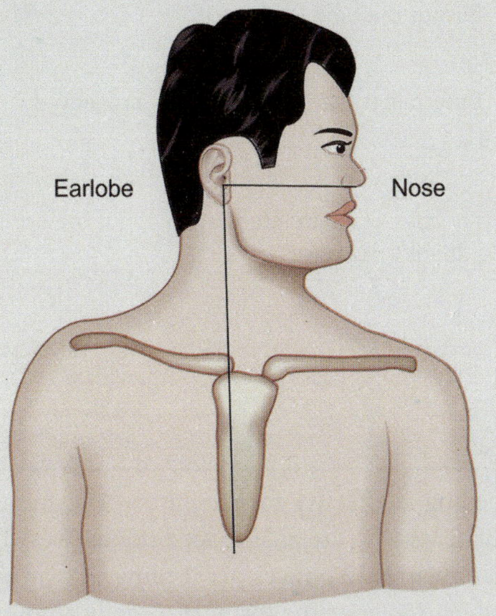	Marking the tube after measurement individualizes the tube length

Earlobe   Nose

Xiphoid process

Fig. 3: Measuring the length of tube

Action/steps	Rationale
6. Chill or warm the tube to the desired stiffness for insertion	A too limp or too stiff tube is difficult to insert. Placing in a basin of ice will stiffen the tube and placing a stiff plastic tube in a basin of warm water will soften it
Implementation	
7. Lubricate the tip of the tube and insert it through the nostril with the patient's head hyperextended, advance the tube down, if you encounter resistance, withdraw the tube and insert it in the other nostril. Do not forcibly push, because this could injure tissue and cause bleeding	For easy insertion, use water or water-based lubricant to moisten the tip of the tube. Do not use oil-based lubricant because of the possibility of liquid aspiration
8. As the tube reaches the back of the throat, have the patient take sips of water through the straw and begin to swallow. Advance the tube each time the patient swallows.	It helps in easy passage of tube
9. Check the position of tube as it passes down the back of the patient's throat by having the patient open mouth and hold down the tongue with tongue depressor. If the tube is coiled up in the mouth, withdraw the tube	Difficulty with the tube entering the esophagus opening sometimes occurs
10. Check the placement of tube by: • Aspirate gastric contents with the syringe • Place stethoscope to the left of the tip of xiphoid and inject 10–20 mL of air into the tube. The air makes "swooshing" sound as it enters the stomach • By measuring the pH of the fluid returned. Gastric pH is 1–4, respiratory pH is >6	When the target point on the tube has reached the nose, the tube should be in the stomach. Either method may be used or X-ray may be needed to confirm the location of tube
11. Tape the tube securely to the face: Cut a 4-inch long piece of tape and split it and tape on the bridge of the nose and split ends down the tube. Be certain the tube is not rubbing the side of the nares because it can cause necrosis.	The tube must be secured so that it is not easily dislodged

Contd...

Action/steps	Rationale
12. Attach the free end of the tube to the connecting tube attached to suction machine or feeding, tube or funnel or syringe.	Low suction pressure is usually ordered to prevent damage to the stomach mucosa
13. Assess residual stomach content in 4 hours and start feeding slowly. Before and after feeding, introduce clear water	Evaluates patient's tolerance of tube feeding, clear water flushes the tube
Evaluation	
14. Ask the patient if nausea is relieved. Assess abdomen for distention. If feeding is started, ask the patient if there is abdominal discomfort	Determines the effectiveness of procedure
Documentation	
15. Document procedure on the nurse's notes and intake and output record. It should include: ■ Reason for tube insertion ■ Time of procedure ■ Type of procedure--suction, feeding ■ Type and size of tube ■ Patient's tolerance of procedure ■ Amount and characteristics of stomach contents	Provides accurate information about the procedure and the patient's response

Tube feedings can be continuous or intermittent. Continuous feeding is effective for patients who cannot tolerate large amounts of fluids at one time. Intermittent feeding is beneficial for patients who are able to feed themselves. The amount of tube feeding is prescribed by the physician and usually ranges from 8 ounces to 12 ounces per feeding. It may be necessary to start with smaller amounts and increase the feeding as the patient is able to tolerate the formula. A daily amount of 2,000 mL is generally sufficient to meet the patient's nutritional requirements. If a syringe is used, it should be 30 mL or 50 mL and the formula should flow in by the gravity; it should not be pushed in as a bolus or in large amounts. Flush tube with 30 mL of water after each feeding to prevent clogging.

Continuous feedings are instilled into the tube drop by drop in the same manner as in intravenous feeding. For this, set similar to intravenous administration is used. The drops are regulated through the drip chamber or set on the pump to control the amount given. Tube feedings contain a high level of glucose to provide the necessary calories. They should be given slowly to prevent diarrhea and glycosuria, over a 24-hour period. When feedings are ordered for 4 or more times a day, the patient is usually given 150–240 mL per feeding.

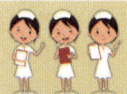

SKILL: NASOGASTRIC TUBE REMOVAL

When the condition for which the tube was inserted has resolved, the tube is discontinued

Action/steps	Rationale
1. Check physician's order for removal of NG tube	Prevents removal of NG tube while still needed
2. Explain procedure to patient	Helps gain patient's confidence
3. Elevate bed to 30 degrees	Position most comfortable for patient
4. Wash hands and put on gloves	Protection against exposure to body fluids
5. Place the emesis basin where the withdrawn tube can be placed into it. Pinch off the tube and pull out gently but quickly	Pinching off the tube keeps gastric contents from spilling into the trachea, which can cause aspiration
6. Offer mouth care	Mouth care removes unpleasant taste from the mouth
7. Remove gloves and wash hands	Prevents spread of microorganisms
8. Assess every 2 hours for signs of nausea, vomiting or abdominal distention. Assess bowel sounds	Provides early recognition of intolerance to removal of NG tube
9. Document the time the tube was removed and the patient's response to the procedure	Documentation provides communication with other health care personnel concerning the care provided to the patient

Contd...

SKILL: GASTROSTOMY/JEJUNOSTOMY TUBE FEEDING

Action/steps	Rationale
Assessment	
1. Check the physician's order for type of feeding, amount and strength of solution	Ensures feeding is given according to physician's order
2. Assess abdomen for distention or tenderness	Identifies discomfort prior to feeding to avoid complications.
Planning	
3. Elevate the head of the bed by 30 degree	Elevation allows gravity to help flow formula into the stomach and helps prevent reflux. This position should be maintained at least 30–60 minutes after the feeding
Implementation	
4. Pinch off the tube and remove the plug, cap, or clamp.	Pinching the tube prevents fluid leaking from the tube. Obtaining gastric contents is the best evidence of proper tube placement
5. Check placement of tube. For NG tube, attach syringe and aspirate small amount of stomach content (5–10 mL).	Obtaining gastric content is the best evidence of proper tube placement
For intermittent feedings	
6. Pinch off the tube and pour the formula in barrel of the syringe, keeping it no more than 18 inches above the level of entry into the stomach.	The formula should be given over 20–30 minutes. Flow can be regulated by raising or lowering the barrel of syringe
7. Add formula to keep the neck of the syringe filled. Continue adding formula to the syringe until the prescribed amount is given. Flush the tube with 30–60 mL of water	If the formula level falls below the neck of syringe, air will enter the tubing and the intestinal tract, causing discomfort as a result of distention. Flushing the tube helps to prevent clogging
For continuous tube feeding	
8. Fill the feeding bag with the prescribed amount of formula, Clear the tubing of air, and attach it to an intravenous pole. Set the rate according to order	Feeding bag can be hung at room temperature for 4 hours. A feeding pump delivers a controlled flow of formula
9. Verify enteral, gastrostomy, or jejunostomy tube placement	Jejunostomy tube sutures must be secure. If the tube is not in place, the feeding could spill into the abdominal cavity causing chemical peritonitis
10. Check the amount of residual from the previous feeding for gastrostomy tube. By aspirating with a syringe, reinstall the fluid	Residual should be checked every 4 hours for gastrostomy tube feedings
11. Attach the tubing from the feeding bag to enteral, jejunostomy or gastrostomy tube using an adaptor as needed. Turn on the pump and check the drip rate. Begin feeding	Drip rate should be checked frequently. Patient tolerance should be checked every hour for distention
12. Pour 1 to 2 ounces of water to clear the tube. Keep the liquid level above the neck of the syringe or bag to prevent air bubbles from collecting in the system	Water helps clear the tubing and prevents clogging
For both continuous and intermittent tube feeding	
13. Remove the syringe or connecting tubing, and clamp the tube by inserting the plug and covering with a cap protector or with a gauze secured with a rubber band	This prevents back flow of the formula or stomach fluid

Contd...

Action/steps	Rationale
14. Wash the bag and tubing or other equipment with soap and water every 8 hours. Change the bag and tubing or syringe every 24 hours	To keep the bag and tubing free from infection
15. Remove gloves and wash hands	Prevents spread of microorganisms
Evaluation	
16. Assess patient for discomfort or complication such as nausea, vomiting and respiratory distress	Provides evidence of patient's tolerance of tube feedings
17. Monitor lab-values and measure weight daily	Assesses for malnutrition
Documentation	
18. It should contain type of formula given, amount, verification of tube placement, amount of residual if obtained, and any signs of intolerance of the feeding	Documents nutritional intake and any problem

TOTAL PARENTERAL NUTRITION

Total parenteral nutrition (TPN) is a method of delivering total nutrition through a catheter placed in a large central vein (e.g., subclavian vein). A large vein with high blood flow is needed to dilute the solution rapidly. The solution may also be infused through a port implanted in the patient's chest wall or a peripherally inserted central catheter (PICC). These options are used for patient receiving long-term therapy such as victims of massive burns, intestinal obstruction, inflammatory bowel disease, acquired immunodeficiency syndrome (AIDS) or cancer chemotherapy.

The TPN is composed of high concentrations of carbohydrates as the main source of energy. Protein is provided through solution of amino acids. Solutions of other essential nutrients are also added to the infusion. Fatty acids are administered through lipid solutions that are infused daily or several times per week. TPN solutions are started slowly to allow the body to adjust to the high level of glucose concentration and the hyperosmolality (increased concentration of solutes within the fluid) of the solution. Usually, 1,000–2,000 mL are administered in the first 24 hours. Later the infusion is increased until the desired amount is given. Monitoring of TPN should be ongoing. The infusion rate should be assessed throughout the shift. Attempts should not be made to catch up if the rate has slowed. The rapid infusion of glucose can be harmful to the patient.

Monitoring Total Parenteral Nutrition

Baseline levels of blood chemistry, vital signs, and nutritional status should be completed prior to beginning TPN infusion. Compare ongoing monitoring to baseline results (Table 4).

TABLE 4: Parameters to monitor Total parenteral nutrition

What to assess	When to assess
IV site (PICC, central line)	Every 4 hours; observe for redness, swelling or drainage from site
Patient response	Every shift, observe for signs of restlessness or discomfort
Blood glucose	Every 6–8 hours; report abnormal levels to physician
Vital signs	Every 4–8 hours; abnormal vital signs may signal development of complication
Weight	Daily or weekly as ordered
Intake and output	Every shift, abnormal urinary output may signal hyperglycemia or altered kidney function
Flow rate	Every 4 hours. Prevents hyperglycemic intolerance to TPN
Electrolytes, CBC, BUN	Daily or as ordered, evaluates patient's response
Nutritional status	Ongoing, include, weight, albumin levels, status of muscle mass

Abbreviations: BUN, blood urea nitrogen; CBC, complete blood count; IV, intravenous; PICC, peripherally inserted central catheter; TPN, total parenteral nutrition.

BIBLIOGRAPHY

1. Taylor CR, Lillis C, LeMone P, et al. *Fundamentals of Nursing – The Art and Science of Nursing Care*, 7th edition. Wolters Kluwer; 2010.
2. DeWit SC. *Fundamental Concepts and Skills for Nursing*. WB Saunders Company. 2000.
3. Berman AT, Snyder S, Kozier BJ, et al. *Kozier & Erb's. Fundamentals of Nursing: Concepts, Process and Practice*, 8th edition. Pearson Education.
4. Sharma S. *Potter and Perry's Fundamentals of Nursing. A South Asian edition*. Elsevier India.   Gurugram; 2013.

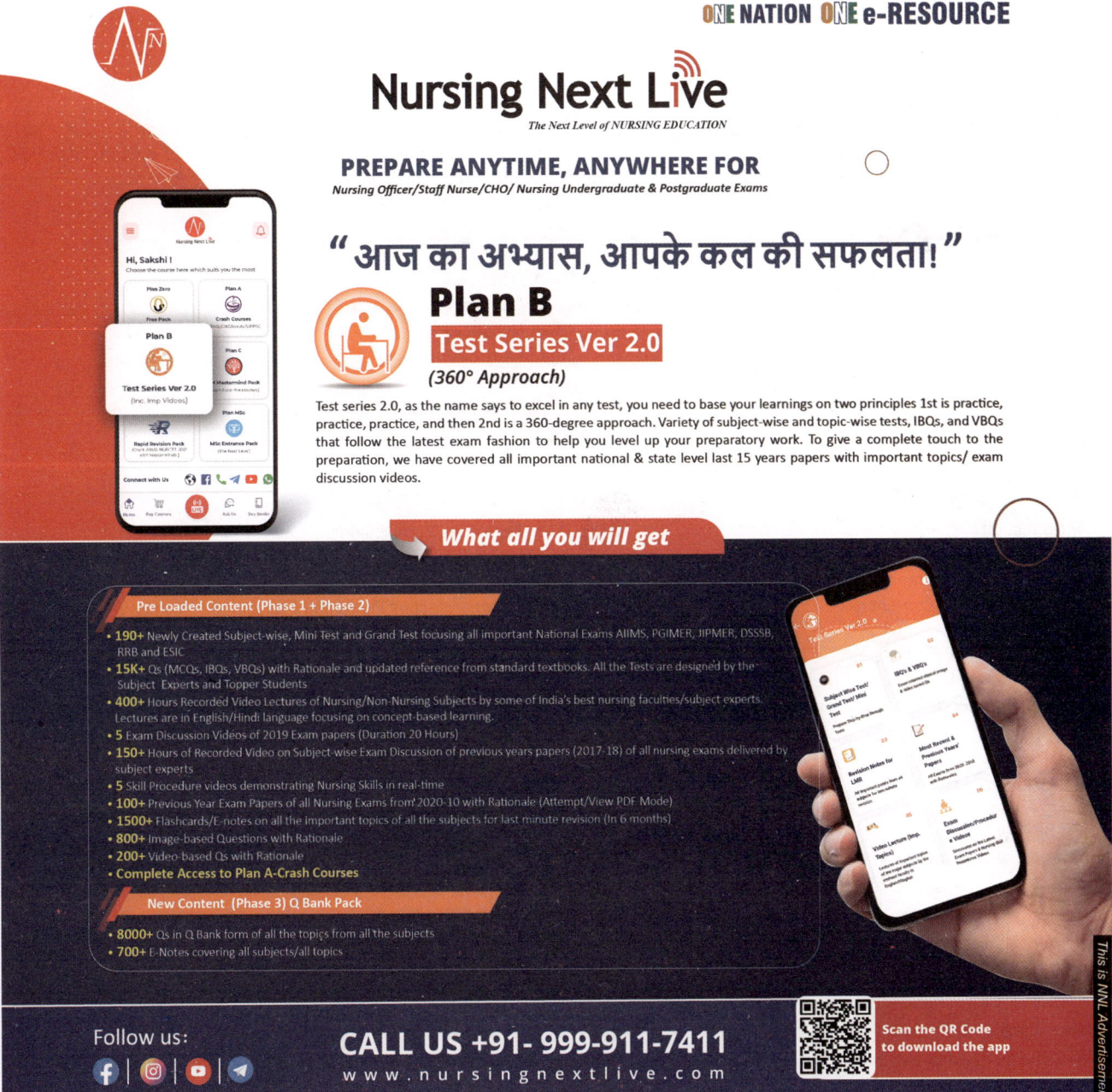

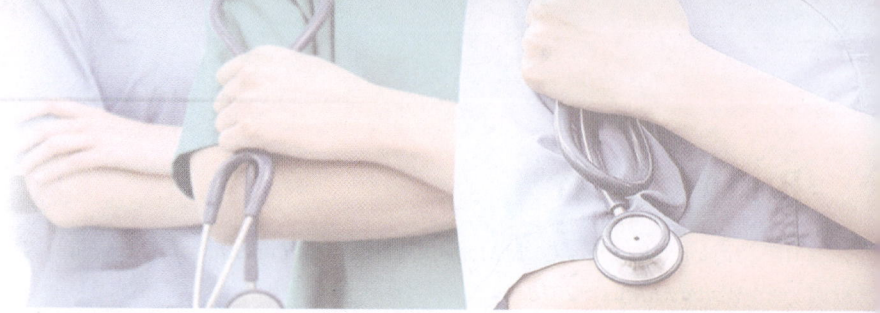

Fluid and Electrolyte Imbalance

INTRODUCTION

In good health, a delicate balance of fluids, electrolytes, acids and bases is maintained in the body. This balance, or physiologic homeostasis, depends on multiple physiologic processes that regulate fluid intake and output and the movement of water and the substances dissolved in it between the body compartments.

Almost every illness has the potential to threaten this balance. Even in daily living, excessive temperatures or vigorous activities can disturb the balance if adequate water and salt intake is not maintained. Therapeutic measures, such as the use of diuretics or nasogastric suction, can also disturb the body's homeostasis unless water and electrolytes are replaced.

BODY FLUIDS

As the primary body fluids, water is the most important nutrient of life. Although life can be sustained for many days without food, humans can survive for only a few days without water. Approximately, 60% of the average healthy adult's weight is water, the primary body fluid. In good health, this volume remains relatively constant and the person's weight varies by less than 0.2 kg (0.5 lb) in 24 hours, regardless of the amount of fluid ingested. Water in the body functions primarily to:

- Provide a medium for transporting nutrients to cells and wastes from cells, and for transporting substances such as hormones, enzymes, blood platelets, and red and white blood cells.
- Facilitate cellular metabolism and proper cellular chemical functioning
- Act as a solvent for electrolytes and non-electrolytes
- Help maintain normal body temperature
- Facilitate digestion and promote elimination
- Act as a tissue lubricant

Age, sex and body fat affect total body water. Infants have the highest proportion of water, accounting for 70–80% of their body weight. The proportion of body water decreases with aging. In people older than 60 years of age, it represents only about 50% of the total body weight. Women also have a lower percentage of body water than men. Women and the elderly have reduced body water due to decreased muscle mass and a greater percentage of fat tissue. Fat tissue is essentially free of water, whereas lean tissue contains a significant amount of water. Water makes up a greater percentage of a lean person's body weight than an obese person's body weight.

BODY FLUID COMPARTMENTS

Body fluids are located in two main compartments, or spaces in the body, the intracellular fluid (ICF) and extracellular fluid (ECF). ICF is the fluid within the cells, constituting about 40% of an adult's body weight or 70% of the total body water. ECF is all the fluid outside the cells. It constitutes about 20% of an adult's body weight, or 30% of total body water. ECF includes intravascular and interstitial fluids. Intravascular fluid, or plasma, is the liquid component of the blood (i.e., fluid found within the vascular system). Interstitial fluid is the fluid that surrounds tissue cells and includes lymph (Fig. 1).

Intracellular fluid is vital to functioning of a normal cell. It contains solutes such as oxygen, electrolytes, and glucose, and it provides a medium in which metabolic processes of the cell take place.

Although extracellular fluid is in the smaller proportion of the two compartments, it is the transport system that carries nutrients to the waste products from the cells. For example, plasma carries oxygen from the lungs and glucose from the gastrointestinal tract to the capillaries of the vascular system. From there, the oxygen and glucose move across the capillary membranes into the interstitial spaces and then across the cellular membranes into the cells. The opposite route is taken for waste products, such as carbon dioxide going from the cells to the lungs and metabolic acid wastes going eventually

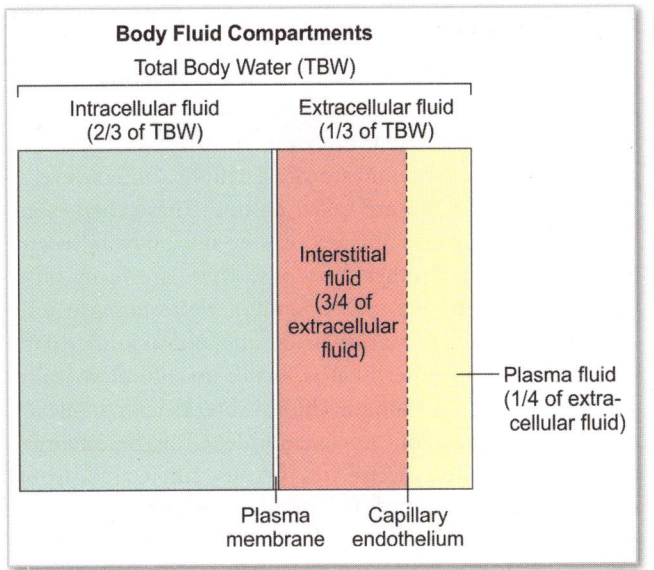

Fig. 1: Body fluid compartments

to the kidneys. Interstitial fluid transports wastes from the cells by way of the lymph system as well as directly into the blood plasma through capillaries.

The term total body water or fluid refers to the total amount of water in the body expressed as a percentage of body weight.

VARIATIONS IN FLUID CONTENT

In a healthy person, total body water constitutes about 50–60% of the body's weight, depending on factors such as the person's age, lean body mass, and sex (Table 1). For example, an infant has considerably more total body fluid and ECF than an adult does. Because ECF is more easily lost from the body than ICF, infants are more prone to fluid volume deficits.

The more obese a person is, the smaller the person's percentage of total body water when compared to body weight. Because women tend to have proportionally more body fat than men, they also have less body fluid than men. Similarly, the decreasing percentage of body fluid in older people is related to an increase in fat cells.

TABLE 1: Water percentage of body weight

Water compartment	Infant (%)	Adult man	Woman	Elderly person
Extracellular				
Intravascular	4	4	5	5
Interstitial	25	11	10	15
Intracellular	48	45	35	25
Total-body water	77	60	50	45

ELECTROLYTES

An **ion** is an atom or molecule carrying an electrical charge. Substances capable of breaking into electrically charged ions when dissolved in a solution are called **electrolytes**. Some ions develop positive charge and are called **cations**. Others develop a negative charge and are called **anions**. These charges are the basis of chemical interactions in the body necessary for metabolism and other functions. There are many other electrolytes in the body such as sodium, potassium, calcium, magnesium, chloride, bicarbonate, and phosphorus. Many salts dissociate in water, that is, break up into electrically-charged ions. The salt sodium chloride breaks up into one ion of sodium (Na^+) and one ion of chloride (Cl^-). These charged particles are called electrolytes because they are capable of conducting electricity. The number of ions that carry a positive charge, called cations, and ions that carry a negative charge called anions, should be equal.

Examples of cations are: sodium (Na^+), potassium (K^+), calcium (Ca^{2+}), and magnesium (Mg^{2+}). Examples of anions include chloride (Cl^-), bicarbonate (HCO_3^{2-}), phosphate (HPO_4^-) and sulfate (SO_4^{2-}).

Sulfate, an anion, is found primarily within cells. The organic acid anions such as lactic acid, which is a major anion, normally has an intermediary role in the cell metabolism. The anion potentiate functions in the process of diffusion to move substances to and from the capillaries. Plasma protein includes albumin, globulin, and fibrinogen. Other electrolytes are required for proper cell functioning but are found only in trace amounts in the body. One example is chromium. A well-balanced diet ordinarily ensures an adequate supply of required trace substances in the body.

Molecules in the body's chemical compounds that remain intact are called nonelectrolytes. In the human body, for example, urea and glucose are nonelectrolytes. **Solvents** are liquids that can hold a substance in solution; **solutes** are substances that are dissolved in a solution. Water is the primary solvent in the body. The solutes are electrolytes and nonelectrolytes.

Fluids in various compartments of the body differ in their constituents. For example, ICF has higher concentrations of certain electrolytes than ECF.

MEASUREMENT OF ELECTROLYTES

Electrolytes are measured in terms of their chemical combining power, or chemical activity. The milliequivalent (mEq) is the unit of measurement that describes the chemical activity of electrolytes. It is the capacity of cations to combine with anions to form molecules. This combining activity is measured in relation to the combining activity of the hydrogen ion (H^+). Thus, 1 mEq of either a cation or an anion is chemically equivalent to the activity of 1 mg of hydrogen. Therefore, 1 mEq of any cation is equivalent to 1 mEq of any anion.

For homeostasis, the total cations in the body are normally equal to the total anions. In healthy people, the mEq per liter for electrolytes in the body vary within a relatively narrow range. When electrolytes are not in balance, the person is at risk for alterations in health because electrolytes regulate water distribution and acid-base balance, and maintain a balanced degree of neuromuscular excitability.

Clinically, the mEq system is most often used. However, nurses need to be aware that different systems of measurement may be found when interpreting laboratory results. For example, calcium levels frequently are reported in mg/dL (1dL = 100mL) instead of mEq/L. It is also important to remember that laboratory tests are usually performed using blood plasma, an extracellular fluid. These results may reflect what is happening in the ECF, but it is generally not possible to directly measure electrolyte concentrations within the cells.

COMPOSITION OF BODY FLUIDS

Extracellular and intracellular fluids contain oxygen from the lungs, dissolved nutrients from the gastrointestinal tract, excretory products of metabolism such as carbon dioxide, and charged particles called ions. The composition of fluid varies from one body compartment to another. In ECF, the principal electrolytes are sodium, chloride, and bicarbonate. Other electrolytes such as potassium, calcium, and magnesium are also present but in smaller quantities (Fig. 2). Plasma and interstitial fluid, the two primary components of ECF, contain essentially the same electrolytes and solutes, with the exception of protein. Plasma is a protein-rich fluid, containing large amounts of albumin, but interstitial fluid contains little or no protein.

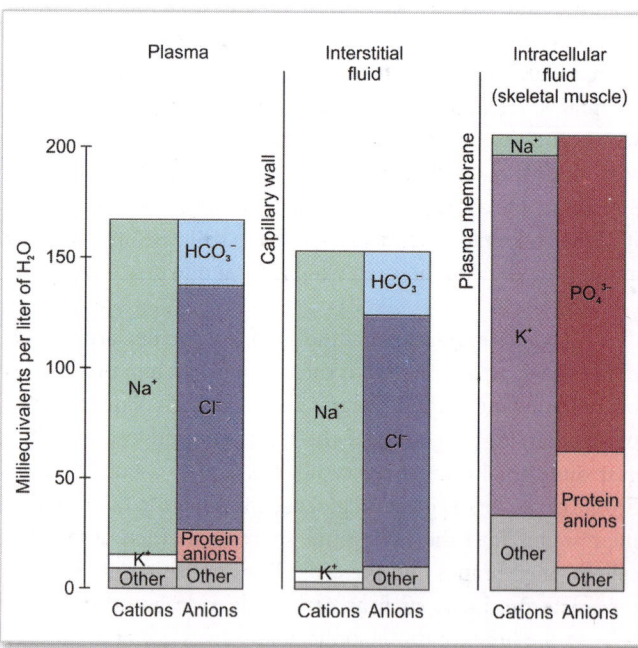

Fig. 2: Composition of body fluids

The composition of ICF differs significantly from that of ECF. Potassium and magnesium are the primary cations present in ICF, with phosphate and sulfate being the major anions. As in ECF, other electrolytes are present within the cell, but in much smaller concentrations.

Maintaining a balance of fluid volumes and electrolyte compositions in the fluid compartments of the body is essential to health. Normal and unusual fluid and electrolyte loss must be replaced if homeostasis is to be maintained.

Other body fluids such as gastric and intestinal secretions also contain electrolytes. This is of particular concern when these fluids are lost from the body. Fluid and electrolytes imbalance can result from excessive loss through these routes.

MOVEMENT OF BODY FLUIDS AND ELECTROLYTES

The body fluid compartments are separated from one another by cell membranes and the capillary membrane. While these membranes are completely permeable to water, they are considered to be selectively permeable to solutes as substances move across them with varying degrees of ease. Small particles such as ions, oxygen and carbon dioxide easily move across these membranes, but larger molecules like glucose and proteins have more difficulty moving between fluid compartments. The methods by which electrolytes and other solutes move are osmosis, diffusion, filtration, and active transport.

Osmosis

Osmosis is the movement of water across cell membranes, from the less concentrated solution to the more concentrated solution. In other words, water moves toward the higher concentration of solute in an attempt to equalize the concentrations (Fig. 3).

Solutes are substances dissolved in liquid. For example, when sugar is added to coffee, the sugar is the solute. Solutes maybe crystalloids (salts that dissolve readily into true solutions) or colloids (substances such as large protein molecules that do not readily dissolve into true solutions). A solvent is the component of a solution that can dissolve a solute. In the previous example, coffee is the solvent for the sugar.

In the body, water is the solvent; the solutes include electrolytes, oxygen and carbon dioxide, glucose, urea, amino acids and proteins. Osmosis occurs when the concentration of solutes on one side of a selectively permeable membrane, such as the capillary membrane, is higher than on the other side. For example, a marathon runner loses a significant amount of water through perspiration, increasing the concentration of solutes in the plasma because of water loss. This higher solute concentration draws water from the interstitial space and cells into the vascular compartment to equalize the concentrations of solutes in all fluid compartments. Osmosis is an important mechanism for maintaining homeostasis and fluid balance.

The concentration of the solutes in body fluids is usually expressed as the osmolality. Osmolality is determined by the total solute concentration within a fluid compartment and is measured as parts of solute per kilogram of water.

Osmolality is reported as milliosmols per kilogram (mOsm/kg). Sodium is by far the greatest determinant of serum osmolality, with glucose and urea also contributing to the same. Potassium, glucose and urea are the primary contributors to the osmolality of intracellular fluid. The term *tonicity* maybe used to refer to the osmolality of a fluid. Solutions may be termed isotonic, hypertonic, or hypotonic. An **isotonic** solution has the same osmolality as body fluids. Normal saline, 0.9% sodium chloride, is an isotonic solution. **Hypertonic** solution has a higher osmolality than body fluids; 3% sodium chloride is a hypertonic solution. **Hypotonic** solution such as one-half normal saline (0.45% sodium chloride), by contrast, have a lower osmolality than body fluids.

Osmotic pressure is the power of a solution to draw water across a semipermeable membrane. When two solutions of different solute concentrations are separated by a semipermeable membrane, the solution of higher solute concentration exerts a higher osmotic pressure, drawing water across the membrane to equalize the concentrations of the solutions. On the other hand, a hypotonic solution administered intravenously will cause the red blood cells (RBCs) to swell as water is drawn into the cells by their higher osmotic pressure. In the body, plasma proteins exert an osmotic draw called **colloid osmotic pressure** or osmotic pressure, pulling water from the interstitial space into the vascular compartment. This is an important mechanism in maintaining vascular volume.

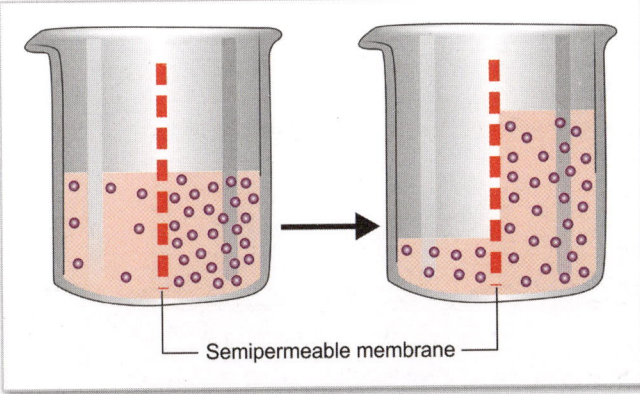

Fig. 3: Mechanism of osmosis

Semipermeable membrane

Diffusion

Diffusion is the continual intermingling of molecules in liquids, gases, or solids brought about by the random movement molecules. For example, two gases become mixed by the constant motion of their molecules. The process of diffusion occurs even when two substances are separated by a thin membrane. In the body, diffusion of water, electrolytes, and other substances occurs through the split pores of capillary membranes.

The rate of diffusion of substances varies according to (a) the size of the molecules, (b) the concentration of the solution, and (c) the temperature of the solution. Larger molecules move less quickly than smaller ones because they require more energy to move about. With diffusion, the molecules move from a solution of higher concentration to a solution of lower concentration (Fig. 4). Increase in temperature increases the rate of motion of molecules and therefore, increase the rate of diffusion.

Filtration

Filtration is a process whereby fluid and solutes move together across cell membrane from one compartment to another. The movement is from an area of higher pressure to one of lower pressure. An example of filtration is the movement of fluid and nutrients from the capillaries of the arterioles to the interstitial fluid around the cells. The pressure in the compartment that results in the movement of the fluid and substances dissolved in fluid out of the compartment is called **filtration pressure. Hydrostatic pressure** is the pressure exerted by a fluid within a closed system on the walls of a container in which it is contained.

The hydrostatic pressure of blood is the force exerted by the blood against the vascular walls (e.g., the artery wall). The principle involved in hydrostatic pressure is that fluids move from the area of greater pressure to the area of lesser pressure. Using the example of the blood vessels, the plasma proteins in the blood exert a colloid, osmotic or oncotic pressure that opposes the hydrostatic pressure and holds the fluid in the vascular compartment to maintain the vascular volume. When the hydrostatic pressure is greater than osmotic pressure, the fluid filters out of the blood vessels. The filtration pressure in this example is the difference between the hydrostatic pressure and the osmotic pressure.

Active Transport

Substances can move across cell membranes from a less concentrated solution to a more concentrated one by **active transport**. This process differs from diffusion and osmosis as metabolic energy is spent in it. In active transport, a substance combines with a carrier on the outside surface of the cell membrane, and they move to the inside surface of the cell membrane (Fig. 5). Once inside, they separate, and the substance is released to the inside of the cell. A specific carrier is required for each substance, enzymes are required for active transport, and energy is spent.

This process is of particular importance in maintaining the differences in sodium and potassium ion concentrations of ECF and ICF. Under normal conditions, sodium concentrations are higher in the ECF, and potassium concentrations are higher inside the cells. To maintain these proportions, the active transport mechanism (the sodium potassium pump) is activated, moving sodium from the cells and potassium into the cells.

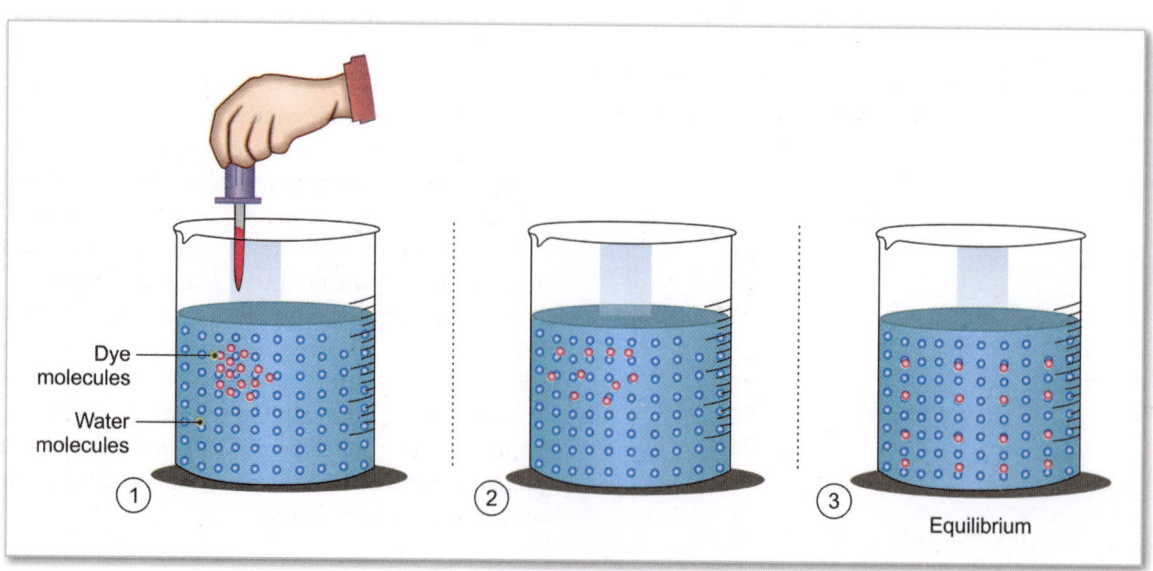

Dye molecules

Water molecules

① ② ③

Equilibrium

Fig. 4: Mechanism of diffusion

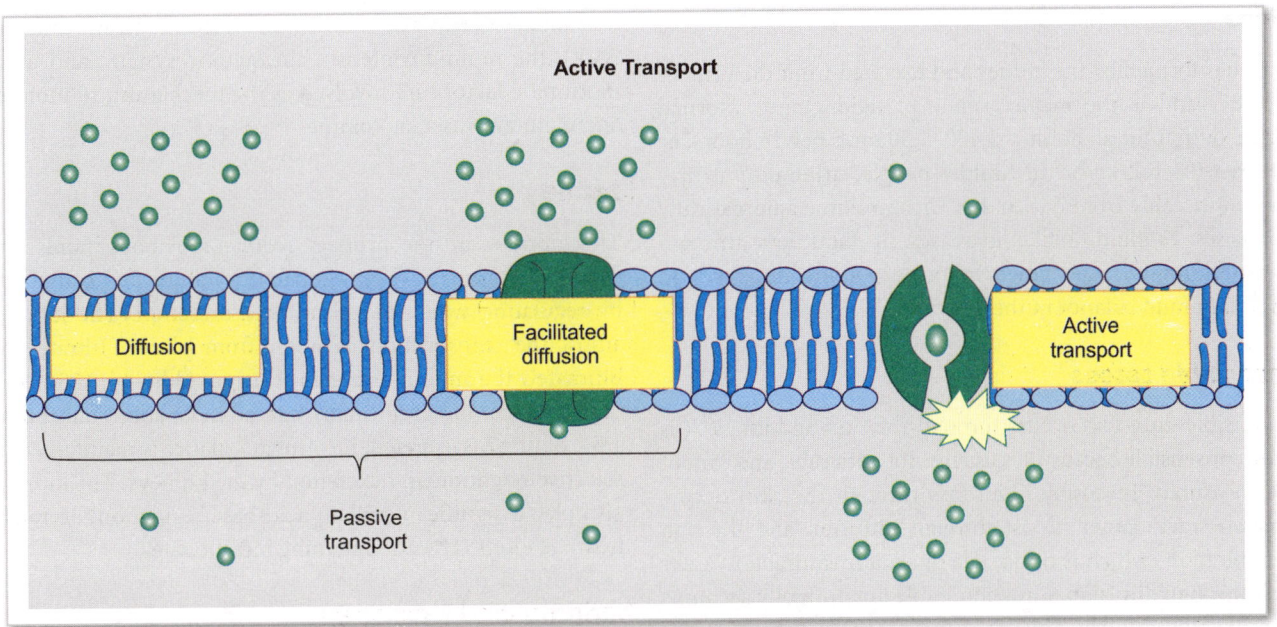

Fig. 5: Mechanism of active transport

REGULATING BODY FLUIDS

In a healthy person, the volumes and chemical composition of the fluid compartments stay within narrow safe limits. Normally fluid intake and fluid loss are balanced. Illness can upset this balance so that the body has too little or too much fluid.

Fluid Intake

During period of moderate activity at moderate temperature, the average adult drinks about 1,500 mL per day but needs 2,500 mL/day, an additional 1,000 mL. This added volume is acquired from foods and from the oxidation of these foods during metabolic processes. Increasingly, the water content of food is relatively large, contributing about 750 mL/day. The water content of fresh vegetables is approximately 90%, of fresh fruits 85%, and of lean meats around 60%.

Water as a by-product of food metabolism accounts for most of the remaining fluid volume required. This quantity is approximately 200 mL/day for the average adult.

The thirst mechanism is the primary regulator of fluid intake. The thirst center is located in the hypothalamus of the brain. A number of stimuli trigger this center, including the osmotic pressure of body fluids, vascular volume, and angiotensin (a hormone released in response to decreased blood flow to the kidney) for example, a long- distance runner loses significant amount of water through perspiration and rapid breathing during a race, increasing the concentration of solutes and the osmotic pressure of body fluids. This increased osmotic pressure stimulates the thirst center, causing the runner to experience the sensation of thirst and the desire to drink to replace lost fluids.

Thirst is normally relieved immediately after drinking a small amount of fluid, even before it is absorbed from the gastrointestinal tract. However, this relief is only temporary, and the thirst returns in about 15 minutes. The thirst is again temporarily relieved after the ingested fluid distends the upper gastrointestinal tract. These mechanisms protect the individual from drinking too much, because it takes from 30 minutes to 1 hour for the fluid to be absorbed and distributed throughout the body.

Fluid Output

Fluid loss from the body counter balance the adult's 2,500 mL average daily intake of fluid. There are four routes of fluid output:

- Urine
- Insensible loss through skin as perspiration and through the lungs as water vapor in the expired air
- Loss through the intestines in feces (Table 2)

TABLE 2: Average daily fluid output for an adult

Route	Amount (mL)
Urine	1,400–1,500
Insensible losses:	
Lungs	300–400
Skin	300–400
Sweat	100
Feces	100–200
Total	**2,300–2,600**

Urine

Urine is formed by the kidney and excreted from the urinary bladder and is the major avenue of fluid output. Normal urine output for an adult is 1,400–1,500 mL per 24 hours, or at least 0.5 mL/kg/hr. In healthy people, urine output may vary noticeably from day to day. Urine volume automatically increases as fluid intake increases. If fluid loss through perspiration is large, however, urine volume decreases to maintain fluid balance in the body.

Insensible Losses

Insensible fluid loss occurs through the skin and lungs. It is called insensible because it is usually not noticeable and cannot be measured. Insensible fluid loss through the skin occurs in two ways. Water is lost through diffusion and through perspiration (which is noticeable but not measurable). Water loss through diffusion is not noticeable but normally accounts for 300–400 mL/day. This loss can be significantly increased if the protective layer of the skin is lost as with burns or large abrasions. Perspiration varies depending on factors such as environmental temperature and metabolic activity. Fever and exercise increase metabolic activity and heat production, thereby increasing fluid loss through the skin.

Another type of insensible fluid loss is the water in exhaled air. In an adult, this is normally 300–400 mL/day. When respiratory rate accelerates, for example, due to exercise or an elevated body temperature, this loss can increase.

Feces

The chyme that passes from the small intestine into the large intestine contains water and electrolytes. The volume of chyme entering the large intestine in an adult is normally about 1,500 mL/day. Of this amount, all but about 100 mL is reabsorbed in the proximal half of the large intestine.

Certain fluid loss is required to maintain normal body functions. This is known as **obligatory loss**. Water lost through respirations, through the skin, and in feces accounts for obligatory loss necessary for temperature regulation and elimination of waste products. The total of all this loss is approximately 1,300 mL/day.

MAINTAINING HOMEOSTASIS

The volume and composition of body fluids is regulated through several homeostatic mechanisms. A number of body systems contribute to this regulation, including the kidneys, the endocrine system, the cardiovascular system, the lungs, and the gastrointestinal system. Hormones such as antidiuretic hormone (ADH; also known as arginine vasopressin or AVP), the renin-angiotensin-aldosterone system, and atrial natriuretic factors are involved as the mechanism to monitor and maintain vascular volume.

Kidney

The kidneys are the primary regulator of body fluids and electrolyte balance. They regulate the volume and osmolality by regulating water and electrolyte excretion. The kidneys adjust the reabsorption of water from plasma filtrate and ultimately the amount excreted as urine. Although 135–180 L of plasma per day is normally filtered in an adult, only about 1.5 L of urine is excreted. Electrolyte balance is maintained by selective retention and excretion by the kidneys. The kidneys also play a significant role in acid-base regulation, excreting hydrogen ions (H^+) and retaining bicarbonate.

Antidiuretic Hormone

ADH, which regulates water excretion from the kidney, is synthesized in the anterior portion of the hypothalamus and acts on the collecting duct of the nephrons. When serum osmolality rises, ADH is produced, causing the collecting ducts to become more permeable to water. This increased permeability allows more water to be reabsorbed into the blood. As more water is reabsorbed, urine output falls and serum osmolality decreases because the water dilutes body fluids. Conversely, if serum osmolality decreases, ADH is suppressed, the collecting ducts become less permeable to water, and urine output increases. Excess water is excreted, and serum osmolality returns to normal. Other factors also affect the production and release of ADH, including blood volume, temperature, pain, stress, and some drugs such as opiates, barbiturates, and nicotine.

Renin-Angiotensin-Aldosterone System

Specialized receptors in the glomerular cells of the kidney nephrons respond to changes in renal perfusion. This initiates the **renin-angiotensin-aldosterone system**. If blood flow or pressure to the kidney decreases, renin is released. Renin causes the conversion of angiotensinogen to angiotensin I, which is then converted to angiotensin II by angiotensin-converting enzyme. Angiotensin II acts directly on the nephrons to promote sodium and water retention. In addition, it stimulates the release of aldosterone from the adrenal cortex. Aldosterone also promotes sodium retention in the distal nephrons. The net effect of the renin-angiotensin-aldosterone system is to restore blood volume (and renal perfusion) through sodium and water retention.

Atrial Natriuretic Factor

Atrial natriuretic factor is released from cells in the atrium of the heart in response to excess blood volume and stretching of the atrial walls. Acting on the nephrons, atrial natriuretic factor promotes sodium wasting and acts as a potent diuretic, thus reducing vascular volume. Atrial natriuretic factor also inhibits thirst that reduces fluid intake.

REGULATING ELECTROLYTES

Electrolytes, charged ions capable of conducting electricity, are present in all body fluids and fluid compartments. Although the concentration of specific electrolytes differs between fluid compartments, a balance of cations (positively charged ions) and anions (negatively charged ions) always exists. Electrolytes are important for:

- Maintaining fluid balance
- Contributing to acid-base regulation
- Facilitating enzyme reactions
- Transmitting neuromuscular reactions

Most electrolytes enter the body through dietary intake and are excreted in the urine. Some electrolyte, such as sodium and chloride, are not stored by the body and must be consumed daily to maintain normal levels. Potassium and calcium, on the other hand, are stored in the cells and bone, respectively. When serum levels drop, ions can shift out of the storage "pool" into the blood to maintain adequate serum levels for normal functioning (Table 3).

TABLE 3: Regulation and functions of electrolytes

Electrolyte	Regulation	Functions
Sodium (Na$^+$)	• Renal reabsorption and/or excretion • Aldosterone increase Na$^+$ reabsorption in collecting ducts of nephrons	• Regulating ECF volume and distribution • Maintaining blood volume • Transmitting nerve impulses and contracting muscles
Potassium (K$^+$)	• Renal excretion and conservation • Aldosterone increases K+ excretion • Movement into and out of cells • Insulin helps move K$^+$ into cells; tissue damage and acidosis shift K$^+$ out of cells into ECF	• Maintaining ICF osmolality • Transmitting nerve and other electrical impulses • Regulating cardiac impulses transmission and muscle contraction • Skeletal and smooth muscle function • Regulating acid-base balance
Calcium (Ca^{2+})	• Redistribution between bones and ECF • Parathyroid hormone and calcitriol increases serum Ca^{2+} levels; calcitonin decreases serum levels	• Forming bones and teeth • Transmitting nerve impulses • Regulating muscle contraction • Maintaining cardiac pacemaker (automaticity) • Blood clotting • Activating enzymes such as pancreatic lipase and phospholipase
Magnesium (Mg^{2+})	• Conservation and excretion by kidney • Intestinal absorption increased by vitamin D and parathyroid hormone	• Intracellular metabolism • Operating sodium-potassium pump • Relaxing muscle contraction • Transmitting nerve impulses • Regulating cardiac functions
Chloride (Cl$^-$)	• Excreted and reabsorbed along with sodium in the kidney • Aldosterone increases chloride reabsorption with sodium	• HCl production • Regulating ECF balance and vascular volume • Regulating acid-base balance • Buffer in oxygen-carbon dioxide exchange in RBCs
Phosphate (PO$_4^-$)	• Excretion and reabsorption by the Kidney • Parathyroid hormone decreases serum levels by increasing renal excretion • Reciprocal relationship with calcium; increasing serum calcium levels decrease phosphate levels; decreasing serum calcium increases phosphate	• Forming bones and teeth • Metabolizing carbohydrate, protein and fat • Cellular metabolism; producing ATP and DNA • Muscle, nerve and RBC function • Regulating acid-base balance • Regulating calcium levels
Bicarbonate (HCO$_3^-$)	• Excretion and reabsorption by the Kidney • Regeneration by the kidney	• Major body buffer involved in acid-base regulation

Abbreviations: ATP adenosine triphosphate; DNA, deoxyribose nucleic acid; ECF, extracellular fluid; ICF, intracellular fluid; RBC red blood cells

Sodium (Na⁺)

Chief electrolyte of ECF that moves easily between interstitial spaces and moves across cell membranes by active transport; influential in many chemical reactions in the body, particularly in nervous tissue cells and muscle tissue cells. Normal serum sodium levels are 135–145 mEq/L. Sodium functions largely in controlling and regulating water balance. When sodium is reabsorbed from the kidney tubules, chloride and water are reabsorbed with it, thus maintaining ECF volume. Sodium is found in many foods, such as bacon, ham, processed cheese and table salt.

Potassium (K⁺)

Potassium is the major cation in intracellular fluids, with only a small amount found in plasma and interstitial fluid. ICF levels of potassium are usually 125–140 mEq/L while normal serum potassium levels are 3.5–5.0 mEq/L. The ratio of intracellular to extracellular potassium must be maintained for neuromuscular response to stimuli. Potassium is a vital electrolyte for skeletal, cardiac and smooth muscle activity. It is involved in maintaining acid-base balance as well, and it contributes to intracellular enzyme reactions. Potassium must be ingested daily because the body can't conserve it. Many fruits and vegetables, meat, fish, and other foods contain potassium (Table 4).

Calcium (Ca²⁺)

The vast majority, 99%, of calcium in the body is in the skeletal system, with a relatively small amount in ECF. Although this calcium outside the bones and teeth amounts to only about 1% of the total calcium in the body, it is vital in regulating muscle contraction and relaxation, neuromuscular function, and cardiac function. ECF calcium is regulated by a complex interaction of parathyroid hormone, calcitonin, and calcitriol, a metabolite of vitamin D. When calcium levels in the ECF fall, parathyroid hormone and calcitriol cause calcium to be released from bones into ECF and increase the absorption of

TABLE 4: Potassium-rich foods

Vegetables	Fruits	Meat and fish	Beverages
Avocado	Dried fruits (e.g., raisins and dates)	Beef	Milk
Raw carrot	Banana	Cod	Orange juice
Baked potatoes	Apricot	Pork	Apricot nectar
Raw tomato	Cantaloupe	Veal	
Spinach	Orange		

calcium in the intestine, thus raising serum calcium levels. Conversely, calcitonin stimulates the deposition of calcium in bone, reducing the concentration of calcium ions in the blood.

With aging, the intestine absorbs calcium less effectively and more calcium is excreted via the kidneys. Calcium shift out of the bone to replace this ECF loss, increasing the risk of osteoporosis and fractures of the wrist, vertebrae, and hips. Lack of weight bearing exercise (which helps keep calcium in the bones) and a vitamin D deficiency because of inadequate exposure to sunlight contribute to this risk.

Milk and milk products are the richest sources of calcium with other foods such as dark green leafy vegetables and canned salmon containing smaller amounts. Many clients benefit from calcium supplements.

Magnesium (Mg²⁺)

Magnesium is primarily found in the skeleton and in ICF. It is the second most abundant intracellular cation with normal serum levels of 1.5–2.5 mEq/L. It is important for intracellular metabolism, being particularly involved in the production and use of adenosine triphosphate (ATP). Magnesium also is necessary for protein and deoxyribonucleic acid (DNA) synthesis within the cells. Only about 1% of the body's magnesium is in ECF; here it is involved in regulating neuromuscular and cardiac functions. Cereal grains, nuts, dried fruits, legumes, and green leafy vegetables are good sources of magnesium in the diet, as are dairy products, meat, and fish.

Chloride (Cl⁻)

Chloride is the major anion of ECF, and normal serum levels are 95–108 mEq/L. Chloride functions with sodium to regulate serum osmolality and blood volume. The concentration of chloride in ECF is regulated secondarily to sodium; when sodium is reabsorbed in the kidney, chloride usually follows. Chloride is a major component of gastric juice as hydrochloric acid and is involved in regulating acid-base balance. It also acts as a buffer in the exchange of oxygen and carbon dioxide in red blood cells (RBCs). Chloride is found in the same foods as sodium.

Phosphate (PO₄⁻)

Phosphate is the major anion of intracellular fluid. It is also found in ECF, bone, skeletal muscle, and nerve tissue. Normal serum levels of phosphate in adults range from 2.5–4.5 mg/dL. Children must have higher phosphate level than adult, with that of new born nearly twice that of an adult. Higher levels of growth hormone and a faster rate of skeletal growth probably account for this difference. Phosphate is involved in many chemical actions of the cell; it is essential for functioning of muscles, nerves, and RBCs. It is also involved in the metabolism of proteins fats and carbohydrates. Phosphate is absorbed from the intestine and is found in many foods such as meat, fish, poultry, milk products, and legumes.

Bicarbonate (HCO$_3^-$)

Bicarbonate is present in both intracellular and extracellular fluids. Its primary function is regulating acid-base balance as an essential component of the carbonic acid-bicarbonate buffering system. Extracellular bicarbonate levels are regulated by the kidneys. Bicarbonate is excreted when it is present in excessive amount; if more is needed, the kidneys both regenerate and reabsorb bicarbonate ions. Unlike other electrolytes that must be consumed in the diet, adequate amounts of bicarbonate are produced through metabolic processes to meet the body's needs.

FACTORS AFFECTING FLUIDS AND ELECTROLYTES BALANCE

Age

Infants and growing children have greater fluid turnover than adults because their higher metabolic rate increases fluid loss. Infant lose more fluids through the kidney because immature kidneys are less able to conserve water than adult kidneys. In addition, infant's respirations are more rapid and the body surface area is proportionally greater than that of adults, increasing insensible water loss.

In elderly people, the normal aging process may affect fluid balance. The thirst response often is blunted. Antidiuretic hormone levels remain normal or may even be elevated, but the nephrons are less able to conserve water in response to ADH. Increased levels of atrial antidiuretic factor seen in older adults may also contribute to this impaired ability to conserve water. These normal changes of aging increase the risk of dehydration. When combined with the increased likelihood of heart diseases, impaired renal function, and multiple drug regimens, the older adult's risk for fluid and electrolyte imbalance is significant.

Gender and Body Size

Total body water is also affected by gender and body size. Because fat cells contain little or no water, and lean tissue has high water content, people with a higher percentage of body fat have less body fluid. Women have proportionately more body fat and less body water than men. Water accounts for approximately 60% of an adult man's weight, but only 52% for an adult woman. In an obese individual, this may even be less, with water responsible for only 30–40% of the person's weight.

Environmental Temperature

People with an illness and those participating in strenuous activity are at risk for fluid and electrolyte imbalances when the environmental temperature is high. Fluid loss through sweating is increased in hot environment as the body attempts to dissipate heat. This loss is even greater in people who have not been acclimatized to the environment.

Both salt and water are lost through sweating. When only water is replaced, salt depletion is at risk. The person who is salt depleted may experience fatigue, weakness, headache, and gastrointestinal symptoms such as anorexia and nausea. The risk of adverse effects is even greater if loss of water is not replaced. Body temperature rises, and the person is at risk for heat exhaustion or heat stroke. Heat stroke may occur in older adults or sick people during prolonged periods of heat; it can also affect athletes and laborers when their heat production exceeds the body's ability to dissipate heat.

Lifestyle

Other factors such as diet, exercise, and stress affect fluid and electrolyte balance.

Regular weight-bearing physical exercise such as walking, running, or cycling has a beneficial effect on calcium balance. The rate of bone loss that occurs in postmenopausal women and older men is slowed with regular exercise, reducing the risk of osteoporosis.

Stress can increase cellular metabolism, blood glucose concentration and catecholamine levels. In addition, stress can increase production of ADH, which in turn decreases urine production. The overall response of the body to stress is to increase the blood volume.

Heavy alcohol consumption affects electrolyte balance, increasing the risk of low calcium, magnesium, and phosphate levels. The risk of acidosis associated with breakdown of fat tissue also is greater in the person who drinks large amount of alcohol.

FLUID IMBALANCE

A number of factors such as illness, trauma, surgery and medications can affect the body's ability to maintain fluid and electrolyte balance. The kidneys play a major role in maintaining fluid and electrolyte balance and renal disease is a significant cause of imbalance. Clients who are confused or unable to communicate their needs are at risk for inadequate fluid intake. Vomiting, diarrhea, or nasogastric suction can cause significant fluid loss. Tissue trauma, such as burns, causes fluid and electrolytes to be lost from damaged cells. Decreased blood flow to the kidneys due to impaired cardiac function stimulates the renin-angiotensin-aldosterone system, causing sodium and water retention. Medications such as diuretics or corticosteroids can result in abnormal losses of electrolytes and fluid loss or retention. Diseases such as diabetes mellitus or chronic obstructive lung disease may affect acid-base balance.

Diabetic ketoacidosis, cancer, and head injury may also lead to electrolyte imbalances.

Fluid imbalance is refined in terms of fluid volume deficit, fluid volume excess, dehydration (hyperosmolar imbalance) and over-hydration (hypoosmolar imbalance).

Fluid Volume Deficit

Isotonic fluid volume deficit (FVD) occurs when the body loses both water and electrolytes from the ECF in similar proportions. Thus, the decreased volume of fluid remains isotonic. In FVD, fluid is initially lost from the intravascular compartment, so it is often called hypovolemia. FVD generally occurs as a result of abnormal losses through the skin gastrointestinal tract or kidney, decreased intake of fluid, bleeding, or movement of fluid into third space.

Risk Factors

- Loss of water and electrolytes from:
  - Vomiting
  - Diarrhea
  - Excessive sweating
  - Polyuria
  - Fever
  - Nasogastric suction
  - Abnormal drainage or wound
- Insufficient intake due to:
  - Anorexia
  - Nausea
  - Inability to access fluids
  - Impaired swallowing
  - Confusion, depression

Clinical Manifestations

- Complains of weight loss and thirst
  Weight loss FVD
  - 2% Loss – Mild
  - 5% Loss – Moderate
  - 8% Loss – Severe
- Fluid intake less than output
- Decreased tissue turgor, dry mucous membrane, sunken eyeballs, decreased tears
- Subnormal temperature, weak and rapid pulse
- Decreased blood pressure, postural hypotension
- Flat neck veins, decreased capillary refill, decreased central venous pressure (CVP), decreased urine volume
- Increased urine specific gravity, hematocrit and blood urea nitrogen (BUN).

Dehydration

Dehydration, or hyperosmolar imbalance, occurs when the water is lost from the body leaving the client with excess sodium. Because water is lost while electrolytes, particularly sodium, are retained, the serum osmolarity and serum sodium levels are increased. Water is drawn into vascular compartment from the interstitial space and cells, resulting in cellular dehydration. Older adults are at particular risk for dehydration because of decreased thirst sensation. This type of water deficit also can affect clients who are hyperventilating or have prolonged fever or are in diabetic ketoacidosis and those receiving enteral feedings with insufficient water intake.

Etiology

Average daily fluid intake for adults is about 1,500–2,000 mL. In addition, about 800 mL of fluid is consumed through solid foods. Fluid balance is maintained in the body because the intake of fluids equals the excretion of fluids. This simple concept can be used to explain common causes of fluid imbalance. A lack of fluid intake, excessive fluid output, or both can lead to dehydration. Conversely, excessive fluid intake and a lack of fluid excretion can lead to overhydration.

Lack of Fluid Intake

Cognitive and physical impairments can quickly reduce water intake. For example, clients who are hospitalized, chairbound, or bedbound may not be able to reach to their water or may be too confused to realize they are thirsty. Clients with dysphagia are at risk for aspiration or may not be able to swallow fluids safely. Tube-fed clients who are not given adequate free water or who are fed hypertonic formulas are also at risk.

Impaired thirst mechanism can also decrease fluid intake. The thirst mechanism is usually triggered by low blood pressure or fluid volume depletion as small as 0.5%. The sensation of a dry mouth arises from salivary gland dysfunction, head or neck radiation, smoking, mouth breathing, oxygen therapy, hyperventilation, and anticholinergic medications.

Osmolality also influences thirst. Hypo-osmolality inhibits the thirst response; conversely, hyperosmolality leads to thirst. It is common to find comatose and confused people with high plasma osmolality, but they are unable to recognize the urge to drink.

Excess Fluid Loss

Unmonitored use of potent diuretics (e.g., furosemide), severe vomiting, and diarrhea are common causes of dehydration. These conditions are commonly associated with changes in levels of electrolytes. Potential causes of fluid loss include fever, diaphoresis, hyperglycemia, gastrointestinal suction, ileostomy, fistulae, burns, blood loss, hyperventilation, hyperthyroidism, decreased antidiuretic hormone (ADH) secretion, diabetes insipidus (nephrogenic and neurogenic), Addison's disease or adrenal crisis, and the diuretic phase of acute renal failure.

Again, older adults are at risk for excessive fluid loss for several reasons, decreased renal concentration of urine, an altered ADH response, and increased body fat and thus a decrease in total quantity of body water in proportion to body weight. Increased drug-drug interactions and multiple chronic diseases potentiate the risk for fluid imbalances.

Pathophysiology

Fluids are normally found in three spaces: inside the cells (intracellular), around the cells (interstitial), and in the blood stream (intravascular). The pathophysiology of dehydration is seen when the normal compensation for fluid loss in the blood stream cannot be corrected by stored fluids elsewhere. When fluids are lost from the intravascular spaces because of lack of intake or excess loss, interstitial fluids move in to restore vascular volume. Because the actual amount of fluid in the interstitial space is limited, other compensation systems are initiated to restore fluid volume. ADH and aldosterone secretion increase to reabsorb water and sodium in the kidney. Fluids are also reabsorbed from the ileum and large intestine. The baroreceptors sense low blood pressure, and the sympathetic nervous system is stimulated to increase peripheral vasoconstriction and the heart rate. Vasoconstriction moves fluids from the periphery into the circulation. Increasing sodium level in the blood is also sensed by the osmoreceptors in the hypothalamus, which signals the thirst mechanism. These compensatory processes occur repeatedly in normal healthy people. When fluid loss continues or when the compensation fails to restore blood volume, the person becomes dehydrated.

If the dehydration is not corrected, fluid is shifted from the cells into the vascular system. The loss of cellular fluid is dangerous because the cells need fluid for cellular function. Less fluid is available for temperature regulation via sweating, and a lowered blood volume decreases the body's ability to transport core heat to the periphery for conductive loss. There is less cerebrospinal fluid and less fluid in the fat pads around the eyes. If cerebral cells become dehydrated, thought processes may be impaired. The cerebral vessels may be stretched and they may bleed or undergo a spasm. If sodium is lost, the muscle and nerve functions that depend on this electrolyte are slowed.

Clinical Manifestations

Loss of Body Weight

Fairly rapid weight loss is an early and common result of fluid loss because water is a major portion of body weight. Mild dehydration exists when the client has lost 2% of body weight. For example, in a client who weighs 150 pounds (68 kg), a 2% loss equals 1.4 L of water. Weight is the most accurate measure of fluid status. Weight-if measured at the same time, on the same scale, and with the same clothes on the client is less subject to errors than is measurement of intake and output.

Changes in Intake and Output

Intake and output measurements provide another means of assessing fluid balance. This data provides insight into the cause of the imbalance (such as decreased fluid intake or increased fluid loss). These measurements are not as accurate as body weight; however, because of relative risk of errors in recording and insensible water loss, it is not measured.

A urine output of 400–500 mL/day (16–20 mL/hr) is considered oliguria and indicates a marked compromise in kidney function. In most people, urine output varies throughout the day. Normally, urine output is low and concentration is higher during the night. Thus the view that urine should flow constantly at 30–40 mL/hr appears to lack justification. Clients who are at risk of becoming dehydrated because they do not have the ability to concentrate urine are those who produce inadequate amount of ADH (e.g., clients with diabetes insipidus), those who do not respond normally to ADH (e.g., older adults), and those with inability to concentrate urine (e.g., clients with kidney failure)

Changes in Vital Signs

Inadequate fluid volume also leads to a decrease in systolic blood pressure, a weak pulse, and a decrease in CVP and pulmonary capillary wedge pressure (PCWP). For every liter of fluid lost, the cardiac output decreases by 1 L/min, the heart rate increases by 8 beats/min, and the core temperature increases by 0.3°C (0.60°F). Postural hypotension is one of the most sensitive indicators of decreased fluid volume. Postural or orthostatic hypotension is a decrease in systolic blood pressure of more than 20 mm Hg or a decrease in diastolic pressure of more than 10 mm Hg accompanied by an increase in pulse rate within 3 minutes of standing.

Sympathetic nervous system stimulation leads to vasoconstriction and increases the heart rate to compensate for the altered tissue perfusion.

Flat jugular veins in a supine position and a prolonged peripheral venous filling time of more than 5 seconds are noted. Because of the inability to cool the body core, an elevated temperature is common and can reach up to 105°F.

Other Manifestations of Dehydration

The mucous membrane of the mouth and eyes become dry even though fluid is received from the interstitial spaces. The lips can crack, and furrows may be seen on the tongue. Swallowing can become difficult.

TABLE 5: Clinical manifestations of dehydration

Clinical manifestations	Mild dehydration	Moderate dehydration	Severe dehydration
Level of consciousness	Alert	Lethargic	Obtunded
Capillary refill time	2 seconds	2–4 seconds	Greater than 4 seconds Cold limbs
Mucous membrane	Normal	Dry	Parched, cracked
Heart rate	Slight increase	Increased	Very increased
Respiratory rate	Normal	Increased	Increased and hyperpnea
Blood pressure	Normal	Normal, but orthostatic	Decreased
Pulse	Normal	Thread	Faint or non-palpable
Skin turgor	Normal	Slow	Tenting
Eyes	Normal	Sunken	Very sunken
Urine output	Decreased	Oliguria	Oliguria/anuria

Testing of the skin (decreased turgor) occurs when the skin tissues tend to stick together because of the decreased interstitial fluid. Soft and sunken eyes may be noted. Muscle weakness from an imbalance of sodium and potassium occurs early and becomes worse as the deficit progresses. Feces becomes hard and less in amount because of compensatory reabsorption of fluid from the colon.

Cerebral signs are always considered serious because it means that ICF compartmental shifting has occurred. Early signs include apprehension, restlessness, and headache. As the fluid deficit progresses, hallucinations, maniacal behavior, and confusion occurs, followed by coma (Table 5).

Diagnostic Findings

In hyperosmolar fluid deficit, more solvent (water in the plasma) is lost than solute (cells and electrolytes in the plasma), which creates hemoconcentration. Plasma sodium concentration is also increased (Hypernatremia). The following elevations are typical findings secondary to a hemoconcentrated state:

- Osmolality greater than 295 mOsm/kg
- Plasma sodium greater than 145 mEq/L
- BUN level greater than 25 mg/dL (in the presence of normal creatinine).
- Plasma glucose level greater than 120 mg/dL

- Hematocrit greater than 55%
- Urine specific gravity greater than 1.030

How to Calculate Plasma Osmolality

To calculate plasma osmolality, you must know the sodium, glucose, and BUN level:

➡ 2 × plasma Na = plasma osmolality
➡ 2 × plasma Na + (BUN ÷ 3) + (Glucose ÷ 18) = plasma osmolality

Outcome Management

A thorough history and physical examination, including collection of demographic variables as age, gender, culture, presence of chronic diseases, and socioeconomic status, is critical in identifying realistic and measurable outcomes. Medical treatment of dehydration depends on the acuteness and severity of the fluid deficit. The goals of treatment are to restore normal fluid volumes by using fluids similar in composition to those lost, to replace ongoing loss, and to correct the underlying problems.

Fluid Restoration

Oral Rehydration

If the fluid loss is mild, the thirst mechanism is intact, and the client can drink fluid and replace the fluids orally. How much is adequate? There are several standard formulas, but the one with the most positive outcomes for the older adult is based on body weight. One formula suggests providing 100 mL for the first 10 kg and 50 mL for the next 10 kg, and adding these numbers to 15 mL for the remaining number of kilograms. Another formula recommends 1.5 mL/kg of intake to meet the increased needs related to sensible losses that occur with activity and other environmental stressors. Oral glucose replacement solutions are palatable, inexpensive, and a good source of fluids, glucose, and electrolytes. For diabetic clients, who need less glucose, Pedialyte is a good alternative. These solutions are quickly absorbed even when the client has diarrhea or is vomiting. Cola drinks should be avoided because they do not contain adequate electrolyte replacement. The sugar content may lead to osmotic diuresis and the caffeine may lead to diuresis.

Intravenous Rehydration

When the fluid loss is severe or life threatening, intravenous (IV) fluids are used for replacement. The volume of fluid is calculated on the basis of the client's weight and the presence of any other comorbidities, such as cardiac, renal, liver, or pulmonary disorders that would decrease the ability of the body to get rid of excess fluids. The type of solution used is based on the type of fluid lost from the body. Generally, isotonic, hypertonic and hypotonic solutions are used.

Monitoring for Complications of Fluid Restoration

Fluid administration is based on the client's overall condition. A client with severe dehydration accompanied by severe heart, pulmonary, liver, or kidney disease cannot tolerate large volumes of fluid or sodium without the risk for development of heart failure. For unstable clients, monitors are used to detect increasing pressures from fluids (e.g., measurement of right atrial and pulmonary artery pressure). If the deficit has existed for more than 24 hours, it is dangerous to correct this deficit too rapidly. Urine output, body weight, and laboratory values of sodium level, osmolality, BUN level, and potassium level are monitored closely. However, it is important to note that BUN level may not be an accurate indicator in someone with protein deficit (lack of intake, kidney or liver disease) and BUN level can be elevated from bleeding or excessive nitrogen breakdown.

Correction of the Underlying Problem

Antiemetic and antidiarrheal drugs may be prescribed to correct problems with nausea and vomiting or diarrhea. Antibiotics may be used in clients with infectious diarrhea. Antipyretic agents may be used to reduce body temperature. Clients who are taking diuretics should have a consultation regarding the benefits versus the risks of continuing the medication.

Nursing Management

Assessment

At the time of admission, obtain the client's history of fluid loss. If the cause is infectious, isolation may be warranted. Determine a history of chronic illnesses that may impair the ability to tolerate fluids at rapid speed. Obtain any advance directives that would rather alter the use or course of fluid resuscitation. Examine the client completely, recording baseline data on lung and heart sounds, skin condition, vital signs, height and weight. Ask the client for height measurement but weigh the client yourself; do not rely on the client's stated weight. Orthostatic hypotension may be present, so help the client onto the scale.

Assess the client's vital signs every 2–4 hours, depending on the severity of the fluid loss; compare them with baseline vital signs and report marked differences. Assess for postural (orthostatic) blood pressure and pulse changes by taking blood pressure and pulse measurement with the client lying down. Then have the client stand up; repeat the blood pressure and pulse measurement after 1 minute. Report a drop in the standing systolic blood pressure of 20 mm Hg or more from the supine blood pressure measurement. Autonomic neuropathy seen in diabetes, dysrhythmias, and some medications (e.g., antihypertensive agents) can also cause hypotension.

Assess the peripheral vein filling time daily. Veins with normal fluid volume should fill in 3–5 seconds when the arm is lowered below the level of the heart.

Monitor intake, output, and daily weights accurately in high-risk clients. Be certain that all sources of intake (including liquids with meals and between meals, with medications, in IV lines, in tube-feedings, and in IV or tube flushes) and all sources of output (including urine, diarrhea, diaphoresis, and hyperventilation) are recorded accurately. If dehydration is mild, assess urine output every 8 hours and compare daily outputs. Instruct the client to report fluids consumed in addition to the fluids on food trays and if urine output is not measured.

Weigh the client daily on the same scale, at the same time of day, with the client wearing clothing of similar weight. Analyze changes in daily weights. A loss of 2.2 pounds is equivalent to 1 L of fluid. Therefore an 8-pound weight loss equals about 3.5 L of fluids, or a moderate fluid volume deficit.

Assess the oral cavity between the gums and cheek for dryness of the mucous membranes and the tongue for dryness and longitudinal furrows. Assess closely for dried and adherent mucus on the soft palate.

Check the skin turgor by gently pinching and lifting the skin. Usually, skin returns to a normal position within 1 or 2 seconds in people younger than 65 years of age. A slower response may indicate loss of interstitial fluids. Generalized weakness may develop because of changes in sodium levels.

Monitor plasma sodium, BUN, glucose, and hematocrit levels to determine plasma osmolality. Assess for confusion, an early manifestation of ICF involvement.

Diagnosis

Deficit in fluid volume related to insufficient fluid intake, vomiting, diarrhea, hemorrhage, or third-space fluid loss such as ascites or burns.

Outcome

The desired outcome is return of normal levels of body fluids. The goal statement may be that the client will have restoration of normal fluid volume, improvement in fluid volume, or no further fluid loss depending on the clinical situation. Indicators of adequate fluid volumes include the following:

- Oral intake between 1500 and 2500 mL or more in 24 hours
- Urine output greater than 0.5 mL/kg/hr
- Stable blood pressure and pulse in the supine and standing positions
- Increasing body weight of about 0.5–1 pound/day
- Absence of crackles (fluid in alveoli), an indicator of pulmonary fluid overload
- Moist tongue and mucous membranes

- Mental status returned to baseline
- BUN, plasma sodium, hematocrit, and osmolality levels approaching normal or baseline ranges over the first 48–72 hours.

Interventions

Restore oral fluid intake

Give small amounts of fluids "of choice" hourly to older, confused, or debilitated clients and to those who require restraints. Keep fluids fresh and within reach. Use orthotic devices as appropriate for those who can assist in their own fluid intake. If a client's lips are dry, he or she may be unable to suck on a straw. Wet the lips and mouth first to facilitate sucking. When medications are given to dehydrated clients, it is helpful to give one-at-a-time, which increases the amount of fluid consumed while taking medications. Because many dehydrated clients are also malnourished, use fluids that provide some nutrient value such as juice or oral supplements. Give antiemetic prophylactically to control nausea before drinking and taking medication that is highly emetogenic. When appropriate, begin with clear fluids, such as oral replacement fluids, broth, or gelatin. Progress to full fluids and then solid foods if tolerated without vomiting or aspiration. Encourage family members to participate in feeding. Interventions include simple verbal cuing, placing fluids/spoons in the resident's hand and with minimal guiding, positive body language, simple praises, limited distractions, and touch.

If dysphagia is present, consult the physician regarding swallowing studies. Once the problem has been identified, a speech pathologist can provide exercises to help the client. Reinforce the speech therapist's prescription during each feeding. You may need to give thickened fluids. Elevate the head rest to 90 degrees before meals and for 1 hour after feeding, and flex the client's head slightly forward at the start of a swallow. Decrease the risk of aspiration by placing small amounts of food on the side of the mouth that has the best sensation and muscle strength. Teaching the client to chew slowly and to swallow two or three times with each mouthful and inspecting the mouth for food pocketing can also decrease the risk of aspiration. Assessing the fit of dentures is also important. If the swallowing problem is not correctable, the client and client's family may need to consider artificial forms of feeding such as tube feeding.

Fluids by intravenous route

Administer IV fluids continuously to clients who are dehydrated. Once fluids are re-established, a larger catheter can be inserted if fluids or an IV access is still needed. Use an IV pump to regulate lV infusion and to decrease the risk of too rapid infusion. Monitor IV solutions, IV sites, and client outcomes hourly. Ensure that the rate of IV fluid via the pump is accurate; significant errors in setting IV pumps have occurred.

Rapid fluid replacement often results in overflow diuresis without cellular replacement. Diuresis compounds dehydration and may result in hypernatremia. In older adults or in those with renal or cardiac disease, rapid fluid administration may also result in pulmonary overload.

Reduce the risk of fluid volume deficit

The goal of fluid promotion and maintenance is to maintain the level of fluid intake at 1.5 mL/kg per 24 hours. If the client is fed hypertonic tube-feedings, give water bolus with them. Recommended dilution is 1 mL of water per 1 kilocalorie (kcal) of feeding formula.

Control the underlying problems

Examine the client's prescription and non-prescription (over the counter, herbal) medication list. lf the onset of the diarrhea was at the same time as a new elixir drug with sorbitol was administered, a common cause of osmotic diarrhea, consult the pharmacist regarding pills rather than the elixir form. Consider viral infections because many infections have been known to result in lactose intolerance. If this is the cause, encourage the client to avoid milk-based products. Avoiding fatty or fried foods also decreases diarrhea and enhances digestion.

Give prescribed antiemetic for nausea, antipyretics for fever, and antibiotics for infections. Besides monitoring for positive responses to treatment, replace sensible fluid losses; for every degree of fever above 38°C, give an additional 500 mL of water above basal needs approximately 1,500 mL.

Monitor for complications

When fluid balance is compromised, a person is at risk for tissue breakdown. Apply a moisturizer or skin barrier to protect the skin from the irritants, enzymes, and microorganisms found in urine and feces. Continue to assess lung sounds for manifestations of fluid overload (crackles).

Diagnosis

Impaired oral Mucous Membrane related to lack of oral intake or other causes is a common problem in client with dehydration.

Outcomes

The desired outcome is that the mucous membranes are restored with expected outcomes of having an improvement in oral score. In addition, the client's tongue, gums, and lips should become moist and the mouth, gums and teeth should be clean and free of accumulation of dried mucus.

Interventions

Provide oral care with a regular toothbrush or a foam toothbrush every 2–4 hours, and apply lip moisturizer. Rinse the client's mouth every 1–2 hours. Examine the client's mouth. Avoid mouthwashes with an alcohol base, which can dry the mucous membranes. The frequency of oral care should be increased to hourly if there is no improvement. Artificial saliva can also be used for the client with a very dry and fissured mouth. Clients who have dysphagia also need oral care; a suction catheter should be used while oral care is provided to reduce the risk of aspiration.

Diagnosis

If orthostatic hypotension is present, risk for injury is another problem that needs to be addressed.

Outcome

The desired outcome is that the client will have a reduced risk for injury as evident by no manifestation of falls (bruises, bumps, abrasions) or reported episodes of falls.

Interventions

Provide safety through stepped-progression position changes. Stepped-progression gives the client's body some time to adapt to changes in position. First, raise the head of the bed. Next, assist the client to sit at the edge of the bed in a "dangling" position until the dizziness has subsided. Make the client stand and assist the client to a chair. Do not progress to the next position until the client tolerates the current one (i.e., without dizziness or marked hypotension). Place alarm monitors on clients who are confused and tend to get out of bed without assistance. Sitters or restraints may be needed if all other measures to control behavior are ineffective.

Evaluation

Mild to moderate fluid deficits should be corrected in 8–24 hours. More severe fluid loss may take several days, especially when they occur in older adults.

Client Teaching on Self-care

Client teaching is one of the primary interventions for promoting and maintaining fluid balance. Teach clients with mild fluid deficit to replace fluid with clear liquids, 30–60 mL or more hourly, as tolerated, to decrease nausea and replace electrolytes. Teach the importance of consulting a physician if an illness lasts longer than 24 hours or if the person is older or has a chronic illness, such as diabetes mellitus or liver, kidney, or heart disease. Teach clients who take diuretics to continue to drink normally to avoid the rebound fluid retention syndrome; if the plasma volume drops too low, the renin

cascade is triggered. Health promotion teaching is critical for those who actively exercise. Teach people who exercise to do the following:

- Understand the importance of exercise and heat acclimatization over several days.
- Avoid exercise during high heat and humidity.
- Wear appropriate clothing (excess clothing decreases evaporation).
- Use more caution to prevent heat exhaustion if the client is obese, because obesity impairs the sweating mechanism.
- Drink cool water before exercise, 150–200 mL every 15 minutes during exercise, and after finishing exercise, and add 500–700 kcal of carbohydrates (for energy and sodium), if exercise is prolonged; do not wait for thirst to appear before drinking.
- Avoid rapid fluid replacement, because this fluid only overflows to the kidneys.
- Use caution when taking medications that interfere with thermoregulation, such as thyroid replacement, amphetamines, beta-blockers, haloperidol, antihistamines, anticholinergic drugs, and phenothiazides.

Fluid Volume Excess

Fluid volume excess (FVE) occurs when the body retains both water and sodium in similar proportions to normal ECF. This is commonly referred to as **hypervolemia** (increased blood volume). FVE is always secondary to an increase in the total body sodium content, which leads to an increase in total body water. Because both sodium and water are retained, the serum sodium concentration remains essentially normal and the excess volume of fluid is isotonic. Specific causes of FVE include, excessive intake of sodium chloride, administering sodium- containing infusions too rapidly, particularly to clients with impaired regulatory mechanism, and disease processes that alter regulatory mechanism, such as heart failure, renal failure, cirrhosis of liver and Cushing's syndrome.

Risk Factors

- Excessive intake of sodium containing intravenous fluids
- Excess ingestion of sodium in diet or medications
- Impaired fluid balance regulation related to
  - Heart failure
  - Renal failure
  - Cirrhosis of the liver

Clinical Manifestations

- Weight gain
  2% gain = mild FVE; 5% gain = moderate; 8% gain = severe
- Fluid intake greater than output

- Full, bounding pulse and tachycardia
- Increased blood pressure and CVP
- Distended neck and peripheral veins; slow vein emptying
- Moist crackles (rales) in lungs; dyspnea, shortness of breath
- Mental confusion

Edema

In fluid volume excess, both intravascular and interstitial spaces have an increased water and sodium content. Excess interstitial fluid is known as edema. Edema typically is most apparent in areas where the pressure is low, such as around the eyes, and in dependent tissues (known as dependent edema), where hydrostatic capillary pressure is high.

Edema can be caused by several different mechanisms. The three main mechanisms are increased capillary hydrostatic pressure, decreased plasma oncotic pressure, and increased capillary permeability. It may be due to FVE that increases capillary hydrostatic pressure, pushing fluid into the interstitial tissues. This type of edema is often seen in dependent tissues such as the feet, ankles and sacrum because of the effects of gravity. Low levels of plasma proteins from malnutrition or kidney or liver diseases can reduce the plasma oncotic pressure so that fluid is not drawn into the capillaries from interstitial tissues, causing edema.

Pitting edema is edema that leaves a small depression or pit after finger is applied to the swollen area. The pit is caused by movement of fluid to adjacent tissue, away from the point of pressure. Within 10–30 seconds, the pit normally disappears.

Water Intoxication Overhydration

It results from either water excess or solute deficit, primarily sodium. In water excess, the number of solutes is normal but they are diluted by excessive water. In solute deficit, the amount of water is normal but there are too few particles per liter of water.

The most common cause of water intoxication is the administration of excessive amount of hypo-osmolar IV fluids, such as 0.45% (half-strength) saline solution or 5% dextrose in water (D5W). Water intoxication occurs in client who receive continuous IV D5W or in older clients who consume excessive amount of tap water without adequate nutrient intake. Syndrome of inappropriate antidiuretic hormone (SIADH) also leads to intracellular fluid volume excess (ICFVE) regardless of whether the SIADH is caused by central nervous system (CNS) trauma, the stress of surgery, pain, or opioid use.

Hypo-osmolar fluids in the vessels move by osmosis to the region of higher concentration of sodium in the cells in an attempt to maintain equilibrium. Too much fluid accumulating in the cells causes cellular edema. Cerebral cells absorb hypo-osmolar fluid more quickly than other cells. Thus, these cell changes often present the earliest warning signs of intracellular shifting.

Because ICF excess is often associated with ECF excess, it is common to see plasma sodium level of less than 125 mEq/L and a decreased hematocrit. However, there is no plasma test to reflect the cell fluid volume. Diagnostic tests, such as computed tomography and magnetic resonance imaging are more helpful in identifying causes underlying water intoxication.

Neurologic cells are vulnerable to fluid excess or deficit. The first priority is to reduce intracranial pressure (ICP) with steroids and osmotic diuretics. Equally important is identifying and addressing the cause of fluid volume excess. Immediate surgical intervention maybe critical.

If SIADH is an impending risk, early administration of IV fluids containing sodium chloride (NaCl) may prevent it. Saline solutions, such as D5/ 0.45% NaCl, increase the osmolality of vascular fluid and prevent or help correct hypo-osmolality.

Perform neurological checks, including level of consciousness, vital signs, reflexes and pupillary responses every hour if cranial changes are present. Cerebral perfusion is altered if systolic blood pressure drops too low or rises too high. Notify the provider if the client's neurologic response deteriorates from the baseline assessment if systolic blood pressure is less than 100 mm Hg or greater than 160 mm Hg, or if other signs persist or worsen.

Monitor IV fluids and input and output hourly, and monitor weight daily. Polyuria is a good sign and indicates that fluid has shifted to the vascular space and to the renal tubules, where it can be excreted. Administer antiemetic prophylactically, as appropriate, to promote food and fluid ingestion and retention and to decrease the risk of vomiting, which worsens the increased ICP.

THIRD SPACE SYNDROME

In **third space syndrome**, fluid shifts from the vascular space into an area where it is not readily accessible as extracellular fluid. This fluid remains in the body but is essentially unavailable for use, causing an isotonic fluid volume deficit. Fluid may be sequestered in the bowel, in the interstitial space as edema, inflamed tissue, or in potential spaces such as the peritoneal or pleural cavities.

The client with third space syndrome has an isotonic fluid deficit but may not manifest apparent fluid loss or weight loss.

Third space is the term used to describe the accumulation of fluids in the interstitial spaces. The third-space fluid is not the fluid in the vessels or cells; it is the fluid around the cells and vessels. Third-space fluid is physiologically useless because it does not circulate to provide nutrients for cells. This abnormal fluid accumulation not only results from pathologic conditions but also reflects an inability of the lymphatic system to compensate. Common sites of third-spacing include the pleural cavity, peritoneal cavity and pericardial sac.

Etiology

Fluids can move into interstitial spaces because of increased hydrostatic pressure, increased capillary permeability, decreased serum protein levels, obstruction of the venous portion of the capillary, or non-functional lymphatic drainage systems.

Any pathological process that triggers the inflammatory or ischemic processes can lead to fluid shifting. For example, massive fluid shifts from the vascular to the interstitial spaces can be seen in crush injuries, major tissue trauma, major surgery, extensive burns, acid-base imbalance, bowel obstruction and sepsis.

Decreased protein intake, production, or storage, or increased protein loss is seen in protein-calorie malnutrition. In liver and kidney disease, it can lead to hypoalbuminemia.

Altered lymphatic function and venous thrombosis impair fluid return to the right atrium, thus promoting third-spacing. The decreased colloidal osmotic pressure from the impaired protein synthesis, as noted earlier, is only compounded by the portal hypertension that accompanies end-stage liver disease, leading to third-spacing in the peritoneal cavity (ascites).

Pathophysiology

Tissue injury causes the release of histamine and bradykinin, resulting in increased capillary permeability, which allows more fluid, protein, and other solutes to move into the interstitial spaces than normal. This form of fluid shift may be time-limited. The early stages of inflammation last about 24–48 hours; the capillary membrane heals and the fluid returns to the venous system. It may take longer in conditions with prolonged inflammatory responses or severe tissue injury.

Protein malnutrition leads to decreased oncotic pressure because protein is not present to pull fluid back into the capillary at the venous end. This form of fluid shifting is usually long term and can be seen in children who are protein malnourished and have large protruding abdomen and pencil-thin legs.

Two phases of fluid shift are associated with tissue injury:

1. Fluids shift from vascular to interstitial spaces, which lead to a risk for fluid volume deficit (hypovolemia). Severe hypovolemia may lead to vascular collapse and death. If cellular damage is severe, a toxic response may occur from intracellular ions, such as potassium that leak into the vascular spaces.

2. As the capillary membrane heals, fluid shifts back from the interstitial to the vascular space, which leads to a risk for fluid volume excess (hypervolemia). If the hypervolemia is severe, it may lead to heart failure. Intracellular potassium ions shift back into the cell during this phase, which increases the risk for hypovolemia.

Clinical Manifestations

Typical manifestations include pallor, cold limbs, weak and rapid pulse, hypotension, oliguria and decreased levels of consciousness. Body weight does not change because fluid has not been lost; it has been redistributed. Severe losses can result in hypovolemic shock.

If fluid collects and obstructs an organ, nerve, or vessel, other clinical manifestations may arise. For example, bowel sounds may change throughout the abdomen. Extremities may become pale, cool and pulseless if fluid obstructs the blood vessels or nerves. Laboratory results may indicate an elevated hematocrit, sodium level, BUN level, and urine specific gravity.

When fluid returns to the blood vessels, the clinical manifestations are similar to those of fluid overload. Signs may include a bounding pulse, crackles, engorgement of peripheral and jugular veins, and an increase in blood pressure. Laboratory results may indicate a decrease in hematocrit and BUN levels.

Management

Medical treatment begins with determining the cause of the fluid volume shift. If the third-spacing has occurred around the heart (pericardial effusion), around the lungs (pleural effusion), or in the peritoneal cavity (ascites), the physician removes the excess fluids by tapping the space with a large bore needle; these procedures are known as pericardiocentesis, thoracentesis, and paracentesis, respectively.

Replace Fluids

When hypovolemia results from tissue injury, such as burns or crush injuries, a large volume of isotonic IV fluid administration is required to replace intravascular volume. When there is an evidence of capillary healing (increase in urine output without additional fluids), albumin may be given to replace the protein lost from the trauma and to promote restoration of capillary oncotic pressures. Because third spacing is a common occurrence after major surgery, maintaining IV fluid intake is essential to maintaining kidney perfusion. During the first 24–72 hours, when there is an increased in ADH and the healing phase is beginning with fluid moving back into the vessels, the client is at risk for fluid overload if the fluid replacement is too rapid.

Stabilize Other Problems

Some etiologies of fluids shifting are life threatening and must be treated aggressively. For example, sepsis causes major increase in capillary permeability and must be treated with IV antibiotics and, usually, vasoactive medications to maintain blood pressure. Bowel obstructions can cause major third-spacing and lead to gangrene, surgical repair is critical. Serious inflammatory disorders require massive doses of steroids to stabilize the mast cell membrane.

Monitor IV Fluids Replacement Needs

If IV fluids are administered too rapidly, fluid overload or hypervolemia may occur. Assess for early signs of fluid overload, such as crackles, difficulty in breathing, and neck vein engorgement. Notify the physician if these signs are present. Anticipate a reduction in IV fluid needs as the third space fluid shift back into the plasma during the capillary repair stage.

If the third spacing is in the abdomen, as with ascites, measure the client's abdominal girth every 8 hours. If a limb is involved, measure the circumference of the limb and assess peripheral pulses every 8 hours. Use preventive measures to prevent skin breakdown of edematous areas.

Monitor urine output every hour, and report an output of less than 0.5 mL/kg/hr. if it persists for more than 2 hours. The client may need more fluids and not diuretics. Urine output is usually reduced after tissue injury because of decreased renal perfusion and a fluid shift into the injured tissue spaces. After one to three days of tissue injury, fluid returns to the circulation and the kidneys excrete excess fluids, unless renal function is impaired, the injury is massive, or the client has impaired adaptive mechanisms. Monitor plasma BUN and creatinine.

ELECTROLYTE IMBALANCES

Sodium

Sodium, the most abundant cation in the ECF, not only moves into and out of the body but also moves in careful balance among three fluid compartments. It is found in most body secretions, for example, saliva, gastric and intestinal secretions, bile, and pancreatic fluid. Therefore, continuous excretion of any of these fluids, such as via intestinal suction, can result in a sodium deficit. Because of its role in regulating water balance, sodium imbalance usually is accompanied by water imbalance.

Hyponatremia

It is a sodium deficit, or serum sodium level of less than 135 mEq/L, and is, in acute care settings, a common electrolyte imbalance. Because of sodium's role in determining the osmolality of ECF, hyponatremia typically results in a low serum osmolality. Water is drawn out of the vascular compartment into interstitial tissues and the cells causing the clinical manifestations associated with this disorder. As sodium level decreases the brain and nervous system are affected by cellular edema. Severe hyponatremia, serum levels below 110 mEq/L, is a medical emergency and can lead to permanent neurological damage.

Risk Factors

- **Loss of sodium**
  - Gastrointestinal fluid loss
  - Sweating
  - Use of diuretics
- **Gain of water**
  - Hypotonic tube feeding
  - Excessive drinking of water
  - Excess IV D5W (dextrose in water) administration
- **SIADH**
  - Head injury
  - Acquired immunodeficiency syndrome (AIDS)
  - Malignant tumors

Clinical Manifestations

- Lethargy, confusion and apprehension
- Muscle twitching
- Abdominal cramps
- Anorexia, nausea and vomiting
- Headache, seizures, coma
- Serum sodium level below 135 mEq/L and serum osmolality below 280 mOsm/kg

Nursing Management

Assessment

- Assess clinical manifestations.
- Obtain thorough diet and medical history, including use of over-the-counter drugs and herbal drugs.
- Monitor daily weight.
- Assess the skin and mucous membrane.
- Monitor lung sounds every 2–4 hours.
- Assess vital signs and peripheral vein filling every 4–8 hours.
- Monitor fluid intake and output.
- Monitor laboratory data (e.g., serum sodium).
- Assess client closely if administering hypertonic saline solutions.

Nursing Diagnosis

Hyponatremia related to vomiting, diarrhea, gastric suctioning, burns, SIADH, surgery, fluid overload.

Interventions

- **Reduce loss in high risk client**
  - If blood plasma sodium is greater than 125 mEq/L, encourage intake of 30–60 mL of clear fluids or more per hour as tolerated.
  - To prevent sodium loss, irrigate nasogastric tubes and wounds with isotonic saline and give only ice chips.
  - Treat nausea with prophylactic antiemetics.
  - Never give more than 3 tap water enema in succession.
  - Consult the physician if plasma sodium is less than 125 mEq/L and if the client is receiving nothing by mouth.
- **Restore sodium balance**
  - Encourage the intake of well balanced diet.
  - Give nutrient rich supplements between diet.
  - Add extra salt to feeding to achieve desired sodium level.
  - To decrease thirst, offer ice chips, cold fluids and frequent oral care.
  - Restricting fluid is contraindicated in clients with subarachnoid hemorrhage because they increase risk for cerebral vasospasm and central pontine myelinolysis.
  - Administer hypertonic IV solutions if plasma level is less than 125 mEq/L.

Hypernatremia

It is excess sodium in ECF or serum sodium of greater than 145 mEq/L. Because the osmotic pressure of ECF is increased, fluid moves out of the cells into the ECF. It is important to note that a person's thirst mechanism protects against hypernatremia. For example, when an individual becomes thirsty, the body is stimulated to drink water which helps correct the hypernatremia. Clients at risk for hypernatremia are those who are unable to access water (e.g., unconscious, unable to request fluids such as infants or elders with dementia, or ill clients with an impaired thirst mechanism).

Risk Factors

- **Loss of water**
  - Insensible water loss (hyperventilation of water)
  - Diarrhea
  - Water deprivation

- **Gain of sodium**
  - Parenteral administration of saline solution
  - Hypertonic tube feedings without adequate water
  - Excessive use of table salt (1tsp contains 2,300 mg sodium)
- **Conditions such as**
  - Diabetes mellitus
  - Heat stroke

Clinical Manifestations

- Thirst with dry and sticky mucous membrane
- Tongue: red, dry and swollen
- Weakness

In Severe Hypernatremia

- Fatigue, restlessness
- Decreased level of consciousness
- Disorientation, convulsions

Laboratory Findings

- Serum sodium above 145 mEq/L
- Serum osmolality above 300 mOsm/kg

Nursing Management

- Monitor fluid intake and output.
- Obtain detailed diet and medical history, including use of corticosteroids, over-the-counter drugs and herbal drugs.
- Monitor daily weight.
- Assess the skin and mucous membrane.
- Monitor lung sounds every 2–4 hours.
- Assess vital signs and peripheral vein filling every 4–8 hours.
- Monitor behavior changes (e.g., restlessness, disorientation).
- Monitor laboratory findings (e.g., serum sodium).

Nursing Diagnosis

- Hypernatremia-related decreased thirst, excessive administration of salt solutions, or impaired excretion of sodium and water

Interventions

- Monitor the client for response to IV fluid replacement of hypo-osmolar electrolyte solutions.
- Offer fluids and water hourly to clients with hypovolemic hypernatremia.
- Consult with the dietician regarding the need for fluid and sodium restriction for clients with hypervolemic hypernatremia.

- Teach the client and family members regarding the food items that should be restricted as well as the rationale for restriction.
- Consult the physician for manifestations that indicate worsening of hypernatremia or fluid overload such as increasing weight or cardiovascular, pulmonary or neurologic manifestations.
- Impaired oral mucous membrane related to lack of body water secondary to hypernatremia.
  - Provide oral care every 2 hours with a non-alcoholic mouthwash.
  - Use a soft toothbrush to prevent injury to the mucosa.
  - Moisten the client's lips every 1–2 hours.
  - Offer low acidic fluids such as apple juice.
  - Teach the client to hold the fluids in mouth for a time to hydrate the mucous membrane.
  - Assess the mouth before and after mouth care.

Potassium

Potassium is vital to normal neuromuscular and cardiac functions. Normal renal function is important for maintenance of potassium balance as 80% of potassium is excreted by the kidneys. Potassium must be replaced daily to maintain its balance. Normally, potassium is replaced in food.

Hypokalemia

It is a potassium deficit or a serum potassium level of less than 3.5 mEq/L. Gastrointestinal loss of potassium through vomiting and gastric suction are common causes of hypokalemia, as well as the use of potassium-wasting diuretics such as thiazide diuretics or loop diuretics (e.g., furosemide). Symptoms of hypokalemia are usually mild until the level drops below 3 mEq/L unless the decrease in potassium was rapid. When the decrease is gradual, the body compensates by shifting potassium from the intracellular environment into the serum.

Risk Factors

- Vomiting and gastric suction
- Diarrhea
- Heavy perspiration
- Use of potassium-wasting drugs, e.g., diuretics
- Poor intake of potassium (as with debilitated clients, alcoholics, anorexia nervosa)
- Hyperaldosteronism

Clinical Manifestations

- Muscle weakness, leg cramps, depressed deep tendon reflexes
- Fatigue and lethargy
- Anorexia, nausea and vomiting
- Decreased bowel sounds and decreased bowel mobility
- Cardiac dysrhythmias
- Weak irregular pulses
- Laboratory findings: Serum potassium level below 3.5 mEq/L and arterial blood gas analysis may show alkalosis
- T-wave flattening and ST segment depression on ECG

Nursing Management

Assessment

- Obtain a history related to dietary intake, condition promoting potassium loss and use of diuretics, cortisone, over-the-counter drugs and herbal medications.
- Assess heart rate and rhythm.
- Assess the apical pulse. If irregular, assess for pulse deficit.
- Review the laboratory potassium level.
- Assess cardiac and renal functions every hour for client with severe hypokalemia and 8-hourly when the conditions improve.
- Assess neuromuscular and bowel functions every 4–8 hours.
- Monitor clients receiving digitalis (e.g., digoxin) closely, because hypokalemia increases risk of digitalis toxicity.

Nursing Diagnosis

- Hypokalemia related to causative factors such as vomiting, diarrhea, Cushing's syndrome, cortisone therapy, decreased intake, and nil per os status.

Interventions

- Monitor the potassium level and report the result to the physician.
- Give oral or IV potassium as prescribed, ensuring that it is diluted in IV fluids; it can be given as an IV push.
- Always irrigate the IV bags containing potassium to prevent giving a loading dose, which can cause cardiac arrest.
- Monitor IV sites hourly for infiltration, phlebitis and confirm the rate of infusion.
- Notify the physician if the signs of hypokalemia persist or worsen in conditions such as:
  - Dysrhythmias of increasing intensity.
  - If urine output is less than 0.5 mL/kg/hr for 2 consecutive hour.
  - If pulse deficit is greater than 20 beats/min.
  - If signs of impaired tissue perfusion are present.
- Administer IV glucose along with potassium as increased insulin moves the potassium back into the cells.

Nursing Diagnosis

- Risk for injury or risk for falls related to muscle weakness and hypotension or seizures secondary to hypokalemia.

Interventions

- Keep the bed in low position with padded side rails up.
- Employ safety and seizure precautions to reduce the risk of injury.
- Before the client walks, clear the path of obstacles and place non-slippery shoes and gait belt on the client.
- Use restraints only if all other alternatives to prevent harm to self and other.

Nursing Diagnosis

- Imbalanced nutrition less than body requirement related to insufficient intake of foods rich in potassium.

Interventions

- Instruct the client to choose and consume potassium rich foods.
  - Instruct the client to take potassium supplements with a glass or more of water or juice and food to decrease GI irritation.

Hyperkalemia

It is a potassium excess or a serum potassium level greater than 5.0 mEq/L. Hyperkalemia is less common than hypokalemia and rarely occurs in clients with normal renal function. It is, however, more dangerous than hypokalemia and can lead to cardiac arrest.

Risk Factors

- Decreased potassium excretion
  - Renal failure
  - Hypoaldosteronism
  - Potassium-conserving diuretics
- High potassium intake
  - Excessive use of K^+ containing salt substitutes
  - Excessive or rapid IV infusion of potassium
  - Potassium shift out of the tissue cells into the plasma (e.g., infections, burns, acidosis)

Clinical Manifestations

- Gastrointestinal hyperacidity and diarrhea
- Irritability, apathy and confusion
- Cardiac dysrhythmias or arrest
- Muscle weakness, areflexia (absence of reflexes)
- Decreased heart rate
- Irregular pulse, paresthesias and numbness in extremities
- Serum potassium above 5.0 mEq/L
- Peaked T wave, widened QRS complex on electro cardiogram (ECG)

Nursing Management

Assessment

- Assess the vital signs, bowel functions, urine output, peripheral edema and lung sounds every 4–8 hours.
- Closely monitor cardiac status and ECG.
- Monitor serum K^+ levels and BUN carefully; a rapid drop may occur as potassium shifts into the cells.
- Assess the apical pulse.

Nursing Diagnosis

Hyperkalemia related to etiology such as renal dysfunction, shock from traumatic injuries, or burn.

Interventions

- Administer IV fluids as ordered to promote renal excretion of potassium.
- Report manifestations indicating the development of hypokalemia and urine output of less than 0.5 mL/kg/hr for two consecutive hours.
- If client is to receive blood transfusion, notify the blood bank for risk of hyperkalemia.

Calcium

Regulating levels of calcium in the body is more complex than the other major electrolytes as calcium balance can be affected by many factors.

Hypocalcemia

It is defined as calcium deficit, or a total serum calcium level of less than 8.5 mg/dL or an ionized calcium level of less than 0.4 mg/dL. Severe depletion of calcium can cause tetany with muscle spasms and paresthesias (numbness and tingling around the mouth and hands and feet) and can lead to convulsions.

Two signs indicate hypocalcemia:

- The Chvostek's sign is contraction of the facial muscles that is produced by tapping the facial nerve in front of the ear.
- Trousseau's sign is a carpal spasm that occurs by inflating a blood pressure cuff on the upper arm to 20 mm Hg greater than the systolic pressure for 2–5 minutes.
- Clients at greatest risk for hypocalcemia are those whose parathyroid glands have been removed This is frequently associated with total thyroidectomy or bilateral neck surgery for cancer. Low serum magnesium levels (hypomagnesemia) and chronic alcoholism also increase the risk of hypocalcemia.

Risk Factors

- Surgical removal of the parathyroid glands
- **Conditions such as**
  - Hypoparathyroidism
  - Acute pancreatitis
  - Hyperphosphatemia
  - Thyroid carcinoma
- **Inadequate vitamin intake**
  - Malabsorption
  - Hypomagnesemia
  - Alkalosis
  - Sepsis
  - Alcohol abuse

Clinical Manifestations

- Numbness, tingling of the extremities and around the mouth
- Muscle tremors, cramps, if severe can progress to tetany and convulsions
- Cardiac dysrhythmias, decreased cardiac output
- Positive Trousseau's and Chvostek's signs
- Confusion, anxiety, possible psychosis
- Hyperactive deep tendon reflexes
- Serum calcium level below 8.5 mg/dL
- Lengthened QT interval and prolonged ST segment on ECG

Nursing Interventions

- Closely monitor respiratory and cardiovascular status
- Take precautions to protect a confused client
- Administer oral or parenteral calcium supplements as ordered when administering intravenously closely monitor cardiac status and ECG during infusion
- Teach clients at risk for osteoporosis about
  - Dietary sources rich in calcium
  - Recommendation for 1,000–1,500 mg of calcium per day
  - Calcium supplements
  - Regular exercise
  - Estrogen replacement therapy for postmeno-pausal women

Hypercalcemia

Hypercalcemia or total serum calcium levels greater than 10.5 mg/dL, or an ionized calcium level of greater than 5.0 mg/dL, most often occurs when calcium is mobilized from the bony skeleton. This may be due to malignancy or prolonged immobilization

Risk Factors

- Prolonged immobilization
- Conditions such as hyperparathyroidism, malignancy of the bone and Paget's disease

Clinical Manifestations

- Lethargy, weakness
- Depressed deep tendon reflexes
- Bone pain
- Anorexia, nausea, vomiting
- Constipation
- Polyuria, hypercalciuria
- Flank pain secondary to urinary calculi
- Dysrhythmias, possible heart block
- Serum calcium greater than 10.5 mg/dL
- Shortened QT interval and shortened ST segments on ECG

Nursing Interventions

- Increase client movement and exercise.
- Encourage oral fluids as permitted to maintain dilute urine.
- Teach clients to limit intake of food and fluid high in calcium.
- Encourage ingestion of fiber to prevent constipation.
- Protect a confused client; monitor for pathologic fractures in clients with long-term hypercalcemia.
- Encourage intake of acid-ash fluids (e.g., prune or cranberry) to counteract deposits of calcium salts in the urine.

Magnesium

Magnesium (Mg^{2+}) imbalance is relatively common in hospitalized clients, although if may be unrecognized.

Hypomagnesemia

It is defined as magnesium deficiency, or a total serum magnesium level of less than 1.5 mEq/L. It occurs more frequently than hypermagnesemia. Chronic alcoholism is the most common cause of hypomagnesemia. Magnesium deficiency may also aggravate the manifestation of alcohol withdrawal, such as delirium tremens.

Risk Factors

- Excessive loss from the gastrointestinal tract (e.g., from the nasogastric suction, diarrhea, fistula drainage)

- Long-term use of certain drugs (e.g., diuretics, aminoglycosides, antibiotics)
- Condition such as chronic alcoholism, pancreatitis, burns

Clinical Manifestations

- Neuromuscular irritability with tremors
- Increased reflexes, tremors, convulsions
- Positive Chvostek's and Trousseau's signs
- Tachycardia, elevated blood pressure, dysrhythmias
- Disorientation, confusion and vertigo
- Anorexia, dysphagia
- Respiratory difficulties
- Serum magnesium below 1.5 mEq/L
- Prolonged PR intervals, widened QRS complex, prolonged QT intervals, depressed ST segment, broad flattened T waves and prominent U waves on ECG

Nursing Interventions

- Assess clients receiving digitalis for digitalis toxicity
- Hypomagnesemia increases the risk of toxicity
- Take protective measures when there is a possibility of seizures.
- Assess the client's ability to swallow water prior to initiating oral feeding
- Initiate safety measures to prevent injury during seizure activity
  - Carefully administer magnesium salts as ordered
- Encourage clients to eat magnesium rich foods if permitted (e.g., whole grains, meat, sea foods and green leafy vegetables)
- Refer client to alcohol treatment program as indicated

Hypermagnesemia

It is present when the serum magnesium level rises above 2.5 mEq/L. It is due to increased intake or decreased excretion. It is often iatrogenic, that is, it occurs as a result of overzealous magnesium therapy.

Risk Factors

Abnormal retention of magnesium, as in
- Renal failure
- Adrenal insufficiency
- Treatment with magnesium salts

Clinical Manifestations

- Peripheral vasodilation, flushing
- Nausea, vomiting
- Muscle weakness, paralysis
- Hypotension, bradycardia
- Depressed deep-tendon reflexes
- Lethargy, drowsiness
- Respiratory depression, coma
- Respiratory and cardiac arrest
- Serum magnesium levels above 2.5 mEq/L
- Prolonged QT interval, prolonged PR interval, widened QRS complexes and tall T wave on ECG

Nursing Interventions

- Monitor vital signs and level of consciousness when clients are at risk
- If patellar reflexes are absent, notify the primary care provider
- Advice clients who have renal disease to contact their primary care provider before taking over-the-counter drugs.

Chloride

Because of the relationship between sodium ions and chloride ions (Cl⁻), imbalance of chloride commonly occurs in conjunction with sodium imbalance. Hypo-chloremia is decreased serum chloride level, in adults a level below 95 mEq/L, and is usually related to excess loss of chloride ion through the GI tract, kidneys, or sweating. Hypochloremic clients are at risk for alkalosis and many experience muscle twitching, tremors, or tetany.

Conditions that cause sodium retention also can lead to high serum chloride level or **hyperchloremia**, in adults a level above 108 mEq/L. Excess replacement of sodium chloride or potassium chloride is an additional risk factor for high serum chloride levels. The manifestations of hyperchloremia include acidosis, and lethargy with a risk of dysrhythmias and coma.

Phosphate

The phosphate anion PO_4^- is found in both ICF and ECF. Most of the phosphorus (P^+) in the body exists as PO_4^-. Phosphate is critical for cellular metabolism because it is a major component of adenosine triphosphate (ATP).

Phosphate imbalance is frequently related to therapeutic interventions of other disorders. Glucose and insulin administration and total parenteral nutrition can cause phosphate to shift into the cells from ECF compartments, leading to hypophosphatemia, defined in adults as a total serum phosphate level less than 2.5 mg/dL. Alcohol withdrawal, acid-base imbalances, and the use of antacids that bind with phosphate in the GI tract are the possible cause of low serum phosphate levels. Manifestations of hypophosphatemia include paresthesias, muscle weakness and pain, mental changes, and possible seizures.

Hyperphosphatemia is defined in adult as total serum phosphate level greater than 4.5 mg/dL and occurs when phosphate shifts out of the cells into extracellular fluids (e.g., due to tissue trauma or chemotherapy for malignant tumors), in renal failure, or when excess phosphate is administered or ingested. Infants who are fed cow's milk are at risk for hyperphosphatemia, as are people using phosphate-containing enemas and laxatives. Clients who have high serum phosphate levels may experience numbness and tingling around the mouth and fingertips, muscle spasms, and tetany.

BIBLIOGRAPHY

1. Black JM, Hawks JH. Medical Surgical Nursing: Clinical Management for Positive Outcome, 8th edition. Mosby's; St Louise, Missouri; 2009. p. 151-66.

2. Bolander VB. Sorensen and Luckmann's Basic Nursing: A Psychological Approach. Pennsylvania; WB Saunders Company; Philadelphia; 1994. p. 1000-46.

3. Leahly JM, Kizilay PE. Foundations of Nursing Practice: a nursing process approach. Pennsylvania: WB Saunders Company; Philadelphia; 1998. p. 1022-6.

4. Smeltzer SC. "Brunner and Siddhartha's Textbook of Medical Surgical Nursing". 11th edition. Lippincott Williams and Wilkins. p. 2184-87.

5. LeMone P, Carol Taylor C, Lillis C. Fundamentals of Nursing: The Art and Science of Nursing Care, 4th edition. Lippincott Williams & Wilkins. 2001 p. 1272-330.

6. Christensen BL, Kockrow EO. Foundations of Nursing, 4th edition. Mosby's; St Louise, Missouri; 1999. p. 544-61.

7. Methany MN. Fluid and Electrolyte balance: The Nursing Consideration. 5th edition. Lippincott Williams and Wilkins. 2010 pp: 524-36.

8. Allen PN. Nurses quick guide to fluid and electrolyte balance. Lippincott Williams & Wilkins. 2010. p. 286-394.

9. Kee JL et al. Manual on Fluid, Electrolyte and Acid-Base Balance. Delmar Publication; New York. 2009. p. 11-74.

10. William SR. Clinical Pocket Manual on Fluid and Electrolyte Balance. Spring House Co-operation. 2008. p. 55-99.

Urinary Elimination

Key Terms

- Micturition
- Polyuria
- Oliguria
- Anuria
- Nocturia
- Dysuria
- Enuresis
- Urinary retention
- Neurogenic bladder
- BUN (blood urea nitrogen)
- Incontinence
- Urinary retention
- Ureterostomy
- Nephrostomy
- Vesicostomy

Chapter Outline

- Anatomy and Physiology of Urinary System
- Factors Influencing Urination
- Alterations in Urinary Elimination
- Nursing Management

ANATOMY AND PHYSIOLOGY OF URINARY SYSTEM

Elimination from the urinary tract helps the body to get rid of the waste products and materials not needed by the body. Urinary elimination depends on effective functioning of the kidneys and ureters; and the urinary bladder, urethra and pelvic floor (Fig. 1).

Kidney

The paired kidneys are situated on either sides of the spinal column, behind the peritoneal cavity. The right kidney is slightly lower than the left due to the position of the liver. Kidneys are the primary regulators of fluid and acid-base balance in the body. The functional units of the kidneys, the nephrons, filter the blood and remove metabolic wastes. In an average adult, 1,200 mL of blood or about 21% of the cardiac output, passes through the kidneys every minute. Each kidney contains approximately 1 million nephrons.

Each nephron has a glomerulus, a tuft of capillaries surrounded by Bowman's capsule (Fig. 2). The endothelium of glomerular capillaries is porous, allowing fluid and solutes to readily move across this membrane into the capsule. Plasma proteins and blood cells, however, are too large to cross the

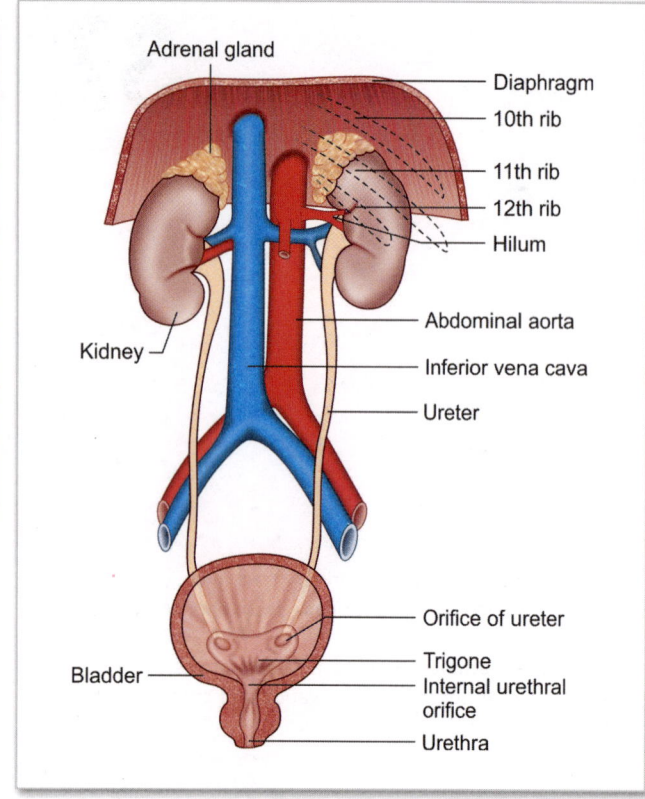

Fig. 1: Anatomic structures of urinary tract

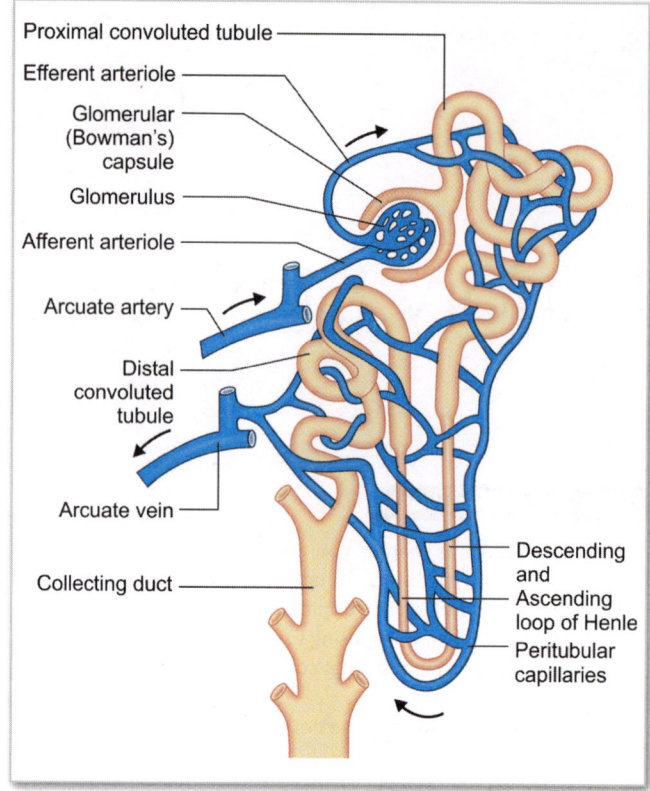

Fig. 2: Structure of nephron

membrane normally. Glomerular filtrate is similar in composition to plasma, made up of water, electrolytes, glucose, amino acids, and metabolic wastes.

From Bowman's capsule, the filtrate moves into the tubule of the nephron. In the proximal convoluted tubule, most of the water and electrolytes are reabsorbed. Solutes such as glucose are reabsorbed in the loop of Henle. In the distal convoluted tubule, additional water and sodium are reabsorbed under the control of hormones such as antidiuretic hormone (ADH) and aldosterone. This controlled reabsorption allows fine regulation of fluid and electrolyte balance in the body. When fluid intake is low or the concentration of solutes in the blood is high, ADH is released from the anterior pituitary, more water is reabsorbed in the distal tubule, and less urine is excreted. In contrast, when fluid intake is high or the blood solute concentration is low, ADH is suppressed. Without ADH, the distal tubule becomes impermeable to water and more urine is excreted. Aldosterone also affects the tubule, when aldosterone is released from the adrenal cortex, sodium and water are reabsorbed in greater quantities, increasing the blood volume and decreasing urinary output.

Ureters

Once the urine is formed in the kidneys, it moves through the collecting ducts into the calyces of the renal pelvis and from there into the ureters. The ureters are 25–30 cm (10–12 inches) long in adults and 0.25 cm (0.5 inch) in diameter. The upper end of each ureter is funnel-shaped as it enters the kidney. The lower ends of the ureters enter the bladder at the posterior corners of the floor of the bladder. At the junction between the ureter and the bladder, a flap like fold of mucous membrane acts as valve to prevent reflux (backflow) of urine up the ureters.

Bladder

The urinary bladder (vesicle) is a hollow muscular organ that serves as a reservoir for urine and as the organ of excretion. When empty, it lies behind the symphysis pubis. In men, the bladder lies in front of the rectum and above the prostate gland and in women, it lies in front of the uterus and vagina. The wall of the bladder is made up of four layers, an inner mucous layer, a connective tissue layer, three layers of smooth muscle fibers, some of which extend lengthwise, some obliquely, and some more or less circularly, and an outer serous layer. The smooth muscle layers are collectively called the **detrusor muscle.** It allows the bladder to expand as it fills with urine, and contract to release urine to the outside of the body during voiding. The **trigone** at the base of the bladder is a triangular area marked by the ureter openings at the posterior corners and the opening of the urethra at the anterior inferior corner.

The bladder is capable of considerable distension because of rugae (folds) in the mucous membrane lining and because of the elasticity of its walls. Normal bladder capacity is between 300 and 600 mL of urine.

Urethra

The urethra extends from the bladder to the urinary meatus. In the adult female, the urethra lies directly behind the symphysis pubis, anterior to the vagina, and is between 3 and 4 cm (1.5 cm) long. The urethra serves only as a passageway for the elimination of urine. The urinary meatus is located between the labia minora, in front of the vagina and below the clitoris.

The male urethra is approximately 20 cm (8 in) long and serves as a passageway for semen as well as urine. The meatus is located at the distal end of the penis.

The urethra has a mucous membrane lining, which is continuous with the bladder and ureters in both men and women. Thus, an infection of the urethra can extend through the urinary tract to the kidneys. Women are more prone to urinary tract infections because of their short urethra and the proximity of the urinary meatus to the vagina and anus.

Pelvic Floor

The vagina, urethra and rectum pass through the pelvic floor, which consists of sheets of muscles and ligaments that provide support to the viscera of the pelvis. They extend from the symphysis pubis to the coccyx forming a sling. The internal sphincter muscle is situated in the proximal urethra and the bladder neck is composed of smooth muscle under involuntary control. It provides active tension designed to close the urethral lumen. The external sphincter muscle is composed of skeletal muscle under voluntary control, allowing the individual to choose when to void urine.

Urination

Micturition, voiding, and urination all refer to the process of emptying the urinary bladder. Urine collects in the bladder until pressure stimulates special sensory nerve endings in the bladder wall called stretch receptors. This occurs when the adult bladder contains between 250 mL and 450 mL of urine. In children, a smaller volume of 50–200 mL stimulates these nerves.

These stretch receptors transmit impulses to the spinal cord, specifically to the voiding reflex center located at the level of the second to fourth sacral vertebrae, causing the internal sphincter to relax and stimulating the urge to void. If the time and place are suitable for urination, the conscious portion of the brain relaxes the external urethral sphincter muscle and urination takes place. If the time and place are not suitable, the micturition reflex usually subsides until the bladder becomes more filled and the reflex is stimulated again.

Voluntary control of urination is possible only if the nerves supplying the bladder and urethra, the neural tracts of the spinal cord and brain, and the motor area of the cerebrum are all intact.

FACTORS INFLUENCING URINATION

Numerous factors affect the volume and characteristics of the urine produced and the manner in which it is excreted.

Developmental Factors

Infants

Urine output varies according to fluid intake but gradually increases to 250–500 mL a day during the first year. Frequency of urination may be 20 times a day. The urine of the neonate is colorless and odorless and has a specific gravity of 1.008 because newborns and infants have immature kidneys, they are unable to concentrate urine very effectively.

Preschoolers

The preschoolers are able to take responsibility for independent toileting. During this period, children often forget to wash their hands or flush the toilet and need instructions in wiping themselves.

School Age Children

The school age child's elimination system reaches maturity during this period. The kidneys double in size between 5 and 10 years. During this period, the child urinates 6–8 times a day.

Elders

The excretory function of the kidney diminishes with age but usually not significantly below normal levels unless a disease process intervenes. With age, the number of functioning nephrons decreases to some degree, impairing the kidney's filtering abilities. The more noticeable changes with age are those related to the bladder complaints of urinary urgency and urinary frequency. In men, these changes are often due to enlarged prostate gland and in women they may be due to weakened muscles supporting the bladder or weakness of the urethral sphincter. The capacity of the bladder and its ability, to completely empty diminish with age.

Psychosocial Factors

For many people, a set of conditions helps stimulate the micturition reflex. These conditions include privacy, normal position, sufficient time, and occasionally, running water.

Circumstances that do not allow for the client's accustomed conditions may produce anxiety and muscle tension. As a result, the person is unable to relax abdominal and perineal muscles and the external urethral sphincter and voiding is inhibited. People may also voluntarily suppress urination because of perceived time pressures.

Fluid and Food Intake

When the amount of fluid intake increases, the output increases in order to maintain balance in a healthy body. Foods that contain caffeine, e.g., coffee, tea, and cola drinks also increase urine production. By contrast, food and fluids high in sodium can cause fluid retention because water is retained to maintain the normal concentration of electrolytes.

Certain foods and fluids can change the color of urine, e.g., beetroot can cause urine to appear red.

Medications

Many medications, particularly those affecting the autonomic nervous system, interfere with the normal urination process and may cause retention. Diuretics increase urine formation by preventing the reabsorption of water and electrolytes from the tubules of the kidney into the blood stream. Some medications may alter the color of urine.

Muscle Tone

Good muscle tone is important to maintain the stretch and contractility of the detrusor muscle so the bladder can fill adequately and empty completely. Clients who require a retention catheter for a long period may have poor bladder muscle tone because continuous drainage of urine prevents the bladder from filling and emptying normally. Pelvic muscle tone also contributes to the ability to store and empty urine.

Pathological Conditions

Some diseases can affect the formation and excretion of urine. Diseases of the kidney may affect the ability of nephrons to produce urine. Abnormal amount of proteins or blood cells may be present in urine, or the kidneys may virtually stop producing urine altogether in renal failure. Heart and circulatory disorders such as heart failure, shock, or hypertension can affect blood flow to the kidneys, interfering with urine production. If abnormal amount of fluid is lost by the body, e.g., in vomiting, water is retained by the kidneys and urine output falls.

Process that interferes with the flow of urine from the kidneys to the urethra affects urinary excretion. A urinary stone may obstruct a ureter, blocking urine from the kidney to the bladder. Hypertrophy of the prostate gland, a common condition affecting older men, may obstruct the urethra, impairing urination and bladder emptying.

Surgical and Diagnostic Procedures

Some surgical and diagnostic procedures affect the passage of urine. The urethra may swell following a cystoscopy, and surgical procedures on any part of the urinary tract may result in some postoperative bleeding. As a result, the urine may have red or pink tinge for some time. Surgery on structures adjacent to the urinary tract can also affect voiding because of swelling in the lower abdomen.

ALTERATIONS IN URINARY ELIMINATION

Despite normal urine production, a number of factors or conditions can affect urinary elimination.

Related to Frequency

- **Polyuria or diuresis:** It is the production of abnormally large amounts of urine by the kidneys. Polyuria can cause excessive fluid loss, dehydration and weight loss.
- **Oliguria and anuria:** Oliguria is low urine output, usually less than 500 mL a day or 30 mL an hour for an adult. It may occur due to less fluid intake or abnormal fluid loss. It indicates impaired blood flow to the kidneys. Anuria refers to lack of urine production which occurs when kidney stops functioning.
- **Urinary frequency:** Voiding at frequent intervals, i.e., more than 6 times per day. It can occur due to increased fluid intake. Conditions such as urinary tract infections, stress and pregnancy can lead to increased urine frequency. Frequent voiding of small quantities (50–100 mL) of urine and total intake may be normal.
- **Nocturia:** It is voiding urine two or more times at night.
- **Urgency:** It is the sudden desire to void. It is due to psychologic stress and irritation of the trigone and urethra.
- **Dysuria:** It means voiding that is either painful or difficult. It can be due to stricture of the urethra, urinary infection, and injury to the bladder and urethra.
- **Enuresis:** Enuresis is involuntary urination in children beyond the age when voluntary bladder control is normally acquired, usually 4 or 5 years of age. Nocturnal enuresis or bedwetting is the involuntary passing of urine during sleep.

Urinary Incontinence

Urinary incontinence, or involuntary urination is a symptom, not a disease. It can have a significant impact on the client's life, creating physical problems such as skin breakdown leading to many psychosocial problems such as embarrassment, isolation and social withdrawal. Common causes of incontinence include urinary tract infections, urethritis, pregnancy, hypercalcemia, volume overload, delirium, restricted mobility, stool impaction and psychologic causes.

Urinary Retention

When emptying of the bladder is impaired, urine accumulates and the bladder becomes over-distended, giving rise to a condition known as urinary retention. Over distention of the bladder causes poor contractility of the detrusor muscle, which further impairs urination. Common causes of urinary retention include prostatic hypertrophy. Clients with urinary retention may experience overflow voiding or incontinence, eliminating 25–50 mL of urine at frequent intervals. On palpation, the bladder is firm and distended and may be displaced to one side of midline.

Neurogenic Bladder

Impaired neurologic functions can interfere with the normal mechanisms of urine elimination, resulting in a neurogenic bladder. The client with neurogenic bladder does not perceive bladder fullness and is unable to control the urinary sphincters. The bladder becomes flaccid and distended or spastic with frequent involuntary urination.

NURSING MANAGEMENT

Assessment

A complete assessment of a client's urinary function includes: Nursing history, physical assessment of genitourinary system, hydration status and examination of the urine and relating the data obtained to the results of any diagnostic tests and procedures.

Nursing History

The nurse determines the client's normal voiding pattern and frequency, appearance of the urine and any recent changes, any past or current problems with urination, the presence of any urinary diversions and factors influencing the elimination pattern.

Physical Assessment

Complete physical assessment of the urinary tract usually includes percussion of the kidneys to detect areas of tenderness, palpation and percussion of the bladder. If there is a need, the urethral meatus of client is inspected for swelling, discharge and inflammation. The skin is also observed for color, texture, turgor as well as excoriation near perineum due to incontinence.

Assessing Urine

Normal urine consists of 96% of water and 4% solute. Organic solutes include urea, ammonia, creatinine and uric acid.

TABLE 1: Characteristics of normal and abnormal urine

Characteristic	Normal	Abnormal
Amount in 24 hours (adult)	1,200–1,500 mL	Less than 1,200 mL or above 1500
Color, clarity	Straw amber, transparent	Dark amber, cloudy, dark orange, red or dark brown, mucous plugs, viscid, thick
Sterility	No microorganisms present	Microorganisms present
pH	4.5–8	Over 8 or under 4.5
Specific gravity	1.010–1.025	Over 1.025 or under 1.010
Glucose	Absent	Present like in type 2 diabetes mellitus
Ketone bodies (acetone)	Not present	Present like in type 1 diabetes mellitus
Blood	Not present	Present, occult or bright red

Urea is the chief organic solute. Inorganic solutes include sodium, chloride, potassium, sulfate, magnesium and phosphorus. Characteristics of normal and abnormal urine are shown in Table 1.

Measuring Urinary Output

Normally the kidneys produce urine at a rate of approximately 60 mL per hour or about 1,500 mL/day. Urine output is affected by many factors, including fluid intake, body fluid losses through other routes such as breathing, perspiration or diarrhea, and the cardio-vascular and renal status of the individual. To measure urine output, instruct the client to keep urine in urine collection container and pour the voided urine into a calibrated container and record the amount on the fluid intake and output sheet.

If the client has a catheter, then follow these steps

- Put on clean gloves
- Take the calibrated container to the bedside
- Place the container under the urine collection bag so that the spout of the bag is above the container because calibrated container is not sterile, but the collection bag is sterile
- Open the spout and permit the urine to flow into the container.
- Hold the container at eye level, read the amount in the container having a measuring scale inside
- Record the output in intake and output sheet

Measuring Residual Urine

Residual urine (urine remaining in the bladder following the voiding) is normally 50–100 mL. Some conditions may interfere with complete emptying of the bladder such as bladder output obstruction due to enlargement of the prostate gland or loss of bladder muscle tone. Manifestation of urine retention may include frequent voiding of small amounts less than 100 mL in adult. Urinary stasis and urinary tract infections are possible consequences of incomplete emptying of bladder.

For measuring residual urine, the client needs to be catheterized. The amount of urine voided and the urine obtained by catheterization is measured and recorded.

Diagnostic Tests

Two metabolically produced substances, urea and creatinine are used to evaluate renal function. Both are eliminated by the kidneys through filtration and tubular secretion. Urea and end products of protein metabolism, are measured as blood urea nitrogen (BUN). Creatinine is produced in relatively constant quantities by the muscles. The creatinine clearance tests use 24-hour urine and serum creatinine levels to determine the glomerular filtration rate, a sensitive indicator of renal function.

Other tests related to the urinary system include urodynamic studies, cystoscopy, intravenous pyelogram, retrograde pyelogram, computed tomography (CT) scans, renal biopsy and ultrasound examination. Nurses are responsible for preparing the patient for the procedure and giving appropriate after care.

Diagnosing

The data collected about the client's urinary functioning may lead to one or more nursing diagnosis. Examples of North American Nursing Diagnosis and Association (NANDA). Nursing diagnosis: Urinary elimination:

- Impaired urinary elimination such as functional urinary incontinence, reflex urinary incontinence, stress urinary incontinence, total urinary incontinence, urge urinary incontinence, over flow urinary incontinence, urinary retention.
- Risk for infection for clients who have urinary retention or undergo invasive procedures such as catheterization or cystoscopic examination
- Low self-esteem or social isolation if the client is incontinent
- Risk for impaired skin integrity-in incontinence
- Self-care deficit in case of functional urinary incontinence, i.e., inability of usually continent person to reach toilet on time.
- Risk for deficient fluid volume or excess fluid volume
- Disturbed body image if patient has a urinary diversion
- Deficient knowledge

- Risk for caregiver role strain related to incontinence of family member
- Risk for social isolation in incontinent client.

Planning

The goals established will vary according to the diagnosis. The overall goals for clients with urinary elimination problems may include:

- Maintain or restore a normal voiding pattern
- Regain normal urine output
- Prevent associated risks such as infection, skin breakdown, fluid and electrolyte imbalance, and lowered self-esteem.
- Contain urine with appropriate device, catheter, ostomy appliance or absorbent product.

Appropriate preventive and corrective nursing intervention that relate to these must be identified. Specific nursing interventions associated with these can be selected to meet the client's individual needs.

To provide for continuity of care, the nurse needs to consider the client's needs for teaching and assistance with **care in the home.** Discharge planning includes assessment of the client and family resources and abilities for self-care, available financial resources and the need for referrals and home health services.

Implementation

Maintaining Normal Urinary Elimination

Most interventions to maintain normal urinary elimination are independent nursing functions. These include promoting adequate fluid intake, maintaining normal voiding habits and assisting with toileting.

Promoting Fluid Intake

Increasing fluid intake increases urine production, which in turn stimulates the micturition reflex. A normal daily intake average 1,500 mL is adequate for adult clients. Many clients have increased fluid requirements necessitating a higher daily fluid intake, e.g., clients who are perspiring excessively or who are experiencing abnormal fluid losses through vomiting, gastric suction, diarrhea, or wound drainage require fluid to replace these losses in addition to their normal daily intake requirements.

Clients who are at risk for urinary tract infection or urinary calculi (stones) should consume 2,000–3,000 mL of fluid daily. Dilute urine and frequent urination reduce the risk of urinary tract infection as well as stone formation.

Increased fluid intake may be contraindicated for client with kidney failure or heart failure. For clients with kidney failure or heart failure, a fluid restriction may be necessary to prevent fluid overload and edema.

Maintain Normal Voiding Habits

Client's normal voiding habits are often interfered with prescribed medical therapies. When client's urinary elimination pattern is adequate, the nurse helps the client adhere to normal voiding habits as much as possible by:

- **Positioning:** Assist the client to a normal position for voiding, standing for male clients and for female clients, squatting or leaning slightly forward when sitting.

  If the client is unable to ambulate to the lavatory, use bedside commode for females and urinal for males.

- **Relaxation:** Provide privacy for the client and allow the client sufficient time to void. Let the client listen to music or read. Pour warm water over the perineum of a female or have the client sit on a warm bed pan to promote muscle relaxation. Applying a hot water bottle to the lower abdomen of both males and females helps muscle relaxation.

  Turn on running water within hearing distance of the client to stimulate the voiding reflex and providing emotional support to decrease muscle tension.

- **Timing:** Assist client who has the usage to void immediately. Offer toileting assistance to the client at usual times of voiding for example, on awakening, before or after meals, and at bed time.

For Clients Who are Confined to Bed

Warm the bed-pan. A cold bed-pan causes contraction of perineal muscles. Elevate the head of the client's bed to Fowler's position. Place a small pillow or rolled towel at the back to increase physical comfort, and make the client flex the hips and knees. This position stimulates the normal voiding position as closely as possible.

- **Assisting with toileting:** Clients who are weak due to disease process require assistance with toileting. The nurse should assist those clients to the bathroom and remain with them if they are at risk for falling.

  For clients unable to use bathroom facilities, the nurse provides urinary equipment close to the bedside and provides necessary assistance to use them.

Preventing Urinary Tract Infections

The urinary tract infections (UTI) is greater in women than men because of the short urethra and its proximity to the anal and vaginal areas. To prevent urinary tract infections, follow these guidelines:

- Drink eight glasses of water per day to flush bacteria out of urinary system.
- Practice frequent voiding every 2–4 hours to flush bacteria out of the urethra and prevent organisms from ascending into the bladder. Void immediately after intercourse.
- Avoid use of harsh soaps, bubble bath, powder or sprays in the perineal area.
- Avoid tight fitting pants that prevents ventilation of the perineal area.
- Wear cotton underclothes to absorb moisture.
- Girls and women, should always wipe the perineal area from front to back following urination or defecation in order to prevent introduction of gastrointestinal bacteria into the urethra.
- If recurrent urinary infections are a problem, take showers rather than baths.

Those at greatest risk for UTI include:

- **Sexually active women:** During intercourse, perineal bacteria can migrate into urethra and bladder.
- **Women who use diaphragm for contraception:** The spermicide used with a diaphragm decreases the amount of normally protective vaginal flora.
- **Postmenopausal women:** Urinary stasis which is common at this age, provides an optimal environment for bacteria to multiply and decreased estrogen contributes to loss of protective vaginal flora
- **Individuals with an indwelling urinary catheter in place:** About half of all patients with an indwelling catheter become infected within 1 week after its insertion.
- **Individuals with diabetes mellitus:** Glucose in the urine acts as an excellent medium for bacteria to proliferate.
- **Elderly people:** The physiologic changes associated with aging predispose older people to the development of UTI.

Managing Urinary Incontinence

Urinary incontinence is any involuntary leakage of urine that is widely under reported and undiagnosed. It is one of the most common chronic health problems. It is more prevalent in women and increases with age. Older adults may experience decreasing control over urination and may find it more difficult to reach a toilet in time to void because of mobility problems or dexterity problems in undressing.

Types of Urinary Incontinence

- **Transient incontinence:** Appears suddenly and lasts for 6 months or less. It is usually caused by infection, as a result of medical treatment, use of diuretics or intravenous fluid administration.
- **Stress incontinence:** Occurs when there is involuntary loss of urine related to increase in intra-abdominal pressure. This commonly occurs during coughing, sneezing, laughing, childbirth, menopause, obesity or straining from chronic constipation.
- **Urge incontinence:** The involuntary loss of urine that occurs soon after feeling an urgent need to void (urgency). These patients experience incontinence before getting to the toilet and an inability to suppress the need to urinate.
- **Overflow incontinence:** The involuntary loss of urine associated with over distension and overflow of

the bladder. The signal to empty the bladder may be underactive or absent, the bladder fills and dribbling occurs. It may occur due to effect of some drugs, fecal impaction, or neurologic conditions.

- **Functional incontinence:** Urine loss caused by the inability to reach the toilet because of environmental barriers, physical limitations, loss of memory or disorientation.
- **Reflex incontinence:** Clients with this incontinence experience emptying of bladder without the sensation of the need to void. Spinal cord injuries may lead to this type of incontinence.
- **Total incontinence:** A continuous and unpredictable loss of urine, resulting from surgery, trauma or physical malformation.

Treatment for Incontinence

- **Bladder training:** Bladder training program requires the involvement of the nurse, the client and support of the people. Clients must be alert and physically able or have caregivers who can assist with implementation of the plan of care. Bladder training requires the client to postpone voiding, resist or inhibit the sensation of urgency, and void according to a timetable rather than according to the urge to void. The goals are to gradually lengthen the intervals between urination to correct the client's frequent urination, to stabilize the bladder and to diminish urgency. Delayed voiding provides larger voided volumes and longer intervals between voiding. Initially voiding may be encouraged every 2–3 hours except during sleep and then every 4–6 hours. A vital component of bladder training is inhibiting the urge-to-void sensation. To do this, the nurse instructs the client to practice deep, slow breathing until the urge diminishes or disappears. This is performed every time the client has a premature urge to void.

- **Habit training:** Also referred to as timed voiding or scheduled toileting, attempts to keep clients dry by having them void at regular intervals. With habit training, there is no attempt to motivate the client to delay voiding if the urge occurs.
- **Pelvic muscle exercises (PME):** PME or Kegel exercises help to strengthen pelvic floor muscles and can reduce or eliminate episodes of incontinence. The client can identify the perineal muscles by stopping urination midstream or by tightening the anal sphincter as if to hold a bowel movement. PME can be performed anytime, anywhere sitting or standing even when voiding.

Maintaining Skin Integrity

Skin that is continually moist becomes macerated (softened). Urine that accumulates on the skin is converted to ammonia, which is very irritating to the skin. Both irritation and maceration predispose the client's skin to breakdown and ulcerate. The incontinent person requires meticulous skin care. To maintain skin integrity, the nurse washes the client's perineal area with mild soap and water, rinses it thoroughly, dries it gently and thoroughly, and provides clean, dry clothing or bed linen. The nurse applies barrier ointment or creams to protect the skin from urine. Sometimes absorbent sheet helps to maintain skin integrity, it does not stick to the skin when wet, decreases the risk of bed sores and reduces odor.

Applying External Urinary Drainage Devices

The application of a condom or external catheter connected to a urinary drainage system can be used for incontinent males. Use of a condom appliance is preferable to insertion of a retention catheter because the risk of urinary tract infection is minimal.

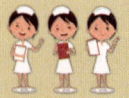 **SKILL: APPLYING A CONDOM CATHETER**

Purposes

- To collect urine and control urinary incontinence
- To permit the client's physical activity while controlling urinary incontinence
- To prevent skin irritation as a result of urine incontinence

Equipment

- Condom catheter
- Gloves
- Drape (sheet or bath blanket)
- Basin of warm water and soap

- Washcloth and towel
- Skin preparatory pads or solution
- Clippers for hair removal if needed
- Urine collection bag with drainage tubing and elastic tape or Velcro strap.

Steps of Procedure

Review and carry out the standard steps as given in Appendix

Action/steps	Rationale
Assessment	
1. Review the client's record to determine a pattern of voiding and other pertinent data. Assess condition of skin on penis	Urine incontinence places the skin at risk for breakdown
Planning	
2. Gather equipment and prepare the working space by raising the bed to proper height	Promotes work efficiency and prevents back strain.
3. Close the door or draw curtains	Protects the client's privacy
4. Explain the procedure	Promotes cooperation and reduces anxiety.
5. Place the client in supine position and drape the upper torso with a bath blanket and then fold the sheet down so it covers the legs and can be lowered to expose the genitalia.	Provides comfort, conserves body heat and prevents unnecessary exposure
6. Prepare the urinary drainage collection system. Roll the wider tip of the condom sheath toward the narrower tip.	Prepares the system for use.
Implementation	
7. Wash hands and put on gloves	Prevents transfer of microorganisms
8. Wash and dry the penis and surrounding skin. Clip the hair at the base of the penis, apply the skin prep and allow to dry.	Cleanses the skin before application of the condom. The skin prep protects the skin against urine and provides an adherent surface on which to apply the condom catheter.
9. Apply the double-sided elastic tape in a spiral fashion from the base of the penis downward.	Provides a surface on which the condom catheter can be attached without impending circulation in the penis.
10. Grasp the penis along the shaft with the non-dominant hand. Hold the condom sheath at the tip of the penis and smoothly roll the sheath onto the penis leaving 1–2 inches of space between the tip of the penis and the drainage tube of the condom sheath.	Positions the condom catheter on the penis. Allows free passage of urine into the collecting tube and drainage bag. Keeps penis away from collecting urine. Adheres the condom sheath to the penis.
11. Position the penis downward and connect the drainage tube to the collection bag (Fig. 3).	Allows urine to flow into the collection bag.

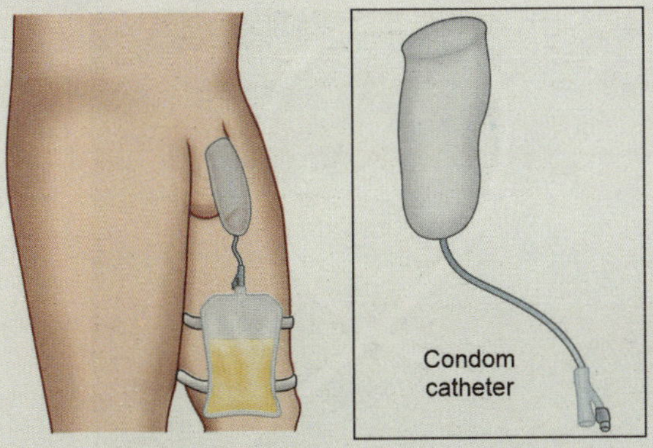

Condom catheter

Fig. 3: Placing the condom catheter

Contd...

Action/steps	Rationale
12. Make patient comfortable; place call bell within reach of client.	Prevents accidents and provides comfort and security.
13. Check the penis after 30 minutes and then every 2 hours and ensure that the catheter is not twisted so that urine can drain freely	Ensure that the catheter is not too tight and impairing circulation; twisting of catheter impedes urine flow
14. Remove gloves and wash hands	Reduces transfer of microorganisms
15. Check if the catheter fits smoothly and firmly adheres to the penis? Is there evidence of irritation to the skin or impaired circulation? Is urine draining into the bag? Is there any leakage of urine?	Determines whether system is functioning effectively without problems
Documentation	
16. Note date, condition of genital area, size and type of catheter applied, amount, color and character of urine and patient's tolerance of procedure.	Documents use of condom catheter

Managing Urinary Retention

If nursing interventions that assist the client to maintain normal voiding pattern fail to initiate voiding, urinary catheterization may be necessary to empty the bladder completely.

Urinary Catheterization

Urinary catheterization is the introduction of a catheter into the urinary bladder. This is usually performed only when absolutely necessary, because there are chances of introducing microorganisms into the bladder. Thus, strict sterile technique is used for catheterizations. Another hazard is trauma with urethral catheterization, particularly the male client, whose urethra is longer and more tortuous. It is important to insert a catheter along the normal contour of the urethra. Damage to the urethra can occur if the catheter is forced through stricture or at incorrect angle. In males, the urethra is normally curved, but it can be straightened by elevating the penis to a position perpendicular to the body.

Catheters are commonly made of rubber or plastics or polyvinyl chloride (PVC), latex or silicone. They are sized by the diameter of the lumen using the French (Fr) scale; the larger the number, the larger is the lumen. Either straight catheters, inserted to drain the bladder and then immediately removed, or retention catheters, which remain in the bladder to drain urine, may be used.

The straight catheter is a single lumen tube with a small eye or opening about 1¼ cm (1/2 inch) from the insertion tip (Figs 4A and B). The coude catheter is a variation of the straight catheter. It is more rigid than other straight catheters and has a tapered, curved tip (Fig. 5). This catheter may be used for men with prostatic hypertrophy because it is more easily controlled and is less traumatic on insertion.

The retention, or Foley catheter is a double lumen catheter (Fig. 6). The larger lumen drains urine from the bladder. A second, smaller lumen is used to inflate a balloon near the tip of the catheter to hold the catheter in place within the bladder. Clients who require continuous or intermittent bladder irrigation may have a three-way Foley's catheter, in which the third lumen through which sterile irrigating fluid can flow into the bladder (Fig. 7). The fluid then exits the bladder through the drainage lumen, along with the urine. The balloons of retention catheters are sized by the volume of fluid used to inflate them. The two commonly used sizes are 10 mL and 30 mL balloons. The size of the balloon is indicated on the catheter along with the diameter, for example, # 18 Fr–10 mL.

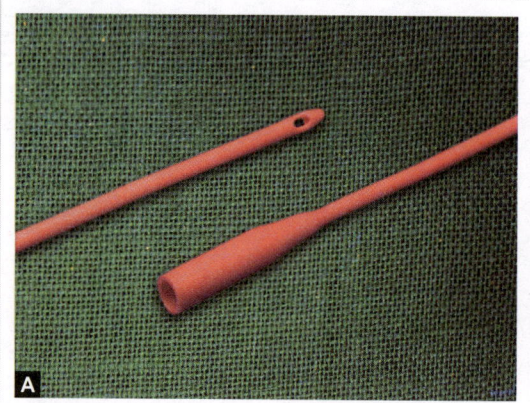
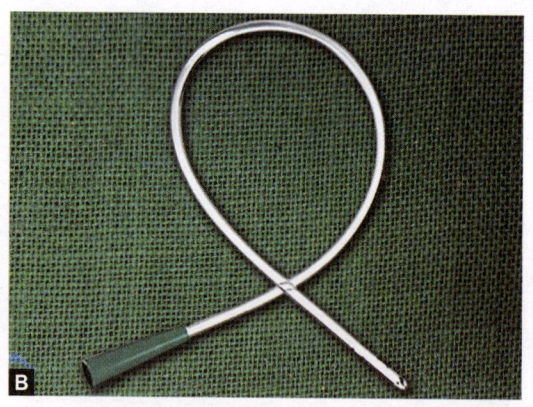

Figs 4A and B: Red-rubber or plastic Robinson straight catheters

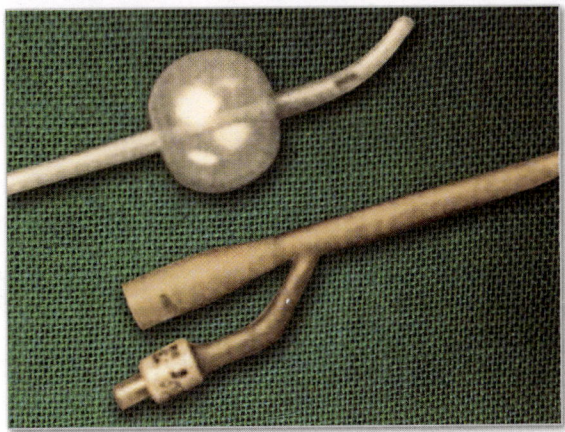

Fig. 5: Coude catheter

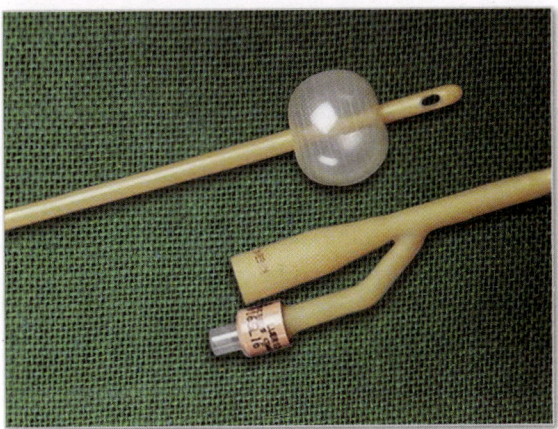

Fig. 6: An indwelling/retention (Foley's) catheter with the balloon inflated

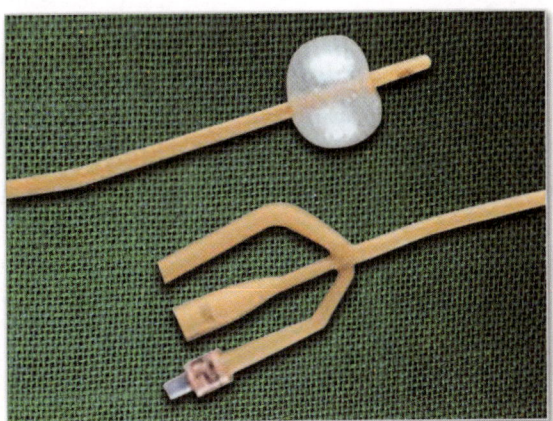

Fig. 7: A three-way Foley's catheter often used for continuous bladder irrigation

Retention catheters are usually connected to a closed gravity drainage system. The system consists of the catheter, drainage tubing, and a collecting bag for the urine. A closed system cannot be opened anywhere along the system, from catheter to collecting bag, thereby they reduce the risk of microorganisms entering the system and infecting the urinary tract.

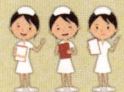 **SKILL: PERFORMING URINARY CATHETERIZATION:**

Purposes

- To relieve discomfort due to bladder distension or to provide gradual decompression of a distended bladder.
- To assess the amount of residual urine if the bladder empties incompletely.
- To obtain a sterile urine specimen
- To empty the bladder completely prior to surgery

Equipment

- Foley's catheter or plain catheter kit with appropriate size
- Sterile gauze
- Bath blanket, basin with warm water, towel and wash cloth
- Mild soap

- Tape, extra light, waste receptacle/paper bag.
- Antiseptic solution
- Lubricant

Steps of Procedure

Review and carry out the standard steps as given in Appendix

Action/steps	Rationale
Assessment	
1. Check the physician's order for type and size of catheter	Catheterization is only done by medical order
2. Assess the patient's knowledge of catheterization and use of a catheter	Consider the patient's knowledge level before beginning the teaching for the same
3. Assess whether patient is allergic to iodine or tape	Povidone iodine is often used to cleanse the perineum before catheterization
Planning	
4. Identify the patient, gather equipment and prepare the working space by raising the bed to proper height and positioning the over bed table for use	Ensures that the procedure is performed on the correct patient; promotes work efficiency and prevents back strain
5. Close the door or draw curtain to maintain privacy	Protects the patient's right to privacy and prevents embarrassment.
6. Explain the procedure	Decreases fear of unknown and prepare the patient
Implementation: For catheterizing female patient	
7. Wash your hands and don gloves	Reduces transfer of microorganisms
8. Assist to assure the dorsal recumbent position and drape with bath blanket or sheet	Positions patient for viewing the meatus and inserting the catheter into bladder
9. In good light, inspect the perineum. Wash the area, if needed. Spread the labia with your non dominant hand and locate the urinary meatus (Fig. 8) 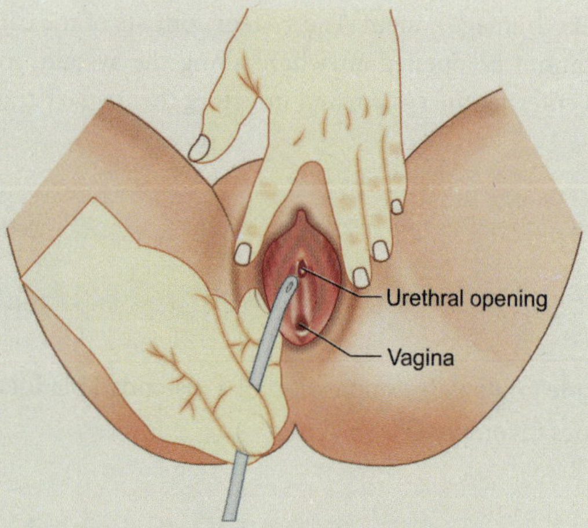	This ensures greater success in placing the catheter into the bladder

Fig. 8: Site of catheter insertion

10. Remove glove and wash your hands	Reduces transfer of microorganisms
11. Remove the paper/cloth wrapped catheter tray and place it on the bed between patient's legs, near the perineum (8–12 inches away)	Provides a work space

Contd...

Action/steps	Rationale
12. Pick up the sterile absorbent under pad by one corner, and while holding two corners turned under, slip it under the patient's buttocks with plastic side down while asking her to lift the buttocks. Touch only the corners and underside of the pad	Keeps solution from soiling; keeps the center of the pad sterile
13. Put on the sterile gloves and place the sterile drape with the opening over the genital area, exposing the labia.	Sterile drape helps prevent catheter from touching the skin on the thighs as the meatus is approached.
14. Soak the cotton balls with the antiseptic solution and remove the plastic sleeve on the catheter by tearing it down the perforated side and place it in a tray for easy access.	Prepares the cotton balls and catheter for use and preventing a break in sterile techniques
15. Test the patency of the balloon by attaching sterile water-filled syringe in the balloon port of the catheter and insert the water	Ensures balloon patency before the catheter is introduced into the bladder
16. After the test, draw the water back into the syringe leaving the syringe attached to the catheter balloon port	Makes it easier to inject the water into the balloon at the right moment.
17. With the forefinger and thumb of the non-dominant hand, separate the labia minora, exposing the meatus	Exposes the urinary meatus so that catheter can be introduced
18. Using the forceps, pick up one saturated cotton ball at a time and cleanse down one side of the labia majora and then the other, discarding each used cotton ball after one stroke. Cleanse one side of the labia minora and then the other. Lastly cleanse the meatus with a slow downward stroke. Do not allow the labia to close over the meatus after cleansing. Discard the forceps.	Removes microorganisms from the perineal area and urinary meatus. Take care not to pass over the sterile field with used cotton balls when discarding them, contaminated forceps must be discarded
19. Pick up the catheter about 3 inches from the tip, lubricate it well and gently insert it into the meatus, pointing slightly toward the umbilicus. Insert it about 2–3 inches or until you visualize urine flow. There may be slight resistance as the catheter passes the internal urethral sphincter. If urine does not flow, rotate the catheter gently and insert it another inch farther. Do not use force. Ask the patient to take deep breath, to relax the sphincter and advance the catheter	Ensures easy insertion into the bladder and collecting urine in sterile waste receptacle
20. Hold the catheter in place with the dominant hand while instilling the water into the balloon with non-dominant hand. Remove the syringe from the port after inflation and discard it. Gently pull on the catheter to see if it is anchored securely, then gently push it into the bladder about ½ inch. Watch the patient's face for expression of discomfort while inflating the balloon to be certain that the balloon is not in urethra	Keeps the catheter from slipping back into the urethra
21. Attach the drainage bag to the stationary part of the bed frame along the side of the bed. Remove the drapes, dry the genital area, remove gloves and wash hands.	Keeps bag from coming into contact with the floor
22. Attach the catheter to the thigh with the tape. Coil the excess drainage tubing on the bed so that last portion hangs straight to the drainage bag and secure it	The secured catheter does not cause tension on the urethral sphincter. The catheter drains better if no tubing is hanging below the level of entry into the urinary bag.
23. Restore the unit, lower the bed, raise the bed rails and place the call-light within reach	Protects the patient; call-light provides sense of security
Evaluation	
24. Ask yourself if sterile technique was maintained. Is urine draining well? Is patient without pain	Determines whether the procedure was done correctly and whether catheter is patent
Documentation	
25. Note date, time, size and type of catheter, amount of water instilled into balloon, color and characteristics of urine and output of urine	Documents catheter insertion and urine output
Implementation: For catheterizing male patient	
Note: For catheterizing male patient follow assessment and planning steps (1–6) as for female patients	
26. Wash your hands	Reduces transfer of microorganisms.

Contd...

Action/steps	Rationale
27. With the patient supine and knees slightly apart, drape by fanfolding the bedcovers down to cover the legs exposing the perineal area. Use a bath blanket to cover the trunk	Draping keeps the patient warm and reduces embarrassment and maintains privacy
28. Place the absorbent pad under the perineum and place the opening of the sterile drape over the penis and onto the perineum without touching the top surface after putting on gloves	Provides a sterile field within which to work
29. Remove the plastic sleeve from the catheter and test the balloon by inflating water	Prepares the catheter for use, to detect leaks in balloon
30. Lubricate 3–4 inches (5–7 cm) of the catheter (xylocaine gel)	Lubricant prevents undue trauma while inserting catheter into the urethra
31. Retract the foreskin, if necessary, to expose the head of the penis	Foreskin interferes with adequate cleansing
32. Using forceps and a saturated cotton ball, grasp the glans below the tip with the non-dominant hand, hold it erect, and cleanse the glans in a circular motion moving outward from meatus	Reduces the number of microorganisms around the meatus.
33. Pick up the catheter with the dominant hand 3–4 inches (8–10 cm) below the tip with the penis at a 90–degree angle to the body, pull it slightly upward and insert the catheter into the meatus about 8 inches (20 cm) using a rotating motion until urine begins to flow	Elevating and putting slight traction on the penis straightens the urethra and makes it easier to insert the catheter into the bladder
34. If resistance is met, twist the catheter and ask the client to take a deep breath. If resistance persists, do not force the catheter. Remove it.	The internal sphincter relaxes when a deep breath is taken. Forcing catheter may cause trauma
35. Gently push the catheter 1–2 inches more after urine starts to flow. Hold the catheter in place and inject the contents of the prefilled syringe into the balloon and detach the syringe while holding the plunger all the way down.	Guides the balloon away from the sphincter, preventing pressure on the neck of the bladder. Filling the balloon ensures that the catheter will remain in the bladder. Holding down the plunger of the syringe that is used to fill the balloon keeps the water from flowing back into the syringe.
36. Pull gently on the catheter to check that the balloon is inflated. Then push it back slightly.	Ensures that the catheter will not fall out. Relieves pressure on the sphincter.
37. Remove the drape and reposition the foreskin if it was retracted	Repositioning of foreskin prevents constricting the penis, swelling and circulation difficulties
38. Tape the catheter to the abdomen if it is to remain in place for an extended period. Alternatively it may be taped to the inner thigh for short-term use	Secures the catheter, so there is no tension on the internal urinary sphincter
39. Attach the drainage bag to the bed frame (not the side rail). Coil the excess drainage tubing on the mattress and secure it.	The drainage bag must be kept below the level of bladder for drainage to occur. Tubing should not hang below the level of entry into the bag.
40. Remove the drape, make the patient comfortable, lower the bed, raise the side rails, and restore the unit, placing the call-light within reach	Provides for patient comfort and safety
41. Remove gloves and wash hands	Reduces transfer of microorganisms
Evaluation	
42. Were sterile methods maintained? Was urine obtained? Were any problems encountered?	Questions help determine success of the procedure
Documentation	
43. Note date, time, size and type of catheter inserted, amount of water in balloon, any problems encountered, amount and character of urine obtained	Documents procedure, catheter size and output of urine.

Nursing Interventions for Clients with Indwelling Catheter

Nursing care of the client with an indwelling catheter and continuous drainage is largely directed toward preventing infection of the urinary tract and encouraging urinary flow through the drainage system. It includes encouraging large amounts of fluid intake, changing retention catheter and tubing, maintaining the patency of the drainage system and preventing contamination of the drainage system.

Fluids

The client with a retention catheter should drink up to 3,000 mL/day if permitted. Large amounts of fluid intake ensure a large output, which keeps the bladder flushed out and decreases the likelihood of urinary stasis and infection. It also minimizes the risk of sediment obstructing the drainage tubing.

Dietary Measures

Acidifying the urine of clients with a retention catheter may reduce the risk of urinary tract infection and calculus formation. Foods such as eggs, cheese, meat and poultry, whole grains, plums and tomatoes tend to increase the acidity of urine.

Perineal Care

Routine hygienic care is necessary for clients with retention catheter as per agency practice.

Changing the Catheter and Tubing

Collection of sediments in the catheter or tubing or impaired urine drainage are indicators for changing the catheter and drainage system. When this occurs, the catheter and drainage system are removed and discarded, and a new sterile catheter and closed drainage system is inserted.

Removing Indwelling Catheters

Indwelling catheters are removed after their purpose has been achieved. If the catheter has been in place for a short time, the client usually has little difficulty regaining normal urinary elimination patterns.

Clients who have had a retention catheter for a prolonged period may require bladder retraining to regain bladder muscle tone. With an indwelling catheter in place, the bladder muscle does not stretch and contract regularly as it does when the bladder fills and empties by voiding. A few days, before removal, the catheter may be clamped for specified periods of time (2–4 hours) then released to allow the bladder to empty. This allows the bladder to distend and stimulates its musculature.

To remove a retention catheter, follow these steps:

♦ Collect supplies: Receptacle for the catheter, a clean disposal towel, clean gloves and sterile syringe to deflate the balloon.

♦ Ask the client to assume a supine position

♦ Remove the tape attaching the catheter to the client, put on gloves and place towel between the legs of the female patient or over the thighs of a male.

♦ Insert a syringe into the injection port of the catheter, and withdraw the fluid from the balloon

♦ Do not pull the catheter while the balloon is inflated, doing so may injure the urethra.

♦ After all the fluid is withdrawn from the balloon, gently withdraw the catheter and place it in the waste receptacle.

♦ Dry the perineal area with a towel.

♦ Remove gloves.

♦ Measure the urine in the drainage bag and record the removal of catheter. Include in the recording: The time the catheter was removed, the amount, color and clarity of the urine, the intactness of the catheter and instructions given to the client.

♦ Provide the client with urinal, bedpan or commode to be used with each subsequent unassisted voiding.

♦ Following removal of catheter, determine the time of the first voiding and amount voided during the first 8 hours and compare the output with client's intake.

Care of Urinary Diversions

A urinary diversion is the surgical rerouting of urine from the kidneys to a site other than the bladder. There are two categories of diversions: Incontinent and continent.

♦ **Incontinent:** With incontinent diversions, clients have no control over the passage of urine and require the use of an external ostomy appliance to contain the urine. Urinary diversions may or may not involve the removal of the bladder (cystectomy) Examples of incontinent diversions include ureterostomy, nephrostomy, vesicostomy and ileal conduits. A **ureterostomy** is when one or both of the ureters may be brought directly to the side of the abdomen to form small stomas providing direct access for microorganisms from the skin to the kidneys, the small stomas are difficult to fit with the appliance to collect the urine and being narrow, impair urinary drainage. **Nephrostomy** diverts urine from the kidney to a stoma. A **vesicostomy** is performed when the bladder is left intact but voiding through the urethra is not possible. The ureters remain connected to the bladder, and the bladder wall is surgically attached to an opening in the skin below the naval forming an incontinent stoma. The most common urinary diversion is the **ileal conduit** or ileal loop. In this, a segment of the ileum is removed and the intestinal ends are reattached. One end of the portion removed is closed with sutures to create a pouch and the other end is brought out through the abdominal wall to create a stoma. The ureters are implanted into the ileal pouch. The ileal stoma is more readily fitted with an appliance.

- **Continent diversion:** With continent diversion, a continence mechanism is created giving clients control over the passage of urine either by intermittent catheterization of the internal reservoir (Koch pouch) or by strained voiding (neobladder). This is used when the bladder is diseased or damaged. This new bladder is sutured to the functional urethra. Clients with these can control voiding.

When caring for clients with a urinary diversion, the nurse must accurately assess intake and output, note any changes in urine color, odor or clarity and frequently assess the condition of the stoma and surrounding skin. Clients who wear a urine collection appliance are at risk for impaired skin integrity. Because of irritation of urine, well-fitting appliance is must. Clients with urinary diversions may experience problems with their body image and sexuality and may require assistance in coping with the changes and managing the stoma. Most clients are able to resume their normal activities and lifestyle.

Bladder Irrigation or Instillation

The flushing of a tube canal or area with solution is called irrigation.

Purposes

- Wash out residual urine or sediment from the bladder
- Remove clots after prostate or bladder surgery
- Soothe irritated bladder tissues and promote healing
- Ensure that the lumen of the indwelling catheter is open and draining
- Instill medications into the bladder.

Irrigation may be intermittent or continuous depending on the need for keeping the drainage system patent.

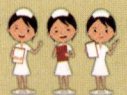

SKILL: PERFORMING INTERMITTENT BLADDER IRRIGATION

Equipment

- Sterile irrigation set
- Clear and sterile gloves
- Absorbent pad
- For open irrigation sterile tubing cap
- Antiseptic swabs

- Sterile normal saline
- Sterile 30–50 mL syringe
- Tubing clamp
- Bath blanket.

Steps of Procedure

Review and carry out the standard steps as given in Appendix

Action/steps	Rationale
Assessment	
1. Check the order about type of irrigation and amount of solution	Provides data about the types and solutions to be used
Planning	
2. Identify the patient	Verifies correct patient
3. Gather the equipment	Promotes work efficiency
4. Explain the procedure to patient	Decreases fear of the unknown and enhances patient's cooperation
Implementation	
5. Wash your hands and lower the side rail	Reduces transfer of microorganisms
6. Have patient assume a dorsal recumbent position and fanfold the linen to expose the catheter without exposing the patient. Use bath blanket to cover the trunk of the patient	Exposes work area and protects patient's dignity. Keeps the patient from becoming cold
7. Check the bladder for distension by palpation	Ensures that fluid will not over distend the bladder

Contd...

Action/steps	Rationale
8. Open the sterile irrigation set and place beside the patient's thigh or between legs. Maintain sterility	Keeps supplies within reach
9. Place the absorbent pad under the catheter drainage tubing connection	Provides a field for work and protects bedding
10. Put on gloves	Reduces transfer of microorganisms
11. For bladder irrigation, clamp the drainage tubing distal to the catheter connection	Clamping directs the solution toward the bladder and prevents the solution from draining into the collection bag
12. Determine the amount of urine in the drainage bag before beginning the irrigation	The amount of urine must be subtracted from the total drainage at the end of the procedure to determine the return of all irrigating solution
13. Pour 100–200 mL of irrigating solution into the sterile container using aseptic technique	Amount depends on medical order
14. Remove the cap from the syringe and draw up to 30–40 mL of solution at a time and remove any air, if present	30–40 mL of solution at a time is normal for irrigation of the adult bladder. Air in bladder causes discomfort
15. With an antiseptic swab, wipe the port on the drainage tubing or the place on the lumen of the catheter for instilling solution	Reduces contamination of the system by microorganisms
16. Insert the needle into the port and gently instill the solution	Gentle instillation prevents injury to the lining of the bladder and helps prevent bladder spasms
17. Remove the needle from the port and cleanse the port with an antiseptic swab. Place the needle and syringe in the sterile container	Keeps the needle sterile so that the procedure can be repeated until the full amount of irrigant has been instilled
18. For an irrigation, immediately unclamp the tubing and lower the catheter so that the fluid runs into the drainage tubing	Allows return of irrigating fluid and any debris that was clogging the catheter
19. For a bladder instillation, leave the tubing clamped for the time ordered, then unclamp it and allow the fluid to run into the drainage container	Allows medicine to remain in contact with bladder wall before draining
20. Repeat the process until all of the ordered solution has been used or until the outflow is clear	Accomplishes purpose of the irrigation or instillation.
21. Empty the urine drainage bag and measure the output. Note the color and characteristics of the drainage and enter the amount on the intake and output record	Irrigation solution must be deducted from the total output. Amount of irrigant is entered as input and drainage is entered as output
22. Dispose of used equipment, remove gloves and wash hands	Reduces transfer of microorganisms.
23. Make the patient comfortable, lower the bed, raise side rails and place the call-light within reach	Demonstrates caring and concern for the patient
Evaluation	
24. Assess for changes in discomfort. Ask yourself, is the catheter draining well? Is the urine clear, free of clots, etc.	Determines whether the procedure was effective
Documentation	
25. Note date, time, how the irrigating solution was used each time, appearance of return flow, how patient tolerated the procedure, whether catheter is now patent.	Verifies ordered procedure was carried out
For open system Irrigation	
26. Follow (1–13 steps above) for patient preparation, wash hands and put on sterile gloves. Make sure that there is written order for performing open irrigation	Reduces transfer of microorganisms. Catheter drainage system should not be opened unnecessarily
27. With an antiseptic swab, disinfect the junction of the catheter and drainage tubing	Reduces chances of contamination of the lumen of the catheter or drainage tubing
28. Placing your fingers at least 1 inch from the junction, separate the catheter and tubing and place a sterile tube cap over the end of the tubing	Keeps the end of the drainage tubing sterile

Contd...

Action/steps	Rationale
29. Draw the 30–40 mL solution into the sterile irrigation syringe and carefully fit the irrigation tip into the end of catheter	Prepares the solution for instillation
30. Gently instill the solution into the catheter by squeezing the bulb of the syringe or pressing the plunger	Too much force may damage the bladder lining or cause bladder spasms
31. Remove the syringe and allow the fluid to run from the catheter into the sterile drainage receptacle. Repeat until the fluid is running freely or the purpose of the irrigation is accomplished	Provides proper drainage of fluid. A clogged catheter may take several irrigations before it is unclogged
32. Carefully remove the cap on the drainage tubing and reattach it to the catheter. Keeping both ends sterile, swab the connection with an antiseptic swab	Restore the closed drainage system without contaminating either the catheter or the tubing
33. Remove gloves and follow the remaining steps as performed for closed irrigation	Reduces transfer of microorganisms

For Continuous or Frequent Bladder Irrigation

Continuous bladder irrigation (CBI) may be ordered when a blood clot or other debris threatens to block the catheter. Closed system irrigation is recommended to prevent entry of pathogens into the bladder (Fig. 9).

For doing continuous bladder irrigation, a triple lumen catheter is used, on which one port is attached to the irrigating fluid with drip chamber, second port is used for inflating the balloon and third port is used for drainage purpose. Hang the bladder irrigant on IV pole and release clamp on irrigation tubing and regulate flow at determined flow rate. If the bladder irrigation is to be done with a medicated solution, use an electronic infusion device to regulate the flow. As the irrigation fluid container nears being empty, clamp the administration tubing. Do not allow drip chamber to empty. Disconnect empty bag and attach a new full irrigation bag. Empty drainage collection bag as each new container is hung and recorded. Document the amount of urine and irrigant is emptied from the drainage bag. Subtract the amount of irrigant solution from the total volume of drainage to obtain the volume of urine output.

Evaluation

Review the expected outcomes written during the planning phase in order to evaluate the effectiveness of interventions for the patient's problems properly. Determine whether the patient can urinate normally, or when a Foley's catheter is removed, indicate whether infection has been eliminated. Noting intake and output records and comparing them from day to day indicates whether fluid intake is sufficient and output is adequate. Noting the condition of skin in the perineal area of the patient who has been incontinent provides information as to whether measures to protect the skin are sufficient. Evidence that the patient has had fewer episodes of incontinence over a period of days indicates that the continence training program is helpful. Checking the appearance of the urine for normal characteristics is an important evaluation tool.

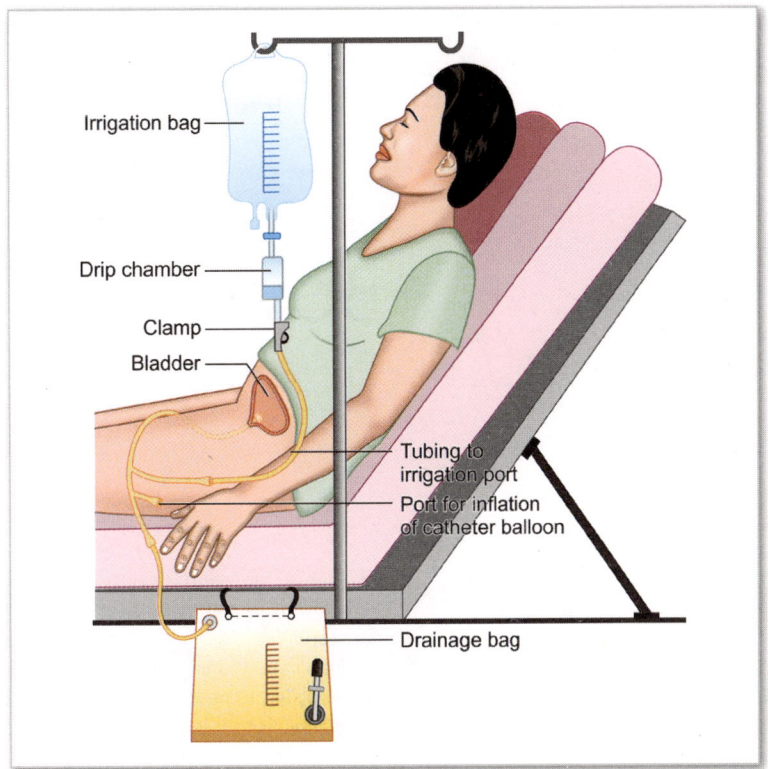

Fig. 9: Continuous bladder irrigation

BIBLIOGRAPHY

1. Taylor C, Lillis C, LeMone P, Lynn P. *Fundamentals of Nursing, 6th edition. Philadelphia: Lippincott Williams and Wilkins. 2008.*

2. Berman AT, Snyder S, Kozier BJ, et al. *Kozier & Erb's. Fundamentals of Nursing: Concepts, Process and Practice, 8th edition. Pearson Education.*

3. Dewit SC. *Fundamental Concepts and Skills for Nursing, 3rd edition. Saunders. 2008. p. 992.*

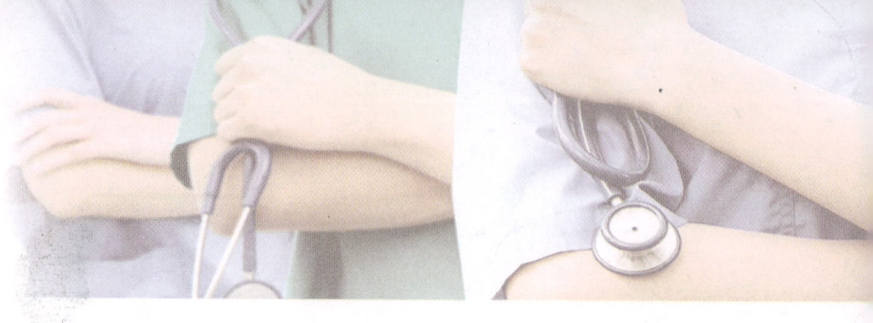

Bowel Elimination

INTRODUCTION

The term *Bowel* refers to the intestine. Bowel elimination, the excretion of solid waste, is the final step in the process of digestion. Many people experience severe or chronic alteration in bowel elimination that affect their fluid and electrolyte balance, hydration, nutritional status, skin integrity, comfort and self-concept. Moreover, many illnesses, diagnostic tests, medication and surgical treatments can affect bowel elimination.

PHYSIOLOGY OF ELIMINATION

The gastrointestinal tract extends from the mouth to the anus. However, the major organ involved with bowel elimination is the large intestine.

Stomach

Stomach is a hollow, J-shaped, muscular organ located in the left upper portion of the abdomen. The stomach stores food during eating, secretes digestive fluids, churns food to aid in digestion, and pushes the partially digested food called chyme, into the small intestine. The pyloric sphincter, a muscular ring that regulates the size of the opening at the end of the stomach, controls the movement of chyme from the stomach into the small intestine.

Small Intestine

The small intestine is about 20 feet (6 meters) long and about 1 inch (2.2 cm) wide. The small intestine is made up of three parts: the first is the duodenum, the middle section is the jejunum and the distal section that connects with the large intestine is the ileum (Fig. 1).

Functions

The small intestine secretes enzymes that digest proteins and carbohydrates. Digestive juices from the liver and pancreas enter the small intestine through a small opening in the duodenum. The small intestine is responsible for digestion of food and absorption of nutrients into the blood stream.

Large Intestine

The connection between the ileum of the small intestine and the large intestine is the ileocecal or ileocolic valve. This valve normally prevents contents from entering the large intestine and prevents waste products from returning to small intestine. The large intestine, the primary organ of bowel elimination, is the lower or distal, part of gastrointestinal tract. The large intestine also known as colon, extends from the ileocecal valve to the anus. It is about 5 feet (1.5 m) long, but variations in length are normal, width also varies from 1 inch to 3 inch. (Fig. 1)

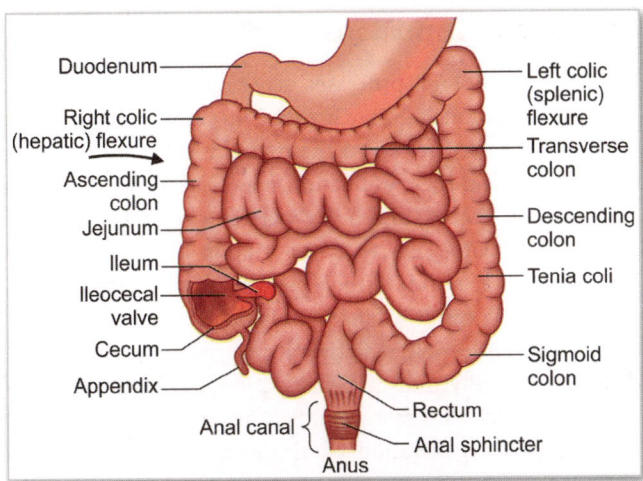

Fig. 1: Small and large intestines

From the cecum, the first part of the large intestine, the digestive contents enter the colon, which consists of several segments. The ascending colon extends from the cecum upward toward the liver, where it turns to cross the abdomen. This turn is called the hepatic flexure. Upon turning, this portion of the colon becomes the transverse colon, crossing the abdomen from right to left. The colon then turns at the splenic flexure to become the descending colon. The descending colon passes down the left side of the body to the sigmoid colon.

The sigmoid colon contains feces, solid waste products that have reached the distal end of the colon and are ready for excretion. Once excreted, feces are called stool. The sigmoid colon empties into the rectum, the last part of the large intestine. The rectum is about 12 cm (5 inches) long and 2–5 cm of which is the anal canal. In the rectum, three transverse folds of tissue are present that may help to hold the fecal material in the rectum temporarily. Vertical folds are also present, each of which contains an artery and a vein. If the vein becomes abnormally distended, **hemorrhoids** occur.

The rectum is empty except immediately before and during defecation (the process of bowel elimination, a bowel movement). Feces are excreted from the rectum through the anal canal, which is approximately 2.5–3.8 cm (1–1.5 inches) long, and out an opening called the anus.

Functions

Functions of large intestine include the absorption of water, the formation of feces and the expulsion of feces from the body. Bacteria that reside in the large intestine act on food residue while it makes its way through the large intestine. Bacterial action produces vitamin K and some of the B complex vitamins.

FACTORS AFFECTING BOWEL ELIMINATION

Various factors can affect bowel elimination. Interference with the normal functioning of elimination from the intestines can occur in health as well as during illness. The factors are:

Developmental Considerations

Age affects, what a person eats and his ability to digest nutrients and eliminate wastes. The stools of an infant are different from those of an older person. **Infant** is being fed on breast milk or formula feed. Breastfeed babies have more frequent stools because breast milk is easier for the intestines to breakdown and absorb; and the stools are yellow to golden and loose and usually have little odor. With formula or cow's milk feeding, the infant's stools vary from yellow to brown, are paste-like consistency and have a strong odor because of the decomposition of protein. Infants have no voluntary control over bowel elimination. The number of stools infants pass varies greatly, e.g., breastfed infants can pass 2–10 stools daily, whereas bottle feed infants pass 1–2 stools daily. At the age of 1 year, all infants commonly pass one to two stools a day. **Diarrhea** is an increase in frequency, and a change in consistency of stool. If **constipation** (dry, hard stool, persistently difficult passage of stool or incomplete passage of stool) occurs, dietary modification is the initial treatment.

In **toddlers** between the ages of 18 and 24 months, the nerve fibers innervating the internal and external anal sphincters become fully developed, and voluntary control of defecation becomes possible. Voluntary defecation requires intact muscular, sensory and nervous structures. Successful bowel training also includes awareness by the toddler of the need to defecate, the ability to communicate this need, the wish to please the significant person involved in bowel training and praise and reinforcement for the toddler's successful behavior. Day time bowel control is normally attained by 30 months of age, but the age varies with each child.

School-aged Child, Adolescent and Adult

From childhood to adulthood, defecation patterns vary in quantity, frequency and rhythmicity. Many people worry needlessly about normal stool characteristics or bowel habits. They need to be made aware of the use of over-the-counter laxatives and enemas, which can have serious consequences.

Older Adult

Older adults experience frequently the problems with bowel elimination, e.g., chronic constipation, diarrhea, fecal impaction (build-up of stool in the colon) or fecal incontinence (involuntary or inappropriate passing of stool or flatus) which can result from physiologic or lifestyle changes.

Food and Fluid

Both, the type and the amount of foods eaten and the amount of fluids ingested affect elimination. A high fiber diet and a daily fluid intake of 2,000–3,000 mL facilitate bowel elimination. High fiber foods such as whole grains and bran, dried peas and fresh fruits and vegetables, increase the bulk in fecal material. Bulkier feces increase pressure on the intestinal wall, which serves as a stimulus for peristalsis. As a result, feces move more quickly through the colon, allowing less water to be reabsorbed. Subsequently the stool is soft and easy to pass. When the stool moves quickly through the colon, there is also less time for toxins to be absorbed from feces by the colon.

Food intolerance may alter bowel elimination, resulting in diarrhea, gaseous distention, and cramping, e.g., lactose intolerance people cannot digest milk due to the lack of enzyme lactose, which helps in the breakdown of the simple sugar lactose found in the milk.

♦ **Constipating foods:** Processed cheese, lean meat, eggs. Foods with laxative effect like fruits and vegetables, bran, chocolate, spicy foods, alcohol, coffee. Gas producing foods like onion, cabbage, beans and cauliflower.

Activity and Muscle Tone

Regular exercise improves gastrointestinal motility and muscle tone, whereas inactivity decreases both. Adequate tone in the abdominal muscle, the diaphragm, and the perineal muscles is essential for defecation.

Lifestyle

Many individuals, family, and sociocultural variables influence a person's usual elimination habits. The long-term effects of bowel training may result in a person's acceptance of bowel elimination as a normal life process, preoccupation with bowel elimination feeling that bowel elimination is 'dirty' process. Rituals associated with bowel elimination, cleanliness considerations, the language used to talk about bowel elimination or reluctance to discuss it, individual responses to involuntary passage of flatus (gas), and so on vary widely among people. A person's daily schedule, occupation, and leisure activities may contribute to a habit of defecating at regular times or to an irregular pattern.

Psychological Variables

Psychological stress affects the body in many ways. In some people, anxiety seems to have a direct effect on gastrointestinal motility, and diarrhea accompanies periods of high anxiety. Persons who chronically worry and those with certain personality types who tend to hold onto problems and negative feelings may experience frequent constipation.

Pathologic Conditions

Numerous pathologic processes may change a person's usual bowel elimination habits. Changes in stool characteristics or frequency may be one of the first clinical manifestations of a disease, and their evaluation may lead to the diagnosis of a disease. For example, if a patient complains that the stool has become narrower or ribbon-like, tumor may be obstructing normal stool passage through the colon. Diarrhea may result from pathologic conditions such as diverticulitis infection, malabsorption syndromes, neoplastic diseases, hyperthyroidism. Constipation may be the result of conditions such as diseases within the colon or rectum and injury to, or degeneration of, the spinal cord, mechanical obstruction resulting from pressure on the intestinal walls, e.g., tumors, etc.

Medications

Medications are available that can promote peristalsis or inhibit peristalsis. Other medications that may affect bowel elimination and stool characteristics are opioids, antacids containing aluminum, iron sulfate and anticholinergic medications decrease gastrointestinal motility with a potential to cause constipation.

Medications may also influence the appearance of the stool, for a variety of reasons, Drugs may cause gastrointestinal bleeding (Anticoagulants, aspirin products) may cause the stool to appear pink to red to black. Iron salts result in black stool from the oxidation of iron.

Patients receiving treatment with antibiotics are at risk for a healthcare, acquired infection with clostridium difficile, which causes intestinal mucosal damage and inflammation, resulting in diarrhea and abdominal cramping. Treatment with antibiotics disrupts the normal intestinal flora and allows microorganisms to flourish within the intestine.

Diagnostic Studies

A patient's bowel elimination pattern may be affected by diagnostic studies. For example, patients may need to fast for diagnostic studies. The ingestion of barium during diagnostic procedures, such as barium enema, may cause constipation. Stress of hospitalization and waiting for the results of studies, changes in food intake, can severely alter a patient's elimination patterns. The use of cathartics or enemas used for bowel cleansing before certain diagnostic studies of the gastrointestinal tract can interfere with the normal timing of a patient's bowel movements.

Surgery and Anesthesia

Direct manipulation of the bowel during abdominal surgery inhibits peristalsis, causing a condition termed paralytic ileus. This temporary stoppage of peristalsis normally lasts 24–48 hours, during this time, food and fluids are withheld.

Inhaled general anesthetic agents also inhibit peristalsis by blocking the parasympathetic impulses to the intestinal musculature.

NURSING PROCESS FOR PATIENTS WITH BOWEL ELIMINATION PROBLEMS

Assessment

Assessment of gastrointestinal tract and bowel elimination includes pertinent patient history, physical assessment, and diagnostic studies.

Nursing History

Include pertinent bowel elimination questions in nursing history (Table 1).

Patients who are critically ill may not be able to report about their bowel accurately, so the nurse or ancillary staff who assist the patient with bowel elimination records any bowel movement.

Physical Assessment

The examination techniques that may be helpful when assessing the functioning of gastrointestinal tract are:

Abdomen

The sequence for abdominal assessment proceed from inspection, auscultation, and percussion to palpation. Inspection and auscultation are performed before palpation because palpation may disturb normal peristalsis and bowel motility. Place the patient comfortably in supine position with the abdomen exposed, the chest and pubic area draped, and the knees slightly flexed. Encourage the patient to urinate prior to the examination so that bladder is empty.

TABLE 1: Nursing history

Factors to assess	Questions
• Usual patterns of bowel elimination	How often do you have bowel movement? Any special time of the day? **What does your stool look like** • Frequency • Time of day • Description of usual stool characteristics
• Aids to elimination	Do you use anything to help your bowel movement? • Natural aids (liquids, foods) • Pharmacologic aids (Laxatives) • Enemas
• Recent changes in bowel elimination	Have you noticed any changes in your stool recently? Have you noticed any blood in your stool? Have you noticed a difference in the appearance of stool?
• Problems with bowel elimination	Are your bowels causing you any problem now? • Nature of disturbance • Onset and frequency • Causes—related to factors • Severity • Symptoms • Interventions attempted and results
• Presence of artificial orifice	What is your routine with your colostomy or ileostomy? Do you have any problem with it?

Inspection

Observe the contour of abdomen, noting any masses, scars, or areas of distention. Significant findings may include the presence of distention or protrusion.

Auscultation

Listen for bowel sounds with the help of diaphragm of a stethoscope in all abdominal quadrants using a clockwise approach. Note the frequency and character of bowel sounds, audible clicks, and gurgles produced by the movement of air and flatus in the gastrointestinal tract. They are usually high pitched, gurgling, and soft. Their frequency may range from 5 to 34 bowel sounds per minute, depending on the rate of peristalsis. Describe bowel sounds as **audible**, **hyperactive**, **hypoactive** or **inaudible**. Hyperactive bowel sounds indicate increased bowel motility, commonly caused by diarrhea, gastroenteritis, or early bowel obstruction. Hypoactive bowel sounds indicate diminished bowel motility, commonly caused by abdominal surgery or late bowel obstruction. Inaudible bowel sounds (evidenced only after listening for 5 minutes) signify the absence of bowel motility, commonly associated with peritonitis, paralytic ileus or prolonged immobility.

Percussion

Percuss all quadrants of the abdomen in a systematic, clockwise manner to identify any masses, fluid or air in the abdomen. Expect a resonant sound or tympany over the abdomen and stomach because these are hollow organs. Areas of increased dullness may be caused by fluid, mass, or a tumor.

Palpation

Both light palpation and deep palpation in each quadrant are performed. Note any muscular resistance, tenderness, enlargement of organs, and masses. If the patient's abdomen is distended, note the presence of firmness or tautness. If patient is in pain, administer medication before proceeding with the palpation.

Anus and Rectum

Perform a superficial examination each time the anal area is washed. Examine the anal area for cracks, nodules, hemorrhoids (distended veins), masses, or polyps. Inspect the perineal area for skin irritation or breakdown secondary to diarrhea or fecal incontinence. Insert a gloved, lubricated finger through the anus into the rectum to assess sphincter tone and smoothness of the mucosal lining, note any masses, polyps, hardened stool, bleeding, pain or abnormal discharge.

Stool Characteristics

Nurses are responsible for reporting and recording information about the patient's stool. Note and record

TABLE 2: Normal characteristic of stool

Characteristic	Normal finding
◆ Volume	Variable
◆ Color	**Infant:** Yellow to brown **Adult:** Brown
◆ Odor	Pungent: may be affected by foods consumed
◆ Consistency	Soft , semisolid, and formed
◆ Shape	Formed stool is about 1 inch in diameter and has the tubular shape of the colon but may be longer or smaller depending on the condition of colon.
◆ Constituents	Waste residues of digestion, bile, intestinal secretions, shed epithelial cells, bacteria and, inorganic material (chiefly calcium and phosphates), seeds, fibers.

anything unusual, including the passage of little or no gas or unusual amounts. Note and record the frequency, amount and characteristics of the patient's bowel movement. Table 2 describes the characteristics of normal stool.

FECAL ELIMINATION PROBLEMS

Four common problems are related to fecal elimination: constipation, diarrhea, bowel incontinence and flatulence.

Constipation

Constipation may be defined as fewer than three bowel movements per week. This infers the passage of dry, hard stool or the passage of no stool. It occurs when the movement of feces through the large intestine is slow, thus allowing time for additional reabsorption of fluid from the large intestine, resulting in difficult evacuation of stool. Person may also have a feeling of incomplete stool evacuation after defecation. Careful assessment of the person's habits is necessary before a diagnosis of constipation is made.

Causes and Factors Contributing to Constipation

- Insufficient fluid intake
- Insufficient fiber intake
- Insufficient activity or immobility
- Irregular defecation habits
- Change in daily routine
- Lack of privacy
- Chronic use of laxatives or enemas
- Irritable bowel syndrome (IBS)
- Pelvic floor dysfunction or muscle damage
- Poor motility or slow transit
- Neurological conditions (e.g., Parkinson's disease), stroke, or paralysis

- Emotional disturbances such as depression or mental confusion
- Medications such as opioids, iron supplements, antihistamines, antacids, and antidepressants

Constipation can cause health problems for some clients. Straining associated with constipation often is accompanied by holding the breath. This is called Valsalva maneuver that can present serious problems to people with heart disease, brain injuries, or respiratory disease. Holding the breath, while bearing down increases intrathoracic pressure and vagal tone, slowing the pulse rate.

Fecal Impaction

Fecal Impaction is a mass or collection of hardened feces in the folds of the rectum. Impaction results from prolonged retention and accumulation of fecal material. In severe impactions, the feces accumulate and extend up into the sigmoid colon and beyond. Fecal impaction can be recognized by the passage of liquid fecal seepage (diarrhea) and no normal stool. The liquid portion of the feces seeps out around the impacted mass. It can be assessed by digital examination of the rectum.

Causes

The causes of fecal impaction are usually poor defecation habits and constipation. The barium used in radiological examinations of upper and lower gastrointestinal tract can also cause this. So removal of a fecal impaction digitally can be done by health care provider. Oil retention enema, a cleansing enema, suppositories or stool softeners are given when fecal impaction is suspected.

Diarrhea

Diarrhea refers to the passage of liquid feces and an increased frequency of defecation. Rapid passage of chyme reduces the time available for the large intestine to reabsorb water and electrolytes. In diarrhea, the stool is relatively not formed and excessively liquid. The person with diarrhea finds it difficult or impossible to control the urge to defecate for very long. Bowel sounds are increased and with persistent diarrhea, irritation of the anal region extending to the perineum and buttocks generally results.

Causes

- Psychological stress
- Medications—antibiotics, iron, cathartics
- Allergy to foods, fluids or drugs
- Intolerance of food or fluid
- Diseases of the colon—Crohn's disease, malabsorption syndrome

The irritating effects of diarrhea stool increase the risk for skin breakdown. Therefore, the area around the anal region should be kept clean and dry and be protected with zinc oxide.

Bowel Incontinence

Bowel incontinence also called fecal incontinence, refers to the loss of voluntary ability to control fecal and gaseous discharges through the anal sphincter. The incontinence may occur at specific times, such as after meals, or may occur irregularly. Two types of bowel incontinence are described: partial and major. Partial incontinence is the inability to control flatus or to prevent minor soiling. Major incontinence is the inability to control feces of normal consistency.

Fecal incontinence is generally associated with impaired functioning of anal sphincter or its nerve supply. Fecal incontinence is an emotionally distressing problem that can ultimately lead to social isolation. Several surgical procedures are used for the treatment of fecal incontinence. These include repair of the sphincter and fecal diversion or colostomy.

Flatulence

Flatulence is the presence of excessive flatus in the intestines that leads to stretching and inflation of the intestines. There are three primary sources of flatus, action of bacteria on the chyme in the large intestine, swallowed air and gas that diffuses between the blood stream and the intestine.

Most gases that are swallowed are expelled through the mouth by eructation (belching). However, large amounts of gas can accumulate in the stomach resulting in gastric distention. The gases formed in the large intestine are absorbed through the intestinal capillaries into the circulation.

Causes

Flatulence can occur in the colon from a variety of causes such as:
- Foods–Cabbage, onions
- Abdominal surgery–Paralytic ileus
- Narcotics

If excessive gas cannot be expelled through the anus, it may be necessary to insert a rectal tube to remove it.

Planning

The major goals for clients with fecal elimination problems are to:
- Maintain or restore normal bowel elimination pattern
- Maintain or regain normal stool consistency
- Prevent associated risks such as fluid and electrolyte imbalance, skin breakdown, abdominal distention, and pain.

Appropriate preventive and corrective nursing interventions that relate to these must be identified. Specific nursing activities associated with each of these can be selected to meet the client's individual needs.

Implementation

Promoting Regular Defecation

The nurse can help clients to achieve regular defecation by attending to:

* The provision of privacy
* Timing
* Nutrition and fluids
* Exercise
* Positioning

Privacy

Privacy during defecation is extremely important to many people. The nurse should therefore provide as much privacy as possible for such clients who are too weak to be left alone. Some clients also prefer to wipe, wash, and dry themselves after defecating. A nurse may need to provide water and washcloth and towel for this purpose.

Timing

A client should be encouraged to defecate when the urge is recognized. To establish regular bowel elimination, the client and nurse can discuss when mass peristalsis normally occurs and provide time for defecation. Many people have well-established routines. Other activities such as bathing and ambulating should not interfere with defecation time.

Nutrition and Fluids

The diet, a client needs for regular normal elimination, varies. Depending on the kind of feces the client currently has, the frequency of defecation, and the types of foods that the client eats assist with normal defecation.

* **For Constipation:** Increase daily fluid intake, and instruct the client to drink hot fluids and fruit juices. Include fiber in the diet such as raw fruit, bran products, and whole grain cereals and bread.
* **For Diarrhea:** Encourage oral intake of fluids and bland diet. Eating small amounts can be helpful because it is more easily absorbed. Excessively hot or cold fluids should be avoided because they stimulate peristalsis. In addition, highly spiced foods and high fiber foods can aggravate diarrhea.
* **For Flatulence:** Limit carbonated beverages, the use of drinking straws, and chewing gum all of which increase the ingestion of air. Gas forming foods such as cabbage, beans, onions and cauliflower should be avoided.

Exercise

Regular exercise helps clients develop a regular defecation pattern. A client with weak abdominal and pelvic muscles may be able to strengthen them with the following isometric exercises:

In a supine position, the client tightens the abdominal muscles as though pulling them inward, holding them for about 10 seconds and then relaxing them. This should be repeated 5–10 times, four times a day, depending on the client's health.

Again in a supine position, the client can contract the thigh muscles and hold them contracted for about 10 seconds, repeating the exercise 5–10 times, four times a day. This helps the client who is confined to bed, gain strength in the thigh muscles, thereby making it easier to use a bedpan.

Positioning

Although the squatting position best facilitates defecation. On a toilet seat, the best position for most people seems to be leaning forward. For clients who have difficulty sitting down and getting up from the toilet, an elevated toilet seat can be attached to a regular toilet.

A bed-side **commode**, a portable chair with a toilet seat and a receptacle beneath that can be emptied, is often used for the adult client who can get out of bed but is unable to walk to the **bathroom**. Some commodes have wheels and can slide over the base of a regular toilet when the waste receptacle is removed, thus providing clients the privacy of a bathroom (Fig. 2).

Clients restricted to bed may need to use a bedpan, a receptacle for urine and feces. Female clients use bedpan for both urine and feces; male clients use a bedpan for feces and a urinal for urine. There are two main types of bedpans; regular high-back pan and the slipper (Fig. 3).

The slipper bedpan has a low back and is used for clients who are unable to raise their buttocks.

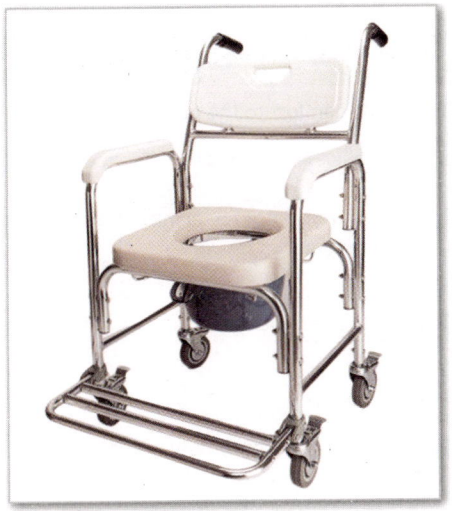

Fig. 2: Commode with overlying seat

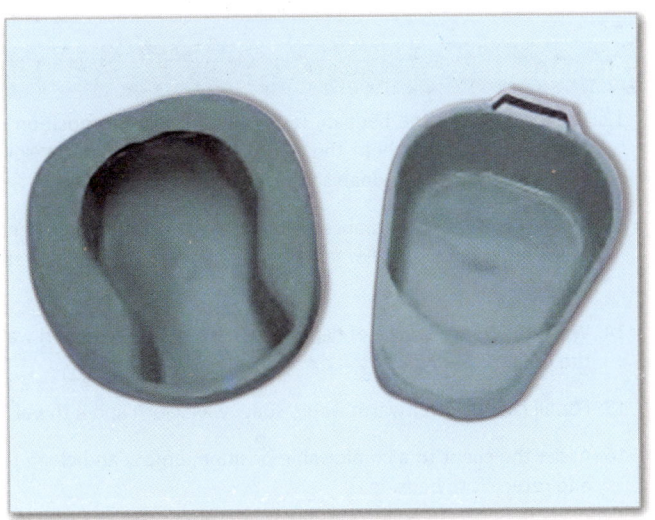

Fig. 3: The high-back or regular bedpan

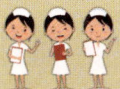 **SKILL: GIVING AND REMOVING A BEDPAN**

Equipment

Gloves, appropriate type of clean bedpan with cover, Toilet tissue/gauze, specimen container labeled with date, patient's name, washcloth, absorbent pads, clean draw sheet, perineal tray with cotton balls and artery clamp, soap and water.

Review and carry out the standard steps as given in Appendix

Action/steps	Rationale
1. Wash hands and apply gloves and provide curtain	To maintain privacy and safety
2. If metal bedpan, warm it by rinsing under warm water	For comfort of patient
3. Adjust the bed to height appropriate to prevent back strain	For comfort of nursing personnel
4. Elevate the side rails on the opposite side	To prevent the client from falling out for bed.
5. Ask the client to assist by flexing the knees, resting the weight on back and heels, and raising the buttocks, or by using trapeze bar	For easy placement of bedpan
6. Place a regular bedpan so that the clients buttocks rest on the smooth, rounded rim. Place a slipper bedpan with the flat, low end under the client's buttocks	To place the bedpan in a right way
7. For the client who cannot assist, obtain the assistance to help lift the client into the bedpan	To prevent back strain for nurse and helping the client
8. Elevate the head end of the bed to a semi-Fowler's position	Helps the client to assume a normal position as possible for defecation
9. Cover the client with bath blanket to maintain dignity	To maintain comfort
10. Provide toilet tissue, place the call light within reach, elevate the side rail and leave the client alone	To make the client self-reliant and to answer call bell promptly
11. Do not leave anyone on bedpan longer than 15 minutes unless the client is able to remove pan himself	Lengthy stay on bedpan can cause pressure ulcers

Contd...

Action/steps	Rationale
12. While removing the bedpan, return the bed to the position used when giving the bedpan, hold the bedpan steady to prevent spillage of its contents cover the bedpan and place it on adjacent chair	To provide comfort to the patient and prevent soiling of linen
13. If the client-needs assistance, put on gloves and wipe the client's perineal area with toilet tissue. For female patients, clean from the urethra toward the anus	To prevent transfer of rectal microorganism into the urinary meatus
14. Wash the perineal area of dependent clients with soap and water and dry the area	To clean the perineal area
15. For all clients, offer warm water, soap, washcloth and a towel	To wash hands
16. Assist the client to a comfortable position, empty and clean the bedpan, and return it to bedside	To make the client comfortable
17. Remove and discard gloves and wash hands	To prevent infection
18. Spray the room with air freshener as needed	To control odor
19. Document color, odor, amount and consistency of feces, and the condition of the perineal area	For documentation

ENEMAS

An enema is the introduction of fluid into the rectum and colon by means of a tube. Enemas are given to stimulate peristalsis and the urge to defecate or to wash out the waste products or feces. The action of an enema is to distend the intestine and sometimes to irritate the intestinal mucosa, thereby increasing peristalsis and the excretion of feces and flatus. Enemas are classified into cleansing and retention enemas.

Cleansing Enemas

Cleansing enemas are given chiefly to:
- Prevent the escape of feces during surgery
- Prepare the intestine for certain diagnostic tests such as X-ray or visualization, e.g., colonoscopy
- Remove feces in case of constipation and impaction

Cleansing enemas use a variety of solutions which are given in Table 3.
- *Hypertonic* solution exerts osmotic pressure, which draws fluid from the intestinal space into the colon. The increased volume in the colon stimulates peristalsis and hence defecation. A commonly used hypertonic enema is the commercially prepared fleet phosphate enema.
- *Hypotonic* solutions, e.g., tap water exert a low osmotic pressure than the surrounding interstitial fluid, causing water to move from the colon into the interstitial space. Before the water moves from the colon, it stimulates peristalsis and defecation.

Retention Enemas

Retention enemas are retained in the bowel for a prolonged period for purpose of:

TABLE 3: Commonly used solutions

Solution	Constituents	Action	Time to take effect
Hypertonic	50–120 mL of solution (e.g., sodium phosphate)	Draws water into colon	5–10 minutes
Isotonic	500–1,000 mL of normal saline	Distends colon, stimulates peristalsis and softens feces	15–20 minutes
Hypotonic	500–1,000 ml of tap water	Distends colon, stimulates peristalsis and softens feces	15–20 minutes
Soap suds	500–1,000 ml/3–5 mL of soap to 1,000 mL of water	Irritates mucosa and distends colon	10–15 minutes
Oil/mineral, olive, cotton seed	90–120 mL	Lubricates the feces and the colon mucosa	½ –3 minutes

- **Oil retention enemas:** To lubricate the stool and intestinal mucosa, making defecation easier. About 150–200 mL of solution is administered to adults.
- **Carminative enemas:** Help to expel flatus from the rectum and provide relief from gaseous distention. Common solutions include the milk and molasses, enema

(equal parts) and the magnesium sulfate—glycerine—water (MGW) enema (30 mL of magnesium sulfate, 60 mL of glycerine, and 90 mL of warm water.

- **Medicated enemas:** Provide medications that are absorbed through the rectal mucosa.
- **Antihelminthic enemas:** Destroy intestinal parasites.

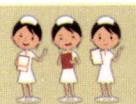

SKILL: ADMINISTERING AN ENEMA

Equipment

Enema container and tubing with clamp, bedpan or bedside commode, lubricant, gloves, enema solution, bath blanket, tissue wipes, mackintosh (plastic sheet) with cover, kidney tray and cotton swabs.

Review and carry out the standard steps as given in Appendix

Action/steps	Rationale
Assessment	
1. Check the physician's order. Determine what patient knows about the enema procedure. Check to see that a bedpan or bedside commode is on hand.	Ensures that an enema order has been written. Determines how much explanation is needed
Planning	
2. Plan time to give a large-volume enemas without interruption	A large volume enema procedure may take as long as 30 minutes if the order is "enemas until clear"
Implementation	
3. If possible, place the patient in the left sim's position and drape with bath blanket (Fig. 4) **Fig. 4:** Left lateral position	Solution travels up easily in the colon when the patient is lying on the left side.
4. Full the enema can (bag) with the correct solution; temperature, of the water. Should be between 100°F and 105°F. Expel air from the tubing by opening the clamp and allowing the solution to run through. Use bedpan or kidney tray to collect the solution, reclamp the tube and put on gloves.	Prevents air from being introduced into colon, which could cause the patient discomfort. Water that is too hot may burn the patients; water too cool may cause cramping. Gloves prevent transfer of microorganism.
5. Position the bedside commode or put the bedpan close at hand: lubricate the end of the enema tube and gently insert it into anal opening about 4 inches in the adult by separating folds of buttocks with the help of cotton swabs. Direct the tube toward the umbilicus. Ask the patient to take deep breath through the mouth to relax the anal sphincter. Twisting the tube gently helps it pass through the sphincter.	Bedside commode or bedpan is needed as soon as all the fluid has been instilled. It is possible to perforate the wall of the rectum with the tube if force is used; gentle pressure and slow advancement are best.
6. With the container about 12–18 inches above the anus, open the clamp on the tube, and allow the solution to flow slowly into the bowel. Lowering slightly and again raising the container (enema can) to this height will regulate the speed of the flow. When the patient expresses discomfort, stop the flow by kinking the tubing or clamping it, and instruct the patient to take deep breaths by mouth until the cramping and urge to expel the fluid pass. Continue until the patient can retain no more or the container is empty. Clamp the tubing and withdraw it asking the patient to squeeze the sphincter shut; place the soiled tube in the kidney tray	Too forceful a flow may damage the bowel. Instilling the fluid slowly prevents cramping and usually obtains the best result with the least discomfort. Some patients can hold only a few hundred milliliters of solution at a time, others can tolerate the entire volume.

Contd...

Action/steps	Rationale
For Disposable Enema	
7. Add extra lubricant to the tip and insert the tip into the anal opening. Gently squeeze the bottle, and roll it up from the bottom as the contents enter the bowel. Squeeze as much of the fluid into the patient as possible. Remove the tip slowly and hold the buttocks together.	The lubricant on the tip sometimes dry up. Disposable enemas contain approximately 120–240 mL of solution. Slow instillation achieves the best result. An **oil retention enema** is given in the same manner but the patient should retain it for 20 minutes to 2 hours. So that it softens the stool
8. Assist the patient onto the bedpan or bedside commode. If the patient uses the toilet, request to see the result before flushing. If a bedpan is used, raise the head of the bed to a sitting position. Place call bell and toilet paper within reach.	This provides a container for collection of enema return and an opportunity to observe the characteristics of stool expelled.
9. Once the bowel contents have been expelled, assist the patient in cleaning the anal area; observe the results of the enema, noting the color, amount, and consistency of the stool. Remove and clean the bedpan or bedside commode.	Results of the enema are judged by the stool expelled.
10. Restore the patient unit, lower the bed, replace the side rails, and place the call bell within reach.	Shows consideration for the patient and provides safety.
Evaluation	
11. Ask yourself, was the patient able to hold sufficient enema fluid to flush the bowel? Did all the fluid return? Was there a normal amount of stool expelled? Does the patient feel relief from fullness and flatulence?	Answers determine whether enema was successful.
Documentation	
12. Note date, time, type of enema and amount of fluid instilled; describe the result and how the patient tolerated the procedure.	Documents the procedure and its results.

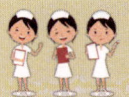

SKILL: REMOVAL OF A FECAL IMPACTION

If a patient has been found to have impacted stool that cannot be flushed out with an oil-retention enema followed by cleansing enema, manual removal of the impaction is required. The patient should be given analgesia before carrying out the procedure as it is a painful process.

Equipment

Gloves, toilet tissue, lubricant, bedpan

Review and carry out the standard steps as given in Appendix

Action/steps	Rationale
Assessment	
1. Assess when the last bowel movement occurred, check risk factors that contribute to constipation, assess the abdomen, and determine if small amounts of liquid stool have been passed.	Assessment data help in determination as to whether facial impaction has occurred.
2. Have patient assume a left lateral or sim's position. Put on gloves and arrange the bedpan and toilet tissue on a chair by the bed within reach. Lubricate the index finger of the gloves.	Lubrication prevents injury to the anal and rectal mucosa as the finger is introduced. An oil-retention enema, 20 minutes to 3 hours prior to impaction removal is helpful.
3. Insert the index finger into the anus along the wall of the rectum in a slightly curving motion. As the finger comes in contact with feces in the rectum, note the consistency; then move the finger into the lower portion of the fecal mass, again note the consistency.	This provides data about the amount and consistency of the stool in the rectum.

Contd...

Action/steps	Rationale
4. With the examining index finger, dislodge or break off a small amount of fecal material and gently remove it. Placing it in the bedpan. Continue removing as much fecal material as you can reach with your finger or until the patient's discomfort, or palpitations or dizziness; warrants discontinuing the procedure. After the patient has rested, reglove and remove the remaining fecal material. Cleanse the rectal area. Remove gloves and dispose them properly.	The stool is broken up so that it can be removed with less discomfort to the patient and without damage to the rectal mucosa.
5. Make the patient comfortable, lower the bed, raise side rails, and restore the unit.	Shows consideration for the patient; provides safety.

SITZ BATH

Sitz bath is a method of applying tepid or warm water to the pelvic or rectal area by sitting in a tub, special chair or basin filled with sufficient water to reach the umbilicus at the desired temperature (Fig. 5). The legs and feet remain out of the water.

Purposes

A sitz bath is recommended to:

- Relieve pain in the rectal or perineal area
- Reduce inflammation
- Relieve painful hemorrhoids
- Encourage voiding
- Decrease congestion of blood in the pelvic area
- Promote drainage from wound
- Relieve renal colic
- Helps to remove slough.

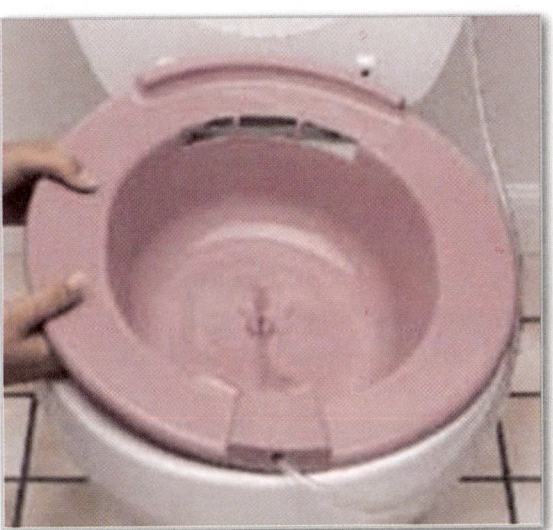

Fig. 5: Bath tub on toilet seat

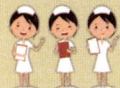 **SKILL: ASSISTING WITH A SITZ BATH**

Equipment

Tub (Preferably sterile), thermometer, hot and cold water, bath blanket, towel, gown, dressing tray, lotions–sterile water, potassium permanganate (1:10,000), boric acid (2.5%), normal saline, soda bicarb (2%), and magnesium sulfate solution, T binder.

Action/steps	Rationale
Assessment	
1. Check the physician's order. Determine what patient knows about the procedure-check to see tub with water is nearby.	Ensure that a sitz bath order has been written. Determine how much explanation is needed.
Planning	
2. Plan time to give a sitz bath without interruption.	Sitz bath procedure may take around 20 minutes.
Implementation	
3. Test the water in a sitz bath with a thermometer before the patient enters the water.	If the purpose of the sitz bath is to apply heat, use water at a temperature of 93–99°F for 15 minutes. If purpose of sitz bath is to produce relaxation or to promote healing of wound by cleansing it of discharge and debris, use water at temperature 93–99°F.

Contd...

Action/steps	Rationale
4. Assist the patient into the tub and position properly with patient's feet flat on the floor without pressure on the sacrum or thighs (Fig. 6).	The patient should be able to sit in the tub comfortably.

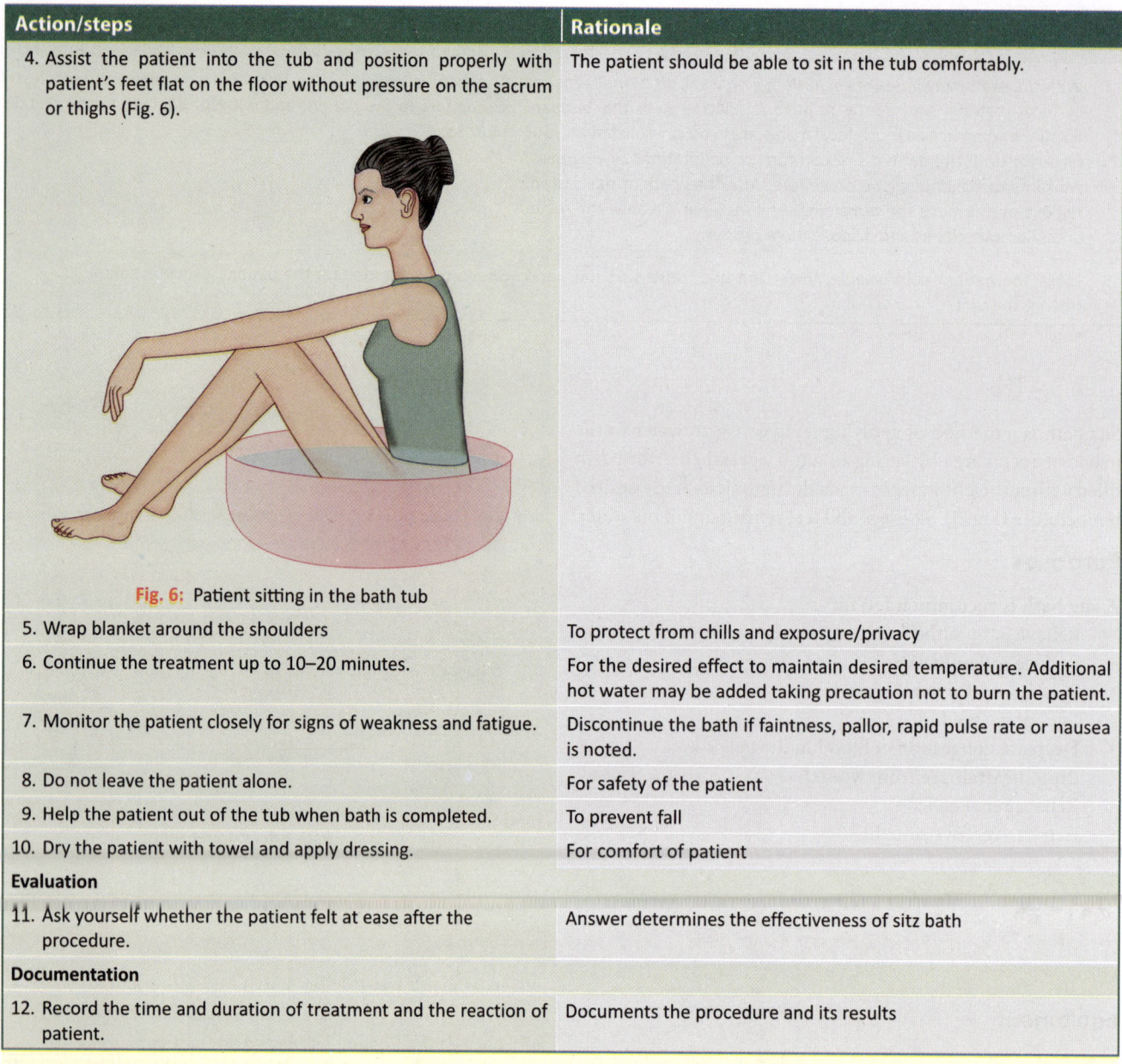

Fig. 6: Patient sitting in the bath tub

Action/steps	Rationale
5. Wrap blanket around the shoulders	To protect from chills and exposure/privacy
6. Continue the treatment up to 10–20 minutes.	For the desired effect to maintain desired temperature. Additional hot water may be added taking precaution not to burn the patient.
7. Monitor the patient closely for signs of weakness and fatigue.	Discontinue the bath if faintness, pallor, rapid pulse rate or nausea is noted.
8. Do not leave the patient alone.	For safety of the patient
9. Help the patient out of the tub when bath is completed.	To prevent fall
10. Dry the patient with towel and apply dressing.	For comfort of patient
Evaluation	
11. Ask yourself whether the patient felt at ease after the procedure.	Answer determines the effectiveness of sitz bath
Documentation	
12. Record the time and duration of treatment and the reaction of patient.	Documents the procedure and its results

BOWEL WASH

A bowel wash involves washing out the colon with large quantities of solution.

Purposes

- To stimulate peristalsis
- To reduce inflammation
- To relieve fecal incontinence
- To dilute and remove toxic agents
- To supply fluid and electrolytes
- Before special investigations such as barium enema

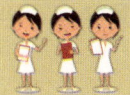

SKILL: BOWEL WASH (COLONIC IRRIGATION)

Equipment

Jugs of hot and cold water, colon lavage set with tubing and glass connection, rectal tube (clean), lubricant, gauze pieces (Tissue wipes). Long waterproof sheet (mackintosh), kidney tray, lotion, thermometer, bedpan, disposable gloves, plastic apron, linen for change.

Review and carry out the Standard Steps as given in Appendix

Action/steps	Rationale
Assessment	
1. Check for physician's order. Make sure equipment is within reach	Ensures that bowel wash order has been written
2. Explain the procedure to the patient and relatives	Helps to gain cooperation and relaxation
3. Place long mackintosh under patient	To protect bed from getting wet
Planning	
4. Place the patient in the left lateral position	Solution travels up easily in the colon
5. Drape the patient	To maintain privacy
Implementation	
6. Prepare the solution at the desired temperature 104°–110°F	Solution should be at right temperature for desired effect.
7. Lubricate the tip of rectal tube up to 4 inches and connect to a funnel and tubing and put on gloves	Lubrication makes insertion easier
8. Fill the funnel with solution and expel air from the tubing by allowing a small quantity of solution to run into kidney tray, then pinch the tube	Air trapped inside will prevent smooth flow of the fluid
9. Separate the patient's buttocks to visualize the anus clearly and insert the tip of tube up to 4–5 inches, while the patient takes deep breathe	Deep breathing through the mouth helps to relax anal sphincter
10. Do not force the tube or if the tube is not going easily	
11. Allow the fluid to run through by raising funnel about 12–18 inches above the anus for 5 – 10 minutes (200–300 mL and lower the funnel before it is completely empty invert it below the level of rectum and empty into bedpan	Allow fluid to run slowly to prevent cramps and discomfort. The funnel should be inverted before it is empty to prevent air entry for siphon to work
12. Repeat the process until the return flow is clear	
13. Remove the rectal tube by using tissue wipes (gauze piece) and discard, remove gloves	Rectal tube is contaminated with fecal matter
14. Restore the patient's unit change linen if soiled	Shows consideration for the patient
Evaluation	
15. Ask yourself, was the patient hold sufficient fluid to cleanse the bowel? Was the return flow clear?	Answers determine whether bowel wash was successful
Documentation	
16. Record time, type and amount of solution used, result of procedure, color, abnormalities in return flow and any discomfort experienced by the patient	Documents the procedure and its results

Contd...

RECTAL SUPPOSITORIES

Rectal suppositories consist of concentrated food, soap, glycerine, plain or medicated cocoa butter, prepared in the shape of a cone. They retain this shape at ordinary room temperature but when introduced into the rectum, these suppositories are dissolved by body heat and the drugs contained in them are then released.

Purposes

♦   Soap and glycerine suppositories are used to stimulate defecation

♦   The presence of suppositories acts as an irritant that stimulates the rectum to expel its contents

Types of Suppositories

♦   Evacuating suppositories such as glycerine
♦   Astringent suppositories such as tannic acid, belladonna and glycerine –used in dysentery and diarrhea
♦   Suppositories containing opium or barbital are used for sedation
♦   Anodyne are used for hemorrhoids, dysentery and diarrhea
♦   Ice suppositories are used to treat local bleeding.

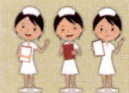

SKILL: INSERTING A RECTAL SUPPOSITORY

Equipment

Suppositories, Gloves, Lubricant, Bedpan.

Review and carry out the standard steps as given in Appendix

Action/steps	Rationale
1. After checking the order, obtain the suppository, gloves, and water-soluble lubricant	Needed supplies are readily available at hand
2. Wash hands, identify the patient, provide privacy, explain the procedure, raise the bed to working height, and lower the near side rail	Ensures correct patient receives suppository. Patient should know the purpose of suppository
3. Place the patient in left lateral (Sims') position and fold the top bedding obliquely back over the hips to expose the buttocks. Visualize the anus	Provide for easier insertion of suppository into rectum
4. Put on gloves and open lubricant, squeezing it on to gauze. Remove foil wrapper from suppository and dip the point into the lubricant	Prepares suppository for insertion
5. Ask patient to take deep breath through the mouth as the suppository is placed into the anus. Gently push the suppository along the wall of the anus up into the rectum with index finger as far as it can reach (Fig. 7). Withdraw finger and hold both buttocks tightly together for a few seconds while the patient breathes deeply and the urge to expel the suppository has passed. 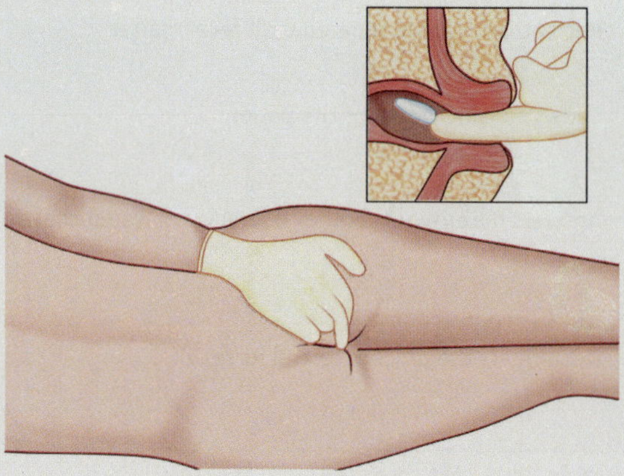	Positions suppository above sphincter so that it cannot expelled immediately. Urge to expel, it will pass in a minute or so.

Fig. 7: Insertion of suppository

Contd...

Action/steps	Rationale
6. Wipe excess lubricant from anus. Instruct patient to try to hold suppository in place for at least 20 minutes.	Suppository melts and allows deposit medication to act and stimulate the bowel.
7. Remove the gloves and discard in proper waste container. Wash hands.	Reduces transfer of microorganisms.
8. Document administration of the suppository and the outcome of its use.	Provides data on success or failure of treatment.

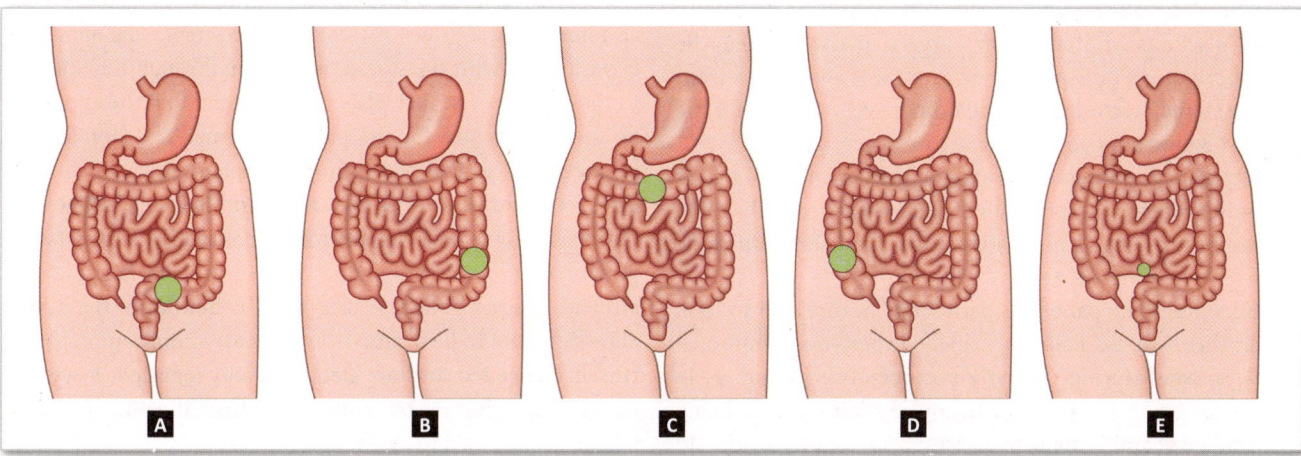

Figs 8A to E: A. Sigmoid colostomy, B. Descending colostomy, C. Transverse colostomy, D. Ascending colostomy, E. Ileostomy. (A–D) Location of various colostomies in large intestine and (E) location of an ileostomy.

MEETING THE NEEDS OF PATIENTS WITH BOWEL DIVERSIONS

Sometimes patients undergo surgical procedures to create an opening into the abdominal wall for fecal elimination. **Ostomy** is a term used for surgical opening from the inside of an organ to the outside. The intestinal mucosa is brought out to the abdominal wall and a **stoma**, the part of the ostomy that is attached to the skin, is formed by suturing the mucosa to the skin.

An **ileostomy** allows liquid fecal content from the ileum of the small intestine to be eliminated through the stoma.

A **colostomy** permits formed feces in the colon to exit through the stoma. Colostomies are further classified by the part of the colon from which they originate (Figs 8A to E).

Colostomy and Ileostomy Care

The patient with an ostomy needs physical and psychological support both preoperatively and postoperatively. This support comes from the family members, members of health care team and from people who have had similar experiences. The articles needed for colostomy irrigation and care are given in (Fig. 9). These guidelines help to promote the patient's physical and psychological comfort:

♦ Keep the patient free from odor as possible. Empty the ostomy appliance frequently.

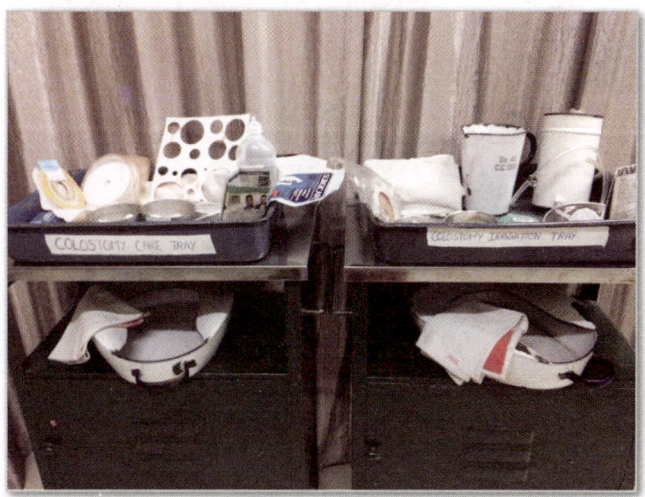

Fig. 9: Articles for colostomy care and irrigation

♦ Inspect the patient's stoma regularly. It should be dark pink to red and moist. A pale stoma may indicate anemia, and a dark or purple–blue stoma reflects compromised circulation or ischemia.

■ Bleeding around the stoma if excessive, if any change in color must be notified to physician.

♦ Note the size of the stoma, which usually stabilizes within 6–8 weeks. Most stomas protrude ½–1 inch from the abdominal surface and may appear initially swollen and edematous. After 6 weeks, the edema gets usually subsided.

♦ Keep the skin around the stoma site clean and dry. If care is not taken to protect the skin around the stoma, irritation or infection may occur with an ileostomy, enzymes in the effluent can quickly cause excoriation. A skin barrier paste (Zinc oxide ointment or karaya) is used to prevent excoriation of skin.

♦ Check the ostomy appliance for the quality and quantity of discharge. Initially after surgery, peristalsis may be inhibited. As peristalsis returns, stool is eliminated from the stoma. Record intake and output every 4 hours for the first 3 days after surgery.

♦ Explain each aspect of care to the patient and explain his or her role in self-care. Patient teaching is one of the most important aspects of colostomy care and should include family members also.

♦ Encourage the patient to participate in care and to look at the ostomy. Patients usually experience emotional depression during the early postoperative period. Help the patient to cope by listening, explaining and being available and supportive. Patients usually begin to accept their altered body image when they are willing to look at the stoma, make neutral or positive statements concerning the ostomy, and express interest in learning self-care.

Applying an Ostomy Appliance

There are many different sizes and types of ostomy appliances. All appliances have a face plate, or disk, that attaches to the abdomen, and a pouch for collecting effluent. The appliance is positioned with the stoma protruding through the opening in the center of the face plate. It is essential that the appliance be the correct size for the patient's stoma. The stoma must be measured so that the right size appliance can be chosen. The pouch attaches over the stoma and is fastened onto the faceplate. Some patients wear a belt that also supports the pouch so that it is not pulled loose from the face plate as effluent fills the pouch. A clamp at the bottom of the pouch allows effluent to be drained. Pouches are simply emptied and rinsed as needed and are detached and replaced every few days (2 days). It is best to empty stool from the pouch when it becomes one-third to one-half full.

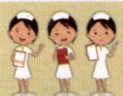

SKILL: CHANGING AN OSTOMY APPLIANCE

Equipment

Gloves, washcloth, plastic stoma measuring template, Clean pouch and face plate, skin barrier paste, pouch closure device, scissors, tissue or gauze pieces, tape or belt.

Review and carry out standard steps as given in Appendix

Action/steps	Rationale
Assessment	
1. Assess the type of ostomy and location. Assess stoma for color and appearance. Assess size of stoma using stoma measuring device. Assess skin condition around stoma	Red or dark-pink color indicates adequate blood supply. Stoma should not be receding or protruding. Provides data regarding stoma size for choice of correct appliance
Planning	
2. Gather appropriate supplies needed to apply the new pouch/appliance	Ensures that all needed items are on hand before beginning
Implementation	
3. Measure the stoma with the stoma measuring device. Prepare the skin barrier or pouch with face plate by cutting an opening in the center approximately ¼ inch larger than the stoma. Smoothen the cut edges with finger to prevent irritation or leakage around the stoma	Ensures more accurate size to fit. The edges of the pouch can injure or irritate the stoma if the opening is too small
4. Put on gloves and empty old pouch	Prevents transfer of microorganisms. Prevents the weight of the pouch contents from loosening and spilling
5. Remove old pouch by stabilizing the skin with one hand and pulling the backing from the skin with the other hand, discard the old pouch in the plastic bag	Readies the area for new pouch application

Contd...

Action/steps	Rationale
6. Clean the stoma and skin gently with warm water and soft cloth. Dry the skin well. Place tissue at stoma opening to prevent leakage	Prepares skin for attachment of new appliance. Tissue absorbs any leakage
7. Change gloves remove paper from skin barrier on back of appliance. Apply skin barrier paste to peristomal area	Reduces transfer or microorganisms. Prepares an adhesive surface on the skin for attachment of pouch appliance
8. Gently press down the skin barrier ring around the stoma while abdomen is pushed out by patient check that seal is wrinkle free	Adheres appliance to skin without causing wrinkles. Good adherence prevents leakage
9. Reinforce ring with tape as needed	Prevents edges from loosening during shower
10. Instruct patient to lie quietly for 5 minutes to allow body heat to seal pouch well	Body heat activates the skin barrier and causes it to adhere to the skin
11. Place deodorant inside pouch if patient desires	Various types of ostomy deodorants are available
12. Attach and secure pouch tail closure so that bow of clip fits curve of abdomen. Allow a 1 inch fold-over of pouch before closing the clip	Closes pouch, when bow fits curve of abdomen, clip is less noticeable through clothing
13. Attach belt to face plate of pouch if belt is to be worn	Belt helps to prevent leakage
14. Remove gloves and wash hands	Reduces transfer of microorganisms
15. Assist patient to replace gown or clothing and make patient comfortable	To make patient comfortable
Evaluation	
16. Ask yourself, is the appliance applied without wrinkles? Is it attached securely? Is the bottom of the pouch closed securely? Was the old pouch disposed of properly? Is there any leakage from pouch?	Determines whether appliance pouch was applied correctly
Documentation	
17. Note date, time, condition of stoma and peristomal area. Indicate type of skin barrier used, size of opening cut for new appliance, treatment of skin and new pouch applied	Documents nursing action and provides data for next pouch change to health care team

Irrigating a Colostomy

Irrigations are frequently used to promote regular evacuation of some colostomies. Various factors, such as the site of the colostomy in the colon (sigmoid colostomy) and the patient's and doctor's preferences, determine whether the colostomy is irrigated.

Ileostomies are not irrigated because the fecal content of the ileum is liquid and cannot be controlled.

Water is inserted into the colostomy, and the water and feces are expelled from the colostomy into the irrigation sleeve and then the toilet. Following a colostomy irrigation, no feces or flatus should pass from a colostomy until the next irrigation.

VAGINAL IRRIGATION

Vaginal irrigation is also called a douche. Topical solution is introduced into the vaginal cavity.

Purposes

- To cleanse the vagina in preparation for surgery.
- To supply antiseptics to reduce bacterial growth.

Solutions Used

- 2% sodium bicarbonate solution.
- Diluted hydrogen peroxide
- Povidone-iodine solution
- A weak solution of acetic acid (1 tablespoon vinegar to 1000 mL of fluid)
- Amount of solution: Range from 1500–2000 mL
- Temperature of solution 100–105°F

Method

Prepare the douche solution as per the directions with the medication.

- Fill the douche bag/Irrigative can and run a small amount of fluid through the tubing to clear the air in the tube and clamp the tube.
- Hang the douche bag not more than 18 inches above the level of the hips so that pressure is less.
- Make the patient sit either in dorsal recumbent position with the bed pan or sitting on a commode.
- Gently insert the irrigating nozzle, directing it downward or backward to the back of the vagina.
- Rotate the nozzle during the irrigation.

- Unclamp the tubing and allow the solution to flow slowly into the vagina and keeping the labia closed until the vagina fills and then ease the grip allowing the solution to flow out of vagina. Hold the labia closed again until the vagina fills: repeat the process until all the irrigating solution has been used.
- The time period for the solution to run through range from 10–15 minutes.
- Close the clamp and remove the nozzle.
- Dry the perineum and make patient comfortable.

Evaluation

The nurse evaluates the effectiveness of the plan of care to promote regular bowel movement by checking to see if the patient has met the individualized patient outcomes specified in the plan. Nursing care is effective if the patient expresses satisfaction with his or her regular pattern of defecation and the ability to pass a soft, formed stool comfortably without the use of medications or laxatives.

BIBLIOGRAPHY

1. *Taylor C, Lillis C, LeMone P, Lynn P. Fundamentals of Nursing, 6th edition. Lippincott Williams and Wilkins. Philadelphia; 2008.*
2. *Berman AT, Snyder S, Kozier BJ, et al. Kozier & Erb's. Fundamentals of Nursing: Concepts, Process and Practice, 8th edition. Pearson Education.*
3. *Dewit SC. Fundamental Concepts and Skills for Nursing, 3rd edition. Saunders. 2008. p. 992.*

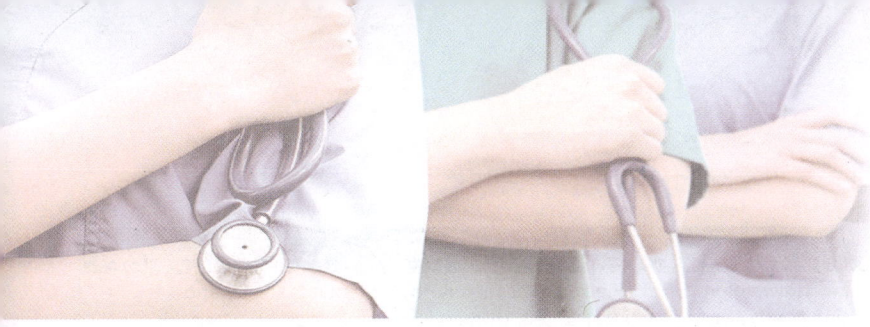

Observation and Collection of Urine, Stool, Vomitus and Sputum

INTRODUCTION

Nutritional and metabolic state of the body is reflected in the composition of body secretions like urine, stool, vomitus, sputum, etc. Observation of these secretions is included in every routine heath assessment when diseases are suspected. These secretions are assessed in laboratory for changes. Collection of these secretions is one of the most important responsibilities of the nurse. The nurse needs to understand the rationale for the specific test ordered, as well as the correct collection procedure associated with the required test in order to ensure obtaining the appropriate sample.

OBSERVATION OF SPECIMENS

Urine

The kidneys remove waste products from blood which are excreted in the form of urine. Assess the urine for color, clarity, odor, and the pressure of any sediment. Note any abnormalities.

In selected patients, monitor the pH and specific gravity of the urine and check the urine for abnormal constituents such as proteins, blood, glucose, ketone bodies and bacteria. The normal characteristics and special considerations of urine are given in Table 1.

Stool

Waste product of gastrointestinal tract is excreted out through feces/stool. Examination of stool helps in diagnosis of gastrointestinal tract problems and infestations. The normal and special considerations to be observed are given in Table 2.

Sputum

It is a material from mucus lining of trachea and bronchi, which is coughed out through mouth. Its observation helps to detect the function of respiratory system and any disease process. The normal and special considerations to be observed are given in Table 3.

TABLE 1: Characteristics of urine

Characteristic	Normal Findings	Special Considerations
Color	A freshly voided specimen is pale yellow, straw-colored, or amber, depending on its concentration	Urine is darker than normal when it is scanty and concentrated. Urine is lighter than normal when it is excessive and diluted. Certain drugs, such as cascara, i-dopa and sulfonamides alter the color of urine. Some foods can alter the color; for example, beets can cause urine to appear red.
Odor	Normal urine smell is aromatic. As urine stands, it often develops an ammonia odor because of bacterial action.	Some foods cause urine to have a characteristic odor; for example, asparagus causes urine to have a strong, musty odor. Urine high in glucose content has a sweet odor. Urine that is heavily infected has a fetid odor
Turbidity	Fresh urine should be clear or translucent; as, urine stands and cools, it becomes cloudy.	Cloudiness observed in freshly voided urine is abnormal and may be due to the presence of red blood cells, white blood cells, bacteria, vaginal discharge, sperm, or prostatic fluid.
pH	The normal pH is about 6.0, with a range of 4.6–8. (urine alkalinity or acidity may be promoted through diet to inhibit bacterial growth or urinary stone development or to facilitate the therapeutic activity of certain medications.) Urine becomes alkaline on standing when carbon dioxide diffuses into the air.	A high-protein diet causes urine to become excessively acidic. Certain foods tend to produce alkaline urine, such as citrus fruits, dairy products and vegetables, especially legumes. Certain foods such as meats tend to produce acidic urine. Certain drugs influence the acidity or alkalinity of urine; for example, ammonium chloride produces acidic urine, and potassium citrate and sodium bicarbonate produce alkaline urine.
Specific gravity	This is a measure of the concentration of dissolved solids in the urine. The normal range is 1.015–1.025.	Concentrated urine will have a higher than normal specific gravity, and diluted urine will have a lower than normal specific gravity. In the absence of kidney disease, a high specific gravity usually indicates dehydration and a low specific gravity indicates over hydration.
Constituents	Organic constituents of urine include urea, uric acid, creatinine, indican, urine pigments, and undetermined nitrogen. Inorganic constituents are ammonia, sodium, chloride, traces of iron, phosphorus, sulfur, potassium, and calcium.	Abnormal constituents of urine include blood, pus, albumin, glucose, ketone bodies, casts, gross bacteria, and bile.

TABLE 2: Normal findings and special considerations while observing stool sample

Characteristics	Normal findings	Special considerations
Volume	Variable	The volume of the stool depends on the amount the person eats and the nature of the diet. For example, the diet high in roughage produces more feces than a soft, bland diet. Consistently large diarrheal stools suggest a disorder in the small bowel or proximal colon; small, frequent stools with urgency to pass suggest a disorder of the left colon or rectum
Color	Infant: Yellow Adult: Brown	The brown color of the stool is due to stercobilin, a bile pigment derivative. The rapid rate of peristalsis in the infant causes the stool to be yellow The color of the stool is influenced by diet. For example, the stool will be almost black if the person eats red meat and dark green vegetables, such as spinach. The stool will be light brown if the diet is high in milk and milk products and low in meat. The absence of bile may cause the stool to appear white or clay-colored Certain drugs influence the color of the stool. For example, iron salts cause the stool to be black. Antacids cause it to be whitish. Bleeding high in the intestinal tract causes a stool to be black owing to the digestion of the blood. Bleeding low in the intestinal tract will result in fresh blood in the stool. The stool darkens with standing

Contd...

Characteristics	Normal findings	Special considerations
Odor	Aromatic; may be affected by foods ingested	The characteristic odor of the stool is due to indole and skatole, caused by putrefaction and fermentation in the lower intestinal tract. The odor of the stool is influenced by its pH value, which normally is neutral or slightly alkaline. Excessive putrefaction causes a strong odor. The presence of blood in the stool causes a unique odor
Consistency	Soft, semi-solid and formed	The consistency of the stool is influenced by fluid and food intake and gastric motility. The less time stool spends in the intestine (or the shorter the intestines), the more liquid the stool. Many pathologic conditions influence consistency
Shape	Formed stool is usually about one inch (2.5 cm) in diameter and has the tubular shape of the colon, but may be larger or smaller, depending on the condition of the colon	A gastrointestinal obstruction may result in a narrow, pencil-shaped stool. Rapid peristalsis thins the stool. Increased time spent in the large intestine may result in hard, marble-like fecal mass.
Constituents	Waste residues of digestion: bile, intestinal secretions, shredded epithelial cells, bacteria, and inorganic material (chiefly calcium and phosphates); seeds, meat fibers, and fat may be present in small amounts	Internal bleeding, infection, inflammation, and other pathologic conditions may result in abnormal constituents. These include blood, pus, excessive fat, parasites, ova, and mucus. Foreign bodies also may be found in the stool.

TABLE 3: Normal characteristics and special considerations of sputum

Characteristic	Normal	Special considerations
Amount	Normally, no sputum very little is expectorated	Amount may vary according to the diseases, e.g., asthma or bronchitis
Color	It is colorless and translucent	• Yellowish color indicates bacterial infection • Blackish color indicates carbon pigment, e.g., smoking • Bright red/dark red, tarry- color indicates blood • Greenish color indicated bronchiectasis; Brown color indicates gangrenous condition of lungs
Odor	Odorless	Unpleasant odor indicates lung abscess, lung cancer, lung gangrene
Consistency		Frothy-watery, tenacious and thick depending on the type of condition.

Vomitus

It is the ejection of the contents of stomach through mouth, it occurs due to gastric and intestinal disorders, poisoning and irritation to vomiting centers due to increased intracranial pressure. The following points should be observed in vomitus:

♦ Relationship to food intake
♦ Relationship to pain whether it increases or is relieved
♦ The frequency and amount—vomitus in 24 hours
♦ Manner of ejection: Projectile significant in pyloric stenosis and if the vomiting is effortless—significant of intestinal obstructions
♦ **Contents of vomitus:**
  ▪ Mucus: Seen in gastritis
  ▪ Undigested food: Seen in pyloric stenosis
  ▪ Presence of bile: Present in abnormal functioning of pylorus
  ▪ Feculent vomitus: Is significant of intestinal obstruction

COLLECTION OF SPECIMENS

A specimen is a small sample or part taken to show the nature of the whole as a small quantity of urine, stool, vomitus or a small fragment of tissue for a microscopic study.

Purposes

♦ To understand the importance of specimen collection
♦ To develop skill in collection of different specimens
♦ To differentiate the variation from normal to abnormal in sickness.

Name of patient: _____		Ward/Bed No. _____
Age: _____	Sex: _____	MRDNo.: _____
Nature of specimen: _____		
Nature of test to be done: _____ _____		
Date of collection: _____		

Fig. 1: Sample of the label

Types of Examination

The specimens collected for various examinations are given in Table 4.

Nurses' Responsibilities in Collection of Specimens

- Collection to be done in a specific container that is clean, sterile, specific quantity for specific tests and labeled for clear identification
- All specimens must be collected fresh usually in the morning
- Follow the correct method of collection
- All specimens should be well labeled with (Figure 1):
  - The patient's name
  - Bed no., ward no., registration no.
  - Date of collection, doctor's unit
  - Name of the specimen
  - Investigation required

Collection of Urine Specimen

Preparation of Patient

- Explain the patient and relatives the need for collection of specimens
- Explain the steps of procedure if the patient has to collect the specimens himself or herself
- Provide privacy, if the patient is bedridden.

Preparation of Articles

Following articles are required:
- A big container: For 24-hour urine collection
- A clean container: For routine examination
- A sterile test tube: For culture and sensitivity
- A bed pan/urinal: For bedridden patient
- Disposable gloves: For self protection
- Waste receptacle: To discard the waste

- Wash down tray with soapy/wet swabs and water-to clean perineum
- Screen-to provide privacy.

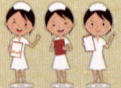

SKILL: COLLECTION OF MIDSTREAM URINE FOR CULTURE AND SENSITIVITY AND ROUTINE EXAMINATION ASSESSMENT

Action/steps	Rationale
Assessment	
1. Assess client's mobility and explain the patient how and what specimens to be collected	Determine the level of assistance required clarify doubts to promote client's cooperation
Planning	
2. Provide privacy to the client by screen	Helps the client to relax and give specimen
3. Wash hands and wear gloves	◆ To protect the nurse's hand ◆ To reduce risk of transmission of infection

Contd...

Action/steps	Rationale
Implementation	
4. Give a bedpan to bedridden patient	To clean the perineum
5. Assist or allow the client to wash the perineum	To clean the perineum
6. After initiating urine stream, pass the urine to the specimen bottle and collect 30–60 mL or urine	Initial stream of urine flushes out the microorganisms from urinary meatus
7. Remove the specimen container before the client empties the bladder	Urine for culture and sensitivity test must be midstream specimen so that it is free from contamination
8. Replace the cap on the specimen container and remove the gloves	To prevent spillage of urine
9. Label and transport the specimen to laboratory within 15 minutes	To prevent misplacing of specimen and sending quickly to laboratory prevents growth of bacteria
Documentation	
10. Record date and time of collection of specimen	Recording avoids duplication of work

Urine Specimen from Indwelling Catheter

- Sterile specimen may be obtained by using:
  - Clean catch technique
  - Catheterizing the client
  - Obtaining the specimen from indwelling catheter

Steps

- Wear sterile gloves clamp catheter and disconnect the urine bag
- Wipe the end of catheter with antiseptic swab
- Hold the sterile specimen container near the end of the catheter, unclamp the catheter and let urine drip into the sterile container
- After collecting the required amount, connect the catheter with the urine bag.
- Label the specimen container and send to laboratory.

24-hour Urine Specimen

- For 24-hour urine specimen, the collection is initiated at a specified time from 6 am to 6 am of next day in a receptacle
- After 24 hours are over, the specimen is collected and preservatives are added as per the institutional policy to prevent decomposition and multiplication of bacteria.
- The specimen is labeled before the start of collection of urine and send to laboratory.

Freshly Voided Urine

- Freshly voided urine is collected to determine the presence of glucose and ketones.

Urine for Pregnancy Test

- Urine is collected after 14 days of missed period preferably morning sample. The urine is tested for human Chorionic Gonadotropin (hCG)

Collection of Stool Specimens

- Explain the procedure to the client to gain cooperation
- Ask the client to pass urine so that stool does not mix with urine
- Ask the patient to defecate into clean bedpan. It is easy to collect and transfer stool into the specimen container by using a wooden spatula.
- Wear gloves and with a clean wooden spatula lift up a portion of the stool from the center of the mass and place it directly into the labeled specimen container.
- Send the specimen to the laboratory
- Specimen and types of examination are given in Table 4.

Stool for Ova and Parasites

- Stool for ova and parasites is collected as per the steps above to detect intestinal infections.
- The client should be instructed to avoid drugs such as mineral oil, castor oil or antidiarrheal compounds, which may alter the feces.
- The client should be informed that stool specimens are to be given for three consecutive days.

TABLE 4: Specimen and types of examination

Specimen	Type of examination
Urine	- Collection of mid-stream urine - Routine examination - Culture and sensitivity - 24-hours urine - Pregnancy test - Double voided specimen
Stool	- Routine microscopic and culture - Occult blood - Ova and cyst
Sputum	- Microscopic acid fast bacilli - Culture

Stool Culture

♦ This is carried out to identify pathogenic organisms in the gastrointestinal tract.
♦ If the client is on antibiotics recently, it has to be reported.
♦ It should be collected using sterile technique in a sterile stool container for three consecutive days.

Stool for Occult Blood

Stool examinations for occult blood help to detect gastrointestinal bleeding and early diagnosis of colorectal cancer. The guaiac or ortho toluidine test is commonly used

♦ If the ortho toluidine test is used, the client is instructed to eat high-fiber diet for 48–72 hours before the collection of stool specimen. The client should avoid red meat, poultry, fish and turnips. This may create a false positive result. The following medications should be withheld for 48–72 hours before the test such as iron preparation, bromides, steroids, colchicine and vitamin C, which can produce a negative result
♦ Usually three specimens over consecutive days are required.

Stool for Lipids

Excessive secretion of fecal fats may occur in various digestive and absorption disorders.

Normally, dietary lipids are completely absorbed in the small intestine.

♦ The client should be instructed to have extra high fat diet and refrain from alcohol for three days before the test and during the collection period
♦ The client should avoid drugs that interfere with the test such as mineral oil, neomycin and potassium chloride.

Collection of Sputum Specimen

♦ The client should be instructed to rinse the mouth with plain water, avoiding the brushing of teeth and food intake.
♦ A wide-mouth container or sputum mug and if possible wax-lined disposable paper cups should be taken.
♦ The client is instructed to cough up the morning specimen in the container after deep coughing.
♦ The outside of the container should not be soiled
♦ Send the labeled container to the laboratory as soon as possible.

URINE ANALYSIS

Urine testing refers to laboratory analysis on a routine or clean voided specimen or a specimen obtained from catheter to perform a routine or microscopic examination of urine.

Purposes

♦ To observe urine color and clarity
♦ To measure specific gravity of urine
♦ To determine the acidity or alkalinity of urine
♦ To determine the presence of glucose, albumin and ketone bodies in urine
♦ To aid in diagnosis of renal disorders
♦ To carry out a microscopic examination of urine for detection of red blood cells, occult blood, pus, casts, crystals and bacteria.

Equipment Required for Urine Testing

♦ Test tube rack with 4–6 test tubes
♦ Test tube holder, spirit lamp and match box
♦ Waste receptacle kidney tray
♦ Red and blue litmus paper
♦ Chemicals: Acetic acid, nitric acid, ammonium sulphate crystals, sodium nitroprusside crystals, weak solution of iodine, sulphur powder, Benedict's solution, Fehling solution A and B
♦ Urinometer, a glass jar
♦ A dropper
♦ Reagent test strip and appropriate color scale (glucose, albumin, ketone bodies).

Urinary pH

♦ Dip one end of blue litmus paper into urine and observe the change in color of blue litmus paper.
♦ If blue litmus paper remains blue, the urine is alkaline.
♦ It blue litmus paper changes to red, the urine is acidic.

Specific Gravity

Pour 20 mL of fresh urine in the glass cylinder or fill it 3/4th and place the urinometer into the cylinder. Allow the urinometer to float in the urine freely. The urinometer should not touch the bottom and side of the jar. Hold the urinometer at eye level and read the measurement at the base of meniscus. Normal specific gravity is 1.016–1.025.

Urine Sugar

Benedict's Test

Take 5 mL of Benedict's test solution in a test tube and bring it to boil, cool it and add 8–10 drops of urine with a dropper into the test tube. Boil it again. Remove the test tube from fire and allow it to cool. The result may be recorded according to the color.

♦ Blue: Absence of sugar
♦ Green: +
♦ Yellow: ++

- Orange: +++
- Brick red: ++++

Fehling's Test

Take an equal quantity of Fehling's solution A and B in two test tubes. Pour together and boil.

In another test tube, take an amount of urine equal to the boiled mixture of Fehling's Solution A and B. Pour urine into the boiled mixture and boil

Formation of typical red or golden yellow precipitate indicates the presence of sugar.

Acetone

Rothera's Test

Take 2 cc of urine in a test tube and saturate it with ammonium sulphate.

- Put a few drops of freshly prepared nitroprusside.
- Add 1/2 cc of concentrated ammonia
- Allow it to stand
- Do not shake.
- If acetone is present in urine, a permanent purple colored ring is formed at the junction of urine and ammonia.

Albumin

Hot Test

- Filter the urine specimen. Fill 2/3 of a test tube with filtered urine.

- Heat the upper 1/3 of urine over a flame.
- If upper 1/3 becomes cloudy, add few drops of acetic acid
- If cloudy appearance disappears, it shows presence of phosphates
- If cloudy appearance is not present, it shows presence of albumin

Cold Test

- Pour 2 cc of concentrated nitric acid in a test tube.
- Pour 2 cc of filtered urine in another test tube
- With a dropper pour the urine gently along the sides of the first test tube
- A white ring at the junction of the two fluids indicates the presence of albumin

Test for Bile

- Take 1/2 test tube of urine and shake it vigorously.
  - If bile is present, the froth will be yellow or greenish
- **Hey's test:** Take urine in a test tube and sprinkle sulfur powder on top of it. If bile is present, the sulfur sinks to the bottom.
- **Iodine test:** Take 1/3 test tube of urine. Add 2 drops of 10% solution of Tr. iodine. If bile is present, a green color will be obtained at the junction of two liquids.

Record the findings in the client's chart and replace the test tubes in test tube rack after washing and discard the left over specimen.

BIBLIOGRAPHY

1. The Trained Nurses Association of India. *Fundamental of Nursing: Procedure Manual. TNAI Publication.*
2. Lindeman CA, Mccathie M. *Fundamentals of Contemporary Nursing. WB Saunders company.*
3. White L. *Basic Nursing. Foundations of Nursing Skills and Concepts. Delmar Thomson Learning;* 2002. p. 919.

Chapter
40

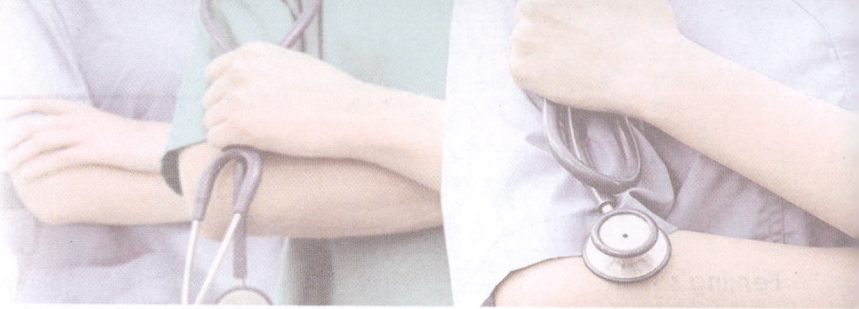

Maintenance of Normal Body Alignment and Mobility

Learning Objectives

After completing this chapter, you will be able to:

- Describe the maintenance of normal body alignment and mobility
- Identify factors affecting movement and alignment
- Differentiate isotonic, isometric, and isokinetic exercise
- Describe the effects of exercise and immobility on major body systems
- Assess body alignment, mobility and activity tolerance, using appropriate interview and physical assessment skills
- Develop nursing diagnosis that correctly identifies mobility problems amenable to nursing interventions
- Utilize principles of body mechanics when appropriate
- Use safe patient handling and movement techniques and equipment (assistive devices) when positioning, moving, lifting and ambulating patients
- Plan, implement and evaluate nursing care related to nursing diagnosis involving mobility problems

Key Terms

- Atrophy
- Body alignment
- Body mechanics
- Contractures
- Dangling
- Flaccidity
- Foot drop
- Gait
- Isokinetic exercise
- Isometric exercise
- Isotonic exercise
- Range of motion
- Osteoporosis

Chapter Outline

- Maintenance of Normal Body Alignment and Mobility
- Factors Affecting Movement and Alignment
- Exercise
- Effects of Exercises on Major Body Systems
- Effects of Immobility
- Nursing Management
- Principles Underlying Body Mechanics
- Equipment and Assistive Devices
- Positioning Patients

MAINTENANCE OF NORMAL BODY ALIGNMENT AND MOBILITY

Purposeful, coordinated movement of the body and maintenance of alignment require the integrated functioning of the musculoskeletal and nervous system. The following concepts are an important part of normal movement and musculoskeletal functioning, and contribute to a person's overall well-being.

Body Alignment or Posture

Good posture or good body alignment is the alignment of body parts that permits optimal musculoskeletal balance and operation and promotes healthy physiologic functioning. A person in correct alignment experiences no under strain on the joints, muscles, tendons, or ligaments while balance is maintained.

Balance

A body in correct alignment is balanced. An object is balanced when its center of gravity is close to its base of support, the line of gravity goes through the base of support and the object has wide base of support. The center of gravity of an object is the point at which its mass is centered. In humans, the center of gravity when standing is located in the center of the pelvis about midway between the umbilicus and the symphysis pubis. The line of gravity is a vertical line that passes through the center of gravity. The base of support is the foundation that provides for an object's stability. The wider the base of support and the lower the center of gravity, the greater the stability of the object.

Body balance increases when individual keeps the feet apart, thereby broadening the base of support and flex the hips and knees, thus lowering the center of gravity. These two simple maneuvers are important interventions that can decrease the musculoskeletal strain that occurs with excessive stretching or overexertion of a muscle or muscle tendon unit.

Coordinated Body Movement

Using major muscle groups, rather than weaker ones and taking advantage of the body's natural levers and fulcrums facilitate the actions of lifting, carrying, pushing, pulling and moving objects. Major muscle groups include the flexors, extensors and abductors of the thighs, flexors and extensors of the knees, flexors and extensors of the upper and lower arms. Use of arm bones as levers and the elbows as fulcrums facilitates lifting a weight against resistance.

Postural Reflexes

Integrated functioning of the musculoskeletal and nervous systems is essential for body alignment and balance. This depends on the functioning of several postural reflexes as described below.

Labyrinthine Sense

The sense of position and movement is provided by the sensory organs in the inner ear, which are stimulated by body movement and transmit these impulses to the cerebellum.

Proprioceptor or Kinesthetic Sense

This informs the brain of the location of a limb or body part as a result of joint movements stimulating special nerve endings in muscles, tendons, and fascia.

Visual or Optic Reflexes

Visual impressions contribute to posture by alerting the person to relationship with the environment.

Extensor or Stretch Reflex

When extensor muscles are stretched beyond a certain point, their stimulation causes a reflex contraction that aids a person to re-establish erect posture.

FACTORS AFFECTING MOVEMENT AND ALIGNMENT

Developmental Considerations

A person's age and degree of neuromuscular development markedly influence body proportions, posture, body mass, movements and reflexes. To facilitate each patient's use of the body to perform self-care actions, nurses need to be familiar with developmental variations in body proportions and neuromuscular development.

Physical Health

Problems in the musculoskeletal or nervous system can have a negative influence on body alignment and movement. Illnesses involving other body systems may interfere with movement. Therefore, be sensitive to how both acute and chronic health problems affect patient's posture, body movements and ability to perform activities of daily living.

Mental Health

Just as an individual's physical health influences body appearance and movement, so does the person's mental health. Body processes tends to slow down in depression, and there is a lack of visible energy. Body posture may also be affected, for example, person with depression often sits with head bowed down and shoulders slumped.

Nutrition

Poorly nourished people have muscle weakness and fatigue. Vitamin D deficiency causes bone deformity. Inadequate calcium intake increases risk of osteoporosis. Obesity can distort movements and can stress joints.

Lifestyle

An individual's lifestyle, whether active or sedentary, is influenced by many variables, including the individual's occupation, leisure activity preferences, and cultural influences. Activities in many occupations are sedentary. Therefore, individuals wishing to exercise regularly need to plan ahead of their leisure activities by preparing to exercise before or after working hours. In addition, person's diet and smoking history are other lifestyle variables that influence mobility. Culture and gender may also play a role, encouraging or discouraging exercise. As a nurse, we need to consider appropriate exercise forms/schedule which is safe and feasible that can have a positive effect in improving the quality of life and reducing fatigue.

Attitude and Values

Attitude and values learned early may be internalized for a lifetime. Individual values also influence the exercise options people make. Individuals who place a high value on physical attractiveness may be highly committed to regular exercise, another individual may exercise because of the desire for physical strength. However, someone may perceive body development as simply wastage of time and that could be better used to develop the mind. Therefore, sometimes, exercise is viewed as too much of a chore and the individuals avoid exercise. We need to offer suggestions on how to incorporate exercise into the person's daily routine, thus making exercise less of a chore.

Fatigue and Stress

Chronic stress may deplete body's energy to the point that fatigue makes the thought of exercise overwhelming. Regular exercise is emerging and can better equip a person to deal with daily stresses. Excessive exercise may stress the body and lead to fatigue.

External Factors

Many external factors can influence activity and mobility. Among these, weather exerts the greatest influence over outside exercise. A clear day invites physical activity. On the other hand, high humidity, very hot and very cold temperature, rain and snow, discourage outdoor exercise. Sufficient financial resources for gym memberships, access to exercise equipment and safe outdoor parks encourage regular exercise.

EXERCISE

Active exertion of muscles involving the contraction and relaxation of muscle groups is termed exercise. There are two types of exercises. One is based on the type of *muscle contraction* occurring during the exercise. The second is based on type of *body movement*.

Muscle Contraction

- **Isotonic exercise** involves muscle shortening and active movement. Examples include carrying out activities of daily living (ADLs) independently performing range of motion exercises, and swimming, walking, jogging, and bicycling. Benefits include: increased muscle mass, tone, and strength, improved joint mobility, increased cardiac and respiratory function, increased circulation and increased osteoblastic or bone-building activity.
- **Isometric exercise** involves muscle contraction without shortening. Examples include contraction of quadriceps and gluteal muscles. Benefits include increased muscle tone, mass and strength, increased circulation to the exercising body part, and increased osteoblastic activity.
- **Isokinetic exercise** involves muscle contraction with resistance. The resistance is provided at a constant rate by an external device. Examples include rehabilitative exercises for knee and elbow injuries and lifting weights.

Body Movement

Types of exercises involving body movement include aerobic exercises, stretching exercises, strength and endurance exercises, and movement and ADLS.

Aerobic exercise refers to sustained muscle movements that increases blood flow, heart rate, and metabolic demand for oxygen over time, promoting cardiovascular conditioning. Examples include swimming, walking, jogging, aerobic dancing, bicycling and jumping rope.

Stretching exercises involve movements that allow muscles and joints to be stretched gently through their full range of motion, increasing flexibility, specific warm-up and cool down exercises. Benefits include increased range of joint movements, improved circulation and relaxation.

Strength and endurance exercises are components of a variety of muscle building programs. Weight training, calisthenics, and specific isometric exercises can build both strength and endurance, increasing the power of musculoskeletal system.

Movement and ADLs include home cleaning, running after playful toddlers and climbing stairs.

Range of Motion

Range of motion (ROM) exercises are those in which a joint is moved through a full range of motion according to its capacity. It includes active exercises which is done by person himself and passive exercises which are carried with help of another person. The main purpose is to improve muscle strength, prevent complications of immobility like contractures and to increase joint flexibility.

Range of motion exercises should start from head to downward. These exercises include, flexion, extension, hyperextension, abduction, adduction, circumduction, external rotation, internal rotation, pronation, supination, etc. (Figs 1A to J).

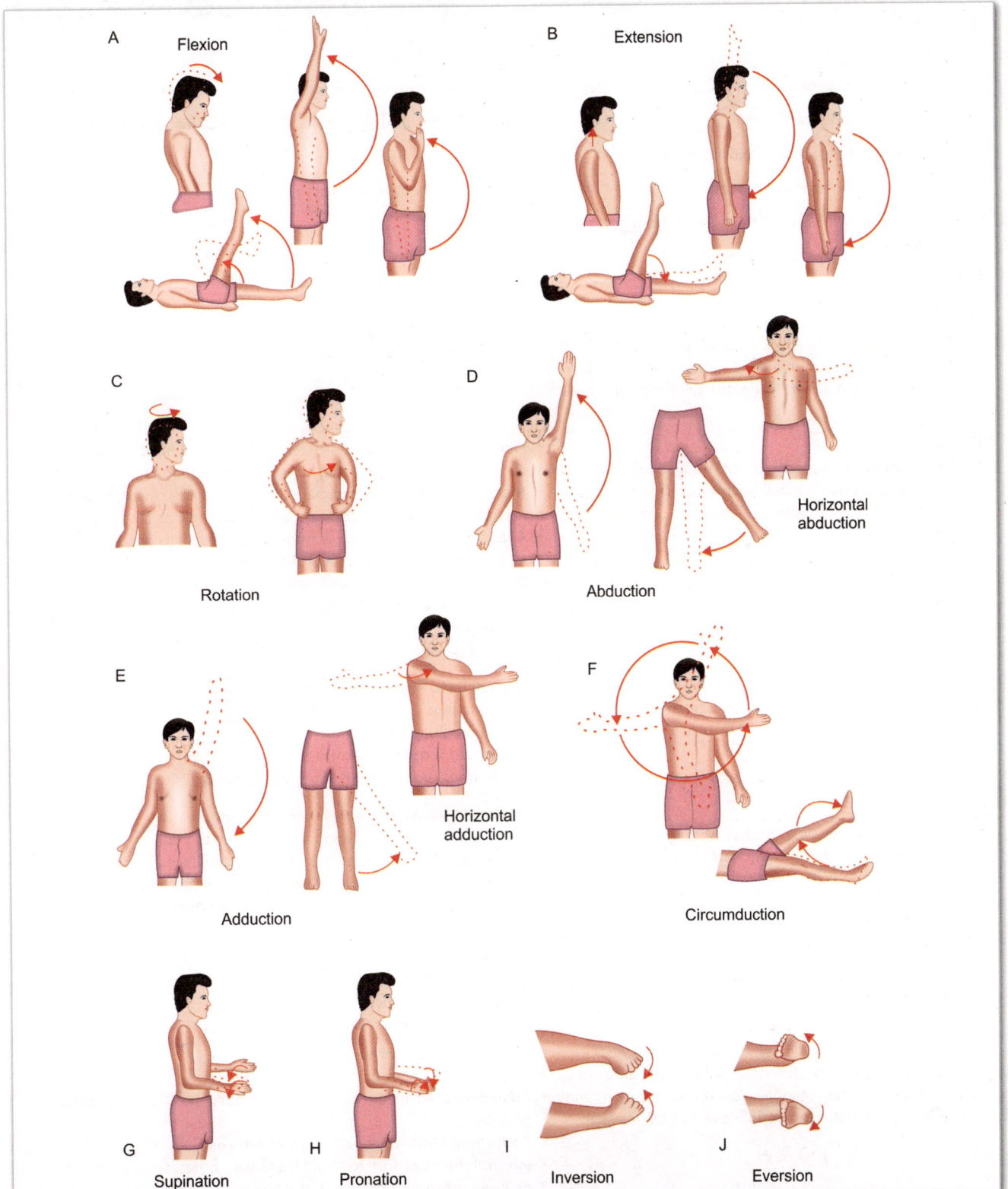

Figs 1A to J: Range of motion exercises

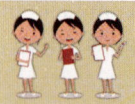

SKILL: PERFORMING RANGE OF MOTION EXERCISES

Action/steps	Rationale
1. Explain the patient the purpose of performing the exercise	Ensures cooperation of the patient
2. Remove rings or other constrictive jewellery, if present	In case of hand exercises, this may impede circulation
3. Provide privacy and wash hands	Reduces patient's anxiety and risk of transfer of microorganisms
4. Expose only the area that is being exercised	Reduces embarrassment of patient
5. Position bed to an appropriate height	Ensures proper body mechanics
6. Start proceeding passive ROM exercise from the head downwards	
Neck 7. Move head through flexion, extension, lateral flexion, rotation, and hyperextension of the neck ▪ Movement of head is contraindicated in spinal surgery, spinal trauma, and other central nervous system trauma and for patients having central venous line	♦ *Flexion:* Bring chin to rest on chest ♦ *Extension:* Return head to erect position ♦ *Hyperextension:* Bend head back as far as possible ♦ *Lateral flexion:* Tilt head as far as possible in circular movement
Shoulder 8. Flexion, extension, hyperextension, adduction, abduction and circumduction, external rotation, and internal rotation. Shoulder should be supported proximally and distally.	♦ *Flexion:* Raise arm from side position to forward position ♦ *Extension:* Return arm to position at the side of body ♦ *Hyperextension:* Move arm behind body, keeping elbow straight ♦ *Adduction:* Lower arm sideways and across body as far as possible ♦ *Abduction:* Move arms away from body as much as possible ♦ *Internal rotation:* With elbow flexed, rotate shoulder by moving arm until thumb is turned inwards and toward back ♦ *External rotation:* With elbow flexed, move arm until thumb is upward and lateral to head ♦ *Circumduction:* Move arm in full circle
Elbow 9. Flexion, extension, pronation, and supination. Support elbow joint both proximally and distally.	♦ *Flexion:* Bend elbow so that lower arm moves toward its shoulder joint and hand is in level with shoulder ♦ *Extension:* Bring elbow straight by lowering hand ♦ *Pronation:* Turn lower arm so that palm is down ♦ *Supination:* Turn lower arm so that palm is up
Wrist 10. Flexion, extension, hyperextension, and lateral flexion (radial and ulnar) position; wrist in functional position	♦ *Flexion:* Move palm toward inner aspect of forearm ♦ *Extension:* Move fingers and hand posterior to midline ♦ *Hyperextension:* Bring dorsal surface of hand back as far as possible ♦ *Radial deviation:* Bend wrist laterally toward fifth finger ♦ *Ulnar deviation:* Bend wrist medially toward thumb
Fingers 11. Move fingers through flexion, extension, hyperextension, abduction, adduction, opposition of the thumb, and circumduction of thumb	♦ *Flexion:* Move across palmar surface of hand ♦ *Extension:* Move straight away ♦ *Abduction:* Extend laterally ♦ *Adduction:* Move back ♦ *Opposition:* Touch to each finger
Hip 12. Move hip through flexion, extension, abduction, adduction, internal rotation and external rotation, and circumduction with support above and below joints	♦ *Flexion:* Move leg forward and up ♦ *Extension:* Move leg back beside other leg ♦ *Adduction:* Move leg back toward medial position and beyond if possible ♦ *Abduction:* Move leg laterally away from body ♦ *Internal rotation:* Turn foot and leg toward other leg ♦ *External rotation:* Turn foot and leg away from other leg ♦ *Circumduction:* Move hip in circle

Contd…

Action/steps	Rationale
Knee 13. Move knee through flexion and extension	• *Flexion:* Bring heel back toward back of thigh • *Extension:* Return leg to floor
Ankle and foot 14. Plantar flexion, dorsiflexion, circumduction, eversion and inversion of foot	• *Dorsiflexion:* Move foot so that toes are pointed upward • *Plantar flexion:* Move foot so that toes are pointed downward. Move ankle in circle. • *Inversion:* Turn sole of foot medially • *Eversion:* Turn sole of foot laterally
Toes 15. Move through flexion, extension, abduction and adduction	• *Flexion:* Curl toes downward • *Extension:* Straight toes • *Adduction:* Bring toes together • *Abduction:* Spread toes apart
16. Wash hands	• To prevent cross-infection
17. Record procedure	• Serves as a legal document
18. Position the patient in a comfortable position	• To enhance comfort

EFFECTS OF EXERCISES ON MAJOR BODY SYSTEMS

Regular exercise is necessary for the healthy functioning of the human body. Individuals who have inactive lifestyles are at a high risk for serious health problems.

Cardiovascular System

Benefits include:
- Increased efficiency of the heart
- Decreased heart rate and blood pressure
- Increased blood flow to all body parts
- Increased circulating fibrinolysin (substance that breaks small clots)
- Increased venous return.

Respiratory System

It helps in improving depth of respiration, respiratory rate, gas exchange at the alveolar level and rate of carbon dioxide release. Over period of time, regular exercise leads to improved pulmonary functioning.

Musculoskeletal System

The rhythmic contraction and relaxation of muscle groups during exercise results in increased muscle mass, tone, strength and increased joint mobility. Regular exercise produces the following benefits:
- Increased muscle efficiency and flexibility
- Increased coordination
- Increased efficiency of nerve impulse transmission

Regular exercise is also believed to slow the effects of aging. Exercise helps in preventing osteoporosis (the process of bone demineralization) associated with aging. Exercise also minimizes bone loss during chemotherapy.

Metabolic Processes

The metabolic rate increases during exercise so that sufficient glucose and fatty acids can be converted to provide the energy needed for increased muscle function. During strenuous exercise, the metabolic rate can increase up to 20 (the normal range). Increased body heat and waste products are also produced with regular exercise. The efficiency of metabolism and body temperature regulation is increased.

Gastrointestinal System

During exercise, blood is shunted away from the stomach and intestines to the exercising muscles.
With regular exercise:
- Appetite is increased
- Intestinal tone is increased, which improves digestion and elimination
- Weight may be controlled.

Urinary System

Regular exercise increases blood circulation, including improved blood flow to the kidneys. This allows the kidneys to maintain the body's fluid balance and acid base balance more efficiently and to excrete body wastes.

Skin

Increased circulation resulting from regular exercise nourishes the skin. Thus, regular exercise aids in promoting the overall general health of the skin.

Psychosocial Outlook

Benefits of regular exercise include:
* Increased energy, vitality and general well-being
* Improved sleep
* Improved appearance (body image)
* Improved self-concept
* Increased positive health behaviors.

EFFECTS OF IMMOBILITY

Each system has a unique response to the stress of immobility.

Integumentary System

* Reduced skin turgor and atrophy of the skin.
* **Skin breakdown:** Immobility interferes with circulation and diminishes supply of nutrients resulting in skin breakdown and formation of pressure sores. Friction and shearing forces also contribute to skin breakdown and the development of bed sores.

Musculoskeletal System

Disuse Osteoporosis

There is a loss of minerals and organic materials. Without the stress of weight bearing activity, the bones demineralize. Regardless of the amount of calcium in a person's diet, the demineralization process occurs with immobility. The loss of bone tissue weakens the bone and makes it more susceptible to fracture. The more osteoporotic the bone becomes; the less trauma is needed to sense the bone to break (pathological fractures).

Loss of Muscle Mass and Strength (Disuse Atrophy)

It is the wasting of any part of the body, due to degeneration of cells, from decreased nourishment or nerve supply. In fact in two months of immobility, a muscle may be reduced to half of its original size.

Contractures

A contracture is a condition, in which the muscle is fixed, shortened and resists stretching. When body muscles are not used, permanent shortening of muscles occur which limits joint mobility. Normally the opposing muscles maintain a state of balance between muscles that serve to contract in opposite direction, e.g., muscles that flex and extend, adduct and abduct. This state of balance is often disrupted in clients of immobilized joints.

Stiffness and Pain in Joints

After a muscle has remained in shortened position for 5–7 days, its loose connective tissue which normally allows full range of motion, begins to shorten and gradually changes to dense connective tissue. In addition, as the bone demineralize, excess of calcium may deposit in the joint contributing to stiffness and pain.

Cardiovascular System

Cardiac Strain

Immobilized person increases cardiac workload by using Valsalva maneuver. It is the name given to the physiologic mechanism that operates when a person attempts to exhale against a closed glottis and traps air in the lungs, greatly increasing intrathoracic pressure.

The immobilized person most frequently uses Valsalva maneuver when using arm and trunk muscles to move in bed, straining during defecation, coughing or vomiting. When the person stops moving or straining, there is sudden drop in the intrathoracic pressure and increase in venous return to heart. These changes may cause dysrhythmias.

Orthostatic Hypotension

An immobilized person when changes position, for example, standing, it leads to drop in blood pressure.

Venous Vasodilatation and Stasis

Due to muscle atrophy, blood pool in the vein increases the blood pressure that leads to vasodilatation and stasis.

Dependent Edema

When the venous pressure is sufficiently great, some of the serous component of the blood is forced out of the blood vessels causing edema. The edema is seen in area below heart level such as distal portions of arms, legs, etc. These are dependent areas and the edema is called dependent edema.

Thrombus Formation

Thrombus formation originates in the large vein of legs because of the low velocity of blood flow and it is called deep vein thrombosis.

Respiratory System

Decreased Respiratory Movement

In an immobile patient, ventilation of the lungs is passively altered. The body presses against the rigid bed and curtails chest movements. The abdominal organs push against the diaphragm restricting the lung movement and making it difficult to expand the lung fully.

Pooling of Respiratory Secretions

Secretions of the respiratory system are normally expelled by changing positions or posture and by coughing. Inactivity allows secretions to pool by gravity, interfering with the normal diffusion of oxygen and carbon dioxide in the alveoli. Often the immobilized person's intake of fluids decreases and this results in sputum that is thick and difficult to expectorate.

Atelectasis

Bed rest decreases the amount of surfactant produced. The combination of decreased surfactant and blockage of bronchiole with mucous can cause atelectasis, it is the collapse of the lung tissue.

Pneumonia

Pooled secretions provide an excellent media for bacterial growth. Under those conditions, a minor respiratory infection can evolve rapidly into severe infections of the lower respiratory tract.

Metabolic System

Decreased Metabolic Rate

In an immobilized client, basal metabolic rate and gastrointestinal mobility decreases as energy requirement of the body decreases.

Negative Nitrogen Balance

Immobility creates a marked imbalance between catabolism and anabolism, and the catabolic processes exceed the anabolic process. Catabolized muscle mass releases nitrogen. Over a period of time, more nitrogen is excreted than is ingested, producing a negative nitrogen balance.

Anorexia

Anorexia occurs because of the decreased metabolic rate.

Negative Calcium Balance

It occurs as a result of greater amount of calcium extracted from bone than replaced.

Urinary System

Urinary Stasis

In a mobile person, gravity plays an important role in the emptying of kidney and the bladder. When the person remains immobile,

gravity impedes the emptying of the kidney and urinary bladder. As a result, urinary stasis occurs.

Renal Calculi

Calcium concentration is increased in urine of an immobilized person because of bone resorption and at the same time, fluid intake is low which will result in concentrated urine. All these contribute to renal calculi.

Urinary Retention

The decreased muscle tone of urinary bladder leads to urinary retention. In addition, the discomfort of using a bedpan or urinal, the embarrassment and lack of privacy and the unnatural position for urination combine to make it difficult for the client to relax the perineal muscles sufficiently to urinate while lying in bed.

Urinary Infection

Static urine provides an excellent medium for bacterial growth. The flushing action of normal frequent urination is absent and also the increased alkalinity of the urine is caused by the hypercalciuria that supports bacterial growth.

Gastrointestinal System

Constipation

Constipation is a frequent problem for immobilized people because of decreased peristalsis and colon motility. The overall skeletal muscle weakness affects the abdominal and perineal muscle used in defecation.

Psychoneurogenic System

Due to less secretion of endorphins, people experience negative effects on mood leading to inability to engage in any physical activities.

NURSING MANAGEMENT

Assessment

Nursing assessment uses both interview and physical assessment skills to elicit data about the patient's mobility status.

Nursing History

Interview patients regarding their daily activity level, endurance, exercise, mobility problems, physical and mental health alteration that affect mobility and external factors that affect mobility.

Physical Assessment

Physical Assessment includes an assessment of general ease of movement and gait, alignment, joint structure, and function, muscle mass, tone and strength; and endurance. During this assessment, direct attention to both structure and function is given. The patient's ability to stand, walk, sit up and grasp are important because these enable the patient to wash, dress and feed himself or herself and perform other basic ADLs.

For older people who make large part of the population, there is functional decline, i.e., inability to care for oneself by bathing, dressing, toileting, eating, transferring and maintaining continence, can have severe consequences. Changes in mobility status contributes to this functional decline.

Gait

Physical assessment of an ambulatory patient begins as he/she walks into the room. Voluntary controlled and coordinated body movements are key to integrated functioning of the skeletal, muscular, and nervous systems. Note whether the patient's body movements are quick or slow and deliberate. Common involuntary movements that may be observed include tremors and tics (irregularly occurring spasmodic movements such as winking, grimacing, or shoulder shrugging).

Note the gait of the patient who is ambulatory. The patient's movement while walking should be coordinated and the posture should be well balanced. The arms should swing freely in a rhythm alternating with the legs. Detection of the gait abnormalities is important because they may place the individual at risk for injury and also may indicate intoxication or a neuromuscular disorder. Note whether the patient uses any assistive devices such as wheelchair, brace, cane, walker, or crutches to aid in ambulation. Also, determine whether this aid is meeting the patient's needs, if the aid is required for mobility, and if the aid is being used safely.

Alignment

Correct body alignment permits musculoskeletal balance and promotes physiologic functioning. Deviations in body alignment may result from chronic poor posture, trauma, muscle damage, or nerve dysfunction. Fatigue and a person's mental and emotional status may also influence alignment. Observe alignment when a patient is standing, sitting or lying. Note whether the patient is able to maintain correct alignment independently.

A patient's body is in correct body alignment while standing when:

- The head is erect
- The face is in forward position, in the same direction as the feet

- The chest is held upward and forward
- The spinal column is upright and the curves of the spine are within normal limits
- The abdominal muscles are held upward and the buttocks downward
- The knees are extended-not bent or hyperextended in the knee lock position
- The feet are at right angles to the lower legs
- The line of gravity goes through the center of the knees and in front of the ankle joints
- The base of support is on the soles of the feet, and weight is distributed equally to the soles and heels

Correct body alignment when sitting is similar to correct alignment when standing except that the hips are flexed, the knees are flexed and not crossed, and the base of support is on the buttocks and upper thighs. The popliteal area should be free of the edge of the chair to prevent circulatory stasis and possible nerve injury.

Joint Structure and Function

Use inspection and palpation to examine joints, their range of motion, and the surrounding tissue. Range of motion is the complete extent of movement of which a joint is normally capable. For example, normal shoulder and upper arm movements are flexion, extension, hyperextension, abduction, adduction and circumduction, inward rotation and outward rotation. The chief muscles involved in these movements are the deltoid (adducts upper arm), pectoralis major (flexes and adducts the upper arm), latissimus dorsi (extends and adducts the upper arm), trapezius (raises and lowers the shoulders), and serratus anterior (pulls the shoulder forward)

The knees and elbows can be flexed and extended. The biceps, quadriceps and hamstring muscles are active in these movements. The forearm can be supinated and pronated. The four principle muscles that move the forearm are the biceps brachii (flexes and supinates), brachialis (flexes and pronates), triceps brachii (extends) and pronator quadratus (pronates).

Thigh movements involve the gluteus muscles and the adductor muscles. The gluteus muscles (maximus, medius and minimus) extend, rotate and abduct the thigh. The adductor muscles adduct the thigh and flex the leg. Flexion, extension, adduction and inward and outward rotation from the hip are usually possible. Circumduction of the hip involves all the movements of the hip. Most hip movements involve the movements of the pelvis as well.

The ankle is a hinged joint that permits plantar flexion and dorsal flexion. Inversion and eversion of the feet takes place in the gliding joints. The joints of the toes permit flexion, extension, abduction and adduction.

The vertebral joints permit flexion, extension, lateral flexion and rotation of the cervical spine and trunk.

The rectus abdominis, the external and internal oblique muscles and the sacrospinalis muscle are involved in these movements. When assessing joint mobility, note the following:

- Size, shape, color and symmetry of joints. Note any masses, deformities or muscle atrophy.
- Range of motion of each joint.
- Any limitation in the normal range of motion or any unusual increase in the mobility of a joint. Range of motion varies among individuals and decreases with aging.
- Muscle strength when performing range of motion exercise against resistance.
- Any swelling, heat, tenderness, pain, nodules or crepitations.
- Compare findings in one joint with those of the opposite joint.

Muscle Mass, Tone and Strength

Muscle Mass, Tone and Strength are prerequisite to body movement and work performance. Mass refers to muscle size. Assess muscle mass throughout the body and compare one muscle group to another using tape measurements. Atrophy describes muscles mass that is decreased through disuse or neurologic impairment. Hypertrophy refers to increased muscle mass resulting from exercise or training. Patients experiencing muscle wasting as a result of a chronic disease process such as cancer may report visible changes in muscle mass.

Assess muscle tone by flexing and extending the elbow, knee and noting the degree of resistance to other movements. Decreased tone, hypotonicity or *flaccidity* results from disuse or neurologic impairments (*spasticity*). Increased tone that interferes with movement, is also caused by neurologic impairments.

Muscle strength varies greatly from one individual to another and within same individual and is affected by muscle use. Test muscle strength by asking the patient to move actively against resistance.

Impaired muscle strength or weakness is termed *paresis*. The absence of strength secondary to nervous impairment is called *paralysis*. Hemiparesis refers to weakness of one half of the body. Hemiplegia is paralysis of one half of the body. Paraplegia is paralysis of the legs, and *quadriplegia* is paralysis of the arms and legs.

Endurance

When assessing endurance, evaluate the patient's ability to turn in bed, maintain body alignment, when sitting or standing, ambulate, and perform self-care activities. When a physical or psychological factor is believed to be affecting endurance, accomplish the following:

- Obtain vital signs when the patient is at rest
- Instruct the patient to perform the activity

- Observe the patient's response during and after the activity
- Take the vital signs immediately after the activity
- Reassess the vital signs after the patient has rested for 3 minutes

Significant findings indicate that a person's exercise tolerance has been reached including noticeably increased pulse, respirations and blood pressure, shortness of breath, dyspnea, weakness, pallor, confusion, and vertigo.

Diagnosis

Diagnosis indicates both potential and actual problems when analyzing data about a patient's mobility status. The plan of a care for the patient with an alteration in mobility should include nursing diagnosis that identifies the complications of immobility for which the patient is at greatest risk.

Planning

If the patient is not experiencing any mobility problems, expected outcomes are directed toward the promotion of physical fitness. Patients at high risk for specific mobility problems require different expected outcomes. For example, adhere to every two hours positioning schedule, demonstrate full range of joint motion, demonstrate adequate muscle mass, tone and strength to perform functional ADLs. Patients who are immobile require outcomes directed toward preventing complications related to inactivity and its effects on body system. For example, the patient will:

- Be free from signs of breakdown
- Change from lying to a standing position safely
- Show signs of adequate venous return
- Be free of contractures

Implementation

Providing patient care places demands on the nurse's musculoskeletal system. Certain principles underlying body movement can serve as guides for the patient and the nurse.

PRINCIPLES UNDERLYING BODY MECHANICS

Muscles tend to act in groups rather than singly. Using a group of large muscles places less strain on the body than using a group of smaller muscles or a single muscle. For example, less strain results when a heavy object is raised by flexing the knees rather than by bending from the waist. The former movement utilizes the large gluteal and femoral muscles, whereas the latter utilizes the smaller muscles such as the sacrospinal muscle of the back.

Active movement results in the contraction of muscles. Active and passive exercises are often prescribed for patients.

Active movement involves the contraction of the muscle; the energy is supplied by the patient. Passive movement does not require muscle contraction; the energy is essentially supplied by a second person. The nurse can assist a patient with both active and passive movements as a part of nursing care.

Muscles are always in slight contraction. This condition is called muscle tone. If the nurse prepares her muscle for action prior to activity, she will protect her ligaments and muscles from strain and injury. For example, she will be better prepared to lift a heavy object if she first contracts the muscle of her abdomen and pelvis and the gluteal muscles of the buttocks.

The stability of an object is greater when there is a wide base of support and a low center of gravity and when a vertical line from the center of gravity falls within the base of support. The nurse can assume a broad stance and bends her knees rather than bending at waist. This practice keeps the vertical line of her center of gravity within her base of support, thus providing her with greater stability.

The amount of effort required to move a body depends upon the resistance of the body as well as the gravitational pull. By utilizing the pull of gravity rather than working against it, the nurse can reduce the amount of effort required in movement.

The force required to maintain body balance is the greatest when the line of gravity is farthest from the center of the base of support. Therefore, the person who holds a weight close to his body uses less effort than the person who holds the weight in his extended arms.

Changes in activity and position help to maintain muscle tone and avoid fatigue. If a person changes his position even slightly while he is carrying out a task, and if he changes his activity from time to time, he will maintain better muscle tone and avoid undue fatigue.

The friction between an object and the surface upon which the object is moved affects the amount of work needed to move the object. Friction is a force that opposes motion. The smoothest surface creates the least friction. Consequently, less energy is needed to move objects on smooth surfaces. The nurse can apply this principle when a patient changes position in bed by providing a smooth foundation upon which the patient can move.

Pulling or sliding an object requires less effort than lifting it, because lifting necessitates moving against the force of gravity. If, for example, the nurse lowers the head of patient's bed before she helps him to move up in the bed, less effort is required than when the head of the bed is raised.

Mechanical devices can reduce the amount of work required in movement. If in lifting heavy objects, the nurse uses her arm as lever whenever possible, she will utilize less energy than she would in direct lifting.

Using one's own weight to counteract a patient's weight requires less energy in movement. If a nurse uses her own weight to pull or push a patient, her weight increases the force applied to the movement.

EQUIPMENT AND ASSISTIVE DEVICES

Many devices and equipment are available to aid in transferring, repositioning, and lifting patients. It is important to use the right equipment and appropriate device based on patient's assessment and desired movement.

Gait Belts

A gait belt is a device used for transferring patients and assisting with ambulation. The gait belt is used to help the patient stand and provide stabilization during pivoting. The belt, which often has handles, is placed around the patient's waist and secured by Velcro fasteners. Gait belts allow the nurse to assist in ambulating patients who have leg strength, can cooperate, and require minimal assistance. Gait belts should not be used on patients with abdominal or thoracic incisions.

Stand Assist and Repositioning Aids

Some patients need minimal assistance to stand up with an appropriate support to grasp, they can lift themselves. These devices can be attached to the bed or wheelchair, which can help the patient to stand.

Lateral Assist Devices

Lateral Assist devices reduce patient-surface friction during side-to-side transfers. Roller boards, slide boards, transfer boards, inflatable mattresses, and friction reducing lateral devices make transfer safer and comfortable for the patient. For example, an inflatable lateral assist device is a flexible mattress that is placed under the patient. An attached, portable air supply then inflates the mattress, which provides a layer of air under the patient. This air cushion allows the nurse to perform the move with much less effort. Another device is transfer board, usually made of smooth, rigid, low friction material (such as coated wood or plastic). The board is placed under the patient that provides a slick surface for the patient during transfers, thereby reducing friction and the force required to move the patient.

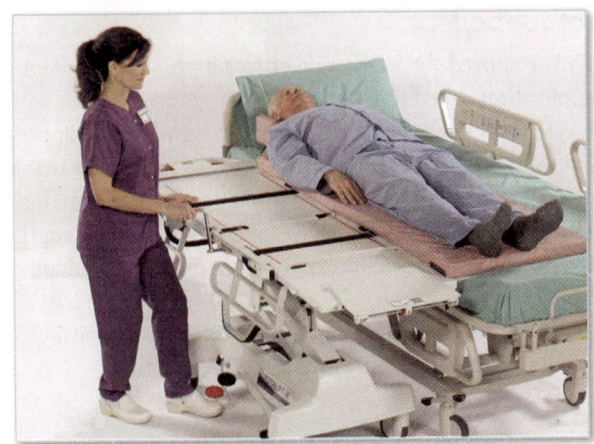

Fig. 2: Mechanical lateral assist device

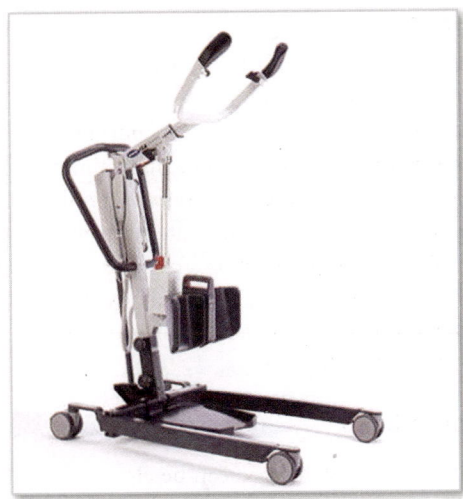

Fig. 3: Stand assist aid

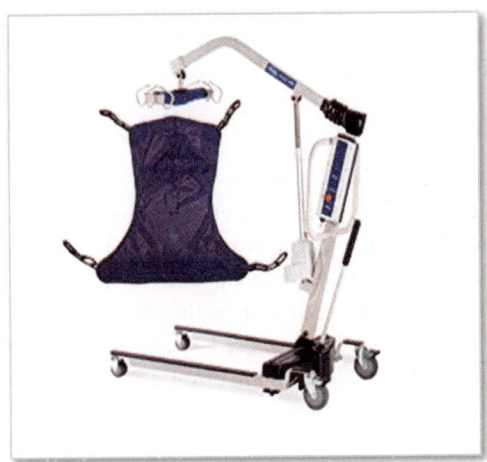

Fig. 4: Powered full-body lift

There are mechanical lateral assist devices (Fig. 2), which include specialized stretchers and eliminate the need to slide the patient manually. A portion of the device moves from the stretcher to the bed, sliding under the patient and effectively moves the patient without any pulling.

Transfer Chairs

Chairs that can convert into stretchers are available. These are useful with patients who have no weight bearing capacity, cannot follow directions and cannot cooperate. The back of the chair bends back and the leg supports elevate to form a stretcher configuration, eliminating the need for lifting the patient.

Powered Stand Assist

Powered stand assist devices can be used with patients who can bear weight on at least one leg, can follow directions, and are cooperative. A simple sling is placed around the patient's back and under the arms. The patient rests his feet on the devices foot rest and places his hands on the handle (Fig. 3).

The device mechanically assists the patient to stand, without any assistance. Once the patient is standing, the device can be wheeled to a chair, the toilet, or bed, some have scales incorporated into the device that can be used to weigh the patient.

Powered Full-body Lifts

Powered full-body lifts devices are used with patients who cannot bear any weight to move them out of bed, into and out of chair, and to a commode or stretcher. A full body sling is placed under the patient's body, including head and torso, then the sling is attached to the lift (Fig. 4). The device slowly lifts the patient. Some devices can be lowered to the floor to pick-up a patient who has fallen.

POSITIONING PATIENTS

Positioning that maintains correct body alignment and facilitates physiologic functioning contributes to the patient's psychological and physical well-being. The force of gravity pulls parts of the body out of alignment unless adequate support is provided. Various positions are protective in nature only when the patient is positioned properly.

Common Devices to Promote Alignment

Pillows

Pillows are used to provide support or to elevate a body part. Pillows of different sizes are useful for different parts. For head, they are usually full-sized pillow and small pillows are ideal for support or elevation of the extremities, shoulders, or incisional wounds.

Mattresses

Mattresses should be comfortable, firm to permit good body alignment. There are different kinds of mattresses available for both therapeutic and comfort purposes. The foam rubber mattresses put less pressure upon the patient's bony prominences. Air or water mattresses are the alternating pressure mattresses, which are alternatively inflated and deflated. With the result, there is a continuous change in the pressure upon the various parts of the body. These alterations of pressure stimulate circulation to the skin, thus facilitating the nourishment of the tissues.

Adjustable Beds

The head of an adjustable bed can be elevated to the desired degree. The foot can also be elevated as desired. The height of the bed can also be adjusted so that the patient can stand with the least amount of effort and health care workers use the higher positions, so that they do not strain their backs while providing care.

Trapeze Bar

A trapeze bar is a hand grip suspended from a frame near the head of the bed. The patient can grasp the bar with one or both hands and then raise the trunk from the bed (Fig. 5).

The trapeze makes moving and turning considerably easier for many patients and facilitates transfers into and out of bed. It can also be used when a patient needs to perform exercises that strengthen some muscles of the upper extremities.

Foot Support

This is required for patient's feet to support and prevent the complication called foot drop.

This occurs when patient's feet, remain unsupported in the dorsiflexion position. The toes drop downward, and the feet are in plantar flexion. If plantar flexion remains for extended periods, it can cause alteration in the length of muscles and the patient experiences extreme difficulty in walking (Figs 6A and B).

So use of foot support or high top canvas sneaker can prevent occurrence of this problem.

Cradle

If top bedding must be kept off the patient's lower extremities, a device called a cradle is used. A cradle is metal frame that supports the bed linens away from the patient while providing privacy and warmth.

Sandbags

In various sizes, it can be used to immobilize an extremity and support body alignment. When properly filled, this should be pliable enough to be shaped according to body's contours

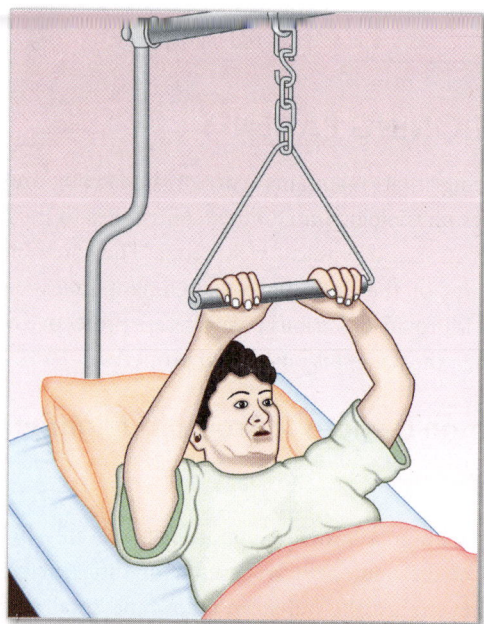

Fig. 5: A trapeze bar

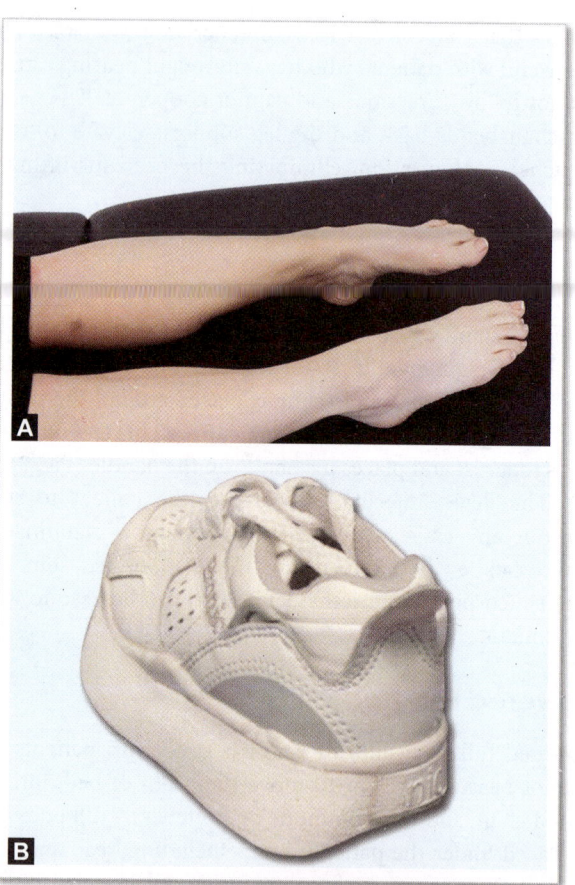

Figs 6A and B: A. Plantar flexion occurs when the foot is not supported. B. When high-top-sneakers support the feet, the dorsiflexion position is maintained

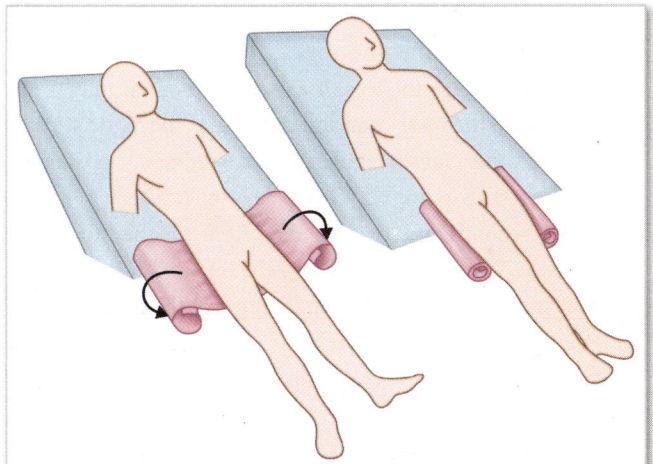

Fig. 7: Trochanter rolls prevent the external rotation of the hips of bedridden patient. The patient is placed on a folded sheet so that the top edge is at the hips and the lower edge is about one third of the way down the thighs. Towels or bath blankets are rolled under each side until the roll is snugly against the patient's hips and thighs. The support cannot unroll, and the weight of the patient keeps it secure.

to provide support. Avoid hard or firmly packed sandbags. Position a sandbag to avoid creating pressure on a bony prominence.

Trochanter Rolls

Trochanter rolls are used to support the hips and legs so that the femur does not rotate outward (Fig. 7). Properly placed pillows can also be used to help prevent the thigh joints from turning outward, but they need frequent adjustment to be effective as they tend to slip out of place.

Side Rails

Side rails can assist the patient in rolling from one side to the other or by sitting up without calling for assistance. Using side rails can help the patient retain or regain muscle efficiency. When using side rails, be sure to explain their use to the families, patients and follow the protocol of the agency.

Positioning

When the patient is unable to change position independently, use a turn schedule posted at the bedside to assist with and document the rotation of positions.

Fowler's Position

Fowler's position is defined as the semi-sitting position with head of the bed raised to 45–60 degrees. This position is often used to promote cardiac and respiratory functioning because abdominal organs drop in this position, thereby providing maximal space in the thoracic cavity. Variations of Fowler's position include high fowler's and low Fowler's or semi-Fowler's position. In the high Fowler's position, the head of the bed is elevated to 90 degrees. When a bedside table with the pillow on top of it is placed in front of the patient in high Fowler's position, the patient can lean forward and rest the arms on the pillow, assuming a posture that allows for maximal lung expansion. In low Fowler's or semi-Fowler's position, the head of the bed is elevated only 30 degrees.

In Fowler's position, the buttocks bear the main weight of the body. In this position, the heels, sacrum, and scapulae are at risk for skin breakdown and require frequent assessment.

Supine or Dorsal Recumbent Position

In this position, patient lies flat on the back with the head and shoulders elevated with a pillow unless contraindicated, such as spinal anesthesia or surgery on the spinal vertebrae.

Side Lying or Lateral Position

In the side lying position, the patient lies on the side and the main weight of the body is borne by the lateral aspect of the lower scapula and the lateral aspect of the lower ileum. This is a comfortable alternative to supine position for the patient on bed-rest. The patient lies on his side with both arms forward and his knees and hips flexed. The upper leg is flexed more than the lower leg.

A pillow to support the patient's arm permits greater chest expansion and enables the nurse to readily observe the character and rate of his respiration. A pillow to support back is placed lengthwise. This position is prescribed in order to take weight off the sacrum of the patient and patient can eat more easily in this position. It also facilitates drainage and many people find it a relaxing position.

Sims' Position (Semi-Prone Position)

The Sims' position is similar to the lateral position except that the patient's weight is on the anterior aspect of the patient's shoulder girdle and hip. The patient's lower arm is behind him and his upper arm is flexed at the shoulder and elbow. The upper leg is acutely flexed at the hip and knee.

A pillow placed laterally and in front of the patient's abdomen will support the patient in this position. Pillows for the patient's upper arm and upper leg will prevent adduction of these limbs, and a small pillow for the patient's head will prevent lateral flexion. If the patient is unconscious, in order to promote mucus drainage from mouth, a pillow under the head is contraindicated. The Sims' position can be established on both left side and the right side. The patient's position should be changed frequently. If he/she is unable to move himself, the nurse can help him/her turn every two hours.

Prone Position

In this position, the patient lies on the abdomen with the head turned to one side. Many people are relaxed and sleep well in this position; some find it more comfortable to flex their arms over their head.

Supportive measures for the patient in this position include a small pillow or roll under the abdomen at the level of the diaphragm in order to give support to the lumbar curvature and in case of female patient, to take weight off the breasts. In addition, a pillow under the lower legs elevates the patient's toes off the bed and permits slight flexion of the knees. If the patient prefers a pillow for head, a small pillow is more comfortable unless it is contraindicated. (Table 1 describes common bed positions and nursing measures to prevent complications associated with these positions).

Antiembolism Stockings and Pneumatic Compression Devices

Venous stasis and development of venous thrombosis are potential complications of immobility. These devices are passive interventions prescribed for prevention of venous stasis and the development of venous thrombosis.

Antiembolism Stockings

Antiembolism stockings are often used for patients at risk for deep vein thrombosis, pulmonary embolism and to help prevent phlebitis. They are made of elastic material and are available in either knee-thigh or thigh-high length. By applying pressure, antiembolism stockings increase the velocity of blood flow in the superficial and deep veins and improve venous valve function in the legs, promoting venous return to the heart. When assisting with use of antiembolism stockings, follow these guidelines:

- Measure the patient's legs to determine the proper size of stocking. Each leg should have a correct fitting stocking: If measurements are different, then two different size of stocking need to be ordered to ensure correct fitting on each leg. Some stockings are marked as right or left. An improperly fitting stocking is uncomfortable and ineffective and possibly even harmful.
- Assess the skin condition and neurovascular status of the legs. Report abnormalities before continuing with the application of the stockings.
- Be prepared to apply the stockings in the morning before the patient is out of bed and while the patient is in supine position. If the patient is sitting or has been up and about, have the patient lie down with legs and feet elevated for at least 15 minutes before applying the stockings. Otherwise,

the leg vessels are congested with blood, reducing the effectiveness of the stockings.

- Do not massage the legs. If a clot is present, it may break away from the vessel wall and circulate in the blood stream.
- Check the legs regularly for redness, blistering, swelling and pain. Check the legs once every 8 hours, some recommend twice a day. Remove the stockings, completely once a day to bathe the legs and feet.
- Get the stockings washed at least every third day. Patient may need two pairs of stockings so that he or she can wear one pair while the second pair is being cleaned.
- Remove antiembolism stockings during morning care and inspect the legs. Then reapply the stockings before the patient is out of bed.

Pneumatic Compression Devices

Intermittent pneumatic compression devices may be used in conjunction with antiembolism stockings. They are composed of air pump, connecting tubes, and extremity sleeves. They require physician's order and are often prescribed for high risk surgical patients, patients with decreased mobility, patients with chronic venous disease, and patients at risk for deep-vein disorder. Pneumatic compression devices apply intermittent sequential pressure to the leg to enhance blood flow and venous return, stimulating the normal muscle-pumping action in the legs.

Turning the Patient in Bed

Many a times, patient cannot turn in bed without assistance. Nurses need to use their knowledge of correct alignment to turn the patient from the back onto the side, from the back onto the abdomen, and from the abdomen onto the back. When turning the patient, the bed should be at the height of the caregiver's elbows to ensure comfortable working height.

- The nurse stands on the side of the bed toward which the patient is to be turned. The patient places his/her far arm across his/her chest and his far leg over his/her near leg. The nurse checks that the patient's near arm is lateral to, and away from his/her body so that he/she does not roll upon it.
- The nurse stands opposite the patient's waist and faces the side of the bed with one foot step in front of the other.
- She places one hand on the patient's far shoulder and one hand on his/her far hip.
- As the nurse shifts her weight from her forward leg to her rear leg, the patient is turned toward her. The nurse's hips come downward during this motion.

TABLE 1: Common bed positions and nursing actions

Positions	Complication to be prevented	Suggested preventive actions
Fowler's position 	◆ Flexion contracture of the neck ◆ Exaggerated curvature of the spine ◆ Dislocation of the shoulder ◆ Flexion contracture of the wrist ◆ Edema of the hand ◆ Flexion contractures of the fingers and abduction of the thumbs ◆ Impaired lower extremity circulation and knee contracture ◆ Pressure on heels ◆ External rotation of the hips ◆ Foot drop.	◆ Allow the head to rest against the mattress or be supported by a small pillow only. ◆ Use a firm support for the back; position the patient so that the angle of elevation starts at the hips. ◆ Support the forearms on pillows to elevate them sufficiently so that no pull is exerted on the shoulders. ◆ Support the hand on pillows so that it is in natural alignment with the forearm. ◆ Support the hand so that it is slightly elevated in relation to the elbow. ◆ Provide hand-wrist splints if necessary. ◆ Elevate the knees for only brief periods; place one or two pillows under the lower legs from below the knees to the ankles; avoid pressure on the knee gatch. ◆ Use trochanter roll. ◆ Support the feet in dorsal flexion. Use foot board; high-top sneakers can also be used.
Supine position 	◆ Exaggerated curvature of the spine and flexion of the hips ◆ Flexion contracture of the neck ◆ Internal rotation of the shoulders and extension of the elbows (hunch shoulders) ◆ Flexion of the lumbar curvature ◆ Extension of the fingers and abduction of the thumbs (claw hand deformities) ◆ External rotation of the femurs ◆ Hyperextension of the knees ◆ Foot drop	◆ Provide a firm supportive mattress; use a bed board if necessary. ◆ Place pillows under the upper shoulders, the neck, and the head so that the head and the neck are held in the correct position. ◆ Place pillows or arm supports under the forearms so that the upper arms are alongside the body and the forearms and pronated slightly. ◆ Place rolled towel or small pillow under lumbar curvature if needed. ◆ Use hand-wrist splints if appropriate. ◆ Place sandbags or a trochanter roll alongside the hips and the upper half of the thighs. ◆ Place a pillow under the lower legs from below the knees to the ankles. ◆ Use a footboard or make an improvised firm foot support to hold the feet in dorsal flexion; high-top sneakers may also be recommended.
Lateral or side lying position 	◆ Lateral flexion of the neck ◆ Inward rotation of the arm and interference with respiration ◆ Extension of the finger and abduction of the thumbs ◆ Internal rotation and adduction of the femur ◆ Twisting of the spine	◆ Place a pillow under the head and the neck. ◆ Place a pillow under the upper arm; lower arm should be flexed and positioned comfortably. ◆ Provide hand-wrist splint if necessary. ◆ Use one or two pillows as needed to support the leg from the groin to the foot. ◆ Ensure that the two shoulders are aligned with the two hips.

Contd...

Positions	Complication to be prevented	Suggested preventive actions
Modified lateral position		• Modified lateral position (Oblique position) is an alternative to the side lying position and results in significantly less pressure on the trochanter area.
Sims' position 	• Lateral flexion of the neck • Damages to nerves and blood vessels in the axillae of the lower arm • Internal shoulder rotation and adduction • Internal rotation and adduction of the hip; lumbar lordosis • Twisting of the spine • Foot drop	• Place a small pillow under the head unless the drainage of oral secretions is desired. • Carefully position lower arm behind and away from the patient's back. • Abduct the upper shoulder slightly so that shoulder and elbow are flexed; place a pillow between the chest and upper arm • Place a pillow under the upper flexed leg from the groin to the foot. • Ensure that the two shoulders are aligned with the two hips. • Support the lower foot in dorsal flexion with a sandbag.
Prone position 	• Flexion on the cervical spine • Hyperextension of the spine; impaired respirations • Foot drop	• Place a small pillow under the head • Place some suitable support under the patient between the end of the ribcage and the upper abdomen if this facilitates breathing and if there is space • Move the patient down in bed so that the feet are over the mattress, or support the lower legs on a pillow just high enough to keep the toes from touching the bed.

• The patient is stopped by the nurse's elbows, which come to rest on the mattress at the edge of the bed.

Helping the Patient Move to the Side of the Bed

The nurse may require to move the patient to side of the bed. For example, if she is changing the dressing. She can follow these guidelines (Figs 8A and B).

• The nurse stands facing the patient at the side of the bed toward which she wishes to move

• She assumes a broad stance with one leg forward of the other and with her knees and hips flexed in order to bring her arms to the level of the bed.

• The nurse places one arm under the shoulders and neck of the patient and the other arm under the small of the patient's back.

• She shifts her body weight from her front foot to her back foot as she rocks backward to a crouched position, bringing the patient toward her to the side of the bed. The nurse's hips come downward as she rocks backward.

• The nurse then moves the middle section of the patient in the same manner by placing one arm under the patient's back and one arm under the thighs. Then the patient's feet and the lower legs are moved with the same motion.

• Care should be taken not to pull the patient off the side of the bed.

Helping the Patient Turn on his/her Side

When a patient needs help in order to turn on his side, the nurse must take particular care that the patient does not fall off the bed.

The nurse stands on the side of the bed toward which the patient is to be turned. The patient places his/her far arm across his chest and his/her far leg over his near leg. The nurse checks that the patient's near arm is lateral to, and away from, his/her body so that he/she does not roll upon it. (Figs 9A to C).

• The nurse stands opposite the patient's waist and faces the side of the bed with one foot a step in front of the other.

• She places one hand on the patient's far shoulder and one hand on his/her hip.

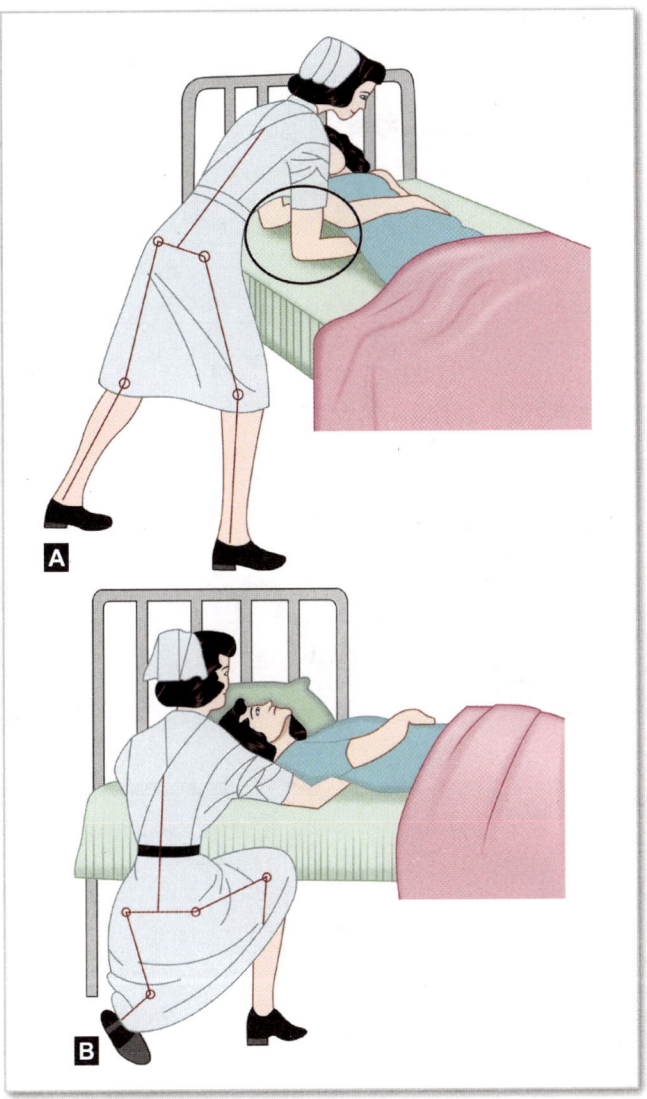

Figs 8A and B: Helping the patient move to the side of the bed

- As the nurse shifts her weight from her forward leg to her near leg, the patient is turned toward her. The nurse's hips come downward during the motion.
- The patient is stopped by the nurse's elbows which come to rest on the mattress at the edge of bed.

Moving the Semihelpless Patient up in Bed

The movement is facilitated if the patient can assist by flexing his knees and pushing with his legs. In assisting the patient to make this movement, the nurse should take precautions that his/her head does not hit the top of the bed. Thus, the nurse can lower the head of the bed and put the patient's pillow at the head of the bed, where it can act as a pad. Helping the patient move up in bed can be done by one or two nurses: in the latter instance one nurse stands at each side of the patient's bed. Follow these steps:

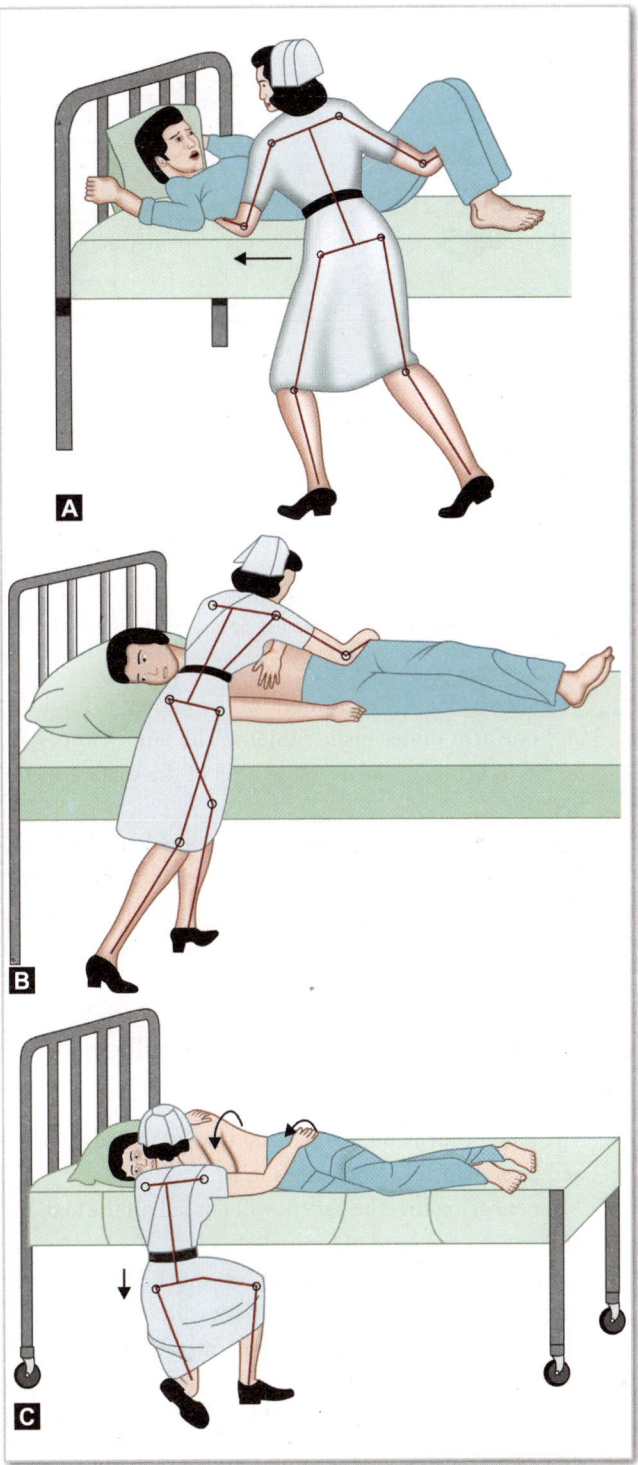

Figs 9A to C: Helping the patient to turn on his/her side

- The patient flexes his/her knees, bringing his/her heels up towards his/her buttocks.
- The nurse stands at the side of the bed, turned slightly toward the patient's head. One foot is a step in front of the other, the foot that is closer to the bed being to the rear; her feet are directed toward the head of the bed.

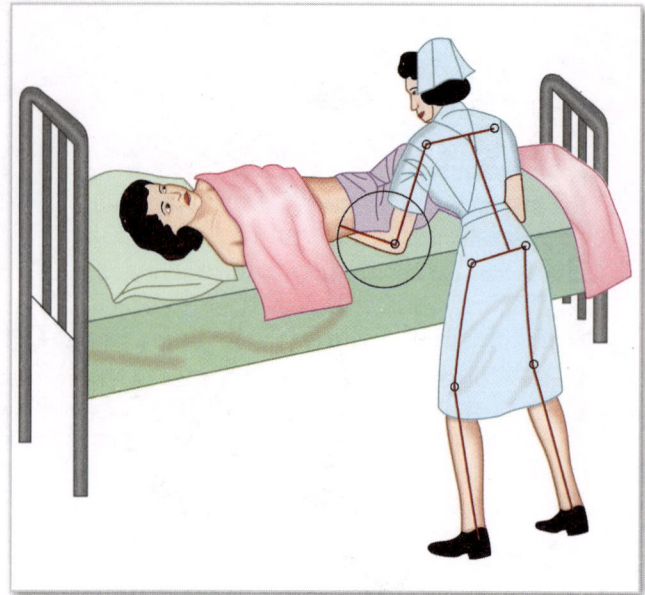

Fig. 10: Moving the semi-helpless patient up in the bed

- The nurse places one arm under the patient's shoulders and one arm under his/her thighs. The nurse's knees are flexed to bring her arms to the level of the surface of the bed.
- The patient places his/her chin on his/her chest and pushes with his/her feet as the nurse shifts her weight from her rear foot to her forward foot. By grasping the head of the bed with his/her hands, the patient can help pull his/her own weight (Fig. 10).

Assisting the Patient to a Sitting Position on the Side of Bed

- The patient turns on his/her side toward the edge of the bed upon which he/she wishes to sit
- After ensuring that the patient will not fall off the bed, the nurse raises the head of the bed
- Facing the far bottom corner of the bed, the nurse supports the shoulders of the patient with one arm, while with the other, she helps the patient to extend his/her lower legs over the side of the bed. The nurse assumes a broad stance, with her foot that is forward the bottom of the bed being to the near of the other foot.
- The patient is brought to a natural sitting position on the edge of the bed when the nurse, still supporting the patient's shoulders and legs, pivots her body in such a manner that the patient's lower legs are swinging downward. The nurse's weight is shifted from her front leg to her rear leg (Figs 11A and B).

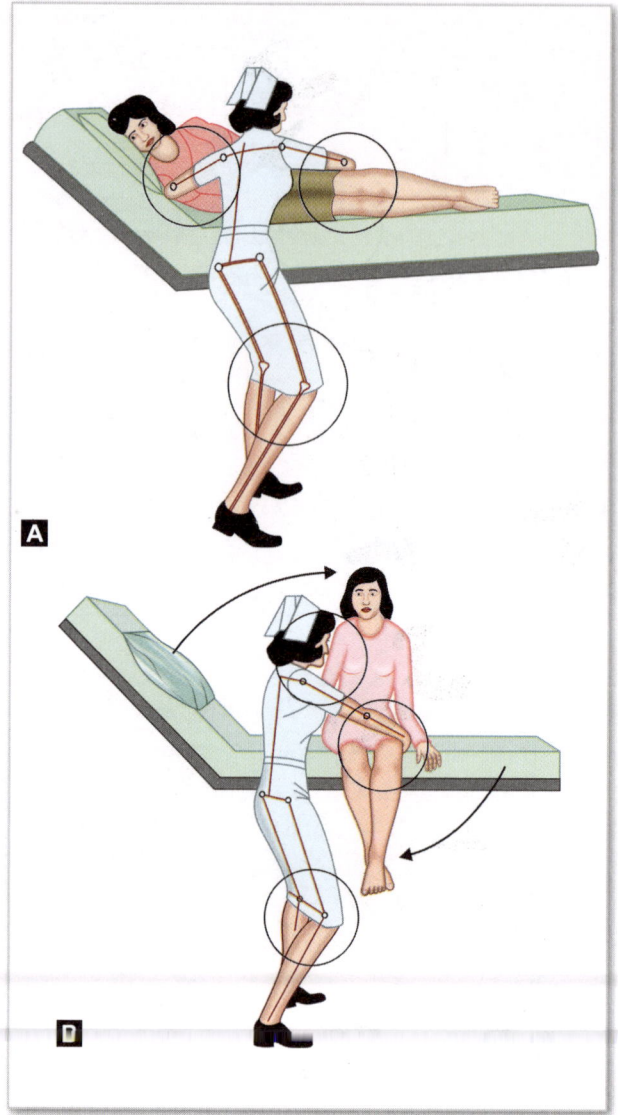

Figs 11A and B: Assisting the patient to a sitting position on the side of the bed

Assisting the Patient to Get Out of Bed and Shift to a Chair

In this procedure, the bed should be at a height from which the patient can step naturally to the floor. If the bed cannot be lowered sufficiently, the nurse should obtain a footstool for the patient. The footstool must be stable and have a surface upon which the patient is unlikely to slip. Also, it is adjustable for the patient to wear low heeled shoes rather than loose slippers. The former enable, the patient to walk comfortably (Fig. 12A to C).

- The patient assumes a sitting position on the edge of the bed and puts on shoes and dressing gown.

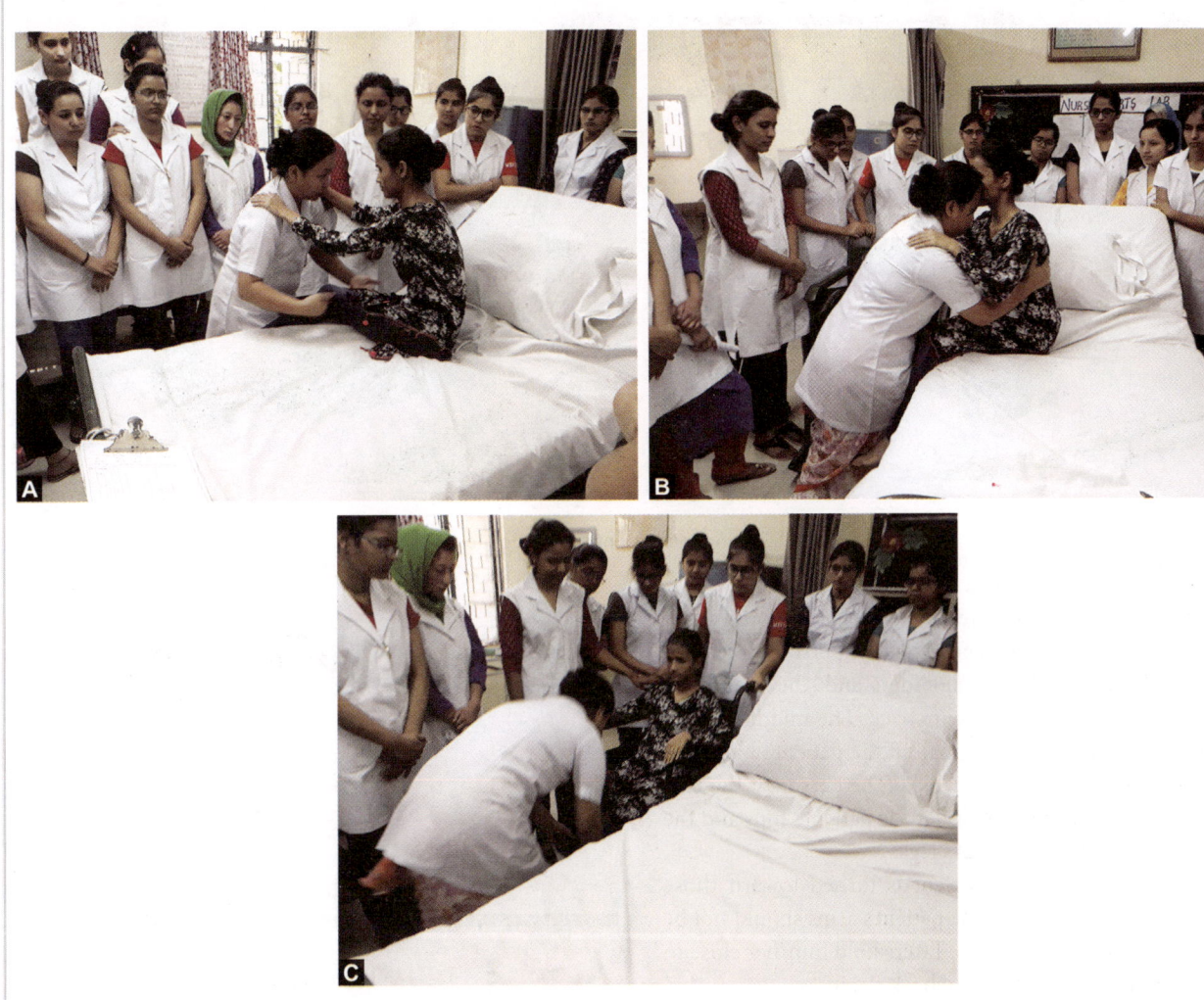

Figs 12A to C: Assisting the patient to get out of bed into a chair

- A chair is placed at the side of the bed with its back toward the foot of the bed.
- The nurse stands facing the patient, her foot that is closer to the chair is a step in front of the other, to give her a wide base of support.
- The patient places her hands upon the nurse's shoulder, and the nurse grasps the patient's waist.
- The patient steps to the floor, and the nurse flexes her knees so that her forward knee is against the patient's knee. This prevents the patient's knee from bending involuntarily.
- The nurse turns with the patient while maintaining her wide base of support. She bends her knees as the patient sits in the chair.

Shifting the Patient from a Bed to a Stretcher (Three Men Carry)

To move a patient who must remain in the horizontal position from one place to another, for example, from a bed to a stretcher, three persons are usually needed (Figs 13A and B). The tallest person should take the top-third of the patient, because she probably has the longest reach and can most easily support the patient's head and shoulders. The second person supports the middle-third of the patient, usually the heaviest part. She will be helped by the first and third person by putting their arms besides her. The shortest person supports the patient's legs.

Before the patient is moved, a stretcher is placed at right angle to the bed, with the head of the stretcher almost touching the foot of the bed. The stretcher wheels should be locked. To coordinate their movement, the three persons must work by the numbers; the person who takes the head of the patient calls the numbers.

- The three who are to move the patient face the side of the patient's bed. Each assumes a broad stance, with her foot that is toward the stretcher being forward.

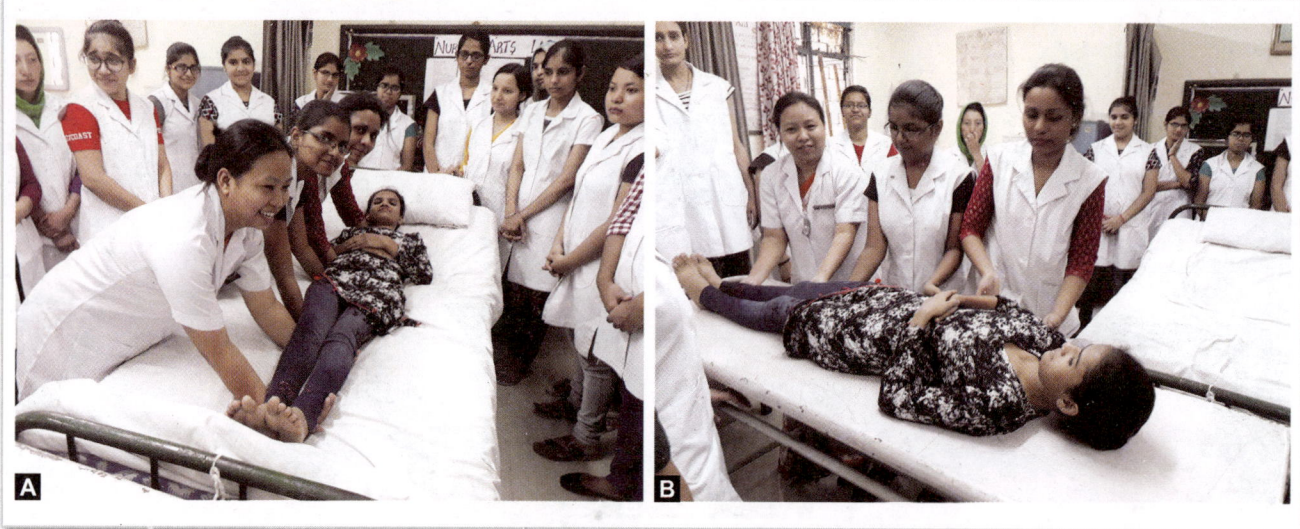

Figs 13A and B: Shifting the patient from a bed to a stretcher

- At the call of 'one', the three bend their knees and place their arms under the patient. The first person places one arm under the neck and shoulders and; the other arm under the small of the patient's back. The middle person places one arm under the small of the patient's back and the other arm under his/her hips. The person at the foot of the bed places one arm under the patient's hips and the other arm under the patient's legs.
- At the call of 'two' the patient is turned toward those who are lifting him/her. The patient's arms should not be allowed to dangle freely. The lifters hold him/her close to their bodies in order to avoid back strain.
- At the call of "three", they rise, step back (with the forward foot) and walk in unison to the stretcher.
- At the call of "four", they bend their knees and rest their elbows on the stretcher.
- At the call of "five", each lifter extends her arms so that the person rolls to his/her back at the middle of the stretcher.
- At the call of "six", each lifter withdraws her arms.
- In lifting the patient, the lifters should hold the patient close to their bodies. It is also important to lift and lower the patient with an easy smooth motion in order not to jar or frighten him/her.

Logrolling a Patient

When a patient has a spinal injury or is recovering from neck, back, or spinal surgery, it is often necessary to keep the body in straight alignment when turning the patient. Two or three nurses can accomplish this safely by logrolling a patient. Do not logroll the patient without enough help. Do not twist the patient's head, spine, shoulders, knees, or hips while logrolling (Fig. 14).

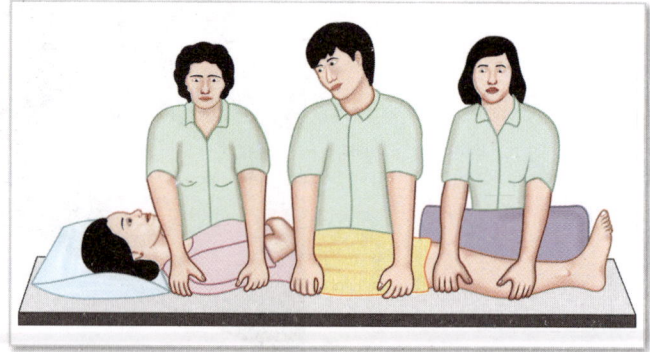

Fig. 14: Logrolling the patient

- Provide privacy by closing door or bedside curtain.
- Explain the procedure to the patient.
- Raise the bed to a comfortable working height and lower the side rails.
- Have the patient cross his/her arms on the chest.
- Place a pillow between the knees.
- Have two nurses stand on one side of the bed opposite the direction the patient will be turned. The third helper stands on the other side.
- Fanfold or roll the draw sheet tightly against the patient and carefully slide him or her to the side of the bed toward the two nurses.
- Have one helper then move to the other side of the bed, so that two nurses are on the side to which the patient is turning.
- Face the patient. Holding the rolled draw sheet taut to support the body, turn the patient as a unit toward the two nurses. The patient's head, shoulders, spine, hips and knees should turn simultaneously.

- Use pillows to support the patient's back, buttocks, and legs in straight alignment in a side lying position.
- Raise the side rails, lower the bed, and place the call bell within patient's reach.
- Document the procedure and patient's response.

Helping Patient Ambulate

Prolonged periods of bed rest are no longer considered necessary during most illnesses. Actively, even a short walk around the room, down the hall, from the bedroom to the living room, is a protective measure for the body.

Physical Conditioning

Patients who are not confined to bed for long periods, who sleep well, who take short periods of rest may not require preparation for ambulation. However, others have to be prepared for ambulation when it has to be resumed. Certain exercises that strengthen the overall efficiency of the musculoskeletal system can be done in bed. Check for physical activity restrictions or other contraindications before beginning any exercises.

Quadriceps and Gluteal Setting Drills

One of the most important muscle groups used in walking is the quadriceps femoris. The muscle group helps extend the leg and flex the thigh. Quadriceps drills are isometric exercises, in which muscle tension occurs without a significant change in the length of the muscle. Encourage bedridden patients to contract this muscle group frequently.

- Have the patient contract or tighten the muscles on the front of the thighs. The patient has the feeling of pushing the knees downward into the mattress and pulling the feet upward.
- Have the patient hold the position just described while counting slowly to four, and then relax the muscles for an equal count. Emphasize the relaxation is important to prevent muscle fatigue.
- Caution the patient not to hold his/her breath during these exercises to avoid straining the heart.
- Teach the patient to do quadriceps drills two or three times each hour, four to six times a day.
- The muscles in the buttocks can be exercised in the same way by pinching the buttocks together and then relaxing them. This is called gluteal setting. Tightening and holding abdominal muscles for 6 seconds and then relaxing them also strengthens this muscle group to facilitate walking.

Push-ups

The muscles of the arms and shoulders may also need strengthening before the patient is out of bed. Exercises should improve the strength needed to hold or get into a chair and to move about with greater ease. They are a part of preparation for patients who must learn to walk on crutches. They are done as follows:

- While sitting up in bed without support, the patient can do push-up exercises to strengthen the triceps. Instruct the patient to lift the hips off the bed by pushing down with the hands on the mattress. If the mattress is too soft, a block of books can be placed on the bed under the patient's hands.
- Push-ups may also be done with the patient lying in bed on the abdomen. Instruct the patient to place the hands near the outstretched body at about shoulder level, with palms down on the mattress and elbows bent sharply. Then, have the patient straighten the elbows to lift the head and shoulders off the bed.
- Push-ups may also be done when the patient sits on arm chair or wheelchair. The patient places the hands on the arms of the chair and then raises the body out of seat.
- Push-ups should be done three or four times a day at first, with the number increased as upper body strength is increased.

Dangling

Dangling refers to the position in which the person sits on the edge of the bed with legs and feet over the side of the bed. This exercise prepares patients for being out of bed.

It is carried out as follows:
- Place the patient in the sitting position in bed for a few minutes. This will accustom the patient to this position and help prevent feeling of faintness.
- Place the bed in the low position or have a foot stool handy on which the patient can rest the feet while dangling.
- Move the patient toward the side of the bed near you so that you do not stretch and strain while turning the patient.
- The patient may place his or her hands on your shoulders and let the patient swing legs over the side of the bed.
- Rest the patient's feet on foot stool to give a sense of security.
- Have the patient move the feet using an up and down, marching motion. This promotes circulation in the legs.
- Remain with the patient and be ready to place the patient back to a lying position if he or she feels faint, to prevent falling out of bed.

Assistance with Walking

Many patients who have been confined to bed for an extended period find that they must learn to walk all over again. Nurses can help the patients to walk after making assessments regarding the patient's ability to walk and need for assistance

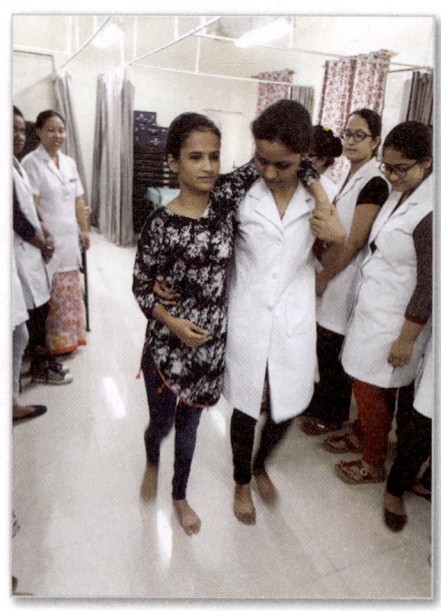

Fig. 15: One-nurse assist

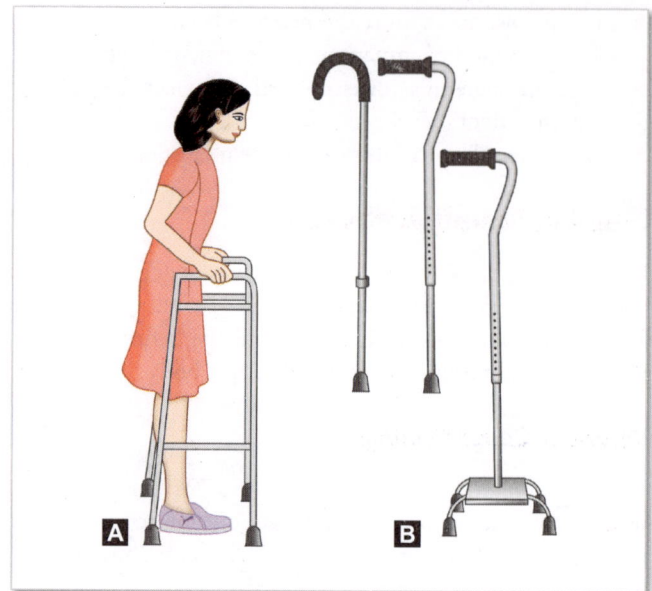

Figs 16A and B: Mechanical aids to walking. A. A walker; B. Three types of canes

(one nurse, two nurses, walker, cane, or crutches). Explain the patient exactly what is to be done: projected distance to be ambulated, assistance available and instructing patient to alert the nurse, immediately if feeling dizzy or weak.

One-nurse Assist

Patients who require minimal nursing assistance may walk well with the nurse walking alongside. Provide support by standing at the patient's side and placing both hands at the patient's waist. Supporting the patient at the waist helps the patients to maintain erect posture and prevents pulling the patient to one side (Fig. 15).

It is necessary to assist the patient with intravenous therapy equipment to walk. The patient walks with the assistance of the nurse and the portable intravenous pole. If a patient has weakness of one side, stand on weaker side and support the patient's weak arm by using one hand to support the patient's forearm and hand.

Two-nurse Assist

It is a safer method to use when there is uncertainty about the patient's ability to walk. Use of a gait belt snugly secured around the patient's waist provides a safe place for the nurse to support the patient.

Walker

A walker is a lightweight metal frame usually aluminium with four legs. Walkers improve balance by increasing the support, enhancing lateral stability, and supporting the patient's weight.

The walker provides a sense of security and support. Some walkers have wheels on the front legs, they are best for patients with a gait that is too fast and for patients who have difficulty lifting a walker, because lifting repeatedly is not required. Energy expenditure and stress to the back and upper extremities is lower than the standard walker. Walkers are also available with wheels on all four legs. These can be used for patients who require a large base of support and do not rely on the walker to bear weight. Wheeled walkers are the best for patients who need minimum weight bearing from the walker (Fig. 16A).

Canes

Canes widen a person's base of support, providing increased balance (Fig. 16B). Three types of canes are used: single-ended canes with half circle handles are recommended for patients requiring minimal support. Single-ended canes with straight handles are recommended for patients with hand weakness. Three or four prong canes are recommended for patients with poor balance. Rubber tips on the cane prevent slipping and accidents. The elbow should be flexed 30 degrees when holding the cane. When walking with a cane, instruct patients to hold the cane in the opposite hand from the leg with the most severe deficit.

Crutches

Patients are advised use of crutches for a while to avoid using one leg or to help strengthen one or both legs. The two types of crutches most commonly used are axillary and forearm crutches. Forearm crutches are used for patients, requiring long-term support for ambulation. Axillary crutches are

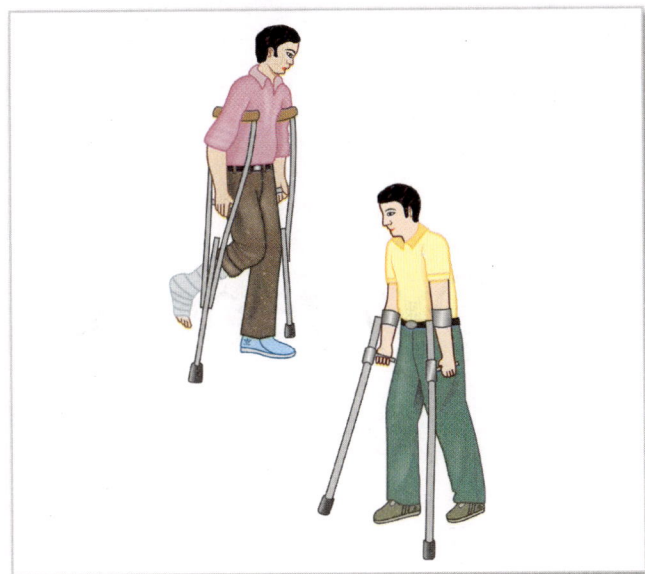

Fig. 17: Axillary (left) and forearm (right) support crutches

used to provide support for patients who have temporary restrictions on ambulation (Fig. 17).

Gait using Crutches

Gait with a Single Cane of Forearm Crutch

A cane or single forearm crutch is recommended to people who need additional support when walking. Oftentimes, such necessity results from a weaker or lesser weight-bearing leg or foot. In this situation, **the crutch or cane should be used in the hand opposite the weaker leg.**

The strong leg can bear the person's weight by itself whereas the weaker lower limb is assisted by the weight placed on the ambulation aid, effectively distributing the user's weight among two support points. The only exception to this rule is if that hand or arm is injured or significantly weaker than the other.

If the person is equally strong (or weak) in both lower extremities and uses a cane or crutch for support, then the cane or crutch should generally be used in the stronger hand or arm—the "dominant" one.

Using a single forearm crutch, the 2-point gait is identical except that the forearm cuff "looks" the arm in place, takes the strain off the wrist and provides more security and stability than a cane.

Gait with Underarm Crutches

A person on underarm crutches can use either the 3-point, swing-to or swing-through gaits.

Due to the much higher pivot point of an underarm or axillary crutch (the axilla versus the wrist), it is our opinion that this fulcrum is too high to maintain correct posture during other gait patterns.

The 2-point and 4-point gaits on underarm crutches cause the body to lean excessively forward compared to the same gait patterns while using forearm crutches.

Gait with Forearm Crutches

A person on forearm crutches (also known as elbow, Lofstrand or Canadian crutches) can use all gait patterns.

BIBLIOGRAPHY

1. Potter PA, Perry AG. Fundamentals of Nursing, 6th edition. Elsevier; New Delhi; 2008.
2. Taylor CR, Lillis C, LeMone P, et al. Fundamentals of Nursing - The Art and Science of Nursing Care, 7th edition. Wolters Kluwer; Gurugram; 2010.
3. Smeltzer SC. "Brunner and Siddhartha's Textbook of Medical Surgical Nursing". 11th edition. Lippincott Williams and Wilkins. pp. 2184-87.

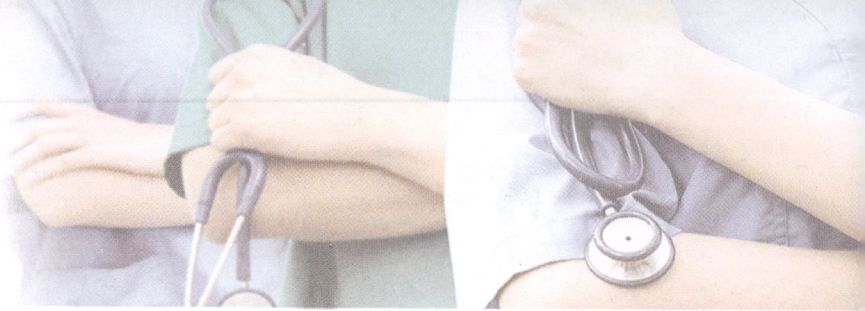

Oxygenation

INTRODUCTION

Oxygen is clear, odorless gas that constitutes approximately 21% of the air we breathe. Oxygen is necessary for proper functioning of all living cells. The absence of oxygen can lead to cellular, tissue and organism death. Although, the delivery of oxygen to body tissues is regulated indirectly by other body system such as cardiovascular system while the respiratory system is directly involved in this process. Impaired function of the system can significantly affect our ability to breathe, transport gases, and participate in everyday activities.

Respiration is the process of gas exchange between the individual and the environment. The process of respiration involves three components.

* Pulmonary ventilation or breathing: The movement of air between the atmosphere and the alveoli of the lungs during the process of inhalation and exhalation.

- Gas exchange, which involves diffusion of oxygen and carbon dioxide between the alveoli of the lungs and pulmonary capillaries.
- Transport of oxygen from the lungs to tissues and carbon dioxide from the tissues to the lungs.

STRUCTURE AND FUNCTIONS OF THE RESPIRATORY SYSTEM

The respiratory system is divided structurally into the upper respiratory system and lower respiratory system. Mouth, nose, pharynx and larynx compose the upper respiratory system. The lower respiratory system includes trachea and lungs, with the bronchi, bronchioles, alveoli, pulmonary capillary network and pleural membranes.

Air enters through the nose, where it is warmed, humidified, and filtered. Large particles in the air are trapped by the hair present in the nares, and smaller particles in the air are trapped as air changes direction or contact with the nasal turbinate and septum. Sneeze reflex is initiated by irritants in nasal passages. A large volume of air rapidly exits through the nose and mouth during a sneeze, helping to clear nasal passages.

Inspired air passes from the nose through the pharynx. Pharynx is a shared pathway for air and food. It includes both the nasopharynx and the oropharynx, which are richly supplied with lymphoid tissue that traps and destroys pathogens entering with the air.

Larynx is a cartilaginous structure that can be identified externally as Adam's apple in males. It plays a major role in production of voice and important for maintaining airway patency from swallowed fluids and food. During swallowing, the inlet to the larynx (epiglottis) closes, routing food to the esophagus.

Epiglottis is open during breathing, allowing air to move freely into the lower airways. Below the larynx, the trachea leads to the right and left bronchi and the other conducting airway of the lungs. Within the lungs, the primary bronchi divide repeatedly into smaller and smaller bronchi, ending with the terminal bronchioles. Together these airways are known as the bronchial tree. The trachea and bronchi are lined with mucosal epithelium that traps the pathogens and microscopic particulate matter. These foreign particles are then swept upward toward the larynx and throat by cilia—tiny hair-like projections on the epithelial cells. The cough reflex is triggered by irritants in the larynx, trachea, or bronchi until air passes through the terminal bronchioles and enters the respiratory bronchioles and alveoli, no gas exchange occurs. Alveoli have very thin walls, composed of a single layer of epithelial cells covered by a thick mesh of pulmonary capillaries. The alveolar and capillary walls form the respiratory membrane (also known as the alveolar capillary membrane), where gas exchange occurs between the air on the alveolar side and the blood on the capillary side.

Outer surface of the lungs is covered by a thin, double layer of tissue known as a pleura. Parietal pleura lines the thorax and surface of the diaphragm. Visceral pleura covers the external surface of the lungs. Between these pleural layers is a potential space that contains a small amount of pleural fluid. The fluid prevents friction during the movements of breathing and serves to keep the layer adherent through its surface tension.

Pulmonary Ventilation

Ventilation of the lungs is accomplished through the act of breathing which involves Inspiration—when air flows into the lungs and Expiration—when air moves out of the lungs. Adequate ventilation depends on several factors:

- Clear airways
- An intact central nervous system and respiratory center
- An intact thoracic cavity
- Adequate pulmonary compliance and recoil.

The number of mechanisms including ciliary action and the cough reflex work to keep airways open and clear. However, these defenses may be overwhelmed, if there is edema, inflammation and excess mucous production which may clog airway, impairing ventilation of distal alveoli.

Respiratory centers, medulla and pons in the brain stem control the breathing. Severe head injury or drugs that depress central nervous system (opiates and barbiturates) can affect the respiratory centers, impairing the drive to breathe.

Expansion and recoil of the lungs occur passively in response to changes in pressures within the thoracic cavity and the lungs themselves. The **intrapleural pressure** is always slightly negative in relation to atmospheric pressure. This negative pressure is essential because it creates the suction force that holds the visceral pleura and the parietal pleura together as the chest cage expands and contracts. The recoil tendency of the lungs is a major factor in creating this negative pressure.

The intrapulmonary pressure always equalizes with atmospheric pressure. Inspiration occurs when the diaphragm and intercostal muscles contract, increasing the size of thoracic cavity, therefore increasing volume and decreasing the intrapulmonary pressure. Air then rushes into the lungs to equalize the pressure with atmospheric pressure. Conversely when the diaphragm and intercostal muscles relax, the volume of the lungs decreases and intrapulmonary pressure rises, air is expelled.

During normal breathing, the degree of chest expansion is minimum, which requires with energy expenditure. In adults, approximately 500 mL of air is inspired and expired with each breath. This is known as tidal volume. Some diseases such as muscular dystrophy or trauma such as spinal cord injury can affect the muscles of respiration, impairing the ability of thoracic cavity to expand and contract. Chest injury may allow intrapleural pressure to equalize with the atmosphere, causing lungs to collapse.

Lung compliance, the expansibility or stretchability of lung tissue, plays a significant role in the case of ventilation. Lung compliance tends to decrease with aging, making it more difficult to expand alveoli and increasing risk of **atelectasis** or collapse of a portion of the lung.

In contrast to lung compliance is **lung recoil**, which is necessary for normal expiration. The elastic fibers in lung tissue contribute to lung recoil, the surface tension of fluid lining the alveoli has the greatest effect on recoil. **Surfactant,** a lipoprotein, produced by specialized alveolar cells acts like a detergent reducing the surface tension of alveolar fluid. Without surfactant, lung expansion is exceedingly difficult and the lungs collapse.

Transport of Oxygen and Carbon Dioxide

Oxygen needs to be transported from the lungs to tissues and carbon dioxide must be transported from the tissues back to the lungs. Normally most of the oxygen (97%) combines loosely with hemoglobin (oxygen carrying red pigment) in the red blood cells and is carried to the tissues as oxyhemoglobin (compound of oxygen and hemoglobin). Several factors that affect the rate of oxygen transport from the lungs to the tissues are as follows:

- Cardiac output
- Number of erythrocytes and blood hematocrit
- Exercise

Any condition that decreases cardiac output (e.g., damage to heart muscle, blood loss, or pooling of blood in the peripheral blood vessels) diminishes the amount of oxygen delivered to the tissues. Heart compensates for inadequate output by increasing its pumping rate or heart rate but in severe blood loss or damage, it may not be possible to restore blood flow and oxygen to the tissues.

In men, the circulating erythrocytes averages about 5 million per cubic milliliter of blood and in women about 4.5 million per cubic milliliter. In men the hematocrit is about 40–54% and in women it is 37–50%. Excessive blood hematocrit raises the blood viscosity, reducing the cardiac output and therefore reducing oxygen transport. Excessive reduction in blood hematocrit as occur in anemia reduces oxygen transport.

Exercise also has a direct influence on oxygen transport. In athletes, oxygen transport is increased up to 20 times the normal rate, due to increased cardiac output and to increased use of oxygen by the cells.

Carbon dioxide, continually produced in the processes of cells metabolism, is transported from the cells to the lungs.

Respiratory Regulation

Respiratory regulation includes both neural and chemical controls to maintain the correct concentrations of oxygen, carbon dioxide, and hydrogen ions in body fluids. A chemosensitive center in the medulla oblongata is highly responsive to increase in blood CO_2 or hydrogen ion concentration. There are special neural receptors which are sensitive to decrease in O_2 concentration. These are located outside the central nervous system in the carotid bodies (just above the bifurcation of the common carotid arteries) and aortic bodies located above and below the aortic arch. Decrease in arterial oxygen concentration stimulates the chemoreceptors, which in turn stimulate the respiratory center to increase ventilation. Of the three blood gases (hydrogen, oxygen and carbon dioxide) that can trigger chemoreceptors, increased carbon dioxide concentration normally has the strongest effect on stimulating respiration.

Note: In client with chronic lung ailments, such as emphysema, oxygen concentrations, not carbon dioxide concentrations, play a major role in regulating respiration. For such clients, decreased oxygen concentrations are the main stimuli for respiration because the chronically elevated carbon-dioxide levels that occur in emphysema "desensitize" the central chemoreceptors. This is called "hypoxic drive". Increasing the concentration of supplemental oxygen depresses the respiratory rate. Therefore, only low concentrations of supplemental oxygen are administered to these clients.

Cardiovascular System and Transport of Respiratory Gases

Oxygen and carbon dioxide must move through the alveoli and be carried to and from body cells by the blood. Thus, an adequately functioning cardiovascular system is vital for exchange of gases. Deoxygenated blood is carried from the right side of the heart to the lungs, where oxygen is picked up and carbon dioxide is released, then returned to the left side of the heart. This oxygenated blood is pumped out to all other parts of the body and back again (Fig. 1).

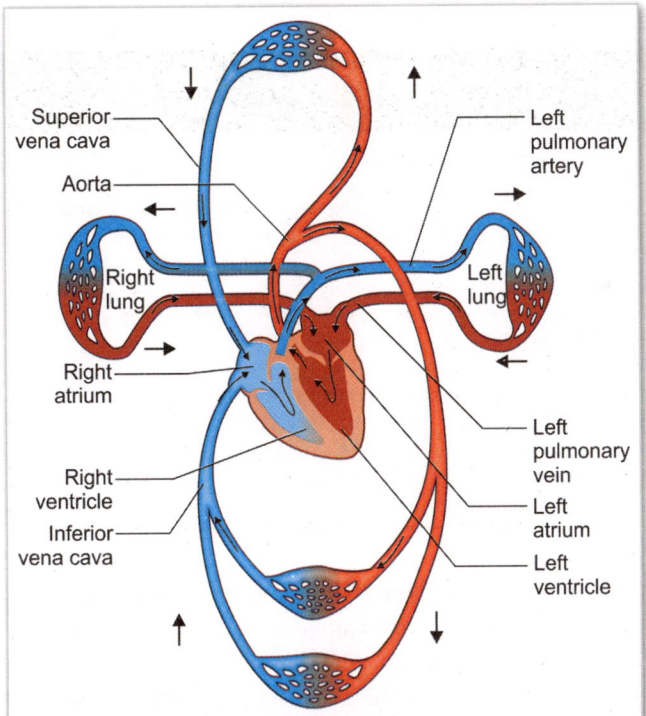

Fig. 1: The right side of the heart pump deoxygenated blood to the lungs, where oxygen is picked up and carbon dioxide is released. The left side of the heart pumps oxygenated blood out to all other parts of the body

Oxygen is carried by plasma and red blood cells. The hemoglobin in red blood cells has a strong affinity for oxygen. Therefore 97% of oxygen is carried in the body by red blood cells as part of hemoglobin in the form of oxyhemoglobin. Hemoglobin also carries carbon dioxide easily in the form of carboxyhemoglobin.

Once the red blood cells, reach the tissues, internal respiration occurs. Internal respiration is the exchange of oxygen and carbon dioxide between the circulating blood and the tissue cells. Any abnormality in the blood's constituents affects internal respiration. For example, hemorrhage or loss of blood can cause a decrease in cardiac output. A decrease in cardiac output causes a reduction in the amount of circulating, blood that is available to deliver oxygen to tissues. Exercise can improve the transport of oxygen because exercise improves pumping of heart effectively.

Factors Affecting Respiratory Functioning

Levels of Health

Acute and chronic illnesses can affect a person's respiratory function drastically. People with cardiac or renal disorders often have compromised respiratory functioning because of fluid overload and impaired tissue perfusion. People with

chronic illnesses often have muscle wasting and poor muscle tone. These problems affect all the muscles, including those of respiratory system. Alterations in muscle functions contribute to inadequate pulmonary ventilation and respiration. Anemia can result in impaired respiratory function due to inadequate supply of oxygen to the tissues of the body. Hemoglobin also carries carbon dioxide to the lungs, anemia results in diminished carbon dioxide exchange. Myocardial infarction causes a lack of blood supply to the heart muscle. Damage to the heart muscle interfere with effective contraction of the heart muscle, leading to decreased perfusion of tissues and decreased gas exchange.

Developmental Considerations

There are many age-related developmental considerations affecting respiratory function (Table 1).

Neonates and Infants

Many changes occur in the lungs of a newborn. In infants, chest is small and the airways are short, therefore aspiration is a potential problem. The respiratory rate is 30–60 breaths/min. As the alveoli increase in number and size, adequate oxygenation is accomplished at lower respiratory rates. Surfactant is formed in utero between 34 and 36 weeks. An infant born before 34 weeks may not have produced sufficient surfactant, leading to collapse of the alveoli and poor alveolar exchange. Respiratory pattern is primarily abdominal in infants.

Toddlers, Preschoolers, School Aged Children and Adolescents

In pre-school children, Eustachian tubes, bronchi and bronchioles are elongated and less angular. Therefore, the average incidence routine colds and infections decrease until the child enters daycare or school where he/she is exposed more frequently to pathogens. Most children at this age have colds or upper respiratory infections, but some have more serious problems of otitis media, bronchitis and pneumonia. At this stage, it is important to encourage good hand hygiene practices. By the end of late childhood and during adulthood, the immune system is prepared to protect the person from most infections.

Older Adults

Specific physical changes occur in older adults such as decreased elastic recoil of the lungs, expiration requiring use of accessory muscles, fewer functional capillaries and more fibrous tissue in alveoli, and reduction in vital capacity and increase in residual volume, all these lead to decreased gas exchange and increased work of breathing. There is decreased

TABLE 1: Respiratory variations in the life cycle

	Infant (birth–1 year)	Early childhood (1–5 years)	Late childhood (6–12 years)	Aged adult (65 + years)
Respiratory rate	30–60 breaths/min	20–40 breaths/min	15–25 breaths/min	16–20 breaths/min
Respiratory pattern	Abdominal breathing, irregular in rate and depth	Abdominal breathing, irregular	Thoracic breathing, regular	Thoracic, regular
Chest wall	Thin, little muscle, ribs and sternum are easily seen	Same as infant's but with more subcutaneous fat	Further subcutaneous fat is deposited, structures are less prominent	Thin, structures are prominent
Breath sounds	Loud, harsh crackles at end of deep inspiration	Loud, harsh expiration longer than inspiration	Clear inspiration is longer than expiration	Clear
Shape of thorax	Round	Elliptical	Elliptical	Barrel shaped or elliptical

ventilation and ineffective cough due to less air exchange; more secretions remain in lungs, drier mucous membranes, altered pain sensation, greater risk of aspiration due to slower gastric motility. Airways collapse more easily. These alterations increase the risk for disease, especially pneumonia and other chest infections.

Medications

Many medications affect the function of the respiratory system. For example, opioids are chemical agents that depress the medullary respiratory center. As a result, the rate and depth of respirations decrease.

Lifestyle

Activity levels and habits can affect a person's respiratory status. For example, sedentary activity patterns do not encourage the expansion of alveoli and the development of pulmonary exercise patterns. People who exercise (aerobics, walking, swimming) three to six times per week can better respond to stressors to respiratory health.

Cigarette smoking, active or passive, is a major contributor to lung disease and respiratory distress.

Environment

There is a high correlation between air pollution and cancer and lung disease. Occupational exposure to asbestos, silica, or coal dust, as well as environmental pollution, can lead to chronic pulmonary disease.

Psychological Health

Many psychological factors and conditions can affect the respiratory system. Individuals responding to stress may sigh excessively or exhibit hyperventilation (increased rate and depth of ventilation, above the body's normal metabolic requirements). Hyperventilation can lead to lowered level of arterial carbon dioxide. Generalized anxiety has been shown to cause enough bronchospasm to produce an episode of bronchial asthma.

NURSING PROCESS FOR OXYGENATION

Assessment

The patient's health history is an essential component for assessing respiratory functioning. Either the patient or a family member can provide this information. The nursing examination combined with laboratory findings can provide information to identify a patient's strength, the nature of the problem, its course, related signs and symptoms, and its onset, frequency and effects on activities of daily living. The nurse decides, based on these findings, what problems can be treated independently by nursing, other problems are referred to the physician and other collaborative professionals for decisions on treatment.

Nursing History

The nursing history, an important clinical tool, helps to identify current or potential health deviations. The information gained provides data about why the patient needs nursing care and what kind of care is required to maintain sufficient intake of air. Before starting the interview, ascertain that the patient is not in acute distress. If in distress, initiate appropriate measures to help relieve symptoms. Ask family members to help answer questions. If the patient is conscious and can give the interview, ask the patient to expand the initial database. Some of the important areas that can be assessed while taking nursing history are:

- Usual patterns of breathing
- Any medications used for breathing
- Health history: Any heart, lung or breathing conditions and any family history of breathing conditions
- Recent changes: Related to breathing, chest pain, respiratory infection, any relief measures used
- Lifestyle and environment: History of smoking, how many packs per day, living with the smoker, pollutants at work place
- Cough: How much and how often, character of cough, (dry or with sputum—color of sputum) any allergies
- Sputum: How much, its color and odor
- Chest pain: Pain with breathing, on a scale of 0 to 10 (10 being very painful), how severe is the pain where is the pain, any radiation of pain.

Physical Assessment

The sequence followed during physical assessment is inspection, palpation, percussion, and auscultation.

Inspection

Inspect the chest contour and shape. Normally the chest contour is slightly convex with no sternal depression. The anteroposterior diameter should be less than the transverse diameter, the ratio of transverse diameter to the anteroposterior diameter is 1:2. Note for symmetrical movement of the chest. Inspect the skin over thorax for temperature and color. It should be warm and dry and cyanosis or pallor in color. Note any scars and observe the respiratory rate and rhythm for full 1 minute. Normally, respirations are quiet and non-labored. Note any flaring of the nostrils, muscular retraction, tachypnea (rapid breathing), or bradypnea (slow breathing).

Palpation

Palpate the trachea, which should be equidistant from each clavicle. Measure thoracic excursion by placing hands on the patient's posterior thorax at the 10th rib, with both thumbs almost touching the vertebrae. Ask the patient to take few deep breaths, and watch the movement of the hands. Usually the thumbs move 5–8 cm symmetrically on maximum inspiration.

Assess tactile fremitus (the capacity to feel sound on the chest wall) by placing your palm to the patient's chest wall, avoiding bony areas (scapula). Ask the patient to repeat some multi-syllable word (e.g., ninety-nine) and feel for the vibration. Normally the vibrations are equal bilaterally in different areas on the chest wall. The greatest intensity is noted at the anterior and posterior base of the neck and along the trachea and lungs. Increased fremitus occurs in patients with pneumonia because solid tissue conducts sound well. Conversely, patients with chronic obstructive pulmonary disease (COPD) have decreased fremitus because air does not conduct sound as well. Note the presence or absence of masses, edema, or tenderness on palpation.

Percussion

Percussion is used to assess the position of the lungs, density of lung tissue, and identify changes in the tissue. The details are already discussed in chapter on General Health Assessment.

Auscultation

Using the diaphragm of a stethoscope, move from apex to base of the lungs, comparing one side with the other side. Normal breath sounds include **vesicular** (low-pitched, soft sounds heard over peripheral lung fields), **bronchial** (loud, high-pitched sounds heard over the trachea and larynx), and **bronchovesicular** (medium-pitched blowing sounds heard over the major bronchi). Auscultate as the patient breathe slowly through open mouth. If abnormal breath sounds are detected, instruct the patient to cough and auscultate again. Record location, change in breath sounds after coughing, and the phase of respiration in which the abnormal sounds are heard.

Adventitious breath sounds or abnormal lung sounds: They include the following:

- **Crackles,** frequently heard on inspiration, are soft, high-pitched intermittent popping sounds. They are produced by fluid in the airways or alveoli and delayed reopening of collapsed alveoli. They occur due to inflammation or congestion and are associated with pneumonia, congestive heart failure, bronchitis, and COPD. There may be fine crackles, which are brief sounds, similar to the sound of hair rubbing together with fingers. It may be coarse crackles, which are somewhat louder, moist, bubbling sounds.
- **Wheezes** are continuous, musical sounds, produced as air passes through airways constricted by swelling, narrowing, secretions or tumors.
- A **pleural friction rub** is a continuous, dry grating sound. Pleural friction rub is caused by inflammation of pleural surfaces and loss of lubricating pleural fluid. It resembles the sound made by rubbing two leather surfaces together.

Diagnosis

After the assessment is completed and the data are examined, the nursing diagnosis indicating alterations in respiratory functions are:

- Ineffective airway clearance
- Ineffective breathing pattern
- Impaired gas exchange
- Activity intolerance.

These nursing diagnoses may also be the etiology of several other nursing diagnoses such as:

- Anxiety related to ineffective airway clearance and feeling of suffocation
- Fatigue related to ineffective breathing pattern
- Fear related to chronic respiratory illness
- Powerlessness related to maintain independence in self-care activities because of ineffective breathing pattern
- Insomnia related to orthopnea and required oxygen therapy
- Sound isolation related to activity intolerance.

Planning

The overall outcomes for a client with oxygenation problems are to:

- Maintain a patent airway
- Improve comfort and ease of breathing
- Maintain or improve pulmonary ventilation and oxygenation
- Improve ability to participate in physical activities
- Present risks associated with oxygenation problems such as skin and tissue breakdown, syncope, acid-base imbalance and feeling of hopelessness and social isolation.

These outcomes provide directions for planning interventions and as criteria for evaluating client progress.

Implementation

Nursing interventions to facilitate pulmonary ventilation may include—ensuring a patent airway, positioning, encouraging deep breathing and coughing, and ensuring adequate hydration. Other nursing interventions helpful in ventilation are—suctioning, lung inflation techniques, administration of analgesics before deep breathing and coughing, postural drainage, and percussion and vibration. Many dependent nursing interventions such as oxygen therapy, tracheostomy care, and maintenance of a chest tube are also to be included in maintaining oxygenation.

Promoting Oxygenation

The interventions which the nurse can take to maintain normal respiration for client include:

- Positioning the client to allow maximum chest expansion
- Encouraging or promoting frequent changes in position
- Encouraging ambulation
- Implementing measures that promote comfort, such as giving pain medications

Positioning

For maximum expansion of lungs, the semi-Fowler's or high Fowler's position is given to clients who are confined to bed, particularly those with dyspnea. The nurse also encourages clients to turn from side-to-side frequently so that alternate sides of the chest can have maximum expansion. An over-bed table can also be used to assist the client in breathing using a pillow for support. The client can lean forward over the over-bed table which presses the abdominal organs downward so that full expansion of chest can take place.

Deep Breathing and Coughing

The nurse can facilitate respiratory functioning by encouraging deep breathing exercises and coughing to remove secretions from the airways. When coughing raises sensations high enough, the client may either **expectorate** (spit out) or swallow.

Breathing exercises are recommended frequently for clients with restricted chest expansion, such as people with COPD or clients recovering from thoracic surgery. Abdominal (diaphragmatic) breathing is the commonly employed breathing exercise, which permits deep full breath with little effort. Pursed lip breathing helps the client by creating a resistance to the air flowing out of the lungs, thereby prolonging exhalation and preventing airway collapse by maintaining positive airway pressure. The client purses the lips as if about to whistle and breathes out slowly and gently, tightening the abdominal muscles to exhale more effectively. The client usually inhales to a count of 3 and exhales to a count of 7.

Hydration

Normally, respiratory tract secretions are thin and are therefore, moved readily by ciliary action. However, when the client is dehydrated or when the environment has a low humidity, the respiratory secretions can become thick and tenacious. Adequate hydration maintains the moisture of the respiratory mucous membranes.

Humidifiers are the devices that add water vapor to inspired air. Room humidifiers provide cool mist to room air. Nebulizers are used to deliver humidity and medications. They may be used with oxygen delivery systems to provide moistened air directly to the client. Their purposes are to prevent mucous membranes from drying and becoming irritated and to loosen secretions for easier expectoration.

Medications

Many types of medications can be used for clients with oxygenation problems. **Bronchodilators,** anti-inflammatory drugs, expectorants and cough suppressants are some medications that may be used to treat respiratory problems. These drugs may be administered orally or intravenously but the preferred route is by inhalation to prevent many systemic side effects.

Since these drugs (bronchodilators) dilate the bronchioles and improve breathing they also enhance the sympathetic nervous system, so clients must be monitored for side effects of increased heart rate, blood pressure, anxiety and restlessness. This is especially important in elders, who may also have cardiac problems.

Anti-inflammatory drugs such as glucocorticoids which can be given orally or intravenously to decrease the edema and inflammation in the airways and allowing a better gas exchange. If both the bronchodilators and anti-inflammatory drugs are ordered by inhaler, then patient should be instructed to use bronchodilator inhaler first and then the anti-inflammatory inhaler. If the bronchioles are dilated first, more tissue is exposed for the anti-inflammatory drugs to act upon.

Expectorants help "break up" mucus, making it more liquid and easier to expectorate.

Other medications can be used to improve oxygenation by improving cardiovascular function. The digitalis glycoside improves strength of contraction of heart and slow the heart rate.

Incentive Spirometry

Incentive spirometers (Fig. 2), also referred to as sustained maximal inspiration (SMI) devices, measure the flow of air inhaled through the mouthpiece and are used to:

- Improve pulmonary ventilation
- Counteract the effects of anesthesia or hypoventilation
- Loosen respiratory secretions
- Facilitate respiratory gaseous exchange
- Expand collapsed alveoli

They offer an incentive to improve inhalation when using an SMI, the client should be assisted into a position, preferably an upright sitting position in bed or a chair, that facilitates maximum ventilation. The process of use of the spirometer is given in Box 1.

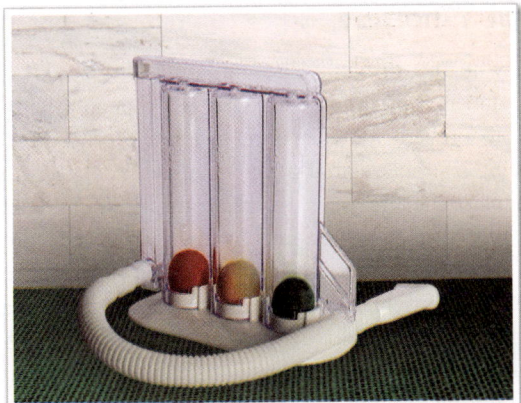

Fig. 2: Incentive spirometer

Box 1

Using an incentive spirometer

- Hold and place spirometer in an upright position
- Exhale normally
- Seal the lips tightly around the mouthpiece
- Take in a slow, deep breath to elevate the balls and then hold the breath for 2 seconds initially, increasing to 6 seconds, to keep the balls elevated.
- Greater lung expansion is achieved with a very slow inspiration then with a brisk, shallow breath, even though it may not elevate the balls or keep them elevated while holding breath. Sustained elevation of the balls ensures adequate ventilation of the alveoli.
- Remove the mouthpiece and exhale normally
- Cough after this because deep ventilation may loosen secretions, and coughing can facilitate their removal.
- Relax and take normal breaths before using the spirometer again.
- Repeat the procedure several times and then four or five times hourly. Practice increases inspiratory volume, maintains alveolar ventilation and prevents atelectasis.
- Clean the mouthpiece with water and shake it dry.

Percussion, Vibration and Postural Drainage

Percussion, vibration and postural drainage (PVD) are performed according to physician's order.

Percussion

Percussion is forceful striking of this skin with cupped hands. Fingers and thumb of the hand are held together and flexed slightly to form a cup. Percussion over congested lung areas can mechanically dislodge tenacious secretions from the bronchial walls. Cupped hands trap the air against the chest. The trapped air sets up vibrations through the chest wall to the secretions.

Steps of Percussion

- Cover the area with a towel/gown to reduce discomfort
- Ask the client to breathe slowly and deeply to promote relaxation
- Alternatively flex and extend the wrists rapidly to slap the chest (Fig. 3A)
- Percuss each affected lung segment for 1 – 2 minutes

Percussion should be avoided over the breasts, sternum, spinal column, and kidneys, when done correctly, it produces a hollow, popping sound.

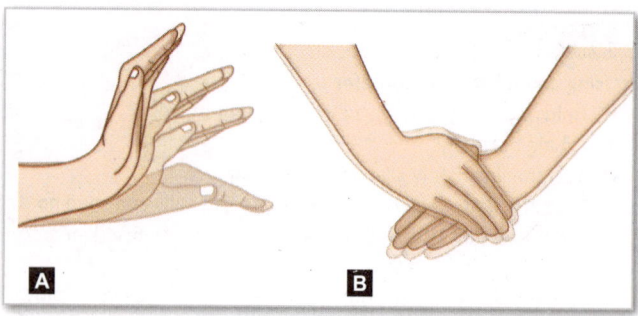

Figs 3A and B: A. The cupping position and action of the hand on manual percussion of the lung area; B. The position and action of the hands are necessary to use vibration to loosen respiratory secretions in the lungs

Vibration

This is a series of vigorous quivering produced by hands that are placed flat against the client's chest wall. It is used after percussion to increase the turbulence of the exhaled air and thus loosen thick secretions-It is often done alternatively with percussion.

Steps of Vibrations

♦ Place hands, palms down, on the chest area to be drained, one hand over the area with the fingers together and extended (Fig. 3B) Alternatively, the hands may be placed side by side.

♦ Ask the client to inhale deeply and exhale slowly through the nose or pursed lips

♦ During the exhalation, tense all the hand and arm muscles, and using mostly the heel of the hand, vibrate (shake) the hands, moving them downward. Stop vibrating when the client inhales

♦ Vibrate during five exhalations over one affected lung segment

♦ After each vibration, encourage the client to cough and expectorate secretions into the sputum container.

Postural Drainage

It is the drainage by gravity of secretions from various lung segments. Secretions that remain in the lungs or respiratory airways promote bacterial growth and infection. They can also obstruct the smaller airways and cause atelectasis. Secretions in the major airways, such as trachea and the right and left main bronchi, are usually coughed into the pharynx, where they can be expectorated, swallowed or effectively removed by suctioning (Fig. 4).

A wide variety of positions is necessary to drain all segments of the lungs, but not all positions are required for every client. Only those positions are used that drain specific affected area. The lower lobes require drainage most frequently because the upper lobes drain by gravity. Before postural drainage, the client may be given a bronchodilator medication or nebulization therapy to loosen secretions. Postural drainage treatments are scheduled two or three times daily depending on the degree of congestion in lungs. The best time includes before breakfast, before lunch in the late afternoon and before bedtime. It is best to avoid hours shortly after meals because it can be tiring and may induce vomiting.

Steps of Postural Drainage

The sequence for PVD is usually:

♦ Positioning, percussion, vibration, and removal of secretions by coughing and suction.

♦ The nurse needs to evaluate the client's tolerance of postural drainage by assessing the stability of client's vital signs particularly the pulse and respiratory rates and by noting the signs of intolerance, such as fatigue, pallor, diaphoresis, dyspnea and nausea.

♦ Have tissue wipes, emesis basin in hand.

♦ Use high Fowler's position to drain the apical sections of the upper lobes of the lungs.

♦ Place the patient in a lying position, half on the abdomen and half on the side, right and left, to drain the posterior sections of the upper lobes of the lungs.

♦ Place the patient lying on the left side with the pillow under the chest wall to drain the right lobe of the lung.

♦ Place the patient in Trendelenburg position to drain the lower lobes of lungs.

♦ Each position is usually assumed for 10 – 15 minutes, although beginning treatments may start with shorter times and gradually increase.

Following PVD, the nurse should auscultate the client's lungs, compare the finding with baseline data, and document the amount, color, and character of expectorated secretions.

Oxygen Therapy

Client who has difficulty in ventilating all areas of his/her lungs, due to impaired gas exchange or people with heart failure to prevent hypoxia need to get the procedure done. Providing a supplemental oxygen supply via oxygen therapy can increase the amount of oxygen transported in the blood.

Oxygen must be ordered by the health care provider. Clients get frightened for oxygen therapy, therefore it is important to provide clear explanations about the procedures and purposes to help reduce anxiety. The health care provider specifies the concentration, method of delivery, and depending on the method, the amount of flow per minute. When administering oxygen as an emergency measure, the nurse may initiate the therapy without a primary care provider's order.

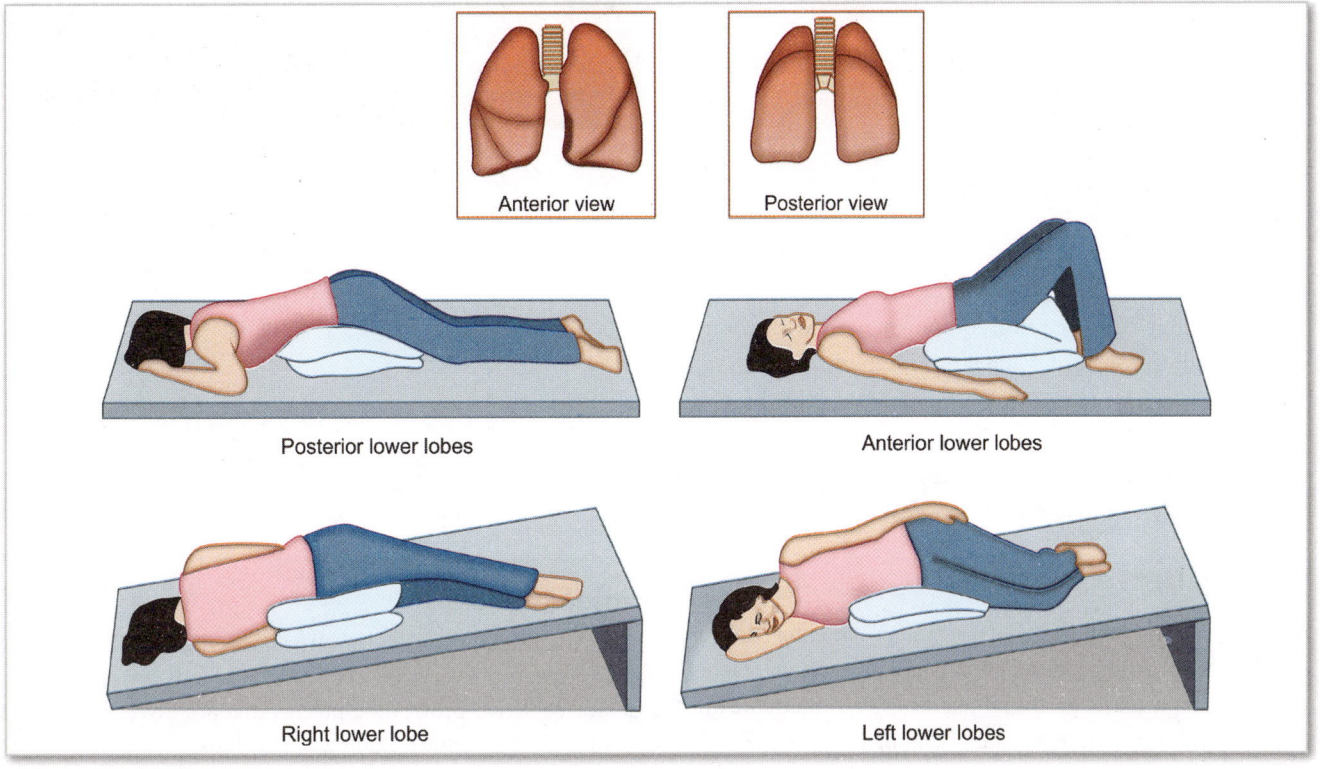

Anterior view

Posterior view

Posterior lower lobes

Anterior lower lobes

Right lower lobe

Left lower lobes

Fig. 4: Postural drainage. Shown are four positions that use the force of gravity to assist the drainage of secretions from the smaller bronchial airways into the bronchi and trachea so the patient is able to cough them up.

Oxygen is supplied in several different ways. In hospitals and long-term care facilities, it is usually piped into wall outlets at the client's bedside, making it readily available for use at all times. Cylinders of oxygen under pressure are also frequently available for use when wall oxygen is either unavailable or impractical.

Oxygen, whether administered from a cylinder or wall outlet system, is dry. Dry gases dehydrate the respiratory mucous membranes. Humidifying devices that add water vapor to inspired air are thus an essential adjunct of oxygen therapy (Fig. 5).

These devices provide 20–40% humidity. The oxygen passes through sterile distilled water or tap water and then along a line to the device through which the moistened oxygen is inhaled (e.g., a cannula, nasal catheter, oxygen mask).

Humidifiers prevent mucous membranes from drying and becoming irritated and loosen secretions for easier expectoration. Oxygen passing through water picks up water vapor before it reaches the client. The more bubbles created during this process, the more water vapor is produced. Clients who are given very low liter flows (e.g., 1–2 L/min) by nasal cannula do not require humidification, as there is enough atmospheric air inhaled (which naturally has water vapor in it) to prevent drying mucosa.

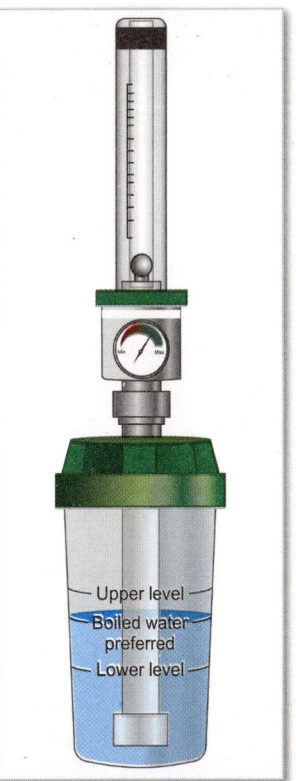

Upper level
Boiled water preferred
Lower level

Fig. 5: An oxygen humidifier attached to a wall outlet oxygen flow meter

Precautions for Oxygen Administration

Oxygen, which constitutes 21% of normal air, is a tasteless, odorless, and colorless gas. It supports combustion. To prevent fire, take the following precautions:

- Avoid open flames in the client's room
- Place 'NO SMOKING' signs in places where oxygen is being administered. Instruct visitors and family members about the hazards of smoking.
- Check to see that electrical equipment used in the room is in good working order and emits no sparks.
- Avoid wearing and using synthetic fabrics that build up static electricity.
- Avoid using oil in the area, oil can ignite spontaneously in the presence of oxygens.

Oxygen Delivery Systems

Oxygen can be administered by many different delivery systems: Nasal cannula, nasopharyngeal catheter, transtracheal catheter, simple mask, partial rebreathing mask, nonrebreather mask, venturi mask, and tent. Table 2 compares several oxygen delivery systems.

TABLE 2: Oxygen delivery systems

Method	Amount delivered FiO$_2$ (fraction inspired oxygen)	Priority nursing interventions
Nasal cannula	Low flow 1 L/min = 24% 2 L/min = 28% 3 L/min = 32% 4 L/min = 36% 5 L/min = 40% 6 L/min = 44%	Check frequently that both prongs are in patient's nares. May be no more than 2–3 L/min to patient with chronic lung disease.
Simple mask	Low flow 6–10 L/min = 35%–60% (5 L/min is minimum setting)	Monitor patient frequently to check placement of the mask. Support patient if claustrophobia is a concern. Secure physician's order to replace mask with nasal cannula during mealtime.
Partial rebreather mask	Low flow 6–15 L/min = 70%-90%	Set flow rate so that mask remains two-thirds full during inspiration. Keep reservoir bag free of twists or kinks.

Contd...

Method	Amount delivered FiO$_2$ (fraction inspired oxygen)	Priority nursing interventions
Nonre-breather mask	Low flow 6–15 L/min = 60%–100%	Maintain flow rate so reservoir bag collapses only slightly during inspiration. Check that valves and rubber flaps are functioning properly (open during expiration and closed during inhalation). Monitor SaO$_2$ with pulse oximeter.
Venturi mask	High flow 4–10 L/min = 24%–55%	Requires careful monitoring to verify FiO$_2$ at flow rate ordered. Check that air intake valves are not blocked.

Nasal Cannula

A nasal cannula, also called nasal prongs, is the most commonly used oxygen delivery device. Cannula is a disposable plastic device with two protruding prongs that are inserted into the nostrils. The cannula is connected to an oxygen source with a flow meter and many times, a humidifier (Fig. 6).

The nasal cannula is easy to apply and does not interfere with the client's ability to eat or talk. It is also relatively comfortable, permits some freedom of movement; and is well tolerated by the client. It delivers a relatively low concentration of oxygen (24–45%) at flow rates of 2–6 L/min. Limitations of the cannula include inability to deliver higher concentration of oxygen and it can be drying and irritating to mucous membranes. Administering oxygen by cannula is given in detail later in this chapter under heading skill of administering oxygen.

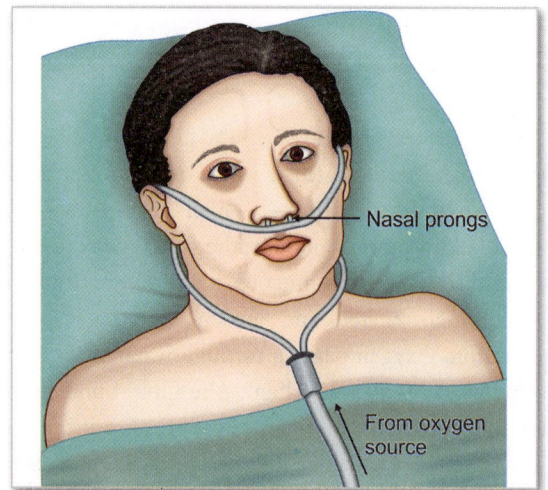

Fig. 6: A nasal cannula

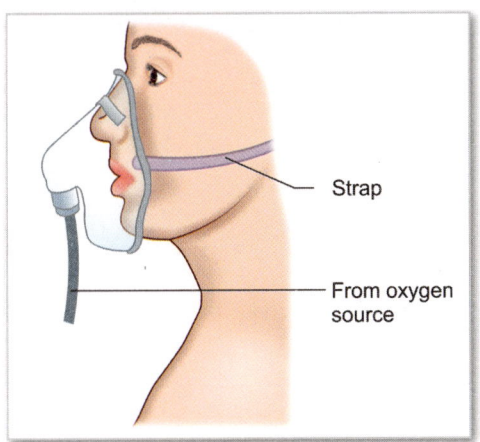

Fig. 7: A simple face mask

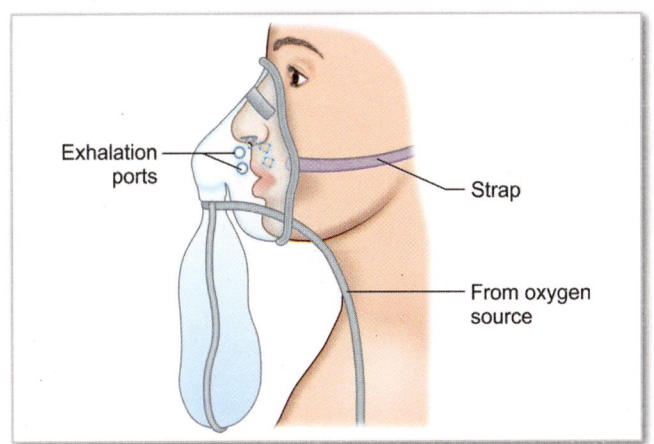

Fig. 8: A non-rebreather mask

Face Mask

Face masks that cover the client's nose and mouth may be used for oxygen inhalation. Exhalation ports on the sides of the mask allow exhaled carbon dioxide to escape. A variety of oxygen face masks are discussed as follows.

Simple Face Mask

The simple face mask delivers oxygen concentrations from 40% to 60% at flow rate of 5–8 L per minute (Fig. 7).

Partial Rebreather Mask

The partial rebreather mask delivers oxygen concentration of 60 – 90% at flow rate of 6 – 10 L/min. The oxygen reservoir bag that is attached allows the client to rebreathe about the first third of the exhaled air in conjunction with oxygen. Thus, it increases the fraction of inspired oxygen (FiO_2), by recycling expired oxygen. The partial rebreather bag must not totally deflate during inspiration to avoid carbon dioxide build up. If this problem occurs, the nurse should increase the liter flow of oxygen.

Non-breather Mask

The non-breather mask delivers the highest oxygen concentration possible, i.e., 95% – 100% by means other than intubation or mechanical ventilation at flow rate of 10 – 15 L/min. One way valves on the mask and between the reservoir bag and the mask prevent the room air and the clients exhaled air from entering the bag so only the oxygen in the bag is inspired. To prevent carbon dioxide build-up, the non-breather bag must not totally deflate during inspiration. If it does, the nurse should correct this problem by increasing the liter flow of oxygen (Fig. 8).

Venturi Mask

Oxygen concentration delivered by the venturi mask varying from 24% to 40–50% at flow rate of 4 – 10 L/min. The venturi mask has wide bore tubing and color-coded jet adapters that

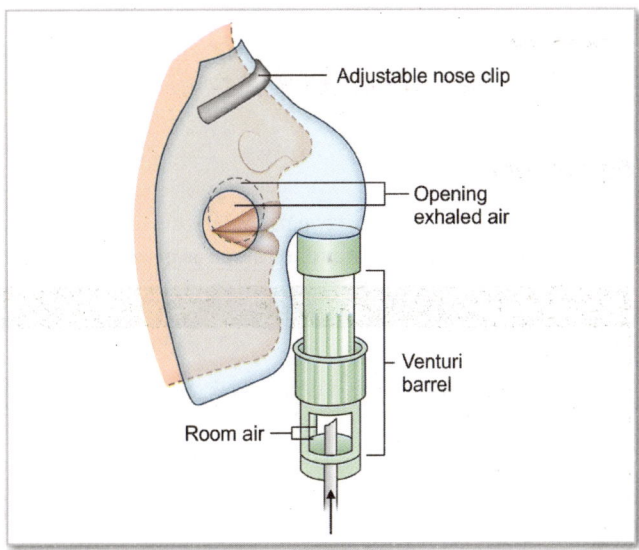

Fig. 9: A Venturi mask

correspond to a precise oxygen concentration and flow rate (Fig. 9).

For example, a blue adaptor delivers 24% concentration of oxygen at 4 L/min and a green adaptor delivers a 35% concentration of oxygen at 8 L/min.

Administering oxygen by mask is similar to administering oxygen by cannula, except that the nurse must choose a mask of appropriate size. Smaller sizes are available for children. Limitations of mask include difficulty in achieving a proper fit and poor tolerance of some clients who may complain of feeling hot or "smothering".

Face Tent

Face tents can replace oxygen mask when masks are poorly tolerated by clients. Face tents provide varying concentrations of oxygen, from 30% to 50%, at flow rate of 4 – 8 L/min. Frequently inspect the client's facial skin for dampness or chaffing, treat as needed. The facial skin must be kept dry (Fig. 10).

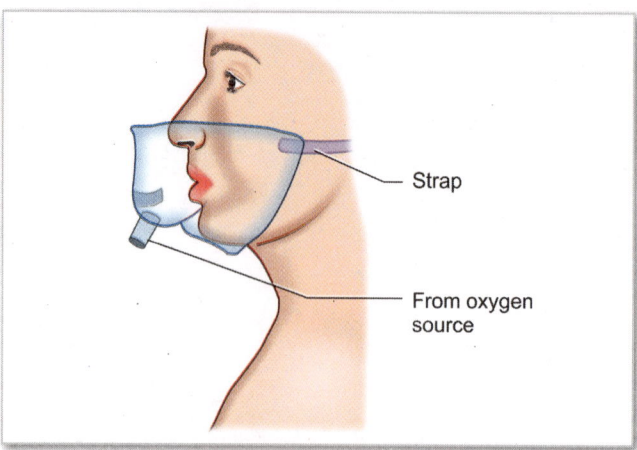

Fig. 10: An oxygen face tent

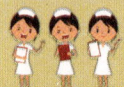

SKILL: ADMINISTERING OXYGEN

Equipment

Oxygen source, humidifier, oxygen delivery device (nasal cannula, face mask, face tent), oxygen flowmeter, connecting tubing.
Review and carry out the standard steps as given in Appendix

Action/steps	Rationale
Assessment	
1. Check the chart for the ordered flow rate and oxygen delivery method	Ensures that patient will receive oxygen therapy as needed
2. Assess patient's breathing and lung sounds	Provides baseline for determination as to whether oxygen therapy is effective
Planning	
3. Plan the length of connecting tubing to the oxygen source needed for the patient	Length of tubing needed depends on activity level and whether oxygen needs to be continuous or intermittent
4. Determine whether oxygen set up will need a humidifier	Low flow oxygen does not need a humidifier to moisten the flow. If patient suffers from sinus problems, it is best to add humidifier. Oxygen dries the mucosa, therefore, humidifier is needed to provide moisture
Implementation	
5. Connect the flow meter to the piped in oxygen outlet on the wall by pressing it firmly into the outlet, or attach the flowmeter to the oxygen cylinder	Prepares the oxygen to be dispensed in a regulated flow
6. Attach the humidifier and the connecting tubing to the oxygen delivery device and turn on the oxygen adjusting the flow to the ordered rate	Readies the delivery system for the patient. By turning the knob on the flow meter, the metal ball rises inside the glass graduated gauge, indicating the rate of flow being delivered
7. Correctly position the oxygen delivery device on the patient and secure it in place	An oxygen cannula should be positioned with the nasal prongs curved downward as they go into the nares. The tubing is looped over the ears and secured in place by raising the device toward the chin. Be certain that the tubing is not causing pressure on the ears. A face mask should fit over the nose and mouth. A face tent fits below the chin and rises to cover the lower part of the face.
8. Instruct patient and visitors regarding safety during oxygen use	Helps prevent fires and injury

Contd...

Action/steps	Rationale
Evaluation	
9. Ask yourself, is the patient able to tolerate the oxygen device? Is the oxygen flow at the level ordered? Is "oxygen in use" sign posted? Is breathing loss labored with oxygen administration? Is oxygen saturation improving?	Answers determine whether patient tolerates the oxygen and whether the procedure is effective
Documentation	
10. Include the reason for the oxygen therapy, the time that oxygen therapy is instituted, the type of oxygen delivery device in use, flow rate, and whether it is continuous or PRN.	Verifies that oxygen is administered as ordered: data support oxygen administration

Artificial Airways

Artificial airways are used to relieve an obstruction, to protect the airway, to facilitate suctioning and to provide artificial ventilation.

There are two types of pharyngeal airways: the **nasopharyngeal airway** and the **oropharyngeal** airway. They are used to keep the tongue from falling back into the throat and frequently required for postoperative patients until they have recovered from anesthesia. These airways are used for patients who can breathe on their own (Fig. 11).

Oropharyngeal Airways

Oropharyngeal stimulate the gag reflex and are only used for clients with altered levels of consciousness due to overdose of general anesthesia or head injury.

Following are the steps to insert the oropharyngeal airway
1. Place the client in a supine or semi-Fowler's position
2. Put on clean gloves
3. Hold the lubricated airway by the outer flange, with the distal end pointing up.
4. Open the client's mouth and insert the airway along the top of the tongue

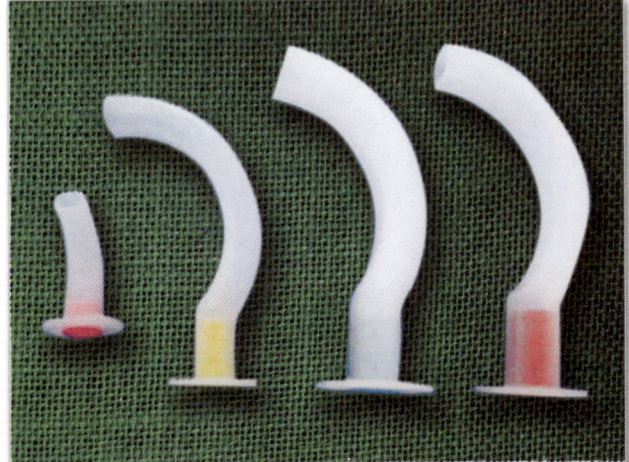

Fig. 11: Types of airways (endotracheal, nasal, oropharyngeal).

5. When the distal end of the airway reaches the soft palate at the back of the mouth, rotate the airway 180 degrees downward, and slip it past the uvula into the oropharynx.
6. If no contraindication is noticed, place the client in a side-lying position or with the head turned to the side to allow secretions to drain out of the mouth.
7. The oropharynx may be suctioned as needed by inserting the suction catheter alongside the airway
8. Do not tape the airway in place, remove it when the client begins to cough or gag
9. Provide mouth care at least 2–4 hours, keeping suction available at the bedside.

As per the patient's condition, remove the airway every 8 hours to assess the mouth and provide oral care. Reinsert the airway immediately once the oral care is done.

Nasopharyngeal Airways

Nasopharyngeal airways are well tolerated by alert patient. Nasopharyngeal airways are inserted through the nares, terminating in the oropharynx. While caring patient on nasopharyngeal airway, provide frequent oral and nares care, repositioning the airway in the other nares every 8 hours or as ordered to prevent necrosis of the mucosa.

Endotracheal Tube

Endotracheal tubes (ETT) are most commonly inserted in clients who have had general anesthetics or in those who are in emergency situations where mechanical ventilation is required. An endotracheal tube is inserted by the primary care provider, nurse respiratory therapist with specialized education. It is inserted through the mouth or nose and into the trachea with the help of laryngoscope. The tube terminates just superior to the bifurcation of the trachea into the bronchi. The tube may have an air filled cuff to prevent air leakage around it. Because an endotracheal tube passes through the epiglottis and glottis, the client is unable to speak while it is in place.

Nursing Intervention for Clients with Endotracheal Tubes

- Assess the client's respiratory status at least every 2 hours, or more frequently, if needed. Assess respiratory rate, rhythm, depth, equality of chest expansion, and lung sounds, level of consciousness and skin color.
- Frequently assess nasal and oral mucosa for redness and irritation. Report any abnormal findings.
- Secure the endotracheal tube with tape or a commercially prepared holder to prevent movement of the tube farther into or out of the trachea.
- Assess the position of the ETT frequently. Notify, if the tube is not in place. If the tube advances into a main bronchus, reposition it to ensure ventilation of both lungs.
- Unless contraindicated, place the client in side lying or semi-prone position as tolerated to prevent aspiration of oral secretions.
- Using sterile technique, suction the endotracheal tube as needed to remove excessive secretions.
- Closely monitor cuff pressure, maintain a pressure of 20–25 mm Hg to minimize the risk of tracheal tissue necrosis. If recommended, deflate the cuff periodically.
- Provide oral and nasal care every 2–4 hours. Use an oropharyngeal airway to prevent the client from biting down on an endotracheal tube. Move endotracheal tube to the opposite side of the mouth every eight hours, taking care to maintain the position of the tube in the trachea. This prevents irritation to the oral mucosa.
- Provide humidified air or oxygen because the endotracheal tube bypasses the upper airways, which normally moisten the air.
- If the client is on mechanical ventilation, ensure that all alarms are enabled at all times because the client cannot call for help in case of emergency.
- Communicate frequently with the client, providing a note pad or picture board for the client to use for communicating.

Tracheostomy Tube

Clients who need long-term airway support may have a tracheostomy. A tracheostomy is an opening into the trachea through the neck. A tube is usually inserted through this opening and an artificial airway is created. Tracheotomy is done by using one of the two techniques: The traditional open surgical method or a percutaneous insertion. The percutaneous method can be done at the bedside in a critical care unit. The open technique is done in the operating room, and surgical incision is made in the trachea just below the larynx. A curved tracheostomy tube is inserted to extend through the stoma into the trachea. Tracheostomy tubes may be either plastic or metal and are available in different sizes.

Tracheostomy tubes have an outer cannula that is inserted into the trachea and a flange that rests against the neck and allows the tube to be secured in place with tape or ties. All tubes also have an obturator, which is used to insert the outer cannula and is then removed. The obturator is kept at the client's bedside in case the tube becomes dislodged and needs to be reinserted. Some tracheostomy tubes have an inner cannula that may be removed for periodic cleaning (Fig. 12).

Cuffed tracheostomy tubes are surrounded by an inflatable cuff that produces an airtight seal between the tube and the trachea. This seal prevents aspiration of oropharyngeal secretions and air leakages between the tube and the trachea.

The nurse provides tracheostomy care to the client to maintain patency of the tube and reduce the risk of infection. Initially, tracheostomy may need to be suctioned and cleaned as often as every 1 – 2 hours. After the initial inflammatory response subsides, tracheostomy care may only need to be done once or twice a day depending on the client.

When the client breathes through a tracheostomy, air is no longer filtered and humidified as it is when passing through the upper airways; therefore, special precautions are necessary. Clients with long-term tracheostomies may wear a 4 in × 4 in gauze held in place over the stoma, to filter the air as it enters the tracheostomy.

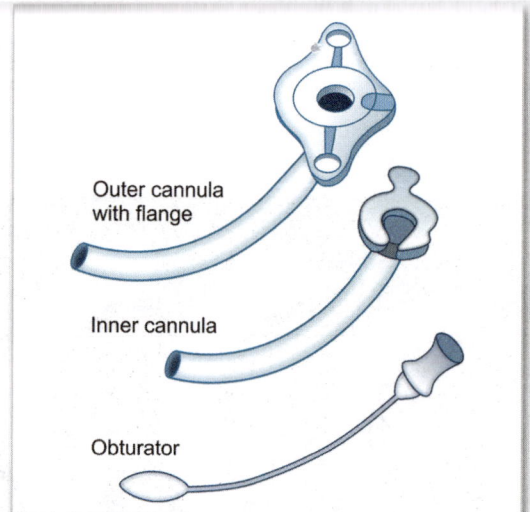

Fig. 12: Components of a tracheostomy tube

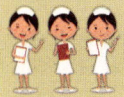

Equipment

- Portable or wall suction unit with tubing
- Sterile suction catheter with Y port size for adult 10 Fr – 16 Fr
- Sterile gloves, sterile water or saline
- Towel mouth wipes
- Disposable clean gloves
- Water-soluble lubricant
- Personal protective equipment (PPE), mackintosh (water proof lining)

Review and carry out the standard steps as given in Appendix

Action/steps	Rationale
Assessment	
1. Auscultate the lungs to locate retained secretions. Assist patient to cough and expectorate, if possible.	Determines the necessity for suctioning. If secretions are cleared suctioning is not necessary.
2. Bring necessary equipment to the bed-side or overbed table	To conserve energy and time.
3. Perform hand hygiene and put on Personal protective equipment (PPE) (Goggles, mask, face shield)	Hand hygiene and PPE prevent spread of microbes. PPE for self-protection.
4. Determine the need for suctioning and verify the suction order. For postoperative patient, administer pain medication before suctioning	To minimize trauma to airway mucosa, suctioning should be done only when secretions have accumulated or adventitious breath sounds are audible. Suctioning stimulates coughing, which is painful for surgical patients.
Planning	
5. Explain the procedure to patient. Reassure patient that the procedure can be interrupted any time in case of respiratory difficulty	Explanation alleviates fears. Even if patient appears unconscious, explain what is happening.
6. Adjust bed to comfortable working height. Lower side rail should be closest to your side. If patient is conscious, place him or her in a semi-Fowlers's position. If unconscious, place the patient in the lateral position	Having the bed at proper height prevents back and muscle strain. A sitting position helps the patient to cough and makes breathing easier. Gravity also helps catheter insertion. The lateral position prevents airway becoming obstructed.
7. Place towel and mackintosh across the patient's chest.	This protects bed linens.
8. Adjust suction to appropriate pressure. For a wall suction unit for adult 100–120 mm Hg and adolescents 80–120 mm Hg For a portable unit for adult 10–15 cm Hg and adolescents 8–10 cm Hg	Higher pressure can cause excessive trauma, hypoxemia, and atelectasis.
Implementation	
9. Put on disposable clean gloves and occlude the end of connecting tubing to check suction pressure.	To check proper functioning.
10. Open sterile package using sterile technique. Open wrapper. Pour normal saline in sterile container	Sterile normal saline or water is used to lubricate the outside of the catheter. It is also used to clear the catheter between suction.
12. Increase the patient's supplemental oxygen level as per policy of facility	Suctioning can cause hypoxemia.
13. Put on face shield or goggles and mask. Put on sterile gloves. Catheter is manipulated by dominant hand therefore it should remain sterile. The non-dominant hand should also remain clean to control the suction on the catheter	Handling the sterile catheter using sterile glove helps prevent introducing organisms into the respiratory tract.

Contd...

Action/steps	Rationale
14. With dominant hand pick up sterile catheter. Pick up the connecting tube with non-dominant hand and connect the tubing and suction catheter.	Sterility of suction catheter is maintained.
15. Moisten the catheter by dipping it into the container of sterile saline. Occlude y-tube to check suction	Checking suction ensures equipment is working properly
16. Encourage the patient to take several deep breaths.	Suctioning removes air from the patient's airway and can cause hypoxemia.
17. Remove the oxygen delivery device. Do not apply suction as the catheter is inserted. Hold the catheter between your thumb and forefinger	Using suction while inserting the catheter can cause trauma to the mucosa and removes oxygen from the respiratory tract. For determining insertion distance-measure from the patient's earlobe to the nose for nasopharyngeal suctioning

Insert the catheter:
- For nasopharyngeal suction, gently insert catheter through the nares and along the floor of the nostril toward the trachea. Advance the catheter approximately 5–6 inches to reach pharynx
- For oropharyngeal suction—insert catheter through mouth toward the trachea. Advance the catheter 3–4 inches to reach the pharynx

Action/steps	Rationale
18. Apply suction intermittently occluding the Y port on the catheter with the thumb of non-dominant hand and gently rotate the catheter as it is being withdrawn. Do not suction for more than 10–15 seconds at a time.	Rotating the catheter as it is withdrawn minimizes trauma to the mucosa. Suctioning for longer than 10–15 seconds robs the respiratory tract of oxygen, results in hypoxemia. Suctioning too quickly may be ineffective in clearing all secretions
19. Replace the oxygen delivery device using your non-dominant hand, have the patient take several deep breaths.	Suctioning removes air from the patient's airway. Hyperventilation can help prevent suction-induced hypoxemia.
20. Flush catheter with saline. Assess effectiveness of suctioning and repeat as needed.	Flushing clears catheter and lubricates it for next insertion.
21. Allow at least 30-second to 1-minute interval if additional suctioning is needed. No more than three times suction at one time is recommended. Suction the oropharynx after suctioning the nasopharynx. Alternate nare, if repeated suctioning is required.	Excessive suction can contribute to complications. Alternating nare reduces trauma. Suctioning the oropharynx after the nasopharynx clear the mouth of secretions. More microorganism are present in mouth so it is suctioned last, for patient safety and comfort.
22. When suctioning is completed, remove gloves from both hands and dispose catheter in appropriate receptacle. Assist patient in comfortable position.	
23. Turn off suction. Remove supplemental oxygen placed for suctioning, if appropriate. Remove face shield or goggles and mask. Perform hand hygiene.	Proper removal of PPE and hand hygiene reduces risk of transmission of microorganisms.
24. Reassess patient's respiratory status, including respiratory rate, effort, oxygen saturation and lung sounds	This assesses effectiveness of suctioning and the presence of complications.

Evaluation

Action/steps	Rationale
25. Auscultate the lungs and listen to see if there is any noise indicating retained secretions	To determine whether procedure was effective.

Documentation

Action/steps	Rationale
26. Document the time of suctioning, your pre- and post-intervention assessment, reason for suctioning, route used, and the characteristic and amount of secretions.	Proper recording helps other health care providers about the intervention.

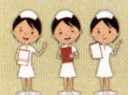

SKILL: ENDOTRACHEAL AND TRACHEOSTOMY SUCTIONING

Equipment

♦ Suction source, face shield, sterile normal saline, sterile suction catheter tray containing, solution container, sterile gloves, sterile suction catheter, resuscitation bag, connecting tubing.

Review and carry out the standard steps as given in Appendix

Action/steps	Rationale
Assessment	
1. Auscultate the patient's lungs to determine if there are retained secretions present.	Moist breath sounds including gurgles and bubbling indicate a need for suctioning.
Planning	
2. Be certain that all equipment are in the reach of the hand and in working condition.	Ensures that the procedure is going smoothly.
3. Pre oxygenate the client with the resuscitation bag if possible	Pre-oxygenation helps in prevention of depletion of oxygen by suctioning.
4. Attach the connecting tubing to suction source and turn on suction, check the pressure.	Verify that the suction is functioning by occluding end of suction tubing with your thumb and set pressure between 80 and 120 mm Hg for wall suction.
Implementation	
5. Wash your hands, open supplies and put on sterile gloves. Pour the sterile water into the container. Hold the catheter and attach to the connecting tube. Make sure that the catheter should not get sterile.	Prepares the water for use and catheter for suctioning.
6. If client is receiving oxygen, increase the concentration to 100% for a short time or give two to three sigh breath with the ventilator.	Pre-oxygenation prevents hypoxia during suctioning.
7. Moisten the catheter tip in the sterile saline solution. Disconnect the ventilator tubing if in use, and immediately introduce the catheter into the endotracheal tube or tracheotomy tube using sterile gloved hand. Do not use suction while placing the catheter. Advance catheter until resistance is met, then pull back 1 cm.	Moisture lubricates the catheter and makes it easier to introduce. Resistance occurs when the catheter reaches carina (junction of main bronchi).
8. Apply suction while rotating and withdrawing the catheter, allow no more than 10 seconds to suction and withdraw the catheter.	Suction draws out secretions. Rotating the catheter between the fingers rotates the catheter openings at the tip so that secretions around the circumference of trachea can be sucked-up. Suctioning more than 10 seconds depletes the client of oxygen.
9. Re-attach the patient's tube to the oxygen source, and allow a rest period before suctioning again. Keep the catheter sterile while waiting. Auscultate the lungs when finished to ascertain that secretions have been adequately cleared.	Suction draws out oxygen as well as secretions and may cause hypoxia. Hyperoxygenation should be done again before each suctioning.
10. Suction the nasopharynx, if needed.	Secretions may collect above the cuffed tracheotomy tube and need to be removed.
11. Discard the catheter by holding it in gloved hand and pulling the gloves off or over it.	A sterile catheter must be used each time the tracheobronchial suctioning is performed. Pulling glove over the used catheter prevents spread of microorganism.
12. Suctioning with sleeved catheter.	
13. Open catheter package without disturbing protective sleeve covering the catheter.	Sleeve maintains sterility of catheter so that it can be used several times.

Contd...

Action/steps	Rationale
14. Attach catheter to endotracheal tube or tracheostomy adaptor and to suction tubing. If secretions are thick, inject sterile saline via saline port as per agency protocol.	Sterile saline helps in thinning secretions.
15. If catheter is inserted via endotracheal tube or tracheostomy, sleeve slides back; advance the catheter as far as possible.	Positions catheter within trachea to carina.
16. Apply suction while rotating and withdrawing the catheter, allow the sleeve to recover the catheter as it is withdrawn, pull it back out of the tube opening.	The sleeve prevents the catheter from becoming contaminated from outside the trachea. Prevents the catheter from occluding the airway. Clears the suction tubing; ensures that airway is clear.
17. Rinse the catheter and connecting tubing with sterile normal saline when finished by injecting it with a syringe into the irrigation port, while applying suction. Auscultate lungs to be certain that secretions have been cleared sufficiently.	
18. Remove gloves and wash hands turn off suction	Reduces transfer of microorganisms
Evaluation	
19. Ask yourself, did patient tolerate the procedure. Are the lungs clear to auscultation? Did suctioning remove secretions? Was sterility maintained?	Answers provide data to determine if procedure was effective
Documentation	
20. Include number of times the patient has received suctioning, type of technique used, characteristics of secretions, and any problems encountered	Documents procedure and any problems encountered

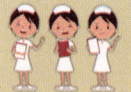

SKILL: PROVIDING TRACHEOSTOMY CARE

Equipment

- Normal saline, forceps
- Sterile gloves
- Hydrogen peroxide tracheostomy dressing
- Tracheostomy tape
- Scissors
- Sterile 4 × 4 gauze pad
- Cotton swabs, bowls and kidney receptacle.

Review and carry out the standard steps as given in Appendix

Action/steps	Rationale
Assessment	
1. Suction as needed before beginning the procedure.	Clears airway. Movement of the tracheostomy tube during cleaning and care may make patient cough and may block the airway.
Planning	
2. Set-up the equipment on a table close to the patient and plan the order in which the tasks to be performed	Planning makes work more efficient.
Implementation	
3. Place the patient in low semi-Fowler's position. Wash the hands, open the supplies, and put on one glove. Pour solutions with ungloved hand. One part hydrogen peroxide to one part normal saline for the wash solution, normal saline is used to rinse	Makes visualization of the tracheostomy site clear, prepares the supplies for use. Gloves prevent transfer of microorganisms

Contd...

Action/steps	Rationale
4. Put on the second glove. Undo the lock of the outer cannula, stabilizing the tube flange with the index finger and thumb, and remove the inner cannula by gently pulling it out toward you.	Latch must be unlocked to remove the inner cannula.
5. Place the reusable inner cannula in the basin of wash solution and clean the lumen thoroughly with brush. Rinse in the normal saline or sterile water.	If second inner cannula is available to place into the tracheostomy tube. Store the inner cannula after cleaning .
6. Re-insert the cannula after excessive moisture has been removed. Using aseptic technique, insert the inner cannula into the lumen of the outer cannula. Lock in place by turning the latch of the outer cannula	Excessive moisture may make the patient cough as the cannula is replaced. Cannula must be firmly locked into place so that it is not coughed out
7. Remove the soiled dressing and discard. Clean around the tube with solution using cotton swabs, rinse with saline	The area around the tube is cleaned every 6–8 hours as per protocol using cotton swabs and hydrogen peroxide
8. Replace soiled tracheostomy ties. Punch a hole in the end of the tie with forceps. Pass the end through the flange on the side of the tracheostomy tube, and thread the tie through the hole, pulling it taut. Repeat for the other side, and tie the tapes at the side of neck.	Ties are replaced when soiled or at least once in 24 hours. Ties are easier to replace, if done before the new dressing is applied.
9. Apply the precut dressing or a V-folded gauze. Place it under and around the outer cannula to soak secretions	Cutting 4 × 4 gauze pad to use as tracheostomy dressing should not be done because the loose gauze may fall into the tracheostomy tube and be aspirated by the patient.
Evaluation	
10. Ask yourself, did the procedure go smoothly? Was the tube moved too much, making the patient cough a lot? Are the ties smooth? Is the dressing in proper place?	Answers to these questions determine whether the procedure was done properly and efficiently.
Documentation	
11. Documentation may be in narrative form or on a flowsheet. Note the care given and the condition of the tracheostomy site.	Recording helps to note that nursing care was administered

CARE OF CHEST TUBES AND CHEST DRAINAGE

Patient with fluid (Pleural effusion), blood (hemothorax), or air (pneumothorax) in the pleural space require a chest tube to drain these substances and allow the compressed lung to re-expand. A chest tube is a firm plastic tube with drainage holes in the proximal end that is inserted in the pleural space. Once inserted, the tube is secured with a suture and tape, covered with an airtight dressing, and attached to a drainage system that may or may not be attached to suction. Other components of the system may include a closed water–seal drainage system that prevents air from reentering the chest once it has escaped and a suction control chamber that prevents excess suction pressure from being applied to the pleural cavity. The suction chamber may be a water filled or a dry chamber. A water filled suction chamber is regulated by the amount of water in the chamber, whereas dry suction has a one-way mechanical valve system that allows air to leave the chest and prevents air from moving back into the chest and is automatically regulated to changes in the patient's pleural pressure.

Most of the health care agencies use a molded plastic, three compartment disposable chest drainage unit for management of chest tubes (Fig. 13).

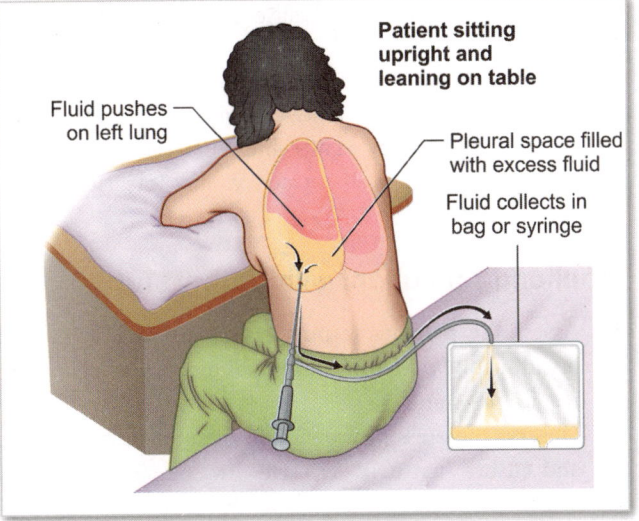

Fig. 13: A chest drainage system attached to a patient

There are also portable drainage systems that utilize gravity for drainage and water seal drainage bottle system (Figs 14A to C).

The placement of the chest tube is determined by the type of drainage. When air is to be drained, the tube is placed higher in the chest. If fluid needs to be drained then the tube

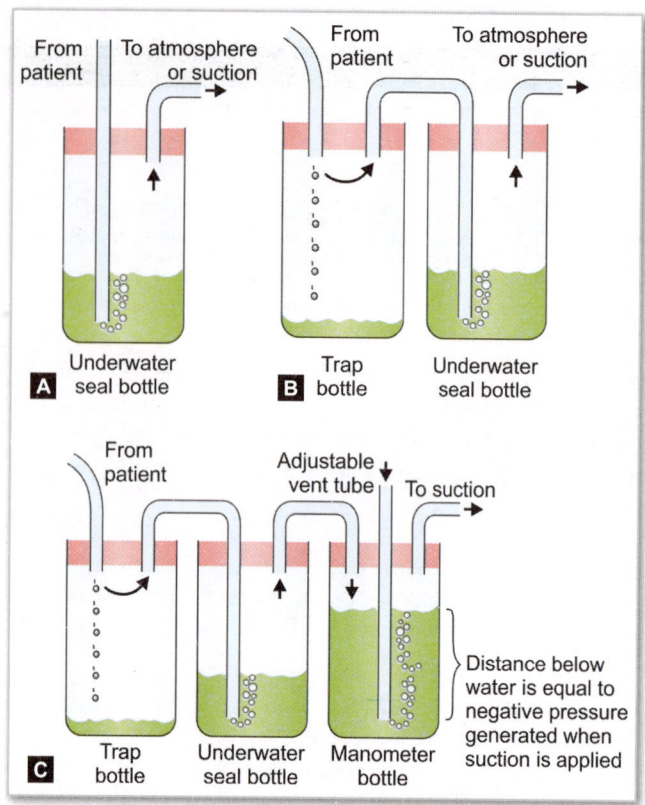

Figs 14A to C: Water-seal closed chest drainage systems.
A. One-bottle system. B. Two-bottle system.
C. Three-bottle system using suction

is inserted lower in the lung because fluids settle at the base of the lung.

Nursing responsibilities include assisting with insertion and removal of chest tube. Once the tube is in place, monitor the patient's respiratory status and vital signs, check the dressing, and maintain the patency and integrity of the drainage system.

Monitoring a Patient with a Chest Tube

- Assess the patient's respiratory status, vital signs, and breath sounds. Monitor for any indication of change in respiratory status.
- Observe the dressing around the chest tube insertion site and ensure that it is occlusive. All connections should also be taped securely.
- Check that the drainage tube has no dependent loops or kinks. The drainage collection device must be positioned below the tube insertion site to facilitate drainage.
- Keep drainage collection device secure so that it does not tip over and below chest level.
- Make sure that two padded Kelly clamps are available at bedside. If the drainage unit requires changing, position one clamp 1½ to 2½ inches from the insertion site, position the second clamp 1 inch down from the first one.

- Assist the patient to remain in high Fowler's position in case of hemothorax or semi-Fowler's position for pneumothorax.
- Avoid milking or stripping the tube to promote drainage. This creates excessive negative pressure that can damage delicate lung tissue.
- Never clamp the tube if the patient leaves the unit for a test or moves away from the bed. Disconnect the suction tubing from the drainage system, allowing the unit to continue to collect drainage by gravity.
- Assess the suction control chamber if suction is in use. If water suction is used, ensure that water is at the appropriate level. Gentle bubbling in the suction chamber indicates that suction is being applied to assist drainage.
- Measure drainage output at the end of each shift by marking the level on the container or placing a small piece of tube of the drainage level to indicate date and time.
- Document color and consistency of drainage. Drainage exceeding 100 mL or bright red color drainage indicates fresh bleeding which requires immediate notification of the physician.

PULSE OXIMETRY

Pulse oximetry is used for any patient who is at risk of hypoxia. With the pulse oximeter (machine to measure oxygen saturation of the blood), changes in arterial oxygen saturation can be continuously monitored. It is one of the valuable tools to measure arterial oxygen saturation. The device measures oxygen saturation by determining the percentage of hemoglobin that is bound with oxygen. A sensor or probe is attached to an appendage of the patient on earlobe, fingertip, toe, through which infrared and red light can reach the capillary vascular bed. Oxyhemoglobin absorbs more infrared than red light. A microprocessor in the monitor receives the information from the sensor-probe, computes the saturation value, and displays it on the monitor screen.

Adhesive sensors can be applied to the nose or the forehead. These are generally disposable, whereas clip on probes may be reusable.

Pulse oximetry is the noninvasive measurement of arterial oxygen saturation done with the help of pulse oximeter.

Purposes

- To monitor the oxygen saturation of arterial blood
- To monitor the effectiveness of oxygen therapy.

Indications

- Patients with impaired gas exchange
- Patients with respiratory illnesses such as Asthma, chronic obstructive pulmonary disease (COPD), etc.

- Patients who are on respiratory depressants
- Patients who are sedated or under the effects of anesthesia

Principles

The light emitting diode emits light in wavelengths that are absorbed differently by the oxygenated and deoxygenated hemoglobin molecules. The amount of light transmitted through the tissues is then converted to a digital value representing the percentage of hemoglobin saturated with oxygen. The more hemoglobin saturated by oxygen, the higher is the oxygen saturation. Normally oxygen saturation (SPO_2) is greater than 90%.

Site for Pulse Oximetry

Site selected should be free from moisture and has adequate circulation. If nail bed is used, it should be free of nail polish. Use forehead or earlobe, in case the patient has tremors and if the patient is obese use disposable probe because clip or probe may not fit properly (Fig. 15).

Nursing Process

Assessment

Assess for alterations in oxygen saturation, i.e., altered respiratory rate, depth and rhythm, restlessness, irritability, confusion and reduced level of consciousness.

Assess for risk factors such as acute or chronic compromised respiratory function, traumatic chest injury, or ventilator dependence. Assess the previous SPO_2 level to have baseline data and determine the site for sensor probe placement.

Nursing Diagnosis

- Impaired gas exchange
- Ineffective airway clearance
- Ineffective breathing pattern

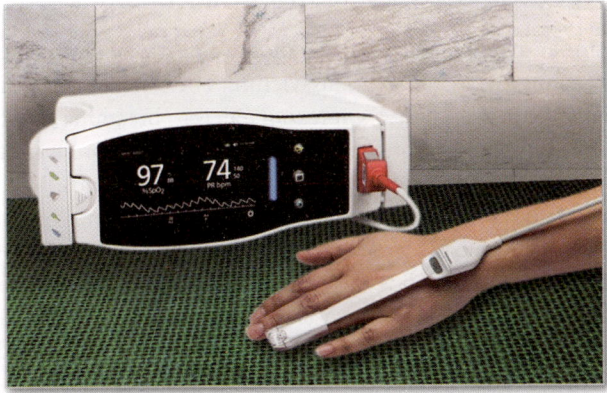

Fig. 15: Pulse Oximetry

Planning

Pulse oximeter with probe or probe with cardiac monitor.

Implementation

Action/steps	Rationale
1. Explain the procedure to patient	To gain cooperation
2. Position comfortably by supporting arm	To enhance comfort
3. Remove nail polish, if present	Nail polish alters the oxygen saturation
4. Attach sensor to monitoring unit	To detect saturation
5. Turn on the oximeter and observe pulse waveform and audible beep and correlate with radial pulse.	Enables detection of valid pulse.
6. Leave sensor in place and set alarm limits as lower limit of 85% and higher limit 100%. Explain to patient about oximeter alarm	Reduces anxiety
7. Record the findings.	For further comparison
8. Position patient comfortably	To enhance comfort.

Evaluation

Compare SPO_2 levels with previous baseline and acceptable levels of SPO_2.

Documentation

Record the date, time, site of probe placement and the reading. Specify the type and amount of oxygen, if the patient is on oxygen flow and report any abnormalities.

NEBULIZATION

Nebulization is a process of administration of medication via inhalation. By this method, the medication is dispersed in the form of mist and delivered into the respiratory tract with the help of device called nebulizer.

Purposes

- To relieve respiratory insufficiency
- To improve the vital capacity of the lungs
- To reduce the inflammatory and allergic responses of the respiratory tract
- To liquefy and remove thick secretions.

Indications

- Bronchospasm
- Excessive and thick secretions of the respiratory tract.
- Respiratory conditions such as pneumonia, atelectasis and asthma.

Nursing Process

Assessment

- Assess for history of allergy to medications
- Assess for symptoms of the patient and illness severity
- Assess the ability to use a nebulizer.

Nursing Diagnosis

- Impaired gas exchange
- Ineffective breathing pattern
- Activity intolerance
- Anxiety.

Planning

Preparation of equipment

- Nebulizer
- Oxygen source
- Nebulizer mask
- Medication
- Sterile water or normal saline
- Cotton balls
- Kidney tray
- Stethoscope
- Medication card
- Sputum mug.

Implementation

	Action/steps	Rationale
1.	Explain procedure to the patient	To gain cooperation
2.	Check the name, dose and frequency of the medication	To prevent medication error
3.	Assemble equipment at bed side	To prevent waste of time
4.	Wash hands	To prevent spread of microorganisms
5.	Connect the plug to check the functioning of equipment and pour medication into nebulizer and clean the mask with cotton balls dipped in normal saline	For dispersal of medication
6.	Position the patient in semi-Fowler's position	For easy lung expansion
7.	Auscultate the lung fields	Serves as baseline data
8.	Connect the oxygen tubing to the nebulizer and regulate the flow of oxygen to 6–10 L/min and ensure that vapor is produced.	To regulate the flow

Contd...

	Action/steps	Rationale
9.	Instruct the patient to breathe through nose deeply and exhale normally	For effectiveness of therapy
10.	Stop the flow once the medicine is over	
11.	Encourage patient to cough and provide sputum cup	To help in bringing out the secretions
12.	Position the patient comfortably Replace articles and wash hands.	To promote comforts for next use

Evaluation

- Monitor the response to the therapy
- Auscultate the lung fields to see the effectiveness of the therapy.

Documentation

- Record the date, time, medication used, dosage and duration of therapy
- Specify the auscultation findings before and after the procedure.

BASIC LIFE SUPPORT

Basic life support consists of a series of actions and skills performed by the rescuer based on assessment findings. The first actions the rescuer performs on finding an adult victim are to assess for responsiveness and to look for signs of breathing. This is done by tapping or shaking the victim's shoulder and asking, "Are you all right?" and seeing the movement of chest for breathing. If the victim does not respond, there is no breathing or abnormal breathing, the rescuer shouts for help, and activates emergency response system and gets automatic external defibrillator (AED) and begins cardiopulmonary resuscitation (CPR).

Cardiopulmonary Resuscitation

Cardiac arrest is characterized by the absence of a pulse and breathing in an unconscious victim. The current approach for CPR is the chest compression–airway breathing (CAB) sequence. The first step in CPR is to perform a pulse check by palpating the carotid pulse for at least 5 seconds. While maintaining a head tilt position with one hand on the forehead, locate the victim's trachea using two or three fingers of the other hand. Slide these fingers into the groove between the trachea and the neck muscles where the carotid pulse can be felt. The technique is more easily performed on the side nearest to you.

If a pulse is felt, give one rescue breath every 5–6 seconds (10–12 breaths/min) recheck the pulse every 2 minutes. If no pulse is felt, initiate CAB.

Chest Compressions

The proper technique for providing chest compressions consists of fast and deep applications of pressure on the sternum. The victim must be in the supine position when the compressions are performed. The victim must be lying on a flat, hard surface, such as a CPR board or if necessary, the floor. Position yourself close to the side of the victim's chest.

Chest compressions are combined with rescue breathing for an effective resuscitation effort of an adult victim of cardiac arrest. The compression ventilation ratio for one or two rescuer CPR is 30 compressions to 2 breaths. If the patient has an advanced airway, e.g., endotracheal tube, do not pause between compressions for breaths.

It is preferable to have two persons performing CPR, one rescuer, positioned at the victim's side, performs chest compressions, while the second rescuer, positioned at the victim's head, maintains an open airway and performs ventilations. To maintain the quality and rate of compressions, rescuers should change roles every 2 minutes. Interruptions in CPR should be limited.

Defibrillation

When the automatic external defibrillator (AED) or advanced cardiac life support (ACLS) team arrives, assess the victim's rhythm. If the victim has a shockable rhythm (e.g., ventricular tachycardia, ventricular fibrillation), deliver one shock followed by five cycles of CPR before checking the rhythm again. (Fig. 16)

If the rhythm is not a shockable rhythm, resume CPR and recheck the rhythm every five cycles. CPR should continue between rhythm checks and shocks, and until the ACLS team arrives or the victim shows signs of movement.

Airway and Breathing

If a victim has a pulse but is gasping or not breathing, establish an open airway and begin rescue breathing, open an adult's airway by hyperextending the head. Use the head tilt-chin lift maneuver. This involves tilting the head back with one hand and lifting the chin forward with the fingers of the other hand. Use the jaw-thrust maneuver, if you suspect a cervical spine injury.

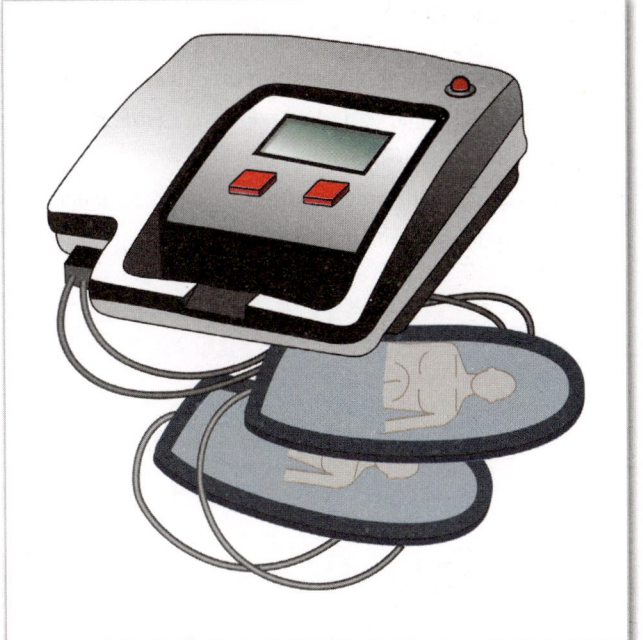

Fig. 16: Automatic external defibrillator

Attempt to ventilate the victim using a mouth-to-barrier device or mouth-to-mouth resuscitation.

For mouth-to-mouth resuscitation give ventilations with the victim's nostrils pinched. Take a regular breath and tightly seal the lips around the victim's mouth. Give one breath and watch for a rise in the victim's chest. Continue rescue breaths at a rate of 10–12 per minute. When the victim has a tracheostomy, give ventilations through the stoma.

Hands only CPR

Hands only CPR can be used to help adult victims who suddenly collapse from cardiac arrest outside health care setting. If such event is witnessed, choose to provide chest compressions only or conventional CPR. Both methods are effective when done in the first few minutes of an out of hospital cardiac arrest.

Evaluation

Evaluation is the final step of the nursing process. The nurse collects data to evaluate the effectiveness of interventions. If outcomes are not achieved, the nurse, client, and support person need to explore the reasons before modifying the care plan.

BIBLIOGRAPHY

1. Potter PA, Perry AG. Fundamentals of Nursing, 6th edition. Elsevier; New Delhi; 2008.
2. Taylor CR, Lillis C, LeMone P, et al. Fundamentals of Nursing - The Art and Science of Nursing Care, 7th edition. Wolters Kluwer; Gurugram; 2010.
3. Smeltzer SC. "Brunner and Siddhartha's Textbook of Medical Surgical Nursing". 11th edition. Lippincott Williams and Wilkins. pp. 2184-87.

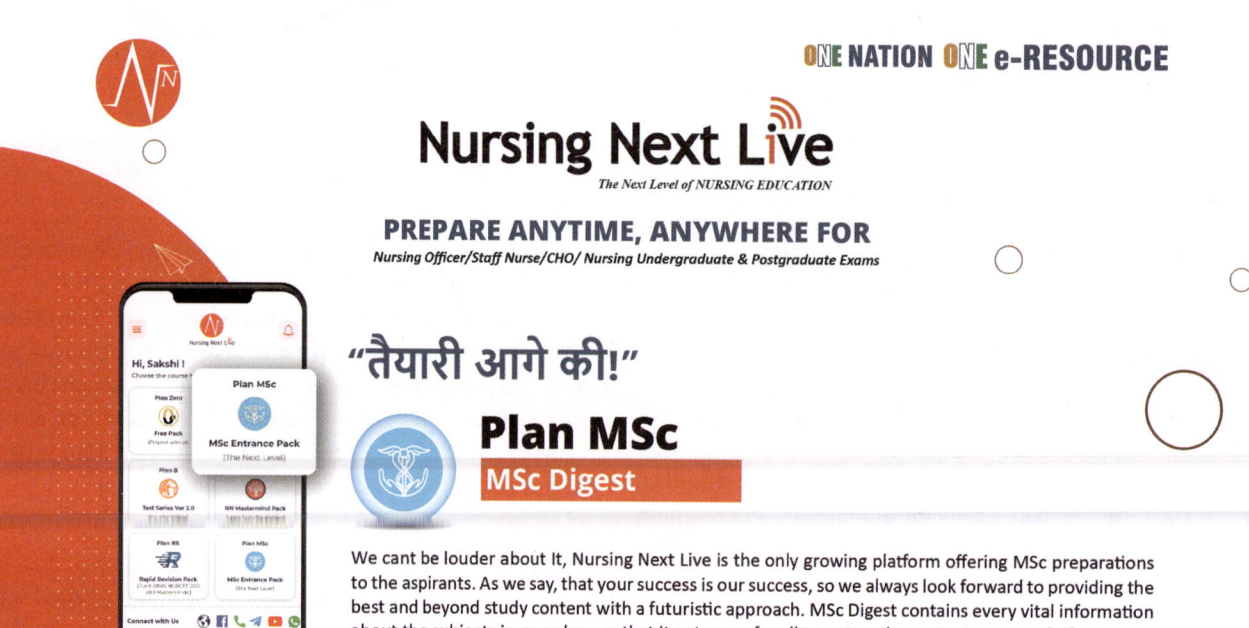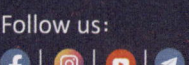

Cardiopulmonary Resuscitation

INTRODUCTION

Cardiopulmonary resuscitation/basic life support is a basic technique for oxygenating brain and heart until appropriate definite medical treatment can restore normal heart and ventilation.

REVIEW OF ANATOMY AND PHYSIOLOGY OF CARDIOVASCULAR SYSTEM

- Cardiovascular system (CVS) includes heart and blood vessels
- Heart pumps blood into the blood vessels
- Blood vessels circulate the blood throughout the body
- Blood transports nutrients and oxygen to the tissue and removes carbon dioxide and waste product from the body.

Heart

- Heart is a muscular organ and located in the left side of the mediastinum.
- The heart consists of three layers.
  - The epicardium is the outermost layer of the heart.
  - The myocardium is the middle layer and is actual contracting muscle of the heart.
- The endocardium is the innermost layer and lines the inner chamber and heart valves.

Pericardial Sac

Encases and protects the heart from trauma and infection. It has two layers:

* The parietal pericardium is the tough, fibrous outer membrane
* The visceral pericardium is thin, inner layer

The pericardial space is between the parietal and visceral layers; it holds 5 – 20 mL of pericardial fluid, which lubricates the pericardial surface and cushions the heart.

Heart Chambers and Valves

There are four heart chambers—right atrium, right ventricle, left ventricle and left atrium.

There are four valves in the heart—mitral valve, tricuspid valve, aortic valve and pulmonic valve.

Action of the Heart

Action of the heart are classified into four types:

* Chronotropic action is the frequency of heart beat or heart rate
* Inotropic action means force of contraction of heart.
* Dromotropic action is the conduction of impulse through heart.
* Bathmotropic action is the excitability of cardiac muscle.

Blood Vessels

* **Artery:** Carries blood from heart to tissues or cells.
* **Vein:** Carries blood from tissues or cells to heart.

Division of Circulation

* Systemic circulation
* Pulmonary circulation

Systemic Circulation

Also known as greater circulation. Blood pumped from left ventricle passes through all body systems for exchange of various substances between blood and the tissues and returns to right atrium of the heart.

Pulmonary Circulation

Also known as lesser circulation. Blood pumped from right ventricle goes to lungs through pulmonary artery for exchange of gases between blood and alveoli of the lungs and returns to left atrium.

IMPORTANT TERMINOLOGIES

Resuscitation

Resuscitation is a method, which includes all measures that are applied to revive patient who has stopped breathing suddenly and unexpectedly due to cardiac or respiratory failure.

Emergency

It is a sudden development of a cardiac/respiratory arrest that is likely to be dangerous for life, and calls for immediate action. In this care, patient needs resuscitation otherwise this will lead to brain hypoxia.

Cardiac Arrest

It is defined as abrupt cessation of cardiac function, which is potentially reversible. The heart may be in state of asystole.

Basic Life Support (BLS)

It is a maneuver that aims at maintaining a certain level of circulation until more definite treatment with **advanced life support** can be given. Management of collapsed client requires prompt assessment and restoration of circulation, airway and breathing.

Advanced Cardiac Life Support (ACLS)

In this, the steps of resuscitation combined with the use of medical equipment and drugs in the hospital setting are used to improve the survival rates. Early CPR coupled with early defibrillation is a very powerful combination.

It refers to a set of clinical intervention for the urgent treatment of cardiac arrest, stroke and other life-threatening medical emergencies as well as the knowledge and skill to deploy those interventions.

The three cardinal signs of cardiac arrest are:

1. Apnea
2. Absence of carotid and femoral pulse
3. Dilation of pupil.

CAUSES OF CARDIAC ARREST

* Coronary heart disease
* Cardiomyopathy
* Congestive heart failure
* Non cardiac cause–any trauma, drowning, suffocation, electric shock and severe allergic reactions.

SIGNS OF CARDIAC ARREST

* Unresponsiveness
* Sudden loss of consciousness
* Absence of carotid pulse
* Cessation of respiration: No chest wall movement
* Dilation of pupils
* Marked cyanosis

INDICATIONS OF CPR

Cardiac Arrest

- Ventricular fibrillation
- Ventricular tachycardia
- Asystole
- Pulseless electrical activity

Respiratory Arrest

It is the cessation of effective respiration.

- Drowning
- Stroke
- Foreign body in throat
- Smoke inhalation (Suffocation)
- Drug overdose
- Electrocution or injury by lightning
- Suffocation
- Accident, injury
- Coma
- Epiglottis paralysis.

PURPOSES OF CPR

- To maintain blood circulation by chest compressions (C).
- To maintain an open and clear airway (A).
- To maintain breathing by artificial ventilation (B).
- To provide basic life support till advanced life support arrives.

STEPS OF BLS/ACLS

Following are the approaches in the emergency.

Scene Safety

Scene should be safe for the rescuer and the victim.

Check Responsiveness

- Tap the person's shoulder and shout, ''Are you ok?''
- Look for normal breathing. Call national helpline number 102 for ambulance if there is no response.

Breathing Assessment

Scan the chest at eye level from head end, sides or foot end to find out chest movements. Take only 5–10 seconds for this.

Check Carotid Pulse

- By doing head tilt, chin lift method
- Find the groove between the thyroid notch and the sternomastoid muscle. Here pulse can be felt
- Check the pulse of only one side at a time.
- Take only 5–10 seconds.

Call for Help

- Call ambulance
- Give all information like:
  - Self-identification
  - Place (venue) from where you are calling, number of patients (single or mass causality)
  - Approximate age of the victim (e.g., middle-aged)
  - Condition of the patient like gasping, no breathing, presence or absence of pulse.
  - Whether you are going to start CPR or not.
  - Ask them to send an emergency medical service (EMS) team with automated external defibrillator (AED).
  - Do not disconnect the call, unless you get the reply or message to do so from the other end.

Do Chest Compressions

- Place the victim on a hard surface in supine position, push the clothes aside, and start with early chest compressions.
- Kneel at victim's side.
- Locate the lower rib margin using index finger of the hand and move the fingers up to the point where rib connects the sternum.
- Place the heel of the hand on the center of the person's chest along the nipple line, lower half of the sternum.
- Place the heel of the other hand on top of the first hand, interlacing fingers together, do not allow them to touch the chest.
- Keep arms straight and the shoulders directly over the hands (chest of the victim). Begin 5 cycles of CPR.
- Compress the chest of adult for 2 – 2.4 inches depth at a rate of 100–120 compressions per minute.
- Allow complete recoil of the chest and do not lift hands off chest.
- Provide 30 chest compressions, followed by two ventilations and evaluate after four cycles.
- Then continue with chest compressions. Do not interrupt chest compressions to check pulse.
- The compression rate is 100–120 per minute and compression ventilation ratio is 30:2 (one or two rescuers).

Airway

- Open airway by head tilt, chin lift or maneuver.
- In trauma patients, jaw thrust method should be adopted.

Breathing (Ventilation)

- Occlude the victim's nostrils with thumb and index finger of the hand with head tilted backward.

- Provide two full breaths for 0.5–2 seconds either with mouth-to-mouth method or Ambu bag.
- Observe for the rise and fall of the chest.
- Provide approximately 6–8 rescue breaths/min
- Recheck pulse every 2 minutes

Automated External Defibrillator (Use an AED)

- AED is a device that automatically analyzes the heart rhythm and can send an electric shock to the heart to restore normal rhythm.
- Turn on the AED
- Wipe chest dry
- Attach the pads, after putting jelly
- Plug in connector, if needed.
- Make sure no one is touching the person. Say "I clear, you clear, everybody clear" so that people know to stay back and not touch the person
- Push the "Analyze" button, if necessary
- If a shock is advised, push the "Shock" button
- Resume compressions and follow AED prompts.

Continue compressions and breaths—30 compressions, two breaths—until help arrives. After a shock, the cycle starts from the beginning.

If pulse is there, give rescue breaths 10–12 bpm.

Note: AEDs are used to treat sudden cardiac arrest (SCA)

Stop only if:
- The person starts breathing normally
- A trained responder or emergency help takes over
- Too exhausted to continue.
- There is an automated external defibrillator (AED) to use.

UNDERSTANDING OF ABC FOR CPR

CPR Consists of Six Main Parts

1. **A**   Airway
2. **B**   Breathing
3. **C**   Circulation
4. **D**   Drugs/Defibrillation
5. **E**   Endotracheal intubation
6. **F**   Fluids

The CPR tray is shown in (Fig. 1).

A

Opening the Airway

The following methods are used:
- Abdominal thrust

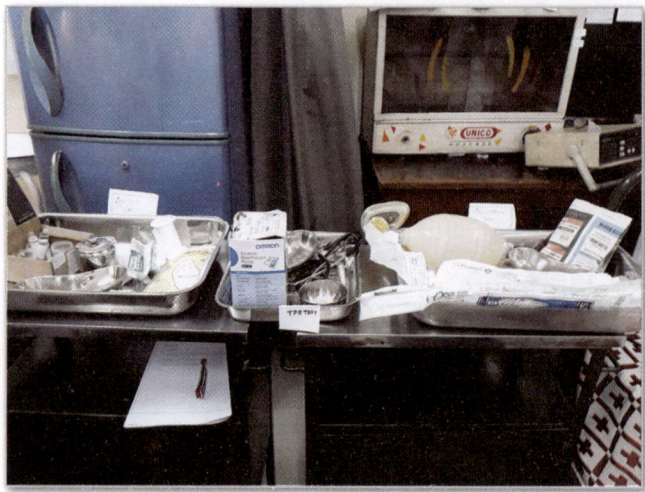

Fig. 1: CPR tray

- Head tilt/chin lift
- Finger sweep
- Jaw thrust

Abdominal Thrust

- Stand or kneel behind the victims and wrap arms around the victim's waist
- Make a fist with one hand
- Place thumb side of the fist against the victim's abdomen, in the midline slightly above the navel and below the breast bone
- Grasp the fist with another hand and press it into victim's abdomen with a quick upward thrust
- Repeat it until the object is expelled
- This is called as Heimlich maneuver.

To Perform Head Tilt/Chin Lift Maneuver

- Place the hand on victim's forehead and push palm to tilt the head back
- Place the finger of the other hand under the bony part of the lower jaw near the chin
- Lift the jaw to bring the chin forward

Finger Sweep

- A gloved finger is swept through the mouth of the victim so as to clear the mouth
- Care should be taken that finger must not go very deep.

Jaw Thrust Maneuver

- Place finger of the other hand under the bony part of lower jaw forward and teeth almost to occlusion (triple maneuver)

- Grasp the angle of patient jaw and lifting with both the hands, one on either side displace the mandible forward, while tilting the head backward
- This is jaw thrust technique and it is the safest method in suspected spinal injury.

B

Giving Breathing

- Mouth-to-mouth breathing
- Mouth-to-nose breathing
- Mouth-to-stoma breathing
- Mouth-to-mask breathing

Mouth-to-Mouth Breathing

- Hold the victim's airway with head tilt and chin lift
- Pinch the nose with thumb and index finger
- Form airtight seal and prevent air from escaping the nose
- Give one breath blow for one second watch for chest for rise
- If chest doesn't rise give the second breath.

Mouth-to-Nose Breathing

- Here the mouth of victim held tightly close with one of rescuer hand and rescuer hand is placed over the nose of victim and breaths are delivered.
- This is done in case when mouth-to-mouth breathing is not possible

Mouth-to-Stoma Breathing

Breaths are given directly into opening made in trachea called tracheostomy

Mouth-to-Mask Breathing

- Position yourself at the side of victim
- Place mask on victim's face
- Place hand along with sides of mask
- Place thumb of the another hand on lower margin of the mask
- Place remaining fingers of other hand closure to victim's neck at the bony portion of jaw and lift the jaw
- While lifting the jaw press firmly around the margin of mask against the face
- Deliver air over 1 second to make the victim's chest rise.

C

Circulation

Pericardial Thump

It is a blow which is delivered to the lower half of sternum with the fleshy part of fist, from 8 inches to 12 inches above patient's chest.

This blow generates a small current of electricity, which transmit shock to the myocardium and stimulates heartbeat and circulation.

To be effective, it should be done within 1 minute of arrest otherwise it can produce ventricular fibrillation

Reasons to discontinuing pericardial thump

- Poor success rate of 20–25%
- Untrained person, if perform can lead to further injury and can produce ventricular fibrillation

Cardiac Compression (Fig. 2)

- Place your hand on the breastbone at nipple line
- Remove all clothing to see patient's chest
- Put the heel of one hand on the center of patient's bare chest between the nipple
- The artificial breathing and cardiac massage should be corresponding to normal respiration and pulse rate. The ratio should be 30:2, i.e., 30 compressions to 2 ventilation. Compress chest 2–2.4 inches, 100–120 times/min
- Ventilate lungs with two slow rescue breaths.
- Reassess the victim after four complete cycle (30:2)

D

Defibrillation/AED

An AED analyzes the heart rhythm to identify the presence of a rhythm that responds to shock therapy (also called shockable rhythm) If ventricular fibrillation (VF) or ventricular

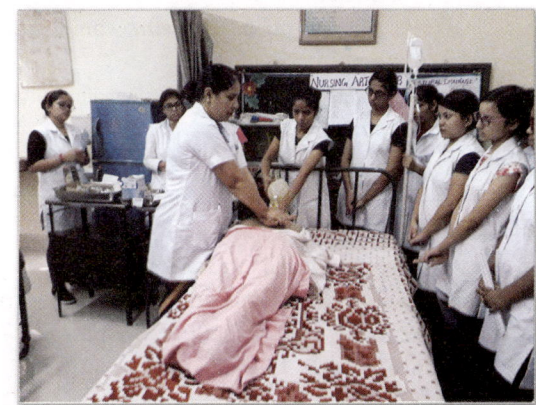

Fig. 2: Cardiac compression administration

tachycardia (VT) is identified, the device prompts the delivery of an electrical shock to the heart. This stops the VF or VT and "resets" the electrical system of the heart, so a normal heart rhythm can return.

Drugs

The main drugs used in CPR are:

- Adrenergics
  - Dopamine hydrochloride
  - Epinephrine
- Antiarrhythmics
  - Adenosine
  - Amiodarone hydrochloride
  - Atropine
- Electrolytes and Buffers
  - Sodium bicarbonate
  - Calcium chloride
  - Magnesium sulfate

General Instructions for Effective CPR

- Cardiopulmonary resuscitation CPR techniques are used in a person whose respirations and circulation of blood have suddenly and unexpectedly stopped.
- There is no need to attempt CPR techniques in a patient in the last stage of an incurable illness and in a person whose heart beat has been absent for more than 6 minutes.
- The immediate responsibilities of a resuscitator are:
  - To recognize the signs of cardiac arrest
  - Protect the patient's brain from anoxia by immediately starting artificial ventilation and cardiac massage
  - Call for help.
- The CPR must be started within 3–4 minutes in order to prevent permanent brain damage.
  - Strike the center of the chest sharply with the side of the clenched fist twice
  - Call for assistance
  - Clear the airway of false teeth, vomitus, food material, etc.
  - Initiate ventilation and external cardiac massage without wasting time
- CPR techniques should not be discontinued for more than 5 seconds before normal ventilation of lung and circulation established, except:
  - When patient is moved to a hard surface.
  - When endotracheal intubation is being carried out (maximum time for these two procedures is 15 seconds)

- Before CPR is attempted in a patient make sure that airway is clear. So keep the neck hyperextended after confirming that he is having any cervical injuries or not.
  - If the food material has been lodged deep into trachea and giving resistance to the entry of air in to lungs
  - To prevent the tongue falling back and obstructing the airway by head tilt chin lift method or jaw thrust manoeuvre.
- The artificial breathing and cardiac massage should be corresponding to normal respiration and pulse rate. The ratio should be 5:1, i.e., 5 cardiac compressions to 1 ventilation
- A nasogastric intubation and aspiration of gastric content are necessary for a patient with full stomach to prevent vomiting and aspiration.

PREPARATION FOR CPR

Preparation of Patient and Environment

- No time should be wasted in explaining the procedure to the patient and relatives.
- If someone is free he/she can explain the procedure in simple and native language
- Ask them to leave the room to lessen distraction and fasten the rescue work.
- The patient may be shifted to hard surface or board
- Remove or push aside the clothing, which covered the patient's chest to observe for cardiac beats and respiration.
- Place the patient on his/her back without any pillow. This position helps in maintaining airway and giving cardiac compression.
- Tight clothing around the chest and neck should be removed.
- Ensure fresh air in room by opening windows and doors.
- External cardiac massage must be started within 4–6 minutes following the cardiac arrest otherwise irreversible brain damage occurs due to oxygen deprivation.

Preparation for Articles

Equipment

A tray containing the following articles
- Endotracheal tubes of various sizes (7, 5, 8)
- An Ambu bag with mask
  - Stillet (in a plastic cover)
  - Megal's forceps (in a plastic cover)
- A suction tube or catheter

- Laryngoscope with different sizes of blades
- Nasal airways
- Oral airways
- Gloves in a cover
- A kidney tray
- A paper bag
- Masks of various sizes
- Local anesthetic agent (xylocaine 2% and 4%)
- Disposable syringes with needles
- An IV set or cut down set
- Syringes with needles, cannulas and cotton pad
- A bowl with gauze pieces
- Lubricating jelly
- Adhesive tape, scissor and torch

Others

- Oxygen inhalation (central supply)
- Suction point (central supply)
- Defibrillation

A tray containing following emergency drugs:

- Injection adrenaline
- Injection atropine
- Injection digoxine
- Injection sodium bicarbonate
- Injection dopamine
- Injection efcorlin
- Injection decadron
- Injection avil
- Injection calcium gluconate
- Injection Lasix
- Injection aminophylline
- Injection calmpose
- Injection 20% dextrose
- Injection deriphyllin

Signs of Effective Resuscitation

- Constriction of pupils, key sign that brain is sufficiently oxygenated
- Distinct carotid pulsation with each cardiac compression
- Blinking upon stimulation of eyelids
- Breathing begins spontaneously
- Movement and struggling
- Decrease in cyanosis

INEFFECTIVE RESUSCITATION DUE TO CPR

- Incorrect resuscitation techniques
- Heart is drained of its blood by hemorrhage and cardiac tamponade
- Blood supply to the heart is obstructed by the presence of pulmonary embolus
- Severe chronic lung disease has destroyed lungs' capacity to oxygenate the blood
- Lungs are filled with vomitus as a result of aspiration during cardiac massage.

CARE FOLLOWING CPR

- Skilled aftercare is needed for the patient after CPR
- The patient should be continuously monitored for 48–72 hours in intensive care unit.
- Give oxygen continuously for 48 hours following resuscitation, this is necessary because respiration is depressed in some patients after CPR
- Monitor ECG, CVP, BP and respiration continuously
- Frequently check victim's head and jaw position because his tongue may fall back and obstruct airway
- Temperature should be taken every hour. A high temperature usually indicates cerebral damage or edema.
- Blood gases and pH to check metabolic/respiratory, acidosis/alkalosis.
- Check the color of skin, persistent cyanosis indicates inadequate oxygenation.
- A portable chest X-ray film is obtained, ribs can be accidently fractured and also to check the location of all the tubes.
- Insert Foley's catheter to monitor hourly urine output, report if less than 30 mL/hr
- Watch for convulsions. It may occur due to brain damage or acidosis.
- Start IV infusion to administer enough fluids to patient
- If patient is not intubated, insert an endotracheal tube, it will help to open airway in unconscious patient
- A nasogastric insertion and aspiration of contents is necessary for a patient with full stomach to prevent vomiting and aspiration of contents.

COMPLICATION DURING CPR

- Fracture of the ribs and xiphoid process
- Pneumothorax
- Damage to cervical spine due to hyperextension of neck
- Intra-abdominal hemorrhage
- Aspiration of vomitus into lungs
- Gastric distension with air
- Hemopericardium

RECORDING

- Record the procedure on the nurse's record with date and time
- Time when the victim was discovered
- Type of arrest (respiratory/cardiac/both)
- Any complication developed during the procedure time at which spontaneous respiration and pulse returned
- Time at which CPR started and discontinued
- Vital signs when CPR team left the patient
- What are the medicines given (with dosage and route of administration)?
- Result of CPR also must be mentioned.

BIBLIOGRAPHY

1. *Sembulingam K, Sembulingam P. Essential of Medical Physiology, 6th edition. Jaypee Brothers Medical Publisher (P) Ltd; New Delhi; pp. 519–24.*

2. *Silvestri LA. Saunder Comprehensive Review for the NCLEX-RN Exams, 5th edition, Elsevier, pp 785.*

3. *Smeltzer SC, Bare BG, Hinkle, et al. Brunner & Suddarth's Textbook of Medical-Surgical Nursing, 12th edition. Lippincott Williams & Wilkins; 2009.*

4. *Black JM, Hawks JH. Medical-Surgical Nursing: Clinical Management for Positive Outcomes, 8th edition. WB Saunders; Philadelphia; 2009.*

5. *Chintamani, M Mrinalini. Lewis's Medical Surgical Nursing, 1st edition. Mosby Publication; 2010.*

Psychosocial Needs

CONCEPT OF CULTURAL DIVERSITY

The society we live in consists of many diverse backgrounds. Cultural diversity includes but is not limited to people of varying cultures, racial and ethnic origin, religions, languages, physical size, gender, sexual orientation, age, disability, socioeconomic status, occupational status and geographic location. The essential knowledge and skills of understanding cultural diversity and providing culturally competent care have become essential components of nursing practice. To be able to provide cultural competent care to people from diverse backgrounds, nurses must be sensitive to these factors. It is also vital to remember that each individual may be a member of multiple cultural, ethnic, and racial groups at one time. Therefore, different cultural values may guide an individual in different situations based on what is most important to them at the time.

CULTURE

Culture may be defined as a shared system of beliefs, values, and behavioral expectations that provides social structure for daily living. Culture defines roles and interactions with others as well as within families and communities and is apparent in the attitudes unique to particular groups. (Andrew and Bowle, 2008). The **characteristics of culture** include the following:

- Culture guides what is acceptable behavior for people in a specific group
- Culture is learned by each new generation through both formal and informal life experiences.
- Language is the primary means of transmitting culture.
- Culture practices and beliefs may evolve over time, but they mainly remain constant as long as they satisfy a group's needs
- Culture influences the way people of a group view themselves, have expectations, and behave in response to certain situations

There are **subcultures** within most cultures. A subculture is a large group of people who are members of an even larger cultural group, but who have certain ethnic, occupational, or physical characteristics that are not common to the larger culture.

Societies include dominant culture groups and minority culture groups.

A dominant group is the group that has the most ability to control the values and sanctions of the society. It is usually the largest group in a society.

Minority groups usually have same physical or cultural characteristic such as race, religion, beliefs or occupation that identifies the people within it as different from the dominant group.

Cultural assimilation occurs when a minority group lives with a dominant group, many of their members may lose the cultural characteristics that once made them different, and their values may be replaced by the values of the dominant group.

Culture shock or the feelings, a person experiences when placed in a different culture perceived as strange culture shock may result in psychological discomfort or disturbances, as the patterns of behavior a person found acceptable and effective in his or her culture may not be adequate or even acceptable to the new one. The person, may then feel inadequate, incompetent, or humiliated. These feelings eventually can lead to frustration, anxiety, and loss of self-esteem.

ETHNICITY

Ethnicity is a sense of identification with a collective cultural group, largely based on the group's common heritage. One belongs to a specific ethnic group either through birth or through adaption of certain characteristics of that group. People within the ethnic group generally share unique cultural and social beliefs and behavior patterns, including languages, religions practices, literature, music, political interests, food preferences, and employment patterns. Ethnicity largely develops through day-to-day life with family and friends within the community.

RACE

The term "Race" is often used interchangeably with ethnicity, these terms are not the same. Racial categories are typically based on specific physical characteristics such as skin pigmentation, body stature, facial features, and hair texture.

CULTURAL INFLUENCES ON HEALTH CARE

The process usually is multidirectional, for example, in a health care setting, the patient evaluates the attitudes and actions of the health care provider, at the same time the health care provider interprets the behavior of the patient, what may seem irrelevant and ridiculous to a nurse. The reverse is also true; practices a nurse perceives as logical and effective may seem senseless to a patient.

Physiologic Variations

Many studies have shown that certain racial and ethnic groups are more prone to developing specific diseases and conditions.

Reactions to Pain

Many of the expressions and behaviors exhibited by people in pain are culturally prescribed as shown by various health researches. Some cultures allow and even encourage the open expression of emotions experienced by a person in pain, whereas other cultures frown on the open and free expressions of emotions

For nurses, the main issue in this area of cultural expression is their attitude toward the patient. Nurses often assume that a patient who does not complain of pain is not having pain and may have his pain reduction needs ignored. To avoid this, be sensitive to other signals of discomfort, such as holding or applying pressure to the painful area, self-restriction of activities that intensify the pain, facial grimacing and moaning. Nurses should also consider-patients who freely express his discomfort as constant complainers whose request for pain relief seems excessive. Pain is a warning from the body that something is wrong, so it needs to be assessed carefully and care must be individualized.

Mental Health

Many people deal with problems related to mental health within the family and would view it as inappropriate to tell problems to a stranger. Many people consider mental illness a stigma, therefore, seeking psychiatric help would be a disgrace to the family. As nurses, they need to be aware of these variations and accept them as culturally appropriate.

Gender Roles

In many cultures, the man is the dominant figure and generally makes decisions for all family members. For example, if approval of medical care is needed, the man gives it regardless of which family member is involved. In male-dominant cultures, women are usually passive. On the other hand, in some cultures like African and American families, the women are often dominant.

Knowing the dominant member of the family is important when planning nursing care.

Language and Communication

When people from different cultures, with different background, with many languages spoken, communication problems can arise during health care activities. Even in different regions of the country, certain dialects or word meanings can cause differences in understanding. Nurses, who work in a geographic area where people speak a language other than English, need to learn pertinent words and phrases in that language. Sometimes a family member or friend can translate for the nurse.

CULTURAL INFLUENCES ON HEALTH AND ILLNESS

People's values and belief, about health, illness and care for an illness develop as a direct result of cultural and ethnic influences. For example, in some groups, illness is classified as natural or unnatural.

"Natural illnesses" are caused by dangerous agents, such as cold air or impure water, air or food. "Unnatural illness" are punishments for failing to follow God's rules, resulting in evil forces or witchcraft causing physical or mental health problems.

In some cultures, the power to heal is thought to be a gift from God bestowed on certain people. People in these cultures believe traditional healers for treatment and think health care providers as incompetent to treat an illness.

People from different cultures may also have different beliefs about best way to treat an illness or disease. For example, use of herbs is common method of treatment. Other types of traditional therapies include the use of cutaneous stimulation, therapeutic touch, acupuncture, acupressure.

CULTURALLY COMPETENT NURSING CARE

Culturally competent nursing care means that care is planned and complemented in a way that is sensitive to the needs of individuals, families, and groups from diverse populations within society (Fig. 1). The nurse who recognizes and

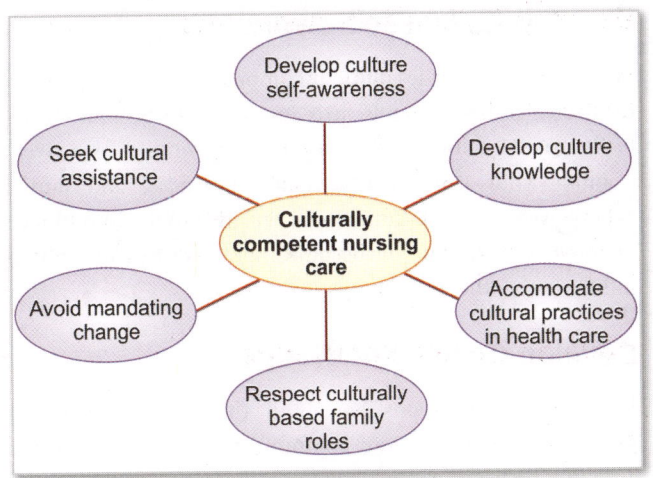

Fig. 1: Culturally competent nursing care

respects cultural diversity will be better equipped to exhibit cultural sensitivity and provide nursing care that accepts the significance of cultural factors in health and illness. National standards issued by the office of Minority Health (2001) were developed in response to the need to ensure that all people entering the health care system be provided equitable and effective treatment in a culturally and linguistically appropriate manner.

Some of the additional guidelines that are useful in providing appropriate nursing care (Table 1).

TABLE 1: Assuring cultural competence in health care

- Ensure that all patients/consumers receive from all staff members effective, understandable, and respectful care that is provided in a manner compatible with their cultural health beliefs and practices and preferred language.
- Implement strategies to recruit, retain, and promote at all levels of the organization a diverse staff and leadership that are representative of the demographic characteristics of the service area.
- Ensure that staff at all levels and across all disciplines receives ongoing education and training in culturally and linguistically appropriate service delivery.
- Offer and provide language assistance services, including bilingual staff and interpreter services, at no cost to each patient/consumer with limited English proficiency at all points of contact in a timely manner during all hours of operation.
- Make available the easily understood patient-related materials and post signs in the language of the commonly encountered groups and/or groups represented in the service area.
- Ensure that data on the individual patient's/consumer's race, ethnicity, and spoken and written language are collected in health records, integrated into the organization's management information systems, and periodically updated.
- Maintain a current demographic, cultural, and epidemiological profile of the community, as well as a needs assessment to accurately plan and implement services

Develop Culture Self-awareness

Before you can provide culturally competent care to the patients from diverse backgrounds, it is important to become aware of the role of cultural influences in your own life, objectively examine your own beliefs, values, practices, and family experiences. As you become more sensitive to the importance of these factors, you will become more sensitive to cultural influences in others' lives.

Develop Culture Knowledge

Learn as much as possible about the belief system and practices of people in your community and of people in the area in which you work. Practice techniques of observation and listening to acquire knowledge of the beliefs and values of patients for whom you are caring.

Accommodate Cultural Practices in Health Care

Incorporate factors from the patient's cultural background into health care whenever possible and when the practices are not considered harmful to health. Modify care to include traditional practices as much as possible and be an advocate for patients from diverse culture groups.

Accommodate the cultural dietary practices of patients as much as possible. Teaching patients and families about therapeutic diets can also be done within the framework of particular cultural practices. Families may be encouraged to bring food from home for patients with particular preferences when this practice does not violate policy.

Respect Culturally Based Family Roles

Take into consideration the cultural role of the family member who takes most of the important decisions. In some cultures, it is the husband or father, whereas in others, it is the grandmother or any other elderly person. To disregard this fact is to proceed with nursing care that is not approved by this person can result in conflict so it is important to involve this person in the nursing care planning.

Avoid Mandating Change

Keep in mind that health practices are part of all cultures and changing them may have widespread implication for the person. Do not force the client to participate in care that conflicts with their values. If the client is forced to accept it the care may become harmful because it will result in feelings of guilt and alienation from a religious or cultural group, which could threaten the patients' well-being.

Seek Cultural Assistance

Seek assistance of a respected family member, member of the clergy, or traditional healer, so that patient is more likely to accept health care services. This may be an important way of building trust, respect and cooperation.

STRESS AND ADAPTATION

Stress is a universal phenomenon. Everybody experiences it. Parents refer to the stress of raising children, working people talk about the stress of their jobs, and students talk about the stress they experience in schools and colleges. Stress can result in both positive and negative experiences. When the equilibrium of the body is disturbed, stress occurs.

Stress is a condition in which the person experiences changes in the normal balanced state.

A stressor is an event or stimulus that causes an individual to experience stress.

Sources of Stress

There are many sources of stress. They can be broadly classified as internal or external stressors, or developmental or situational stressors.

- *Internal stressors* originate within a person, for example, infection or feelings of depression.
- *External stressors* originate outside the individual, for example a move to another city, a death in the family, or pressure from peers.
- Developmental *stressors* occur at *predictable* times throughout an individual's life. *Situational stressors* are unpredictable and may occur at any time during life.
- *Situational stress* may be positive or negative, e.g., death of a family member, marriage or divorce, birth of a child, new job, illness, etc.

The degree to which any of these events has positive or negative effects can depend to some extent on an individual's developmental stage as shown in Table 2.

Effects of Stress

Stress affects the whole personality of a person as it can have physical, emotional, intellectual, social, and spiritual consequences (Table 3). Physically, stress can threaten a person's physiologic homeostasis. Emotionally, stress can produce negative feelings about the self. Intellectually, stress can influence a person's perceptual and problem-solving abilities. Socially, stress can alter a person's relationships with others. Spiritually, stress can challenge one's beliefs and values. Stress disturbs the homeostasis of the organism and it results in the person's disability to adapt himself or herself according to situation.

TABLE 2: Selected stressors associated with developmental stages

Developmental stage	Stressor
Child	◆ Beginning school ◆ Establishing peer relationships ◆ Peer competition
Adolescent	◆ Changing physique ◆ Relationships involving sexual attraction ◆ Exploring independence ◆ Choosing a career
Young adult	◆ Marriage ◆ Leaving home ◆ Managing a home ◆ Getting started in an occupation ◆ Continuing one's education ◆ Children
Middle adult	◆ Physical changes of aging ◆ Maintaining social status and standard of living ◆ Helping teenage children to become independent ◆ Aging parents
Older adult	◆ Decreasing physical abilities and health ◆ Changes in residence ◆ Retirement and reduced income ◆ Death of spouse and friends

TABLE 3: Common signs and symptoms of stress

Physical effects	Psychological effects
◆ Dry mouth ◆ Rapid pulse ◆ Rapid shallow breathing ◆ Increased perspiration ◆ Shakiness and tremors ◆ Increased blood pressure ◆ Frequent urination ◆ Muscle lesion ◆ Inability to sit still ◆ Talking rapidly, stammering ◆ "Butterflies" in stomach ◆ Inability to control tears	◆ Confusion and forgetfulness ◆ Anxiety ◆ Irritability ◆ Labile moods ◆ Quick to anger ◆ Depression

Adaptation

To adapt is to respond to change. The systems of the body have self-regulatory mechanisms to maintain homeostasis. These mechanisms require pathways of communication between the brain and the various body systems. Coordination of the central nervous system, autonomic nervous system, and the endocrine system is required for the body to adjust, adapt and maintain equilibrium.

The central nervous system consisting of the brain and spinal cord, coordinates adaptation within the body. Cortex, the thinking part of the brain, communicates with the midbrain and brain stem, which contains many of the structures involved in adaptation and maintenance of physiologic functions. Along with the action of the endocrine glands these structures regulate breathing, heart action, blood pressure, body temperature, hunger and sleepiness.

The reticular activating system (RAS), a bundle of nerve fibers in the brain stem, transmits messages to the cortex from the sensory receptors of the body and carries messages back to the hypothalamus in the midbrain to regulate physiologic functions. The hypothalamus helps regulate the autonomic nervous system and the secretion of hormones by the endocrine system.

The autonomic nervous system regulates physiologic functions that are essentially automatic and beyond voluntary control. It is divided into the sympathetic and parasympathetic nervous systems. When the brain perceives a stimulus as threatening, the sympathetic nervous system stimulates the physiologic functions needed for fight or flight. Once the threatening situation is over the parasympathetic nervous system works to restore equilibrium. The glands of the endocrine system produce hormones that act on other organs or systems of the body. Initiation of a stimulus for hormone production comes from the cortex of the brain and travels to the hypothalamus. The hypothalamus activates the pituitary gland, which in turn secretes hormones that stimulate the other endocrine glands. As long as the body's capacity is not over-taxed, the central nervous system, autonomic nervous system, and endocrine systems regulate body systems to maintain homeostasis.

General Adaptation Syndrome (GAS)

Hans Selye, a Canadian physician in 1950, published his research-based theories on stress. He found that no matter what the nature of the stressor was, the same nonspecific physical response occurred. The body attempted to deal with stressors by secretion of hormones that caused adaptive responses. Selye concluded that stress plays a role in every disease process because of faulty adaptation (maladaptation) by the body. If the body overreacts in defending itself, there is surplus of hormones that are favorable to the development of inflammation, etc. may develop. When the body underreacts, too many inflammatory hormones are circulating and serious infection or peptic ulcers may result. Selye states that a general adaptation syndrome (GAS) occurs in response to long-term exposure to stress. The stages are the: **alarm stage**, the **stage of resistance** and the **stage of exhaustion**. Brief stress responses result in adjustment by homeostatic mechanisms and equilibrium is restored. During the alarm stage, hormone released mobilizes the body's defences. Nonspecific signs of illness such as slight rise on temperature, a loss of energy, decreased appetite and a general feeling of malaise occur.

During the second stage, the stage of resistance, the body is battling for equilibrium. If this stage is excessive or prolonged, the response becomes maladaptive and a pathologic condition occurs, which may be in the form of a stress-related disorder.

The stage of exhaustion occurs if the stressor is severe enough or is present over a long enough period of time to deplete the body's resources for adaptation. Critical illness or death results. Stressor that causes the GAS includes trauma, burns, infection, severe cold, and emotional upsets.

The body adapts to local stressors also in similar ways. The local response is called the local adaptation syndrome (LAS). This takes place within a single organ or area of the body, such as injury or cut finger become inflamed.

Coping

Coping means adjusting to or solving challenges. Coping mechanisms helps us to resist and master stressors. Coping mechanisms are learned and once used successfully, they become part of our psychological defence armor. Common patient stressors are enlisted in Table 4.

TABLE 4: Common patient stressors

• Having to wear an ill-fitting gown that opens down the back • Sharing a room with a stranger • Being dependent on others for toileting or bathing • Sleeping in a different bed with a different pillow • Eating meals at different times than usual • Being awakened at odd hours and many times • Too many or too few visitors • Worrying about medical costs, home bills, family needs • Being uncertain of the diagnosis and what will happen • Not understanding medical terms	• Have to deal with many health care people who are strangers • Not being able to obtain desired foods, drinks or objects • Being left on a stretcher in a hall without sufficient warm covers • Have to wait for tests to be done or for the doctor to come • Being pieced with a needle repeatedly for laboratory specimens or intravenous (IV) therapy • Having other health care workers barge in during toileting or cleansing • Having different personnel providing care each day

There are three types of coping responses:

1. Actions or thoughts that change the situation so it is no longer stressful
2. Alteration of thoughts to control the meaning of the situation before it triggers a stress response
3. Control of thoughts and actions to stop a stress reaction. Ways to achieve these responses are:
   - Seeking information (eliminates fear of unknown)
   - Taking direct action (taking yourself away from a dangerous situation)
   - Stopping an unhelpful reaction (refraining) from shouting or throwing things when angry

   - Discussing the situation with someone from your social support system
   - Using defence mechanisms to perceive the situation differently.

Defence mechanisms are strategies that protect us from increasing anxiety. Defence mechanisms both reduce anxiety and the secretion of stress hormones. Defence mechanisms are used to maintain and improve our self-esteem. Unconsciously using defence mechanism gives us time to solve the problems and adopt in a positive manner. Using defence mechanisms relieves tension and lessens anxiety. They can be overused in a maladaptive way as well. (Table 5)

TABLE 5: Common defense mechanisms

Defense mechanism	Characteristics	Example
Repression	Blocking a wish or desire from conscious expression	You forget the name of someone for whom you have intense negative feelings
Projection	Attributing an unconscious impulse, attitude or behavior to someone else (blaming or scapegoating)	A man who is attracted to his friend's wife on an unconscious level accuses his own wife of flirting with his friend
Reaction-formation	An intense feeling regarding an object, person, or feeling is out of awareness and is unknowingly acted out consciously in an opposite manner	You treat someone whom you unconsciously dislike intensely in an overly friendly manner

Contd...

Defense mechanism	Characteristics	Example
Regression	Returning to an earlier level of adaptation when severely threatened	A child resumes bed-wetting after having long since stopped when his baby brother is born and fussed over at home
Rationalization	Unconsciously falsifying an experience by giving a contrived, socially acceptable and logical explanation to justify an unpleasant experience or questionable behavior	A student who did not study for an examination blames his failure on the teacher's poor lecture material and the unfairness of the examination
Identification	Modeling behavior after someone else	A 6-year-old girl dresses up in her mother's dress and high-heeled shoes
Displacement	Discharging intense feelings for one person onto another object satisfying an impulse with a substitute object	A child who has been scolded by her mother hits her doll with a hairbrush
Sublimation	Rechanneling an impulse into a more socially desirable object.	A student satisfies sexual curiosity by conducting sophisticated research into sexual behaviors

STRESS REDUCTION TECHNIQUES

There are various stress reduction techniques that help reduce stress and anxiety in patients (Table 6).

TABLE 6: Measures to help reduce stress and anxiety in patients

• Explain everything– hospital routine, TV, lights, curtains, procedures, and diagnostic tests	• Provide uninterrupted rest and sleep periods; coordinate care and treatments
• Listen carefully to the patient; answer questions.	• Keep visitors within acceptable numbers and time limits per patient's desire
• Provide privacy	
• Treat the patient with respect	• Keep noise to a minimum
• Answer call-lights promptly	• Insist that roommates respect each other's rights
• Protect confidentiality	• Try to keep patient advised as to when to expect diagnostic tests to be performed and when the doctor usually makes rounds
• Check on the patient frequently	
• Make certain that dietary needs and wants are satisfied as much as possible	• Allow the patient some control; give choice for time of bathing, ambulating, etc.
• Return to the patient's bedside when you say you will	• Keep the room temperature adjusted to patient's comfort
• Bring requested as-needed (PRN) medication promptly; do not allow pain to go untreated	

Other measures that help to control the degree of anxiety and reaction to stressors include progressive relaxation, imagery, massage, biofeedback, yoga, and meditation. Another method of stress reduction is regular physical exercise. Exercise causes release of endorphin which promotes a feeling of well-being and tranquility.

SELF-CONCEPT

Self-concept is one's mental image of oneself. A positive self-concept is essential to a person's mental and physical health. Individuals with a positive self-concept are better able to develop and maintain interpersonal relationships. An individual possessing a strong self-concept should be better able to accept or adapt to changes that may occur over the lifespan. How one views oneself self affects one's interaction with others.

Self-concept involves all of the self-perceptions appearance, values and beliefs that influence behavior and referred to when using the word I for me: self-concept is complex that influences the following:

- How one thinks, talks and acts
- How one sees and treats another person
- Choices one makes
- Ability to give and receive love
- Ability to take action and to change things.

Dimensions of Self-concept

There are four dimensions of self-concept.

Self-knowledge

Self-knowledge is the knowledge that one has about oneself, including insights into one's abilities, nature and limitations.

Self-expectation

Self-expectation is what one expects of oneself; may be a realistic or unrealistic expectation.

Social Self

Social self is how a person is perceived by others and society.

Social Evaluation

The appraisal of oneself in relationship to others, events or situations.

Many people are "me centered", i.e., they value "how I perceive me" they try hard to live up to their own expectations and compete only with themselves, not with the others. On the other side, there are people who value "how other perceive me," they are other centered people who have a high need for approval from others, competing, and evaluating themselves in relation to others. They are unable to assert themselves, and fear disapproval. The positive self-concept, therefore, is me centered and is formed with minimal reference to others opinions.

It is important for the nurse to promote a positive self-concept on the client. A nurse's own self-concept is also important. Nurses who understand the different dimensions of themselves are better able to understand the needs, desires, feelings, and conflicts of their clients. Nurses who feel positive about themselves are more likely to help clients meet their needs.

Self-awareness refers to the relationship between one's perception of himself or herself and others perceptions of him or her. Becoming more self-aware has perceptions that are very congruent. The nurse gains insight into the self through working with other nurses who serve as mentors and acting on the feedback obtained during regular performance reviews. Once the nurse has developed a clear understanding and awareness of self, the nurse can respect and avoid projecting his or her own beliefs on others.

Formation of Self-concept

A person is not born with a self-concept; rather, it develops as a result of social interactions with others.

According to Erikson (1963), throughout life people face developmental tasks associated with eight psychosocial stages, (Table 7). The success with which a person copes with these developmental tasks largely determines the development of self-concept. Difficulty in coping results in self-concept problems at the time and, often, later in life.

TABLE 7: Examples of behavior associated with Erikson's stages of psychosocial development

Stage: Developmental tasks	Behaviors indicating positive resolution	Behaviors indicating negative resolution
Infancy: Trust vs mistrust	Requesting assistance and expecting to receive it expressing belief of another person sharing time, opinions, and experiences	• Restricting conversation to superficialities • Refusing to provide a person with personal information • Being unable to accept assistance
Toddlerhood: Autonomy vs shame and doubt	• Accepting the rules of a group but also expressing disagreement when it is felt • Expressing one's own opinion • Easily accepting deferment of a wish fulfillment	• Failing to express needs • Not expressing one's own opinion when opposed • Over concern about being clean • Imitating others rather than developing independent ideas • Apologizing and being very embarrassed over small mistakes • Verbalizing fear about starting a new project
Early school years: Industry vs inferiority	• Completing a task once it has been started • Working well with others • Using time effectively	• Not completing tasks started • Not assisting with the work of others • Not organizing work
Adolescence: Identity vs role confusion	• Asserting independence • Planning realistically for future roles • Establishing close interpersonal relationship	• Failing to assume responsibility for directing one's own behavior • Accepting the values of others without question • Failing to set goals in life
Early adulthood: Intimacy vs isolation	• Establishing a close, intimate relationship with another person • Making a commitment to that relationship, even in times of stress and sacrifice • Accepting sexual behavior as desirable	• Remaining alone • Avoiding close interpersonal relationships
Middle-aged adults: Generativity vs stagnation	• Being willing to share with another person • Guiding others • Establishing a priority of needs, recognizing both self and others	• Talking about oneself instead of listening to others • Showing concern for oneself in spite of the needs of others • Being unable to accept interdependence
Older adults: Integrity vs despair	• Using past experience to assist others • Maintaining productivity in some areas • Accepting limitations	• Crying and being apathetic • Not accepting changes • Demanding unnecessary assistance and attention from others

- Lists examples of behaviors indicating successful and unsuccessful resolution of their development tasks.
- People are thought to base their self-concept on how they perceive and evaluate themselves in the following areas:
  - Vocational performance
  - Personal appearance and physical attractiveness
  - Intellectual functioning
  - Sexual attractiveness and performance
  - Being liked by others
  - Ability to cope with and resolve problems
  - Independence
  - Particular talents.

Self-concept in these areas also extends to the choices people make and perception they have about their health. Persons with strong positive self-concept about appearance are likely to value healthy behaviors and take action to maintain the health of their skin, hair, and body. Person with negative self-concept may be less proactive about health promotion and illness prevention activities. Maintaining and evaluating one's self-concept is an ongoing process. Events or situations may change the level of self-concept overtime. Having self-concept includes how we see ourselves and how we are seen by others.

Components of Self-concept

There are four components of self-concept: Personal identity, body image, role performance and self-esteem.

Personal Identity

Personal identity is the conscious sense of individuality and uniqueness that is continually evolving throughout life. People often view their identity in terms of name, sex, age, race, ethnic origin or culture, occupation or roles, talents and other characteristics such as marital status and education. Personal identity may also include beliefs, values, personality and character, e.g., the person is outgoing, friendly, reserved, generous, selfish. Identity is what distinguishes self from others. The individual with a strong sense of identity sees himself or herself as a unique person.

Body Image

The image of physical self is body image that how a person perceives the size, appearance, and functioning of the body and its parts. Body image has both cognitive and affective aspects. The cognitive is the knowledge of the material body; the affective includes the sensations of the body, such as pain, pleasure, fatigue, and physical movement. Body image is the sum of these attitudes, conscious and unconscious, that a person has toward his or her body. Body image includes clothing, makeup, hairstyle, jewelry, and other things intimately connected to the person. It also includes body prosthesis, such as artificial limbs, dentures, as well as devices required for functioning such as wheelchairs, canes and eyeglasses.

Body image of a person develops partly from other's attitudes and responses to that person's body and partly from the individual's own exploration of the body. Body image develops in infancy as the parents or caregivers respond to the child with smiles, holding, and touching, and as the child explores its own body sensations during breastfeeding, thumb sucking, and the bath. Cultural and societal values also influence a person's body image.

If a person's body image closely resembles with one's body ideal, the individual is more likely to think positively about self. A person with a healthy body image will normally show concern for both health and appearance. This person will seek for help if ill and will include health promoting practices in daily activities. A person who has an unhealthy body image is likely to be concerned about minor illness and neglect activities like sleep and a healthy diet that are important to health.

The person who has a body image disturbance may hide or not look at or touch a body part that is significantly changed in structure by illness or trauma. Some individuals may also express feelings of helplessness, hopelessness, powerlessness, and vulnerability, and may exhibit self-destructive behavior such as over- or under-eating, neglecting oneself or suicidal attempts.

Role Performance

A role is a set of expectations about how the person occupying one position or behaves. **Role performance** relates what a person in a particular role does to the behaviors expected of that role. Each person usually has several roles, such as husband, parent, brother, son, employee, friend, and nurse. Some roles are assumed for only limited periods such as client, student, and ill person.

Role mastery means that the person's behaviors meet social expectations. Expectations or standards of behavior of a role, are set by society.

Role development involves socialization into a particular role.

To act appropriately, people need to know who they are in relation to others and what society expects for the positions they hold.

Role ambiguity occurs when expectations are unclear, and people do not know what to do or how to do it and are unable to predict the reactions of others to their behavior. Failure to master a role creates frustration and feelings of inadequacy, often with consequent lowered self-esteem.

Self-concept is also affected by role strain and role conflicts. People undergoing role strain are frustrated because they feel or are made to feel inadequate or unsuited to a role. It is often associated with sex role stereotypes, for example, women in occupations traditionally held by men might be treated as having less knowledge and competence than man in the same roles.

Role conflicts arise from opposing or incompatible expectations. In an interpersonal conflict, people have different expectations about a particular role. For example, a grandparent may have different expectations than the mother about how she should care for her children. Role conflicts can lead to tension, decrease in self-esteem and embarrassment if needs for achievement, independence and recognition are unmet.

Self-esteem

Self-esteem is one's judgment of one's own worth, that is, how that person's standards and performances compare to others and to one's ideal self. If a person's self-esteem does not match with the ideal self, then low self-concept results. These are two types of self-esteem: global and specific.

- **Global self-esteem** is how much one likes oneself as a whole.
- **Specific self-esteem** is how much one approves of a certain part of oneself.

Global self-esteem is influenced by specific self-esteem. Self-esteem is derived from self and others. In infancy, self-esteem is related to the caregiver's evaluations and acceptances. Later the child's self-esteem is affected by competition with others. As an adult, a person who has high self-esteem has feelings of significance, competence, the ability to cope with life, and control over one's destiny.

The foundation for self-esteem is established during early life experiences, usually within the family structure. However, an adult's level of overall self-esteem may change markedly from day-to-day and moment to moment. Severe stress can substantially lower a person's self-esteem, for example, stress related to prolonged illness or unemployment. It is important that both strengths and weakness be identified.

Factors that Affect Self-concept

Many factors affect a person's self-concept. Major factors are—stage of development, family and culture, stressors, resources, history of success or failure, and illness.

Stage of Development

As an individual develops, the conditions that affect the self-concept change. For example, an infant enquires a supportive, caring environment, while a child requires freedom to explore and learn. Elder's self-concept is based on their experiences in progressing through life stages.

Family and Culture

A young child's values are largely influenced by the family and culture. Later on peers influence the child and thereby affect the sense of self. When the child is confronted by differing expectations from family, culture, and peers, the child's sense of self is often confused. For example, child may realize that his parents expect he will not drink alcohol and attend religious services every Sunday. At the same time, his peers drink beer and encourage him to spend Sundays with them.

Stressors

Stressors can strengthen self-concept as an individual copes successfully with his/her problems. On the other hand, overwhelming stressors can cause maladaptive responses including substance abuse, withdrawal and anxiety. The ability of a person to handle stressors will largely depend on personal resources.

Resources

An individual's resources are internal and external. Examples of internal resources include confidence and values, whereas external resources include support network, sufficient finances, and organizations. Generally the greater the number of resources a person has and uses, the more positive the effect on the self-concept.

History of Success or Failure

People with a history of success will have a more positive self-concept whereas people who have a history of failures see themselves as failures. People with positive self-concept tend to find contentment in their level of success while a negative self-concept can lead to viewing one's life situation as negative.

Illness

Illness and trauma can also affect the self-concept. A woman who has mastectomy may see herself as less attractive, and the loss may affect how she acts and values herself. People respond to stressors such as illness and alterations in function related to ageing in a variety of ways. Acceptance, denial, withdrawal, and depression are common reactions.

Many researches have shown that self-concept and health-related behavior are interwoven. People with positive self-concept may enhance their health and are likely to follow health care plan.

NURSING MANAGEMENT

Assessment

A thorough assessment includes a psychosocial assessment of the client and the family support to provide clues to actual or potential problems. The nurse assessing self-concept focuses on the four components, personal identity, body image, role performance and self-esteem. Before conducting a psychosocial assessment, the nurse must establish trust and a working relationship with the client. Identify the stressor and coping style of the client. (Table 8)

Diagnosing

Nursing diagnosis that may apply for clients with problems of self-concept include the following:
- Disturbed body image
- Ineffective role performance

TABLE 8: Stressors affecting self-concept

Personal identity stressors
• Change in physical appearance (e.g., facial wrinkles)
• Declining physical, mental, or sensory abilities
• Inability to achieve goals
• Relationship concerns
• Sexuality concerns
• Unrealistic ideal self
Body image stressors
• Loss of body parts (e.g., amputation, mastectomy, hysterectomy)
• Loss of body functions (e.g., from stroke, spinal cord injury neuromuscular disease, arthritis, declining mental or sensory abilities)
• Disfigurement (e.g., through pregnancy, severe burns, facial blemishes, colostomy and tracheostomy)
• Unrealistic body ideal (e.g., a muscular configuration that cannot be achieved)
Self-esteem stressors
• Lack of positive feedback from significant others
• Repeated failures
• Unrealistic expectations
• Abusive relationship
• Loss of financial security
Role stressors
• Loss of parent, spouse, child or close friend
• Change or loss of job or other significant role
• Divorce
• Illness
• Ambiguous or conflicting role expectations
• Inability to meet role expectations

- Low self-esteem
- Disturbed personal identity
- Anxiety related to changed physical appearance, e.g., amputation, mastectomy
- Impaired adjustment to changed physical functioning
- Ineffective coping with role change
- Hopelessness
- Powerlessness
- Parental role conflict
- Readiness for enhanced self-concept
- Disturbed sleep pattern
- Social isolation

Planning

The nurse develops plan in collaboration with the client and support people. The nurse and client set goals to enhance the client's self-concept.

Implementing

Nursing interventions to promote positive self-concept include helping a client to identify areas of strength. The strategies to reinforce strength are:

- Stress on positive thinking rather than self-negation
- Notice and verbally reinforce client strengths
- Encourage the setting of attainable goals
- Acknowledge goals that have been attained
- Provide honest, positive feedback.

Evaluation

To determine whether client outcomes have been achieved, the nurse uses data collected during interactions with the client. The nurse, client and significant others need to understand that to change beliefs, feelings, and behaviors affecting self-esteem requires time and ongoing effort. Improving one's self-concept can be a continuing concern and is not so easily evaluated. Example:

Nursing diagnosis	Nursing activities
Disturbed body image (permanent colostomy)	Assist patient to discuss changes caused by illness/surgery
	Assist patient in identifying parts of his body that have positive perceptions associated with them
	Facilitate contact with individuals with similar changes in body image
	Encourage independence but interference when patient is unable to perform

SPIRITUAL HEALTH

Meeting the client's spiritual needs can decrease suffering and aid in physical and mental healing. To implement spiritual care, nurses need to be skilled in establishing a trusting nurse-patient relationship and possess a healthy spiritual self-awareness. This will help the nurse to identify and be empathetic towards the spiritual concerns of clients. Nurses also need to be aware of the diverse spiritual beliefs and practices that their clients may possess. Because spiritual beliefs and practices are coping resources for persons, understanding how such beliefs and practices help or hinder a client's health is vital. Thus, each client needs to be approached in light of these unique needs. Whether the client presents with a need to relieve spiritual distress or to enhance spiritual health, nurses can implement spiritual care therapeutics and promote spiritual and emotional health, help with coping and adjustment, or assist one to face a more peaceful death.

Spiritual well-being or Spiritual Health

Spiritual health or spiritual well-being is manifested by a feeling of being "generally alive, purposeful, and fulfilled" (Ellison, 1983, p. 332). According to Pitch (1998), spiritual wellness is "a way of living, a lifestyle that views and lives life as purposeful and pleasurable, that seeks out life-sustaining and life-enriching options to be chosen freely at every opportunity, and that sinks its roots deeply into spiritual values and/or specific religious beliefs."

Indicators of spiritual health are shown in Table 9 and examples of spiritual needs are depicted in Table 10.

People nurture or enhance their spirituality in many ways. Some focus on development of the inner self, others focus on the expression of their spiritual energy with others or the outer world. Relating to one's inner self or soul may be achieved by conducting an inner dialogue with a higher power or with oneself through prayer or meditation, by analyzing dreams, by communing with nature, or by experiencing the inspiration or art. The expression of person's spiritual energy to others is manifested in loving relationship with and service to others, joy and laughter, participation in religious services, and expression of compassion, empathy, forgiveness, and hope. Nurses who attend to their own spirituality are better able to work with clients who have spiritual needs (Taylor, 2005). Therefore, it is important to be comfortable with one's own spirituality.

TABLE 9: Indicators of spiritual health

- Faith
- Hope
- Meaning and purpose in life
- Achievement of spiritual world
- Feelings of peacefulness
- Ability to love
- Ability to forgive
- Ability to pray
- Ability to worship
- Spiritual experiences
- Participation in spiritual rites and passages
- Participation in meditation
- Participation in spiritual reading
- Interaction with spiritual leaders
- Expression through song/music
- Expression through writing
- Connectedness with inner-self
- Connectedness with others
- Interaction with others to share thoughts, feelings, and beliefs

TABLE 10: Examples of spiritual needs

Needs related to the self:
- Need for meaning and purpose
- Need for express creativity
- Need for hope
- Need to transcend life challenges
- Need for personal dignity
- Need for gratitude
- Need for vision
- Need to prepare for and accept death

Needs related to others:
- Need to forgive others
- Need to cope with loss of loved ones

Needs related to the ultimate other:
- Need to be certain there is a god or ultimate power in the universe
- Need to believe that God is loving and personally present
- Need to worship

Needs among and within groups:
- Need to contribute or improve one's community
- Need to be respected and valued
- Need to know what and when to give and take

Spiritual Distress

Spiritual distress refers to a challenge to the spiritual well-being or to the belief system that provides strength, hope, and meaning to life. Some factors that may be associated with or contribute to a person's spiritual distress include physiologic problems, treatment related concerns, and situational concerns.

Physiological problems include having a diagnosis of terminal disease, experiencing pain, experiencing the loss of a body part or function, etc. Treatment-related factors include recommendation for blood transfusions, abortion, surgery, dietary restrictions amputation of body part or isolation. Situational factors include the death or illness of a significant other, inability to practice one's spiritual rituals, etc. (Carpenito-Moyet, 2006). NANDA International (2007) offers the following as defining characteristics of spiritual distress:

- Expresses lack of hope, meaning and purpose of life, forgiveness of self
- Expresses being abandoned by or having anger toward God
- Refuses interaction with friends and family
- Sudden changes in spiritual practices
- Requests to see a religious leader
- No interest in nature, reading spiritual literature.

Concepts Related to Spirituality

They include religion, faith, hope, transcendence and forgiveness.

Religion

Religion is an organized system of beliefs and practices. It offers a way of spiritual expression that provides guidance for believers in response to life's questions and challenges. Religious development of an individual refers to the acceptance of specific beliefs, values, rules of conduct, and rituals. Religious development may or may not parallel spiritual development. An **agnostic** is a person who doubts the existence of God. An atheist is one without belief in God. **Monotheism** is the belief in the existence of one God while **polytheism** is the belief in more than one God.

Faith

Faith is to believe in or be committed to something or someone. Faith gives meaning to the life and providing the individual with strength in times of difficulty. For the client who is ill, faith in a higher authority (e.g., God, Allah), in oneself, in the health care team, or in a combination of all—provides strength and hope.

Hope

Hope is a concept that incorporates spirituality. It is a process of anticipation that involves the interaction of thinking, acting, feeling, and relating, and is directed toward a future fulfillment that is personally meaningful. In the absence of hope, the client gives up, losing spirit, and illness is likely to progress more rapidly.

Transcendence

This term is used interchangeably with self-transcendence which means the capacity to reach out beyond oneself, to extend oneself beyond personal concerns and to take on broader life perspectives, activities, and purposes, Transcendence is also thought to involve a person's recognition that there is something other or greater than the self and is seeking and valuing of that greater other, whether it is an ultimate being, force, or value.

Forgiveness

The concept of forgiveness is receiving increased attention among health care.

Professionals

For many clients, illness or disability brings a sense of shame or guilt. The health problem is interpreted as a punishment for past sins. Clients facing imminent death may seek forgiveness from others as well as from God.

LOSS, GRIEF, AND THE DYING PATIENT

Loss, grief and death are well known and universal parts of life. People adjust to loss through the grieving process, and coping with loss is learned from childhood onwards. A person's reaction to loss is influenced by the importance of what was lost and the culture in which the person is raised.

Death is a universally shared event. In all cultures and religions there are beliefs and rituals to explain and cope with death, loss, and grief.

Nurses and other health care professionals may have similar fears and anxieties about the end of life. They are responsible for providing the best care possible to their dying patients. But to meet the emotional and physical needs of patients and their significant others, nurses first take the time to look at their own view of death and come to terms with its reality.

Loss and Grief

Loss

Loss means to no longer possess or have an object, person, or situation. It is a familiar occurrence in everyday life, for example, losing money, a job, one's health or life. A loss can be physical, such as amputation of a leg, or inability to speak, or walk after a stroke. A loss can also be psychosocial. Disfiguring surgery, or scarring from burns may result in altered self-image and emotional problems. A person may lose the ability to carry out the role of homemaker or wage earner due to illness. Very often loss consists of both physical and psychosocial aspects. Loss can be viewed as ranging from minor to catastrophic. A person's reaction to loss depends not so much on the size of the loss but on the person's value of what has been lost plus the influence of previous experiences and the ability to cope. Only the person experiencing the loss can define the value of the loss.

Grief

Grief is the total emotional feeling of pain and distress that a person experiences as a reaction to loss. The grieving process occurs over a period of time. A person adapts to the feelings and moves through the pain and associated symptoms toward recovery or acceptance. Both of them, who is dying and his loved ones experience loss and grief when faced with a terminal diagnosis.

Bereavement is the state of having suffered a loss by death. A person who is grieving may experience both physical and emotional symptoms, such as crying, fatigue, changes in appetite, sleep disturbances, loneliness, and sadness. When a person thinks or knows that a loss is going to occur in the future, anticipatory grieving may occur before the loss actually happens. This happens when patients and their families face a serious or life-threatening illness, and it is believed to improve coping with the loss when it occurs.

Stages of Grief

The grieving person goes through stages; shock and disbelief, protest, disorganization, and reorganization (Parkes, 1986).

Each stage has identifying behaviors and feelings, and each person moves through the stages at his own pace, and may skip or return to an earlier stage. It is important for the nurse to recognize the great individuality of the grieving process and offer supportive care for the symptoms or behavior the person demonstrates, rather than anticipating what grieving response is the right one.

Nurses can assist persons who are grieving by accepting their feelings and behaviors and validating their loss. To validate the loss is to reassure the grieving person that the loss was important and that you understand the loss. Quiet presence, a warm caring concern for the person's well-being, and the ability to listen to the person speak about his or her pain and loss are supportive. Observe the non-verbal communication of the patient, and be aware of and use appropriate nonverbal language such as a smile or a gentle touch. Crying may be embarrassing for the patient, and is simple act of handling the issue through weeping, a patient acknowledges that he/she feels sad for loss, but should avoid saying that I know just how you felt.

As a person moves through the stages of the grieving process, there is a continuing decline in function as the person attempts to adjust to the loss, with the stage of reorganization,

there is gradual improvement in the level of daily function. Successful movement through the grieving stages allows the person to emerge with realistic memories of the event and the decreased, renewed energy, a sense that life has meaning, and ability to gain experience pleasure, social relationship, and activities. The time it takes to move through the stages depends on the loss and its meaning to the person.

Death and Dying

The Nature of Death

Death is an event marked in different ways. The absence of a heartbeat and breathing, was accepted definition of death earlier but in today's high tech hospital environment, a ventilator can support the patient's breathing and heartbeat. So, a definition of death that has been used since 1980s is **brain death** (the permanent stopping of integrated functioning of a person as a whole).

Death may be sudden, unexpected, and instant, as when a person is killed in an accident or dies of a massive heart attack or stroke. Death may also be the end of long battle against a chronic disease such as cancer or heart disease, or old age. Death is also encountered in situations where the outcome could be either death or survival, as in an acute severe infection or trauma. Nurses who work in an emergency room, intensive care unit, med-surgical unit, nursing home, or hospice generally have different experiences of patients' death and dying. In these different situations, the individual who die and those who care about them experience different emotions and physical reactions. Each death and dying experience is unique, although there are some common features that can help you to provide truly satisfying care to the patient and the family.

The Dying Process

Kubler-Ross and the Five Stages of Dying

In the late 1960s, Dr Elisabeth Kubler-Ross, a psychiatrist, began talking with terminally ill patients and identifying their needs. She also began educating medical students, nurses, and doctors about death and stages through which she saw the terminally ill patients' progress. She transformed the health care community and much of the public view about death, and she promoted additional research into the areas of loss and death. As a result of her pioneering work, nurses and doctors are much more sensitive to the needs of the dying patients and families. According to Dr Kubler-Ross's identification of the stages, a dying person moves through various stages and that has been the foundation for understanding the dying process. Five stages are described as characteristics of dying: denial, anger, bargaining, depression, and acceptance (DABDA) (Table 11).

The stage overlaps, and as with the grieving process, the patient may move back and forth or even skip stages. In some cases, the patient may "get stuck" in one stage and not move through to acceptance. Family members are often at different stages from the patient and each other. Nurses too move through the stages when they care for patients who are dying. Standards of care for the terminally ill patient are given in Table 12.

TABLE 11: Kubler-Ross's stages of coping with death

Denial	"No, not me." The person cannot believe the diagnosis or prognosis. It serves as a buffer to protect the patient from an uncomfortable and painful situation. A patient may seek other opinions or believe there has been an error
Anger	"Why me?" The person looks for cause or fixes blame. Doctors and nurses are often the target of displaced anger, as well as family and even God. Powerlessness to control the disease and events are the underlying issue
Bargaining	"If I'm good, then I get a reward. "The wish is for extension of life, or later for relief from pain, and the person knows from past experience, that "good behavior" is often rewarded.
Depression	"It's hopeless". There is a sense of great loss, of the impending loss of being. People mourn losing family, possessions, responsibilities, all they value
Acceptance	"I'm ready." The pain is gone, the struggle is over, the patient has found peace and there is withdrawal from the engagement of everyday activities and interests. Verbal communication is less important, touch and presence most important.

TABLE 12: Standards of care for the terminally ill patient

- You must consider the terminally ill patient's preferences, personality, and lifestyle when planning care. Rigid rules, routines, and agency regulations should not be automatically applied.
- Every effort is made to maintain functional capacity and to relieve discomfort through the control of symptoms, regardless of the expected length of time until death.
- Pain control is a major goal of treatment.
- The patient's preferences and intentions regarding health care as set out in an advance directive, or by durable power of attorney, take precedence as far as the law allows
- The patient should feel safe and secure with the care that is provided and with the level of communication regarding this care.
- The patient has ample opportunities to finish business with loved ones and to say goodbyes.
- Opportunities are provided for the dying individual to spend final moments in a personally meaningful way with people who are important to the patient.
- Family members and significant others have opportunities to discuss the patient's imminent death and their emotional needs with the staff.
- Family members and significant others are provided with private time with the patient before and after death as desired.
- Family members are allowed to perform rituals and carry out cultural customs regarding the body after death.

NURSING AND THE DYING PROCESS

Patients express many fears when they know they are dying: fear of pain, loneliness, abandonment, the unknown, loss of dignity, loss of control. There may also be unfinished business that occupies the patient's thoughts. The concept of comfort care is focused on identifying symptoms that cause the patients distress, and adequately treating these symptoms. Palliation is the relief of symptoms when cure is no longer possible, and treatment is provided solely for comfort.

Application of Nursing Process

Assessment

A baseline assessment and continuing data collection are essential to identify the problems and needs of the patient and his family. An admission history should determine what they have been told by the physician regarding the illness and its expected course.

Questions about advance directives regarding treatment options, resuscitation, advanced life support, and organ donation can provide information about the patient's attitude toward death and the stage of his grief or dying reaction.

An assessment of the patient's physical condition would include such measures as weight, mobility, ability to perform ADL, weakness or energy level, appetite, bowel and bladder function and respiratory function. Special attention should be paid to assessing pain: Location, nature and what makes it better or worse. Pain should be assessed using 0–10 scale.

The patient's emotional condition can often be observed during the interaction, and symptoms such as anxiety, agitation, confusion or depression may be obvious. Spiritual assessment can begin with questions about the patient's religious affiliation, and whether he would like to meet with a spiritual advisor.

Planning

Planning is very important to include the patient and his family in the planning of care, and in establishing the goals or outcomes. Planning should be a team effort, by making all members of the team aware of the patient's goals and needs. Giving the patient control is a first priority at a time when it seems that he has no control. The goal is to provide comfort. Measures include relaxing restrictive visiting hours, eliminating routine vital signs and laboratory work, and avoiding rigid schedules for getting up, bathing or sleeping.

Nursing Diagnoses

Nursing diagnosis for the dying patient generally varies, depending on the disease process. Certain nursing diagnoses are common at some point to most dying patients:

- Activity intolerance
- Death anxiety
- Fear
- Anticipatory grieving
- Altered nutrition: Less than body requirements
- Risk for loneliness
- Pain
- Impaired physical mobility
- Fatigue
- Impaired skin integrity
- Knowledge deficit
- Self-care deficit

Implementation

The nurse promotes self-care as long as the patient is able. Family members can derive much satisfaction in learning to provide physical care when the patient is no longer able to be independent. Be sensitive to patient and family member reluctance to provide what is uncomfortable for either one, such as performing perineal care for a patient.

Common Problems of the Dying Patient

Pain Control

Research has demonstrated safe and effective principles of pain control, but many terminally ill patients die with uncontrolled pain. Pain can be controlled in almost all cases when the medical and nursing team work together. Regular scheduled pain medication with PRN (as needed) back up for pain is most effective. Carefully assess pain location, intensity, and response to medication every 2 – 4 hours or more often, if needed. There is no concern for addiction or of reaching a safety or effectiveness limit when narcotics are increased in response to pain. Patients with several pain can receive huge doses of narcotics without respiratory depression or tolerance when the dose has been increased in response to increasing pain. The oral route is preferred, and long-acting transdermal patches can also avoid the necessity of injections.

Non-pharmacological approaches to pain relief may include visualization, guided imagery, relaxation and breathing exercises, massage, music therapy, meditation, religious healing, biofeedback, hypnosis, use of TENS (transcutaneous electrical nerve stimulation), and hydrotherapy (Whirlpool), Teach the patient these simple techniques as an adjunct to drug therapy.

Constipation

Constipation is common among patients who are receiving opiates, decreased fluid intake and mobility, and having certain abdominal diseases. To prevent constipation, the nursing measures to be employed are increasing fiber, fluids, and exercise. Consult physician for stool softeners and a laxative, suppositories and enemas or manual removal.

Anorexia, Nausea, Vomiting

Anorexia may be due to nausea, drug's side effects, disease process or the slowdown that occurs naturally in the dying process. Antiemetics are given to eliminate nausea and vomiting. Small servings, eliminating unpleasant sights and odors at meal time may stimulate poor appetite. A bad taste can be improved by frequent oral care, mouth washes. Moistening the mouth with fluids or artificial saliva may be helpful.

Dehydration

As death nears, patient spend more time in sleeping. Research has shown that dehydration results in less distress and pain and that hydration does not improve comfort. Dry mouth and thirst are the most common complaints and these can be alleviated by small sips of fluids, ice chips, and lip lubrication. Resulting decreased urine output means less effort to use a commode or less incontinence. It is an emotional issue and families often have a difficult time accepting that withholding fluids is more comforting than administering them. Families can be confronted with an explanation of how the dying person is indeed made more comfortable by withholding fluids.

Dyspnea

Difficulty in breathing may be seen early in the dying process in certain lungs and heart disorders. It is also seen shortly before death when respirations may become noisy, irregular or labored. Secretions in the lungs accumulate and block the airways to contribute to noisy or rattling respirations. The patient is usually not responsive, or aware of the dyspnea but it is very upsetting for the family members. Suction is not effective in clearing secretions. Administering oxygen by nasal prong may provide comfort.

Impaired Skin Integrity

Skin breakdown occurs due to weight loss, decreased nutrition, incontinence, and inactivity in a dying patient. Turn and position the patient, use protective measures such as an air pressure mattress, heel or elbow protectors and keeping the skin clean and dry. An indwelling or condom catheter may be used to prevent skin breakdown.

Weakness, Fatigue and Decreased Ability to Perform ADL

Increasing weakness results in the patients becoming bedridden. Accept the patient's wishes regarding walking, sitting up in a chair, or remaining in bed. Allow the patient to do as much as possible for himself, and provide physical care when he is no longer able to perform. The dying patient is not going to get stronger or better; he gets weaker and weaker, not because he is lying in bed, but because he is dying.

Anxiety, Depression, Agitation

Emotional or psychological symptoms may be treated with appropriate drugs with good effect. Listen and use good therapeutic communication skills to allow the patient to express his fears, feelings and needs and to convey nonjudgmental acceptance.

Spiritual Distress, Fear of Meaninglessness

Each person needs to believe that his life has a meaning, and this is the essence of the spiritual nature of the dying process. A life review allows the patient to put his life in perspective. It is more important to listen then to talk.

Evaluation

Evaluation is based on the specific expected outcomes for the patient. These depend on which nursing diagnosis are pertinent to the patient's situation in most cases, the degree of comfort obtained for the patient by the nursing interventions needs to be evaluated. Is pain adequately controlled? Is tissue integrity protected? The actions to facilitate the patient's and family's grieving process effective? Is the patient's fear alleviated? Do interventions for a self-care deficit make the patient more comfortable? Answers to these questions help determine whether expected outcomes have been met. If the plan of care is not effective, the plan must be revised.

Signs of Impending Death

Physical Signs

As death approaches, the patient grows physically weaker and begins to spend more time sleeping. Bodily functions slow down, appetite decreases and the patient may refuse even favorite foods and later fluids as well. Explain to the patient and family what to expect. Moistening the patient's lips and mouth, and providing oral hygiene, are more comfortable than "pushing" food or fluids.

Urine output decreases and urine becomes more concentrated. There may be edema of the extremities or over the sacrum. Incontinence may occur as patient becomes less aware of his surroundings. However, be alert to the possibility of urinary retention and the need for catheterization.

Vital signs change as death approaches. The pulse increases and becomes weaker and thready. Blood pressure declines, and the skin of the extremities becomes mottled, cool and dusky. Respirations become shallow and irregular. There may be pooling of secretions in the lungs and causes respirations to sound moist "death rattle". Cheyne Stoke respirations may be noted, i.e., periods of apnea (no breathing) followed by shallow breathing. Body temperature may rise, and the patient may complain of feeling hot or cold.

Psychosocial and Spiritual Aspects of Dying

As death draws closer, the patient reaches the stage of acceptance. It is during this time that the patient talks about making funeral arrangements. To say good bye to those people and things that are important. It may also involve saying "I am sorry, forgive me", "I forgive you," and "I love you". It is a time when the patient may give to family and friends special memories or possessions.

As individuals approach death, their spiritual needs take on greater importance. As patient ponder the meaning of his life, his beliefs about what happens to him in death take on new meaning. Religious practices and rituals have great significance for some patients. It is important for you to be familiar with those beliefs. You must not impose your own religious beliefs on dying patient and family, but assist patients to find comfort and support in their own belief systems.

As death approaches, the patient becomes less verbal and more withdrawn. Everyday activities and news are not of interest and nonverbal communication becomes most important. Sitting with patient and using touch, such as holding his hand or stroking his hair, are most meaningful. Always be aware of remarks you make in the presence of unresponsive patients because they do hear. Hearing is believed to be one of the last senses to be lost before death, and dying patient has awakened to report conversations by family and health care workers that they were not meant to overhear.

Dying patient may exhibit confusion and disorientation. He may report dreams or visions of deceased relatives. Often this is comforting and he may speak of preparing for a journey to join loved ones. At times patient may become restless and agitated. Adequate pain and anxiety medication can ease the distress of these symptoms.

BIBLIOGRAPHY

1. *Craven RF, Hirnle JC. Fundamental of Nursing, 3rd edition, Lippincott Williams & Wilkins. 2000. pp. 307, 1227-1245, 1295-1314.*
2. *Lindeman CA, Marylon M. Fundamentals of Contemporary Nursing Practice, 1st edition. WB Saunder's Company; 1999. pp. 903-929, 1033-1051.*
3. *White L. Basic Nursing. Foundations of Nursing Skills and Concepts. Delmar Thomson Learning; 2002. p. 919.*
4. *Taylor C et al. Fundamentals of Nursing. 1st edition. JB Lippincott Company. 1989. pp. 227-236.*

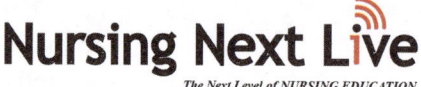
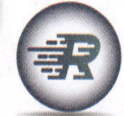
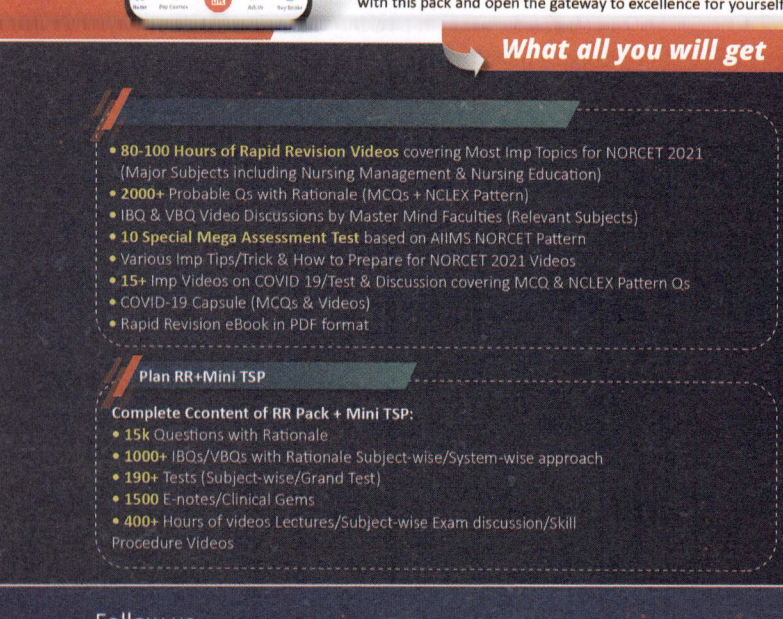
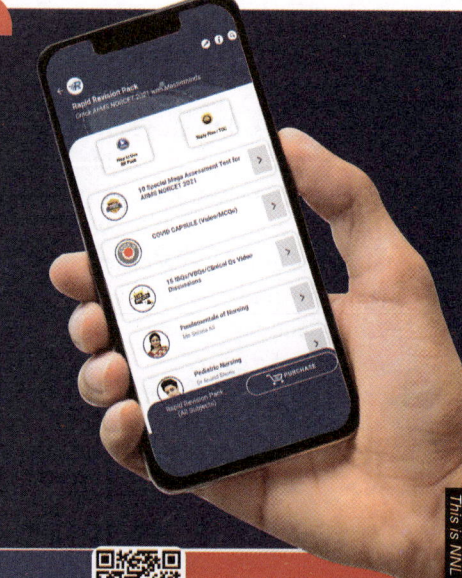 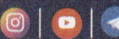

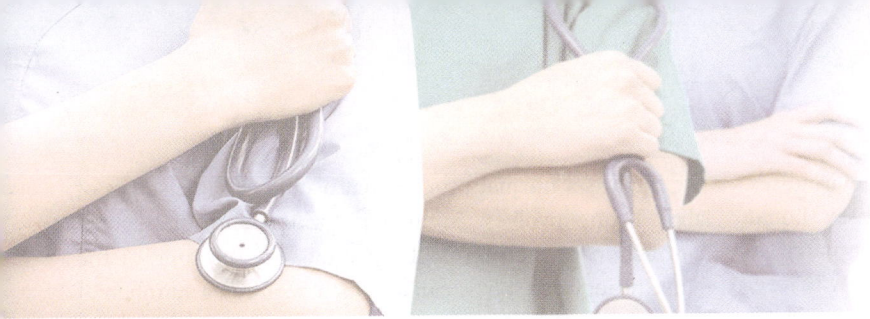

Sexuality

INTRODUCTION

During last 30–50 years, knowledge about sex has been recognized as an important and necessary aspect for human development. Change in sexual functioning can affect quality of life. Sexuality and sex are two different things. Sex is often used in two ways. One is physical part of relationship and another is genital sexual activity. It is also used to label gender, whether one is female or male.

Sexuality on the other hand is expressed through interactions and relationship with people of the opposite sex and or same sex and includes person's thoughts, experiences, learnings, ideas, values and emotions. It is related to how people feel about themselves and how they communicate those feelings to others.

DIMENSIONS OF SEXUALITY

Sociocultural Dimensions

Every society plays a powerful role in shaping sexual values and attitudes. Each social group has its own set of rules and norms that guides the behavior of its members. Sexual lives are embedded in social lives that offer opportunities and constraints, e.g., partners are approved or disapproved by each other. As a result, people tend to marry those who resemble them in age, education, race, religion, social status.

Religious and Ethical Dimensions

Sexual decisions are based on religion; what people consider to be right or wrong. Different categories take their sex in different ways like—traditional category says pre and extramarital sex were always wrong. Rational category believes that sex should be a part of a loving relationship and not reserved for marriage. Recreational category said that sex has nothing to do with love.

Psychological Dimensions

Here, parents treat their children differently, based on gender, like—the attitudes of male and female children are different from each other.

NORMAL HUMAN SEXUALITY

Functions of the Sexuality and Reproductive System

Reproduction is only one component of sexuality. Human being can be sexually engaged and find sexual expression without reproducing. The female reproductive system is responsible for cyclic maturation and release of an ovum and preparation for implantation of fertilized ovum. Male reproductive system is responsible for the generation and maturation of spermatozoa.

Sexual Expression

Sexual expressions may vary among different individuals, which are discussed as follows:

Menstruation and Ovulation

Menstruation is the cyclic and periodic discharge of blood from the uterus through the vagina during woman's reproductive age. The cycle repeats every 28 days. The menstruation cycle consists of ovarian cycle, divided into follicular phase, ovulatory phase and luteal phase. Uterine cycle or menstrual cycle is divided into proliferative and secretory phase.

Conception, Pregnancy and Birth

For reproduction and conception to occur, several complicated factors must fully operate. First, man must produce fully mature spermatozoa in sufficient numbers and with enough motility to penetrate woman's cervix and ascend to the uterus and fallopian tube.

Fertilization of one ovum with one spermatozoa normally occurs in the outer third of the Fallopian tube. After fertilization, the fertilized ovum undergoes several cell divisions and moves toward the uterine wall.

The average length of pregnancy is approximately 267 days or 38 weeks, but may vary by about 2 weeks in either direction.

Birth is a normal process that occurs in three stages of labor. Labor involves stimulation by hormones that causes contraction of the uterus. This results into pushing of the fetus through the birth canal, which requires a number of hours.

Many women experience symptoms at the time of ovulation or during the postovulatory phase of menstrual cycle. Some symptoms are partially due to effect of estrogen or progesterone that may lead to lower abdomen pain, discomfort at time of ovulation, breast fullness or hardness, fluid retention, irritability or depression. For some women, these symptoms remain consistent and severe and are included under premenstrual syndrome (PMS). Cessation of menstruation takes place around 45–60 years.

NORMAL SEXUAL PATTERN

Masters and Johnson (1996) have defined the sexual response cycle with the following phases—Excitement, plateau, orgasm and resolution. These phases are the result of vasocongestion and myotonia, which are the basic physiologic responses of sexual arousal.

Excitement

This phase involves gradual increase in sexual arousal. The earliest signs of sexual arousal are vaginal lubrication and penile erection. The vaginal wall secretions provide lubrication and in men, testicles become elevated and enlarged and scrotum becomes elevated and thickened.

Plateau

The responses of the excitement phase are heightened in the plateau phase. Increase in vasocongestion and myotonia leads to an increase in blood pressure, pulse rate and respiration.

Orgasm

Orgasm is the sudden release of the pooled blood and tension in the muscles at the climax of sexual excitement. It can be a highly pleasurable event involving the feeling of physiological and psychological release.

Resolution

Resolution involves a physiological and psychological return to an aroused state. During the resolution phase, there is a rapid loss of genital vasocongestion, nipple erection and the sex flush. As vitals turn to normal, the palms or sole may start to sweat. The experience is a feeling of relaxation.

FACTORS AFFECTING SEXUALITY

Relationships

The quality of a person's relationship can strongly influence the quality of his or her sexual experience. Love and trust may be the key factors in facilitating comfort with sexuality and several relations.

Cognition and Perception

Psychological factors include such aspects as certain mental images triggered in the mind, leading to sexual arousal. Emotional state may greatly influence sexual response. For example, a person who is happy and content. In addition, the degree of knowledge or misconception about sexuality influences the sexual functioning.

Cultural Values and Beliefs

Cultural factors include society's predominant views of sexuality and the social content within which people experience it. Values and morals are additional influences. Religious beliefs or personal values may shape views concerning contraception, abortion, sex education and sex outside marriage.

Self-concept

People who are comfortable with themselves are likely to experience pleasure and comfort with sexual relations. A person who feels decreased self-esteem and self-confidence may experience negative effects in sexual functioning. The person may have a decreased sexual drive or conversely, may attempt to compensate for this negative self-concept by over emphasizing in sexual relations.

Previous Experience

Previous experience with sexuality or ideas about sexuality influence current sexual functioning, for example, a person who was sexually abused in the past is likely to experience repercussions that negatively affects current sexual functioning.

Pregnancy

Pregnancy clearly influences the sexual functioning. Many women find their sexual drive decreased during the first trimester.

During the second trimester, many women experience a surge of energy and a corresponding increase in sexual drive.

The third trimester may again be a time of decreased sexual drive.

Environment

Environment can largely impact several functioning. Hospitalized clients, particularly those undergoing long-term treatments, may have inhibition to have sexual relations with partner.

Illness

Illnesses pose a threat to normal sexual functioning. A person with cardiac problem may feel overexertion from engaging in sexual relations. A person with a sexually transmitted disease (STD) may feel transmitting the disease to a partner or vice versa. Pain and disorders of joint also affect sexual relations.

Medication

Some medications affect the ability to perform sex, which include antihypertensives, antipsychotic tranquilizers, antidepressants, neurotransmitters, and hormones, social drugs, alcohol, opiates, marijuana, cocaine sedatives hypnotics, lysergic acid diethylamide (LSD). Methyldopa decreases libido in men and women, antidepressant increases libido.

Surgery

Examples of surgical procedures that affect sexuality are cesarean birth, hysterectomy and mastectomy. Women who undergo cesarean deliveries may experience longer recovery period than women who deliver vaginally and may feel less desire to resume sexual relations.

Altered Human Sexuality

Certain conditions are directly related to sexuality which influence a person's ability to engage in mutually satisfying sexual relations.

Manifestations of Altered Sexuality

Alteration in normal pattern of sexuality can be seen in following manifestations:

Sexual Abuse

Some people manifest altered sexual functions by being sexually abusive to others, whether it is children, spouses' acquaintances or strangers. Sexual abuse results in sexual problems for abused people as well.

Inhibited Sexual Desire

Lack of or inhibited sexual desire is subjective because there is no "normal" frequency of sexual relations, determining the frequency that reflects inhibited sexual desire is difficult. Key features may be partner's dissatisfaction with frequency of sexual relations.

Impotence

The inability to attain and maintain an erection long enough for satisfactory sexual intercourse. There are two types of impotencies:

Primary

Primary impotency refers to a man who has never been able to achieve an erection necessary for intercourse.

Secondary

Secondary impotency refers to a man who was once successful in attaining and maintaining erection but who subsequently experiences difficulty.

Ejaculatory Dysfunction

Premature Dysfunction

It is a condition in which the man is unable to maintain an erection long enough for satisfactory intercourse to occur.

Orgasmic Dysfunction

It is the difficulty or inability of a woman to reach orgasm during sexual stimulation. This disturbance can lead to decline in sexual desire and sex occurs less often because sex is not enjoyable for both partners.

Dyspareunia

Dyspareunia or painful intercourse, is thought to occur regularly in 1% to 2% of adult women. Common causes of dyspareunia or organic problems include lack of adequate lubrication, vaginal infection and pelvic disease.

Vaginismus

Vaginismus is involuntary contraction of the muscles surrounding vaginal orifice such that penetration may be impossible and very painful.

ROLE OF NURSE

Assessment

Assessment involves collecting subjective and objective data regarding normal sexual function, risk factors for sexual dysfunction and any present sexual dysfunction.

Subjective Data

Collect the data by taking a careful history mostly include sex-related questions.

- Allow adequate time to conduct an uninterrupted interview
- Assure confidentiality and privacy
- Use of warm and empathetic approach
- Assume that all clients are uncomfortable talking about their sexuality.
- Carefully observe nonverbal gestures of the client.
- Adapt the interview to the client's lifestyle and attempt to overcome cultural and language barrier.
- Have a rationale for each question and be willing to share with your client.
- Avoid pressurizing client to respond to the questions asked.
- Use open ended questions that encourage more than yes or no response. It is sometimes useful to ask how or when questions than do you question.

Objective Data

Physical Assessment

Complete systematic head to toe examination:

- Provide privacy: Use careful draping
- Instruments should be warm
- Be sure to wear gloves during examination of client's genitals.

Examination of Male Genitalia

- Helping male client into a position for proper examination
- Having the man lie on his back with the knees bent or standing

Inspection and Palpation

- Check and observe distribution of hair
- Careful attention to any skin masses, skin lesion, discharge from the penis or anal/rectal abnormalities.
- Note the absence or atrophy of testicles and presence of the foreskin or of circumcision.
- Location of urethra
- Observe male breast for deviations from normal.

Examination of Female Genitalia

- Help client in lithotomy position.
- Ensure comfort.
- Inspect her genitalia for hair distribution.
- Assist in complete pelvic examination to check pelvic masses, pelvic tenderness, vaginal discharge, any sign of infection

Speculum Examination

It allows visualization of the vagina and cervix. The speculum should be warm before insertion.

As the speculum is withdrawn, the clinicians view the vaginal wall.

Bimanual Palpation

The clinician places the index and the middle finger of one hand into the vagina while placing the other hand on the lower abdomen. The cervix, ovaries and uterus are palpated by this method.

Examine breast for size, symmetry, contour, color, lesion and nipple discharge.

Diagnostic Test and Procedure

Test/procedure	Description
• Venereal disease Research laboratories (VDRL) • Chlamydia culture • Gonorrhea culture • Wet preparation (KOH-Potassium hydroxide) (NS-Normal Saline) • Pap smear test	• Blood test to detect syphilis • Cervical culture to detect *Chlamydia* and gonorrhea • Slide preparation from vaginal secretion to detect *Candida* (monilia) and *Trichomonas*. • Slide preparation from endocervix to detect cellular changes in cervix, and cervical cancer.

NURSING DIAGNOSIS

The North American Diagnosis Association (NANDA) approved Nursing Diagnosis.

Sexual Dysfunction

Sexual dysfunction is related to the following conditions:
* Spinal cord injury
* Chronic illness
* Pain

Altered Sexuality Pattern

Altered sexuality patterns are related to the following:
* Death of spouse
* Illness of spouse
* Depression
* Decreased self-esteem

Impaired Adjustment

Impaired adjustment is related to the following:
* New role as parent
* Diagnosis of life-threatening illness
* Change in body image

Rape Trauma Syndrome

Rape trauma syndrome are related to the following:
* Forceful sexual activity with stranger
* Date rape

Knowledge Deficit

Knowledge deficit is related to the following:
* Unfamiliarity with birth control
* Sexual inexperience

Body Image Disturbance

Body image disturbance is related to the following:
* Surgical mutilation
* Sexual dysfunction
* Sexually transmitted diseases

PLANNING

After the nursing diagnosis and related factors are identified, client's goal and nursing interventions are planned.
* The client/couple recognizes symptoms of sexual dysfunction
* The client/couple have decreased symptoms of altered sexual functioning.
* The client/couple expresses satisfaction with level of sexual functioning.
  - Planning revolves around the client's motivation to be healthy.
  - Use education interventions to teach clients about self-care and responsible sex.

IMPLEMENTATION

Nurses play a key role in assisting clients with any of the diagnosis. At times, however, they must refer client to other health care providers, if a major sexual dysfunction is noted.

Self-awareness

Assist the clients to become more aware of their bodies and how they function.

Self-examination

As part of developing awareness of own bodies, men and women need assistance in learning technique of self-examination. Men should learn to perform testicular self-examination and women to perform self breast examination.

Kegel's Exercise

Kegel's exercises involve contraction and release of pubococcygeous muscle, which contracts when one prevents urine flow or a bowel movement. Muscle tone can be restored in about 6 weeks of regular practice of Kegel's exercise.

Sex Education

Parents and caregivers of preschool need guidance in becoming comfortable answering questions as well as in volunteering information that their children may not directly ask.

- Assist parents in dealing with the mood swings and unpredictability of their adolescents.
- Give reassurance and support regarding their approach toward children.
- Teaching men and women to participate in responsible sex. As a part of responsible sex teaching, teach client about the prevention of sexually transmitted diseases (STDs). Some STDs are easily treatable whereas others are not (e.g., herpes). Use of condoms, limiting number of sexual partners and various methods to limit size of families are to be told to the client.

NURSING INTERVENTIONS FOR ALTERED FUNCTION

A holistic approach addresses both psychological issues related to sexual dysfunction.

- Counseling and education regarding a specific problem area.

- Making referrals to appropriate resource.
- Assist in home management
- Assist clients in achieving and maintaining a level of daily living that maximizes their potential.

Evaluation

Specific outcome criteria help to evaluate attainment of client's goals related to sexuality possible outcome criteria.

Goals

- The client/couple recognizes symptoms of sexual dysfunction.
- The client has decreased symptoms of sexual diseases.
- Clients describe male and female reproductive anatomy after teaching session.
- Client identifies some symptoms
- Client verbalizes to nurse that symptoms are decreasing.

CONCLUSION

Sexuality is an integral component of personhood and therefore, may impact on or be affected by health status. Sex always remains as controversial issue because of ethical values systems. With sensitivity and insight; nurses can assist their clients in assuming responsibility for decision about sexuality, thus enhancing their total health.

BIBLIOGRAPHY

1. Potter PA, Perry AG. Fundamental of nurse concepts, Process and Practice, 2nd edition Mosby; St Louis: 1989, pp. 751-89.
2. Leahy JM, Patricia EK. Foundation of Nursing Practice, 1st edition, W B Saunders Company; Philadelphia: 1998. pp. 114-39
3. Craven RF, Hirnel CJ, Henshaw CM. Fundamentals of Nursing-Human Health and Function. Lippincott Williams and Wilkins; Philadelphia: 2000. pp. 1322-45
4. Wong DL, Perry SE. Maternal Child Nursing Care, 1st edition, Mosby co. USA; 1998. pp. 1093-5.
5. Taylor C, Lillis C, LeMone P, Lynn P. Fundamentals of Nursing, JB Lippincot co; Philadelphia: 1989. pp. 1061-95.
6. I am, "sexuality and sexual health promotion for the older person", British journal of Nursing. 2004, 13(4)

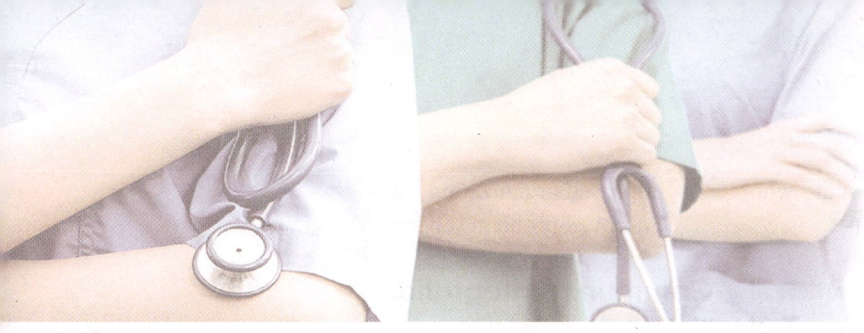

Recreational and Diversional Therapies

INTRODUCTION

"All work and no play make Jack a dull boy".
People have been saying it for years; and for good reasons. Life is not all about work. One should have a steady balance of work and play; and that is where recreation comes in. Recreational therapy embraces a definition of health, which includes not only the absence of illness, but also extends to enhancement of physical, cognitive, emotional, social and leisure development so that the individual may participate fully and independently in chosen life pursuits. Recreational therapy weaves the concept of healthy living into treatment to ensure not only improved functioning, but also to enhance independence and successful involvement in all aspects of life.

DEFINITION

Recreation is anything which diverts, stimulates or refreshes our mind and body.

COMMON RECREATIONAL ACTIVITIES

Reading a book or magazine, watching TV, playing musical instrument, swimming, walking on the beach, art and crafts, meditation, gardening, etc.

Recreational therapy is a treatment service designed to restore, remediate and rehabilitate a person's level of functioning and independence in life activities, to promote health and wellness as well as reduce or eliminate the activity limitations and restrictions to participate in life situations caused by an illness or disabling condition.

- Recreation therapy, or therapeutic recreation, strives to improve the functioning and independence to the individuals who are ill or disabled.
- Recreational therapy services are delivered by qualified professionals with training and education in therapeutic recreation and professionally certified by the National Council for Therapeutic Recreation Certification.

- Recreational therapists are certified professionals who work with doctors and rehabilitation specialists to assess a person's abilities and design a plan of activities.
- Recreation therapy services are delivered in a variety of settings of rehabilitation hospitals, rehabilitation units in general hospital, long-term care, skilled nursing facilities, substance abuse rehabilitation facilities, home health care services and residential facilities for persons with disabilities.

GOALS OF RECREATIONAL THERAPY

- Promoting social interaction among patients to improve quality of life
- Increasing activity tolerance
- Cognitive stimulation
- Providing opportunities to learn new skills and maintain current level of functioning
- Offering leisure education opportunities
- Community resource planning for patients being discharged home
- Provide opportunities for community involvement while in hospital
- Opportunities for self-expression

BENEFITS OF RECREATIONAL THERAPY

Physical Outcomes

- Increased immune system activity
- Reduced pain
- Increased muscular strength
- Improved flexibility and balance
- Improved cardiovascular functioning
- Developed consistent activity routine for maintenance
- Reduced urinary tract complications
- Increased endurance

Psychosocial Outcomes

- Enhanced body image perceptions
- Changed attitude toward disability
- Improved sense of self
- Achieved control over stress
- Enhance self-efficacy
- Developed sense of mastery

Cognitive Outcomes

- Increased mental alertness
- Increased attention span
- Enhanced memory skills

- Improved organization skills
- Improved problem solving

Community Integration

- Prevention of social isolation
- Development/maintenance of social skills
- Building of skills to minimize disability stigma
- Increased knowledge of community resources
- Increased overall activity level
- Improved cooperation skills
- Increased self-assertiveness
- Increased skills in conversation

FACTORS AFFECTING RECREATIONAL THERAPY

- **Age:** The recreational needs of children, adult and old age may differ as the patient of different age groups need different kinds of recreation.
- **Experience:** A person's interest can be affected by his experience. New experiences are more recreating to the patient.
- **Type and duration of illness:** According to the nature and duration of illness, the recreation given to patient may change.
- **Cultural prejudices:** The patient may have her own principles, cultural and religious prejudice, etc. so, accordingly we have to plan the recreational activities.
- **Ability of the patient:** It is necessary to plan activity according to what the patient is able to do. There are various types of recreation for the chronically ill patient or bedridden patient.
- **Physical condition**
- **Emotional state and attitudes:** The type of recreational activity may change according to the emotional state of the patient.

WHO BENEFITS FROM RECREATION THERAPY?

Recreation therapy interventions address the areas of restoration of function, health maintenance, reduction of health risk factors, and psychosocial competence.

Benefits for Persons with Physical Disabilities

Therapeutic recreation specialists work with individuals with diverse diagnoses, including but not limited to spinal cord injury; stroke; traumatic brain injury; cardiovascular disease; diabetes; chronic pain; visual and hearing impairment, multiple sclerosis; post-polio syndrome; amputation; burns, asthma, cystic fibrosis; and HIV/AIDS.

Benefits for Persons with Developmental Disabilities

Therapeutic recreation specialists work with individuals with developmental disabilities in a variety of setting including developmental disabilities, substance abuse programs, supported employment programs, community residential agencies, schools, and other community inclusion programs.

Benefits for Persons with Psychiatric Disabilities

- Helps in improving symptoms like anxiety, depression, sleep disturbances, hallucinations, negative thinking, etc.
- Helps in improving social skills and communication skills.

Benefits to Older Adults

- Therapeutic recreation specialists work with older adults with diagnosis as stroke, cardiac dysfunction, cancer, diabetes, Alzheimer's disease, and other degenerative cognitive disorders, and psychiatric disorders.
- Frail older adults who received exercise programs experienced significantly increased cardiovascular fitness, decreased blood pressure, and increased flexibility, strength, and improved ambulatory skills.
- Frail older adults in both psychiatric hospitals and nursing homes who participated in social, expressive, artistic, or nature-based recreation therapy programs demonstrated decreased loneliness and increased affiliation with others.
- Improved verbal interaction, improved morale and life satisfaction, decreased levels of depression, enhanced perception of personal control and competence.

Benefits for Children

- Structured games improve mobility and range of motion, decreases loss of function, and increased rates of healing.
- Recreation plays a critical role in the rehabilitation of children undergoing medical treatment for acute, chronic, or rehabilitative needs.

Benefits for Persons with Addictions

- Therapeutic recreation specialists work with persons with addictions in hospital, residential, or outpatient settings.
- They typically concentrate their efforts on strengthening those skills which enhance the process of recovery and prevent relapse.

NATURE OF RECREATIONAL THERAPY

- The recreational therapy process begins with an individual assessment of one's:
  - Strengths, interests, and values
  - Previous leisure activities and expectations
  - Available resources in your home and community
  - Social needs and relationships
  - Economic and other potential problem areas in participating in recreational and leisure activities
  - Lifestyle adjustments necessary for healthy leisure functioning.
- Recreational activities are used to increase or maintain motor skills and improve reasoning function.
- Most activities are done in a social environment to assist the patient with confidence building and reduce emotional and mental difficulties such as anxiety and depression.
- Community-based activities help the patients to actively participate in their communities in an attempt to increase independence and confidence.
- Dance, music, and arts and crafts are popular activities that help keep the mind sharp while improving fine and gross motor skills. Movement activities other than dance may be used.
- Stretching and relaxation techniques that use gentle movement improve both physical function and emotional.
- Structured group activities encourage social interactions decreasing the effects of depression and isolation.
- Many of the activities may be designed to prevent future medical problems by helping the patients maintain a level of functioning that helps extend their well-being.
- Working closely with a team of other health professionals, plan and implement activities that facilitate the patient's improvement in all areas—physical, mental, and emotional.
- At each step in the therapeutic activities, the recreational therapist works with medical records and assessments.
- Careful observations and recording of data about the patient's condition and progress are an integral part of the job. Recreational therapists must be capable of creating, understanding, and maintaining records.

RECREATIONAL NEEDS OF ELDERLY

Recreational activities for the elderly are essential for maintaining good physical and mental health. There are some general guidelines to be kept in mind while selecting the appropriate recreational activities for the elderly.

- **Consider their interests:** Designing activities that involve their past interests are of the utmost importance.

For example, if they love to garden, foster that passion with stimulating gardening activities.

- **Re-establish old routines:** It is very common for seniors to feel as if they have lost their sense of purpose. Design activities in which they can be together with their children.
- **Provide opportunity for social interaction:** The children should carry their parents with them once they go to any grocery shop, market, outings, etc.
- **Avoid physical hazards:** When elderly people are engaged in physical activities, utmost care to be taken to avoid any injuries.

The various activities in which the adults can get engaged are discussed as follows:

Church Groups

These groups go out for dinner, meet at each other's homes, plan fun outings, and just enjoy fellowship together.

Centers and Clubs

They organize team sports and club activities like volunteer-participation at various medical and rehab camps, hobby classes and competitions and even weekend activities that could ripple through the week.

The core function and focus of such community centers is to enable every senior member to identify some activity to fill the void that comes along with retirement and age.

The arts and crafts competitions and workshops, cultural activities and day trips assure the elderly members to develop a feeling of belonging to other places in the area. The resultant fellowship generates a rejuvenated spirit and renewed pride.

Dedicated Volunteering

Senior citizens can also take up dedicated volunteering at venues like schools, colleges, local community centers and other similar project venues.

The services and talents that they have to offer enhance the quality of interaction with the youth and other professionals.

In schools, seniors can volunteer as teachers, coordinators and counselors for various school activities. There are summer camps and programs that are consistently on the lookout for volunteers to enrich the environment with love, guidance and self-esteem. The one-to-one situations help the exchange of expertise and quality assurance to any indoor or outdoor bound activity.

Art and Craft Activities

Arts and crafts are fun for people of all ages but they can be therapeutic recreation for the elderly. Craft activities can be adjusted to fit the needs, and abilities of the disabled, and they are a fun group project that can help the elderly socialize and visit while creating with their hands.

Picture Magnet

- For the elderly individual, choose a favorite photo, like—one of family members or pets. Assist him with drawing a circle or oval around the main focal point of the picture, then cutting it out with scissors.
- Give him a long piece of lace or other decorative border and help him to glue it around the picture like a frame.
- Use tacky glue to secure the picture to a flat magnet. He can stick his picture magnet on his refrigerator or give it as a gift to a loved one.

Scrapbooks

- Help the elderly individual search through and pick out favorite old photographs. Provide a variety of construction paper and glue, and allow him to paste the pictures on the paper as he/she wishes.
- Those with strong memory may want to divide the scrapbook into sections by year or decade.
- Allow the individual to use markers to label each picture, encouraging him to make notes about what he remembers about the people or place it features. When he is finished, laminate each page, if possible and then assist him with stapling or binding the pages together in order.

Other forms of recreational activities are:

- Singing
- Dancing
- Chatting with friends
- Gardening
- Babysitting
- Reading
- Fishing
- Cooking
- Having a pet

RECREATIONAL NEEDS OF CHILDREN

- In children, recreational activities include those activities performed for self-amusement that have behavioral, social, and psychomotor rewards.
- It is child-directed, and the rewards come from within the individual child; it is enjoyable and spontaneous.
- **Play** is one of the most important parts of recreational activities of the childhood development.
- Through play, children learn about shapes, colors, cause and effect, and themselves. Besides cognitive thinking, play helps the children learn social and psychomotor skills. It is a way of communicating joy, fear, sorrow and anxiety.

Common Recreational Activities of Children

Games, playing with toys, arts and crafts (cat sock puppet, colorful butterflies, modeling clay, etc.), nursery rhymes, science experiments, drawing, athletic activities, gardening, nature activities (planting a tree, listen to the world, nature hunt, etc.), photography, etc.

Importance of Recreational Activities for Children

Sensorimotor Development

- Active play is essential for muscle development and serves a useful purpose in release of surplus energy.
- Through sensorimotor play, children explore the nature of the physical world. Infants gain impressions of themselves and their world through tactile, auditory, visual, and kinesthetic stimulation.

Intellectual Development

- Through exploration and manipulation, children learn colors, shapes, sizes, textures, and the significance of objects.
- They learn the significance of numbers and how to use them; they learn to associate words with objects; and they develop an understanding of abstract concepts and spatial relationships, such as up, down, under, and over.
- Activities such as puzzles and games help them develop problem-solving skills. Books, stories, films, and collections expand knowledge and provide enjoyment as well.
- Play helps children comprehend the world in which they live and distinguish between fantasy and reality.

Socialization

- Through play and various activities with other children, they learn to establish social relationships and solve the problems associated with these relationships.
- They learn to give and take.
- Children learn right from wrong, the standards of the society, and assume responsibility for their actions.

Creativity

- Children can experiment and try out their ideas in play through every medium including raw materials, fantasy and exploration.
- Creative thinking is often enhanced in group settings where listening to others' ideas stimulates further exploration of one's own ideas. After children feel the satisfaction of creating something new and different, they transfer this creative interest to situations outside the world of play.

Self-awareness

- Children learn who they are and their place in the world. They become increasingly able to regulate their own behavior, to learn what their abilities are, and to compare their abilities with those of others.
- Through play, children are able to test their abilities, to assume and try out various roles, and to learn the effect their behavior has on others.

Therapeutic Value

- Recreational activities provide a means for release from the tension and stress encountered in the environment.
- Children are able to experiment and test fearful situations and can assume roles and master the roles and positions that they are unable to perform in the world of reality.
- Throughout their play, children need the acceptance of adults and their presence to help them control aggression and to channel their destructive tendencies.

Moral Value

- Although children learn about the right or wrong behaviors at home and at school, in the culture, the interaction with peers during play contributes significantly to their moral training.
- If they are to be included as acceptable members of the group, children must adhere to the accepted codes of behavior of the culture (fairness, honesty, self-control, consideration for others).

Precautions to be Taken for the Recreational Activities of Children

- Select toys that suit the skills, abilities, and interests of children.
- Select toys that are safe for the specific child and age group.
- Remember toys that are safe for one age may not be safe for another.
- Maintain a safe play environment.
- Remove and discard plastic wrappings on toys immediately; they could suffocate a child.
- Supervise young children closely during play and other recreational activities.
- Instruct older children to keep their toys away from younger brothers, sisters and friends.
- Keep children away from stairs, hills, traffic and swimming pools who are playing with riding toys.
- Instruct not to put toys in the mouth as the paint may harm them.

- Insist that children wear helmets when using bicycles, skate board or in-line skates.
- Instruct children on electrical safety. Teach children the proper way to unplug an electric toy-pull on the plug, not the cord.
- Teach children to beware of electrical appliances and even electrically operated playthings; often children are unfamiliar with the hazards of electricity in association with water.

CONCLUSION

Incorporating client's interests, and the client's family and/or community makes the recreation therapy process meaningful and relevant. Recreational therapy is extremely individualized to each person, his past, present and future interests and lifestyle. Recreational therapists weave the concept of healthy living into treatment to ensure not only improved functioning, but also to enhance independence and successful involvement in all aspects of life.

BIBLIOGRAPHY

1. *Sr. Nancy. Stephanie's Principles and Practice of Nursing, 6th edition. Vol: 1; pp. 281-82.*
2. *Potter PA. Potter-Perry Fundamentals of Nursing, 7th edition. Mosby Publication; 2009. pp. 361-72.*
3. *Mary. C. Townsend; Psychiatric Mental Health Nursing, 5th edition. Jaypee Brothers, New Delhi; pp. 207-10.*

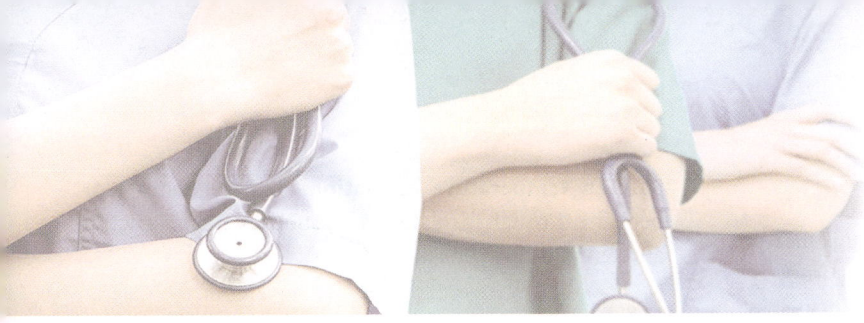

Care of Patient having Alterations in Temperature

Learning Objectives

After completing this chapter, you will be able to:
- Explain the regulation of body temperature
- Enlist the factors affecting temperature
- Provide care to patient having fever

Key Terms

- Conduction
- Connection
- Radiation
- Hyperpyrexia
- Hypothermia

Chapter Outline

- Introduction
- Regulation of Body Temperature/Thermoregulation
- Factors Affecting Temperature
- Temperature Alteration
- Classification of Temperature
- Nursing Management of Patient with Hyperthermia and Hypothermia

INTRODUCTION

Despite extremes in environmental conditions and physical activity, temperature-control mechanisms of human beings keep the body's core temperature (temperature of the deep tissues) relatively constant. However, surface temperature fluctuates depending on blood flow to the skin and amount of heat lost to the external environment. The measurement of body temperature is aimed at obtaining a representative average temperature of core body tissues. Sites reflecting core temperature are more reliable indicators of body temperature than sites reflecting surface temperature. In addition, the temperature value obtained may differ depending on the site of measurement. No single temperature is normal for all people.

- The average normal oral temperature is 37°C.
- The acceptable temperature ranges from 36°C to 38°C (96.8°–100.4°F)

- The normal range of oral temperature is 36.1°–37.5°C
- The normal range of rectal temperature is 36.1°–38.1°C
- The normal range of axillary temperature is 35.5°–36.4°C
- The normal range of tympanic temperature is 36.4°–38.1°C

REGULATION OF BODY TEMPERATURE/ THERMOREGULATION

Temperature may be defined as the degree of heat maintained by the body. It is a balance between heat produced and heat lost from the body. It is the difference between the amount of heat produced by body processes and the amount of heat lost to external environment. For the body temperature to stay constant and within an acceptable range, body mechanisms must maintain the relationship between heat production and heat loss.

Neural and Vascular Control

The hypothalamus, located between the cerebral hemispheres, controls body temperature. It senses minor changes in body temperature. The anterior hypothalamus controls heat loss and posterior hypothalamus control heat production.

Heat Production/Thermogenesis

Thermogenesis is the chemical regulation of heat production. It is done by the following ways:

- **Oxidation of food:** During metabolism of food, heat is produced as a by-product. As metabolism increases, additional heat increases and as metabolism decreases, less heat is produced.
  - 1 gram of carbohydrates gives 4 kcal of heat
  - 1 gram of proteins gives 4 kcal of heat
  - 1 gram of fat gives 9 kcal of heat
- **Muscle activity:** During muscle activity, the stored glycogen is converted into sugar causing heat production. Shivering of skeletal muscle also increases heat production. Non-shivering thermogenesis occurs primarily in neonates.
- **Hormonal effect:** Increased activity of thyroid and adrenal glands increases basal metabolic rate (BMR) by breaking down glucose and fats
- **Sympathetic stimulation:** Epinephrine and norepinephrine stimulate the nervous system to increase metabolism and thus, heat production.

Heat Loss/Thermolysis

Thermolysis is the physical regulation of heat by heat loss. The heat in the body is lost by the following ways:

- **Radiation:** It is the transfer of heat from the surface of one object to the surface of another without direct contact between the two objects. For example, standing exposes a greater radiating surface area.
- **Convection:** It is the transfer of heat by air movements. Convective heat loss increases when moistened skin comes in contact with slightly moving air (using of fans, open doors and windows)
- **Evaporation:** It is the transfer of heat energy when water in liquid state changes to gaseous state. For example, sweating, sponging of patient.
- **Conduction:** It is the transfer of heat from an object to another object by direct contact between them. For example, when skin is in contact with environmental objects like air, water, clothes and chair.
- **Behavioral control:** It involves the voluntary acts the person takes to maintain comfortable body temperature when exposed to temperature extremes. For example, change in clothing, sitting with arms folded, taking cold shower/baths, etc.

- **Skin in temperature regulation:** Skin regulates temperature through insulation of the body, vasoconstriction and temperature sensation.

FACTORS AFFECTING TEMPERATURE

- **Age:** Temperature regulation is unstable and immature until children reach puberty. Normal temperature gradually decreases as an individual approaches adulthood to old age.
- **Exercises:** Any form of exercise increases metabolism and will increase heat production and thus, body temperature.
- **Hormones level:** Women experience greater fluctuation than men due to the hormonal variations during menstrual cycle, an elevated progesterone level and even during menopause.
- **Circadian rhythm:** Body temperature normally changes from 0.9°–1.8°F (0.5°–1°C) during 24-hour period; lowest in the morning, rises steadily during the day with maximum in the evening.
- **Stress:** Physical and emotional stress increases body temperature through hormonal and neural stimulation, which increases metabolism and thus, heat production.
- **Environment:** It influences body temperature. When placed in a warm room, a client may be unable to regulate body temperature by heat loss mechanism

TEMPERATURE ALTERATION

- Fever
- Hyperthermia
- Heat stroke
- Heat exhaustion
- Hypothermia

CLASSIFICATION OF TEMPERATURE

- **Core** (rectal, esophageal, etc.)
- **Hypothermia:** <35.0°C (95.0°F)
- **Normal:** 36.5°–37.5°C (97.7°–99.5°F)
- **Hyperthermia:** >37.5° or 38.3°C (99.5 or 100.9°F)
- **Hyperpyrexia:** >40.0 or 41.5°C (104.0 or 106.7°F)

Hypothermia

Definition

Hypothermia is a life-threatening condition that may result in death. It occurs as a result of heat loss during prolonged exposure to cold, which overwhelms the body's ability to produce heat. A drop in the core body temperature below 95°F indicates hypothermia.

TABLE 1: Types of hypothermia

Accidental hypothermia	Results from unintentional exposure to cold (cold, wet or windy climate) with an ambient temperature of below 16°C and also from accidental immersion in cold water.
Therapeutic hypothermia	It refers to deliberate reduction of core body temperature (32°–34°C) for a specific duration of time in an effort to improve health outcomes. Example: cold application, cardiac and neurosurgery.
Spontaneous hypothermia	It sometimes develops following a high fever; body temperature remains low for several days after defervescence to normal. It may also accompany cerebrovascular diseases, infections, liver or renal failure.

This temperature is below what is required for normal body metabolism and bodily functions. Three types of hypothermia are given in Table 1.

Stages

1. **Stage 1: Mild (32°–35°C):** Awake and shivering hypertension, tachycardia, tachypnea, vasoconstricton
2. **Stage 2: Moderate (28°–32°C):** Drowsy and not shivering, pallor, cyanosis, polyuria/oliguria, stupor, poor coordination of toes and fingers
3. **Stage 3: Severe (20°–28°C):** Difficulty in speaking, amnesia, immobility, hypotension, bradycardia, bradypnea, unconscious, not shivering
4. **Stage 4:** Profound (<20°C) no vital signs.

Causes

- Excessive heat loss intentional, e.g., in surgery or accidental exposure to cold climate
- Diminished heat production
- Impaired thermoregulation

Hyperpyrexia

Hyperpyrexia is an elevated body temperature related to the body's inability to promote heat loss or reduce heat production is hyperthermia.

Fever/Pyrexia

Pyrexia is an elevation in core body temperature above 98.6°F up to 102.2°F.

Phases and Degree

1. **Onset or invasion:** In this stage, there is a sudden or gradual rise in temperature.

TABLE 2: Types of fever

Intermittent fever	Temperature rises from normal or subnormal to high fever and back to normal. Regular intervals which may vary from few hours to three days.
Remittent fever	Temperature fluctuates more than 2°C above normal between morning and evening but does not reach normal (example: inflammation of endocardium, typhoid fever).
Constant fever	Temperature that vary by more than 2°C between morning and evening but does reach normal for a specific period of weeks or days.
Relapsing fever	It is one in which there are brief febrile periods followed by one or more days of normal temperature (example malaria).
Irregular fever	When fever is entirely irregular in its course and cannot be classified in any of the categories.
Inverse fever	In this the higher range of temperature is recorded in the morning and evening which is contrary to that found in normal fever.
Rigor	It is a severe sudden attack of shivering in which body temperature rises rapidly to a stage of hyperpyrexia (example malaria).

2. **Fastigium or stadium:** In this stage, body temperature has reached its maximum and remains constant at a high level.
3. **Defervescence/decline:** In this stage, elevated temperature returns to normal. Fever may decline suddenly (crisis) or gradually (lysis).

Causes

- Exposure to hot environment
- Vigorous activity
- Medications
- Anesthesia
- Dehydration

Types of Fever

Types of fever are given in Table 2.

NURSING MANAGEMENT OF PATIENT WITH HYPERTHERMIA AND HYPOTHERMIA

Nursing Assessment

- Assess the vital signs every two hourly or depending on the condition of the patient

- Inspect and palpate skin for color, turgor and dehydration and oral mucosal lesions
- Take a detailed history about common symptoms
- Observe for vomiting, diarrhea and behavioral changes
- Assess the status of nutrient intake and nutrient requirement
- Assess the level of fatigue and anxiety
- Assess the level of sleep pattern
- Assess the level of self-care activities
- Monitor electrolyte level (sodium, potassium and chloride).

Hyperthermia

- Heat cramps
- Heat syncope
- Level of consciousness
- Thirst fatigue
- Nausea
- Delirium
- Moist skin
- Tachycardia
- Temperature more than 104°F (37.8°C)

Hypothermia

- Shivering
- Tachycardia
- Deep breathing
- Rigid muscles
- Decreased blood pressure
- Poor coordination
- Slurred speech
- Cyanosis
- Weak irregular pulse
- Dilated pupil
- Loss of consciousness

Risk Factors for Hypothermia

- Poor accommodation/inadequate heating
- Malnourishment
- Exposure to a cold environment, for example, immersion in cold water, exposure to cold environment for long period
- Burns, which can lead to excessive heat loss
- Overdose of medication that leads to coma and immobility. The drugs that may cause or exacerbate hypothermia include: Phenothiazines, benzodiazepines, morphine, barbiturates and vasodilators
- Underlying illness, for example, hypothyroidism, diabetic ketoacidosis, hepatic encephalopathy and cerebrovascular accident
- Alcohol abuse: Ethanol is a vasodilator that produces anesthesia and depresses the central nervous system

Nursing Diagnosis

- Ineffective thermoregulation related to infectious disease/exposure to low external temperature
- Imbalanced nutrition less than body requirement related to loss of appetite
- Fluid volume deficit and electrolyte imbalance related to excessive sweating
- Fatigue related to disease process
- Disturbed sleeping pattern related to change in environment
- Altered skin integrity related to skin disorders secondary to hypothermia

Planning

- To maintain normal body temperature
- To maintain adequate nutrition
- To maintain the fluid and electrolyte balance
- To promote comfort and rest
- To maintain the skin integrity

Nursing Interventions

Maintaining Normal Temperature

Hyperthermia

- Assess the body temperature
- Provide cold compress, cold sponge bath and ice bags
- Provide cool environment
- Remove extra clothing and patient from hot environment
- Administer antipyretics as advised

Hypothermia

- Assess the body temperature
- Rewarm the client by using room heaters, supplying warm humidified oxygen, applying warm blankets, infusing warm fluids, giving hot foot bath or warm soaks (104°F) applying heat pads or water bottles, placing radiant lamps over the client, performing warm fluid lavage
- Remove all cold and wet clothing replacing them with warm clothing
- Avoid exposure of body parts
- Provide adequate nutrition and fluid intake

Maintaining/Improving Nutritional Status

- Assess the nutritional status and fluid intake
- Assess the severity of anorexia or nausea
- Monitor the vital signs
- Encourage patient to increase intake of fluids
- Encourage to take small and frequent meals. Take high caloric diet
- Insert Ryle's tube if advised

- Administer intravenous fluids as directed
- Maintain an input/output chart
- Provide mouth care

Maintaining Fluid and Electrolyte Balance

- Assess the vital signs
- Assess skin turgor and mucous membranes for signs of dehydration
- Assess color and amount of urine
- Maintain input and output chart
- Change cold and wet clothing and replace with warm clothes
- Provide sweet drinks and plenty of fluids
- Administer intravenous fluids as advised
- Monitor the electrolyte levels (sodium, potassium and chloride)

Maintaining Activity Level within Capabilities

- Assess the severity of fatigue
- Assess the ability to perform daily activities
- Monitor the vital signs
- Assist patient in performing activities of daily living
- Provide adequate rest and sleep
- Assist patient in performing active and passive exercises
- Administer intravenous fluids as advised
- Take measures to prevent sweating (provide warm environment, warm drinks, hot water bottle, warm soaks or immersions, warm blankets)
- Provide relaxation therapies (music therapy)
- Encourage family support

Promoting Optimal Amount of Sleep

- Assess the sleeping pattern
- Assess patient's perception of cause of sleep difficulty and possible relief measures
- Review the daily schedule of sleep to determine period of sleep

- Advise patient to wake up at the same time daily
- Provide dark, calm and soothing environment. Limit noise
- Restrict visitors during sleep period
- Provide back rub, warm foot bath, comfortable position and relaxation technique for stimulating sleep
- Avoid strenuous activities and fluid intake before bedtime

Maintaining Skin Integrity

- Assess the general skin condition
- Assess the nutritional status of patient
- Provide meticulous skin care
- Avoid rubbing of skin vigorously
- Provide a clean, dry and wrinkle-free bed
- Change wet clothing. Keep patient's body dry
- Rapid rewarming should be done
- Advise patient to change positions every two hourly
- Advise to take adequate amount of fluids
- Inform physician if any problem arises (rashes, ulcers, etc.)
- Administer medications as prescribed

Evaluation

- Body temperature to be maintained within normal limits
- Nutritional status to be maintained
- Fluid and electrolyte balance to be maintained
- Improved activity tolerance and fatigue is reduced
- Improved sleep pattern
- Skin integrity to be maintained

CONCLUSION

Temperature management is a significant area of clinical practice particularly within nursing. Maintaining a constant body temperature is important and especially in the neonatal population. Hypothermia and hyperthermia should be avoided as they can have severe outcomes, increasing morbidity and mortality.

BIBLIOGRAPHY

1. *Potter PA, Perry AG. Fundamentals of Nursing, 7th edition. Mosby: Elsevier; 2009.*
2. *Black MJ. Medical Surgical Nursing: Clinical Management for Positive Outcomes, Vol 2, 8th edition. Saunders Elsevier. pp 2212-13.*
3. *The Trained Nurses Association of India. Fundamental of Nursing: Procedure Manual. TNAI Publication, 1st edition. 2005. pp. 308-15.*
4. *Sr. Nancy. "Stephanie's Principles and Practice of Nursing Senior Nursing Procedure and Nursing administration", vol. 2, 4th edition. NR Brothers; 2005. pp. 461-82.*

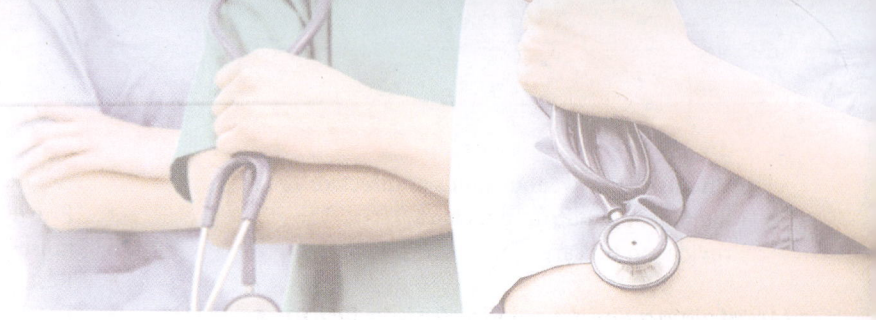

Chapter 47

Care of Patient having Alterations in Respiration

INTRODUCTION

Good patient outcomes rely on ability to assess ventilation, oxygenation, work of breathing (WOB), lung function, airway resistance and air flow. The number of treatment choices is increasing and they're becoming more complex. Nurses have a pivotal role in managing the patient's respiratory functions. Timely and appropriate management of the patient's respiratory function can have a tremendous impact on the experience of illness and eventual outcomes for patients and their families.

ANATOMY AND PHYSIOLOGY

The respiratory system (also referred to as the ventilator system) is a complex biological system comprising several organs that facilitate the inhalation and exhalation of oxygen and carbon dioxide in living organisms or in other words, breathing.

For all air-breathing vertebrates, respiration is handled by the lungs, but these are far from the only components of the respiratory system. In fact, the system is composed of the following biological structures: nose and nasal cavity, mouth, pharynx, larynx, trachea, bronchi and bronchioles, lungs and the muscles of respiration.

A properly functioning respiratory system is a vital part of our good health. Respiratory infections can be acute and sometimes life-threatening. They can also be chronic, in which case, they place tremendous long-term stress on the immune system, endocrine system and much more. The respiratory system is divided into two main components.

Upper Respiratory Tract

The upper respiratory tract is composed of the nose, the pharynx, and the larynx.
- Nasal cavity is lined with epithelial tissue containing serous glands, mucus-secreting goblet cells, and hair-like projections called cilia which help to filter the air.

The nasal passage is richly supplied with blood vessels that warm and moisten the air.

- Pharynx connects the nasal passages and mouth to the lower parts of respiratory tract. It serves as a passageway for both food and air. Inspired air goes to larynx and ingested food goes to esophagus.
- The larynx is essential to human speech. It contains vocal cords and is a passageway for air entering and leaving the trachea.

Lower Respiratory Tract

The lower respiratory tract is composed of the trachea, the lungs, and all segments of the bronchial tree (including the alveoli). The organs of the lower respiratory tract are located inside the chest cavity.

- **Trachea:** Located just below the larynx, the trachea is the main airway to the lungs and is also called windpipe. It is 2–2.5 cm wide and 10–12 cm long. It terminates into two tubes: the right and left bronchi.
- **Bronchi:** The bronchi branch from the trachea into each lung. Right bronchus is wider and more vertical than the left. Within lungs, the bronchi branch off into increasingly smaller diameter tubes, until they become terminal bronchioles.
- **Diaphragm:** The diaphragm is the main respiratory muscle that contracts and relaxes to allow air into the lungs.

Functions of Respiratory System

- It helps in carrying out the exchange of oxygen and carbon dioxide in the lungs and tissue.
- It helps to maintain the metabolism of tissue.
- The first part of respiratory system also serves as olfactory function.
- It is involved in mechanism of temperature regulation, oxygen and other necessary substance absorption.
- It regulates acid-base balance.
- It regulates blood pressure and circulation in the body.

Respiration

The process of interchange of gases between the living organisms and environment is called respiration. There are two phases of gas interchange:

1. **External respiration:** It is the exchange of gases between the inhaled air and the blood in the pulmonary capillaries.
2. **Internal respiration:** It is the exchange of gases at the cellular level between cells and blood in system capillaries.

RESPIRATORY DISTRESS

Respiratory distress is generally referred to as labored breathing or difficulty in breathing. The sensation of respiratory distress is called shortness of breath or dyspnea.

Five Key Signs

The signs that suggest severe respiratory distress include:

1. Retractions and the use of accessory muscle to breathe
2. Inability to speak full sentences (or difficulty in speaking between breaths)
3. Inability to lie flat
4. Extreme diaphoresis
5. Restlessness, agitation or declining level of consciousness.

In respiratory distress, there will be severe difficulty in achieving adequate oxygenation in spite of significant efforts to breathe. It is usually associated with increased breathing rate and the use of accessory muscles in the chest wall. It occurs in approximately 20–74% of patients. Respiratory distress often occurs as a part of the terminal events in dying process.

Signs and Symptoms

The signs and symptoms are varied and depend on the age.

- Abnormal respiration
- Tachypnea
- Bradypnea
- Clubbing
- Apnea
- Retractions/accessory muscle use
- Nasal flaring
- Grunting
- Color change: pale or cyanotic
- Poor aeration
- Altered mental status

Factors Affecting Respiratory Function

- **Body position:** An upright posture (standing or sitting erect) allows for the greatest ease of lung expansion. Breathing requires more effort when lying down because the abdominal content pushes against the diaphragm.
- **Environment:** People's reaction to weather conditions is highly personalized. Some tolerate heat and humidity while others may complain of difficulty in breathing under these conditions. People who move to different climates may experience slight changes in breathing patterns until they become acclimatized to their new surroundings.

  People with chronic respiratory diseases often find breathing more difficult when the weather is hot and humid because humidity contributes to air viscosity.
- **Occupational chemicals and dust:** Industrialized urban areas may have elevated levels of air pollutants, e.g., hydrocarbons and oxidants, interfere with oxygenation by directly damaging lungs. Prolonged exposure to dust, vapors, irritants, fumes at workplace causes the respiratory distress. Workers in industrial plants or in certain

occupations may be exposed to strong concentrations of specific pollutants and harmful dust. These workers may be prone to development of respiratory problems.

- **Pollens and allergens:** Specific substances that cause allergic responses can affect respiration, sometimes severely.
- **Air pollution:** High level of urban air pollution is harmful to persons with existing lung diseases. Fossil fuels that are used for indoor heating and cooking increase risk for respiratory disease especially in poor ventilated areas.
- **Smoking:** The most important lifestyle choice that affects respiration is smoking. Smokers are far more likely to acquire emphysema, chronic bronchitis, lung cancer, and oral cancer as well as cardiovascular disease than non-smokers. Smoking inhibits mucus removal and causes airway blockage, promoting bacterial colonization and infection.
- **Drugs and alcohol:** Barbiturates, narcotics and some sedatives can depress the central nervous system, which results in decreasing respiration.
- **Nutrition:** Without proper diet, the body cannot effectively produce plasma proteins and hemoglobin. In addition, sufficient calories and protein are required for respiratory muscle strength.
- **Restricted lung movement:** Certain conditions and diseases may cause the lungs to stiffen or may restrict expansion of the chest.
- **Airway obstruction:** Any process that reduces the diameter of the conducting airways causes increased airway resistance. Breathing then requires more effort because air must be drawn through a narrower passageway.
- **Infection:** Severe recurring respiratory tract infection impairs normal defense mechanisms, making bronchioles and alveoli more susceptible to injury. Most common causative organisms are *Streptococcus, Haemophilus influenzae,* etc.
- **Aging:** Aging results in changes in lung structure and some degree of emphysema that is common in older adults, even in nonsmoker. Thoracic cage changes result from osteoporosis. It becomes rigid and the ribs are less mobile. As a result, decreased chest compliance and elastic recoil occurs, which increases the work of breathing.

Diagnostic Tests and Procedures

The most commonly used tests for assessing respiratory status are chest X-ray, pulmonary function tests, sputum culture, and analysis of arterial blood gases.

- **Pulmonary function tests:** Spirometer is the most common instrument for the pulmonary function test measuring the lung function, especially the amount (volume) or speed (flow) of air that can be inhaled and exhaled. It is

an important tool used for assessing conditions such as asthma, pulmonary fibrosis, cystic fibrosis and chronic obstructive pulmonary disease (COPD).

- **Chest X-ray:** It is used to identify abnormalities in chest structure and lung tissue. It is done to detect infection, effusion and foreign body.
- **Arterial blood gas analysis:** It is used to determine degree of oxygenation in blood and also used to determine acidic or alkaline state of blood.
- **Sputum specimen for Gram stain and culture:** It is done to identify the organism causing infection.
- **Pulse oximetry:** It uses an infrared light to determine the percentage of hemoglobin that has combined with oxygen. It helps in knowing the oxygen saturation in the blood.
- **Complete blood count:** It is used to check the presence of infection.
- **Bronchoscopy:** It allows the physician to visualize the larynx, trachea and bronchi to identify lesions, remove foreign bodies and secretion. It is also used to obtain tissue for biopsy.
- **Skin tests:** Skin test can be performed to identify a client's allergies to specific substances.

Medical Management of Patient with Respiratory Distress

The goal of the management is to relieve symptoms, prevent disease progression, reduce mortality, improve exercise tolerance, improve health status and prevent and treat complications and exacerbations.

- Smoking cessation is essential to stop injury to respiratory epithelium.
- Inhaled bronchodilators reduce dyspnea and bronchospasm; delivered by meter dose inhaler, dry powder inhalers or hand held or mask nebulizer devices.
- Anticholinergic, short and long acting beta-adrenergic agonists can be given.
- For retained secretions, chest physiotherapy, including postural drainage for secretion, clearance and breathing retraining may be used for improved ventilation and control of dyspnea.
- Supplemental oxygen therapy for patients with hypoxemia. Carbon dioxide must be monitored to determine increased carbon dioxide retention.
- Pulmonary rehabilitation to improve function, strength, symptom control, disease self-management techniques, independence and quality of life.
- Antimicrobial and antibiotic agents for episodes of respiratory infection.
- Influenza (annual) and pneumococcal vaccination
- Self-management strategies such as management of exacerbations.

- Physical therapy and respiratory therapy
  - Breathing retraining, e.g., pursed lip breathing
  - Effective coughing, e.g., Huff coughing
  - Chest physiotherapy
  - Postural drainage

Nursing Management of Patient with Respiratory Distress

As nurses, they need to meet this challenge and strengthen their skills in caring for patients.

- The nurse should also assess dyspnea or respiratory distress by observing the depth and rate of respirations, the color of person's skin, amount of respiratory effort and facial changes such as pursing of lips or flaring of the nostrils.
- Medication can decrease the effort of breathing and reduce dyspnea. The administration of bronchodilators, theophylline and corticosteroids can help relieve dyspnea and may be administered in and attempt to manage respiratory distress.

Improving Patient Airway Clearance

- Eliminate pulmonary irritants, particularly cigarette smoking
- Keep patient's room dust free
- Administer bronchodilators to control bronchospasm and dyspnea
- Assess for adverse effects: Tachycardia, cardiac dysrhythmias, central nervous system stimulation and hypertension
- Auscultate the chest after administration of bronchodilators
- Mobilize the patient when stable and use postural drainage positions to aid in clearance of secretions if present
- Encourage fluid intake within level of cardiac reserve

Improve Breathing Pattern

- Teach diaphragmatic, lower costal and abdominal breathing using a slow and relaxed breathing pattern to reduce respiratory rate.
- Discuss and demonstrate relaxation exercises to reduce stress, tension and anxiety.

Control the Infection

- Obtain the sputum for Gram stain and culture and sensitivity.
- Administer prescribed antimicrobials to control secondary bacterial infections.

Improve Nutrition

- Encourage for frequent small meals, if patient is dyspneic
- Offer liquid nutritional supplements to improve calorie intake and counteract weight loss.

- Avoid gas producing food and abdominal discomfort.
- Encourage pursed-lip breathing between bites if patient is having shortness of breath; rest after meal, supplemental oxygen while patient is eating to relieve dyspnea as described.
- Employ good oral hygiene before meals

Increase Activity Tolerance

- Reemphasize the importance of graded exercise and physical conditioning programs
- Train patient in energy conservation techniques and pacing of activities.

Improve Sleep Pattern

- Maintain balanced schedule for activity and rest.
- Use nocturnal oxygen therapy when appropriate.
- Avoid use of sedatives and hypnotics that may cause respiratory depression. Morphine is an effective medication to help decrease dyspnea by suppressing respiration and also providing sedation. Studies show that morphine was able to decrease the intensity of dyspnea without statistically modifying the oxygen saturation level in the blood, the respiratory rate or overall exchange of air.
- Administration of oxygen may also reduce respiratory distress
- The use of oxygen and nebulized morphine has shown some therapeutic benefits in chronic obstructive pulmonary disease (COPD).
- Relaxation and psychophysical techniques have been found helpful in relieving respiratory problems.
- Other psychophysiological techniques include meditation, visual imagery and yoga.
- Fresh air and fan are simple interventions that can be helpful.
- Optimizing the effectiveness of respiratory effort and reducing the work of breathing can be achieved by encouraging and helping patient to cough and expectorate sputum.
- Giving prescribed bronchodilators or passing a nasogastric tube to relieve gastric gas.
- Minimizing the patient oxygen demands and carbon dioxide production can be achieved by reducing the amount of work a patient has to do to ventilate his lungs effectively. The more work an individual has to do, the more oxygen is used by respiratory muscles and carbon dioxide produced.
- The aim is to build close and therapeutic relationship with your patient.
- Help the individual to achieve the optimum position. Safe and appropriate positioning of the patient can contribute to improve comfort and ease the work of breathing.

It influences lung function, inspiratory and expiratory lung volume.

- Sitting upright in a chair
- Sitting upright in bed
- Side lying in bed

- Monitor the rate and rhythm of respiration. It provides valuable information about the patient's clinical condition.
- Administer prescribed pharmacological agents and monitor for their effects and complications.

Monitor the amount of oxygen patient requires and how this impacts on oxygen saturation when pulse oximetry monitoring is used.

Health Education

- Advise patient to avoid respiratory irritants.
- Encourage patient involvement in self-management techniques such as identification and prompt reporting of respiratory infection or respiratory deterioration.
- Warn patient to stay out of extremely hot or cold weather and to avoid aggravating bronchial and sputum obstruction.
- Warn patient to avoid excessive fatigue, which is a factor in producing respiratory distress.
- Advise patient to adjust activities as per individual fatigue patterns.
- Advise to cope with emotional stress as positively as possible.
- Warn patient to avoid persons with respiratory infections and to avoid crowds and areas with poor ventilation.

- Teach the patient how to recognize and report the evidence of respiratory infection promptly such as chest pain, changes in character of sputum (amount, color and consistency), increasing difficulty in raising sputum, increasing coughing and wheezing and increasing shortness of breath.
- Tell patient to drink plenty of fluids and non-caffeinated beverages each day to keep mucus thin and easier to cough.
- Instruct patient to avoid overeating and eating of foods that cause gas or bloating. A full stomach or bloated abdomen might make breathing uncomfortable.
- Instruct patient to stick to treatment regimen and for strict follow up even after symptoms subside.

CONCLUSION

Respiratory distress is a common and often serious emergency. Good patient outcomes require rapid and skilled assessment of the airway, breathing and oxygenation. Caring for the patient with altered respiratory function is a significant challenge for nurses. If shortness of breath is used as a simple example, this has the potential to lead the patient into a vicious cycle of events that have extremely serious consequences. Timely and appropriate management of the patient's respiratory function can have a tremendous impact on the patient's condition and eventual outcome.

BIBLIOGRAPHY

1. Chintamani, Mrinalini M. Lewis's Medical Surgical Nursing. Mosby; 2011. pp. 637–47.
2. Bassett C. Essentials of Nursing Care. Whur Publication; 2004. pp. 47–92.
3. Ruth FC, Constance JH. Fundamentals of Nursing: Human Health and Function, 3rd edition. Lippincott Williams & Wilkins; pp. 784-800.
4. Smeltzer SC, Bare B, Hinkle JL, et al. Brunner and Suddarth's Textbook of Medical-Surgical Nursing, Vol 1, 11th edition. Lippincott, pp. 601–620.

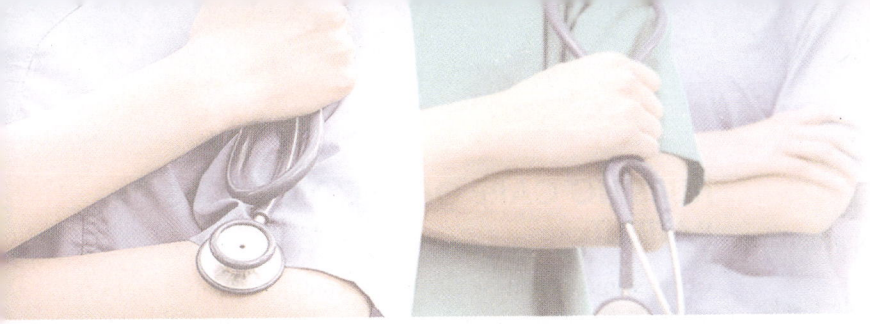

Care of Patient having Alterations in Sensorium

INTRODUCTION

Consciousness

Consciousness is defined as a state of awareness of self, time and of environment, as well as a state of responsiveness to that environment or adaptation to the external stimuli.

Unconsciousness

Unconsciousness is a condition in which the patient is unresponsive and unaware of environmental stimuli.

It can be brief, lasting for few seconds, hours, days or longer.

CAUSES OF UNCONSCIOUSNESS

- Head injury (traumatic brain injury)
- Skull fracture
- Brain hypoxia (e.g., due to a brain infarction or cardiac arrest)
- Extremes of body temperature
- Cardiac arrest
- Blood loss
- Cerebrovascular accident
- Epilepsy
- Hypoglycemia
- Hyperglycemia
- Drug overdose
- Encephalitis
- Meningitis
- Fluid and electrolyte imbalance
- Hypothermia
- Poisonous substances and fumes (that depress the activity of the central nervous system)

LEVELS OF UNCONSCIOUSNESS

- **Lethargy:** Sleepy, slow to respond but appropriate response; opens eyes to stimuli; oriented.
- **Stupor:** Aroused by painful stimuli, never fully awake, confused and unclear conversation
- **Semi-coma stage:** Moves in response to painful stimuli, no conversation, protective blinking and pupillary reflex patient.
- **Coma:** Unresponsive except to severe pain, no protective reflexes, fixed pupil and no voluntary movement.

GLASGOW COMA SCALE

Level of consciousness is assessed through Glasgow coma scale (Table 1)

Client's response is rated from 3 to 15. Less than 3 indicates unconsciousness due to neurological impairment.

TABLE 1: Glasgow coma scale

Eye opening
Spontaneous = 4
To speech = 3
To pain = 2
None = 1
Verbal response
Oriented = 5
Confused = 4
Inappropriate = 3
Incomprehensible sound = 2
None = 1
Motor response
Obeys = 6
Localizing = 5
Normal flexion = 4
Abnormal flexion (decorticate) = 3
Extension (decelerate) = 2
None = 1
Total = 15

NURSING CARE OF UNCONSCIOUS PATIENT

Unconscious comatose clients are completely dependent on others because their consciousness and protective reflexes are impaired. Therefore, requires aggressive nursing intervention. Nurses are responsible for meeting basic needs and preventing the complications associated with unconsciousness.

For the effective care, nurse should perform frequent assessment of comatose client, plan the care and implement the care.

Assess vital signs (temperature, pulse, blood pressure respiration) of the patient 4 hourly or as required to plan the care, prevent complications and manage early signs of any deviation in normal functioning.

Priority Wise Nursing Care of Unconscious Patient

- **Ineffective airway clearance related to upper airway obstruction by tongue and soft tissue**
  Nursing care for maintaining patent airway
  - Assess respiratory rate pattern, lung sound, hypoxia and cyanosis, presence of secretion because of inability to clear respiratory secretions to plan the care.
  - Elevating the head end of the bed to 30 degrees to prevent aspiration
  - Positioning the patient in lateral or semi-prone position to prevent aspiration
  - Insert airway if tongue is paralyzed or obstructing the airway
  - Suction airway intermittently to prevent accumulation of secretion in posterior pharynx and upper trachea and prevent aspiration.
  - Administer humidified oxygen before suctioning and prevent hypoxia.
  - Initiate chest physiotherapy and postural drainage to promote pulmonary hygiene.
  - Prepare client for endotracheal intubation or tracheostomy and connect to mechanical ventilation as needed to maintain respiration, efficient removal of tracheobronchial secretion, protect from aspiration and maintain oxygen level.
  - Increase amount of fluid administered; at least 2.5 liters a day to loosen airway secretion and promoting easy removal.

- Auscultate chest at least every 8 hours to detect adventitious breath sound or absent breath sound.
- Monitor arterial blood gas (ABG) measurement to detect complications of respiration

- **Risk of injury related to unconscious state**
  Nursing care for protecting the client from injury
  - Assess the risk factors for injury: Lack of side rails, seizures, invasive lines and equipment, restraints and tight dressing.
  - Keep side rails up and bed in lowest position whenever the client is not receiving any direct care to prevent fall.
  - Observe seizure precaution for clients with history of seizure episodes.
  - Use padded side rails to prevent injury during seizure activity.
  - Keep client's nails short to prevent scratching.
  - Use caution when moving the client, give adequate support to limbs and head to prevent dislocation.
  - Always turn the client towards the nurse to prevent fall.
  - Protect from external sources of heat such as hot water bags. Unconscious client cannot voice pain.
  - Release restraints every 2 hours. It helps in providing range of motion exercise and prevent complications of immobility.
  - Avoid restraints as far as possible. Allow one family member to be with the client.
  - Keep bed and bedding free from moisture, dust and debris to prevent skin excoriation.
  - Avoid speaking negatively about the client or his conditions the last sense to go is the sense of hearing for psychological integrity.

- **Risk of fluid volume deficit related to inability to ingest food, dehydration from osmotic diuretics.**
  Nursing care for maintaining optimum fluid volume state
  - Assess hydration status by examination of skin turgor, mucus membrane, intake and output changes and analyzing laboratory data electrolytes, creatinine and blood urea nitrogen (BUN).
  - Hydrate the client with use of intravenous (IV) fluids as prescribed to meet fluids needs.
  - Avoid over hydrating the client with IV fluids or blood transfusion because excessive or rapid administration of fluid may lead to cerebral edema and increased intracranial pressure (ICP).
  - Administer fluids slowly to prevent injury to veins.
  - Continue fluid administration with use of Ryle's tube to allow long-term fluid administration.
  - Administer corticosteroids and diuretics in suspected cerebral edema to maintain normal volume of fluids.

- Maintain intake and output and do proper documentation to detect abnormality.
- Evaluate peripheral pulse and blood pressure at regular intervals to measure circulatory adequacy.

- **Imbalanced nutrition less than body requirement related to inability to eat swallow as evidenced by weight and other nutritional parameter less than normal.**
  Nursing care for maintaining nutritional status
  - Assess nutritional status through skin and mucus membrane.
  - Administer IV fluids to meet nutritional mucous.
  - Administer fluid diet in the form of juices, shake, soup, water, milk and protein lactose through Ryle's tube feeding, as unconscious patient cannot take oral feed. Increase the quantity as prescribed because metabolic need increases due to immunodeficiency, protein wasting and lung tissue catabolism.
  - Provide high calorie, high protein and vitamin-rich liquid diet.
  - Initiate total parenteral nutrition if the client cannot tolerate Ryle's tube feed, or according to need.

- **Ineffective thermoregulation due to damage to hypothalamus center as evidenced by persistent elevation of body temperature, warm and dry skin.**
  To maintain body temperature
  - Regularly assess the temperature.
  - Look for possible site of infection.
  - Control persistent elevation of temperature with use of antipyretics, cooling blankets, adequate fluid intake, tepid sponge, cold compress and good ventilation of room. Fever increases metabolic demand of brain, decreases circulation and oxygenation resulting in cerebral deterioration.
  - Control shivering in fever with use of blanket, warm environment and heat application.
  - Prevent infection by using aseptic technique during procedure.

- **Altered oral mucous membrane related to mouth breathing, absence of pharyngeal reflex, inability to ingest fluids as evidenced by dryness, inflammation, crusting and halitosis**
  To maintain oral hygiene
  - Assess oral mucous membrane regularly. Inspect mouth every 8 hourly using flash light and tongue depressor to detect problems in early stage.
  - If denture is present, remove them to prevent choking and other complication.
  - Provide oral care. Cleanse mouth carefully with appropriate solution (potassium permanganate, listerine) every 2–4 hours to prevent halitosis and infection.

- Provide oral care after suctioning to clean oral cavity adequately.
- Apply thin coat of petroleum jelly after oral care to moisten the lips and prevent drying and cracking.
- Clean airway to remove secretions to maintain patent airway.
- Change endotracheal tube bandage as soaked bandage increases the chance of infection and maintain/grooming of the client
- Move endotracheal tube to the opposite side of the mouth to prevent ulceration of mouth and lips.
- Do tracheostomy care, suctioning to remove secretions followed by oral care.
- Avoid lemon or alcohol containing agent for cleaning to prevent dryness.
- Gently swab nose with wet cotton applicator and apply water soluble lubricant to remove encrustation from nose, facilitate nose breathing to prevent dryness of mouth.

- **Risk of impaired corneal integrity related to absence of corneal blink reflex and dryness of eyes.**
  To maintain eyes integrity:
  - Assess signs of impaired corneal integrity (corneal drying, irritation, ulceration). Look for presence of corneal blink responses to plan the care.
  - Protect eyes with shield. If eyes remain open for long period, corneal ulceration will develop.
  - Apply eye patches when indicated to ensure that eyes remain closed.
  - Make sure the client's eyes are not rubbing against anything such as bedding or clothing.
  - Inspect the condition of eyes with flash light at regular intervals to detect corneal irritation at early stage.
  - Irrigate eyes with sterile saline or prescribed solution as ordered. Removal of discharge and debris prevents inflammation.
  - Provide regular eye care with proper sterile technique to prevent eye infection and clean the eyes.
  - Instill prescribed ophthalmic ointment in each eye to prevent corneal ulceration.
  - Instill artificial tears as prescribed to keep eyes moist and prevent dryness of eyes.

- **Self-care deficit (bathing, feeding, grooming and toileting) related to unconscious state.**
  To maintain hygiene:
  - Assess self-care needs to perform self-care activities.
  To maintain skin hygiene or skin integrity:
  - Perform bed bath daily or as required (upon soiling of bed with stool, urine, sweat or dirt). Clean skin prevents bacterial growth and promote overall well-being.

- Regularly change the position.
- Provide passive exercise.
- Provide a range of motion exercises to prevent contracture.
- Apply oil/cream to prevent dryness.
- Provide back care and back massage.
- Provide special beds or air or water cushions to prevent pressure on bony prominences to prevent bed sores.
  - Oral hygiene: Do oral care 4 hourly
  - Perform hair wash twice a week and comb hair as needed
  - Clean the extremities and cut nails short.
  - Perform foot care to prevent ulcer. Use splints, rings, air cushion or sand bag to prevent foot drop.
  - Give perineal care and catheter care twice a day with antiseptic solution to prevent the infection. Watch signs of urinary tract infection (increased body temperature, cloudy urine, hematuria and presence of bad odor as early detection prevents complication).

Preventing urinary retention:
Palpate for full bladder. Empty urinary bladder by inserting an indwelling catheter or use absorbent pads placed under the buttocks in females. Use condom catheter in males.

- Change the dressing (cannula dressing, central venous line dressing, tracheostomy dressing) as needed or daily.
- Change the tubing of ventilator, change the humidifier of ventilator and change sterile water according to protocol.

- **Risk of complications: Pressure sore, contracture, deep vein thrombosis, hypostatic pneumonia, constipation and related to immobility.**
  For prevention of complications:
  Assess initial sign of bedsore (redness on pressure prone areas), deep vein thrombosis (DVT) (redness and swelling in lower extremities), pneumonia (tachypnea, retraction, noisy breathing), contractures (stiff joints, muscle and tendons), constipation (distended hard abdomen, infrequent, emptying of bowel and hard stool).
  Prevention of bedsore:
  - Keep skin clean, dry, free of pressure
  - Use pressure relieving devices (air cushion, air/water mattresses, pillows, foam pads, etc.) to take off pressure from pressure prone area.
  - Change position every 2 hourly.
  - Avoid dragging and pulling the client while changing position, prevent shear force which induces sore.

- Give skin care to pressure prone areas 4 hourly. Massage increases circulation. Skin cleaning is needed to prevent pressure sore from moisture and excessive dryness.
- Avoid vigorous massage of bony prominences (vigorous massage causes skin excoriation over bony prominences).
- Provide high calorie, high protein, vitamin rich diet with more amount of fluid. Adequate nutrition prevents pressure sore formation

Prevention of contracture and joint deformity and muscle wasting:

- Keep the body in the anatomical position with the use of devices like foot rest, trochanter rolls, sand bags, rolled cloth, water filled gloves. Body alignment helps to prevent joint deformity and contracture.
- Give protein-rich diet. It helps to maintain positive nitrogen balance.
- Perform range of motion exercises every 4 hourly after removing the support devices. Passive exercise helps to strengthen the weak muscles, loosens spastic muscles, promotes joint flexibility and increases overall well-being of the client.

Prevention of deep vein thrombosis:

- Elevate lower extremities above the heart level intermittently for 20 minutes. It increases venous return, thus preventing thrombus formation.
- Perform passive range of motion exercise to extremities every 4 hourly.
- Use elastic stockings as required.
- Monitor the presence of redness, swelling and increased temperature of legs.

Prevention of hypostatic pneumonia/aspiration pneumonia:

Pulmonary congestion occurs due to the stagnation of blood in the dependent portions of the lungs in persons who are ill and lie in the same position for long periods.

Aspiration pneumonia is an inflammation (usually due to an infection) of lungs and bronchial tubes by inhaling materials such as vomitus, food, or liquid.

- Suction the airway at regular interval, unconscious client is unable to remove oral and airway secretion and accumulation of secretion leads to pneumonia.
- Change position 2 hourly, prevent pooling of secretion in the lungs and thus hydrostatic pneumonia is prevented.
- Initiate chest physiotherapy and postural drainage unless contraindicated.
- Feed the client in a head elevated.
- Aspirate Ryle's tube before feeding.
- Watch for regurgitation and vomiting.
- Keep head turned to one side.

- Give fluids to loosen airway secretions to facilitate easy removal.

Prevention of constipation:

- Provide adequate fluid. Increased fluids are required for softening the feces.
- Administer stool softener and enema to help in bowel evacuation.
- Change position every 2 hourly. It increases bowel movement.

- **Impaired sensory stimulation related to improper neural functioning**

Providing sensory stimulation:

- Provided at proper time to avoid sensory deprivation.
- Efforts are made to maintain the sense of daily rhythm by keeping the usual day and night patterns for activity and sleep.
- Maintain the same schedule each day.
- Orient the client to the day, date and time accordingly.
- Touch and talk in reassuring voice.
- Proper communication should be done.
- Always address the client by name and explain the procedure each time.

- **Interrupted family process related to chronic illness of family members as evidenced by anger, grief and non-participation in client care.**

- Assess family's response toward the client's illness, severe anxiety, denial, anger, remorse, grief, usual use of coping mechanism, role of client in the family, communication pattern, social support available, financial status and relationship between family members provide baseline data about family and helps in planning the care to help them accordingly.
- Develop a supportive and trusting relationship with the family or significant others to develop good interpersonal relationship
- Provide information and frequent updates on client's condition and progress. It helps to alleviate anxiety.
- Family needs should be maintained.
- Family support should be given. Involve family in routine care. Teach procedure that they can perform at home.
- Demonstrate and teach methods of sensory stimulation to be used frequently. This intervention helps family to understand that client is having internal awareness of what is going on around, though he is not responding to stimuli, helps them to better cope with client's condition and reduce their anxiety to a greater extent and increases their participation in client's care.
- Educate them about the needs of client, care of client, treatment plan, prognosis of treatment and don't provide any false assurance

- Teach them to report unusual restlessness in the client. It indicates cerebral hypoxia or metabolic imbalance.
- Help the family members to verbalize their doubts and cope with the situation.
- Enlist help of social worker, home health agency, or other resources to assist family with financial concern and need for medical equipment in home.

CONCLUSION

Kindness comes in many forms but it has to be always from the heart. Therefore, be kind and caring on your part to promote health and prevent illness in unconscious patients as they are fully dependent on you.

BIBLIOGRAPHY

1. Smeltzer SC, Bare BG, Hinkle, et al. Brunner & Suddarth's Textbook of Medical-Surgical Nursing, 11th edition. 2008. pp. 1281-82.
2. Black MJ. Medical Surgical Nursing: Clinical Management for Positive Outcomes, Vol 2, 8th edition. Philadelphia: Saunders. pp 1006-16.
3. Nettina. Lippincott Manual of Nursing Practice, 9th edition. Lippincott William and Wilkins. pp. 785-9.
4. Basin BS, Cooke JL. Depressed consciousness and Coma. In: Medical Surgical Nursing, 8th edition, Elsevier publication: 2009. pp. 1792-1804.
5. Taylor C, Lillis C. Fundamental of Nursing, 5th edition. Lippincott Williams & Wilkins pp. 785-9.
6. Smeltzer SC, Bare B, Hinkle JL, et al. Brunner and Suddarth's Textbook of Medical-Surgical Nursing, 12th edition. Lippincott, pp. 136-48.

Assessment of Self-care Ability

INTRODUCTION

Activities of daily living (ADL) comprise the basic activities that involve caring for one's self and body, including personal care, mobility, and eating. ADL include the fundamental skills typically needed to manage basic physical needs, comprised of following areas: grooming, personal hygiene, dressing, toileting/continence, transferring/ambulating, and eating. The ability to perform ADL is dependent upon cognitive (e.g., reasoning, planning) and motor (e.g., balance, dexterity, and perceptual (including sensory) abilities.

In many settings, ADL are assessed directly by occupational, physical or speech therapists or by nurses and other members of the health team. ADL capacity assessment is requested during the middle or later stages of dementia but may also occur during the course of recovery from a disease such as stroke. Referral for evaluation of ADL ability may include questions of cognitive, emotional, or behavioral factors that can be interfering with functioning in these basic skills and how their barriers may be overcome to enhance independence.

Salf-care ability of client with intellectual sub-normality can be assessed based on six main domains like assessment of personal care and appearance, dietary and food management, household tasks and responsibility, community and leisure work, sexuality and social communication.

PERSONAL HYGIENE AND APPEARANCE

- Assess the client with the present baseline self-care abilities
- Educate and assist the client regarding self-care abilities
- Activities of daily living:
  - **Oral hygiene:** Check with the brushing ability of the client.
  - **Bathing:** Supervise the client's level of bathing competencies.

- **Dressing and grooming:**
  - ○ Capacity to dress and groom self
  - ○ Dressing style: Type of clothing and footwear's that should be decided and used based on the time of the day, existing weather conditions and special occasions like festivals and weddings
- Able to perform appropriate level of activities like exercising for minimum of 20–30 minutes, at least 3–4 times a week
- Capable to sleep for minimum 6–8 hours at night without disturbing others
- Ability to follow the dosage and timing of prescribed medications as per the physician/psychiatrist
- Tell at least one negative effect of the hazardous substances or situations, e.g., alcohol intoxication is dangerous for liver or smoking can lead to cancer.

DIETARY AND FOOD MANAGEMENT

- Able to consume sufficient quantity of food as per requirements
- Capable to maintain appropriate level of appetite
- Prepares the table for breakfast, lunch or supper
- Nutrition requirement
- Able to remove unwanted particles, dirt or stones from the food (rice/vegetable/fruits, etc.)
- Ability to serve food to self or others
- Clean and wash the used utensils and table after breakfast, lunch or supper
- Capable of cleaning the kitchen after cooking or using

HOUSEHOLD TASKS AND RESPONSIBILITY

- The individual should be able to use various strategies in cleaning their washrooms after use (flushing the toilets and cleaning self).
- Should be able to dust the bed, arrange the bed sheet/bed cover and pillow in order as per house norms.
- Perform household activities on a regular basis as part of responsibility.
- Should recite minimum of 4 lines or 10 words of prayer
- Should verbally state or list down in writing personal activities of whole day with timings on an hourly basis.

COMMUNITY AND LEISURE ACTIVITIES

The individual should be able to:
- Access existing community resources and include in leisure activities independently.
- Travel the predetermined destination within the city by using available means of transportation.

- Make a detailed plan of tour within the city or outside the city like: schedule of travel, destination places, the distance, travel time, mode of transport/conveyance, accommodation for stay and approximate total expenditure.
- Verify the quality and quantity of the desired items as per instructions to be purchased with the given money
- Mail letters, with the given money, purchase stamps/ inland letters/ envelop and collect the receipt.
- Check amount in his account using the passbook, should be able to deposit and withdraw money by using deposit and withdraw forms and ATM card.
- Select from available items from the restaurant by asking or using from menu card, place order, eat the food ordered and pay the bills. Should be able to order for a minimum of two persons.
- Go on tour as per predetermined plans of place/persons of visit and return home as per scheduled travel plans.

FUNCTIONING OF SENSORY ORGANS: VISUAL AND HEARING IMPAIRMENT

Visual Impairment

Visual impairment refers to a significant functional loss of vision that cannot be corrected by medication, surgical operation, or optic lenses.

The person may be **totally blind** when the person is absolutely without sight but may have light and movement perception and travel vision. The degree of blindness includes:

- **Light perception:** Can differentiate light and dark/day and night.
- **Movement perception:** Can detect if an object or a person is in motion or in still position.
- **Travel vision:** Field of vision is enough to travel safely in familiar area.
- **Field of vision:** Refers to the area that normal eyes cover above, below and on both sides when looking at an object or when gazing straight ahead. The normal vision covers approximately a range of 180 degrees.
- **Low vision:** A level of vision that with standard correction hinders an individual in the visual planning and execution of tasks but which permits enhancement of the functional vision through the use of optical or non-optical aids.

Causes

The inability of the eyes to function efficiently is due to:

- Errors of refraction
- Imbalance of the eye muscles
- Diseases
- Trauma or accidents

Levels of Impairment

- **Mild visual impairment:** In this, person can read relatively larger characters and have no difficulty in identifying shapes, colors and brightness.
- **Moderate visual impairment:** In this, person can tell shapes and colors of objects and can distinguish between brightness and darkness and can only read characters with larger size and broader strokes.
- **Severe visual impairment:** In this person can only distinguish more obvious changes in brightness and darkness or may not see anything (completely blind).

Problems Associated with Visual Impairment

Daily Activities

- Squinting to get an object in focus
- Trouble locating familiar objects in a familiar environment
- Wearing mismatched clothing.

Mobility

Leaning against the wall when walking, running into objects, difficulty walking on uneven surfaces.

Eating/Drinking

Difficulty in getting food onto utensils and serving and spilling food.

Reading/Writing

Difficulty writing on the lines of a piece of paper and frequently complaining that the light is inadequate for reading or writing.

Communication Barriers

Many people are uncomfortable with communicating with the blind.

Ways to reduce risk of visual impairment

- Protect your eyes from the sun. Ultraviolet rays from the sun can damage eyesight, so wear a pair of good-quality sun-glasses.
- Find out whether there is a history of glaucoma or eye disease in your family.
- Hypertension
- Pain is a warning sign that the organ needs care.
- Regular eye examinations: Drivers and those who work on computers should get themselves checked regularly.

Hearing Impairment

Hearing impairment is also called deafness or hearing loss and occurs when there is a problem with or damage to one or both parts of the ear. It is a serious problem among older adults and affects their functional ability, which in turn significantly affects their quality of life.

Assessment

- **Observation:** Does the patient cups his/her hand behind the ear? Does she tilt his/her head or lean toward you when listening? Does he/she keep the volume of television very high? Does he/she complain of ringing, roaring or buzzing in his/her ears? Does he/she misinterpret questions or comments or not respond at all? All these signs prompt further assessment and evaluation.
- **The patient's own report:** Ask the patient whether he/she has difficulty hearing in specific situations such as in noisy room, a restaurant, at a lecture, on the telephone or during normal conversations.
- **Audiometry:** It is considered the gold standard of hearing assessment.
- **Whispered voice test:** Done by standing 2 feet behind the patient, covering and rubbing the untested ear (rubbing helps in masking of sound) and whispering three random letters and numbers. The patient than repeats the three letters and numbers. An incorrect response requires the test to be repeated using different letters and numbers.
- **Rinne's and Weber's tuning fork tests**

Interventions

When a patient has hearing impairment, a combination of adaptive techniques, environmental modification and assistive devices including hearing aids are necessary to ensure effective communication.

Communicating with People with Hearing Loss

Successful communication requires the efforts of all people involved in a conversation. Even when the person with hearing loss utilizes hearing aids and active listening strategies.

These communication strategies are:
- Face the hearing impaired person directly.
- Do not talk from another room.
- Speak clearly, slowly, distinctly but naturally, without shouting or exaggerating mouth movements.
- Call the person's name before beginning a conversation.
- Avoid talking too rapidly or using sentences that are too complex.
- Keep your hands away from your face while talking.
- If the hearing impaired listener hears better in one ear than the other, try to position yourself accordingly.
- Try to minimize noise in the background.

- Acquaint the listener with the general topic of conversation.
- Whenever possible provide pertinent information in writing.
- Remember that hearing impaired person has a harder time hearing and understanding when ill or tired.
- Pay attention to the listener so that message is understood.

ASSESSMENT OF SELF-CARE ABILITY AMONG PHYSICALLY CHALLENGED PERSON

Physically challenged people are grouped according to affected part of the body, e.g., orthopedically handicapped (having a plaster cast or traction), sensory handicapped, neurologically handicapped and handicapped due to systemic diseases.

- **Physically challenged** who have a problem with their body that makes it difficult for them to do things that others can do easily.
- Physically disabled in a way that prevents one from using part of their body properly e.g., absence of a limb in a body.

Several rating scales help the nurse to assess the patient's capabilities and define the degree of the patient's current functional abilities.

North-American Nursing Diagnosis Association (NANDA) provides rating scales for five major activities of daily living (ADL). These are: bathing/hygiene, dressing/grooming, feeding, toileting and mobility. Others are urinary continence, bowel continence, ambulating, using a wheelchair, transferring (in and out of bed, from bed to chair and back) communicating and self medicating.

These activities may be further categorized into dependency ratings whether the patient is independent, partially dependent or totally dependent. The nurse assesses the needs to determine the exact nature of help required and how it is to be achieved whether by family, friend, health professional or through specialized equipment. For example, patient is able to eat, comb the hair, brush the teeth, but not able to move out of bed and unable to go to toilet. So, some of the needs are to be attended by others either by family members or by health professionals.

ASSESSMENT OF SELF-CARE ABILITY AMONG MENTALLY CHALLENGED PERSON

Mentally challenged/mentally disabled/intellectual disability (ID) once called mental retardation is characterized by below average intelligence or mental ability and a lack of skills necessary for day to day living. People with intellectual disability can and do learn new skills, but they learn them move slowly.

Mentally challenged condition is very common, there are more than 10 million cases per year in India. ID is chronic and can last life-long. Treatment can help, but and cannot it be cured. The main symptom is difficulty in thinking and understanding. Life skills that can be imparted upon include certain conceptual, social and practical skills.

These persons can be helped by special education and behavioral therapy which helps them to live their life at the fullest.

Causes

- **Genetic factors:** Chromosomal defects, for example, Mongolism syndrome.
- **Causes related to the pregnancy and childbirth:**
- **Prenatal:** Lack of adequate nutritional diet to mother, viral infection in the first trimester of pregnancy such as mumps, rubella infection and premature birth.
- **Natal:** Birth trauma, mechanical injury to the child during forceps delivery. Birth asphyxia leads to 25–30% mental retardation.
- **Postnatal:** Bacterial encephalitis, meningitis which is the most common cause of mental feebleness.
- **Infection:** Congenital rubella, influenza to mother, congenital syphilis.
- **Trauma/head injury**
- **Malnutrition:** In the first-two years of development, leads to mental retardation.
- **Disorders of metabolism:** Phenylketonuria, Hypothyroidism.
- **Intoxication:** Bilirubin encephalopathy, lead poisoning.
- **Sociocultural:** Prolonged isolation during the develop mental period leads to sensory and social deprivation, cultural familial retardation in which the child finds it difficult to interact with others.

Levels of Intellectual Disability

The different levels of intellectual disability are given in Table 1.

TABLE 1: Levels of intellectual disability

Degree	IQ level	Deficit
Mild	52–69	Problem in reading and writing. Difficulty in complex idea. Can learn motor skills than verbal skills. Education up to the 6th grade.
Moderate	36–51	Education up to 2nd grade Intelligence level similar to 4–7 years old child. Require supervision for self care
Severe	20–35	Minimal speech and marked degree of motor impairment. Complete supervision for self-care.
Profound	19 and below	Immobile, incontinent, and rudimentary form of nonverbal communication. No ability to care for their basic needs

Barthal Index

Barthal index is a tool for assessment of self-care ability among mentally challenged individual.

Maximum score is 100. Low scores on individual items highlight area of need.

Patient's Name:	
Rater's Name:	
Date:	
Activity	*Score*
Feeding 0 = unable 5 = needs cutting, spreading butter or required modified diet 10 = independent	—
Bathing 0 = dependent 5 = independent	—
Grooming 0 = Needs help with personal care 5 = independent in grooming of face/hair/teeth/shaving	—
Activity	*Score*
Dressing 0 = dependent 5 = need help but can do half unaided 10 = independent (including button, zip, laces, etc.)	—
Bowel 0 = incontinent 5 = occasional, accidentally 10 = continent	—
Bladder 0 = incontinent or catheterized 5 = occasional, accidental 10 = continent	—
Toilet use 0 = dependent 5 = needs some help, but can do something alone 10 = independent (on and off, dressing, wiping)	—
Transfers (bed to chair and back) 0 = unable, no sitting balance 5 = major help (one or two, people physical), can sit 10 = minor help (verbal or physical) 15 = Independent	—
Mobility (on level surfaces) 0 = immobile or <50 yards 5 = wheel chair independent, including corners >50 yards.	—
Stairs 0 = unable 5 = need help 10 = independent	—
Total	0–100

BIBLIOGRAPHY

1. *White L. Basic Nursing: Foundation of Skills and Concepts, 1st edition. Delmar/Thomson Learning; 2002.*
2. *Kockrow EO, Christensen BL. Foundations of Nursing, 4th edition. Mosby; 2003.*
3. *Brill EL. Down F. Foundations of Nursing, 2nd edition. Appleton-Century Crofts Publications. 1986.*
4. *Taylor CR, Lillis C, LeMone P, et al. Fundamentals of Nursing – The Art and Science of Nursing Care, 7th edition. Wolters Kluwer; 2010.*
5. *Dewit SC. Fundamental Concepts and Skills for Nursing WB Saunders Company; 2001.*
6. *Potter PA, Perry AG. Fundamental of nurse concepts, Process and Practice, 2nd edition St Louis: CV Mosby; 1992.*
7. *Sarkhel S. Kaplan and Sadock's Synopsis of Psychiatry: Behavioral Sciences/Clinical Psychiatry, 10th edition. Indian J Psychiatry. 2009;51(4):331.*

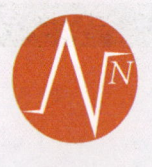
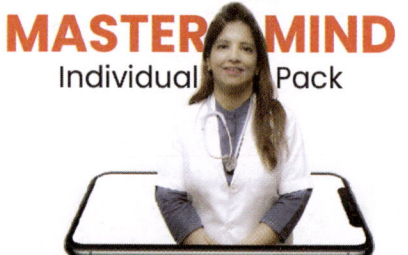

Meeting Needs of Perioperative Patients

INTRODUCTION

The treatment of many diseases includes some type of surgical intervention. Surgery may be performed for a variety of reasons; to cure or minimize disease, to diagnose the specific presence of a disease or condition, to reconstruct or eliminate a defect, to enhance form and function, to prescribe appropriate postoperative treatment and prognosis, to palliate or offer comfort, when cure is not possible, to follow up or monitor an incurable disease process, and to offer a preventable option when disease is inevitable, such as an elective mastectomy for a women at high risk for breast cancer. Surgery may be planned or unplanned, elective or optional, or major or minor and may involve any body part or system.

PHASES OF THE PERIOPERATIVE PERIOD

The patient who is having surgery progresses through distinct phases, called the perioperative period. The three phases of perioperative period are as follows:

- **The preoperative phase:** Begins when the decision to have surgery is made and ends when the patient is transferred to the operating table. The nursing activities associated with this phase include assessing the client, identifying potential or actual health problems, planning specific care based on the needs of the individuals and providing preoperative, teaching for the patient, family and significant others.

- **The intraoperative phase:** Begins when the patient is transferred to the operating table and ends when the patient is admitted to the post-anesthesia care unit (PACU), also called the recovery room. The nursing activities related to this phase include a variety of specialized procedures designed to create and maintain a safe therapeutic environment for the patient. These activities include interventions that provide for the patient's safety, maintaining an aseptic environment, ensuring proper functioning of equipment and providing the surgical team with the instruments and supplies needed during the procedure.

- **The postoperative phase:** Begins with the admission of the patient to the post-anesthesia area and ends till complete recovery from surgery and the last follow- up physician visit. The nursing activities during this phase include assessing the patient's physiologic and psychological response to surgery, performing interventions to facilitate healing and prevent complications, teaching and providing support to the patient and planning for home care.

TYPES OF SURGERY

Surgical procedures are commonly grouped according to urgency, risk and purpose.

- **Surgery based on urgency:** Surgery is classified by its urgency and necessity to preserve the life of patient, body part or body function. They are:
    - **Elective surgery:** It is a procedure that is preplanned and based on the patient's choice and availability of scheduling for the patient, surgeon, and facility. This is a non-urgent procedure that does not have to be done immediately. Examples of elective surgeries are cholecystectomy for chronic gall bladder disease, hip replacement surgery and plastic surgery.
    - **Emergency surgery:** It is performed immediately to preserve function, life or body part, surgeries to control internal hemorrhage or repair a fracture.
    - **Urgent surgery:** It must be done with in a reasonably short time frame to preserve health, but is not an emergency. It is usually done within 24–48 hours.
    - **Optional surgery:** It is not critical to survival or function.

- **Surgery based on degree of risk:** Surgery is also classified as major or minor according to the degree of risk to the patient.
    - **Major surgery:** Involves a high degree of risk: It may be complicated or prolonged, huge loss of blood may occur, vital organs may be involved or postoperative complications may be likely. Examples are, etc. open heart surgery, removal of kidney.
    - **Minor surgery:** Involves little risk, produces few complications and is often performed in an outpatient setting, Examples are: breast biopsy, removal of tonsils.

- **Surgery based on purpose:** Surgery based on purpose includes, diagnostic, ablative, palliative, reconstructive, transplantation and constructive
    - **Diagnostic:** To make or confirm a diagnosis, for example, breast biopsy, laparoscopy, bronchoscopy, exploratory laparotomy, etc.
    - **Ablative:** To remove a diseased body part for example, subtotal thyroidectomy, appendectomy, partial gastrectomy, amputation, etc.
    - **Palliative:** To relieve or reduce intensity of an illness and is not curative. For example, colostomy, nerve root resection, debridement of necrotic tissue, arthroscopy, balloon angioplasty, etc.
    - **Reconstructive:** To restore function of traumatized or malfunctioning tissue and to improve self-concept. For example, plastic surgery, skin graft, internal fixation of a fracture, breast reconstruction, etc.
    - **Transplantation:** To replace organs or structures that are diseased or malfunctioning. For example, kidney, liver, cornea, joint, heart, etc.
    - **Constructive:** To restore function in congenital anomalies. For examples, cleft palate repair, closure of atrioseptal defect, cleft lip, etc.

NURSING PROCESS FOR PREOPERATIVE CARE

Patients who require surgical interventions and nursing care enter the healthcare setting in a wide variety of situations, ranging from healthy people who have planned elective procedures to emergency admissions for treatment of trauma or serious illness such as cardrice arrest or stroke. Surgical patients may be of any age and at any point of health-illness continuum. It is the nurse's responsibility to identify factors that affect the risk of surgical procedure. This includes assessing the physical and psychosocial needs of the patient and family and establishing a plan of care based on appropriate nursing diagnosis. Interventions are based on meeting the patient's needs that facilitate recovery of the patient.

Assessment

Preoperative assessment identifies factors that may place the patient at greater risk for complications during and after surgery.

Assessment of the surgical patient includes:

- Obtaining a health history and performing a physical assessment to establish a baseline database
- Identifying risk factors and allergies that could pose surgical complications
- Identifying medications and treatments, the patient is currently receiving
- Determining the teaching and psychosocial needs of the patient and family
- Determining postsurgical support and referral needed for recovery.

The assessment is conducted several days before surgery. It may be conducted in the hospital, a surgical clinic, outpatient or even in patient's home. Preoperative nursing assessments and teaching are key care activities for patients who will be having outpatient or same day surgery. Preoperative screening tests are usually done up to 30 days before the scheduled surgery.

Health History

Health history identifies risk factors and strengths in the patient's physical and psychosocial status. Health history information significant to the surgical experience includes the patient's developmental level, medical history, medications, previous surgeries, perceptions and knowledge of the surgery to be done, nutrition, use of alcohol, illicit drugs or nicotine, activities of daily living and occupation, coping patterns and support system and sociocultural needs.

Developmental Considerations

Infants and older adults are at a greater risk from surgery than children and young or middle-aged adults. The infant has a lower total blood volume, making even a small loss of blood at risk for hypovolemic shock and the inability to respond to the need for increased oxygen during surgery. The infant also has difficulty in maintaining stable body temperature during surgery because the shivering reflex is not well developed, making hypothermia or hyperthermia a more likely consequence. The effects of muscle relaxants and narcotics may be prolonged in infants because their liver is immature.

Physiologic changes associated with aging increase the surgical risk for older patients. Older adults also have decreased ability to respond to the stress of surgery, effects of preoperative and postoperative medication and altered wound healing processes. With an increasing older adult population, assessing physiologic changes is crucial to providing knowledgeable, safe and holistic nursing care to older surgical patients.

Medical History

It provides information about past and current illness. Pathologic changes associated with past and current illnesses increase surgical risk as well as risk for post-operative complications. Preoperative assessment and documentation are necessary to provide a database and indicate the patient is at higher risk for complications after surgery (Table 1).

TABLE 1: Surgical risk factors

Factor	Key points	Factor	Key points
1. Diabetes mellitus and other chronic diseases	Stress of surgery may cause swings in blood glucose levels that are difficult to control. Patient may receive intravenous insulin during and after surgery. Wound healing tends to be delayed in the diabetic patient, making the risk of dehiscence greater. There is a higher incidence of infection in surgical wounds of diabetic patients. Liver and kidney disease makes it more difficult to metabolize and eliminate anesthesia and waste products.	7. Cardiovascular problems	Patients with hypertension, left ventricular hypertrophy, cardiac arrhythmias, or history of congestive heart failure are at a higher risk for myocardial infarction from the stress of surgery and anesthesia.
2. Advanced age with inactivity	Healing is slower in elderly patients. The risk of disuse syndrome, hypostatic pneumonia, and thrombus formation is higher in an inactive elderly person.	8. Peripheral vascular disease	Poor circulation in the extremities predisposes the patient to possible thrombus formation and pressure sores on the lower legs and feet. Antiembolic stockings or devices are generally prescribed for use during and after surgery.

Contd...

Factor	Key points	Factor	Key points
3. Very young age	Infants have difficulty with temperature control and in maintaining normal circulatory blood volume; they are at risk of dehydration.	9. Substance abuse or alcohol dependence	May alter reaction to anesthetic agents. Alcohol dependence may cause withdrawal symptoms if the use of alcohol is discontinued abruptly.
4. Malnutrition	Inadequate nutritional stores lead to poor wound healing and skin breakdown.	10. Smoking	Causes increased lung secretions from anesthesia and predisposes the patient to atelectasis and pneumonia postoperatively. Smokers are more prone to thrombus formation.
5. Dehydration	Reduced circulating volume reduces kidney perfusion and predisposes to a reduced urine output and thrombus formation. Dehydration also alters electrolyte values. The dehydrated patient is more at risk for problems with pressure areas during surgery.	11. Regular use of certain drugs	Aspirin and anticoagulants make the patient more prone to excessive bleeding. Corticosteroids reduce the body's response to infection and delay the healing process.
6. Obesity	The extremely heavy patient does not breathe as deeply and is at risk of hypostatic pneumonia. Excessive fatty tissue also is a factor in poor wound healing.	12. Excessive fear	Stimulates the sympathetic nervous system and causes the release of hormones, causing swings in the body's chemistry and vital signs. Increased muscle tension makes surgery more difficult. Physical manifestations of fear can interfere with achieving the desired state of anesthesia.

Medications

Surgical risk is increased by drugs in the following categories:

♦ Anticoagulants (may precipitate bleeding)
♦ Diuretics (may cause electrolyte imbalances with resulting respiratory depression from anesthesia)
♦ Tranquilizers (may increase the hypotensive effect of anesthetic agents)
♦ Adrenal steroids (abrupt withdrawal may cause cardio-vascular collapse)
♦ Antibiotics (when combined with certain muscle relaxants used during surgery, may cause respiratory paralysis)
♦ Oral hypoglycemic medications (such as metformin may react with radiologic contrast dyes, and cause acute renal failure)

Many medication are discontinued before the surgery, specific medications may be given the morning of surgery with sips of water.

Previous Surgery

It is important to have data about previous surgeries for meeting physical and psychological needs throughout the preoperative period. The patient's past experiences with surgery also affect the plan of care in preoperative phase, especially if a past experience was negative. The patient's questions about the surgery are important for meeting psychological and family needs when preparing the patient for surgery.

Nutritional Status

Both malnutrition and obesity increase surgical risk. Surgery increases the body's needs for nutrition necessary for normal tissue healing and resistance to infection. A patient, who is malnourished, is at higher risk for alterations in fluid and electrolyte balance, delay in wound healing, and wound infection. Obese patients are at an increased risk for respiratory, cardiovascular, deep vein thrombosis and gastrointestinal problems. Overweight patients may have obstructive sleep apnea, putting them at risk for reduced respiratory function. Fatty tissue has a poor blood supply and therefore, has less resistance to infection, as a result, postoperative complications of delayed wound healing, wound infection, and disruption in the integrity of the wound are common.

Use of alcohol, Illicit Drugs or Nicotine

Patient with a longer habitual intake of alcohol requires larger doses of anesthetic agents and postoperative analgesics, increasing the drug-related complications. Patients who use illicit drugs may render veins hardened, inflamed and unusable for anesthesia administration if they are on IV drug use. Patient who smoke are at a higher risk for respiratory complications after surgery. They are at risk for hypoxia and postoperative pneumonia due to increased mucous secretion and decreased ciliary action in the tracheobronchial tree. Smoking affects healing by constricting blood vessels and impairing blood flow to the tissues for healing.

Activities of Daily Living and Occupation

Exercise, sleep and rest are important in preventing postoperative complications and facilitating recovery. A patient with a well-established exercise program has improved cardiovascular, respiratory, metabolic and musculoskeletal functions, thereby, lowering the risk of surgery. Rest and sleep are essential for recovery from stress of surgery. Many surgical procedures require a delay in returning to a occupation. Therefore, knowledge about this helps the nurse to plan necessary teachings and referrals.

Coping Patterns and Support System

Assessing the patient's psychological, sociocultural, and spiritual dimension is very important as surgery itself is a major psychological stressor and affects coping patterns and support systems. Any surgery whether planned or unexpected, major on minor, causes anxiety and fear. While obtaining health history, the nurse can use cues from the patient's and family's verbal and nonverbal communication to identify fear and concerns and to plan intervention to provide the necessary information and emotional support necessary to successful recovery from surgery.

Anxiety and fear may be expressed in many ways such as anger, withdrawal, apathy, confrontation or questioning. Patients often have fear of unknown, pain or death, and changes in body image and self-concept. The patient has fears about the surgery itself, the anesthesia, the diagnosis, the future, financial and family responsibilities, response to pain, or possible disfigurement or disability. Surgical procedures often leave the patient with permanent changes in body's structure, function, or appearance, from which patient commonly fear alterations in physical appearance, social relationship, lifestyle and sexuality.

It is necessary to develop therapeutic communication skill to identify and resolve fear. Encourage the patient to identify and verbalize fears. At the same time, incorrect knowledge can be identified and corrected, strengths are identified, and teaching can be done. The reduction of fear is of major importance in preoperative preparation.

Coping with stress can be facilitated through the support system identified in the assessment phase of preoperative nursing care. Encourage family members to provide support before and after surgery. Identify the patient's spiritual beliefs as it aids in meeting patient's spiritual needs. These needs can be met through acceptance, participation in prayer, or other rituals.

Sociocultural Needs

A person's perceptions and reactions to the surgical experience are influenced by individual factors, including family health beliefs and practices, economic factors, and cultural or ethnic background. A patient who requires surgery but has grown up in a family that believes that surgical intervention is the last option for treating illness may be hesitant about the surgery. The resulting anxiety may make this patient even more susceptible to surgical risk. Cultural and ethnic influences also affect the patient's responses and perceptions of the surgical experience.

Physical Assessment

Assessing the patient's current physical status provides data for interventions to decrease surgical risk and potential postoperative complications. Physical assessment is conducted as described before.

Preoperative Assessment Form

Directions: Form should be completed 1–24 hours before surgery. Kindly fill in the blanks, circle the appropriate descriptors, and add comments as necessary.

General Information

Name _____ Age _____ Sex _____ Ward _____ Bed No. _____

Height _____ Weight _____ Religion _____ Occupation _____

Allergies _____ Medications _____ Family Support _____

Smoker (Yes/No) packs/day _____ years Recent illness/ or infection _____

Previous Hospitalization _____ Abnormal lab results _____

Past illness Diabetes/Hypertension/Cardiac disease or any other specify _____

Assessment Factors

1. Chief Complaint _____
2. History of present illness:
   2.1 **Onset:** Sudden, Gradual
   2.2 **Duration:** Occasional, Gradual
   2.3 **Severity:** Interferes with activity, tolerable
   2.4 **Location:** _____
   2.5 Precipitating Factors _____
   2.6 Relieving Factors _____
3. Temperature _____ oral/rectal/axilla
4. Pulse _____ regular/irregular/bounding/feeble
5. Blood Pressure _____ sitting/standing/lying
6. Respiration _____ normal/noisy/orthopneic/dyspneic/irregular
7. Vital Capacity _____
8. Breath Sounds: Normal/Abnormal (describe) _____
9. Cough: None/occasional/Frequent/dry, productive (describe) _____
10. Edema: None/present/(describe location and extent) _____
11. Skin color: pink/pale/cyanosis/jaundiced/(comments) _____
12. Skin condition: intact/elastic/smooth/rash/bruises/redness (comments) _____
13. Paralysis/weakness: None/present/(describe) _____
14. Deformities: None/present, (describe) _____
15. Mobility: No impairment/impairment (describe) _____
16. Consciousness: Oriented/disoriented to place/person and time _____
17. Comprehension: understands/doesn't understand/forgetful _____
18. Vision: normal/decreased (Rt., Lt.)/Blind (Rt., Lt.,), glasses/contact lenses _____
19. Hearing: normal/decreased, (Rt., Lt.)/Deaf (Rt., Lt)/Hearing aid (Rt., Lt) _____
20. Speech: clear/slurred _____
21. Language: Speaks hindi/English, any other _____
22. Abdomen: pain/nausea/vomiting, distension/flatulence/indigestion/diarrhea/constipation/bowel movement

Appropriate specimens are collected. The results are documented in the patient's record before surgery, and abnormal findings are reported.

Presurgical screening tests include chest X-ray, electrocardiography, complete blood count, electrolyte levels and urinalysis. Significant abnormal findings include an elevated white blood cell count (presence of infection), decreased hematocrit and hemoglobin levels (presence of bleeding, anemia), hyperkalemia or hypokalemia, elevated blood urea nitrogen (BUN) or creatinine levels (possible renal failure).

Diagnosis

Nursing diagnosis for patients in the preoperative phase may be identified for various actual or potential problems, for which a patient is at risk. These are derived from the analysis of subjective and objective data obtained from the health history and physical examination as well as information from other health team members and screening tests. Examples of common nursing diagnosis are:

- Anxiety related to the surgical experience and outcomes
- Fear related to risk of death, effects of impending surgery or loss of control due to anesthesia
- Anticipatory grieving related to impending loss of a body function or body part
- Knowledge deficit related to preoperative and post-operative routines
- Sleep pattern disturbance related to stress or unfamiliar environment
- Ineffective individual coping related to lack of adequate support
- Altered role performance related to inability to care for children during hospitalization

Planning

Planning for the entire perioperative period is done in the preoperative phase and includes expected outcomes that are discussed and mutually agreed upon by the nurse, the patient, and the family. Specific appropriate outcomes include that the patient:

- Is physically and emotionally prepared for surgery
- Demonstrates turning, coughing, and deep breathing exercises
- Verbalizes understanding of postoperative pain management
- Maintains fluid intake and oral balance to meet needs.

Implementation

Preoperative nursing interventions provide the patient with the necessary psychological and physical preparation for surgery and the postoperative phase.

Psychological Preparation

One of the nurse's responsibility is to teach about postoperative activities. Patients and families need to know about surgical events and sensations, how to manage pain, and how to perform the physical activities necessary to decrease the risk for postoperative complications and facilitate recovery. Patients and their families need to know when surgery is scheduled, about how long the surgery and post anesthesia care will last, and what will be done before, during and after surgery. An explanation of surgical events includes a description of the various members of the health care team, where and when to report for admission, instructions for preoperative fasting and bowel preparation if ordered; and instructions for taking special medications.

Preparation should also include sensory information patient may experience during the perioperative period. Teaching should include information about dry mouth and drowsiness from preoperative medications, a sore-throat from the insertion of an endotracheal tube, a gradual return of feeling and movement after spinal anesthesia and pain from the surgical incision. Patients should also be made aware of the coldness of the environment, the sounds and lights.

Pain Management

The nurse is responsible for assessment, implementation and evaluation of a pain management plan and for teaching the patient preoperatively how to communicate and report pain. Teach the patient and family that medications to relieve pain will be ordered by the physician and administered by the nurse. Physician may order pain medication to be given on a regular basis or on as needed (parenteral, PRN) basis. If medication is ordered PRN, there is restriction between doses every 2 or 4 hours. The patient needs to ask for the medication and should not do so before the pain becomes severe. Many surgeons will order a patient-controlled analgesia (PCA) pump for their patients postoperatively. In this case, patients should receive instructions about the pump and how to operate it prior to surgery.

Nutrition and Fluids

Patient needs to be well-nourished and hydrated before surgery to counterbalance fluid, blood, and electrolyte loss during surgery and to facilitate anesthesia delivery and tissue healing after surgery.

A patient who is undernourished may require parenteral nutrition and intravenous (IV) electrolyte replacement. If the patient screening tests show a hemoglobin level less than 10 g/dL, and a hematocrit of less than 33%, blood or blood component therapy may be given preoperatively to maintain volume and increase the oxygenation of tissue during surgery.

Maintaining nothing by mouth, nil per os (NPO) status for at least 8 hours prior to surgery has been the standard for many years. The American Society for Anesthesiologists (1999) revised the practice guidelines for preoperative fasting. The diet order depends on the type of surgery and type of anesthesia to be used. Current practice is to allow patients to drink liquids or eat food up to 2 hours before surgery depending or the type of surgery and with permission of physician. If clear fluids are allowed, they should be clearly defined for the patient and include water, fruit juices without pulp, carbonated beverages, clear tea and black coffee.

Patient is explained by the nurse about being NPO and she removes all food and fluids from the bedside and places a sign board over the bed about NPO status for all health team members and visitors. It the patient eats or drinks, the physician need to be informed and procedure has to be delayed or concealed.

Hygiene and Skin Preparation

The nurse minimizes skin contamination by organisms evening before surgery the patient takes thorough bath, which may be repeated in the morning of surgery.

Preparation of the site as prescribed. The part is prepared by cleaning, shaving or clipping (as per institutional policy) and application of any prescribed antiseptic such as (Betadine) on operative site.

Preparation of the Part of Surgery

This will include shaving of the part to be operated and its skin preparation (Figs 1A to F).

Preoperative Teaching Program

Preoperative teaching is an important component in the patient's operative experience. Preoperative teaching has

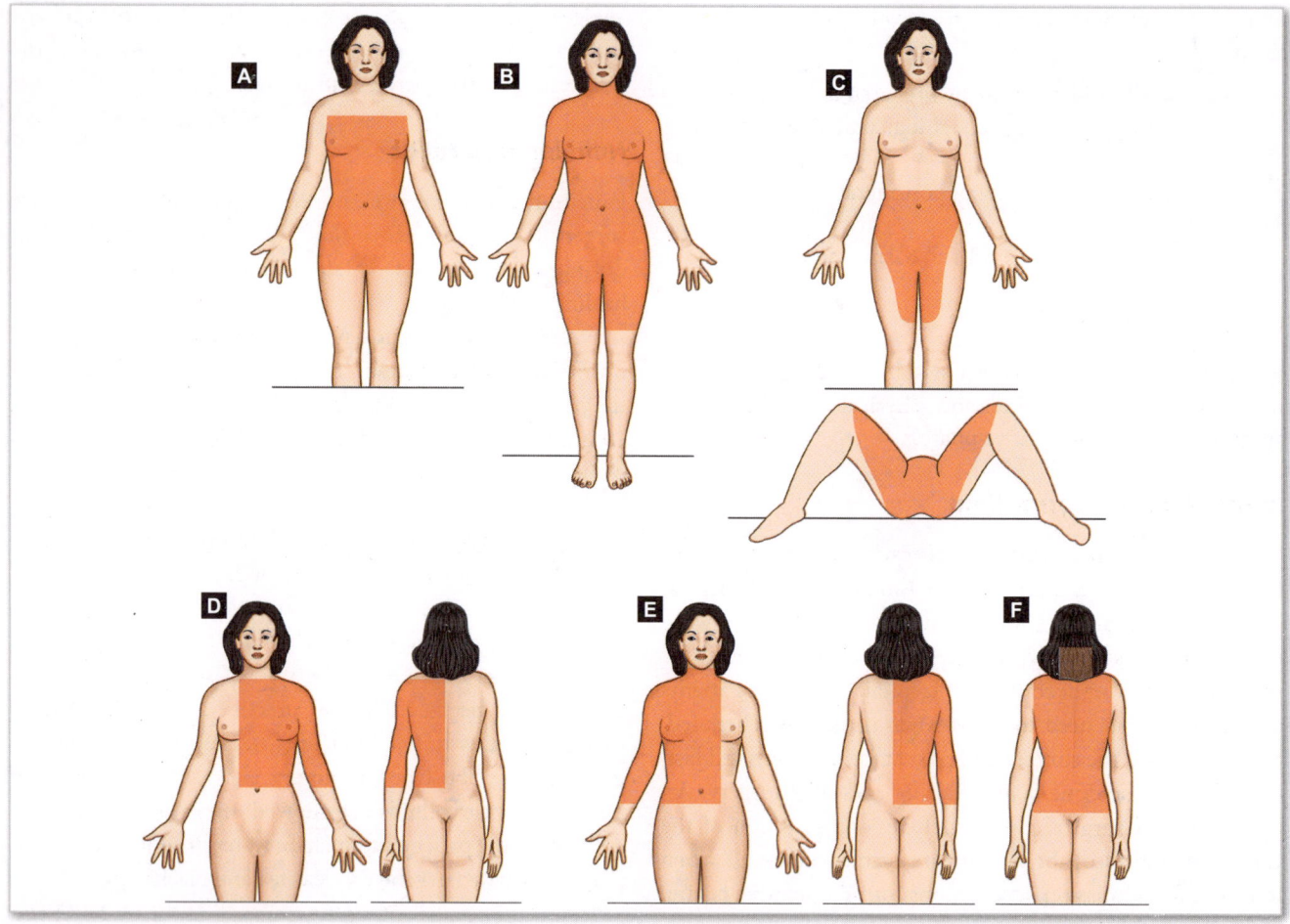

Figs 1A to F: Skin preparation for surgery on various body areas. A. Abdominal and pelvic area, B. Upper anus, thorax, abdomen, pelvic, region and upper things, C. Pelvic region and perineum, D. Front and back on left-side, E. Front and back on right-side; F. Back

proven benefits. It has a positive influence on the patient's recovery. Preoperative teaching allays anxiety and encourages patients to participate actively towards self-care. Structured preoperative teaching has benefits in terms of:

- **Ventilatory function:** Teaching improves the ability to cough and deep breathe effectively
- **Physical functional capacity:** Teaching improves the ability to ambulate and resume activities of daily living early.
- **Sense of well-being:** Patients who are prepared for surgery experience less anxiety and report a great sense of psychological well-being
- **Length of hospital stay:** Structured preoperative teaching can reduce the length of hospital stay
- Prevent the occurrence of postoperative complications.

Preoperative teaching helps the patient to anticipate the steps of procedure and this helps them form realistic images of the surgical experience. When events occur as predicted, clients are better able to cope and attend to the experiences.

It is best to begin preoperative teaching well in advance of the scheduled surgery. If the nurse can teach a client one or two days before surgery, the client will be alert and more

receptive and willing to cooperate. The nurse assesses the surgical client's readiness and ability to learn. If the client is capable of and receptive to learning, the nurse presents information in a logical sequence.

When a client is under general anesthesia, the lungs do not ventilate fully. After surgery, the patient has a reduced lung volume and needs greater effort to breathe. During surgery, venous blood flow to the lungs slows down. Stasis of circulation may lead to thrombi or clots. A clot can break off and travel to the brain, heart or lungs to cause fatal complications. Every preoperative teaching program includes explanation of these postoperative exercises:

- **Deep-breathing exercises:**
  - Diaphragmatic breathing
  - Incentive spirometer
  - Coughing
  - Pursed lip breathing
- **Turning in bed**
- **Leg exercises**
- **Ambulation**

Deep-breathing Exercises

- **Diaphragmatic breathing:** Improves lung expansion and oxygen delivery without using excess energy. The patient learns to use the diaphragm during deep breathing to take slow, deep relaxed breaths and eventually, the client's lung volume improves. Deep breathing also helps to clear out anesthetic gases remaining in the airways. Deep breathing exercises help prevent the accumulation of thick secretions in the respiratory tract by getting air to the smallest of alveoli to assist with reinflating these tiny air sacs. For best results, following steps need to be followed:
  - Assist patient in comfortable position, sitting or standing
  - Instruct patient to place palms of hands along lower border of anterior rib cage.
  - Instruct patient to take slow, deep breaths, inhaling through nose.
  - Explain patient not to use chest and shoulders while inhaling.
  - Explain patient to hold deep breaths for 3 seconds and slowly exhale through mouth.
  - Instruct patient to take 10 slow deep breaths every 2 hours while awake during postoperative period until he/she resumes mobility.

- **Incentive spirometer:** It is a mechanical device that promotes sustained mechanical inspiration by which the client is able to see the results of his/her efforts simultaneously as it gets registered on the spirometer (Fig. 2). This device encourages the client to continue to take deep breaths to maximize lung expansion. The incentive spirometer has three graduated chambers. Each chamber contains movable ball that is pushed up by the

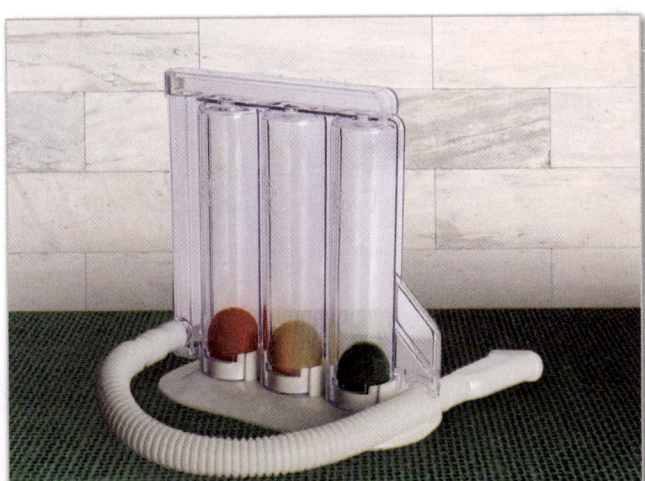

Fig. 2: Incentive spirometer

force of breath and held suspended in the air while the client inhales. The chambers are graduated up to 600 cc., 900 cc. and 1200 cc. The amount of air inhaled and the flow of air are estimated by how long and how much high the balls are suspended. The patient should take a deep breath, sustain, exhale and repeat.

Steps:
- Place the patient in semi Fowler's or Fowler's position
- Exhale normally and place the lips tightly around the mouthpiece
- Inhale slowly and maintain constant flow
- Hold breath for 2–3 seconds and exhale slowly
- Breath normally for short period
- Have patient repeat till goals are reached.
- Record the level of the raise of ball in each graduated chamber

- **Coughing:** Coughing is the natural automatic method for cleansing the airways of secretions. Cilia, which are hair-like structures, that line the mucous membrane of the respiratory tract, move the secretions in an upward motion. Each cough moves the secretions closer to expectoration. Deep breathing is sometimes enough of a stimulus to produce a cough. A deep productive cough is more beneficial than merely cleaning the throat. Postoperative incisional pain makes coughing difficult. The nurse teaches the patient to splint an incision to minimize pain during coughing. The nurse also teaches the patient to cough and deep breathe at least every 2 hours while awake.

Steps:
- Assist patient to assume upright position
- Instruct patient to take two slow breaths and third time hold breath to count of three
- Instruct patient to cough fully
- Instruct patient to place one hand over incisional area and other hand on to top of first or use pillow to support
- Instruct patient to cough 2–3 times every 2 hours while awake.
- Instruct patient to observe sputum for consistency, amount and color change.

- **Pursed lip breathing:** It is helpful to improve expiratory reserve volume.

Steps:
- Assist patient to sit up in bed slightly bending forward
- Instruct patient to take deep breath by pulling abdominal muscles in (Fig. 3A)
- Ask patient to hold breath for 3 seconds.
- Instruct patient to breath out slowly through pursed lips (Fig. 3B)
- Instruct to continue this 6–8 times every 2 hours per day.

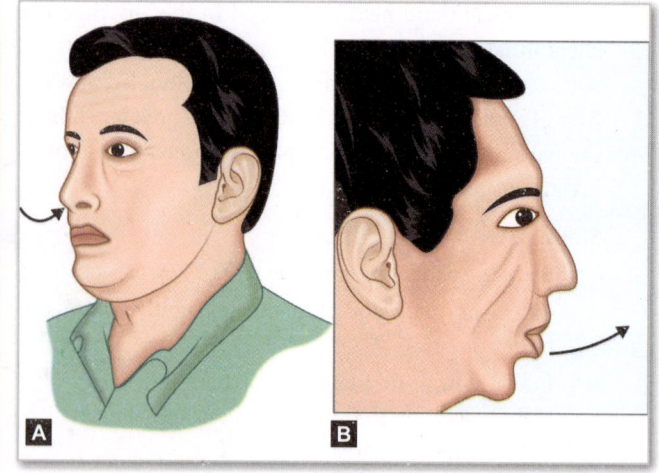

Figs 3A and B: Pursed lip breathing excercise. A. Inhale; B. Exhale

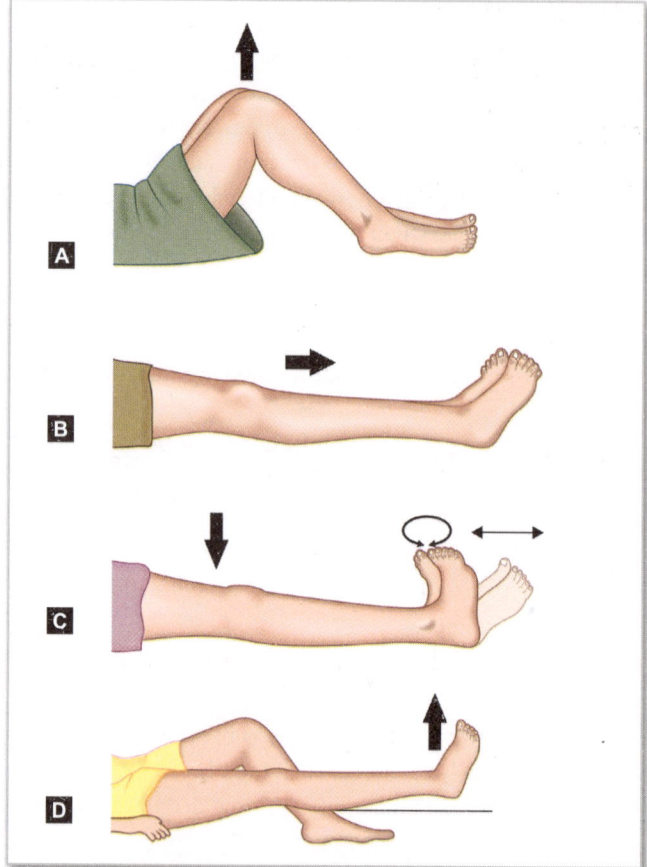

Figs 4A to D: Postoperative leg exercises

Turning in Bed

During surgery, venous blood flow to legs slows down. This stasis of circulation may lead to thrombi formation. A clot may break off and travel to the brain, heart or lungs to cause fatal complications. It is necessary for the patient to turn frequently and perform leg exercises to improve blood flow and thus, reduce stasis. It will also help in improving venous return and maintain joint mobility.

Steps:

- Assist patient to assume supine position to right side of bed.
- Instruct patient to place left hand over incisional area to splint
- Instruct patient to keep left leg straight and flex right knee up and over left leg
- Instruct patient to pull towards left and roll on to left side
- Instruct patient to turn every 2 hours while awake

Leg Exercises

Leg exercises improve venous return and prevent thrombophlebitis (Figs 4A to D).

Steps:

- Assist patient to assume supine position in bed
- Rotate each ankle in complete circle
- Instruct patient to draw imaginary circles with big toe. Repeat 5 times.
- Instruct patient to alternate dorsiflexion and plantar flexion of both feet and direct patient to feel calf muscles contract and relax alternatively
- Instruct patient to continue leg exercises alternatively flexing and extending knees. Repeat five times
- Instruct patient to alternatively raise each leg straight up from bed surface, keeping legs straight. Repeat 5 times.

- Instruct patient to practice at least every 2 hours while awake. Instruct patient to coordinate turning and leg exercises with diaphragmatic breathing, incentive spirometry and coughing exercises.
- Record exercises demonstrated and patient's ability to perform them independently.

Ambulation

Steps:

- Instruct patient to sit on the edge of bed with feet supported
- Ask patient to get down from the bed and walk few steps
- Instruct patient to support the wound while walking.

Elimination

The nurse facilitates/assist in bowel movement, she administers cleansing enema for bowel preparation in gastrointestinal surgery. The enema helps to prevent postoperative constipation because of absence of peristalsis for 24 hours or longer after gastrointestinal surgery. It also helps is preventing contamination of the surgical area by feces. She administers laxative as per order.

She facilitates patient to void. To ensure that bladder is empty, sometimes retention catheter is put. This helps in preventing injury to the bladder, particularly in surgery of large bowel.

Rest and Sleep

The nurse promotes rest and sleep because rest is essential for normal restoration and healing of the body. Anxiety about surgery can interfere with the patient's ability to relax and sleep.

- She provides comfortable bed and linen.
- She provides calm and quiet environment
- She sedates the patient at night as per order for calming effect and relieving client's apprehension
- She provides emotional support to relieve anxiety and fears.

Preparation of Patient on the Day of Surgery

It includes:

- Checking vital signs; provides baseline data with which to compare patient's condition postoperatively. Any deviation from normal should be reported immediately as surgery may have to be postponed

- Meeting hygienic needs by having bath in the morning and attending mouth care. Instruct the patient not to swallow water while providing mouthwash
- She makes sure that consent is signed
- She checks hair for hairpin and clips. Long hair can be braided to keep them in place. Use of head tie or cap to cover hair can be done
- She removes any dentures, contact lens, nail polish and ornaments
- She safeguards valuables
- She checks reports and case sheet for completion
- Checks for special procedures–starting of IV fluids, insertion of nasogastric tube, insertion of Foley's catheter etc.
- Encourages patient to put on hospital dress
- Make sure that the patient is nil per or (NPO)
- Make sure that identification slip is on the patient's dress, and easily accessible.
- Administers preoperative medications as per order, when patient leaves for operating room and records it in case sheet.
- Assists patient in moving from bed to operating room stretcher
- Keeps ready the unit to receive patient postoperatively.

Preoperative Checklist

Patient's Name _____ Ward _____

		Yes	No	Remarks
1.	PAC done (Preanesthetic check)			
2.	Operative area prepared			
3.	Operative area approved by inchange Nurse or ward supervisor			
4.	Jewellery, bangles etc. removed? Tied on			
5.	False teeth removed			
6.	Hair prepared			
7.	A. Voided or catheterized? B. Enema given result			
8.	Premedication given and charted?			
9.	Vital signs are checked and recorded by the ward Nurse			
10.	Consent is taken			
11.	All order and investigation report are			
12.	All X-ray film counted and sent with patient?			
13.	Patient fasting			
14.	Identification tag tied on Patient's hand?			
15.	Check whether patient has any drug allergy			
16.	Whether patient is HbsAg or HIV+ ve			

Signature.........................
Date..................................

Evaluation

Evaluation is based on the expected outcomes. The plan is effective if the patient is physically and emotionally prepared for surgery, verbalizes expected events and sensations of the perioperative period and demonstrates postoperative exercises and activities.

NURSING PROCESS FOR INTRAOPERATIVE CARE

The intraoperative phase of surgery begins with admission of the patient to the surgical area and lasts until the patient is transferred to the post-anesthesia care unit (PACU).

Assessment

Nurse in this unit identifies the surgical patient, assesses the patient's physical and emotional status and verify the information on the preoperative checklist including lab reports, consent for surgery, including skin preparation, starting IV fluids and giving preoperative medications.

Alert

The Joint Commission 2010, an independent accrediting agency, has established a standard of universal protocol to ensure patient's safety, when having surgery by preventing wrong site, wrong procedure and wrong person surgery.

The universal protocol has three components, preoperative verification process, marking the operative site, and a final verification just prior to beginning a procedure.

When the operative room is ready, a perioperative nurse helps transport the patient to the operating room. In the operating room, the patient is positioned is operating table/bed, identified again with the operating team using at least two identifiers (such as name, birth date, medical record number), and then anesthetized and draped. The perioperative nurse assesses the patient and reviews preoperative data, paying special attention to factors that increase surgical risk. To maintain safety, the nurse also assesses the patient during positioning and monitors supplies used.

Diagnosis

During intraoperative period, patient problems are related to the position of patients during surgery, due to effects of anesthesia, equipment used, disruption of tissues during surgery and the incision Nursing diagnosis during intraoperative period includes:

* Risk for imbalanced fluid volume
* Risk for perioperative positioning injuries

Planning

Some of the expected outcomes during this phase focus on identifying intervention for preventing complications, resolving patient's problems and ensuring patient safety. Some of the expected outcomes are:

* Patient will remain free from neuromuscular injury
* Patient will remain free from wrong site, wrong side, wrong procedure surgery
* Maintain fluid and electrolyte balance
* Maintain skin integrity (related to position)
* Patient will have symmetric breathing pattern
* Free from injury, from burns, retained foreign objects (inaccurate count of supplies) and medication errors
* Maintain normothermia
* Remain free from surgical site infection.

Implementation

During surgery, circulating nurse identifies and assesses the patient on admission to the operating room, provides additional supplies, maintains environment safety, and counts the number of instruments, needles, and sponges used during the surgery. Scrub nurse is a member of surgical team who maintains surgical asepsis while draping and handling instruments and supplies. Registered nurse actively assists the surgeon by exposure of the operative area, maintaining hemostasis, and wound closure.

Positioning

The patient is placed in a specific operative position after anesthesia has produced loss of consciousness and reflexes. The skin injury is avoided by lifting, rather than rolling or pulling the patient into the surgical position. Perioperative nurses need to know the position to be used for operative procedure.

Draping

Drapes are used to create and maintain a sterile field around the operative site. The only area left exposed is the incision site.

Documenting

The perioperative nurse documents patient's assessment, sponges count, instruments, sharps, vital signs, urine output, blood loss, pulse oximetry, medications, dressing and drains and specimens throughout surgery.

Transfer to Post-anesthesia Care Unit (PACU)

After the surgery, the patient is moved from the operating bed/table to stretcher or bed and transported to the PACU and the operation theater (OT) nurse verbally communicates relevant preoperative and intraoperative assessments and interventions to the PACU nurse to ensure continuity of care.

Evaluation

Evaluation of the effectiveness of the plan of care for the intraoperative phase is based on the expected outcomes. If they are met, plan was effective.

POSTOPERATIVE NURSING CARE

The postoperative phase can be divided into stages: Immediate care provided in the PACU and ongoing care lasting from return to unit through convalescence.

Immediate Postoperative Care

Care in PACU involves assessing the postoperative patient, with emphasis on preventing complications from anesthesia or the surgery. The assessments made in the PACU include respiratory status, cardiovascular status, central nervous system status, fluid status, wound status and general condition. These assessments initially are made every 10–15 minutes. The average PACU stay is about 1 hour, but varies depending on the type of surgery, length of anesthesia and patient's response. Outpatient or same day surgery patients return home after recovery in the PACU. The critical role functions of the PACU nurse includes monitoring during first hours after surgery, pain management, fluid and electrolyte balance and stabilization of physiologic parameters.

Respiratory Status

Respiratory function is assessed by monitoring respiratory rate, rhythm and depth; auscultating breath sounds; noting the oxygen saturation level, assessing the skin color, and monitoring the cardiovascular and mental status. During a surgical procedure with general anesthesia, an endotracheal tube may be inserted to administer the anesthetic gases and maintain patent air passages. The airway is not removed until the laryngeal and pharyngeal reflexes return, allowing the patient to control the tongue, cough and swallow. The airway is assessed for patency, humidified oxygen is administered and pulse oximetry is initiated.

Ineffective respiratory function is indicated by restlessness and anxiety; unequal chest expansion and use of accessory muscles; shallow, noisy respirations, cyanosis, and tachycardia. Respiratory obstruction is the most common PACU emergency. It may occur as a result of secretion accumulation, obstruction by the tongue, laryngospasm or laryngeal edema. Respiratory obstruction is indicated by assessments of ineffective respiratory function plus observing for wheezing with respiratory effort.

Positioning, administering humidified oxygen, encouraging the patient to take deep breaths, and suctioning may be used to maintain a patent airway and tissue oxygenation.

Cardiovascular Status

Cardiovascular function is assessed by taking vital signs, monitoring electrocardiogram rate and rhythm, and observing skin color and condition, blood pressure findings are compared with base line data from the preoperative period. Transient hypertension can occur as a result of anesthetic effects, respiratory insufficiency, the surgical procedure, or the excitement phase of recovery from anesthesia.

Hypotension may be the result of varied factors, including anesthetic agents, preoperative medications, position changes, blood loss, respiratory alterations, and peripheral blood pooling, Oxygen administration, deep breathing, leg exercises, verbal stimulation (to help expel anesthetic gases and facilitate increasing level of consciousness), and maintaining accurate IV flow rates can increase low blood pressure.

Patients are at risk for altered body temperature related to the surgical procedure, its length, anesthetic agents, a cool surgical environment, age, and use of cool irrigating fluids. This can lead to complications of poor wound healing, hemodynamic stress, coagulopathy, cardiac disturbances and shivering. Measure the patient's body temperature, usually by temporal or tympanic route and initiate interventions, if the patient complains of being cold or is hypothermic. Warm blankets placed on the patient's body are used for rewarming.

All pulses are assessed for bilateral equality, rhythm, rate and character. Tachycardia, an early symptom of shock, must be carefully evaluated. Other assessment for shock include decreasing blood pressure, cyanosis, a cool skin temperature and a decrease in urine output.

Central Nervous System Status

The return of central nervous system function is assessed through the patient response to stimuli and orientation. Consciousness return in reverse order with the pattern being:

- Unconsciousness
- Response to touch and sounds
- Drowsiness
- Awake but not oriented
- Awake and oriented.
- Nurse in the PACU reorients the patient

Fluid Status

Fluid imbalance may result from factors such as preoperative fluid restriction, fluid loss during surgery, wound drainage, surgical stress response (with retention of sodium and water). Imbalanced fluid volume is a risk for all surgical patients. Assessing fluid status includes skin turgor, vital signs, urine output, wound drainage, and IV fluid intake. IV fluid administration assessments include the type of fluid, the rate, location of lines, condition of the IV insertion site, and the patency of the tubing.

Wound Status

The nurse in the PACU assesses the dressing over the incision for amount, consistency, and color of drainage as well as for any tubes or drains the amount and type of drainage by that route. Large amounts of bright red drainage and other assessments such as restlessness, pallor, cold moist skin, decreasing blood pressure, increasing pulse and respiratory rate may indicate hemorrhage and hypovolemic shock, which must be reported immediately.

Pain Management

Pain is both a subjective and an objective experience. Assessment of pain can be done by use of scale. The rating scale may be verbal ranging from no pain to worst possible pain or numerical pain rating scale ranging from 0 to 10. Administration of analgesia, using nonsteroidal anti-inflammatory drugs (NSAIDs) and opiates in PACU. Non-pharmacologic methods to decrease pain and improve comfort include positioning, verbal reassurance, and touch.

General Condition

Ensuring physical comfort, emotional comfort and safety. constant reorientation and reassurance that the surgery is completed provides psychological comfort. Careful assessment, proper positioning, and use of side rails maintains physical safety. The patient is transferred from PACU when physical status and level of consciousness are considered stable. The family is notified that the patient is being transferred back to the room, and the PACU nurse gives a verbal report to the unit nurse about the assessments and intervention during the intra operative and immediate postoperative phases.

NURSING PROCESS FOR ONGOING POSTOPERATIVE CARE ASSESSMENT

The nurse assists PACU personnel in transferring the patient to the bed in the unit and makes initial assessments. The initial assessment is often combined with the implementation of postoperative physician's orders.

Document the time of arrival and all assessment data. Common time frames for assessment are every 15 minutes, until stable, changing to every 1–2 hours for the first 24 hours and every 4 hours thereafter depending upon the agency polices (Table 2).

Diagnosis

Nursing diagnosis in the postoperative phase may represent actual problem or those which the patient is at risk. It will vary depending on the surgery. Examples of North American Nursing Diagnosis Association (NANDA) nursing diagnosis appropriate to the postoperative period are:

TABLE 2: Postoperative assessment and interventions after return to the unit

Assessments	Interventions
Vital signs and oxygen saturation	◆ Temperature, blood pressure, pulse and respiratory rate, oxygen saturation ◆ Note report, and document deviations from preoperative and PACU data as well as symptoms of complications
Color and temperature	◆ Skin color (pallor, cyanosis), skin temperature, and diaphoresis
Level of consciousness	◆ Orientation to time, place and person ◆ Reaction to stimuli and ability to move extremities
Intravenous fluids	◆ Type and amount of solution, flow rate, security and patency of tubing ◆ Infusion site
Surgical site	◆ Dressing and dependent areas for drainage, (color, amount, consistency) ◆ Drains and tubes: be sure they are intact, patent, and properly connected to drainage systems
Other tubes	◆ Assess indwelling urinary catheter, gastrointestinal suction, and others for drainage, patency and amount of output ◆ Be sure dependent drainage bags are hanging properly and suction drainage is attached and functioning ◆ If oxygen is ordered, ensure placement of ordered application and flow rate
Comfort	◆ Assess pain (location, duration, intensity) and determine whether analgesics were given in the PACU ◆ Assess for nausea and vomiting ◆ Cover the patient with a blanket ◆ Reorient to the room as necessary ◆ Allow family members to remain with the patient after the initial assessment is completed
Position and safety	◆ Place the patient in the ordered position or ◆ If the patient is not fully conscious, place in the side-lying position ◆ Elevate the side rails and place the bed in low position

- Risk for infection
- Disturbed body image
- Acute pain
- Urinary retention

Planning

The plan of care in the postoperative phase begins in the preoperative phase, when nursing activities to reduce stress and postoperative activities are taught. Specific expected outcomes are individualized based on risk factors, the surgical procedure and the patient's unique needs. Examples of desired outcomes for a patient after surgery are:

The patient will:

- Deep breathe and cough effectively every 2 hours
- Carry out leg exercises every 2–4 hours
- Verbalize decreasing level of pain
- Have a balanced intake and output
- Regain normal bowel and bladder elimination
- Exhibit a healing of surgical incision
- Remain free of infection
- Verbalize any concerns about appearance of wound
- Verbalize and demonstrate wound self-care

Implementation

Nursing interventions designed to promote patient recovery and complications include:

- Pain management
- Appropriate positioning
- Incentive spirometry and deep breathing and coughing exercises
- Leg exercises
- Early ambulation
- Adequate hydration
- Diet
- Promoting urinary and bowel elimination
- Suction maintenance
- Wound care

Pain Management

Pain is usually greatest from 12 to 36 hours after surgery, decreasing after the second or third postoperative day. During the initial postoperative period, patient-controlled analgesia (PCA) through an intravenous route is often prescribed. Parenteral (PRN) or oral analgesics should be administered on a routine basis every 2–6 hours, depending on the drug, route and dose for the first 24–36 hours.

Positioning

Position the patient as ordered. Patients who have had spinal anesthesia usually lie flat for 8–12 hours. An unconscious or semi-conscious patient is placed on one side with head slightly elevated, if possible, that allows fluids to drain from the mouth.

Deep breathing and coughing exercises, Leg exercises and moving and ambulation are encouraged postoperatively so that recovery is faster. (All those exercises are discussed is preoperative care in preoperative teachings)

Hydration

Maintain intravenous infusion as ordered to replace body fluids lost either before or during surgery. When oral intake is permitted, initially offer only small sips of water. The patient who cannot take fluids by mouth, may be allowed as per surgeon's orders to suck ice chips. Provide mouth care at frequent intervals because postoperative patients often complain of dry and sticky mouth. Measure the intake and output for at least 2 days or until fluid balance is stable and patient is without intravenous infusion.

It is important to ensure adequate fluid balance because sufficient fluids keep the respiratory mucous membranes and secretions moist, thus, facilitating the expectoration of mucus during coughing. An adequate fluid balance is also important to maintain cardiovascular and renal functions.

Diet

Depending on the extent of surgery and the organs involved, the patient may be nil per os (NPO) for several days or may be able to resume oral intake when nausea is no longer present. When "diet as tolerated" is ordered, offer clear fluids initially. If the patient tolerates these with no nausea, the diet maybe switched to full liquids and then to regular diet, provided the gastrointestinal functioning is normal. Assess the return of peristalsis by auscultation of abdomen. Gurgling and rumbling sounds indicate peristalsis. Bowel sounds should be carefully assessed every 4–6 hours so that oral fluids can be started. Note the passage of flatus or abdominal distension.

Urinary Elimination

Provide measures that promote urinary elimination. For example, help male patients stand at the bedside or female patients to a bedside commode. Ensure that fluid intake is adequate. Assess for bladder distension and report to surgery if the patient does not void within 8 hours following surgery. If surgery is done in the pubic area, vagina and rectum, there may be urinary retention. If all measures to promote voiding fails, catheterization is often ordered. Measure all the intake and output for postoperative patients for at least 2 days or until the client reestablishes fluid balance without IV or catheter in place.

Suction

Some patients return from surgery with a gastric or intestinal tube in place and orders to connect the tube to suction. The suction ordered can be continuous or intermittent. Fluids and electrolytes must be replaced intravenously when gastric suction is being done.

Suction may also be applied to other drainage tubes such as chest tubes or a wound drain. Check the receptacle frequently to prevent excess drainage from interfering with the suction apparatus. Note the contents of the drainage and record it.

Wound Care

Most patients return from surgery with a sutured wound covered by a dressing, although in some cases, the wound may be left unsutured. Dressings are inspected regularly to ensure that they are clean, dry and intact. Excessive drainage may indicate hemorrhage, infection or an open wound.

When dressings are changed, the nurse assesses the wound for appearance, size, drainage, swelling, pain and the status of a drain or tubes (Table 3).

The surgical incisions heal by primary intention the following sequential signs of healing can be expected:

- Absence of bleeding and the appearance of a clot binding the wound edges are well approximated and bound by fibrin in the clot within the first few hours after surgical closure
- Inflammation (redness and swelling) is present at the wound edges for 1–3 days

TABLE 3: Assessing surgical wounds

Appearance	Inspect color of wound and surrounding area and approximation of wound edges
Size	Note size and location of dehiscence, if present
Drainage	Observe location, color, consistency, odor and soakage in the dressing
Swelling	Observe the amount of swelling. Minimal to moderate swelling is normal in early stages of wound healing
Pain	Expect severe to moderate postoperative pain for 3–5 days. Persistent severe pain or sudden onset of severe pain may indicate internal hemorrhage or infection
Drains or tubes	Inspect drain security and placement amount and character of drainage and function of drainage apparatus if present

- Reduction in inflammation occurs when the clot diminishes, as granulation tissue starts to bridge the area. The wound is bridged and closed within 7–10 days. Increased inflammation associated with fever and drainage is indicative of wound infection. The wound edges then appear brightly inflamed
- Scar formation: Collagen synthesis starts 4 days after injury and continues for 6 months or longer
- Scar size diminishes a period of 6 months or an year. An increase in scar size indicates keloid formation

A wound that is extensive and involves considerable tissue loss, and in which the edges cannot or should not be approximated, heals by secondary intention healing. An example of wound healing by secondary intention is a pressure ulcer. It differs from primary intention healing in three ways:

1. The repair time is longer
2. The scarring is greater
3. Susceptibility to infection is greater.

Those wounds that are left open for 3–5 days to allow edema or infection to resolve or exude to drain and are then closed with sutures, staples or adhesive skin closures, heal by **tertiary intention**.

Factors Affecting Wound Healing

Characteristics of the individual such as age, nutritional status, lifestyle and medications influence the speed of wound healing.

- **Developmental considerations:** Healthy children and adults often heal more quickly than elders, who are more likely to have chronic diseases that hinder healing. In elders, vascular changes such as atherosclerosis and atrophy of capillaries in the skin can impair blood flow to the wound, cell renewal is slower, leading to delayed healing. Suffering from diabetes or cardiovascular disease increases the risk of delayed healing due to impaired oxygen delivery to these tissues.
- **Nutrition:** Wound healing places additional demands on the body. Patients require a diet rich in protein, carbohydrate, lipids, vitamins A and C, and minerals such as iron, zinc, and copper. Malnourished clients may require time to improve their nutritional status before surgery. Obese clients are at an increased risk of wound infection and slower healing because adipose tissue usually has a minimal blood supply.
- **Lifestyle:** People who exercise daily tend to have good circulation and because blood brings oxygen and nourishment to the wound, they are more likely to heal quickly. Smoking reduces the amount of functional hemoglobin in the blood, thus limiting the oxygen carrying capacity of the blood and constricts arterioles.

- **Medications:** Anti-inflammatory drugs (steroids, aspirin) and antineoplastic agents interfere with healing. Prolonged use of antibiotics may make a person susceptible to wound infection by resistant organisms.

Types of Wound Exudate

Exudate is a material, such as fluid and cells, that has escaped from blood vessels during the inflammatory process and is deposited on tissue surfaces. The nature and amount of exudate varies according to the tissue involved, the intensity and duration of the inflammation, and the presence of microorganisms. There are various types of exudate:

- **Serous exudate:** It consists chiefly of serum (the clear portion of the blood) derived from blood and serous membrane of the body, such as peritoneum. It looks watery and has few cells. An example is the fluid in a blister from a burn.
- **Purulent exudate:** It is thicker than serous exudate because of the presence of pus, which consists of leukocytes, liquefied dead tissue debris, and dead and living bacteria. The process of pus formation is referred to as suppuration and the bacteria that produces pus are called pyogenic bacteria. Not all microorganisms are pyogenic. Purulent exudates vary in color, some acquiring tinge of blue, green or yellow depending on the causative organisms.
- **Sanguineous (hemorrhagic) exudate:** It consists of large amount of red blood cells, indicating damage to capillaries that is severe enough to allow escape of red blood cells from plasma. The type of exudate is frequently seen in open wounds.
- **Serosanguinous:** It consists of clear and blood tinged exudate and is commonly seen in surgical incision.
- **Purosanguinous:** Discharge consists of pus and blood is seen in a new wound that is infected.

Complications of Wound Healing

Several untoward events can interfere with the healing of a wound. These include hemorrhage, infection, dehiscence and evisceration.

Hemorrhage

Some escape of blood from a wound is normal. Hemorrhage i.e. massive bleeding, however is abnormal. A dislodged clot, a slipped stitch, or erosion of a blood vessel may cause severe bleeding. Internal hemorrhage may be detected by swelling or distention in the area of wound. Some patients may have a hematoma, a localized collection of blood underneath the skin that may appear as a reddish blue swelling (bruise). The risk of hemorrhage is greatest during the first 48 hours after surgery. It is an emergency; the nurse should apply pressure dressing to the area and monitor the client's vital signs. In many instances, the patient must be taken to the operating room for surgical intervention.

Infection

Contamination of wound surface with microorganism, leads then to complete with new cells for oxygen and nutrition. It can impair wound healing. When the microorganisms colonizing the wound multiply excessively or invade tissues, infection occurs. Infection is suggested by the presence of a change in wound color, pain or drainage is confirmed by performing a culture of the wound. Severe infection cause fever and elevated white blood cell count. Patients who are immunocompromised, those suffering from cancer, human immunodeficiency virus (HIV) are especially susceptible to wound infections. A wound can be infected with microorganisms at the time of injury, during surgery or postoperatively. Surgical infection is most likely to become apparent 2–11 days postoperatively.

Dehiscence and Evisceration

Dehiscence is the partial or total rupturing of a sutured wound. Dehiscence usually involves an abdominal wound in which the layers below the skin also separate. Evisceration is the protrusion of the internal viscera through an incision. A number of factors, including obesity, poor nutrition, multiple trauma, failure of suturing, excessive coughing, vomiting, and dehydration, increases client's risk of wound dehiscence. Wound dehiscence is more likely to occur 4–5 days postoperatively. It may precede sudden straining such as coughing or sneezing. When dehiscence or evisceration occurs, the wound should be quickly supported by large sterile dressings soaked in sterile normal saline. Place the patient in bed with knees bent to decrease pull on the incision. The surgeon is notified immediately because surgical repair may be necessary.

Surgical Dressings

All surgical dressings do not require change. Sometimes surgeons in the operating room apply a dressing that remains in place until the sutures are removed and no further dressings are required. In many situations, however, surgical dressings are changed regularly to prevent the growth of microorganisms.

In some instances, a client may have a penrose drain inserted. In this situation the main surgical incision is considered cleaner than the surgical stab wound made for the drain insertion, because there is usually considerable drainage. The main incision is, therefore, cleaned first and under no circumstances are materials that were used to clean the stab wound used subsequently to clean the main incision. In this way, the main incision is kept free of the microorganisms.

Wound Drains and Suction

Surgical drains, a penrose drain, are inserted to permit the drainage of excessive serosanguinous fluid and purulent material and to promote healing of underlying tissues. These drains may be inserted and sutured through the incision line, but they are most commonly inserted through stab wounds a few centimeters away from the incision line so that the main incision is kept dry without a drain, some wounds would heal on the surface and trap the discharge inside and an abscess might form.

A closed wound drainage system consists of a drain connected to either an electric suction or a portable drainage suction, such as hemovac. The closed system reduces the possible entry of microorganisms into the wound through the drain. The drainage tubes are sutured in place and connected to a reservoir. These portable wound suctions also provide for accurate measurements of the drainage. The surgeon inserts the wound drainage tube during surgery. Generally, the suction is discontinued from 3 to 5 days, postoperatively or when the drainage is minimal. Nurses are responsible for maintaining the wound suction, which hastens the healing process by draining excess exudate that might otherwise interfere with the formation of granulation tissue.

Sutures

A suture is a thread used to sew body tissues together. Sutures used to attach tissues beneath the skin are often made of an absorbable material that disappears in several days. Skin sutures, by contrast, are made of a variety of nonabsorbable materials, such as silk, cotton, linen, wire, nylon and dacron, silver wire clips or staples are also available. Usually skin sutures are removed 7–10 days after surgery.

There are various methods of suturing. Skin sutures can be broadly categories as either interrupted (each stitch is tied and knotted separately) or continuous (one thread runs in a series of stitches and is tied only at the beginning and at the end). Retention sutures are very large sutures used in addition to skin sutures for some incisions (Fig. 5). They attach underlying tissues of fat and muscle as well as skin and are used to support incisions in obese individuals or when healing may be prolonged. They are frequently left in place for longer than skin sutures (14–21 days). To prevent these large sutures from irritating the incision, the surgeon may place rubber tubing over them.

Regarding removal of sutures, agency policies vary. In some places primary care provider removes sutures and in other places registered nurses can also remove. The nurse should verify whether sutures are to be removed and who may remove them.

Sterile techniques and special suture scissors are used in suture removal. The scissors have a short, curved cutting tip that readily slides under the suture. Wire clips or staples are removed with a special instrument that squeezes the center of the clip to remove it from the skin (Figs 6 and 7).

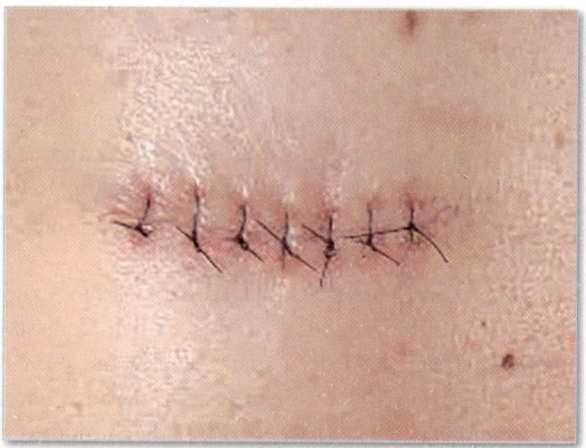

Fig. 5: A surgical incision with retention sutures

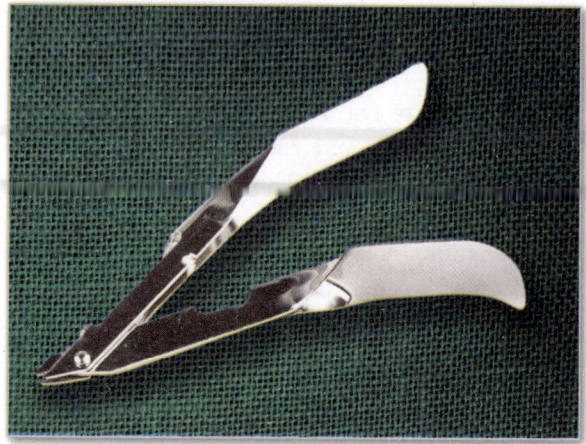

Fig. 6: Staple remover

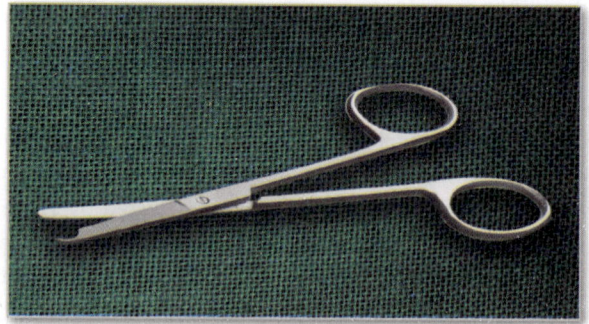

Fig. 7: Suture scissors

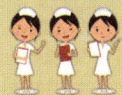

SKILL: STERILE DRESSING CHANGE

Sterile dressing changes are performed for surgical wounds, open wounds, and pressure ulcers, The physician orders the frequency of the dressing change.

Purposes

- To promote wound healing by primary intention
- To prevent infection
- To assess the healing process
- To protect the wound from mechanical trauma

Articles Required (Fig. 8)

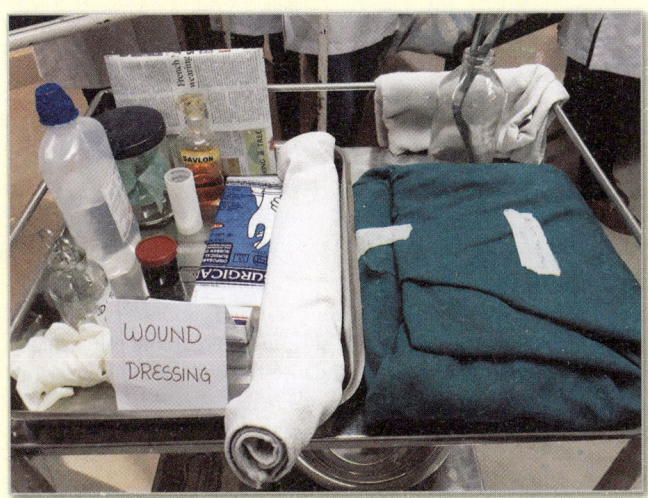

Fig. 8: Articles tray for sterile dressing change

Steps of Procedure

Review and carry out the standard steps as given in Appendix

Action/steps	Rationale
Assessment	
1. Check the orders for direction for wound care and dressing Change	A physician's order is required for dressing change
2. Determine if the patient is ready for the procedure	Saves time if the patient is not involved in other activity
Planning	
3. Check the nurses notes for the types of supplies needed for the dressing change and assess the dressing that is in place	Ensures that the proper supplies will be on hand during the sterile procedure
Implementation	
4. Wash your hands. Loosen the binder or tape, put on clean gloves and remove the old dressing. Pull off the tape toward the wound. Assess the drainage on the dressings and place in the discard bag	Pulling tape toward the wound prevents disruption of the wound. Prevents spread of microorganism and allows visual assessment of the wound and drainage
5. Inspect the wound, noting degree of healing, presence of pus, and necrosis, check for odor, drainage and condition of sutures or drain. Remove gloves and discard them	Provides data for determining progress of wound healing or presence of infection
6. Set up sterile field placing items in the order in which they will be used	Assists in maintaining a sterile field during the procedure and allows the procedure to be done efficiently

Cotnd...

Action/steps	Rationale
7. Put on sterile gloves and clean the area around the wound using alcohol swabs or disinfectant. Cleanse by one of the following methods (Figs 9A and B)	Sterile technique prevents contamination of the wound. The top of the wound is considered the cleanest area. Cleansing by these methods prevents contaminating the wound. If considerable drainage is present in the wound itself, it is gently cleansed using a fresh swab for each single stroke

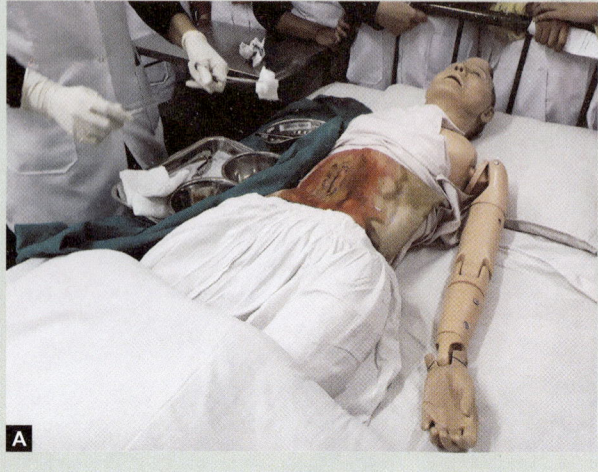 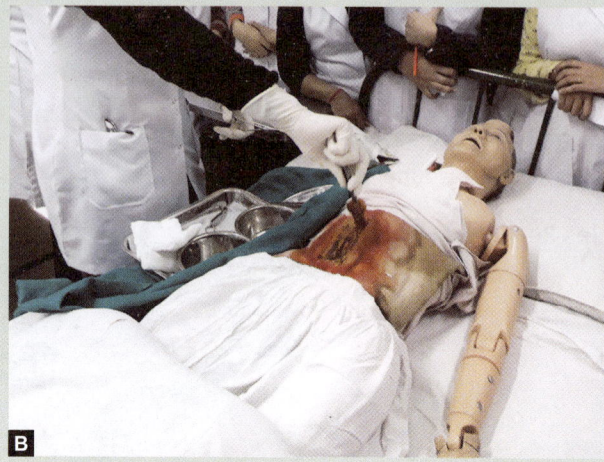

Figs 9A and B: Wound cleaning

- Use a circular motion from the wound outward in a circle
- Use a separate swab from top to bottom on each side of the incision and continue outward
- Use a separate swab from the wound edge outward on one side and then on the other side from top to bottom. Do not cleanse directly over the wound unless there is excessive drainage. Cleanse the drain sites using a circular motion from the drain outward

8. Apply ointment or medication using applicators, if ordered	An order is essential for any medication. Using applicators decreases the chance of contamination of the tube
9. Apply the dressing lightly over the wound. Cover the entire wound and do not move the dressing once it is placed over the wound. Remove and discard the gloves. Secure the dressing in place with tape. A binder or montgomery straps may be used to hold the dressing in place (Figs 10 to 12).	Moving the dressing from one area to another may transfer microorganisms and this action ensures that the wound stays covered

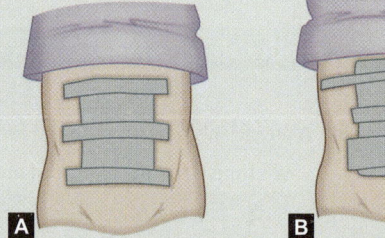

Figs 10A and B: The strips of tape should be placed at the ends of the dressing and must be sufficiently long and wide to secure the dressing. The tape should adhere to intact skin

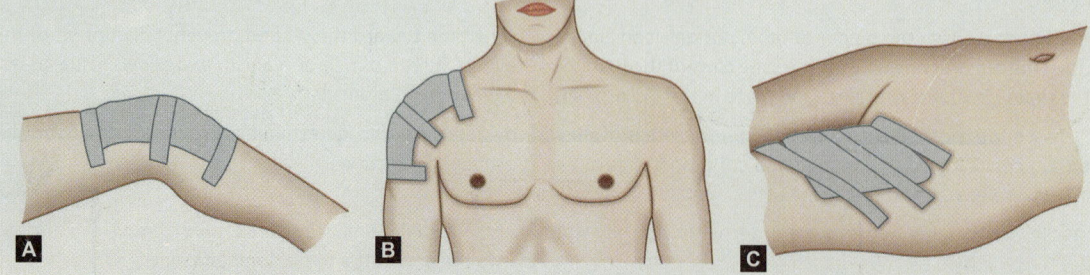

Figs 11A to C: Dressings over moving parts must remain secure in spite of the client's movement. Place the tape over a joint at a right angle to the direction the joint moves

Cotnd...

Action/steps	Rationale

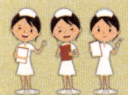

Nonadhesive portion

Adhesive portion

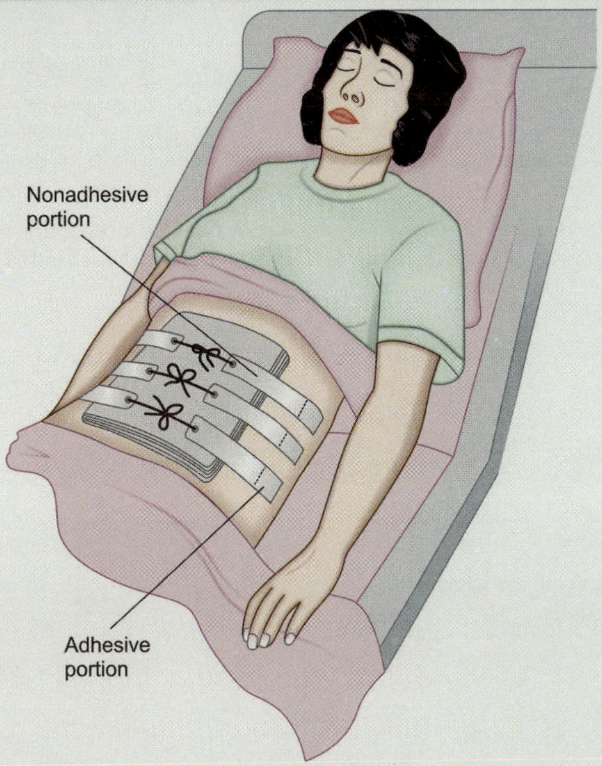

Fig. 12: Montgomery straps

Evaluation

10. Ask yourself: Are there any signs of infection such as redness and warmth around the wound edges there thick or colored exudate present? Is the amount of drainage decreasing? Is the wound drain still in place? Had drainage soaked through the dressing? Did the dressing stay intact?	Answers to these questions provide data regarding wound healing and whether the dressing was sufficient to cover the wound and contain the drainage
11. Document the condition of the wound including subjective statements of the patient as well as objective observations. Include health teachings performed for wound care	Provides data regarding wound healing. Documents use of supplies

Removing Sutures or Staples

Sutures or staples are removed when the wound is well sealed and connective tissue has formed. This occurs in 7–10 days, although the time for suture removal may vary. An order is required for removal of sutures or staples.

SKILL: REMOVING SUTURES OR STAPLES

Steps of Procedure

Action/steps	Rationale
Assessment	
1. Wash hands, put on gloves and remove the dressing, discard it in a plastic discard bag	Exposes the sutures or staples, prevents transfer of microorganisms
2. Open the suture removal or staple removal set	Prepares the equipment for use

Cotnd...

Action/steps	Rationale
For sutures	
3. Pick up the forceps with your non-dominant hand and the suture scissor with the dominant hand	This allows good control of the instruments
4. Lift the knot of the suture away from the skin with the forceps, and slip the curved tip of the scissors under the suture beneath the knot	The suture is cut beneath the knot and pulled from the skin to one smooth motion. Prevents pulling exposed suture back through the skin. The entire suture must be pulled free
5. As long as the skin stays well approximated, remove every other suture. If wound shows no signs of separation, remove the remaining sutures (Figs 13 and 14)	Removing every other suture provides a safeguard in case the wound begins to be separated

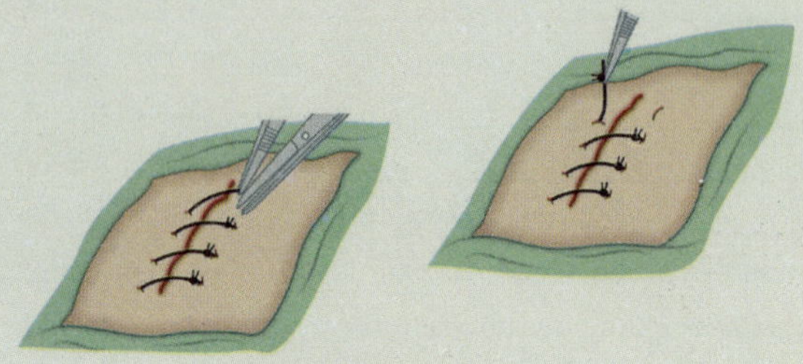

Fig. 13: Clip beneath the knot with the scissors to remove the suture

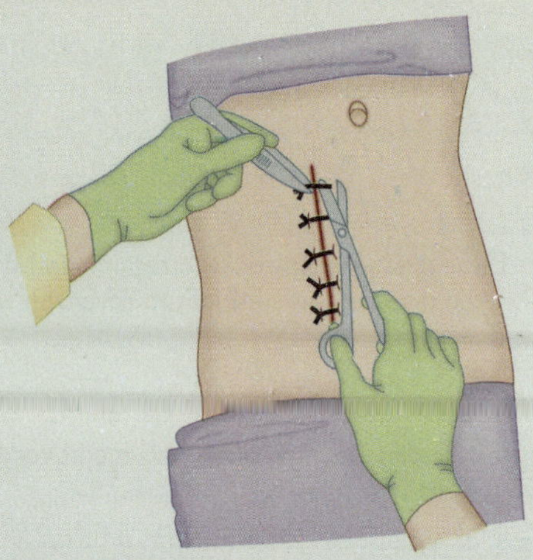

Fig. 14: Removing a plain interrupted skin suture

For staples	
6. After opening the equipment, place the lower jaw of the staple remover under the staple. Be certain the tip is all the way under the staple (Fig. 15)	Positions the tool to crimp the staple

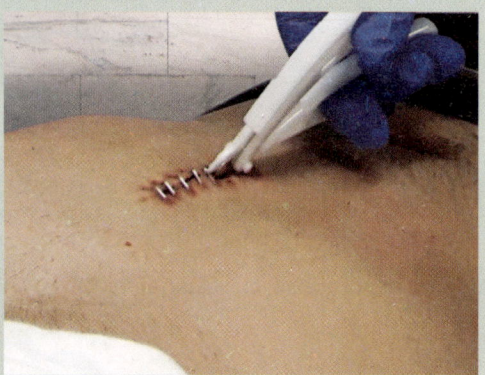

Fig. 15: A special equipment is used for staple removal

Cotnd...

Action/steps	Rationale
7. Press the handles of the staple remover together all the way to depress the center of the staple	The staple must be firmly pressed between the two parts of the staple remover to allow it to be pulled free of the skin
8. When both ends of the staple are visible, lift it up and away from the skin. Drop the staple into the discard bag	Removes the staple, prevents transfer of microorganism and injury by a sharp object
For sutures and staples	
9. Gently cleanse any dried blood from the suture or staple sites with an antiseptic sponge	Suture holes are open to the atmosphere and can admit bacteria. Dried blood may contain microorganisms
10. Place sterile strips or a dressing over the incisional area as ordered	Often the incision will simply be left open to the air
11. Place all used supplies in the discard bag. Remove gloves and discard them. Wash your hands	Prevents transfer of microorganisms

POSTOPERATIVE COMPLICATIONS (TABLE 4)

TABLE: 4 Postoperative complications

Problems	Signs and symptoms	Preventive interventions
Atelectasis	Decreased breath sounds over areas not aerating, dyspnea	Deep breathing and coughing; use of incentive spirometer; early ambulation
Pneumonia, (hypostatic, aspiration, or bacterial)	Fever, malaise, increased sputum, purulent sputum, cough, flushed skin, dyspnea, pain on inspiration; abnormal breath sounds, crackles, rhonchi	Deep breathing, coughing, and frequent turning; early ambulation; incentive spirometer use; range-of-motion exercises if unable to ambulate, medication if bacterial
Paralytic (adynamic) ileus	No bowel sounds 24–36 hours after surgery or fewer than 5 sounds per minute	Monitor bowel sounds; encourage early ambulation; nothing by mouth as ordered. Do not feed until bowel sounds return
Thrombophle-bitis	Pain or warmth in calf of leg, swollen leg, warm, area to touch on leg; possible temperature elevation	Encourage leg exercises; keep the patient well hydrated; encourage ambulation; antiembolic stockings or devices
Urinary retention	Distended bladder; inability to void spontaneously	Palpate bladder; encourage voiding, catheterize if unable to void within 8 hours per order; medicate to increase urinary sphincter tone as ordered
Urinary tract infection	Dysuria, frequency, foul-smelling urine	Force fluids when allowed; encourage frequent voiding; keep catheter clean and patent; use aseptic technique to empty drainage bag
Wound infection	Redness, swelling, pain, warmth, drainage, fever, increased leukocytes, rapid pulse and respiration (fever 72 hours after surgery indicates infection in some system or in the wound)	Use aseptic technique for wound care; encourage adequate nutrition and fluids; encourage activity
Pulmonary embolus	Shortness of breath, anxiety, chest pain, rapid pulse and respirators, cyanosis, cough, bloody sputum	Antiembolism stockings, adequate fluid intake, frequent turning or ambulation, preventive anticoagulant if ordered
Hemorrhage and shock	Evidence of copious bleeding; decreased blood pressure, elevated pulse, cold and clammy skin, decreased urinary output	Give blood or volume expander; Try to stop bleeding. Place in shock position with feet and legs elevated and head flat; administer ordered medications to raise blood pressure; administer oxygen; frequent vital signs measurement

Cotnd...

Problems	Signs and symptoms	Preventive interventions
Wound dehiscence or evisceration	Discharge of serosanguineous drainage from wound and sensation that "something gave"; separation of wound edges with intestines visible through abdominal incision	Teach to splint properly for coughing. Place patient supine; cover wound with sterile saline-soaked gauze or towels
Fluid imbalance	Signs of overhydration: crackles in lungs, edema, weight gain. Signs of dehydration: weight loss, diminished pulse, dry mucous membranes, decreased tissue turgor	Control IV flow rate. Monitor intake and output; correct imbalances. Output will be less than intake first 72 hours after surgery with general anesthesia. Auscultate lungs each shift. Monitor weight; check for edema

EVALUATION

The achievement of desired outcomes for postoperative recovery and rehabilitation may be evaluated in number of ways: The final resolution of some desired outcomes may not be apparent or measurable at the time of discharge, many institutions use follow-up telephone calls or surveys that are mailed to patients. Whatever mechanism is selected, important outcomes, such as the absence of the surgical site infection, the patient's satisfaction with the pain management measures, return to former levels of mobility and activity, and the absence of postoperative nausea and vomiting and other complications for which the patient was at risk should be included as part of evaluative criteria.

BIBLIOGRAPHY

1. *Potter PA, Perry AG. Fundamentals of Nursing, 6th edition. Mosby Inc; 2004.*

2. *Carol Taylor, Carol Lillis. Fundamentals of Nursing—The Art and Science of Nursing Care.*

3. *Berman AT, Snyder S, Kozier BJ, et al. Kozier & Erb's. Fundamentals of Nursing: Concepts, Process and Practice, 8th edition. Pearson Education.*

4. *Craven RF, Hirnle CJ. Fundamentals of Nursing Human Health and Function, 3rd edition. Lippincott Publishers. 2000.*

Bandaging

Learning Objectives

After completing this chapter, you will be able to:
+ Gain knowledge regarding principles of bandaging
+ Apply bandage to various parts of the body

Key Terms

+ Circular turn
+ Spiral turn
+ Reverse spiral turn
+ Recurrent turn
+ Figure of eight turn

Chapter Outline

+ Introduction
+ Purposes
+ Classification of Bandaging
+ Principles for Applying Bandages
+ Various Turns used in Bandaging
+ Special Bandages

INTRODUCTION

Bandage

It is a piece of material that is used to wrap a part of the body.

Binders

These are special bandages used to support larger parts of the body and large dressings in place.

PURPOSES

Bandages

+ To limit movement
+ To hold dressing in place
+ To provide support
+ To keep splints in position
+ To apply warmth
+ To apply pressure in order to control bleeding and promote absorption of tissue fluids.

Binders

+ To support the abdomen.
+ To prevent or reduce wound dehiscence after surgery of abdomen.
+ To hold the dressing in place.
+ To maintain intra-abdominal paracentesis.
+ T-binder is used to hold rectal and perineal dressings.

CLASSIFICATION OF BANDAGING

+ Simple
+ **Special:** Related to which organ to be bandaged.

PRINCIPLES FOR APPLYING BANDAGES

+ Stand in front of the part to be bandaged.
+ Bandages should not be too tight or loose.
+ Prevent contact between two skin surfaces.
+ Use bandage of suitable length and width.
+ Apply the bandage with firm and even pressure throughout.

- Bandage form distal to proximal and from within outwards.
- Pad the axilla or groin when bandaging is to be done near these parts.
- Cove two-thirds of the previous turn of the bandage leaving one-third uncovered.
- The drum of the bandage must be held on the top.
- Start and finish with two circular turns.
- Ensure that the bandage applied is neat and firm.
- Secure the bandage with a safety pin pointing up or with a small strip of adhesive tape.

VARIOUS TURNS USED IN BANDAGING

- **Circular turns:** These are used to anchor bandages and to terminate them. These turns usually are not applied directly over a wound because of the discomfort caused by the bandage (Fig. 1).
- **Spiral turns:** These are used to bandage parts of the body that are fairly uniform in circumference, for example the upper arm or upper leg (Fig. 2).
- **Reverse spiral turns:** These are used to bandage parts, which are not uniform in circumference, e.g., forearm, lower leg (Fig. 3).
- **Recurrent turns:** These are used to cover distal parts of the body, for example tip of the finger, the skull or the stump of an amputation (Fig. 4).
- **Figure of eight turns:** These are used to bandage an elbow, knee or ankle because they permit some movement after they are applied. The spica bandage is a variation of the figure of eight turns, e.g., thumb spica (Fig. 5).

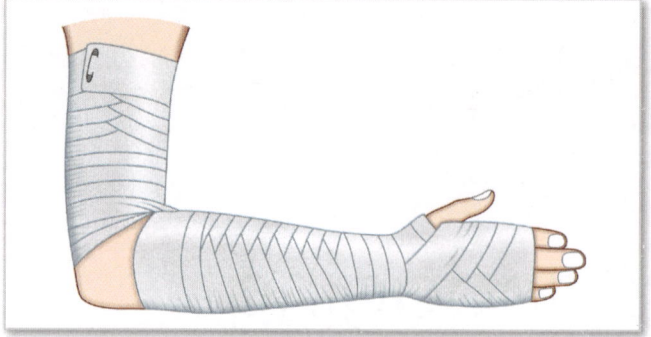

Fig. 3: Reverse spiral turns

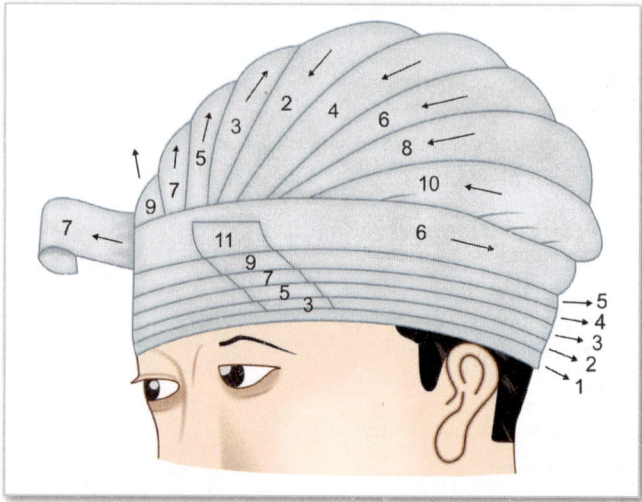

Fig. 4: Recurrent turn (Capline bandage)

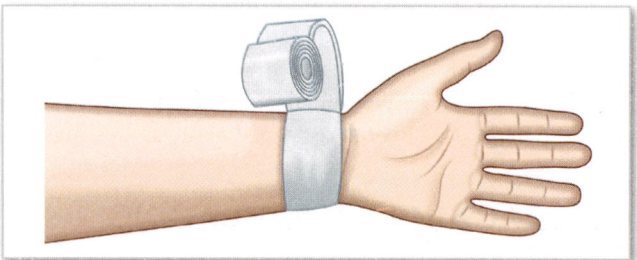

Fig. 1: Circular turns

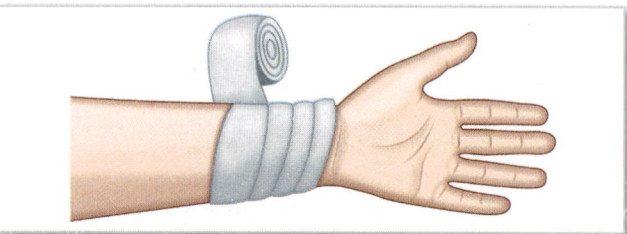

Fig. 2: Spiral turns

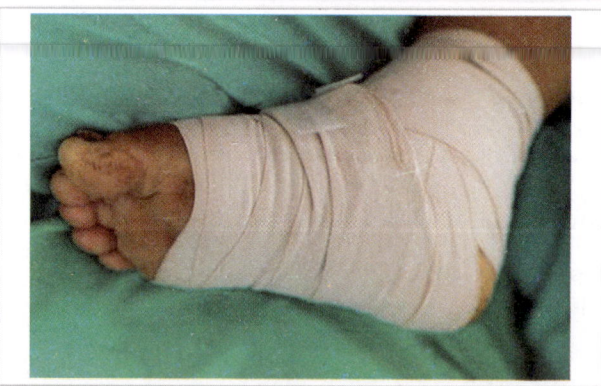

Fig. 5: Figure of eight turn

Technique

Circular Turn

- Hold the bandage in your dominant hand, with the roll on the upper side and unroll the bandage about 8 cm.
- Apply the end of the bandage to the body parts to be bandaged.

- Encircle the body part, each turn covering the previous turn, secure the end of the bandage with tape, metal clip or a safety pin.

Spiral Turn

- Start with two circular turns and cover two-third and continue to wrap the bandage
- Finish with two circular turns
- Secure the bandage using safety pins, tape, or metal clip

Reverse Spiral Turn

- Start with two circular turns around the affected area
- Turn the bandage over so that side on top is now the bottom
- Continue to wrap around the affected area and finish with two circular tums
- Secure the bandage using safety pins or tape

Recurrent Turns

- Start with two circular turns
- Then turns are made over and back
- Subsequent turns are folded alternatively
- Keep your fingers in place at the top to secure the bandage until a circular turn or two can be made to complete the bandage
- Secure the bandage using safety pins or tape

Figure of Eight Turns

- Anchor the bandage with two circular turns.
- Carry the bandage above the joint, around it and then below it making a figure eight.
- Continue above and below the joint, overlapping the previous turn by two third the width of the bandage.
- Terminate the bandage above the joint with two circular turns and secure it with tape, metal clips or safety pin.

SPECIAL BANDAGES

Eye Bandage (Fig. 6)

- Pad the affected eye. Take two circular turns around the head bandaging away from the injured eye.
- Carry the bandage, around the head until it reaches the eye on the affected side.
- Take it obliquely to the back of the head and from there, bring it upwards beneath the eye of the affected side
- Take it further over the pad of the eye to a circular turn and continue over the head to a starting point.

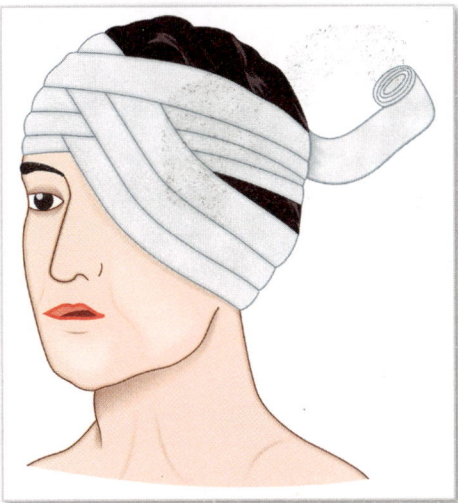

Fig. 6: Eye bandage

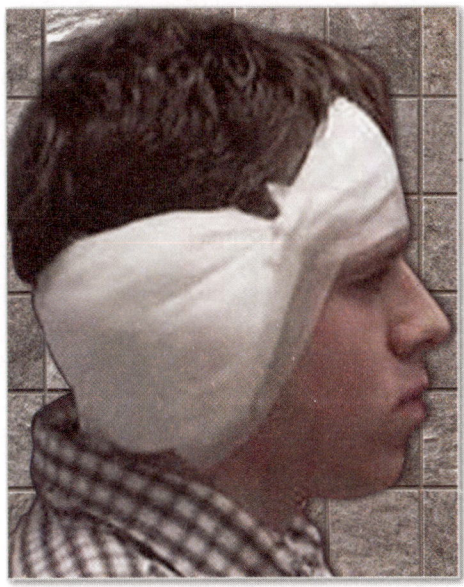

Fig. 7: Ear bandage

- Repeat this turn two or three times until the dressing is covered.
- Secure the bandage with a tape.

Ear Bandage (Fig. 7)

- Secure the roller bandage with two circular turns around the forehead, and then down the nape of the neck.
- Repeat the turns with each turn being slightly higher than the previous one, continue the turns until the whole ear, on the affected side is covered and complete the bandage by two circular turns around the forehead.
- Secure it with adhesive tape or safety pin.

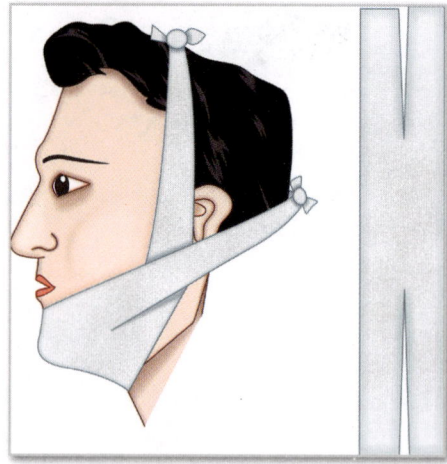

Fig. 8: Jaw bandage

Jaw Bandage Center: Four-tailed (Fig. 8)

- Keep the center of the bandage at the chin.
- Take the upper tails on both the sides above the pinna and secure them at the occiput.
- Take the lower tails behind the ears and secure them on top of the head.

Jaw Bandage: Two-tailed

- Make a small slit at the center of the gauze and place it over the chin, take two ends above the head
- Keep the bandage at the chin at the center slit and ears in the lateral slits
- Secure the bandage at the top of the head.

Shoulder Spica (Fig. 9)

- Stand on the side where the bandage is to be applied; pad the axilla.

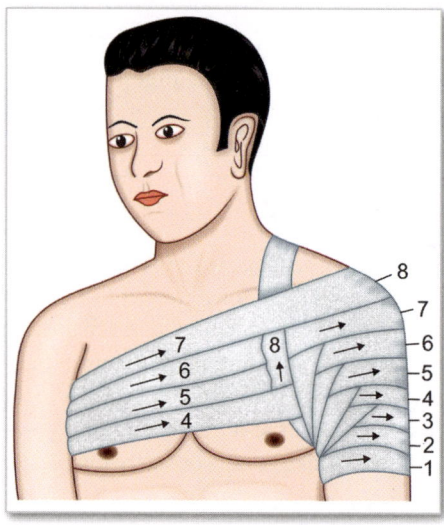

Fig. 9: Shoulder spica

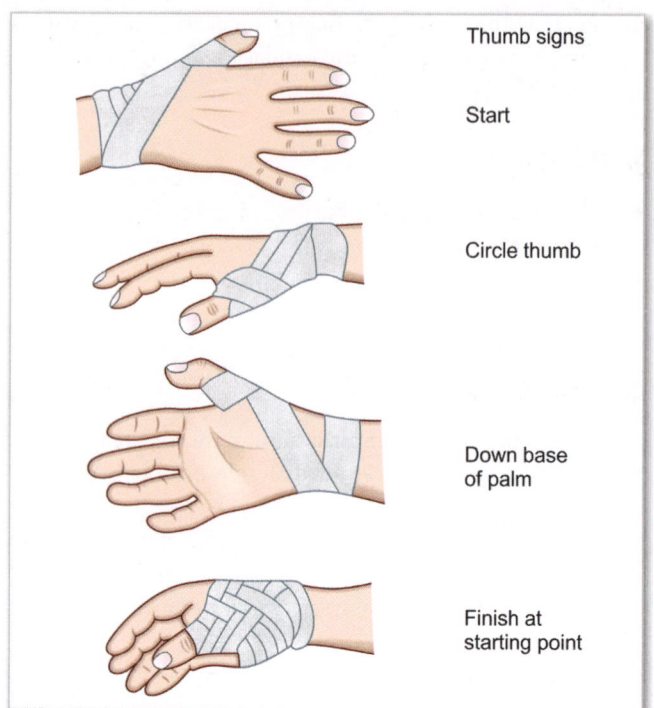

Fig. 10: Thumb spica

- Anchor the bandage around the upper arm near the axilla with two circular turns.
- For injury on the right side, carry around the arm and across the chest. For injury on the left side, take across the chest and through the opposite axilla and across the back to the injured arm, where it crosses the previous turns in mid line.
- Repeat the previous turns by overlapping one half to two-third width crossing it exactly in the midline and ascending towards the shoulder until covered.
- Secure the bandage in the front.

Thumb Spica (Fig. 10)

- Anchor the bandage around the wrist with two circular turns.
- Bring the bandage obliquely across the back of the hand and carry it by quick spiral turns to the tip of the thumb without overlapping the previous turns.
- Make a circular turn near the tip of the thumb and carry the bandage down the thumb by two to three spiral reverse turns, followed by figure of eight till the base of the thumb. Carry it to the dorsum of the thumb and then to the lateral aspect of the wrist and finish with two circular turns at the wrist.

Triangular Bandage (Fig. 11)

- This is used to support the arm, elbow and forearm and to prevent swelling of a hand.

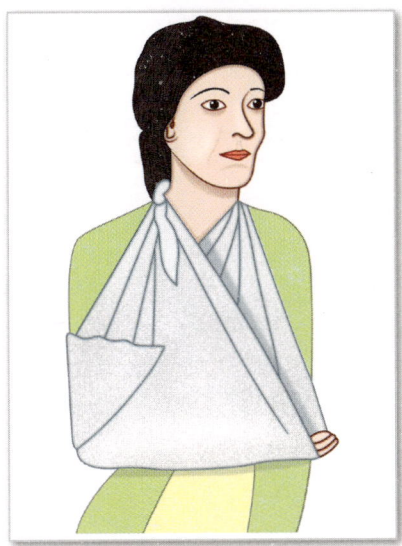

Fig. 11: Triangular bandage

- Triangular bandages can be used for the head, feet and as a sling for the arm.

- Folded triangular bandage can be used around the elbows and the knee.

Binders: Abdominal Binder (Figs 12A and B)

- Position the patient in supine position with the binder in the middle and both straps should extend equally on both the sides.
- Begin at the lower end of the binder, bring alternate right and left straps tightly with slightly upward slant over the abdomen, covering half of the preceding strap, crossing at the midline.
- Hold the free end of the strap until the opposite strap secures them. Overlap final straps horizontally and secure with a clip or safety pin.

'T' Binder (Fig. 12C)

- Secure the waist strap of the binder in the front with a pin.
- Bring double or single T straps between the patients legs and secure over waist strap in the middle using a pin.

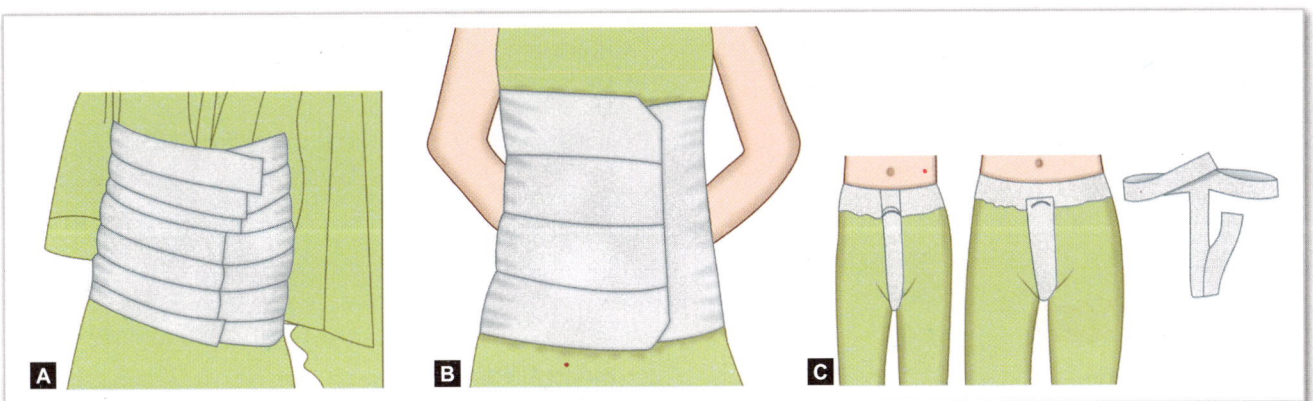

Figs 12A to C: 'T' Bandage. A and B. Abdominal binders; C. T-bandage

BIBLIOGRAPHY

1. *Potter PA, Perry AG. Fundamentals of Nursing, 6th edition. Mosby Inc; 2004.*
2. *Carol Taylor, Carol Lillis. Fundamentals of Nursing—The Art and Science of Nursing Care.*
3. *Berman AT, Snyder S, Kozier BJ, et al. Kozier & Erb's. Fundamentals of Nursing: Concepts, Process and Practice, 8th edition. Pearson Education.*
4. *Craven RF, Hirnle CJ. Fundamentals of Nursing Human Health and Function, 3rd edition. Lippincott Publishers. 2000.*

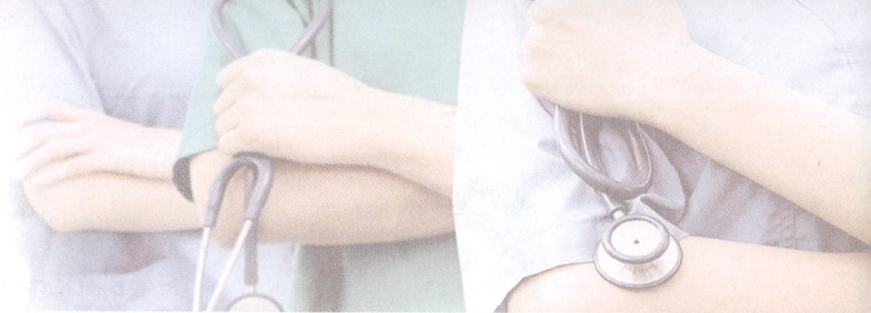

Chapter 52

Pain

INTRODUCTION

Pain is a complex multifactorial phenomenon. It is an individual, unique experience that may be difficult for clients to describe or explain and is often difficult for others to recognize, understand and assess.

Pain is an unpleasant sensory and emotional experience associated with actual or potential tissue damage, or described in terms of such damage. It is the feeling common to such experiences as stubbing a toe, burning a finger, putting iodine on a cut and bumping the "funny bone".

Pain motivates us to withdraw from potentially damaging situations, protect a damaged body part while it heals, and avoid those situations in the future. It is initiated by stimulation of nociceptors in the peripheral nervous system, or by damage to or malfunction of the peripheral or central nervous system.

Most pain resolves promptly once the painful stimulus is removed and the body has healed, but sometimes pain persists despite removal of the stimulus and apparent healing of the body; and sometimes pain arises in the absence of any detectable stimulus, damage or pathology.

Pain is the most common reason for physician consultation. It is a major symptom in many medical conditions and can significantly interfere with a person's quality of life and general functioning. Social support, hypnotic suggestion, excitement in sport or war, distraction and appraisal can all significantly modulate pain's intensity or unpleasantness.

A person's pain experience is influenced by a number of factors including past experience with pain, anxiety, culture, age, gender and expectation about pain relief. These factors may increase or decrease the perception of pain, increase or decrease tolerance for pain and affect the responses to pain.

DEFINITION

The International Association for the Study of Pain (IASP) offers the accepted medical definition of pain as "An unpleasant sensory and emotional experience associated with actual or potential tissue damage or described in terms of such damage.

PERCEPTION OF PAIN

Pain perception or interpretation is an important component of the experience of pain. Because we perceive pain and it is based on our own individual experience, it is different for each person. Some of the factors that affect our pain perception are:

- Physical stimuli or physical damage
- Psychosocial factors
- Cognitive factors such as distractions
- Pain threshold (the lowest intensity of pain stimuli that is perceived by a person as pain). The pain threshold may vary according to physiologic factors such as inflammation or injury near pain receptors, but essentially it is similar for all people if the central nervous system and peripheral nervous system are intact.
- Tolerance is defined as the amount of pain a person is willing to endure. It is different for each person who experiences pain, based on the subjective factors such as the meaning of the pain and the setting. Some people have a high tolerance; that is, they can tolerate a lot of pain without distress, whereas others have a very low tolerance. Tolerance also varies for a given person, depending on a variety of factors associated with each specific pain incidence such as:
  - Nausea
  - Fatigue
  - Meaning of the pain
  - Coping ability
  - Sensory input
  - Genetic make up

Only the person, not the health team, can determine the person's tolerance levels.

MISCONCEPTIONS AND MYTHS

Misconceptions and myths regarding pain along with their facts are given in Table 1.

TABLE 1: Misconceptions and myths about pain

Sl. No.	Myth or misconception	Fact
1.	Addiction occurs with prolonged use of morphine or morphine derivatives.	The incidence of addiction is less than 0.1%.
2.	The physician or nurse is the best judge of client's pain.	Only the client can judge the level and distress of the pain; pain management should be a team approach that includes the client.
3.	Pain is a result, not a cause.	Unrelieved pain can create other problems such as anger, anxiety, immobility, respiratory problems, and delay in healing.
4.	It is better to wait until a client has pain before giving medication.	Playing "catch-up" is not an effective way to manage pain; it is better to routinely administer analgesia, thus maintaining a low pain level.
5.	Real pain has an identifiable cause.	There is always a cause for pain, but it may be very obscure and must be assessed carefully. Pain of a psychological origin is just as real as pain of physiologic origin.
6.	The same physical stimulus produces the same pain intensity, duration, and distress in different people.	Intensity, duration and distress vary with each individual.
7.	Some clients lie about the existence or severity of their pain.	Very few people lie about pain.

Contd...

Sl. No.	Myth or misconception	Fact
8.	Very young or very old people do not have as much pain.	All clients with an intact neurologic system experience pain; age is not a determinant of pain, but it may influence expression of pain.
9.	Pain is a part of aging	Pain does not accompany aging unless a disease or ailment is present.
10.	If a person is asleep, that person is not in pain.	People in pain become exhausted and may truly be asleep or merely trying to sleep. Some people sleep as an escape mechanism.
11.	If the pain is relieved by nonpharmaceutical pain relief techniques, the pain was not real anyway	Nonpharmaceutical pain relief methods can be effective. A client's method of relief should be acknowledged as long as it does not harms.
12.	Nurses should rely on their own definitions of pain and cultural beliefs about pain.	It is a mistake to impose one's own definitions, cultural beliefs, and values to another person's pain. Let the client tell you what the pain means.

TYPES OF PAIN

Acute Pain

- Acute pain is usually of short duration (less than 6 months) and has an identifiable, immediate onset, such as incisional pain after surgery. Acute pain is often described in sensory terms such as "sharp", "stabbing" and "shooting".
- It is also regarded as having a limited and often predictable durations.
- Acute pain may be accompanied by observable physical responses, including:
  - Increased or decreased blood pressure
  - Tachycardia
  - Diaphoresis
  - Tachypnea
  - Focusing on the pain
  - Guarding the painful part
- The cardiovascular and respiratory responses are due to stimulation of the sympathetic nervous system as part of the fight or flight response.
- These responses are often interpreted as positive evidence of a person's pain. Such interpretation is not reliable, however, because these sympathetic responses are temporary and may not be present in client with continuing acute pain.
- Unrelieved pain leads to chronic pain stress.

Chronic Pain

- Chronic pain is a major health concern. The pain may seem originally acute in nature or may have been so obscure that the person does not know when it first developed.
- Chronic pain may be divided into three types:
  - Chronic non-malignant pain, such as from low back pain or rheumatoid arthritis.
  - Chronic intermittent pain, such as from migraine headache.
  - Chronic malignant pain, such as from cancer.
- Sources and causes of chronic pain are enlisted in Table 2.
- A person's response to pain depends on its duration and intensity. Pain that is constant, continuous, and moderate is often described as even more difficult to bear than pain that is intense but relatively short in duration.
- The course of pain includes months and years of pain, not minutes or hours.
- Characteristics of clients experiencing chronic pain syndrome include the following:
  - Depression
  - Increased or decreased appetite and weight
  - Drastically restricted activity level, leading to reduced work capacity, poor physical tone, and increased depression.

TABLE 2: Sources and causes of chronic pain

Source of stimuli	Cause
Cell destruction	<ul><li>Chemotherapy</li><li>Cell necrosis</li><li>Ulceration</li><li>Tissue invasion</li><li>Tissue injury</li></ul>
Inflammation	<ul><li>Products of cell destruction.</li></ul>
Infection	<ul><li>Bacterial invasion</li></ul>
Nerve injury	<ul><li>Direct injury through incising nerve structures</li><li>Tumor invasion of peripheral nerves, plexus, spinal cord and brain</li><li>Chemotherapy/radiation injury</li></ul>
Ischemia/hypoxia	<ul><li>Edema</li><li>Hematoma</li><li>Occlusion of vessels by tumor</li></ul>

Contd...

Source of stimuli	Cause
Noxious stretch or pressure	◆ Distention of thoracic and abdominal viscera, fascia and periosteum ◆ Occlusion of gastrointestinal and genitourinary structures. ◆ Obstruction of ducts and viscus

- Social withdrawal and life role change.
- Preoccupation with physical manifestations
- Poor sleep and chronic fatigue, which may result from inactivity, analgesics and depression as well as from pain.
- Decreased concentration.

Chronic Non-malignant Pain

- It is usually the pain that lasts for more than 6 months (or 1 month beyond the normal end of the condition causing the pain) and has no foreseeable end unless it is associated with very slow healing, as with burns.
- It is continuous or persistent and recurrent.
- Chronic pain may or may not have an identifiable cause, or the cause may be difficult to determine.
- Chronic pain is frequently associated with concomitant disability as a result of the pain experience. For example, a client immobilized by the pain of severe rheumatoid arthritis may be further compromised by the effects of immobility.
- They may seem fearful, tense, fatigued and tend to become withdrawn and isolated. Their pain is exhausting both physically and emotionally for themselves and their families.

Chronic Intermittent Pain

- It refers to the exacerbation or recurrence of the chronic condition.
- The pain occurs only at specific periods, at other times, the client is free from pain.
- Typical conditions include migraine, cluster headache, sickle cell crisis, and the intermittent abdominal pain associated with chronic gastrointestinal disorders, such as irritable bowel syndrome and Crohn's disease.
- Pain management is same as for individual acute pain episodes.
- Chronic recurrences render the condition more difficult to manage as the client anticipates continual exacerbation of the situation and is intensely influenced by psychosocial factors that are difficult to manage.

Chronic Malignant (Cancer-Related) Pain

- Malignant pain has qualities of both acute and chronic pain.
- This category contains neuropathic, deep, visceral, and bone pain, etc.
- Each type of pain is managed specifically, therefore, the nurse needs to carefully assess each type of pain and treat it appropriately.
- A diagnosis of cancer adds an additional psychological component associated with physical deformity and the potential for impending death, preceded by agonizing suffering. It may intensify the pain.

SOURCES OF PAIN

Systems involved in pain production include the following:

- Superficial cutaneous regions encompassing skin and subcutaneous tissues.
- Somatic tissues of the body wall, including muscle, bone, periosteum, cartilage, tendons, deep fascia, ligaments, joints, blood vessels and nerves.
- Visceral structures, including organs and their capsules.

The characteristics of a person's pain experience depends on the source of the stimulation.

Nociceptive Pain

Nociceptive pain is caused by stimulation of peripheral nerve fibers that respond only to stimuli approaching or exceeding harmful intensity (nociceptors), and may be classified according to the mode of noxious stimulation; the most common categories being "thermal" (heat or cold), "mechanical" (crushing, tearing, etc.) and "chemical" (iodine in a cut, chili powder in the eyes).

Nociceptive pain may also be divided into "visceral," "deep somatic" and "superficial somatic" pain.

Cutaneous (Superficial) Pain

It is characterized by an abrupt onset and a sharp or stinging quality or by a slower onset and a burning quality, depending upon the type of nerve fiber involved. Cutaneous pain tends to be easily localized. The skin surface is readily divided into areas called dermatomes. Each dermatome is served by one spinal and dorsal root. When the skin is stimulated by a noxious stimulus, the nerve serving that dermatome is activated. The signal is transmitted to one specific area of the sensory cortex serving the dermatome. As a result, the stimulus is perceived to occur within the dermatome.

The boundaries of dermatomes may appear to be distinct in anatomic drawings, but nerve distribution actually overlaps. Excitation of one nerve may produce pain that is perceived to originate from adjacent dermatomes.

Deep Somatic Pain

Somatic structures are the structures of the body wall, such as muscle and bone. Deep somatic pain is poorly localized, may produce nausea, and may be associated with sweating and blood pressure changes. Deep somatic pain is generally diffuse and less localized than cutaneous pain. Pain from deep structures frequently radiates from the primary site (e.g., pain from a lumbar disc is felt along the sciatic nerve).

Somatic structures vary in their sensitivity to pain. Highly sensitive structures include tendons, deep fascia, ligaments, joints, bone, periosteum, blood vessels, and nerves. Skeletal muscle is sensitive only to stretching and ischemia. Bone and cartilage respond to extreme pressure and chemical stimulation (e.g., rheumatoid arthritis, osteomyelitis).

Visceral Pain

Visceral pain refers to pain coming from body organs. It tends to be a diffuse, poorly localized, vague and dull pain. Nerve fibers innervating the body organs follow the sympathetic nerves to the spinal cord. This may be the reason why autonomic manifestations, (e.g., diarrhea, cramps, sweating, hypertension) frequently accompany visceral pain. Visceral pain typically includes acute appendicitis, cholecystitis, and inflammation of the biliary and pancreatic tracts, gastroduodenal disease, cardiovascular disease, pleurisy, and renal and ureteral colic. It is manifested by sweating, restlessness, nausea, emesis, pallor and agitation.

Referred Pain

It is a pain that is felt in an area distant from the site of the stimulus. It occurs when nerve fibers serving an area of the body distant from the site of the stimulus pass in close proximity to the stimulus. It may be intense. For example, myocardial ischemia is not felt as pain in the heart as most often as pain in left arm, shoulder, or jaw pain. Pain arising from a deep structure, has a referred segmental distribution, or a pattern of pain, determined according to the spinal cord segment supplying to the structure. Examples of common patterns are pleural pain from the diaphragm referred to the shoulder and that of the cholecystitis referred to the back of the scapula.

Neuropathic Pain

It is caused by damage or injury to nerve fibers in the periphery or by damage to the central nervous system (CNS). Noxious electrical impulses are generated at the site of the injury. The pain is felt as numbness, burning, stabbing, like "needles" and electric shock. Client's may experience allodynia, "pain due to a stimulus that does not normally provoke pain". The pain is perceived to occur in the area served by the nerve. For example, an injury to a nerve that serves the hand would be perceived as pain in the hand even though the injury would be at the spinal cord level. As there is no pathophysiologic change at the site, the person may not be believed. It responds poorly to pain medications like nonsteroidal anti-inflammatory drugs (NSAIDs).

Phantom Pain

Phantom pain is pain from a part of the body that has been lost or from which the brain no longer receives physical signals. It is a type of neuropathic pain. Phantom limb pain is a common experience of amputees. Some amputees experience continuous pain that varies in intensity or quality; others experience several bouts a day, or it may occur only once every week or two. It is often described as shooting, crushing, burning or cramping. If the pain is continuous for a long period, parts of the intact body may become sensitized, so that touching them evokes pain in the phantom limb, or phantom limb pain may accompany urination or defection. Phantom body pain is initially described as burning or tingling but may evolve into severe crushing or pinching pain, fire running down the legs, or a knife twisting in the flesh. Onset may be immediate or may not occur until years after the disabling injury.

Psychogenic Pain

Psychogenic pain, also called psychalgia or somatoform pain is caused, increased, or prolonged by mental, emotional, or behavioral factors. Headache, back pain, and stomach pain are sometimes diagnosed as psychogenic. Sufferers are often stigmatized, because both medical professionals and the general public tend to think that pain from a psychological source is not "real". However, specialists consider that it is no less actual or hurtful than pain from any other source.

PATHOPHYSIOLOGY

In the past, it was thought that a sensory input, such as a pinprick, would cause a pain "signal" to be sent directly to the brain via a single nerve. Although still not completely understood till date, the science of pain reveals a much more complex process, and theories are still continuing to evolve. New receptors, pathways, and hypotheses are being investigated every day. In addition to identifying new pathways, genetic variations have been discovered at the receptor level that can further complicate treatment. It is important to have a basic knowledge of the physiology to treat pain effectively. The physiology of pain has been shown in (Fig. 1).

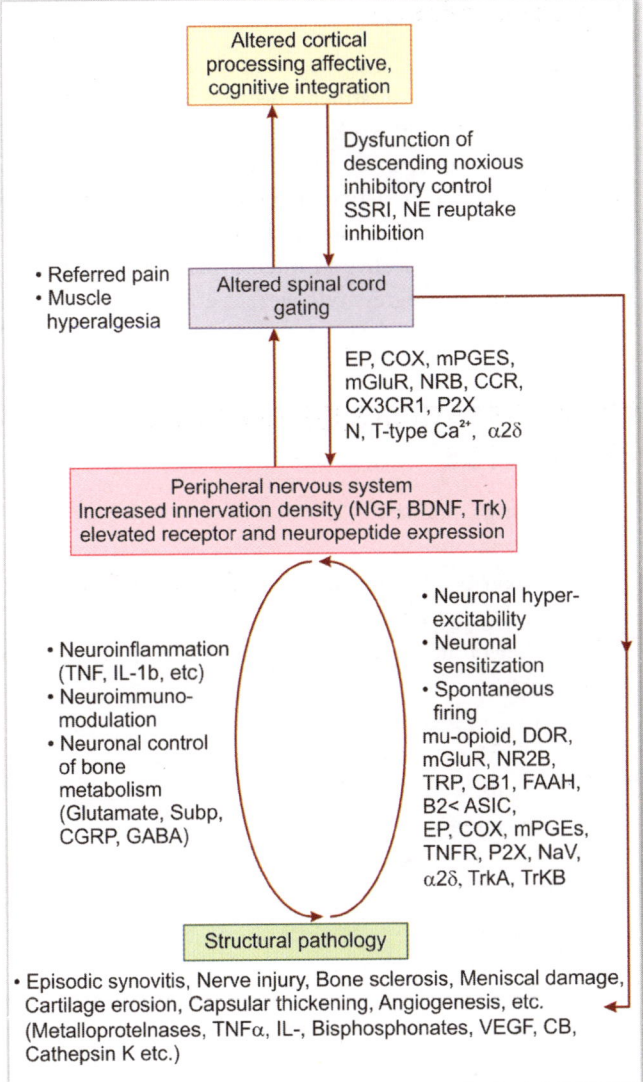

Fig. 1: Physiology of pain

Abbreviations: GABA, gamma aminobutyric acid; IL, interleukin; NGF, nerve growth factor; SSRI, selective serotonin reuptake inhibitor necrosis factor; TNF, tumor calcitruim gene-related peptide; Trk, tyrosine kinase receptor; VEGGF, vascular endothelial growth factor.

The following is a brief review of the four basic concepts that are important to begin to understand the physiology of pain. The concepts are transduction, transmission, modulation, and perception.

1. **Transduction is the process by which afferent nerve endings participate *in translating noxious stimuli* (e.g., a pinprick) into nociceptive impulses.**

   Noxious stimulation is first carried by the faster A-delta fibers, and then by the slower C fibers. "Silent nociceptors," also involved in transduction, are afferent nerves that do not respond to external stimulation unless inflammatory mediators are present. The peripheral nervous system contains primary sensory afferent neurons that have an important role in pain signaling. The axons of these afferent diverge from the cell body in the dorsal root ganglion near the spinal cord and send a short fiber centrally into the cord and a long fiber down the peripheral nerve into the tissues. Their receptors detect mechanical, thermal, proprioceptive, and chemical stimuli.

2. **Transmission is the process by which impulses are sent to the dorsal horn of the spinal cord, and then along the sensory tracts to the brain.**

   The primary afferent neurons are active senders and receive chemical and electrical signals. Their axons terminate in the dorsal horn of the spinal cord, where they have connections with many spinal neurons. In turn, spinal neurons have input from many primary afferents. These spinal neurons project axons to the contralateral thalamus, which in turn projects to the somatosensory pathway, frontal cortex, and other areas. The somatosensory cortex is thought to be involved in the sensory aspects of pain, such as the intensity and quality of pain, whereas the frontal cortex and limbic system are thought to be involved with the emotional responses to it.

3. **Modulation is the process of *dampening or amplifying* these pain-related neural signals. Modulation takes place primarily in the dorsal horn of the spinal cord, but also elsewhere, with input from ascending and descending pathways.**

   The gate control theory is a popular model of pain modulation proposed by Melzack and Wall in 1965, later revised by Melzack and Casey in 1968. These investigators proposed the existence of an endogenous ability to reduce or increase the degree of perceived pain through modulation of incoming impulses at a gate located in the dorsal horn of the spinal cord. The gate acts on signals from the ascending and descending systems and weighs all the inputs. The integration of these inputs from sensory neurons, the segmental spinal cord level, and the brain determines whether the gate will be opened or closed by either increasing or decreasing the intensity of the ascending pain signal. The role of psychological variables in the perception of pain, including motivation to escape pain and the role of thoughts, emotions, and stress reactions in increasing or decreasing painful sensations, is evident in the gate control theory. An example is when patients report more pain at night, when they are isolated and less distracted from their pain than they might be during the day. The proposed gate can be opened or closed by pharmacologic manipulation, transduction, transmission and modulation, and psychological intervention.

4. **Perception refers to the subjective experience of pain that results from the interaction of transduction, transmission modulation, and the psychological aspects of the individual.**

As research continues furthering the understanding of this complex process, there is hope that pain treatments can be developed to target specific parts of the physiologic pathway and become more effective than current treatments.

FACTORS AFFECTING PAIN

Past Experience

It is tempting to expect that a person who has had multiple or prolonged experiences with pain would be less anxious and more tolerant of pain than one who has had little pain. However, this is not true. Often the more experience a person has had with pain, the more frightened he/she is and wants relief from pain as soon as possible. This person may be less able to tolerate pain, that is, he/she wants quicker relief from pain before it gets more severe.

Anxiety and Depression

It is commonly believed that depression and anxiety increase pain. Anxiety that is unrelated to pain may actually decrease the pain. The routine of anti-anxiety drugs may prevent the person from reporting pain because of sedation and may impair the patient's ability to take deep breaths, get out of bed and cooperate with the treatment plan.

Culture

Cultural factors also influence the response to pain. These beliefs vary from one culture to another; therefore people from different cultures who experience the same intensity of pain may not report it in the same ways. Cultural factors must be taken into account while managing pain.

Age

If pain perception is diminished in the elderly, then it is due to disease process and not ageing. Although many elderly people seek medical care for pain, some are reluctant because they take pain to be a normal process in ageing. Response to pain is also different in old age and young people. Some elderly people are reluctant to go for medical care when in pain for fear of being diagnosed with a serious illness.

Gender

Various studies are done. Women reported higher pain intensity, pain unpleasantness, frustration and fear as compared to men. There are also some studies where no difference has been reported in pain perception, on gender basis. There was however, a difference in anxiety and gender, with men being more anxious about their pain.

PLACEBO EFFECT

The placebo effect occurs when a person responds to the medication or other treatment because of an expectation that the treatment will work rather than it actually does so. The placebo effect is more pronounced in people who are prone to anxiety, so anxiety reduction may account for some of the effect, but it does not account for all of the effect. Placebos are more effective in intense pain than mild pain; and they produce progressively weaker effects with repeated administration.

CONSIDERATIONS OF THE PAIN EXPERIENCE

- **Physiologic factors:**
  - Organic origin
  - Integrity of the nervous system including all endogenous opioids.
  - Concomitant physical influences (stress, fatigue)
  - Age
  - Type of pain
  - Location
  - Intensity
  - Duration
  - Frequency
  - Quality
  - Threshold
  - Tolerance
  - Genetics
- **Affective factors:**
  - Distress of pain
  - Depression
  - Mood
  - Anxiety, fear, worry
- **Psychosocial influences:**
  - Family and occupational roles
  - Personal beliefs
  - Spiritual belief system
  - Cultural/social influences
  - Sexual identity and stereotypes
  - Demographic factors
- **Cognitive factor:**
  - Past experience
  - Meaning of pain experience
  - Attention paid to sensation/distraction
  - Expectations
  - Coping mechanisms
  - Knowledge
  - Values/attitudes
  - Communication skills

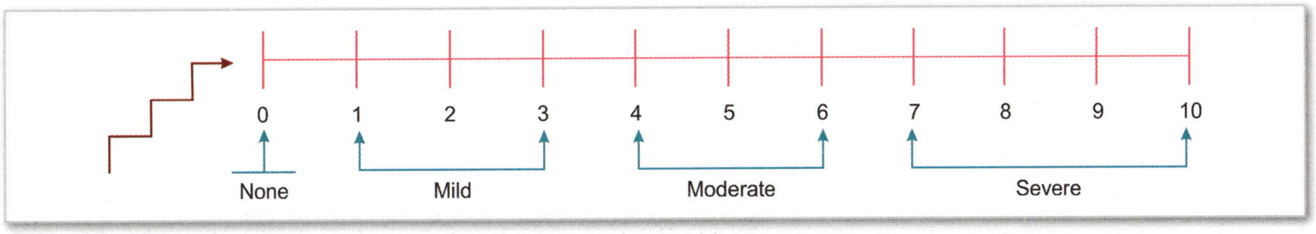

Fig. 2:   Numerical pain rating scale

PAIN ASSESSMENT TOOLS

Numerical Pain Rating Scale (Fig. 2)

Perhaps one of the most commonly used pain scales in healthcare, the numerical rating scale offers the individual in pain to rate their pain score. It is designed to be used by those over the age of 9. In the numerical scale, the user has the option to verbally rate their scale from 0 to 10 or to place a mark on a line indicating their level of pain. 0 indicates the absence of pain, while 10 represents the most intense pain possible.

The numerical rating pain scale allows the healthcare provider to rate pain as mild, moderate or severe, which can indicate a potential disability level.

Wong-Baker Faces Pain Scale (Fig. 3)

The Wong-Baker Faces Pain Scale combines pictures and numbers to allow pain to be rated by the user. It can be used in children over the age of 3, and in adults. The faces range from a smiling face to a sad and crying face. A numerical rating is assigned to each face.

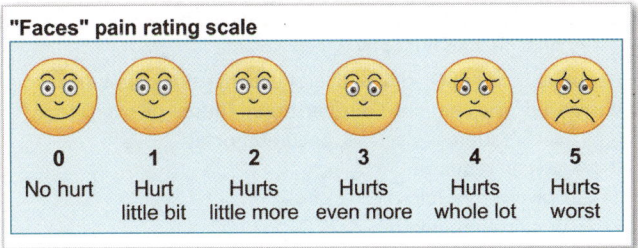

Fig. 3: Wong-Baker FACES pain rating scale

FLACC Scale

FLACC stands for face, legs, activity, crying and consolability. It is an observed rated pain scale, performed by a healthcare practitioner such as a doctor or a nurse. The FLACC pain scale was designed for children between the ages of 2 and 7. However, some practitioners in adult setting may use the FLACC pain scale for people, who are unable to communicate their pain. FLACC provides a pain assessment scale between 0 and 10.

DATE/TIME						
Face 0–No particular expression or smile 1–Occasional grimace or frown, withdrawn, disinterested 2–Frequent to constant quivering chin, clenched jaw						
Legs 0–Normal position or relaxed 1–Uneasy, restless tense 2–Kicking or legs drawn up						
Activity 0–Lying quietly normal position, moves easily 1–Squirming, shifting back and forth, tense 2–Arched, rigid or jerking						
Cry 0–No cry (awake or asleep) 1–Moans or whimpers; occasional complaint 2–Crying steadily, screams or sobs, frequent complaints						
Consolability 0–Content, relaxed 1–Reassured by occasional touching, hugging or being talked to, distractible 2–Difficult to console or comfort						
TOTAL SCORE						

CRIES Pain Scale

The CRIES pain scale is often used in the neonatal healthcare setting. CRIES is an observer-rated pain assessment tool, which is performed by a healthcare practitioner such as a nurse or physician. CRIES assesses crying, oxygenation, vital signs, facial expression and sleeplessness. The CRIES pain scale is generally used for infants that are 6 months old and younger.

DATE/TIME						
Crying– Characteristic cry of pain is high pitched. 0–No cry or cry that is not high-pitched 1–Cry high pitched but baby is easily consolable 2–Cry high pitched but baby is inconsolable						
Requires O₂ for SaO₂ <95%– Babies experiencing pain manifest decreased oxygenation. Consider other causes of hypoxemia, e.g., oversedation, atelectasis, pneumothorax) 0–No oxygen required 1–<30% oxygen required 2–>30% oxygen required						
Increased vital signs (BP* and HR*)—Take BP last as this may awaken child and will make other assessments difficult 0–Both HR and BP unchanged or less than baseline 1–HR or BP increased but increase in <20% of baseline 2–HR or BP is increased >20% over baseline.						
Expression—The facial expression most is often associated with pain is a grimace. A grimace may be characterized by brow lowering, eyes squeezed shut, deepening nasolabial furrow, or open lips and mouth. 0–No grimace present 1–Grimace alone is present 2–Grimace and non-cry vocalization grunt is present						
Sleepless—Scored based upon the infant's state during the hour preceding this recorded score. 0–Child has been continuously asleep 1–Child has awakened at frequent intervals 2–Child has been awake constantly						
TOTAL SCORE						

Purpose of Pain Scales

Most scales make pain measurable, and can tell providers whether your pain is mild, moderate or severe. They can also set baselines and trends for your pain, making it easier to find appropriate treatments. If your pain rating decreases after you take a certain medication, for example, then clearly that medication worked for you. If there was no change, or if the number increased, then your doctor knows, it is time to try something else.

This is also true in the case of a verbal rating scale. Even though there is no numerical rating, doctors can look for a change in the intensity of pain words. You may initially describe your pain using more words from a high-intensity group. A treatment could be considered effective if you choose more moderate pain descriptors afterward.

PAIN MANAGEMENT

Role of Nurse in Pain Management

- **Identifying goals for pain management:** The information obtained rom the patient can help in identifying the goals for management. The goals are shared with the patient. For some patients, elimination of the pain might be the goal, whereas for some others this may seem unrealistic. Another goal can be to reduce the intensity of pain. The goal for the patient may be accompanied by pharmacological or non-pharmacological means.
- **Establishing nurse-patient relationship and teaching:** A positive nurse patient relationship and teaching are keys to manage analgesia in the patient with pain,

because open communication and patient cooperation are essential to the success of pain management. The nurse also provides information by explaining how pain can be controlled.

- **Providing physical care:** The patient in pain may be unable to participate in the usual activities of the daily routine or usual self care and may need assistance to carry out these activities. The patient is usually more comfortable when the physical and self-care needs have been met and efforts have been made to ensure as comfortable a position as possible.

- **Managing anxiety related to pain:** Anxiety may affect a patient's response to pain. The patient who anticipates pain may become very anxious. Teaching the patient about the nature of the impending painful experience and the ways to reduce it often decreases anxiety. Learning about the measures to reduce pain may lessen the threat of pain and give the person a sense of control.

Pain Management Strategies

Acute pain is usually managed with medications such as analgesics and anesthetics. Management of chronic pain, however, is much more difficult and may require the coordinated efforts of a pain management team, which typically includes medical practitioners, clinical psychologists, physiotherapists, occupational therapists, and nurse practitioners.

Inadequate treatment of pain is widespread throughout surgical wards, intensive care units, accident and emergency departments, in general practice, in the management of all forms of chronic pain including cancer pain, and in end of life care. This neglect is extended to all ages, from neonates to the frail elderly.

Pharmacological Intervention

Drug name	Dose and route	Action	Special considerations
Paracetamol	500 mg oral bid/tid. 60, 125, 250 mg suppositories, 500 and 1000 mg IV vials	Analgesic and antipyretic. Exact action not known	Fatty liver is possible when overdose occurs
NSAIDs (ibuprofen, naproxen, indomethacin, piroxicam, diclofenac)	200–400 mg qid oral	Inhibit the enzyme cyclooxygenase, which aids in the production of prostaglandins. Analgesic, antipyretic, anti- inflammatory, anti-platelet	Can cause renal impairment, and gastric ulceration, and increased wheeze in asthmatic patients
Strong opioid (morphine, diamorphine/heroin, hydromorphone, oxycodone, fentanyl, pethidine)	Morphine–10 mg every 4 hours. Diamorphine, oxycodone–5 mg. Hydromorphone–1.3 mg. Fentanyl–1000 mcg. Pethidine–100 mg	Strong analgesic action for visceral pain, musculoskeletal pain, nerve pain, sympathetic pain	Kidney and liver failure. Habit forming. Withdrawal should not be sudden otherwise it may produce withdrawal symptoms like restlessness, muscle spasm, backache and head ache
Weak opioid (codeine, tramadol)	Codeine–30–60 mg od, tramadol–50–100 mg every 4 hours.	Used for musculoskeletal and visceral pain. Inhibits dorsal horn of the spinal cord.	Slow withdrawal should be done. Tramadol when used with other drugs such as anti-depressants can cause reactions.
Muscle relaxants (diazepam, baclofen)	Diazepam–2–5 mg bid or tid. Baclofen–3–80 mg tid.	Used to treat muscle spasm by stimulating GABA receptors in the brain.	Can cause sleep and the patient will get up feeling unfresh. Sleep disorder will persist for up to 6 weeks after withdrawal of the drug.
Antidepressants (amytripitiline)	10–25 mg at night.	It is an unauthorized analgesic used for nerve pain	Can produce cardiac rhythm disturbances so be careful in patients with cardiac diseases
Anticonvulsants (gabapentin, pregabalin, carbamazepine, phenytoin, sodium valproate)	Gabapentin–1800 mg/day Pregabalin–150 mg/day. Carbamazepine–200 mg tid Phenytoin–100 mg bid Sodium valproate–200 mg od	Nerve calcium channel blockers; used to treat nerve pain	May cause alterations in liver enzymes hence hepatic monitoring has to be done

Contd...

Drug name	Dose and route	Action	Special considerations
Antiarrhythmics (lignocaine)	300 mg over 30 minutes	Local anesthetic which blocks sodium channels in the nerves	Must be used under full vital sign monitoring because it may cause cardiac fluctuations
Topical agents (capsaicin, lignocaine 5% medicated plaster)	Apply the cream to the affected area four times daily	Used to treat post-herpetic neuralgia after shingles. The cream is absorbed through the skin to reduce substance P (a neuro- transmitter), which is associated with inflammatory processes	Use only a small amount of cream to avoid redness and heat. Wash hands after applying the cream
Intrathecal drugs (midazolam, ziconotide)	Directly injected into the spinal fluid via an external infusion pump. 2–20 µg/24 hrs	Intrathecal route is preferred for rapid action and pain relief by sedation. Ziconotide is a toxin derived from the marine snail conus magus, which blocks the calcium channels of the nerves	Carries risk of infection and injury because of direct access to the spinal cord

Abbreviation: NSAIDs, nonsteroidal anti-inflammatory drugs

Non-pharmacological Management

Cutaneous Stimulation and Massage

Massage which is generalized cutaneous stimulation of he body specially concentrates on the back and shoulders. Massage improves blood circulation to the muscles and relaxes the muscles spasms.

Ice and Heat Therapies

For greatest effect, ice should be placed on the site of injury immediately after the injury. Ice therapy after joint surgery can significantly reduce the amount of analgesic medications required after surgery. Assess the skin prior to application of ice. It should not be applied for more than 20 minutes, otherwise the rebound phenomena will occur as the body will heat up. Long term application of heat or cold therapy may result in nerve or skin injury.

Application of heat increases blood flow to an area and contributes to pain by speedy healing. Both dry and moist heat applications may provide analgesia.

Infrared heat therapy penetrates deep into soft tissue, making it an ideal source of arthritis pain relief. Athletes and the elderly will benefit from an effective means of loosening sore muscles and stiff joints without the use of ointments or creams that can burn and have an unpleasant odor. Those who suffer from rheumatoid arthritis, amyotrophic lateral sclerosis, and Parkinson's disease can enjoy an easy to use form of pain relief. In addition to making you perspire and removing toxins from your body, infrared heat therapy serves as a means of weight loss and cellulite reduction for those who cannot exercise due to health concerns or mobility issues.

Transcutaneous Electrical Nerve Stimulation (TENS)

It uses a battery-operated unit with electrodes applied to the skin to produce a tingling, vibrating or buzzing sensation to the area of pain. It has been used in both acute and chronic pain. When TENS is used in a postoperative patient, the electrodes are applied around the surgical wound. It is thought to decrease pain by stimulating the non-pain receptors in the same areas as the fibers that transmit the pain.

Distraction

Distraction means turning your attention to something other than the pain. Many people use this method without realizing the pain when they watch television or listen to the radio to "take their minds off" the pain. Distraction may work better than medicine if pain is sudden and intense or if it is brief, lasting only 5–45 minutes. Distraction is useful when you are waiting for pain medicine to start working. If pain is mild, you may be able to distract yourself for hours. Some people think that a person who can be distracted from pain does not have severe pain. This is not necessarily true. Distraction can be a powerful way to temporarily relieve even the most intense pain.

Relaxation Techniques

Relaxation relieves pain or keeps it from getting worse by reducing tension in the muscles. It can help you fall asleep, give you more energy, make you less tired, reduce your anxiety, and make other pain relief methods work better. Some people, for instance, find that taking a pain medicine or using a cold or hot pack works faster and better when they relax at the same time. Relaxation may be done sitting up or lying down. Choose a quiet place wherever possible. Close your eyes. Do not cross your arms and legs because that may cut off circulation and cause numbness or tingling. If you are lying down, be sure you are comfortable. Put a small pillow under your neck and under your knees or use a low stool to support your lower legs.

Ask your doctor or nurse to recommend commercially available relaxation CDs. These CD recordings provide step-by-step instructions in relaxation techniques.

- Temporarily increase number of immune system cells to keep the rest of your body health
- Help reduce feelings of depression
- Increase feeling of well-being.

Guided imagery can be practiced at home with a book or audio recording or with a trained therapist. Guided imagery can be done in group or one-to-one sessions and can last an average of 20–30 minutes. In a typical guided imagery session:

- The therapist will use one of a variety of guided imagery techniques that will lead you through imagined experiences in your mind.
- Usually, the therapist will guide your imagination to places or situation that will make you fell peaceful, safe, relaxed and secure.
- The therapist may use gentle background music to create a relaxed atmosphere and help you avoid distractions.
- You'll be asked to imagine something, such as a warm healing light on the area where the cancer was or images of your immune system attacking cancer cells. One popular exercise involves picturing tiny Pac-Man characters chasing and eating cancer cells.
- The therapist will describe sounds, smells, tastes, or other sensations that might accompany what you're imagining.
- While you focus on the imagined situation, you might start to experience sensation and feelings, such as warmth, lightness, contentment, or strength.

Hypnosis

Hypnotherapy is a term to describe the use of hypnosis in a therapeutic context. Many hypnotherapists refer to their practice as "clinical work". Hypnotherapy can either be used as an addition to the work of licensed physicians or psychologists, or it can be used in a stand-alone environment where the hypnotherapist in question usually owns his or her own business. There is no evidence that 'incurable' diseases are curable with hypnosis (such as cancer, diabetes, and arthritis), but pain and other body functions related to the diseases are controllable.

Physical Therapy

Physical therapy (PT) can be an important part of the treatment strategy. PT techniques are useful in teaching patients to control pain, to move in safe and structurally correct ways, to improve range of motion, and to increase flexibility, strength and endurance. "Active" and "Passive" modalities can both be used, but active modalities, such as therapeutic exercise, are particularly important when the goal is to improve both comfort and function.

Cognitive-behavioral Therapy

Cognitive-behavioral therapy (CBT) has proven to be effective in reducing pain and disability when it is used as part of a therapeutic strategy for chronic pain. CBT addresses the psychological component of pain, including attitudes and feelings, coping skills and a sense of control over one's condition. It can provide educational information and diffuse feeling of fear and helplessness. CBT may include training in various types of relaxation approaches, which can help people in chronic pain, lower their overall level of arousal, decrease muscle tension, control distress, and decrease pain, depression and disability. CBT has been found to be effective as part of a treatment regimen for a variety of pain conditions including episodic migraine and chronic daily headache, chronic musculoskeletal pain, pain in the healthy elderly, chronic cancer pain, rheumatoid arthritis and osteoarthritis, fibromyalgia, myofascial temoromandibular disorders, chronic low back pain, carpal tunnel syndrome pain, and chronic pelvic pain.

Acupuncture

When needles are inserted into acupuncture points, regional increase in blood flow occurs (measured by skin temperature recordings, laser Doppler flow values and electromagnetic impulses). The nerve stimulation sends messages to the spinal cord, brain stem and hypothalamus. These stimulate the release of endogenous opioids such s beta-endorphins, metencephalin, and dynorphin. In addition, acupuncture affects the release of neurotransmitters and neuropeptides such as serotonin and melatonin. These may explain the relaxing effects seen after acupuncture.

Foot Reflexology

Reflexology is an alternative medicine healing system in which specific points on the feet or hands known as reflex points, are manipulated to bring about changes in other parts of the body. These reflex points are believed to correspond to every major organ, gland, and area of the body. By stimulating reflex points on the feet or hands, reflexology is thought to restore the energy flow and one's own natural ability to heal.

Reflexology is viewed primarily as a general healing therapy that helps the body regain natural balance, harmony and health. It claims to stimulate circulation and is considered useful for pain, migraine, sinusitis, and constipation. During a reflexology session, the therapist uses the fingers, thumbs, and palms to stroke or lightly press the reflex points on each foot. Reflexology sessions generally last about 50 minutes.

Neurologic and Neurosurgical Management of Pain Relief

Stimulation Procedures

It uses a battery-operated unit with electrodes applied to the skin to produce a tingling, vibrating or buzzing sensation to the area of pain. It has been used in both acute and chronic pain. When transcutaneous electrical nerve stimulation (TENS) is used in a postoperative patient, the electrodes are applied around the surgical wound. It is thought to decrease pain by stimulating the non-pain receptors in the same areas as the fibers that transmit the pain.

Cordotomy

It is the division of certain tracts of the spinal tract of the spinal cord. It may be performed percutaneously, by the open method after laminectomy, or by other techniques. It is performed to interrupt the transmission of pain. Care must be taken to destroy only the sensation of pain, leaving motor functions intact.

Rhizotomy

Sensory nerve roots are destroyed where they enter the spinal cord. A lesion is made in the dorsal root to destroy neuronal dysfunction and reduce nociceptive input.

NURSING MANAGEMENT OF PAIN

Nursing Assessment

- **History:**
  - Age
  - State of consciousness

- Medications currently being taken/medication for allergies
- Physical state (fatigue, disability, lack of sleep and prolonged suffering reduce a client's ability to tolerate pain)
- Pain apprehension (generalized desire to avoid pain)
- Pain anxiety (because of its associated mystery, loneliness, helplessness, threat)
- Effects on activities and quality of life
- Methods of pain relief: What do you do to relieve the pain? What has not worked to relieve the pain?

- **Physical examination**
  Sympathetic responses:
  - Pallor
  - Increased blood pressure
  - Increased pulse
  - Increased respiration
  - Skeletal muscle tension
  - Dilated pupils
  - Diaphoresis

  Parasympathetic responses:
  - Decreased blood pressure
  - Decreased pulse
  - Nausea, vomiting
  - Weakness
  - Pallor
  - Loss of consciousness

- **Behavioural characteristics:**
  - Assumes a posture that minimizes pain (lying rigidly, guarding, drawing up the legs, or assuming the fetal position)
  - Moans, sighs, grimaces, clenches the jaws or fist, becomes quiet or withdraws from others.
  - Blinks rapidly
  - Crying, appears frightended, exhibits restlessness
  - Has a drawn facial expression
  - Has twitching muscles
  - Withdraws when touched
- Holds or protects affected area or remains motionless.

NURSING DIAGNOSIS

Goal: Relief of pain or decrease in the intensity of pain.

Interventions	Rationale	Outcomes
Reassure the patient that you know that the pain is real and will assist him/her in dealing with it	Fear that pain will not be accepted as it increases tension	Reports relief that pain is accepted as real and that he/she will receive assistance in pain relief
Use pain assessment scale to identify intensity of pain.	Provides baseline for assessing changes in pain level and evaluating interventions	◆ Reports lower intensity of pain and discomfort after interventions implemented ◆ Reports less disruption from pain and discomfort after use of intervention

Contd...

Interventions	Rationale	Outcomes
Assess and record pain and its characteristics: location, quality, frequency and duration.	Data assists in evaluating pain and pain relief and identifying multiple sources and types of pain	Uses pain medication as prescribed
Administer balanced analgesics as prescribed.	Administer early in pain cycle for more effectiveness	Identifies effective pain-relief strategies
Re-administer pain assessment scale.	Permits assessment of effectiveness of analgesia and identifies need for further action, if required	Demonstrates use of new strategies to relieve pain and reports their effectiveness
Document severity of patient's pain on chart.	Assists in demonstrating need for additional analgesics or alternative approach to pain relief	◆ Experiences minimal side effects of analgesia without interruption to treat side effects ◆ Increases interactions with family and friends
Obtain additional prescription as needed.	Inadequate pain relief results an increased stress response, suffering and prolonged hospitalization	
Identify and encourage patient to use strategies that have been successful with previous pain.	Encourages use of pain relief strategies familiar to and accepted by the patient	
Teach patient additional strategies to relieve pain and discomfort: distraction, relaxation etc.	Use of these strategies along with analgesia may produce more effective pain relief	
Instruct patient and family about potential side effects of analgesics and their prevention and management.	Anticipating and preventing side effects enable the patient to continue analgesia without interruption because of side effects	

CONCLUSION

Pain is a feeling triggered in the nervous system. Pain may be sharp or dull. It may come and go, or it may be constant. One may feel pain in one area of your body, such as the back, abdomen or chest or it may be felt all over, such as when the muscles ache from the flu.

Pain can be helpful in diagnosing a problem. Without pain, one might seriously hurt himself/herself without knowing it, or one might not realize that he/she has a medical problem that needs treatment. Once it is taken care , pain usually goes away. However, sometimes pain goes on for weeks, months or even years. This is called chronic pain. Sometimes chronic pain is due to an ongoing cause, such as cancer or arthritis. Sometimes the cause is unknown.

Fortunately, there are many ways to treat pain. Treatment varies depending on the cause of pain. Pain relievers, acupuncture and sometimes surgery are helpful.

BIBLIOGRAPHY

1. *Brunner, Sholtis L, Suddarth, et al. Brunner & Suddarth's Textbook of Medical-Surgical Nursing, 10th edition. Philadelphia: Lippincott Williams & Wilkins; 2004. pp. 217-46.*

2. *Black JM, Hawks JH. Medical Surgical Nursing: Clinical Management for Positive Outcome, 7th edition. Mosby's; St Louise, Missouri; pp. 440-48.*

3. *Sharma S. Potter and Perry's Fundamentals of Nursing. A South Asian edition. Gurugram: Elsevier India. 2013.*

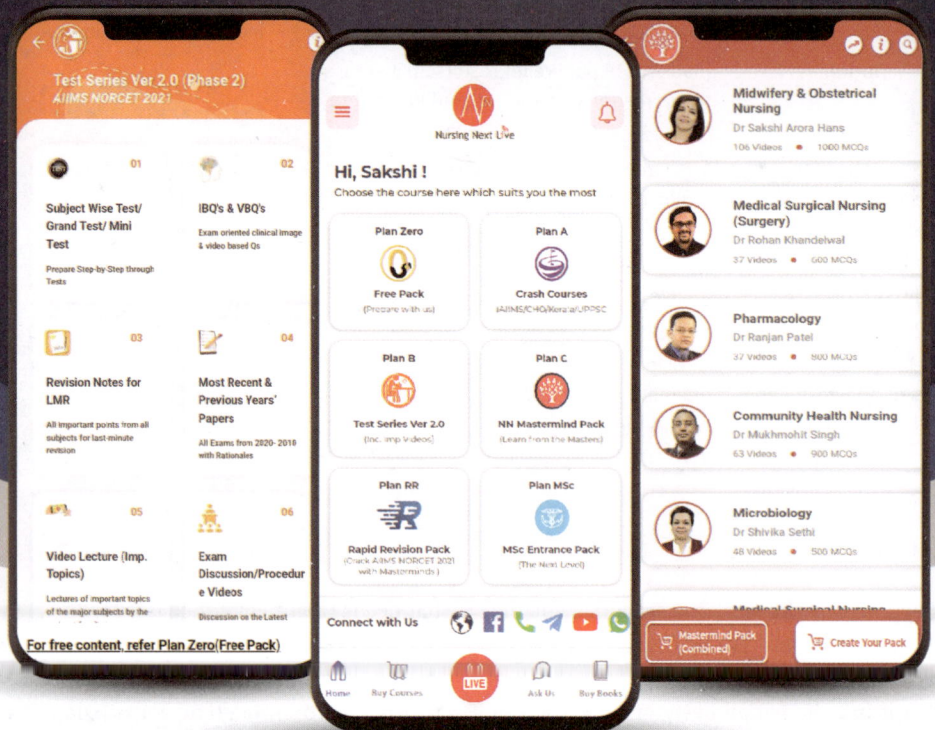 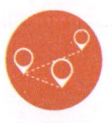

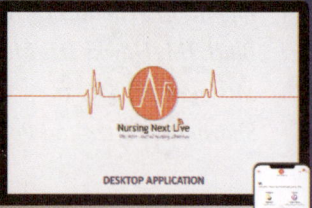
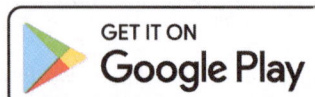

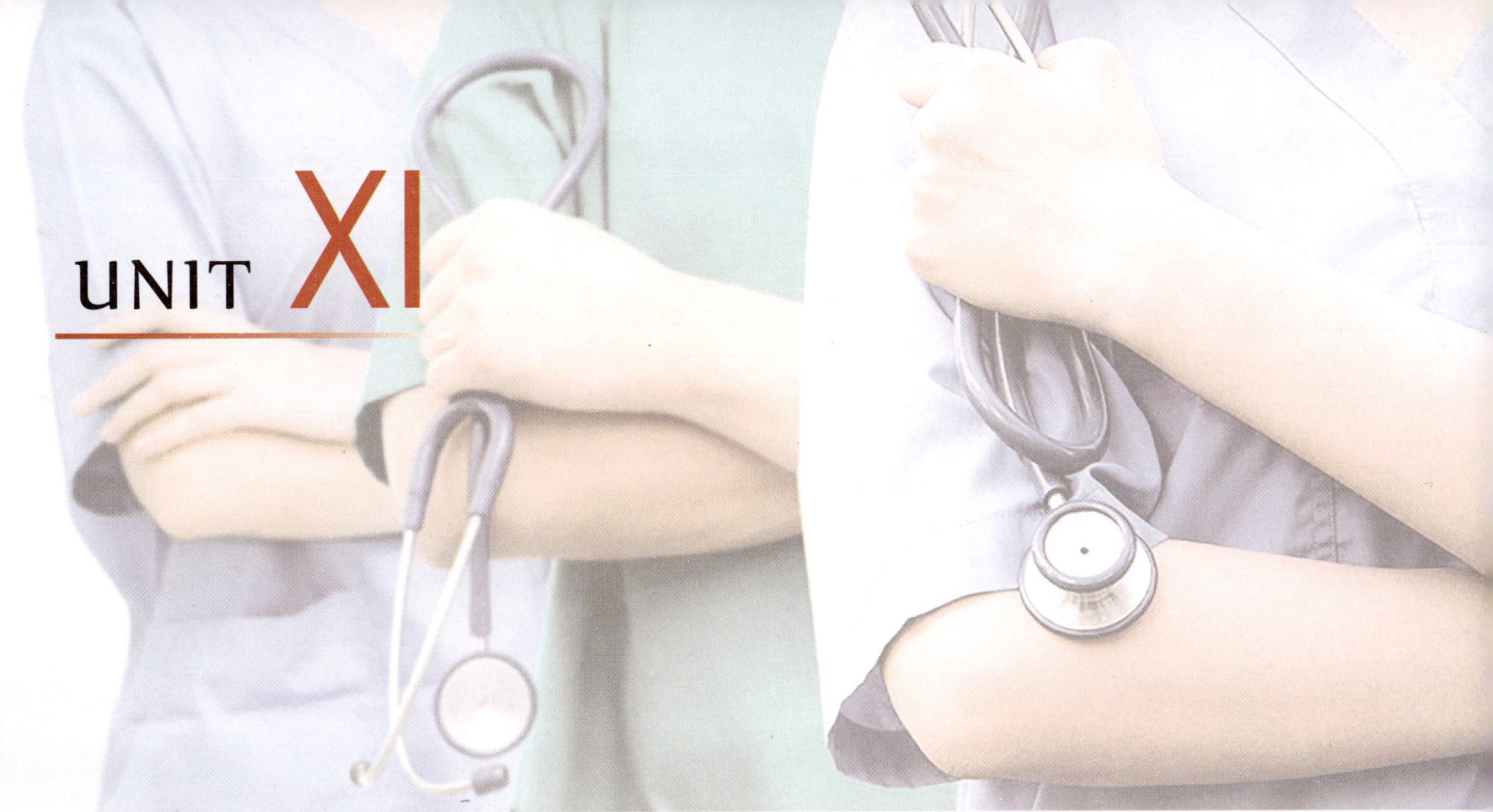

UNIT XI

THERAPEUTIC USE OF HEAT AND COLD APPLICATIONS

Unit Outline

Hot Application

INTRODUCTION

Hot application is the application of hot agent, warmer than skin either in a moist or dry form on the surface of the body. Application of heat is commonly used in the hospital and home as therapeutic measure. Hot application also serves as comfort measure. The nurse, therefore, needs knowledge of the physiological reactions resulting from this measure and also to any untoward reaction, which may occur.

RELATED ANATOMY OF THE SKIN

Skin is one of the sensory and excretory organs. It has important functions like protection, secretion, excretion, temperature regulation and sensation. Skin consists of three layers: epidermis, dermis and subcutaneous layer.

The epidermis is the outer layer and is composed of several layers of cells undergoing different stages of maturation. The innermost layer of epidermis generates new cells that migrate slowly toward the epidermal surface, that is stratum corneum. The epidermis also contains melanocytes which produce melanin, or dark pigment of the skin.

The dermis is the thicker layer containing collagen and elastic fibers to support the epidermis. It contains the nerve fibers, blood vessels, sweat glands, sebaceous glands and hair follicles. Sebum from sebaceous glands lubricate the skin and hair. There are two types of sweat glands: Eccrine glands (present throughout the skin, but more in forehead, palms and soles) and apocrine glands (found in axillary and genital area). The subcutaneous tissue contains blood vessels, lymph and loose connective tissue filled with fat. The fatty tissue serves as a heat insulator.

Appendages

Hairs nails and sebaceous glands are the appendages of skin.

EFFECTS OF HEAT APPLICATION

Local Effect of Heat

- Vasodilatation and increase of blood flow to the affected area.
- Increases inflammation bringing oxygen, nutrients, antibodies, and leukocytes.
- Promotes soft tissue healing and reduces tissue swelling. When applied, blood vessels dilate, causing increased blood flow, increasing oxygen and nutrition to area and removing excess fluid from tissues.
- Decreases joint stiffness, relieves pain and relaxes muscles.
- Sedative effect.

Systemic Effects of Heat

The effect of heat application depends on a number of factors (Fig. 1).

Heat and cold are relative degrees of temperature dependent, to some extent, on the perception of the individual. The temperature at the surface of the skin of the torso is generally 33.9°C (93°F). Local tolerance is thought to range between 41.4°C (105°F) and 43.3°C (110°F). Hot applications that are 11.1°C (20°F) below or 8.3°C (15°F) above this level excite cutaneous nerve fibers.

Purposes

- To promote circulation
- To relieve congestion, reduce edema or inflammation
- To increase suppuration

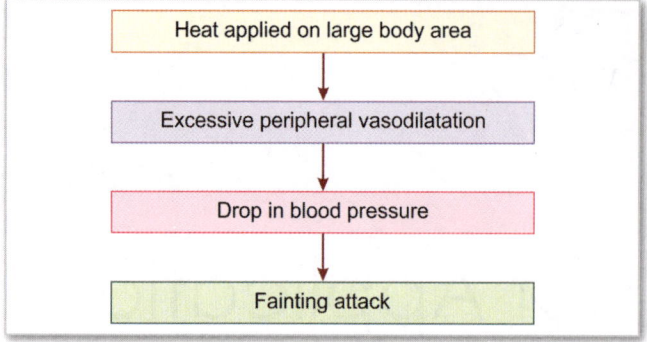

Fig. 1: Systemic effects of heat application

- To promote tissue relaxation
- To relieve pain
- To soften exudates
- To provide warmth and comfort
- To stimulate peristalsis

Classification

Classification of hot application is shown as in Figure 2.

Therapeutic Effect of Heat Application

Vasodilatation (by increased blood supply)	Relieves pain caused by ischemia and local congestion
Reduces blood viscosity	Improves the supply of leukocytes, antibodies and nutrients to the injured area of the body.
Reduces muscle tension	Heat relieves the stiffness or spasm of the muscles by relaxing the muscles and stimulating blood circulation and relieves fatigue.
Increased capillary permeability and tissue metabolism	It provides local warmth and promotes movement of waste products and nutrients.

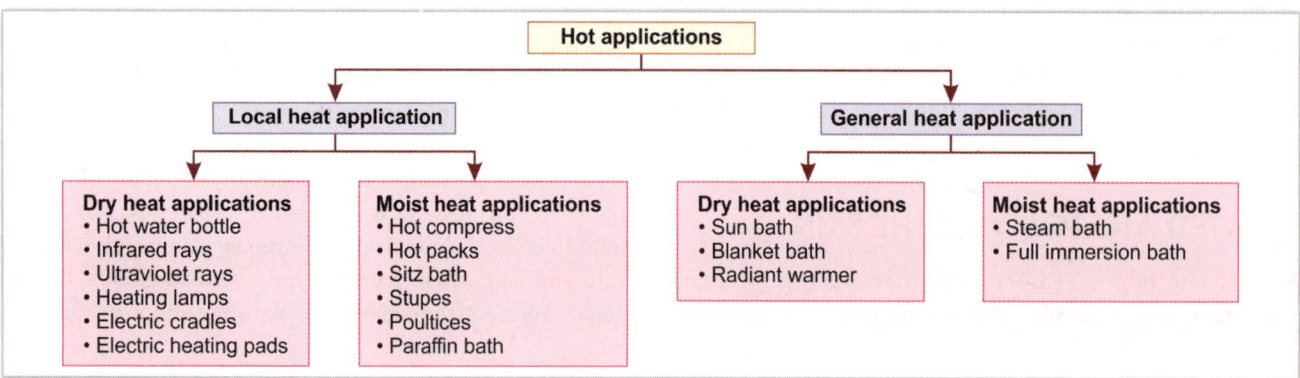

Fig. 2: Classification of hot applications

PRINCIPLES OF APPLICATION OF HOT THERAPY

- Heat is a form of energy resulting from the internal vibration of the molecules of which the body is composed.
- Heat is always passed from a hotter body to a cooler one.
- Heat causes expansion and change of state. Any chemical action capable of being accelerated is increased by rise of temperature.
- Heat is distributed throughout the body by the circulating blood and by direct conduction throughout the tissue.
- Heat is lost from the body through conduction, convection, radiation and evaporation.
- The amount of heat loss from the body is directly proportional to the amount of blood circulating close to the skin's surface. This is influenced by the dilatation and constriction of the peripheral arterioles.
- Moisture conducts heat better than air.
- People vary in their ability to tolerate heat or cold. People at both extremes of age spectrum (very old and very young) are particularly more sensitive to heat and cold.
- People become less sensitive to repeated application of heat and cold.
- The length and time of exposure to extremes in temperature affects the body's tolerance to the temperature.

GENERAL INSTRUCTIONS

- Assess the patient's condition prior to, during and after the therapy.
- Maintain correct temperatures for the entire duration of application.
- Never use any equipment unless you know its operation completely.
- There must be a recovery period between application of heat because it is detrimental to health and tissues.
- Expose patient only to a safe temperature.
- Don't allow patients to adjust temperatures of appliances such as short-wave diathermy, electric heating pads, etc.
- Never ignore even small complaints of patients.
- Ensure that patient is in a position to remove application or to remove devise, if it is causing a discomfort
- The patient must have a calling signal within his reach.
- Since water is a good conductor of heat, squeeze off water from moist heat application to prevent scalding.
- Apply a thin layer of oil to the skin prior to moist heat application. This protective layer reduces soaking of the skin and therefore prevents maceration.
- Do not use electrical appliance close to open oxygen or near water and other fluids. Badly maintained equipment with signs of deterioration should never be used.

- Be extremely careful when patient is unconscious, anesthetized or unable to respond to pain.
- Any signs of complication should be early recognized, stop the procedure, and report immediately.
- After the procedure, dry the part gently by patting and not by rubbing to remove the moisture thereby preventing maceration of the skin and further cooling by evaporation.
- During the procedure protect the patient from chills. Shivering can raise the temperature. It also allows patient to catch a cold.

CONTRAINDICATIONS

- In malignancy, heat increases metabolism of both normal and abnormal cells.
- When heat involves a large body area, blood supply of vital organs gets reduced. This may pose a serious problem to patients of renal impairment, heart and lung diseases.
- Edema associated with venous and lymphatic disease e.g., arteriosclerosis, atherosclerosis which is common in diabetes mellitus patients.
- Cutaneous injuries (e.g., stomas or scar tissues).
- Patients with paralysis.
- Heat is not applied in areas where diffusibility of heat is limited e.g., in abscess of tooth or in an inflamed appendix as heat might cause these areas to rupture, spreading infection in the blood stream.
- It should not be applied to very young or very old or debilitated patients.

PROCEDURES RELATED TO HEAT APPLICATION

LOCAL DRY HEAT APPLICATION

The application of dry heat means the use of an agent warmer than the skin, which is applied in dry form to produce local effect.

Hot Water Bottle

- Hot Water Bottle is the commonest and inexpensive method of applying dry heat locally to the body as a therapeutic and comfort measure
- *Objective:* To supply heat to the area, to provide comfort, a feeling of general warmth and to promote healing
- *Indications:* To relieve pain (rheumatoid arthritis backache, dysentery and dysmenorrhea), to relieve muscle spasm, to reduce inflammation and congestion, and to relieve retention of urine.

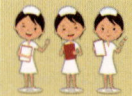

SKILL: HOT WATER BOTTLE APPLICATION

Preparation of Articles

Articles	Rationale
A hot water bag with cover/towel-1	To provide treatment
Jugs-2	One to keep hot water and the other to keep cold water
Duster-1	To wipe outside of the bottle
Lotion thermometer	To check the temperature
Vaseline/oil	To apply on the skin
A kidney tray and paper bag	To receive waste

Preliminary Assessment

♦ Check for the diagnosis and physician's instructions

♦ Inspect the body part that is to receive treatment for any lesion or injury

♦ Check the general condition of the patient and ability to follow commands

♦ Determine the duration and frequency of treatment as instructed

Preparation of the Patient (Planning)

♦ Explain the purpose of the procedure to build rapport

♦ Maintain privacy of the patient, drape the patient if needed

♦ Provide a comfortable position to the patient

♦ Prevent chills by covering patient with blanket or bed cover

Steps of Procedure

Action/steps	Rationale
1. Wash hands	To prevent cross-infection, pathogens can transfer from the source to the new host
2. Screen the patient	To maintain privacy. It helps in giving relaxation and comfort to the patient
3. Collect supplies from the equipment room	To economize time, energy and material. Organization facilitates performance of task
4. Mix hot and cold water and check the temperature (120–149°F or 49–65°C) or keep boiling water till steam disappears	To prepare application within the acceptable range
5. Pour some water into the hot water bottle and empty it	To warm the hot water bottle and minimize heat lost through conduction and convection
6. Pour water to fill the half or two-third of the capacity of hot water bottle	To avoid unnecessary weight on body parts, especially if applied on abdomen and allows to mould over the area to provide even heat
7. Expel the air by placing the bag over a flat surface. Cork it tightly (Fig. 3).	Air in the bag will interfere with the conduction of heat and it will not mould easily to the patient's body

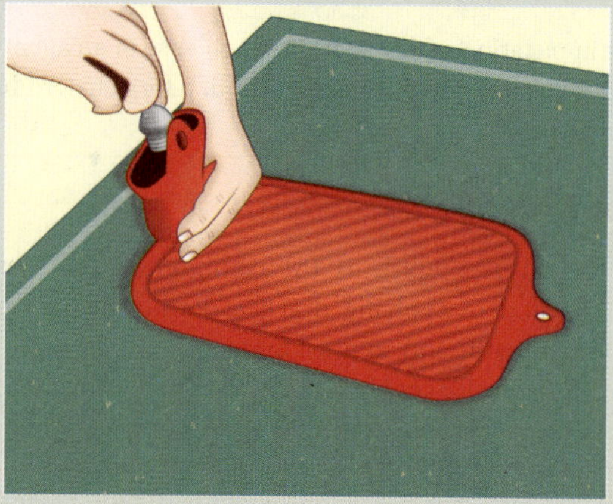

Fig. 3: Expelling air from hot water bag

Contd...

Action/steps	Rationale
8. Dry the outside of the bottle and hold it upside down for checking leakage	To prevent scalding of the patient To ensure that the bottle is not leaking
9. Cover the bag with a bottle cover or other protector and apply to the prescribed area	Protects the skin from direct contact with hot rubber
10. Keep bottle in place for 20–30 minutes, change position if needed and inspect area for redness, pain and swelling	Maximum therapeutic effects from application of heat occur within 20–30 minutes. Extended use of heat causes tissue congestion and vasoconstriction. Inspection and changing position prevent burns

After Care of Patient and Articles

- Remove the bag when treatment is over.
- Inspect area for redness. If present, apply vaseline or oil.
- Note the patient's response and make him comfortable.
- Take all articles to utility room and remove the bag cover. Empty the bag and wash its outside with soap and water.
- Dry the bag by hanging upside down. When dried, fill with some air, cork it and store in a proper place.
- Wash the cover of the bag, dry it and put it in a proper place.
- Wash hands.

Documentation

- Record the procedure with date, time, the area to which it is applied, the purpose and reaction, if any.

Evaluation

- Observe for its therapeutic effectiveness.

Heating Lamp

Flexible necked lamps are used to supply dry heat to the body part and are placed 18–30 inches from the area to be treated. The distance between the exposed part and the lamps depends on the voltage of the light bulb, the pigmentation of the skin and heat tolerance by the patient. The duration of treatment is 20–30 minutes.

The recommended distances are:

- **25 watt bulb:** 35 cms away from the body part
- **40 watt bulb:** 45 cms away from the body part
- **60 watt bulb:** 60 cms away from the body part

Objectives/indications

- To provide dry heat to increase circulation to a small area such as in decubitus ulcer
- To reduce inflammation

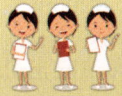

SKILL: HEATING LAMP APPLICATION

Articles Required

Articles	Rationale
A lamp with required voltage	To apply heat
Measuring tape	To check proper distance of the lamp and the body
Screen	To maintain privacy
Vaseline	To prevent skin burning
An extra bed-sheet	To drape the patient

Preliminary Assessment

- Assess the patient's condition.
- Check the diagnosis and doctor's instruction.
- Inspect, clean and dry the body area.
- Determine the distance of the lamp and frequency of treatment.
- Check the working condition of the instrument.

Preparation of the Patient (Planning)

- Explain the purpose of the procedure to build rapport.
- Maintain proper privacy. Drape patient as needed.
- Provide a comfortable position.

Steps of Procedure

Action/steps	Rationale
Implementation	
1. Screen and drape the patient	To maintain privacy
2. Wash hands and dry properly	To prevent cross-infection
3. Measure the proper distance from the lamp to the body	To get the maximum benefit of treatment
4. Focus the lamp at a proper angle	To supply heat
Evaluation	
5. Inspect the area for redness	To observe for any injury

After Care of Patient and Articles

- Switch off the lamp, cool it and keep it back in the inventory.
- Make the patient comfortable.
- Wash hands and record procedure.
- Apply Vaseline or oil if there is any redness.

Heat Cradles

Heat cradles are metallic half circle frames (bed cradle), in which several electrical light sources and sockets for luminous bulbs and a thermometer are installed. They are used when a large body part is to be heated such as abdomen, chest or legs.

Purposes

- To dry large plaster body casts
- To dry the wounds in burns or when patient's condition does not allow covering of the skin with gown or sheets.
- To take the weight off the body of top clothes

Steps of Procedure

- Place the cradle with electric light bulbs over the required area. Often this is covered by top bedding in order to hold in the heat and to prevent cooling by the circulatory air. Temperature should not exceed 52°C or 125°F.
- After the prescribed duration (20–30 minutes), cool the cradle and remove and replace. It may be used continuously, provided a low temperature is maintained.

Electric Pads

Electric pads and electric blankets are frequently used as a means of providing dry heat. These are composed of an electric coil with a waterproof rubber covering and heat control switch to maintain temperature at a desired level.

Precautions

- It should be covered with a flannel cloth to absorb the perspiration and to insulate the pad.

- No wet dressing should be applied while using heating pad.
- Do not apply heating pad with pressure since this reduces the number of air spaces between patient and appliance. It increases chance of burns.
- Instruct patient not to lean or lie against the heating pads

Infrared Lamp

Infrared lamp supply radiant heat or infrared rays (invisible heat rays beyond the red end of the spectrum). Infrared lamp is used to provide heat to a localized area of the body. It penetrates 3 mm of tissue at the most. Thus, it provides surface heat only.

The advantages over other forms of heat application:

- Dosage can be regulated easily.
- The application has no weight and the patient can be made comfortable and undisturbed throughout the procedure.

Uses

- Frequently used in treatment of decubitus ulcers.
- Used in obstetrical and gynecological cases to promote healing of suture area of the perineum.

Cautions

- Check that the patient's skin is dry
- Ask patient to wear cotton clothes
- The lamp should be placed 18–24 inches above the skin area
- The rays should strike the skin at right angle
- Observe patient frequently, note his reaction and terminate application at first sign of redness or pain

Duration of Treatment

♦ It is from 15 to 45 minutes. The length of time depends on the amount of erythema present during treatment.

Ultraviolet Lamps

Ultraviolet lamps are exposure of the body to the ultraviolet portion of light spectrum. A mercury vapor lamp or a cold quartz lamp is used for producing ultraviolet rays.

Uses

♦ The effects of exposure to ultraviolet lamps are pigmentation of the skin, production of vitamin D and bactericidal effects. It is mostly used for a number of skin conditions.

♦ The lamp is placed 30–36 inches away from the skin and the duration is 20–30 minutes.

Caution

♦ Patient and therapist must wear protective goggles as it may cause conjunctivitis.

Diathermy

Shortwave or diathermy is a method of heating to convert electrical or vibrational energy into thermal energy to provide heat, deep in the tissues. In preparation of a client for diathermy, the nurse must see that all forms of metals are removed from patient's body.

LOCAL MOIST HEAT APPLICATION

Application of moist heat means the use of an agent warmer than the skin which is applied in moist form to produce local heat.

Fomentations

Fomentations are local application of moist heat to the skin by means of double thickness of flannel or other soft material. They are of two types:
♦ Medical fomentation
♦ Surgical fomentation

Medical Fomentation

Medical fomentation is done by using only hot water with or without medicine.

Purposes

♦ To stimulate circulation and relax muscle tissue
♦ To relieve pain and congestion in inflamed areas
♦ To relieve retention of urine
♦ To promote suppuration
♦ To stimulate absorption of serous exudates and effusion from body cavities

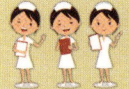

SKILL: FOMENTATION APPLICATION

Preparation of Articles

Articles	Rationale
A kettle with boiling water	To have boiling water at required temperature
Wringer with wringer rods placed in a basin/two artery forceps	To wring out the hot compress
Three pieces of flannel large enough to cover the area/fomentation pads	To apply warmth
Cotton balls in a container	To apply oil
Forceps	To hold cotton balls
Paper bag Kidney tray	To receive used swabs To receive used compress
Waterproof cover and cotton	To insulate the compress and to prevent heat loss
An abdominal binder and safety pin	To keep the compress in position
A hot water bag with cover	To keep over the compress
Screen, if necessary	To provide privacy

Preliminary Assessment

- Identify the patient
- Check diagnosis and physician's order
- Inspect body parts
- Determine the duration and frequency of treatment
- Check the patient's general condition
- Check the available articles

Preparation of Patient and Unit (Planning)

- Identify patient and explain procedure
- Screen the patient. Drape according to the need and expose only the needed part
- Switch off the fan
- Place the patient slightly off the center of the bed towards the edge of the bed for better proximity for treatment
- Place a mackintosh and a towel under the patient
- Keep the abdominal binder in place ready for application
- Prepare the part and apply oil or Vaseline

Steps of Procedure

Action/steps	Rationale
1. Wash hands	To prevent cross-infection
2. Screen and drape patient	To maintain privacy
3. Prepare hot compresses at bedside	To prevent heat loss to air. Moisture causes rapid cooling
4. Place the wringer and fomentation cloth in the basin with the free end outside.	Wringer helps to remove excess water from fomentation cloth without burning the nurse's hands
5. Test the temperature by applying at the back of the hand	To ensure that it will not cause a burn
6. Apply compress over the area. Change the compress frequently or cover with heating agent (hot water bottle, heating pad). Cover with waterproof cover and a cotton pad	Cover maintains constant temperature Also protects bed clothes from getting wet
7. Secure the binder with bandage	To get the maximum benefit of the treatment

After Care of Patients and Articles

- Change compress every 3 minutes for 15 minutes if a hot water bottle is not used. If single application is made and kept warm by hot water bottle, remove the last fomentation after 20 minutes.
- Dry the skin, observe for redness and blister. Report if any, and apply vaseline.
- Cover the patient and provide comfortable position.

Documentation

- Report and chart the procedure.
- Wash all articles. Disinfect pads and replace them in proper place.

Special Points

- Avoid chilling in between fomentations
- Report any redness and take immediate steps
- Always apply fomentation after ascertaining patient's sensitivity to heat

Evaluation

Observe for its effectiveness

Surgical Fomentation

Surgical fomentation is local application of moist heat requiring surgical asepsis when the skin is broken.

Purposes

- To promote suppuration by circulation
- To reduce swelling around a wound
- To hasten separation of slough
- To help in drainage of exudates

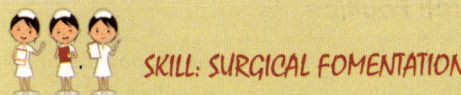

SKILL: SURGICAL FOMENTATION

Articles Required

- A kettle of boiling water
- Tray containing 2 sterile basins, 2 sterile fomentation pads, 2 sterile forceps, 2 sterile small bowls, a piece of plastic cover binder, a kidney tray and paper bag
- Dressing trolley
- Screen

Steps of Procedure

Action/steps	Rationale
Implementation	
1. Assess area for any circulation impairment (numbness, tingling, impaired sensation, cyanosis)	Circulatory impairment may interfere to perceive heat and place the patient at risk of burns
2. Check physician's order and explain the procedure	Explanation encourages patient's cooperation and redness apprehension
3. Gather equipment	Provides for an organized approach to the task
4. Wash hands	To prevent cross–infection
5. Close doors and switch off the fan. Expose the area	To provide privacy and warmth
6. Place mackintosh with waterproof lining under the patient	To protect the bed clothing
7. Assist patient to a comfortable position that provides easy access	To provide comfort and care of application
8. Open the dressing, observe the amount and nature of discharge. Discard dressing in kidney tray	Document the condition of the wound prior to the application
9. Clean the wound. Place sterile fomentation pad into the sterile basin	To maintain aseptic technique
10. Pour boiling water over sterile fomentation and squeeze moisture from it with the help of forceps and apply carefully and gently mould around the wound	Excess moisture may contaminate the surrounding area and is uncomfortable. Moulding compress to the skin promotes retention of warmth around the wound
11. Cover with sterile towels followed by a plastic cover, fix in place with a binder	Towels provide additional insulation
12. Check frequently for any sign of burns	Impaired circulation may affect sensitivity to heat
13. After 30 minutes, remove warm compress. Observe skin condition and patient's response	Maximum therapeutic effect of heat occurs within 20–30 minutes
14. Apply sterile dressing	Protects wound from infection
15. Make patient comfortable	To give comfort to the patient
16. Wash equipment and replace them	To keep it ready for reuse
Documentation	
17. Record with date, time, duration of treatment and condition of wound	Provides accurate documentation of procedure

Evaluation

Observe for its effectiveness.

Stupes

Stupes are medicated local application of moist heat where turpentine is used locally to augment the effects of the hot compress used. These are commonly used to relieve abdominal distention or tympanites. Heat stimulates contraction of intestinal muscle, thereby increasing peristalsis and relaxing muscle spasm

Articles Required

- Same as for medical fomentation
- A drachm glass containing turpentine mixed with olive oil or sweet oil 1:2–3 in adults and 1:6 for children
- A swab stick in a container
- Articles for insertion of a flatus tube

Steps of Procedure

- Adopt same procedure as done for hot compress.
- Take turpentine and olive oil in correct proportion, mix well and warm the mixture by keeping the container in a bowl of hot water.
- Apply warm oil over the part with the help of swab stick.
- Apply hot compress and follow same procedure.
- After 10–15 minutes, insert flatus tube for expulsion of flatus.
- Report and chart time, duration and result of treatment.

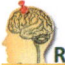

Remember

- Mix turpentine and oil thoroughly
- Avoid blistering of the skin by carefully watching the area in every 15 minutes
- Avoid chills
- Be sure to report the effect of the treatment carefully

Poultices (Cataplasm) and Plasters (Emplastrum)

A poultice is an application of moist heat in the form of a soft spongy mass that retains its heat for a length of time. According to the ingredients used, its effect depends on the heat they supply. The types of poultices are artiphlogestine, linseed, mustard, charcoal, starch, etc. As these are not used, details are not given. Detailed preparation of starch poultice is given below.

Making a Starch Poultice

Take starch and sodium bicarbonate in the proportion of 1:8. Make a paste with cold water. Add more boiling water when the mixture is being stirred. Cook the mixture and make a jelly mass. Spread the jelly on a lint piece with spatula to thickness of one fourth of half an inch. Cover it with another piece (leaving sufficient margin to turn it neatly). Take it to the patient, keeping it in hot plates. Apply on the area as in case of hot compress. It is left in place for half an hour to 1 hour.

Plaster (Emplastrum)

Plaster is made up of substance containing drugs which may be either irritating or soothing in character. The examples are belladonna and opium plaster applied for a soothing effect and a mustard plaster used as a counter-irritant. Application is similar to poultice.

Local Bath (Warm Soaks)

Local bath is a simple method of applying moist heat to the extremity or any part of the body by immersing the body part in warm water/medicated solution or to wrap a part in gauze dressing and then suturing the dressing with the solution. Soaks may employ either a clean or sterile technique. Sterile technique is indicated for open wounds.

Purposes

- To increase blood supply to locally infected area, thus hastening suppuration and softening the exudates.
- To apply medications.
- To aid in cleaning large sloughing wounds such as burns.
- To relieve edema, ischemia and muscle spasm.

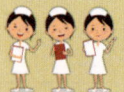 **SKILL: LOCAL BATH**

Articles Required

- A bathtub with required solution at a correct temperature (105–110°F), arm bath tub, foot bath tub
- A mackintosh with cover
- A bath thermometer
- A hot water bottle with cover (for foot and arm bath)
- A screen and extra blanket (for foot and sitz bath)
- A dressing tray, if required
- A kidney tray and paper bag

Solutions Used

- **Sodium bicarbonate:** To relieve itching
- **Boric acid:** To sooth irritated skin, add 3 ounces of boric acid to a gallon of water at a temperature of 35.5°C
- **Potassium sulfate:** To destroy parasites. Add ½–3 oz of potassium sulphate to ½ gallon of water
- **Potassium permanganate:** To treat fungal infection and athlete foot, add one gram of potassium permanganate to one quarter of water

Contd...

Steps of Procedure

- Steps are the same as for hot compress
- Prepare the solution in a bathtub at a correct temperature and take to the bedside
- Explain the procedure and screen the patient
- Loosen top cover at the foot of the bed for giving foot bath
- Place the folded extra blanket at the foot of the bed
- Turn back the bed clothes above the knees, covering the unaffected foot with a blanket.
- Remove soiled dressing, if any
- Flex the knees or raise the patient to a sitting position
- Place the mackintosh and towel under the feet and test the temperature again
- Place the foot tub on the towel. Raise the feet, draw the tub in place and slowly lower the feet into the water

Paraffin Bath/Wax Bath

The paraffin bath is commonly used for painful hands and knees especially for patients with rheumatoid arthritis. The mixture for this treatment consists of 15–30 mL of mineral oil to 1 pound of paraffin wax. It is also used for patients having leprosy.

There are two common methods for use:

1. **Immersion bath:** The patient dips the body part in the wax and removes it so that it dries, then re-dips 6–12 times while allowing it to dry between dips. Then the patient immerses the body part for 5–10 minutes, with care being taken to avoid burning.
2. **Pack glove method:** This method is safer than the immersion bath because there is less chance of burning. With this, the patient dips the body part in the wax and lets it dry. This is repeated 7–12 times. After the last dip,

- Place the folded towel between the legs and the edge of the tub (or bring the bath towel up to cover the edge of tub where the back of the patient's legs is pressing against the tub). The patient's own towel can also be used.
- Hold the blanket in position while drawing down the cover. Keep the feet in water for 20–30 minutes. Keep the jug with water nearby and add from the side of the bath as required.
- Uncover the tub at one corner only when pouring water. Raise the foot and pour in gradually and not near the patient to prevent scalding.
- Turn back the top clothes leaving the blanket over the knees.
- Remove the towel from the edge of the tub.
- Raise the leg, hold over the tub to drain water and then lower the legs over the towel.
- Same steps are followed for giving **arm bath** using **arm bath** tub.

the body part is covered with a plastic bag and then a heat pack is placed over the injury to keep it in the heat.

Sitz Bath

Sitz bath is a local application of moist heat to the pelvic organs. The patient is usually immersed from the mid-thigh to the iliac crest. The temperature should be 110–115°F. Duration of bath is 15–30 minutes.

Purposes

- To relieve congestion of the pelvic organs, e.g., in treating dysmenorrhea
- To relieve pain following cystoscopy
- To relieve inflammation and pain (hemorrhoids, cystitis)
- To relieve pain in retention and painful micturition
- To promote wound healing by cleaning off the discharge and debris

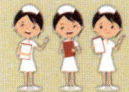 **SKILL: SITZ BATH**

Solutions Used

- Potassium permanganate solution 1:5000
- Boric acid 1 dram to 1 pint
- Eusol solution
- Dettol 1:40

Equipment

- A bed-screen if treatment is to be done at bedside
- A suitable bathtub or basin/sitz bath tub
- A bath thermometer
- A jug with warm water

Contd...

- A bedside stool
- Gown
- Towel for drying

Steps of Procedure

- Explain the purpose of the procedure.
- Fill the tub with water about half full at a temperature of 100°F.
- Screen the patient if at bedside or wheel him to the bathroom in a chair if his condition permits.
- Assist the patient to undress and avoid unnecessary exposure. Stand directly at the patient's back; help the patient to sit down in the tub with the feet flat on the floor. There should be no pressure on the sacrum or thighs.
- Be sure that the thighs, buttocks and lower abdomen are immersed in the solution.
- Drape the patient's legs and thighs. Wrap a bath blanket around the patient's shoulder to protect him/her from chill.

- Observe closely for any sign of weakness or fatigue. Discontinue the bath if the patient has signs of faintness, pallor, rapid pulse and nausea
- Test the water in the tub several times and keep it at the desired temperature 105°F. Additional hot water may be added by pouring it slowly from the jug
- Allow the patient to remain in the basin for 15–30 minutes
- Do not leave the patient alone unless it is absolutely certain that it is safe to do so
- Help the patient to come out of the basin when the bath is completed. Stand in front of him. Place hands under the axilla and partially lift him from the tub to the stool
- Dry the patient with the bath towel and cover him adequately. Assist him into the bed
- Avoid chill
- Rinse the basin, scrub well with soap, rinse, dry and replace
- Leave the patient comfortable. Leave the bathroom in order. Remove the bedside stool
- Record time, duration, type of solutions used and reaction of the patient

Aquathermia Pads

Aquathermia pads come in various sizes. Instructions should be followed according to the manufacturer. These are waterproof pads used for treating muscle sprains, areas of mild inflammation or redness. It consists of a waterproof plastic or rubber pad connected by two hoses to an electrical control unit that has a heating element and motor. Distilled water circulates to the control unit where water is heated or cooled depending on setting of the temperature. Setting is fixed by inserting a plastic key into the temperature regulator. Mostly the temperature is maintained between 105°F and 110ºF. Plain tap water is never added to the unit as it might leave mineral deposits. The pad is never applied directly on the skin. A thin towel or pillow cover should be fitted over this heating pad and later secured with the tape or gauze roll. Any type of pin is never used as it may cause a leak. Duration of total application is 20–30 minutes. Frequent observation of the skin is done for redness and burning. The patient should not be allowed to lie on the bed.

GENERAL APPLICATION OF DRY HEAT

Hot Dry Packs

Purposes

- To prevent chilling
- To relieve retention of urine

- To provide a warm bed with blankets and hot water bottles, thus preventing and treating surgical shocks.

Steps of Procedure

- The hot dry pack frequently follows a hot bath
- Wrap the patient in hot dry blankets
- Keep 2–3 hot water bottles surrounding the blanket
- Give hot drinks like hot soup
- Cold application may be done at the head if the patient has headache or throbbing pain

GENERAL MOIST HEAT APPLICATIONS

Hot Moist Packs

It is the application of hot moist blankets or flannel pieces to a larger area (sometimes whole body is covered). The hot packs may be used to relieve muscle spasms in poliomyelitis.

Whirlpool Bath or Full Immersion Bath

It is helpful in promoting sedation, relieving pain and encouraging debridement of widespread surface burns. When immersed in water, the body becomes buoyant and exercises are, therefore, performed with less efforts. It is expensive and inconvenient to use a warm whirlpool. Despite this, it is good for covering large, irregular surface areas. The temperature should range from 105°F to 110°F, and the duration of treatment should last from 15 to 20 minutes.

Counter-Irritants

These are drugs used to augment the desired effect of heat application to induce vasodilation in the superficial tissues. When the skin absorbs counter-irritants, they irritate the sensory nerve endings and produce vasodilatation by reflex action.

Types of Counter-irritants

They are classified according to their effects and degree of irritation produced:

- **Rubefacients:** It is a simple form of counter-irritant, which causes only reddening of the skin. The effect is immediate and lasts only for a short period. Common rubefacients are mustard plaster, iodine, turpentine, camphor, etc.
- **Vesicants:** These counter–irritants cause blister formation and are not practiced commonly.
- **Pustulants:** They are counter-irritants which when applied on the skin, form pustules.

Steam Inhalation

Inhalation of warm steam to liquefy the secretions and to relieve congestion in the lungs is called steam inhalation.

Purposes

- To loosen the secretion and for easy expectoration
- To moisten the mucous membranes
- To relieve irritation and congestion
- To relax muscles and thus, relieve cough

Assessment

- Assess the patient's ability for self care
- Assess the level of consciousness
- Assess the general condition of the patient
- Auscultate the lungs to assess for the presence of secretions

Nursing Diagnosis

- Impaired gas exchange
- Ineffective breathing pattern
- Activity intolerance
- Anxiety
- Ineffective therapeutic regimen

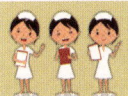

SKILL: STEAM INHALATION

Planning

Articles Required

Articles required for steam inhalation are shown in Figure 4.
- A tray lined with towel containing
  - Enamel or steel bowl (big in size)
  - Nelson's inhaler wrapped with towel
  - Mouth piece which snugly fits Nelson's inhaler or electric inhaler
  - Cotton balls and gauze pieces in a bowl
  - Kidney tray and paper bag
- Kettle with boiling water (120°–160°F)
- Sputum cup
- Medications as per order such as:
  - Tincture benzoin 5 mL/500 mL of water
  - Eucalyptus 2 mL/500 mL of water
  - Methyl salicylate few drops in water
  - Few crystals of menthol in water

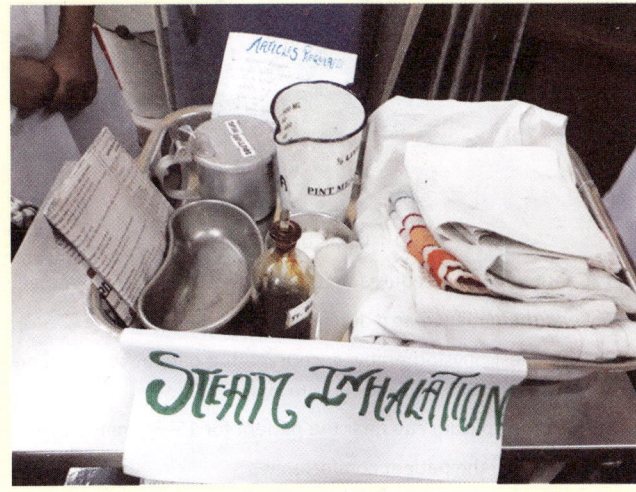

Fig. 4: Articles for steam inhalation

Contd...

Steps of Procedure

Action/steps	Rationale
Implementation	
1. Check for the doctor's order	To plan the care
2. Explain the procedure to the patient	Enhances cooperation and removes fear
3. Rinse the Nelson's inhaler with hot water	
4. Pour hot water into the inhaler from the kettle till the level of the spout (two third of the inhaler)	To prevent injury (scald)
5. Add medicine, if ordered. Close the inhaler with the mouth piece	To prevent heat loss
6. Switch off the air conditioner/fans and close windows and doors	To avoid draughts and chills to patient
7. Wrap the inhaler with towel and keep it in a bowl. Wrap the mouth piece with gauze piece and plug cotton balls into the spout of the inhaler	To prevent heat loss
8. Take it to bed-side and position the patient in Fowler's position and support with cardiac table or extra pillows.	To provide support
9. Keep the sputum cup within easy reach of the patient	To expel the sputum as need arises
10. Place the inhaler and ask the patient to inhale deeply with mouth, hold it to a count of three, exhale through the spout during expiration and remove it during inspiration (Fig. 5) 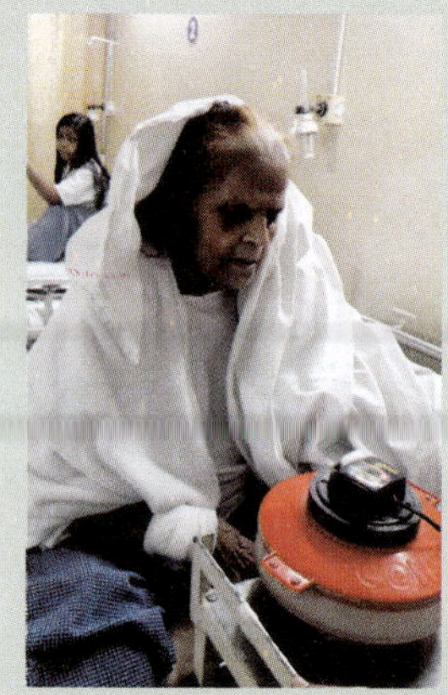	To liquefy the secretions and loosen the secretions To promote atmospheric air entry through spout.

Fig. 5: Inhalation of steam

Action/steps	Rationale
11. Continue the procedure for 10 minutes or till the steam remains	For effectiveness
12. Keep the patient warm during and after the procedure	To prevent chills
13. Give chest physiotherapy, encourage the patient to cough and spit the sputum into the sputum cup	To mobilize the secretions
14. Keep the sputum cup near the patient for 15–30 minutes	To expel the sputum
15. Reposition the patient comfortably	To promote comfort
16. Replace the articles	For the next time
17. Document the procedure done: Date, time, duration and medication added	To prevent duplication of care and serves as legal evidence

Evaluation

- Evaluate the patient's response
- Auscultate the lungs to assess the lung sounds
- Evaluate the color, thickness and odor of sputum
- Monitor the respiratory rate

CONCLUSION

The safe use of heat therapy requires an assessment of the patient's sensory function, identification of risk factors and understanding the physiological effect of heat. Different parts of the body differ in tolerance to heat and cold and so does the physiological tolerance of individual. Warm applications are effective for improving circulation to wound sites and promoting muscle relaxation.

BIBLIOGRAPHY

1. The Trained Nurses Association of India. Fundamental of Nursing: Procedure Manual. TNAI Publication. pp. 412-29.
2. Sr. Nancy. "Stephanie's Principles and Practice of Nursing senior Nursing Procedure and Nursing administration", vol. 2, 4th edition. NR Brothers; 2005. pp. 461-82.
3. Lindeman CA, McAthie M. Fundamentals of contemporary nursing practice, 1st edition. Saunders: Philadelphia; 1999.
4. White L. Basic Nursing: Foundation of Skills and Concepts. Delmar/Thomson Learning, 2002.

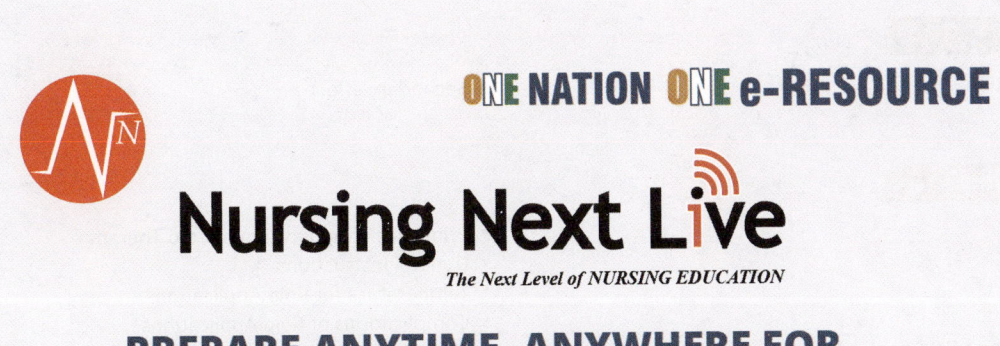

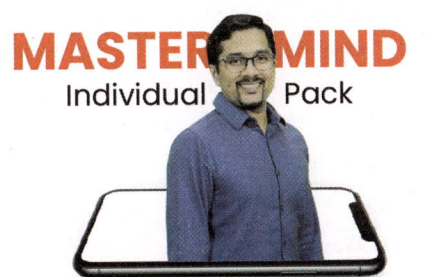

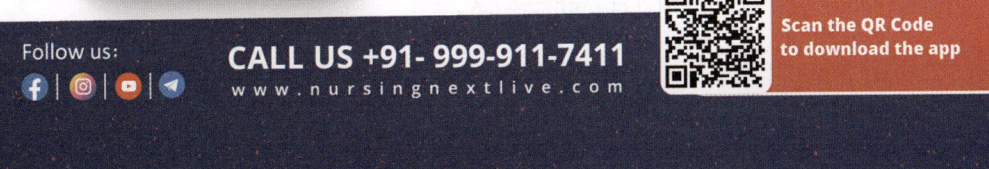

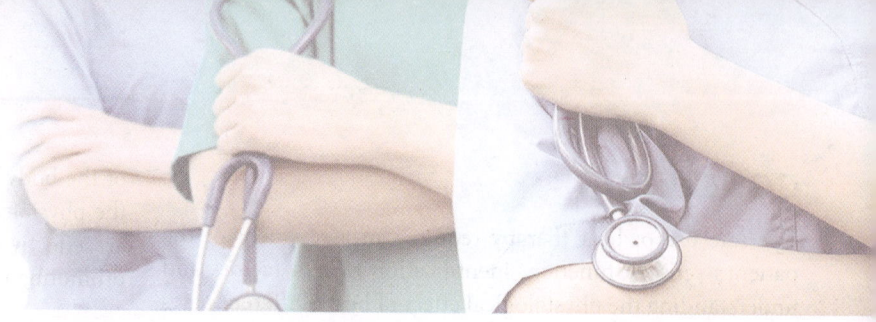

Cold Application

INTRODUCTION

Application of cold is commonly used in the hospital and home as a therapeutic measure. Cold applications also serve as comfort measures. It is also used in the course of physical medicine as part of a rehabilitation program.

DEFINITION

Application of cold means using an agent on the skin that is cooler than the skin. The application is either moist or dry. It can be applied to produce a local or systemic effect or both.

PURPOSES

- To reduce inflammation.
- To relieve pain
- To prevent edema
- To control hemorrhage
- To decrease metabolism and thus, prevent gangrene
- To reduce body temperature
- To anesthetize an area for a short period
- To inhibit bacterial growth and prevent suppuration

CLASSIFICATION

Cold applications are classified as given in (Fig. 1).

FACTORS AFFECTING COLD APPLICATION

- The purpose of the application
- The age of the patient and the condition of the skin

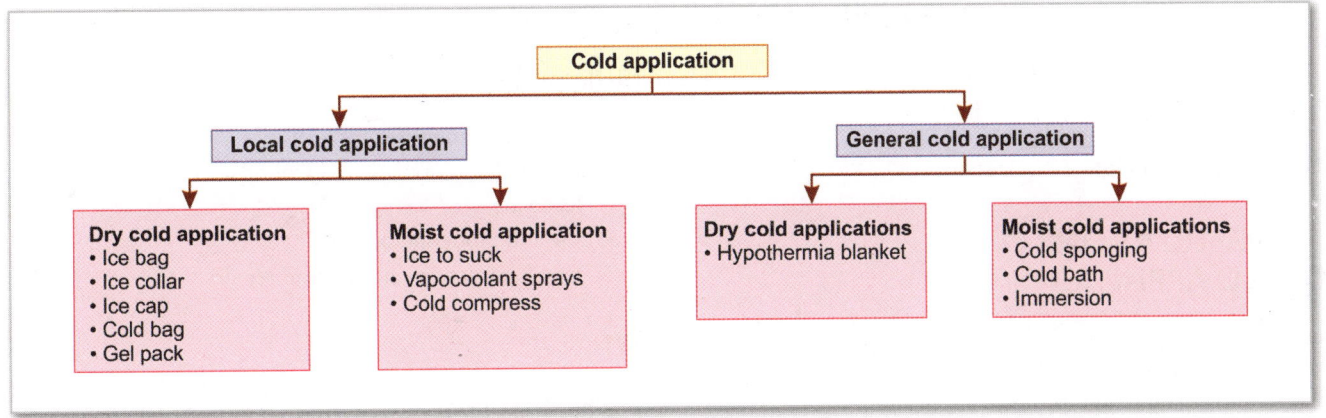

Fig. 1: Classification of cold applications

- The general physical health of the patient
- The area of the body that is affected
- The duration of the treatment
- The intensity of the temperature and its application (moist or dry).

EFFECTS OF COLD APPLICATIONS

- **Physiological changes:**
  - Vasoconstriction: Decreased capillary permeability, decreased local metabolism and decreased oxygen requirement.
  - Increased blood viscosity, decreased blood flow, decreased lymph flow, decreased mobility of leukocytes and reduced muscle tension.
- **Secondary effects:** If the cold application is prolonged, it results in reflex vasodilatation to prevent tissue ischemia, which occurs due to inability to receive an adequate flow of blood and nutrients in the cells.
- **Therapeutic effects of cold applications**
  - Vasoconstriction
  - Increased blood viscosity
  - Reduced cell metabolism
  - Checks the growth of bacteria

CONTRAINDICATIONS

- Disorders which have resulted in impaired circulation. e.g., diabetes mellitus
- Infected wounds
- Patients with decreased sensation in the affected area. e.g., paralyzed patients
- Cold may be applied initially to a burnt area to reduce pain and to decrease the effect of hypoxia but after 24 hours it may be contraindicated as it may retard the healing process
- Patient in shock or collapse

PRINCIPLES OF APPLICATION OF COLD THERAPY

- Cold therapy, also known as cryotherapy, works on the principle of heat exchange.
- This occurs when you place a cooler object in direct contact with an object of warmer temperature (ice against skin). The cooler object will absorb the heat of the warmer object.
- The exposure time should be reduced in moist application.
- Length of time of exposure affects body's tolerance to temperature.

GENERAL INSTRUCTIONS

- Assess the condition of the patient prior to, during and after the application of cold therapy.
- Maintain the correct temperature for the entire duration of the application.
- Always make sure that the patient is in a position to remove the application.
- The patient must have a calling signal within his/her reach.
- Do not use electrical appliances near water or other fluids or handle them with wet hands. Water is a good conductor of electricity and short circuit may occur, giving shock to the patient as well as the operator.
- Any sign of complications should be recognized early, procedure should be stopped and it should be reported immediately.
- During the application, protect the patient from getting chills. Shivering can raise the temperature.
- Recovery period should be given in between the application.

In hyperpyrexia, the temperature of the body should be brought down gradually and steadily. Sudden cooling is dangerous to the patient.

TEMPERATURE FOR COLD APPLICATIONS

- **Tepid:** 27°–37°C; alcohol sponge bath
- **Cool:** 18°–27°C; cold compress
- **Cold:** 15°–18°C; cold pack
- **Very cold:** Below 15°C; ice packs

COMPLICATIONS OF COLD APPLICATIONS

- Pain
- Blisters and skin breakdown
- Maceration with moist cold application
- Bluish discoloration
- Redness as a secondary effect
- Hypothermia

PROCEDURES RELATED TO COLD APPLICATION

LOCAL COLD APPLICATIONS

The local application of cold to small areas may be given in different ways, e.g., ice chips by mouth, ice soaks to an injured extremity.

Purposes

- To relieve pain, burning or irritation.
- To control bleeding.
- To prevent gangrene by decreasing the tissue metabolism.
- To prevent or reduce inflammation and edema.
- To reduce body temperature.

- To provide a sedative effect.

Indications

- Sprains and fractures
- Localized hemorrhage and wounds
- Headache
- Low and moderate pyrexia
- Dental extraction and surgical repairs

Types

Ice Bag and Ice Collar (Local Dry Cold)

- The ice bag or ice chip and ice collar are commonly used for applying dry cold to the body.
- An ice collar is a long narrow rubber or plastic bag, which fits around the neck. The bags are usually made with an opening through which small pieces of ice are inserted.

Nurses' Responsibility

Preliminary Assessment of the Patient

- Check the patient's name, bed no. and other identification parameters
- Check the diagnosis and the general condition of the patient
- Explain the purpose and procedure to the patient
- Maintain a comfortable position
- Prevent draughts by covering the patient with a blanket or a bed cover
- Assemble and check the articles required

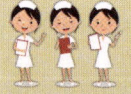

SKILL: ICE BAG AND ICE COLLAR APPLICATION

Articles	Rationale
A big bowl	To keep ice cubes
An ice bag with cover	To provide cold application
A mackintosh with towel	To protect the bed
A roll of tape or bandage	To secure the bag
A jar containing hot water/wooden spatula	To smoothen the ice cubes
A small container with salt	To sprinkle on ice
A small spoon	To take ice pieces form the bowl
A bath blanket	To cover the patient
A hammer	To crush the ice cubes.
A big bowl with small ice cubes	To fill in the bag
A duster/cloth	To wipe the bag after filling
A kidney tray and a paper bag	To discard wastes

Contd...

Steps of Procedure

Review and follow the standard steps as given in Appendix

Action/steps	Rationale
Planning	
1. Wash hands.	To prevent cross-infection.
2. Break the ice into small pieces and leave the pieces in a bowl for a while.	For easy insertion of ice into bags, makes it easier to mould the bag to a body part; to smoothen the sharp edges.
3. Smoothen the sharp edges by touching with wooden spatula dipped in hot water.	
4. Sprinkle salt over the ice.	Salt lowers the melting point and prevents the ice from melting.
5. Check the ice bag for leakage by pouring water into it.	To ensure that the bag is in a good working condition.
6. Empty the bag and fill it about one-third with ice.	This makes the bag light in weight.
7. Keep the bag on a flat surface and squeeze out the air.	Air is removed in order that the ice bag can be moulded according to the patient's body.
8. Screw the cap well and wipe it. Invert and check for any leakage.	To ensure that the bag is not leaking. Dries the excess moisture.
9. Put on a flannel cover.	The cover retains cold for more gradual application and it absorbs the water formed by atmospheric condensation.
Implementation	
10. Spread the mackintosh and the towel over the pillow. Apply the ice cap/collar on the area ordered.	To protect the pillow.
11. The ice bag is applied for about 20 min and then it is discontinued for at least an hour for the recovery period.	To prevent the effect of prolonged exposure to cold and to prevent the secondary effect.
12. Wash hands before and after doing the procedure.	To prevent cross-infection.
Documentation	
13. Record the procedure with date, time and the area on which it is applied.	

Evaluation

Observe for its therapeutic effectiveness.

Cold Compress (Local Moist Cold)

This is a local moist cold application made out of folded layers of gauze, lint piece or old soft linen. The gauze is cooled over ice chips, wrung out and applied. It is replaced as it becomes warm.

Purposes

+ To treat epistaxis
+ To supply moist cold to the eyes
+ To apply on forehead to reduce fever and headache

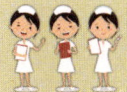 **SKILL: COLD COMPRESS APPLICATION**

Articles Required

A tray containing:

+ A bowl of water containing ice
+ 8 pieces of lint or gauze
+ A bowl with cotton plugs for ears

+ A bowl containing ice cubes
+ A bath blanket
+ An ice cap with cover
+ A hot water bag with cover
+ A small mackintosh and a towel to protect the bed
+ A kidney tray

Contd...

Procedure

- Explain the procedure to the patient.
- Carry equipment to the bedside and screen the patient, if necessary.
- Place a mackintosh and a towel under the area to be treated.
- Remove clothings of the patient and cover the patient with a bath blanket.
- Bring out the compress and apply on head (1), neck (1), both axillae (2), abdomen (2), groin (2) and one for changing. Replace the compress as necessary to maintain coolness.

- Do not cover a cold compress, as it would soon reach the body temperature. Apply cold compress for 15–20 minutes at a time.
- Plug the ears with cotton plugs.
- Place ice cap with cover on the head and hot water bag with cover under the feet.
- Observe for numbness and mottled bluish appearance.
- On completion of treatment, remove and clean the equipment and replace the articles. Leave the patient comfortable and document the treatment.

Cold Pack (Local Moist Cold)

The pack could be a wash cloth, towel, flannel or a sheet depending on the size of the body part to receive the application. A basin of cold water is prepared with a small amount of ice chips and packs are immersed into it. When cooled, excess water will wring out and the pack is applied to the body area. The temperature of the water is maintained at 75°F. Replacing the packs is necessary to maintain coolness.

GENERAL MOIST COLD APPLICATIONS
Cold Sponging (Moist)

It is used to reduce temperature in a patient with hyperpyrexia. It is given to cover a larger area of the body.

Indications

- To soothe the nerves and promote sleep
- To relieve discomfort
- To reduce temperature

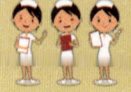 **SKILL: COLD SPONGING**

Articles Required

Articles	Rationale
A basin containing water, jug of cold water	To provide cold compress
A long Mackintosh with 2 bath blankets	To protect the bed and mattress
Ice with ice cap	To apply on head to reduce temperature
A bottle of spirit	For therapeutic use
A bath towel	To wipe the body
3 sponge clothes and 2 treatment towels as compress	To wipe the body
A bath thermometer	To measure the temperature
An ice cap with cover	To give a cooling effect
A hot water bottle with cover	To apply on feet to prevent any untoward effect
A bowl with cotton plugs	To prevent seepage of water into the ear canal
Extra clothes	For patient use
A back care tray	To provide back care
A temperature, pulse and respiration tray	To monitor vitals
Extra ice in a bowl	To maintain the temperature of the body

Contd...

Steps of Procedure

Review and follow the standard steps as given in Appendix

Action/steps	Rationale
Planning	
1. Wash hands.	To prevent cross-infection.
2. Screen the patient and explain the procedure.	To provide privacy. To provide comfort and relaxation to the patient.
3. Offer the bedpan.	To avoid interruption of procedure.
Implementation	
4. Fold the bed clothes at the foot of the bed and cover the patient with a top sheet.	To prevent chill.
5. Remove the patient's clothes and cover with a top sheet.	To make the patient ready for procedure.
6. Place a long Mackintosh and a bath blanket under the patient.	To prevent the mattress from becoming wet.
7. Place an ice cap on the patient's head and hot water bag for feet.	To give a cooling effect and prevent patient going into shock.
8. Sponge the face and dry with a towel.	Sponging cools the skin.
9. Fanfold the bath blanket and expose the farthest part.	To start from farthest to nearest.
10. Continue the bath. Follow the course along with light sweeping strokes, leaving droplets of water on the body.	Friction produces heat, so little or no friction is used during the bath. Evaporation cools the body.
11. Leave sponge clothes on forehead, axilla and groin and treatment towel on abdomen.	Leaving wet cool sponges in these areas help in losing more heat.
12. Replace the articles and wash hands.	For reuse.
13. Record the procedure with date and time.	

Evaluation

Observe for its therapeutic effectiveness.

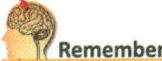 **Remember**

While giving cold sponge use the strokes as follows

- **Stroke 1:** Take a piece of sponge cloth. Wipe the face bringing it down from behind the ear, to the neck. Rest, turn and bring down over the shoulder and outside of the arm to the groin. Turn, bring it down over the inside of the leg, replace it in water. This should be completed within 8 minutes.
- **Stroke 2:** Take the second piece of sponge cloth, place it at the neck, turn, take it over the shoulder to the axilla, rest and turn. Continue on the inside of the arm and then to the outside of the leg. Replace the sponge cloth in water. This should be completed within 8 minutes.
- **Stroke 3:** Take the first piece of sponge cloth, rest at the neck, turn and take it around the breast, place in axilla, turn. Go down at the lateral part of the body and top of the leg. Replace after washing in water. This should be completed within 4 minutes.
  - At the completion of each stroke, mop up water in the bed.
  - Complete the strokes on one side of the body and repeat the same or the other side.
  - After each set of strokes, change the compress on the abdomen and sponge the back.
  - Turn the patient to one side, sponge from neck to heel, long even strokes on either side of the spine, buttocks, and then sponge down the spine.
  - Sponge the back.
  - Dry the patient's back with a towel and rub it with spirit.
  - Remove the wet sheet and mackintosh.
  - Replace the wet top sheet with the bath blanket, rub the body with spirit leaving the abdomen.
  - Help the patient to put on clothes. Remove the bath blanket and replace bed clothes.
  - After 30 minutes, check the TPR and the effect of sponge on the patient.
  - Observe the patient carefully during and after the procedure.
  - Avoid unnecessary exposure.
  - Do not use friction.
  - Give sponge for 20 minutes; discontinue in case of any untoward reactions.

After Care

- Documentation: Document the treatment and its effects; record the date, time, duration of application, or any untoward reaction in the nurse's note.
- Make the patient comfortable.
- Wash the articles (ice cap, ice collar) with soap and water and dry it for reuse.
- Dry and then powder between the layers of the rubber and store after filling it with air.

Cold or Tepid Pack (Moist)

To reduce body temperature, wet sheets and towels are applied to the body and patient is left exposed to air to allow heat loss. Exposed area is rubbed briskly to allow more blood to surface and aid in heat loss from the surface.

HYPOTHERMIA

The term "hypothermia" means a decrease in the body temperature as well as the metabolism of the body. The method used for therapeutic hypothermia are:

- **Surface cooling method:** Here the patient lies below cooling blanket and a cooling liquid circulates through the coils of hypothermia blanket. It reverts body temperature by cooling the surface of the body. It can also be given by:
  - Cooling the body with wet sheets and the fan on
  - Cooling the body surface area with ice bags
  - Immersing the whole body in cold water
- **By using heart lung machine:** This machine cools blood, thereby reducing body temperature, as in cardiac surgeries.

BIBLIOGRAPHY

1. *Perry AG, Potter PA. Basic Nursing Essentials for Practice, 5th edition. Elsevier Publications; 2003. pp. 1618, 1624.*

2. *The Trained Nurses Association of India. Fundamental of Nursing: Procedure Manual. TNAI Publication, 1st edition. pp. 412, 16, 36.*

3. *Lewis LW. Fundamental Skills in Patient Care, 2nd edition. Lippincott Williams and Wilkins. pp. 308-10.*

4. *Christensen BL, Kockrow EO. Foundations of Nursing, 4th edition. Mosby's; St Louise, Missouri; 1999. pp: 435, 439, 442.*

5. *Ruth FC, Constance JH. Fundamentals of Nursing: Human Health and Function, 3rd edition. Lippincott Williams & Wilkins; pp. 989, 922.*

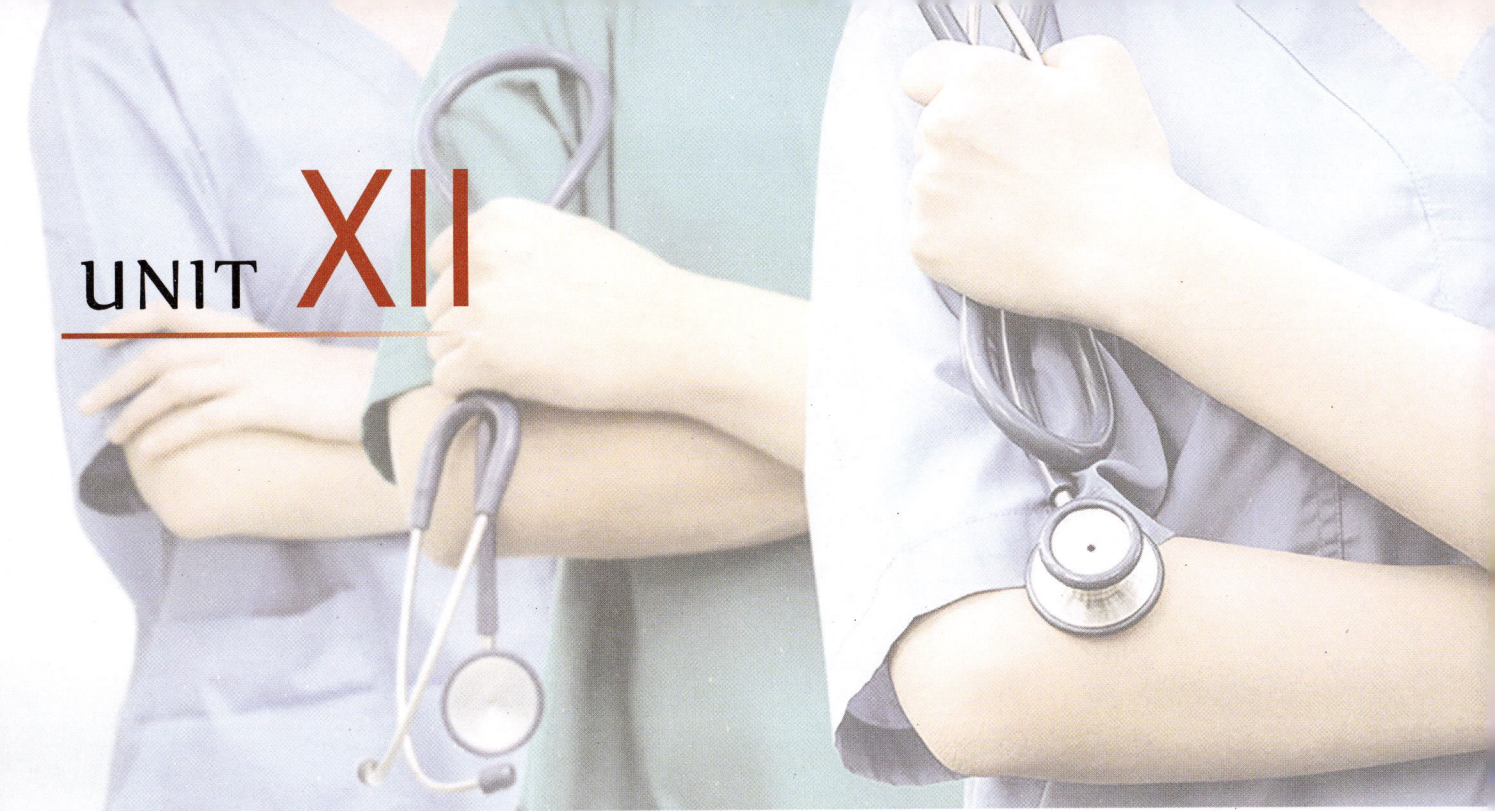

UNIT XII

ADMINISTRATION OF MEDICATIONS

Unit Outline

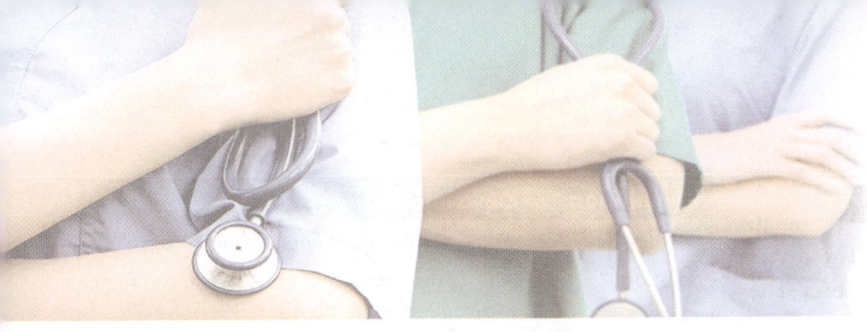

Administration of Medications and Oral Administration

After completing this chapter, you will be able to:
- Describe drug names, types of preparation and types of drug orders
- Identify drug classification and actions
- Discuss adverse effects of drugs
- Calculate drug dosages, using the various systems of equivalents
- Describe the principles used to prepare and administer medications safely by oral route

Key Terms

- Absorption
- Adverse effects
- Anaphylactic reaction
- Idiosyncratic effect
- Infusion
- Injection
- Instillation
- Intradermal
- Intramuscular
- Intravenous
- Intra-arterial
- Intracardiac
- Intrathecal
- Intrapleural
- Epidural
- Intra-articular
- Subcutaneous
- Sublingual
- Synergistic effect

Chapter Outline

- Administration of Medications
- Drug Nomenclature
- Types of Drug Preparations
- Drug Classification
- Mechanisms of Drug Action
- Adverse Drug Effects
- Factors Affecting Drug Action
- Routes of Administration
- Principles of Medication Administration
- Medicine Supply System
- Dosage Calculations
- Using Safety Measures while Preparing Drugs
- Application of Nursing Process in Administration of Medications
- Equivalents

ADMINISTRATION OF MEDICATIONS

One of the basic nursing functions is the medication administration that involves skillful technique and consideration of the patient's development, health status, and safety. The nurse administering medications needs a knowledge base about drugs, including drug names, preparations, classification, adverse effects, and physiologic factors that affect drug action.

DRUG NOMENCLATURE

A drug or medication is any substance that modifies body functions when taken into the body. One drug can have as many as four kinds of names: Its generic name, official name, chemical name, and trademark or brand name. The **generic name** is given before a drug becomes officially an approved medication. The generic name is generally used throughout the drug's use. The **official name** is the name under which it is listed in one of the official publications, e.g., pharmacopeia. The **chemical name** is the name by which a chemist knows it; this name describes the constituents of the drug. The drug's **trade name** is the name given by the drug manufacturer. The trade name is also called the brand name.

The study that deals with chemicals that affect the body's functioning is called **Pharmacology**. A **pharmacist** is a person licensed to prepare and dispense drugs. Physicians, dentists, psychiatrists, podiatrists, physician assistants and advance practice nurses have prescriptive authority. Prescriptive authority for advance practice nurses (clinical nurse specialists, nurse practitioners certified nurse anesthetists, nurse midwives) and physician assistants varies in the degree of independence and varies from state to state. Nurses must be familiar with the laws relative to prescriptive authority in their state of practice.

TYPES OF DRUG PREPARATIONS

Drugs are available in many forms, or preparations. The form in which the drug is prepared may determine the route of administration. Drug preparations are available for oral, topical, and parenteral administration. Some drugs, may be prepared in only one form, can be administered by a certain route. Others may be supplied in several preparations, allowing them to be given through various routes (Table 1).

TABLE 1: Common types of drug preparations

Preparation	Description
Capsule	Powder or gel form of an active drug enclosed in a gelatinous container, may also be called liquigel
Elixir	Medication in a clear liquid containing water, alcohol, sweeteners and flavor
Enteric coated	A tablet or pill coated to prevent stomach irritation
Extended release	Preparation of a medication that allows for slow and continuous release over a predetermined period.
Liniment	Medication mixed with alcohol, oil, or soap, which is rubbed on the skin
Lotion	Drug particles in a solution for topical use
Lozenge	Small oval, round, or oblong preparation containing a drug in a flavored or sweetened base, which dissolve in the mouth and releases the medication; also called troche
Ointment	Semisolid preparation containing a drug to be applied externally; also called an inunction
Pill	Mixture of a powdered drug with a cohesive material; may be round or oval

Contd...

Preparation	Description
Powder	Single or mixture of finely ground drugs
Solution	A drug dissolved in another substance (e.g., in an aqueous solution)
Suppository	An easily melted medication preparation in a firm base such as gelatin that is inserted into the body cavity (vagina, rectum)
Suspension	Finely divided, undissolved particles in a liquid medium, should be shaken before use
Syrup	Medication combined in a water and sugar solution
Tablet	Small, solid dose of medication compressed or molded into hard disc may be any color, size, or shape; enteric-coated are coated with a substance that is insoluble in gastric acids to reduce gastric irritation by the drug
Transdermal patch	Unit dose of medication applied directly to skin for diffusion through skin and absorption into the blood

DRUG CLASSIFICATION

Drug classification or drug classes, are group of drugs that share similar characteristics. Drugs are classified in several ways:

- As per effect on body systems: Drugs that affect respiratory system, drugs that affect the cardio vascular system, etc.
- As per chemical composition
- As per clinical indication for the drug or therapeutic action (analgesic, antibiotic)

MECHANISMS OF DRUG ACTION

- **Pharmacokinetics:** It is the effect of the body on the drug. It is the movement of drug molecule in the body in relation to the drug's absorption distribution, metabolism, and excretion.
- **Absorption:** Is the process by which a drug is transferred from its site of entry into the body to the blood stream. Absorption of a drug is influenced by several factors, which are:
  - **Route of administration:** The rate of absorption depends on the route of administration. Drugs given orally usually take the longest to be absorbed. Injected medications are usually absorbed more rapidly than oral medications. Drugs administered intravenously are placed directly into the blood stream and take effect quickly.
  - **Lipid solubility:** Cell membranes have a fatty and acid layer. A drug that is more lipid soluble can be

absorbed more readily and pass more easily through the cell membrane

- **pH:** Acidic drugs are well absorbed in the stomach. Drugs that are basic remain ionized or insoluble in an acid environment. These drugs, are not absorbed before reaching the small intestine.
- **Blood flow:** Absorption is increased with increased blood flow. Patients with impaired circulatory function absorb drugs less rapidly than do patients with normal circulatory function.
- **Local condition of the site of administration:** The more extensive and absorbing surface, the greater the absorption of the drug and more rapid the effect. For example, a patient with burns would have poor absorption from an intramuscular injection. Food in the stomach can delay the absorption of some medications or enhance the rate of absorption of other drugs. Drug absorption can be manipulated with sustained release preparations or enteric coated preparations which are resistant to the digestive action of the stomach.
- **Drug dosage:** A loading dose, or a larger than normal dose, is usually given when a patient is in acute distress and the maximum therapeutic effect is desired as quickly as possible. A maintenance dose is a lower dosage that becomes the usual or daily dosage.

Distribution

After drug has been absorbed into the blood stream, it is distributed throughout the body. Distribution depends on blood flow to the tissues, the drug's ability to leave the blood stream and is ability to enter the cells. Certain other factors may also influence distribution. The drug may bind to plasma protein, which cause unequal distribution and prevent the drug from reaching its intended site of action. Another factor affecting distribution is the blood brain barrier. Many drugs cannot penetrate the barrier, influencing distribution. Some drugs fail to penetrate central nervous system as readily as others. The placenta, on the other hand is not a barrier like the blood brain barrier. Drugs readily move across the placenta and many drugs produce harmful effects to the fetus. These factors must be considered when planning and implementing drug therapies.

Metabolism

Metabolism is the change of a drug from its original form to a new form. The liver is the primary site for drug metabolism. Various processes and enzymes are involved in metabolism. Physiologic changes associated with aging, the presence of liver disease or other factors that impair the functioning of the liver decrease the ability of the liver to metabolize drugs. Other tissues such as those of the gastrointestinal tract, lungs, kidney and skin, have a role in drug metabolism.

Excretion

After the drug is broken down to an inactive form, excretion of the drug occurs. Excretion is the process of removing a drug, or its metabolites, from the body. The kidneys excrete most drugs. The lungs are the primary route for the excretion of gaseous substances such as inhalation anesthetics. Many drugs are excreted through bile in the gastrointestinal tract. The sweat, salivary and mammary glands are also the routes of drug excretion. Some medications may be contraindicated, or dosages may need to be adjusted if renal excretion is impaired. Changes associated with aging, disease or the presence of other factors that impair the functioning of the kidneys can decrease their ability to excrete drugs.

ADVERSE DRUG EFFECTS

Although therapeutic effect is the desired outcome in administration of medicine sometimes secondary undesirable effects occur. Undesirable effects other than the desired effects of a drug are known as adverse side effects. It is important to monitor for adverse effects from drug therapy.

The adverse effects include allergic effects, drug tolerance, toxic effects, idiosyncratic effects, and drug interactions. It is important to monitor for adverse effects of drug therapy. Serious adverse reactions must be documented according to agency policy and should be reported.

Allergic Effect

An allergic effect is an immune system response that occurs when the body interprets the administered drug as a foreign substance and forms the antibodies against it. Drug allergies can be manifested in a variety of symptoms ranging from minor to serious. The reaction can occur immediately after the patient receives the drug or be delayed for hours and days. Some of the signs and symptoms of a drug allergy are rash, urticaria, fever, diarrhea, nausea and vomiting. The most serious allergic effect is called an **anaphylactic reaction** (anaphylaxis). It is life threatening and results in respiratory distress, sudden severe bronchospasm, and cardiovascular collapse. This reaction is treated with vasopressors, bronchodilators, corticosteroids, oxygen therapy, intravenous fluids, and antihistamines.

Drug Tolerance

Drug tolerance occurs when the body becomes accustomed to the effects of a particular drug over a period of time. Larger doses of the drug must be taken to produce the desired effect.

Toxic Effect

Toxic effects are specific groups of symptoms related to drug therapy that carry risk for permanent damage or death. The organ or system affected by the toxicity is used to name the toxicity as in hepatotoxicity, or damage to the liver. Toxicities can occur from a cumulative effect. A cumulative effect occurs when the body cannot metabolize one dose of a drug before another dose is administered. The drug taken frequently is more than it is excreted, and each new dose increases the total quantity in the body.

Idiosyncratic Effect

An idiosyncratic effect is an unusual or peculiar response to a drug that may manifest itself by over response, under response, or even the opposite of the expected response.

Drug Interactions

Drug interactions occur when one drug is affected in some way by another drug, a food or another substance that is taken at the same time. Drug interactions may be advantageous when a medication is given to decrease the adverse effects of a drug or increase its therapeutic effects. In a drug-drug interaction, the combined effect of two or more drugs acting simultaneously produces an effect either less than that of each drug alone (antagonist effect) or greater than that of each drug alone (synergistic effect). Alcohol and barbiturates when taken together create an non-beneficial synergistic effect with the potential for significantly increased central nervous system depression. Drug interactions in older adults are dangerous because they are likely to take more than one drug and they often see more than one physician and do not always remember to bring the medications that they are taking to show to physician they consult. This leads to polypharmacy (the taking of more than two medications at a time), which can result in serious drug interactions.

Drug interactions can also occur, if someone is taking dietary supplements and herbal and 'natural' remedies. Health care providers need to be aware of the intended benefits, possible adverse effects and potential drug interactions.

FACTORS AFFECTING DRUG ACTION

A number of factors other than the drug itself can affect its action. A person may not respond in the same manner to successive doses of a drug. In addition, the identical drug and dosage may affect different clients differently.

Developmental Factors

Drug taken during pregnancy poses a risk throughout the pregnancy, but poses the highest risk during the first trimester due to the formation of vital organs and functions of the fetus during this time. Most drugs are contraindicated because of the possible adverse effects on the fetus.

Infants usually require small dosage because of their body size and the immaturity of their organs, especially the liver and kidneys. Differences in gastric acidity and liver enzymes required during metabolism may require different medication choices and dosages than adults.

Older adults have different response to medication due to physiologic changes that accompany aging. These changes include decreased liver and kidney function, which can result in the accumulation of the drug in the body. In addition, the older person may be on multiple drugs and incompatibilities may occur. Older adults often experience decreased gastric motility and decreased gastric acid production and blood flow, which can impair drug absorption. Increased adipose tissue and decreased total body fluid proportionate to the body mass can increase the possibility of drug toxicity. Older adults may also experience a decreased number of protein-binding sites and changes in the blood-brain barrier.

Gender

Differences in the way men and women respond to drugs are chiefly related to the distribution of body fat and fluid and hormonal differences.

Culture, Ethnic and Genetic Factors

A client's response to a drug is influenced by genetic variations such as gender, size and body composition. This variation in response is called **pharmacogenetics**. Drug metabolism and variations in enzymes are genetically determined and as a result, may affect a drug response. For example, the genes that control liver metabolism vary. Some clients may have slow liver metabolism and not achieve an adequate response to a medication whereas others are rapid metabolizers and may require lower doses of a medication to avoid adverse reactions.

Ethnopharmacology is the study of the effect of ethnicity on response to prescribed medication. Research has shown that certain medications may work well at usual therapeutic dosage for certain ethnic groups but toxic for others. Pharmacogenetics can also vary in race or ethnic groups.

Cultural factors and practice (Values and beliefs) can also affect a drug's action. For example, a herbal remedy (e.g., Chinese herb, ginseng) may speed up or slow down the metabolism of prescribed medications.

Diet

Nutrients can affect the action of a medication for example vitamin K in green leafy vegetable can counteract the effect of an anticoagulant such as warfarin.

Environment

The client's environment can affect the action of drugs, particularly those that can alter behavior and mood. Therefore, nurses while assessing the effects of a drug need to consider the drug in context of the client's personality and milieu. Environmental temperature may also affect drug activity. When environmental temperature is high, the peripheral blood vessels dilate intensifying the action of vasodilators. In contrast, the cold environment and the consequent vasoconstriction inhibits the action of vasodilators but enhances the action of vasoconstrictors. A client who takes a sedative or analgesic in a busy, noisy environment may not be benefited completely than if the environment is quiet and peaceful.

Psychological Factors

A client's expectations about the action of the drug may affect the response of the medications accordingly. For example, a client who believes that codeine is ineffective as an analgesic may experience no relief from pain after it is given.

Illness and Disease

Illness and disease can also affect the action of drugs. For example, aspirin can reduce the body temperature of a client with fever but has no effect on the temperature of client without fever. Drug action is altered in clients with circulatory, liver or kidney dysfunction.

Time of Administration

The time of administration of oral medication affects the relative speed with which they act. Orally administered medications are absorbed more quickly, if the stomach is empty. Thus, oral medications taken 2 hours before meals act faster than those taken after meals. Some medications. for example iron preparations irritate the gastrointestinal tract and are given after a meal, so that it can be tolerated well.

ROUTES OF ADMINISTRATION

The route of administration should be indicated when the drug is ordered. When administering a drug, the nurse should ensure that the pharmaceutical preparation is appropriate for the prescribed route.

Oral

Oral administration is the most common, least expensive and most convenient route for most clients. In oral administration, the drug is swallowed, therefore, the skin is not broken as in case of injection. Oral administration is also a safe method.

The major disadvantages are possible unpleasant taste of the drugs, irritation of gastric mucosa, irregular absorption from the gastrointestinal tract, slow absorption, and in some cases harm to the client's teeth. For example, the liquid preparation of ferrous sulfate (iron) can stain the teeth.

Sublingual

In sublingual administration drug is placed under the tongue where it dissolves. In a relatively short time, the drug is largely absorbed into the blood vessels on the underside of the tongue. The medication should not be swallowed.

Buccal

Buccal means "pertaining to the cheek". In buccal administration, a medication is held in the mouth against the mucous membranes of the cheek until the drug dissolves. The drug may act locally on the mucous membranes of the mouth or systemically when it is swallowed in the saliva.

Parenteral

The parenteral route is defined as other than through the alimentary or respiratory tract that is by needle. The following are some of the most common routes for parenteral administration:

- Subcutaneous (hypodermic): Into the subcutaneous tissue just below the skin.
- Intramuscular: Into a muscle
- Intradermal: Under the epidermis (into the dermis)
- Intravenous: Into a vein
- Intra-arterial: Into an artery
- Intracardiac: Into the heart muscle
- Intraosseous: Into a bone
- Intrathecal or Intraspinal: Into the spinal canal
- Intrapleural: Into the pleural space
- Epidural: Into the epidural space
- Intra-articular: Into a joint

Topical

Topical applications are those applied to a circumscribed surface area of the body. They affect only the area to which they are applied. Topical applications include the following:

- Dermatological preparations applied to the skin, e.g., applying transdermal patch.
- Instillations and irrigations applied into body cavities or orifices, such as urinary bladder, eyes, ears, nose, rectum and vagina.
- Inhalations: Administered into the respiratory tract by a nebulizer or positive pressure breathing apparatus. Air, oxygen, and vapor are generally used to carry the drug into the lungs.

PRINCIPLES OF MEDICATION ADMINISTRATION

Medication Orders

No medication may be given to a patient without a medication order from a licensed practitioner. Each health agency has its own policies. Usually the order is written, although telephone and verbal orders are also acceptable in number of agencies. Nursing students need to know the policies by the different agencies about the medication order. In some instances, orders are written on a form designed specifically for a primary care provider's order. This becomes part of a patient's permanent record. Many health care facilities use a computer-generated pharmacy order system. Some facilities are beginning to use computer prescriber order entry system (CPOE). CPOE systems allow the prescriber to enter medication orders in a standard format CPOE's guide the prescriber in complete, accurate, and appropriate ordering. Computer sends the order directly to the pharmacy and enters the order into the patient's permanent record. This prevents any guessing when hand writing is illegible. Some of the informations, provided by this system include recommended dose of medications, drug specific information, current patient information, laboratory tests that monitor the action of drug and potential interactions that may occur with other medications or food. A computerized orders entry system can make medication administration safer and reduce adverse drug events.

For safer practice, the nurse should follow only a written or typed order or an order entered into a computer order entry system as these types of orders are less likely to result in error or misunderstanding. Under certain circumstances, such as in emergency a verbal order from the physician may be given to a registered nurse or a pharmacist.

Types of Medication Orders

There are four common medication orders which are as follows:

1. A stat order indicates that the medication is to be given immediately and only once.
2. The single order or one time order is for the medication to be given once at a specified time.
3. The standing order may or may not have a termination date. A standing order may be carried out indefinitely until the order is written to cancel it, or it may be carried out for a specified number of days.
4. A PRN or as needed order permits the nurse to give a medication when she feels it is necessary to give. The nurse must use her good judgment still about when the medication is needed and when it can be safely administered.

Essential Parts of a Drug Order

The medication order consists of seven parts:

1. Patient's name
2. Date and time the order is written
3. Name of the drug to be administered
4. Dosage of the drug
5. Route by which the drug is to be administered
6. Frequency of administration of the drug
7. Signature of person writing the order.

Patient's Name

The patient's full name is used. The middle name or initial should be included to avoid confusion with other patients. Be extremely careful while administering medications in case there is more than one patient in the unit with the same last name. Not only can the nurse give the wrong patient the wrong medication, but, also a prescriber may write an order in the wrong patients chart.

Date and Time the Order is Written

It is important to write the date and time of the order because the nursing staff in inpatient units changes several times during each 24-hour period, it prevents error as different nurses take charge of the patient care. When an order is to be followed for a specified number of days, the date and time are important so that the discontinuation date and time can be determined accurately.

Name of the Drug to be Administered

The name of the drug is stated in the order, either by the brand name or by the generic name.

Dosage of the Drug

The dosage of a drug can be stated in either the metric or the apothecary system. The metric system has been adopted internationally, is the most widely used, and is the safest measurement system for drug dosages. Apothecary measurements are used less frequently. Self-administered drugs are commonly labeled in household measurements to facilitate administration.

Route by which the Drug is to be Administered

The route to be used while administering a medicine is stated clearly because some drugs can be given in more than one way and others may be used safely through only one route.

Frequency of Administration of the Drug

The time and frequency with which a drug is to be administered are usually stated in standard abbreviations in the medication order (Table 2).

The nursing service, facility policy, and pharmacy departments of inpatient facilities usually determine the hours at which routine drugs are given. If the drug is to be given only once or twice a day, it is important to decide the hour that what time it should be given. It depends on the nature of the drug and the patient's plan of care, as well as standard facility administration times. Whenever possible, the patient's choice of time should be considered.

TABLE 2: Standard abbreviations pertaining to medications

Abbreviation	Meaning	Abbreviation	Meaning
Ad.	Up to	Inj.	Injection
a.a.	of each	I.M.	Intramuscular
a.c.	Before meals	I.V.	Intravenous
p.c.	After meals	Subq. Or S.C.	Subcutaneous
b.d. (b.i.d.)	Twice a day	Ung.	Ointment
t.d. (t.a.d.) (t.d.s.)	Three time a day	Pulv.	Powder
q.i.d.	Four times a day	Mist.	Mixture
h.s.	At bed time	Gtt. (Gutt)	Drop
q.o.d.	Every other day	Gtts.	Drops
q.o.n.	Every other night	amp.	Ampule
o.d.	Each day or once in a day	amt.	Amount
h.n.	To night	Aq.	Water
o.n.	Each night	Cap.	Capsule
o.m.	Each morning	dil	Dilute
C.m.	Tomorrow morning	dos	A dose
q.h.	Every hour	elix	elixir
q.2.h.	Every 2 hours	ext.	Extract
q.3.h.	Every 3 hours	H.Hr.	Hour
q.6.h	Every 6 hours	R.X.	Take
Alt. hor.	Every other hour	Tr. (Tinct)	Tincture
Alt. Dieb	Every other day	S.V.M.	Methylated spirit
Alt. noe.	Every other night	S.V.R	Rectified spirit
Ad. Lib.	As desired, at pleasure	Cont.	Continuously
Noet.	Night	U.	Unit
Non.rep.	Not to be repeated	tbsp.	Table spoon
N.P.O.	Nothing per mouth	tsp.	Tea spoon

Contd...

Abbreviation	Meaning	Abbreviation	Meaning
P.r.n.	Whenever necessary	O	Pint
S.O.S.	If necessary in emergency	M	Minim
Stat	At once	Dr.orz.	Dram
rep.	Repeat	fl. Dr.	Fluid dram
s.s. (f.s.)	Half	f1.oz.	Fluid ounce
C	With	Gr.	grain
S	Without		

Drugs should be administered punctually as ordered. A nurse administering drug to several patients, however, cannot give all of the drugs exactly on the hour indicated. Agency policies vary, but a common practice is that the drug should be administered within half an hour before or after the indicated hour. Thus, a drug to be administered at 9 am can be administered any time between 8.30 am and 9.30 am using this policy. This policy does not apply to all the drugs, for example preoperative medication ordered to be given at 7.30 am should be administered at the same here because this time is planned in relation to the time of surgery. This also holds true when patients are given drugs before certain diagnostic procedures.

Signature of Person Writing the Order

Signature, with title of the person writing the order is important for legal reasons because the authority to prescribe drugs is defined by state laws. Also, if there is a question about the order, the signature indicates who should be contacted.

Checking the Medication Order

Agency policy specifies the manner in which the medication order is checked. Various systems are used, and nurses should be familiar with the system used in the agency where they work and should implement it correctly to minimize errors. In many institutions, the order is copied into the patient's medication record, often called a (MAR) medication administration record. Increasing numbers of health care facilities are computerizing patient's records, including medication record (CMAR). The nurse is responsible for checking that the medicines ordered are transcribed correctly by comparing it with the original order. The nurse is also responsible for double checking the dosage and appropriateness of the medication.

Questioning the Medication Order

Nurses are legally responsible for the drugs they administer. Any drug order suspected to be an error should be questioned. The suspected error may be in any part of the order.

On certain occasions, the nurse may not think that there is an error in the order but may not understand reason of describing medicine. In such instances, ask the prescriber, how the order relates, to the patient's plan of care. Such practice may prevent a medication error, if wrong medication has been ordered.

Confusion over the decimal point can lead to medication error. A zero should always precede by a decimal point (e.g., 0.1 mg) for clarity.

A drug to which the patient is allergic may be prescribed inadvertently. Best practice is to question the patient, if they have ever received the medication and if they are aware of any reaction to the medicine. It is general practice to indicate clearly on the patient's chart for any drug allergies. An allergic reaction can be life threatening to the patient.

A drug may be ordered that would potentially interact with another drug the patient is taking. All the medications that a nurse is unfamiliar with, should be verified before administration to avoid possible drug interactions. If the nurse has difficulty reading an order, guessing is gross carelessness; checking with the person who wrote the order is the only safe procedure.

Based on the knowledge and experiences nurses have the right to refuse any medications to avoid any harm to the patient. It is important to understand that the patient's safety is a primary objective in the administration of medication.

MEDICINE SUPPLY SYSTEM

Medicine are supplied in a number of ways. Many facilities make use of one or more systems in conjunction with each other. A new technology based on stock supply of unit dose medication in computerized automated dispensing cabinets (ADCs). A large cabinet containing stock medications for the unit is used.

The nurse accesses the system with a user name and password, calling up a medication list for a specific patient or a list of available medications. In many systems, only medications entered for a specific patient are available for withdrawal at any one time.

Some nursing units use a medication cart for the administration of medications. The standard cart contains individual drawers into which the medications for each patient are placed. The drawer is labeled with the patient's name. The nurse moves the cart from room to room when dispensing medications.

Another medication delivery system uses barcode-enabled medication administration (BCMA). BCMA technology can improve patient's safety and the accuracy of medication administration and documentation. The nurse scans his or her ID, the patient's ID, and each package of medication to be administered. The system confirms the nurse's dispensing authority and the patient's ID, matching the patient with this medication profile. If any of the information is incorrect or does not match, an alert message will appear on the screen, notifying the nurse of the discrepancy.

DOSAGE CALCULATIONS

Systems of Measurement

Nurses need to be proficient in the use of weight and measures as well as system of measurement to calculate drug dosage and prepare medication for administration. Three systems of measurement are used for administering medications. The metric system, the apothecary system, and the household system. The nurse may be called on to convert dosages from one system of measurement to another system of measurement. It is important to be able to calculate commonly used equivalents.

Metric System

The metric system is the most widely accepted and convenient system. The basic units of measurement are the meter (linear), the liter (volume), and the gram (weight). The metric system is a decimal system, in which each unit can be divided into multiples of 10 (10,100,1000). Calculation of the metric system often involves moving the decimal point to the right or left.

Weight

- 1 Kilogram = 1,000 grams
- 1 gram = 1,000 milligrams
- 1 milligram = 1,000 micrograms

Volume

- 1 Liter = 1,000 milliliters or cubic centimeters

It may be necessary to convert drug dosages to different units in the metric system. To convert a larger unit into a smaller unit, move the decimal point to the right. To convert a smaller unit into a larger unit, move the decimal points to the left, e.g., 0.5 g equal to 500 mg and 900 mg equal to 0.9 g.

Apothecary System

The apothecary system is less convenient and precise than the metric system and is infrequently used. The basic unit of weight is the grain. The minim, dram, ounce, pint and quart are used for volume. In this system, Roman numerals are used to express numbers (grains X) and quantities less than 1 are written in fraction form (grains 1/4).

Household System

This system is the least accurate system of measurement and is not widely used except in home setting. Teaspoon, tablespoon, teacup, and glass are commonly used household measures.

Methods of Computing Drug Dosages

Sometimes drugs are prepared and supplied in the amount ordered by the prescriber, and the nurse can see while checking the medication label that no calculation is necessary. At other times, drugs are not prepared and supplied in the exact quantities called for in the medication order, and the nurse must do a dosage calculation to determine what quantity of medication the patients is to receive.

Calculating Dosages

Several formulas can be used to calculate drug dosages. Formula to calculate the ratio

$$\frac{\text{Dose on hand}}{\text{Quantity on hand}} = \frac{\text{Desired dose}}{\text{Quantity desired (x)}}$$

For example erythromycin 500 mg is ordered.

It is supplied in a liquid form containing 250 g in 5 mL. To calculate the dosage, the nurse used the formula

$$\frac{\text{Dose on hand (250) mg}}{\text{Quantity on hand (5 mL)}} = \frac{\text{Desired dose (500 mg)}}{\text{Quantity desired (x)}}$$

$$250\,x = 5\ \text{mL} \times 500\ \text{mg}$$

$$x = \frac{5\ \text{mL} \times 500\ \text{mg}}{250\ \text{mL}}$$

$$x = 10\ \text{mL}$$

Therefore, the dose ordered is 10 mL. The nurse can also use this formula to calculate dosages:

$$\text{Amount to administer (x)} = \frac{\text{Desired dose}}{\text{Dose on hand}} \times \text{Quantity on hand}$$

For example, heparin is in prepared dilution of 10,000 units per milliliter. If the order is 5,000 units, the nurse uses above formula to calculate.

$$x = \frac{5,000}{10,000} = 0.5\ \text{mL}$$

Therefore, the nurse injects 0.5 mL for 5,000 unit dose.

Dosages for Children

For children dosages are calculated as per the body surface area of the body according to weight and height of the patient. Surface area of body is determined by using a nomogram which is considered to be the most accurate method of calculating a child's dose Fig. 1. The formula is the ratio of the child's body surface area to the surface area of an average adult (1.7 square meters, or 7.7 m^2), multiplied by the normal adult dose of the drug:

$$\text{Child's dose} = \frac{\text{Surface area of child (m}^2)}{1.7\ \text{m}^2} \times \text{normal adult dose}$$

For example, a child weigh 10 kg and is 50 cm tall has a body surface area of 0.4 m^2. Therefore, the child's dose of tetracycline corresponding to an adult dose of 250 mg would be:

$$\text{Child's dose} = \frac{0.4\ \text{m}^2}{1.7\ \text{m}^2} \times 250\ \text{mg}$$
$$= 0.23 \times 250 = 58.82\ \text{mg}$$

USING SAFETY MEASURES WHILE PREPARING DRUGS

Safety is of the utmost importance in preparing and implementing drug administration. Medication errors are defined as the preventable inappropriate use of medications. These errors occur when medications are ordered, transcribed, dispensed, administered, and monitored. Medication errors can occur with almost any type of drug. There are many interventions that can minimize the risk for medication errors. These are:

Three Checks and the Rights of Medication Administration

Observe the three checks and the rights of medication administration while administering medications to ensure medications are being administered safely: Check the label on the medication package of container three times during medication preparation and administration Box 1. The label should be read:

- When the nurse reaches for the container or unit dose package.
- After retrieval from the drawer and compared with the computerized medication administration record (CMAR) and before pouring from a multi-dose container
- While replacing the container to the drawer or shelf or before giving the unit dose medication to the patient.

Box 1

Check three times for safe medication administration

First check
- Read the medication administration record (MAR)
- Compare the label of the medication against the MAR
- Check the expiry date of the medication

Second check
- While preparing the medication (e.g., pouring, drawing up, or placing unopened package in a medication cup), look at the medication label and check against the MAR

Third check
- Recheck the label on the container (e.g., vial, bottle) before returning to its storage place

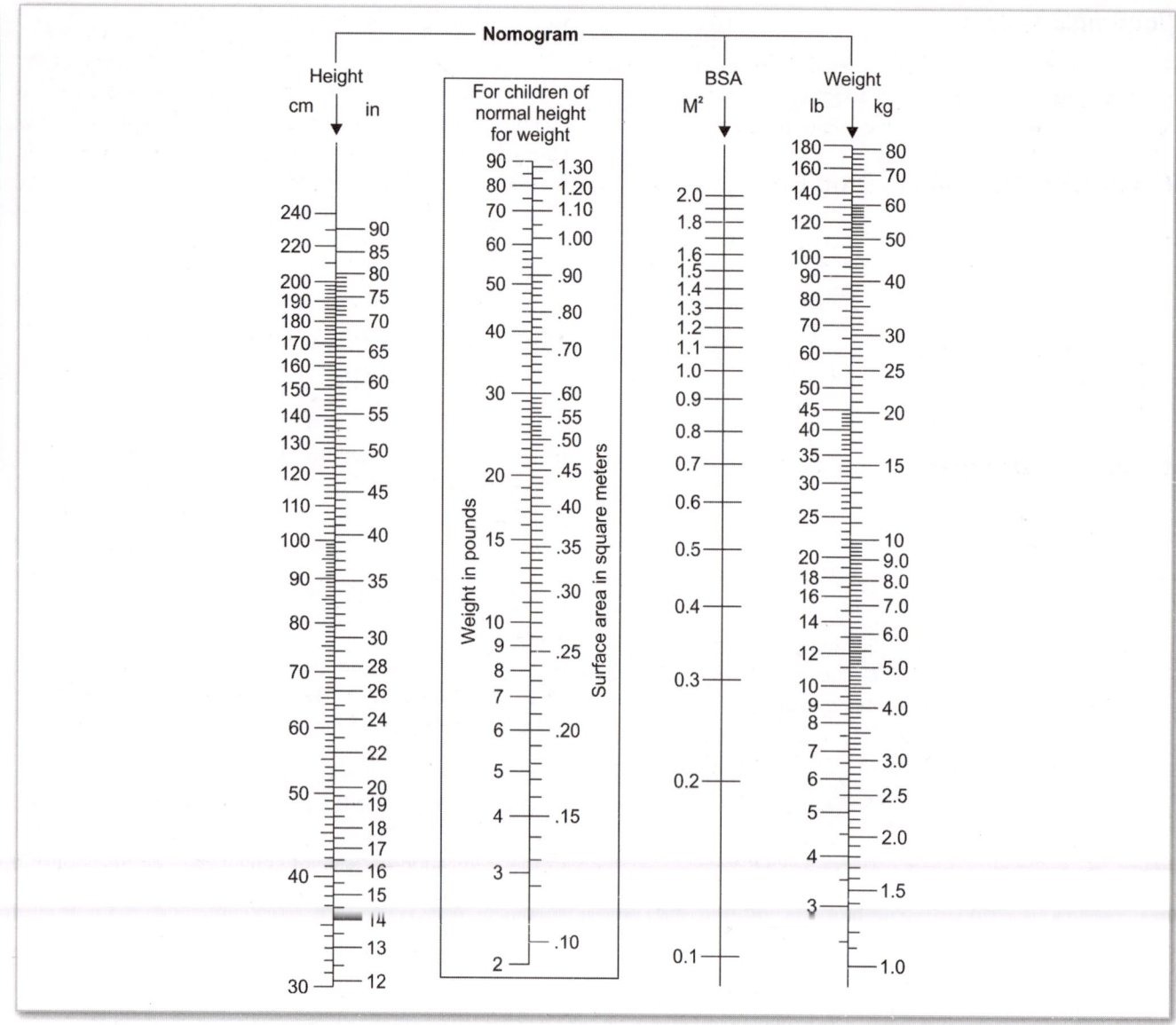

Fig. 1: Nomogram with estimated body surface area. A straight line is drawn between the child's height (on the left) and the child's weight (on the right). The point at which the line intersects the surface area column is the estimated body surface area

The rights of medication administration can help to ensure accuracy while administering medications Box 2. Ensure that the

1. Right medication is given to the
2. Right patient in the
3. Right dosage through the
4. Right route at the
5. Right time
   Additional rights have been suggested to include ensuring
6. The right reason and
7. The right documentation. Validating the right reason requires the nurse to understand the rationale for

administration and answer the question. "Does it make sense". The right documentation refers to accurate and timely documentation of administration.

These seven rights are principles that nurses have been taught as part of their nursing education, however, nurses may not always adhere to the rights and may also lack knowledge about the medication, including the indication, usual dose, route, actions, adverse effects, contraindications and drug-drug or food-drug interactions. Recently three more rights have been introduced.

8. Right to refuse
9. Right assessment
10. Right evaluation

Box 2

Ten 'Rights' of Medication Administration

Right medication
- The medication given was the medication ordered

Right dose
- The dose ordered is appropriate for the client
- Double-check calculations that appear questionable
- Know the usual dosage range of the medication
- Question a dose outside of usual dosage range

Right time
- Give the medication at right frequency and at the time ordered according to agency policy
- Medication given within 30 minutes. Before or after the scheduled time are considered to meet the right time standard

Right route
- Give the medication by the ordered route
- Make Certain that the route is safe and appropriate for the client.

Right client
- Check the client identification bond with each administration of a medication

Right client education
- Explain information about the medication to the client

Right documentation
- Document medication administration after given it, not before.
- If time of administration differs from prescribed time note the time on the MAR and give reason
- If medication is not given, document the reason why

Right to refuse
- Adult clients have this right to refuse the medication
- Nurses role is to communicate the client's refusal to health care provider

Right assessment
- Some medications require specific assessments of vitals prior to administration, e.g., pulse, BP, etc.

Right evaluation
- Conduct appropriate follow-up-to know whether the desired result is achieved or not.

Maintaining a Safe Environment

An environment that promotes safety and good working habits contributes to accuracy in the preparation of drugs for administration. Good lighting must be present when preparing drugs. Increased noise can decrease the ability to concentrate. So medication should be prepared in a relatively quiet location. The nurse who is preparing drugs should work alone to avoid distractions and interruptions, which may lead to errors.

After beginning to prepare drugs for administration do not leave them unattended. If it is imperative to leave for a short time, place the drugs that have been prepared in a locked area, such as the medication cart. The nurse who prepares the medication should also administers the drug and maintains the records of drug administration.

Handling Controlled Substances Safely

Medication dispensing rooms should be locked. Controlled substances are kept in a locked drawer or container as an added safety measure, providing for a "double locked" system. Narcotics or controlled substances may be ordered only by physicians, and in some states nurse practitioner, who are registered with Department of Justice, Bureau of Narcotics, and Dangerous Drugs. According to federal law, a record must be kept for each narcotic drug that is administered. The following information are required in the record:

- Name of the patient receiving the narcotic drug
- Amount of the narcotic drug used
- Hour of administering the narcotic drug
- Name of the physician who prescribed the narcotic
- Name of the nurse who administered the narcotic

It is a common practice to check narcotics daily at specified intervals for example at each shift change. The amount of narcotics on hand is counted, and each used narcotic must be accounted for on the narcotic record. A narcotic count that is not checked properly must be reported immediately. The law requires these special precaution to aid in the control of drug abuse by patients and health care workers.

If for any reason narcotic drug prepared for administration has to be discarded, a second nurse should act as a witness and that person should also sign the narcotic sheet. Document with a witness any time a full dosage is not given or some of the narcotic needs to be disposed off.

Identifying the Patient

Identification of the patient is essential to safe drug administration. Before administering the drug, check carefully to see that the right drug is being given to the right patient. Patient in inpatient health care units usually wear identification bracelets. Identify the patient by checking the identification bracelet, validate the patient name and identification number, medical record number and birth date, comparing with the CMAR. Also ask patient to state his or her name or call the patient by name.

APPLICATION OF NURSING PROCESS IN ADMINISTRATION OF MEDICATIONS

Assessment

Check the order for each medication, noting the patient's name, drug name, dosage route, time, and the date the order was written to be certain it is still valid. Check the patient's record for any allergies. Determine, why the patient is receiving the drug. If previous doses have been given, assess for therapeutic effects. Assess for interactions among the drugs the patient is receiving. Determine, if there is any contraindication to taking the drug. Assess the patient's health status, current and past illnesses, laboratory tests results.

Assess for learning needs of patients regarding what the patient knows about each medication. Assess for side effects of the drug if previous doses have been given. Decide whether the route in which the drug is ordered will be effective for the patient. If the patient is nauseated, an oral dose may not be retained. Assess for drugs that must be given with food or on an empty stomach so that timing of the dose will be appropriate.

If antihypertensive drug is to be administered, always check the blood pressure. The apical heart rate is assessed before giving a digitalis preparation. When topical medications are to be applied assess for adverse effects such as inflammation, swelling, redness, or discharge.

Nursing Diagnosis

Data collected by the nurse may lead to the development of several nursing diagnosis related to medication administration. Each nursing diagnosis statement identifies a patient problem and suggests expected patient outcomes. The following are examples of appropriate nursing diagnosis:

- Ineffective health maintenance related to lack of knowledge about anticoagulant medications
- Anxiety related to daily self-injection of insulin
- Disturbed body image related to effects of chemotherapy
- Constipation related to use of narcotics
- Risk of aspiration related to impaired swallowing of oral medications
- Risk for poisoning related to confusion about medication dosage
- Deficient knowledge related to interaction between herbal remedies and prescribed medications
- Disturbed sleep pattern related to consistent use of sedative hypnotics

Planning

Careful planning and incorporation of the medication administration schedule into the daily shift work schedule is essential for the medications to reach the patient's on time. The overall goals of medication administration are:

- All medication ordered should safely administered to each patient on time
- The medication will be effective
- No allergic reaction to the medication should occur.
- The patient must understand why the drug is prescribed, adhere to the medication schedule, and report serious side effects.

Expected outcomes from the above nursing diagnosis might be:

- Pain is relieved for 3 hours after administration of analgesics
- Blood pressure is controlled within normal limits by antihypertensive medication within 1 week.
- Heart rate is regular while taking antiarrhythmic medication
- Wound culture will be negative at the end of antibiotic therapy
- Patient verbalizes the reason for the medication and the side effects that might occur before discharge

Implementation

While preparing any medication remember to check the label three times and to follow the five rights of medication administration. Always check for patient allergy to the medication before giving it, and document after administering the drug.

Oral Medication

Medication is administered for the diagnosis, cure, treatment or relief of a symptom or for prevention of disease

Oral drugs may be supplied as a tablet capsule, lozenge, or a liquid in the form of syrup, elixir, or suspension. While giving a drug in tablet or capsule form, be sure to offer sufficient water with which to swallow the medication. Some people want to take all their pills at once; others would want to take them one at a time. Remember, any amount of water that is used must be entered in the intake sheet if the patient is on intake and output recording. It is important to assess for side effects of the drug before giving another dose of the medication.

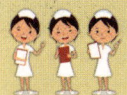

SKILL: ADMINISTERING ORAL MEDICATIONS

Supplies: Unit dose cart stocked with medications, medication cups, straws, drinking cups, water

Steps of Procedure

Review and carry out the standard steps in Appendix

Action/steps	Rationale
Assessment	
1. Verify that the medication record has been compared with the physician's orders within the past 24 hrs. Check each patient's allergies.	Mistakes are sometimes made when transcribing orders on to the medication administration record (MAR). Ensure that no patient is given a medication to which the patient is allergic.
2. Determine that MAR's are present at the cart for all patients to receive medications.	To ensure safety in administration of medication.
3. Assess for side effects of previously given doses of drugs	Prevents potential side effects of the drug
Planning	
4. Assess supplies on cart and restock as necessary	Drinking cups, medication cups for liquid medication
5. Determine which patients are NPO status and which are for certain procedures or surgery	Patients who are NPO must not receive oral medications
6. Calculate any doses that are not individual unit doses	Ensures that the correct amount of drug will be administered as ordered.
Implementation	
7. Wash hands	Medications must be administered using aseptic technique
8. Take the medication cart to the patient room	Unit-dose medication are administered one patient at a time, with the cart at the door of the room.
9. Verify that the patient is present to receive medications	This could delay the taking of oral medications
10. Remove the patient's drawer containing medications, and place it on the top of cart. Check with medication administration record (MAR) for each medication and check the package label with MAR order. Note the following ■ Drug name ■ Dosage ■ Date and time to be given ■ Expiration date of the drug and the order. Proceed to the next medication ordered. Review signs and symptoms of adverse effects	Legally you must know the action, normal dosage, adverse effects, interactions and nursing implication for every drug you give
11. Carefully check each medication second time with the MAR, check the following: ■ Drug name ■ Dosage ■ Route ordered ■ Date and time to be given Place each package into the medicine cup, closed, as the second check is finished.	This completes the second check of medications using the five rights counting the number of medication on the MAR to be given at the designated time. Medication are not opened until third medication check when you are with the patient
12. Pour the liquid medication dose into the medication cup. To pour a liquid medication from a multi bottle, read the dosage from the bottom of the meniscus, the lowest point and pour away from the label.	Do not pour liquid medication over the MAR sheet because spill on MAR sheet will require that the sheet be recopied.
13. Take the medications and the MAR sheet to the patient. Identify the patient by comparing the information on arm band with MAR and explain the procedure, thereby completing the five rights check.	Comparing of the patient name and hospital number is the safest method of identification

Contd...

Action/steps	Rationale
14. Check each medication for the third time as you prepare to open it to give to the patient. Tell the patient what the medication is and check the following: ■ Drug name ■ Dosage ■ Route ordered ■ Date and time	The third check provides an added, safety check for following the five rights of medication administration. Many errors are made because the date and time were not always charted along with drug name and dosage.
15. Pour water for the patient to take pills and perform any assessment necessary before the patient takes medication. Assess for adverse effects and see if any PRN medications are needed.	Liquid is necessary for the swallowing of pills. The heart rate and rhythm must be known before digitalis is administered.
16. Initial the doses given and sign your name on the MAR according to agency policy.	Documentation of an administered dose is done after the patient has taken medication.
17. Proceed to prepare and administer medication to the next patient.	Each patient should receive medications within 30 minutes of the time scheduled.
18. Return the unit dose cart and supplies to the central area.	Retaining the cart makes it available for use later.
Evaluation	
19. For each medication given, ask yourself whether patient had any signs and symptom of adverse effects whether medication appears to be effective in treating the condition.	If a medication is not effective, the use needs to be questioned.
Documentation	
20. Record the medication given	For making sure that the medication is administered

APPENDIX

EQUIVALENTS

Metric Units

The metric system, developed by the French, uses the meter as the basic unit. The metric system is a decimal system, with prefixes that designate the various multiples or divisibles of 10. The most commonly used prefixes in medicine are:

Milli, which means one-thousandth (0.001)

Centi, which means one-hundredth (0.01)

Kilo, which means one thousand (1000)

These prefixes may be affixed to any of the three basic units of measurements, which are:

Meter (m), the unit of length

Gram (g), the unit of weight

Liter (L), the unit of volume

Therefore,

1 millimeter (mm) = 0.001 m

1 milligram (mg) = 0.001 g

1 milliliter (mL) = 0.001 L

1 kilometer (km) = 1000 m

1 kilogram (kg) = 1000 g

1 kiloliter (kL) = 1000 L

Length

The meter (a little longer than a yard) and the kilometer (about 0.6 mile) seldom are used in medicine or nursing. The commonly used measure of length is

1 centimeter (cm) = 0.01 m = about 0.4 inch

Volume

The most frequently used measures of volume are the liter and the milliliter. Some useful equivalents to know are:

1000 milliliters (mL) = 1 liter (L)

1000 cubic centimeters = 1 liter (L)

Weight

The gram designates the weight of 1 mL of distilled water at 4°C. The most frequently used units of weight are:

1,000,000 micrograms (mcg) = 1 gram (g)

1000 micrograms (mcg) = 1 milligram (mg)

1000 milligrams (mg) = 1 gram (g) 1000 grams (g)

= 1 kilogram (kg)

= 2.2 pounds (lb)

Metric Units and their Household Equivalents

Household measurement is inaccurate, with wide variations in the size of teaspoons, teacups, and so forth. The generally accepted household measures are:

60 drops (gtt) = 1 teaspoon (tsp or t)

3 tsp = 1 tablespoon (Tbs or T)

12 Tbs = 1 teacup

16 Tbs = 1 glass (or a standard measuring cup)

Apothecary Units

In the apothecary system:

The unit of weight is the *grain*.

The unit of volume is the *minim*.

Of the many units of measure in the apothecary system, you should know the following units, abbreviations, and equivalents.

Weight

60 grains (gr) = 1 dram (dr or ʒ)

8 drams (dr or ʒ) = 1 ounce (oz or ʒ)

Volume (Table 3)

60 minims (min) = 1 fluid dram (fl dr or fʒ)

8 fl dr = 1 fluid ounce (fl oz or fʒ)

16 fl oz = 1 pint (pt)

2 pt, = 1 quart (qt)

4 qt = 1 gallon (gal)

In the apothecary system, when the symbol or abbreviation is used, the quantity is written in lowercase Roman numerals and follows the symbol. Arabic numerals are used, however in preference to large Roman numerals. For example

5gr = gr v

8 dr = ʒviii

TABLE 3: Metric and household equivalents

Metric unit	Household unit
5 mL	1 tsp
15 mL	1 tbs
180 mL	1 full teacup
240 mL	1 full glass

The quantity one-half may be indicated by the symbol ss.

1 ½ , gr = gr iss

7 ½ gr = gr viiss

Other fractional parts are expressed as common fractions, for example. gr 1/250, gr 1/10.

When pint quart, and gallon are written, the quantity is expressed in Arabic numerals, (e.g., 11/2 pints or 71/2 quarts) 1.

Apothecary Units and Their Household Equivalents (Table 4)

1 drop = 1 minim (m i)

1 tsp = 1 dr (ʒ i)

1 Tbs = 1/2 oz (ʒ ss)

2 Tbs = 1 oz (ʒ i)

1 teacup = 6 oz (ʒ vi)

1 glass or measuring cup = 8 oz (ʒ viii)

2 measuring cups = 1 pt

TABLE 4: Most commonly used approximate equivalents

Metric	Apothecary	Household
0.06 g	Gr i gri	
0.06 mL	Min i	1 drop
1.0 g	Gr xv	
1.0 mL	Min xv	1/5 tsp
5 mL	(1 oz) ʒ i	1 tsp
15 mL	(1/2 oz) ʒ ss	1 tbs
30 mL	(1 oz) ʒ i	2 tbs
500 mL	(16 oz) ʒ16	1 pt
1000 mL	(32 oz) ʒ32	1 qt

*There are many discrepancies among these approximate equivalents. for example, 30 mL is the accepted equivalent for 1 oz (29 .57 mL is the exact equivalent). Such discrepancies are inevitable when two system are used whose equivalents are not exact If the discrepancies are within a 10% margin of error, they usually are acceptable in pharmacology.

BIBLIOGRAPHY

1. Taylor CR, Lillis C, LeMone P, et al. *Fundamentals of Nursing – The Art and Science of Nursing Care, 7th edition.* Wolters Kluwer; 2010.

2. DeWit SC. *Fundamental Concepts and Skills for Nursing. WB Saunders Company.* 2001.

3. Berman AT, Snyder S, Frandsen G. *Kozier & Erb's Fundamentals of Nursing: Concept Process and Practice, 8th edition.* Pearson.

4. Sharma S. *Potter and Perry's Fundamentals of Nursing. A South Asian edition.* Gurugram: Elsevier India. 2013.

5. Brillel. *Foundations for nursing, 2nd edition Appleton century crofts publications.*

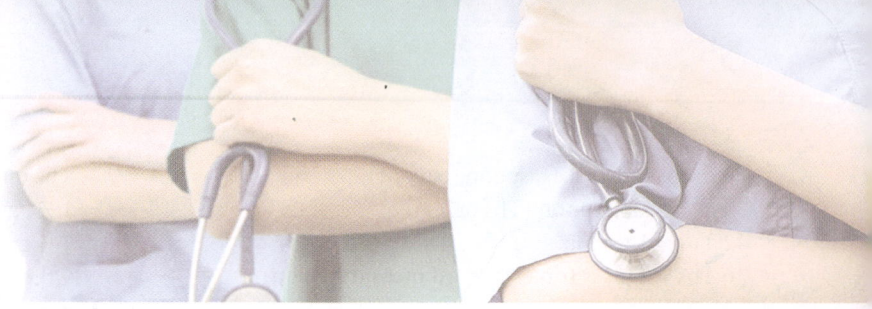

Chapter 56

Parenteral Therapies

INTRODUCTION

The word 'parenteral' means outside the intestines or alimentary canal. It requires the use of syringe and needle, or intravenous catheter, to introduce medications into the body tissues or fluids. Medications that are given parenterally must be sterile, nonallergenic to the patient and readily absorbable. Injections are given for the following **purposes**:

- When the patient cannot take medications by mouth
- To hasten the action of the drug
- When digestive juices would counteract the effects of the drug given through oral route.

Once drugs are injected into the body, they cannot be retrieved. It is therefore essential to observe the following for precaution.

- Ensure that the dose is accurate
- Select the correct site to prevent damage to the tissue
- Use sterile equipment and aseptic technique to prevent infection/sepsis.

The parenteral routes involve injecting medications into various layers of the skin or into veins. The skin is the body's protective covering acting as a barrier between the person and the environment. The outer layer or epithelium is continuously sloughing off dying cells. Below the epidermis is the dermis which contains hair follicles, sweat glands, sebaceous glands, blood vessels and nerve endings. Combined together, these layers of the skin are 1–2 mm in the thickness. Directly below the dermis is the subcutaneous or hypodermal layer of connective tissue, which contains fat cells. The skin has an extensive lymphatic and capillary system, the latter plays a major role in the absorption of medications. The more vascular the tissue, the quicker the medicine is absorbed.

PRINCIPLES FOR SAFE AND EFFECTIVE ADMINISTRATION OF PARENTERAL MEDICATION

- Use only sterile needles and syringes.
- Select the appropriate length of needle to deposit the medication in the proper tissue layer.
- Select the injection site carefully to avoid major nerves, blood vessels and underlying organs.
- Select the injection site that is relatively free of hair, lesions, inflammation, rashes, moles, freckles, etc.
- Rotate injection sites for patients receiving repeated injections.
- Obtain assistance as needed in giving an injection when the patient is a frightened child or uncooperative adult.
- Check for drug allergies before administering an injection
- Aspirate by pulling back the plunger to avoid injecting into the blood vessel.
- Know the medication before administering and observe for side effects and therapeutic action.

ROUTES FOR PARENTERAL MEDICATION

Intradermal, subcutaneous, intramuscular and intravenous routes are used for parenteral medication administration (Fig. 1).

Intradermal Route

The intradermal (ID) route, which deposits small amount of drug solution into the dermal layer, is used extensively for skin testing, such as tuberculin, on the inner surface of the fore arm. The tuberculin syringe with graduated measurement to 1 m^2 is used to measure these small dosages. A fine 24, 27 or 29 gauge (scale of measurement) needle is used at a 15 degree angle of insertion. This creates a pool of medication under the thin layer of skin that forms a bleb (visible elevation of epidermis).

Subcutaneous Route

The subcutaneous (SC) route is used for injecting medication into the tissues below the dermal layer of the skin usually in the upper portion of the upper outer arm, the anterior surface of the thigh, or the abdomen where there are no major vessels or nerves. Small amounts of solution (0.05–1.0 ml) are injected subcutaneously with either a tuberculin or insulin syringe. A 25-gauge or 27-gauge needle is used which is inserted at a 45 or 90 degree angle depending on the needle length and the size of the individual. An obese person requires a longer needle than one who is normal weight, a very thin person requires a shorter needle. Absorption time is slower than with an intramuscular injection owing to the lack of blood vessels in this area as compared with muscle. These sites are used for medications that are to be absorbed slowly for sustained action.

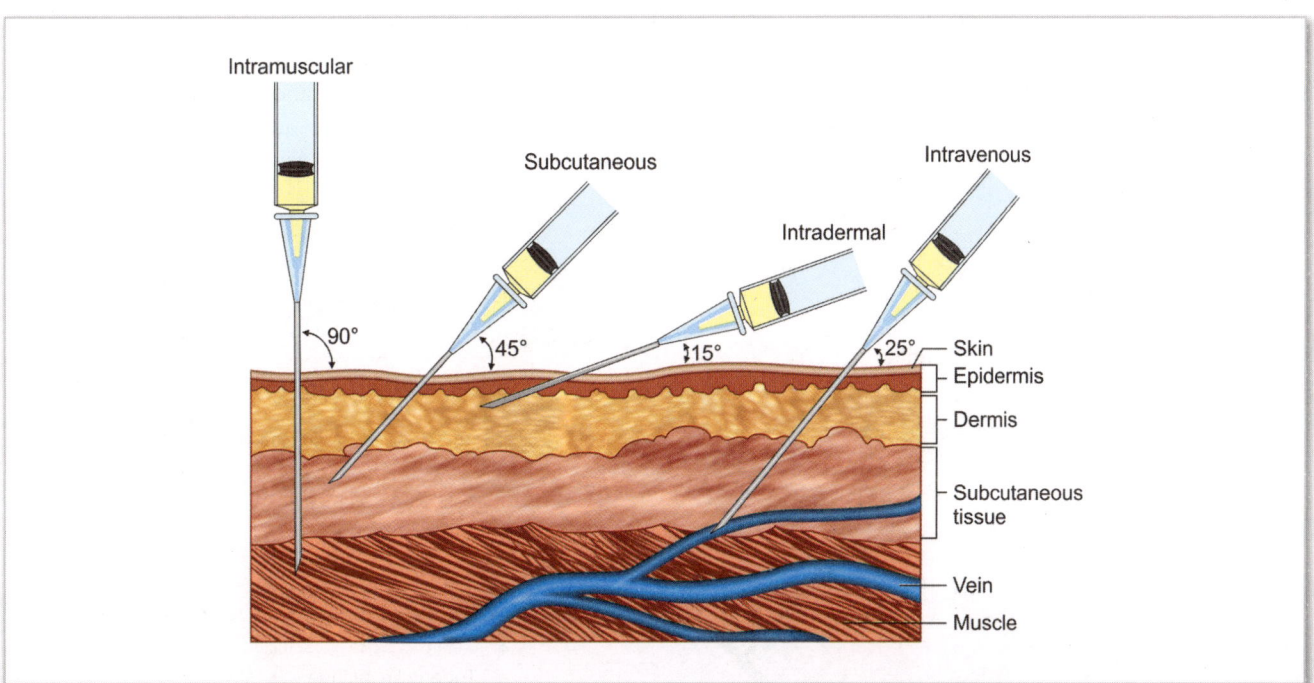

Fig. 1: Angles of various types of injection

Intramuscular Route

The intramuscular route (IM) means medication is injected in the muscular layer. The most frequently used IM sites are the deltoid, dorsogluteal, ventrogluteal, vastus lateralis, and rectus femoris of the thigh. The angle of injection is 90 degrees, and depending on the size of the patient, a needle from 1 to 3 inches in length is utilized. Up to 3 mL can be safely injected in these sites in any patient. The absorption time for IM medications chiefly depends on the form of drug; aqueous solutions are absorbed more rapidly than those in an oil suspension.

Intravenous Route

The intravenous route (IV) is the main method of supplying the patient with fluids and medications when the patient is unable to take them orally. The solution is directly injected through a vein into the circulation. IV fluids are given to supply the body with needed substances or drugs that cannot be supplied as rapidly or efficiently by other means. These substances may be fluid and electrolytes, medications, blood, plasma or other blood components and nutritional formulae containing glucose, amino acids and lipids.

INJECTION EQUIPMENT

Types of Syringes

Syringes are composed of a barrel that has a tip to which the needle is attached and a plunger that fits inside the barrel. The needle, the tip, the inside of the barrel, and the sides of the plunger must be kept sterile. Syringes are made of plastic or glass. The plastic ones are disposable whereas glass syringes can be resterilized and reused.

There are several kinds of syringes, differing in size, shape and material. The three most commonly used types are the standard hypodermic syringe the insulin syringe and the tuberculin syringe (Fig. 2).

A hypodermic syringe comes in 2 mL, 3 mL and 5 mL sizes. The syringe may have two scales marked on it minimum and the milliliter. The milliliter scale is the one normally used. The minimum scale is used for very small dosages.

An insulin syringe is similar to hypodermic syringe but the scale is specially designed for insulin. A 100-unit calibrated scale intended for use with U-100 insulin. This is the only syringe that should be used to administer insulin.

The tuberculin syringe was originally designed to administer tuberculin solution. It is a narrow syringe, calibrated in tenths and hundredths of milliliter (up to 1 mL) on one scale and in sixteenths of a minimum (up to 1 minimum) on the other scale. This type of syringe can only be used for administering other drugs, particularly when small or previous measurement is indicated.

Needle Gauge and Length

A needle is metal tube through which liquid medication flows. It consists of hub fitting onto the end of a syringe, a hollow shaft (also called a cannula) and a bevel (Slanted part of the needle tip) ending in a sharp point (Fig. 3).

The inner part of the cannula is the lumen (opening or interior diameter). Most needles are available in standard sizes measured in gauge from 13 to 30. The larger in the gauge number, the smaller the needle. For intradermal injection 25, 27 or 29 gauge needle works best. For subcutaneous injection 25 gauge needle is strong enough to reach the dermis. For intramuscular injections 21, 22 and 23 gauge needles are needed to penetrate muscle layers.

The length of the needle is measured from its beveled tip to the junction of the shaft and the hub. Most often 1 or 1½ inch needles are used for adult parenteral injections. Adult IM injections frequently use 22–23 gauge needles and

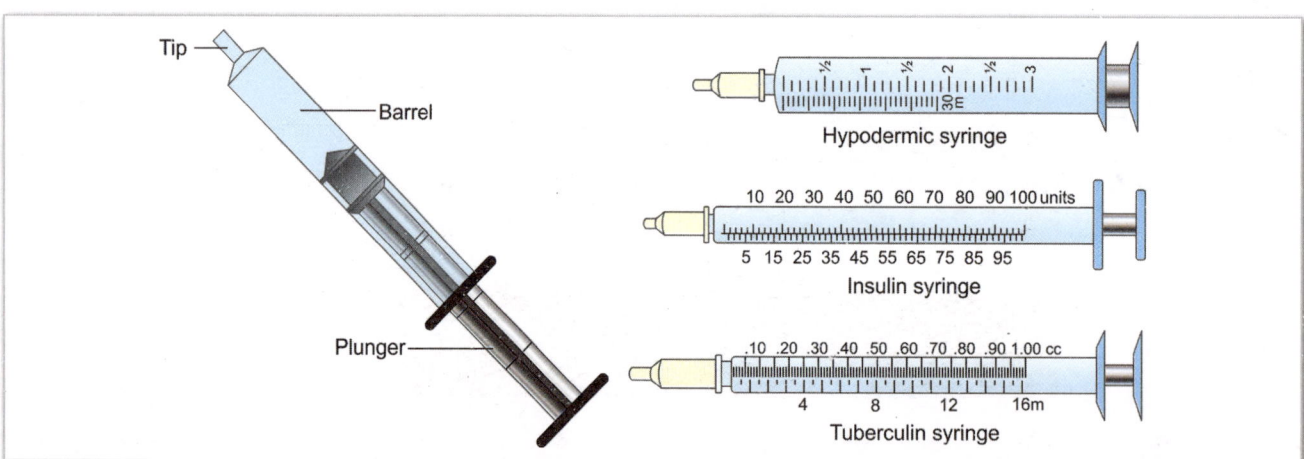

Fig. 2: Various types of syringes

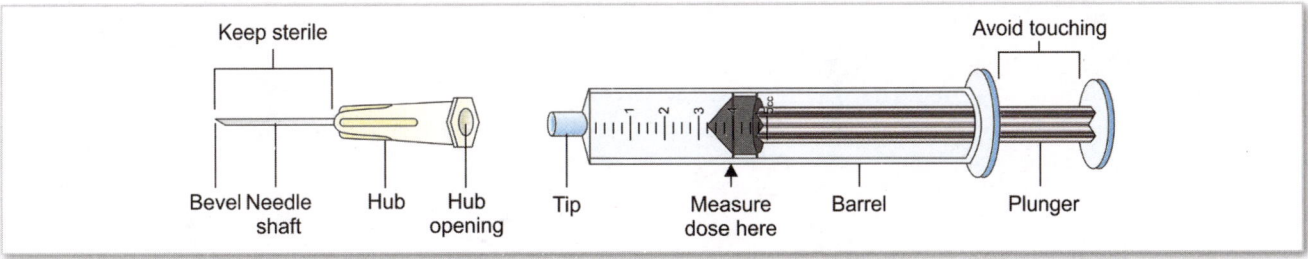

Keep sterile

Avoid touching

Bevel Needle Hub Hub Tip Measure Barrel Plunger
shaft opening dose here

Fig. 3: Parts of needle

21 gauge is preferred for viscous solutions or medications in oil suspension.

PREVENTING NEEDLE STICK INJURIES

One of the most potential hazardous procedure that health care personnel face is using and disposing of needles and sharps. Needle stick injuries present a major risk for infection with hepatitis B virus, human immuno- deficiency virus (HIV), and many other pathogen. Standards have been set by occupational safety and health administration (OSHA) to prevent such injuries.

- Use puncture-proof containers which are disposable to dispose uncapped needles and sharps. These are provided in all client areas. Never throw sharps in wastebaskets. Sharps include any items that can cut or puncture skin such as needles, surgical blades, lancets, razors, broken glass, broken capillary tubes and exposed dental wires.
- Never bend or break needles before disposal
- Never recap used needles, i.e., has been inserted into a client.
- When recapping a needle (i.e., drawing up a medication, into a syringe prior to administration)
  - Use a safety mechanical device that firmly grips the needle cap and holds it in place until it is ready to recap.
  - Use one-handed 'scoop' method. This is performed by (a) placing the needle cap and syringe with needle horizontally on a flat surface, (b) inserting the needle into the cap, using one hand and than (c) using other hand to pick up the cap and tighten it to needle hub. Be careful not to contaminate the needle.

PREPARING INJECTABLE MEDICATIONS

Injectable medications can be prepared by withdrawing the medication from an ampule or vial into a sterile syringe using prefilled syringes, or using needleless injection systems.

Ampules and Vials

Ampules and vials are frequently used to package sterile parenteral medication. An ampule is a glass container usually designed to hold a single dose of a drug. It is made of clear glass and has a distinctive shape with a constrictive neck. Ampules vary in size from 1 mL to 10 mL or more. To access the medication in an ampule the ampule must be broken at its constricted neck. Traditionally files have been used to score the ampule. Today plastic ampule openers are available that prevent injury from broken glass. The device consists of a plastic cap that fits over the top of an ampule. The head of the ampule, when broken, remains inside the cap and is placed into a sharp container. If the ampule opener is not available, the neck should be filed with a small file, and then broken off at that point. Once the ampule is broken, the fluid is aspirated into a syringe (Figs 4A to D).

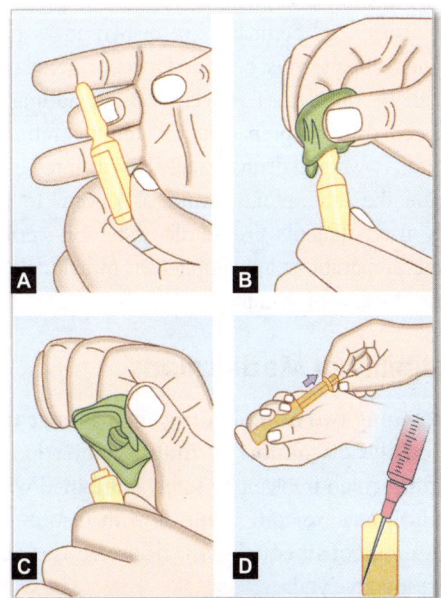

Figs 4A to D: Removing medication from ampule. A. Tapping moves fluid down neck, B. Gauge pad placed around neck of ampule, C. Neck snapped away from hands; D. Withdrawing medicine from ampule

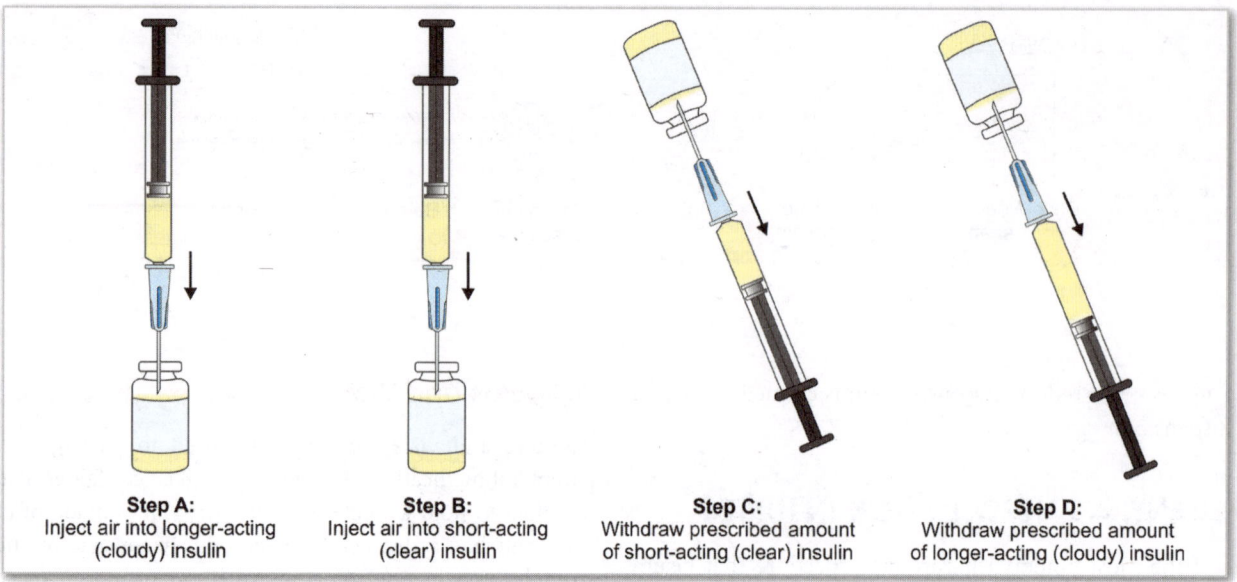

| Step A:
Inject air into longer-acting
(cloudy) insulin | Step B:
Inject air into short-acting
(clear) insulin | Step C:
Withdraw prescribed amount
of short-acting (clear) insulin | Step D:
Withdraw prescribed amount
of longer-acting (cloudy) insulin |

Fig. 5: Mixing dose of insulin from multi-dose vials

A vial is a small bottle with a sealed rubber cap. Vials come in different sizes, form a single to multi-dose vials. They usually have a metal or plastic cap that protects the rubber seal and must be removed to access the medication. To access the medication in a vial the vial must be pierced with the needle. In addition, air must be injected into a vial before the medication can be withdrawn. Failure to inject air before withdrawing the medication leaves a vacuum within the vial that makes withdrawal difficult.

Many drugs, e.g., penicillin are dispensed as powders in vials. A liquid (diluent) must be added to a powdered medication before it can be injected. The technique of adding a diluent to a powdered drug to prepare it for administration is called reconstitution. Powdered drugs usually have printed instructions that describe the amount and kind of solvent to be added. Commonly used diluents are sterile water or sterile normal saline. Some preparations are supplied in individual dose vials; others come in multi-dose vials.

Compatibility of Medications

Before combining two or more drugs in a syringe to save the patient from the discomfort of multiple injections, consult doctor to find which one can be safely combined with others. When medications are compatible as with insulin, the nurse injects an amount of air equal to the desired dose of each drug into their respective vials.

Air is placed in the longer acting insulin vial first. After injecting the air into the second vial, the desired dose is withdrawn. The needle is again inserted into the first vial into which air has already been injected and the exact desired dose of the drug is withdrawn. If too much is drawn up, the contents of the syringe must be discarded and the medications

redrawn because there is no way to separate one drug from the other when already mixed in the syringe in order to discard the excess. Care must be taken not to inject any of the already drawn up medications into the second multidose vial (Fig. 5).

Assessment

Check, the physician's order for the medication. Note the patients name, generic/trade medication name, dosage, route and time. Careful checking prevents medication errors. The identity of the patient who is to receive the injection is carefully assessed to prevent medication errors and harm to the patient. Check the chart for drug allergies and ask the patient about allergies and ask about allergies each time a parenteral medication is given.

Therapeutic effects of previous doses need to be assessed. This may include review of the patient's symptomatic response as well as checking laboratory data such as white blood cell count. If no improvement is seen within 2–3 days, the physician need to be notified.

It is imperative to know what the medication is supposed to do (therapeutic action) and what adverse/side effects may occur. Assess the patient for desired action of the drug, potential side effects, precautions and recommended nursing interventions. If harmful side effects have occurred, the medication must be discontinued and the physician should be consulted.

Check the expiration date on the label of the medication container before drawing it up. All multi-dose vials of medications are dated when opened.

Determine the reason for which the patient is receiving the medication. If the reason is not evident, always question an order if the dosage or particular medication, does not seem appropriate.

Determine the previous injection sites by consulting the medication administration record and the patient. It is best to rotate injection sites to promote the best absorption of the medication. Assess the patient's size and anatomy, and locate the appropriate land marks at the chosen injection site. Determine if the blood circulation is adequate. The needle size and length is determined by the type of injection to be given and the size of muscle tissue and the amount of fat at the injection site of the patient. Adequate circulation is essential for drug absorption.

Nursing Diagnosis

Injections are given for various reasons. The nursing diagnosis that would cover the administration of a particular medication would depend on the purpose of the drug. Few possible nursing diagnosis are:

- Pain related to inflammation or surgery
- Risk for infection related to surgical procedure
- Altered nutrition, less than body requirement, related to inability to utilize glucose properly (insulin)
- Activity intolerance related to postoperative discomfort (pain medication)
- Fluid volume deficit related to vomiting (antiemetic).

Planning

The goals/expected outcomes from the above nursing diagnosis are:

- Pain is relieved for 3 hours by medication
- No signs of infection are present at discharge
- Blood glucose level is maintained within normal limit.
- Patient demonstrates willingness to ambulate, cough, and deep breathe within 30 minutes of injection for pain.
- Nausea and vomiting is controlled by antiemetic medication.

Implementation

Giving injection, involves checking and preparing the medications as well as skillful administration of injection. It is necessary to choose the correct needle size and syringe for the type of injection to be given. Maintaining asepsis while drawing up and giving injections is important. Always follow the 5 'rights' when administering a medication. (right drug, right route, right dose, right time and right patient).

Once used do not recap needles. After use, place needles and syringes in puncture-proof containers, without being recapped because most needle stick injuries occur during recapping. Many acute care facilities are required to provide needles with needle guards to prevent accidental injury. After the injection is given, push the guard into place, preventing injury. Other needle and syringe combinations have a retractable needle that locks and seals inside the syringe barrel. Prefilled syringes are manufactured with retractable needle sheath covers. With these syringes, once the needle is contaminated, the top slides forward and over the needle to prevent a needle stick injury.

INTRADERMAL INJECTIONS

Intradermal injections are most frequently used for tuberculosis or allergy testing. For the intradermal route the amount of solution to be injected is very small. Extreme care must be taken to measure the dose accurately because the solutions are capable of producing severe reactions. A tuberculin syringe and a short needle ¼th to ½ inch length are used. The ventral aspect of the forearm is the site, but when this site is not available for use, the dorsal and lateral side of the upper arm can also be used. The needle is inserted at an angle of about 15 degrees between the upper layers of the skin. The injected solution raises the epidermis to form a bleb. It is then slowly absorbed from the site because the blood vessels are located in the deeper structures of the skin. The dosages given intradermally is small, usually less then 0.5 mL.

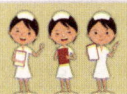 **SKILL: ADMINISTERING AN INTRADERMAL INJECTION**

Intradermal injections are used for various skin tests such as the Mantoux test for tuberculosis and for sensitivity tests. The object is to inject an antigen to determine if the person has an inflammatory reaction, indicating that previous exposure to the antigen has caused antibodies to be manufactured by the body.

Equipment and Supplies

Tuberculin syringe with ¼ inch to ½ inch needle, or 26 or 27 gauge (1 mL calibrated in 0.01 mL units)
- Gloves
- Medication to be injected

Contd...

- Medication administration record or order
- Spirit/alcohol swabs.
- Waste receptacle

Steps of Procedure

Review and follow the standard steps as given in Appendix

Action/steps	Rationale
Assessments	
1. Assess if patient understands the procedure for the intradermal injection and its purpose. Assess for any previous reaction to agent to be injected	Helps to know what all information needs to be given and alerts to possible contraindication to injection
Planning	
2. Determine the completion of 48–72 hours after the injection and assures the availably of person at that time to read the result.	For proper reading it is must that the results of the test are observed within the time period.
Implementation	
3. Wash hands and draw up the medication keeping the five rights in mind	Prepares medication for injection and helps prevent a medication error
4. Identify the patient and select the site cleanse the site with antiseptic swab and allow the skin to dry.	The inside of the forearm is used for intradermal injection
5. Put on gloves and with the index finger and thumb, pull the skin at the selected site on the forearm taut. Insert the needle bevel up at a 5–15 degree angle for the medication to form a bleb.	Positioning the bevel up minimizes resistance of the skin when the needle is inserted decreasing discomfort.
6. Lift up the needle point slightly and inject solution slowly, a bleb should form.	If the bleb is not formed the medication has been deposited in subcutaneous tissue and the test will not be valid.
7. Carefully withdraw the needle and wipe the skin very gently with antiseptic swab, but do not apply pressure.	Applying pressure forces the medications back out the needle track
8. Dispose of the syringe and needle into sharps container, remove gloves and wash your hands.	Prevents needle stick to self or others. Prevents transfer of microorganisms.
9. Circle the injection site with a skin pencil.	Facilitates locating site at time of reading the reaction.
Evaluation	
10. Verify that the bleb remains.	Procedure will have to be repeated, if bleb is not visible.
11. Read the result of the skin test at the proper interval	Different antigens used for testing require different intervals before reading the result.
Documentation	
12. Document the dose and record the exact site and time	Documenting time and site shows where and when to read in 48–72 hours.
13. When result is read, record the findings on patient's record	For future reference.

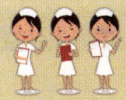

SKILL: ADMINISTRATION OF SUBCUTANEOUS INJECTION

Certain drugs must be injected subcutaneously rather than intramuscularly in order to be absorbed properly and at desired speed. Heparin, Insulin, allergy extract and certain types of immunizations are given subcutaneously.

Equipment and Supplies

- Syringe with needle preferably ½ -5/8 inch in length. (1 mL Calibrated 40 or 80 units for insulin administration)
- Medication to be administered
- Gloves
- Medication administration record (MAR) or order
- Spirit/alcohol swabs
- Waste receptacle

Steps of Procedure

Review and carryout standard steps as given in Appendix

Action/steps	Rationale
Assessments	
1. Check the medication order and determine the availability of medication in the unit and check for presence of allergies	Ensures that time is not lost acquiring the medication. Indicates if patient is allergic to medication
Planning	
2. Plan in which site to give the injection choose an appropriate syringe and needle (Fig. 6).	Consider the size and weight of the patient and the condition of the various sites.
Implementation	
3. Wash your hands and prepare the medication following the five rights	Helps to prevent medication errors.
4. Identify the patient by checking identification band	Prevents medication errors and injury to patient
5. Put gloves, select the site for the injection and expose the area for good visibility cleanse the area gently with spirit swab by using circular motion until 2 inches in diameter is cleansed. Place the swab between the index and middle fingers of nondominant hand. Allow the skin to dry	Cleanses the area, positions the swab for use after the injection vigorous rubbing increases blood flow and could increase rapidity of absorption.
6. Pick up the prepared syringe in one hand and remove the needle guard by pulling it straight off the needle with the other hand to avoid contaminating the needle	Asepsis must be maintained

Fig. 6: Common sites for subcutaneous injections

Contd...

Action/steps	Rationale
7. Support the skin at the site by gently bunching up the tissue between thumb and index finger	Picking up the tissue helps you assess the thickness of the subcutaneous layer into which you will inject the drug.
8. Hold the barrel of the syringe in hand between the thumb and index finger, bracing with the remaining three fingers. Insert the needle into the skin at 45 or 90 degree angle with a firm quick forward thrust release the pinched-up skin.	Stabilizes the tissue so that the needle pierces cleanly. A shorter needle uses a 90-degree angle, a longer needle uses a 45-degree angle to stay in subcutaneous tissue.
9. Press the plunger with a smooth, slow motion until all of the medication is injected	Places medication in the tissue
10. Remove the needle by pulling it out on the angle of insertion while stabilizing the skin with the other hand	Pulling the needle quickly while stabilizing the skin causes the least discomfort. Rub the area.
11. Dispose of the needle and syringe in the sharps container. Remove gloves and wash hands.	Prevents needle stick injury to self or others. Reduces transfer of microorganism
Evaluation	
12. Check with the patient in 30–60 minutes to evaluate the therapeutic effect of the medication	Different medication are to be evaluated for their effects accordingly
Documentation	
13. Document the injection on the medication administration record (MAR) or patient record, noting the location in which the injection was given	Verifies that the injection was given as ordered.

Special Considerations

- If 2 inches (5 cm) of tissue can be grasped insert the needle at a 90 degree angle; if only 1 inch of tissue can be grasped use a 45-degree angle for the injection.
- Heparin injections are given in the abdomen on both sides and below the umbilicus outside of a 2 inch radius around the umbilicus from the costal margins of the iliac crests. Do not aspirate before injecting the heparin. Because heparin (anticoagulant) can increase bruising and needle movement could cause tissue damage.
- Do not massage the site after heparin has been injected because it may cause bruising of the tissue, bleeding and severe ecchymosis (Purplish area under the skin caused by bleeding).
- Insulin injection are given on the lateral surfaces of the upper arm or the anterior and lateral aspects of the thigh. It can also be given in the abdominal subcutaneous sites also but rotation of sites within one anatomic area is important.

INTRAMUSCULAR INJECTIONS

Intramuscular injections are used if the patient can not take medicine orally, or a faster action is desired. IM injections can provide onset of action within 15 minutes because muscle tissue is highly vascular, and drug absorption is faster than the subcutaneous route. Drugs introduced into a large skeletal muscle mass cause less tissue irritation than when drugs are administered intradermally or subcutaneously.

Injection site selection is a critical decision one has to make because improper site selection can result in damaged nerves, abscesses, necrosis, and sloughing of skin as well as pain. Therefore, the individual's stage of development, body build and physical condition as well as the viscosity and amount of the drug to be administered must be considered in giving an injection.

Site for Intramuscular Injection

- **Mid-deltoid muscle:** It is a common location for IM injection. The correct site for injection can be located by placing four fingers across the deltoid muscle with the little finger on the acromion process; the site is three-finger breadths below the acromion process. This site is convenient because it is usually easily accessible. One milliliter of medication can be safely injected into this site (Fig. 7).
  Damage to radial nerve and artery is a risk with use of deltoid site.
- **Dorsogluteal and ventrogluteal:** When using the dorsogluteal and ventrogluteal site in the gluteal (buttocks) area for IM injection, care must be taken to avoid injury to the sciatic nerve and blood vessels located in these areas to locate a safe area for dorsogluteal injection, the head of the trochanter and the posterior iliac spine are palpated (Fig. 8).

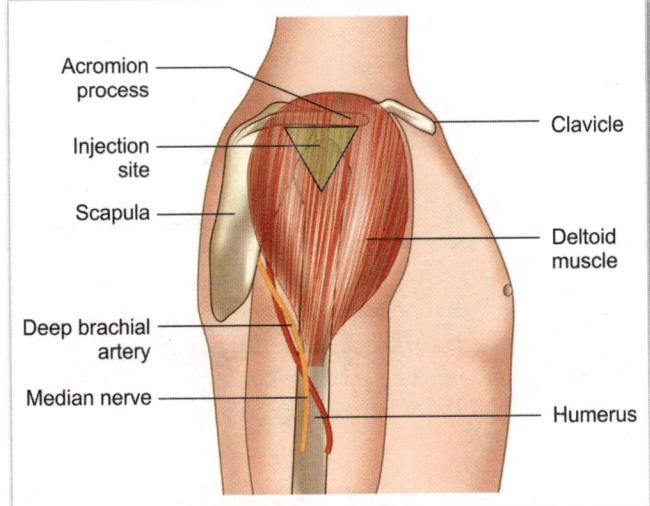

Fig. 7: Site of injection on deltoid muscle

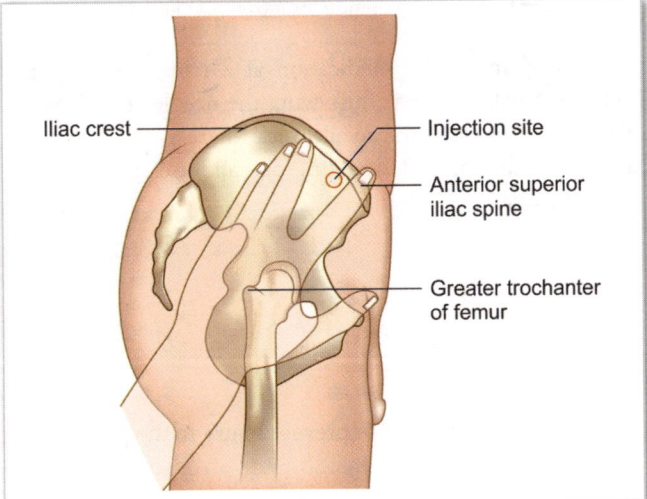

Fig. 8: Anatomical view of ventrogluteal muscle injection site

An imaginary line is drawn between the two bony landmarks. The injection is given above and lateral to the line in the gluteal medius muscle. This avoids the dangerous insertion of a needle into the sciatic nerve.

The ventrogluteal area is the safest IM injection site involving the gluteus medius and minimus muscles. The muscle layer is thick and this site has a very small fatty layer. The site can be used both for adults and children and is especially helpful if patients are only able to lie on their back or turn to one side or the other. To locate the injection site, the palm is placed over the greater trochanter, the index finger is put on the anterior superior iliac spine, and the middle finger is spread as far as possible toward the posterior iliac crest. The center of the V (triangle) bounded by the fingers is the precise injections site to be used.

Flexing of the knee and hip helps the person to relax the muscles.

The vastus lateralis muscle is also a preferred IM injection site for adults, children and infants. Vastus lateralis involves the quadriceps femoris muscle and is located along the anterolateral aspect of the thigh. There are no large nerves or vessels in its proximity, and it does not cover a joint. To locate the site, divide the thigh into thirds horizontally and vertically and administer the injection in the outer middle third. This space provides a large number of injection sites. This site is particularly desirable for infants and children whose gluteal muscles are developed poorly (Figs 9 and 10).

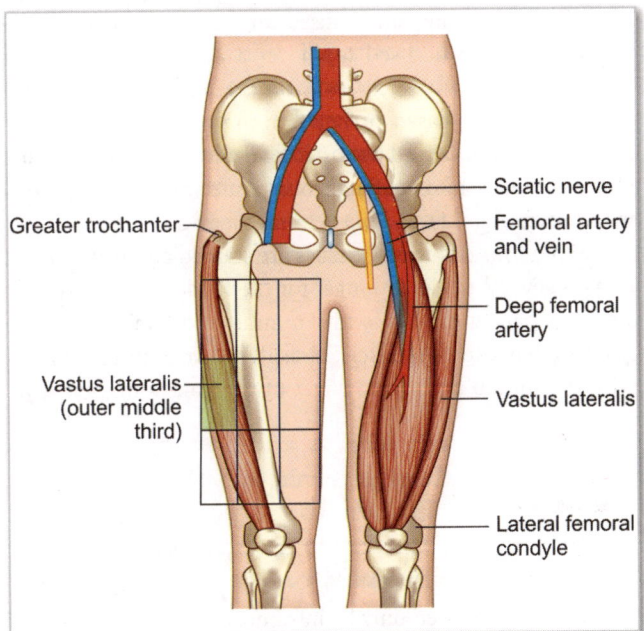

Fig. 9: Anatomical view of the site for intramuscular (IM) injection into the vastus lateralis muscle

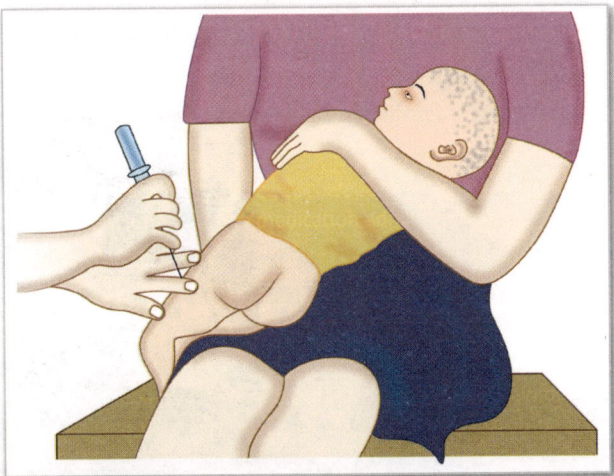

Fig. 10: Giving intramuscular injection to child. Vastus lateralis is preferred site for intramuscular injection

Technique

Air lock technique: An air lock can be used when giving an IM injection to clear the needle of medication and to seal the track so that the medication does not flow back up into the subcutaneous tissues. To use an air lock, after drawing up the exact amount of medication ordered, draw up a further 0.2 mL of air. When preparing to give the injection, be certain that the needle is at a 90 degree angle and the air is behind the medication so that it will be injected last.

The Z-track Technique

The Z-Track (causing a needle track, or pathway, in the shape of a "Z") technique can be used any time an IM injection is given. It must be used whenever a deep IM injection of irritating solutions such as Iron preparations penicillin preparations, oil based preparation are given. This method reduces the pain caused by irritating drugs that leak or escape along the track into subcutaneous tissue when the needle is withdrawn (Fig. 11).

When this occurs the tissues are stained and bruised and it takes several weeks or longer for the tenderness to subside. After preparing the site with an antiseptic swab, inject the needle deep into the muscle. Grasp the barrel of the syringe with the thumb and index finger of the non-dominant hand and slowly inject the medication at a rate of 10 seconds. Release the skin after withdrawing the needle. This leaves a zigzag path that seals the needle track where tissue planes slide across one another. The medication cannot escape from the muscle tissue.

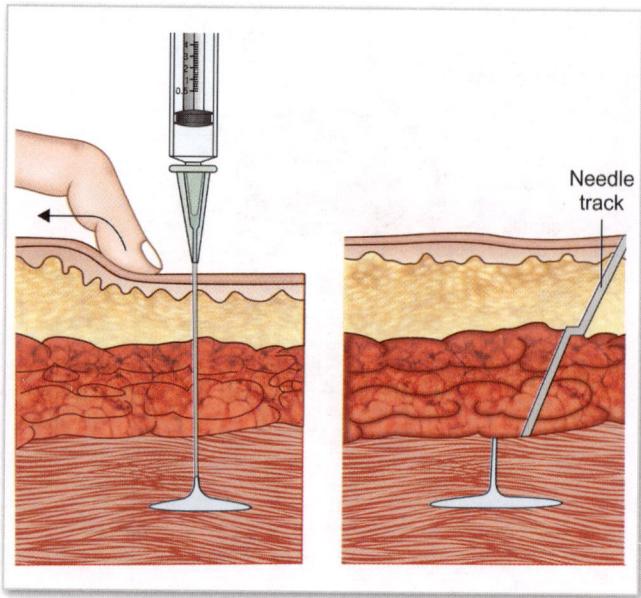

Fig. 11   Z track technique for intramuscular injection

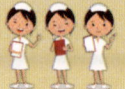

SKILL: ADMINISTERING AN INTRAMUSCULAR INJECTION

Many drugs are given only by intramuscular injection. The site must be carefully selected to prevent injury to the patient. The use of an air lock to be used as per the agency's policy.

Equipment and Supplies (Fig. 12)

- Syringe and needle 1–2 inches in length (18–21 gauge)
- Medication as prescribed

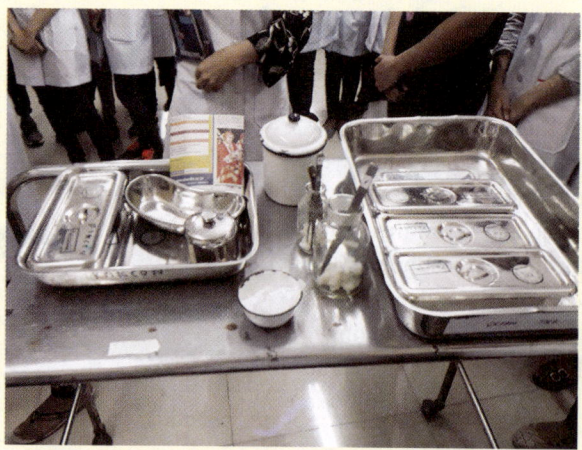

Fig. 12   Articles for intramuscular injection

Contd...

- Gloves
- Medication administration record (MAR)
- Fluid (sterile water) for dissolving powdered medicine
- Alcohol/spirit swabs
- Waste receptacle.

Review and carry out the standard steps as given in Appendix

Action/steps	Rationale
Assessment	
1. Prepare the patient for injection assess for any allergies to drug.	Prevents time wastage between preparation of injection and giving of injection alerts nurse for any allergy.
Planning	
2. Plan the site at which the injection is to be given	The deltoid, dorsogluteal, ventrogluteal, vastus lateralis sites may be used.
Implementation	
3. Verify the medication label with the medication administration record (MAR)	Adhering to the five rights of medication administration and checking each medication three times for drugs, dose, route, date and time prevents medication errors.
4. Select and expose the injection site so that the view is unobstructed. For the ventrogluteal site the patient may be supine or turned to the side. If the dorsogluteal site is used, have the patient on the side or prone with the toes turned slightly inward, Palpate the bony landmarks.	The ventrogluteal site is the safest site. The intramuscular (IM) site chosen must be within defined landmarks. Turning the toes medially with the patient prone relaxes the dorsogluteal muscles.
5. Wash hands and put on gloves, remove alcohol swab and cleanse a space 2 inches in diameter using circular motion. Place the swab between the fingers of the non dominant hand for later use. Allow the area to dry.	Prevents transfer of Microorganisms. Cleanses the site. Makes swab available after the injection
6. Pick up the syringe and verify that the correct dose is taken. If an air bubble is to be used as a lock add 0.2 mL of air. Invert the syringe so that bubble rises to a position behind the fluid in the syringe	An air bubble is thought to seal the needle track, keeping the medication from leaking back.
7. Spread the skin at the site with the nondominant hand, pressing firmly around the site to compress the subcutaneous and muscle tissues.	Taut skin reduces resistance to the needle when it enters the tissues and causes less pain.
8. Grasp the barrel of the syringe firmly between your thumb and index finger, and plunge the needle firmly into the muscle at a 90-degree angle with a quick, firm, forward thrust until the desired depth is reached.	Holding the skin taut and the syringe steady while introducing the needle to the desired depth in one stroke causes the least discomfort to the patient.
9. Steady the barrel of the syringe with the nondominant hand and pull the plunger back with the dominant hand to aspirate for blood. If blood returns in the syringe, withdraw the needle and dispose of the syringe and medication. Prepare a new injection	A medication prepared for IM injection can be harmful if it is injected intravenously. Blood should not be reinjected into tissue.
10. Inject the medication by pushing the plunger into the barrel with a slow, continuous motion, if an air lock is being used, inject the air bubble. Be careful not to displace the needle from the original position while injecting (Figs 13A and B). 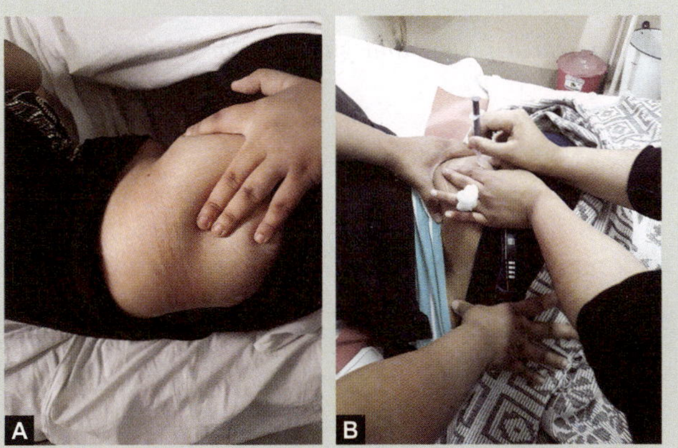	Injecting slowly is less painful because tissue has time to absorb the medication; a medication prepared for IM absorption may cause local tissue reaction, if left in the fatty subcutaneous or intradermal tissue.

Figs 13A and B   A. Site of IM injection; B. Injecting the medicine

Contd...

Action/steps	Rationale
11. Apply pressure with the alcohol swab at the needle site as you quickly remove the needle, drawing it straight up with a quick motion.	Pressure also helps prevent the medication from leaking backup the needle track. Removing the needle with a quick motion is less painful than removing it slowly.
12. Massage the injection site with a gentle, but firm circular motion	Massage increases circulation and helps to disperse the medication so that it is absorbed more quickly.
13. Discard syringe needle and remove gloves and wash hands	Decreases transfer of microorganisms.
Evaluation	
14. Determine how the patient tolerated the injection. Check the therapeutic effect of the drug at proper interval.	If adverse effects to the medication occur, document them and inform physician promptly.
Documentation	
15. Document the dose and the site on MAR and nurses notes for PRN medication	For further reference and patients response to PRN medication must be documented

Evaluation

Administration of an injection is evaluated in terms of whether it was given properly and whether it achieved the purpose for what it was given. Assess for any adverse effects to the medications and check the injection site for signs of inflammation.

Documentation

Injection documentation should include the medication, the dosage, the route and the site at which the injection is given. The testing substance is noted for intradermal injections. Routine injections are recorded on the MAR only. The PRN (as needed) and STAT doses may also be recorded in the nurses notes, along with the reason the medication was given and the result and duration of effect of the injection.

BIBLIOGRAPHY

1. Berman AT, Snyder S, Kozier BJ, et al. Kozier & Erb's. Fundamentals of Nursing: Concepts, Process and Practice, 8th edition. Pearson Education.
2. Dewit SC. Fundamental Concepts and Skills for Nursing, 3rd edition. WB Saunders. 2008.
3. Sharma S. Potter and Perry's Fundamentals of Nursing. A South Asian edition. Gurugram: Elsevier India. 2013.
4. Taylor CR, Lillis C, LeMone P, et al. Fundamentals of Nursing – The Art and Science of Nursing Care, 7th edition. Wolters Kluwer; 2010.
5. Nicoll LH, Hesby A. Intramuscular injection: an integrative research review and guideline for evidence-based practice. Appl Nurs Res. 2002;15(3):149-62.

Administering Intravenous Solutions and Medications

INTRODUCTION

Intravenous route is the main method of supplying the patient with fluids and medications if the patient is unable to take them orally or rectally. The drug or solution given by the intravenous (IV) route has the advantage of making the drug or solution instantly available for circulation to all tissues. The disadvantage is that the material cannot be retrieved, if an error has been made, because the solution is injected directly through the vein into the circulation. All materials must be sterile to avoid introducing bacteria.

Intravenous are given to supply the body with needed substances or drugs that cannot be supplied as rapidly or efficiently by other means. These substances may be:
*   Fluids and electrolytes that the patient is unable to take orally in sufficient amounts.
*   Medications that are more effective by this route or cannot be given by any other way.
*   Blood, plasma, or other blood components
*   Nutritional formulae containing glucose, amino acids, and lipids.

The average adult needs 1500–2000 mL of fluids in a 24-hour period to replace those eliminated by the body. Patients whose fluid intake has decreased or who experience an excessive loss of body fluids require fluid replacement. Fluids are lost by:

- Hemorrhage
- Severe or prolonged vomiting or diarrhea
- Moderate to excessive drainage from wounds, especially from burn wounds
- And by profuse perspiration

Accurately maintaining the record of the patient's intake and output is needed to determine the amount of fluids necessary for daily replacement. The laboratory tests of electrolytes serve as guides to the physician while ordering replacements of sodium, potassium, and chloride, which are the more commonly administered electrolytes.

TYPES OF INTRAVENOUS SOLUTIONS

There are many types of solution available, and others can be prepared to meet the specific needs of the individual patient. The solutions most frequently used are those containing glucose, saline, electrolytes, vitamin, and amino acids. In addition to these, blood and blood products are given intravenously. IV solutions, are either isotonic, hypotonic or hypertonic (Table 1).

Isotonic solutions have the same concentration, or osmolality, as blood and are used to expand the fluid volume of the body.

Hypotonic solutions contain less solute than extravascular fluid and may cause shift out of the vascular compartment.

Hypertonic solutions have a greater tonicity than blood. They are used to replace electrolytes and when given as concentrated dextrose solutions, produce a shift in fluid from the intracellular compartment. Due to greater osmotic pressure it draws water out of the cells.

Solutions that are given intravenously must be sterile and free of contaminating particles. They are supplied in plastic bags

TABLE 1: Common intravenous therapy solutions and tonicity

Solution	Tonicity
0.9% saline	Isotonic
0.45% saline	Hypotonic
5% dextrose	Isotonic
10% dextrose	Hypertonic
5% dextrose in 0.9% saline	Hypotonic
5% dextrose in 0.45% saline	Hypertonic
5% dextrose in 0.25% saline	Isotonic
Ringers lactate	Isotonic
5% dextrose in ringer's lactate	Hypertonic

in 250, 500 and 1000 mL amounts. Glass and plastic bottles are still used for a few solutions and some IV drugs. Smaller bags of sterile water and normal saline are used to dissolve or dilute various drugs for parenteral use. The IV bag is marked with calibrations along the sides to determine the amount of fluid in the hanging position of the bag. A plastic cover on the tubing port is pulled off to allow the tubing spike to be inserted. A plastic or foil tab also covers the port used to add medication to the bag. The bag has a tab with a hole in it that fits on the hanger of an IV pole. Some IV bottles contain a tube that acts automatically as an air vent, for others a vented tubing set must be used to let air in.

ADMINISTRATION SETS

There are many different types of administration sets available for IV use, some of which must be used with a particular brand of IV solution or type of bag or bottle. Administration sets can be classified as:

- Primary infusion sets
- Piggyback sets
- Controlled volume sets
- Parallel or Y sets.

Primary Intravenous Set

The primary IV infusion set up consists of a bottle or bag of solution, a regular tubing set a needle and an IV stand to hold the bottle. A filter may be added. Tubing is either vented or nonvented. The IV tubing set consists of the spike end, which is inserted into the bottle, the drip chamber, the tubing and a flow regulator or clamp. The spike and the needle adapter at the end of the tubing are covered with plastic protectors to keep them sterile. The primary IV infusion set-up is used for any type of IV therapy, except the administration of blood products, which requires a special set with a filter in the drip chamber.

The primary IV tubing set is selected according to the size of the drop to be delivered into the drip chamber. There are three major sizes:

- Regular drops (10–20 gtt/mL) of fluid are used for administering IV therapy to most adult patients.
- Macro drops (10 gtt/mL) are used for viscous (sticky or gummy) fluids such as blood.
- Microdrops (60 gtt/mL) are used when small amounts of fluids are required or when extreme care must be used to measure the exact amounts most often used for giving IV fluids to infants and children.

Secondary or Piggyback Intravenous Set

Medications to be given intravenously are often added to an existing IV line by using the piggyback method. Primary administration sets have one or two inlet ports for adding medications or a second IV. When this is used, the primary infusion is interrupted to infuse medications such as antibiotics and antineoplastic drugs at regular scheduled times. Because these drugs are diluted in amounts of 50–150 mL of solution they must be given by infusion, not by bolus. The advantage of the piggyback system is that when the solution in the smaller bag has been infused the primary IV begins to flow again without further adjustment. The secondary bottle containing the medication is hung slightly higher than the level of fluid in the primary IV so that gravity forces it to empty first. Do not clamp or alter the flow of the primary bag. It will not run until all fluid higher than its level has infused, then it will begin to flow (Fig. 1).

Controlled Volume Set

This is another way of interrupting a primary infusion to give a dose of diluted medication in a controlled volume administration set. This set contains a burette (tube- like

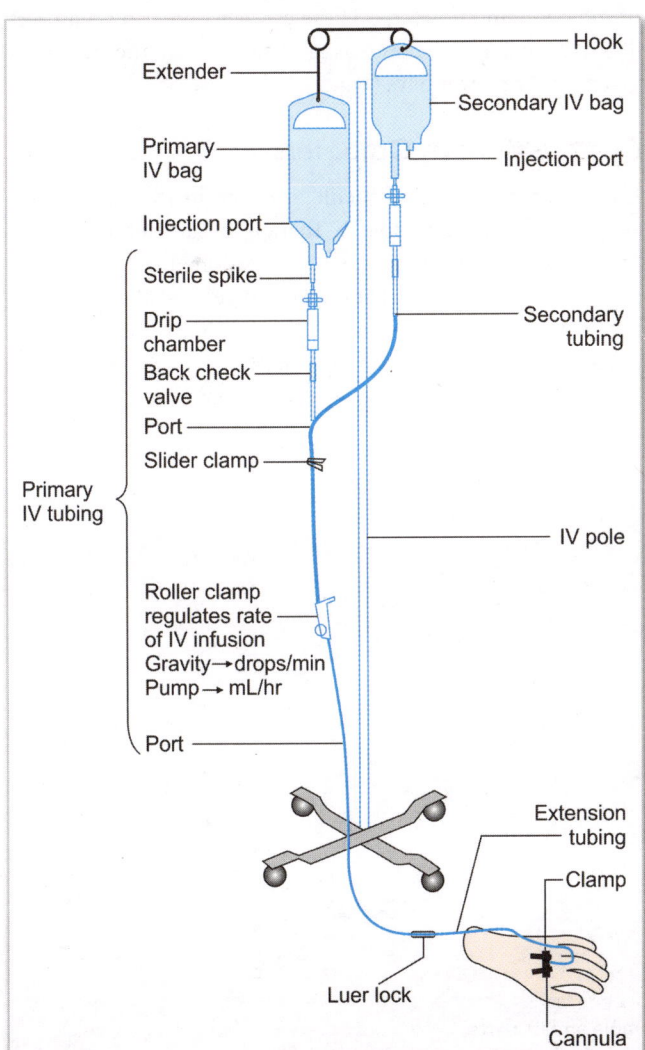

Fig. 1: Infusion set

chamber that holds 150 mL of fluid) into which the medication is injected along with a specified volume of fluid from the primary bag, which is then clamped off. The medicine from the burette goes into the drip chamber and the flow is regulated by a clamp on the IV tubing. The burette set is attached to the primary IV line beneath the bag of fluid. These can also be used when a small amount of fluid is to be infused over a long period. It is often used for administration of fluids to infants, children and the elderly. Using a controlled volume set ensures that a fluid overload cannot occur because only a specified amount of fluid is available to be infused at any one time, i.e., 50–100 mL over 1–2 hours.

Parallel or Y Intravenous Set

A Y-type administration set is used to infuse certain blood products. The blood product is placed on one side and a bag of normal saline is placed on the other side. Saline is the only solution used in conjunction with infusion of a blood product. The saline is started first and then the blood administration is begun. The saline is stopped during blood transfusion, once the transfusion is complete, tubing should be flushed with the normal saline solution.

Intermittent Intravenous Devices (Saline Heparin) or Parenteral Nutrition Lock

Some patients do not require large amounts of fluid by the IV route but may need to receive IV medications at intervals or have an IV access in case emergency medications are needed quickly. An intermittent access device is preferred for patients who receive antibiotics, heparin, corticosteroids, antimetabolites and other drugs. An intermittent IV device is established by inserting an IV cannula that has a cap to prevent blood from leaking out of the vein. The peripheral device is called a saline lock, parenteral nutrition (PRN) lock, or intermittent (INT) lock.

A butterfly IV needle, which has a short piece of tubing attached, may also be used as an intermittent device when it is capped. Because no solution is constantly infusing through the lock, saline or a dilute heparin is periodically infused to maintain patency by preventing clot forming at the tip of the cannula. Often an IV line is converted to an intermittent device in case the patient no longer needs fluids but is still receiving IV medications. The is done by removing the IV tubing and attaching a cannula cap.

Filters trap small particles such as undissolved medication or salts that have precipitated from solution. Filters prevent such particles from entering a vein. A 0.22-micron filter is used for most solutions. For lipid or albumin solution, a 1.2 micron filter is used. A special filter is needed for blood components.

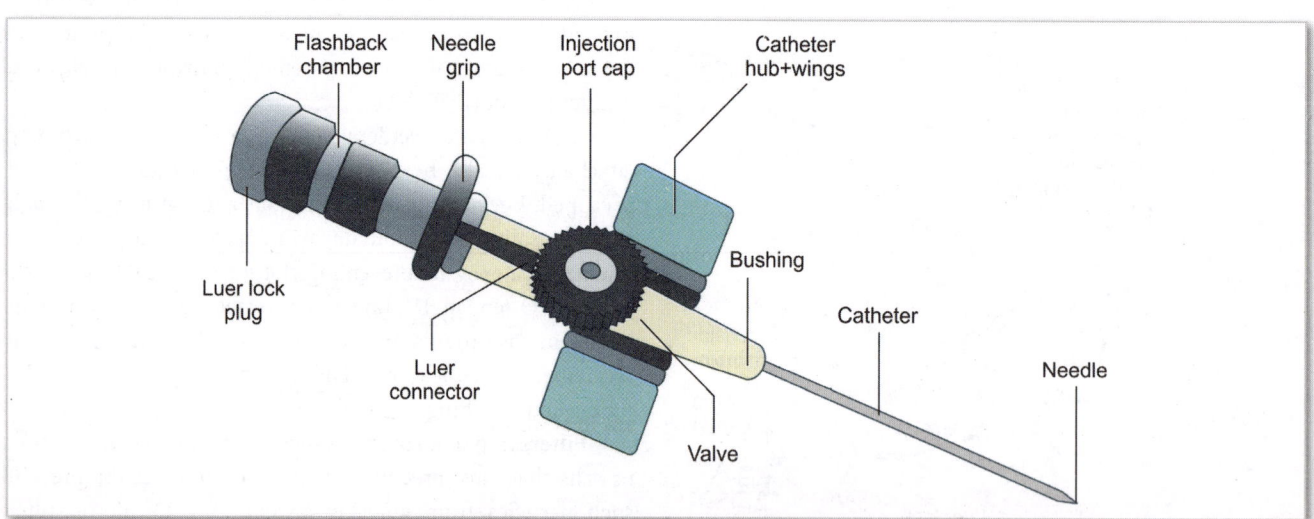

Intravenous Infusion Pumps

Infusion pumps may be used to regulate the flow of IV fluids especially when patients receive total parenteral nutrition or medications for which it is essential that a certain amount be accurately infused over a set period. These pumps deliver IV fluids automatically at a preset rate. In some hospitals they are used in intensive care units to control the amount of heparin and cardiovascular drugs accurately, in labor rooms while inducing labor, and in oncology units to administer chemotherapy drugs, and for the administration of total parenteral nutrition (TPN).

Programmed infusion pumps are more accurate and provide better control over the amount of solution being infused. They have alarms that warn if the IV container is empty, if air is present in the tubing, or if the line is infiltrated or occluded. Disadvantages of pumps include—they exert pressure on the vein, they are expensive and certain types of pumps require special administration sets.

Controllers reduce the risk of infusing fluid too rapidly, assist with detection of infiltration and maintain an accurate flow rate. Rate controller devices operate by gravity flow, which is regulated by a drop sensor and electronic feedback mechanism. Rate controllers are not used for blood or viscous solutions.

Patient-controlled analgesia pumps are used in hospitals and at home for pain control. This type of pump is used for pain control and it has a remote control button by which the patient can administer a controlled bolus of pain medication from time to time. The pump is programmed to allow only a certain limit of medication to be delivered during a particular period.

VENOUS ACCESS DEVICES

Intravenous Needle and Catheters

There are various types of IV needles and catheters used for peripheral IV fluid administration. The winged tip or butterfly needle is meant for short-term therapy, such as to give single dose IV medication or to obtain blood samples. After insertion, the wings are taped to the skin. The butterfly needle is supplied in odd number gauges (17, 19, 23 and 25) and is frequently used for pediatric infusions or for the elderly. Because these needles are rigid they may cause more discomfort than do other types of cannulas, and mobility may be restricted to prevent dislodgement of the needle.

Over-the-needle catheters consist of a needle with a catheter sheath over it. After the device is placed into the vein and the cannula (catheter sheath) is threaded, the needle is removed, leaving the flexible cannula in the vein. Cannulas of this type cause less irritation, thereby decreasing the incidence of infection and phlebitis. These catheters are replaced every 48–72 hours. These cannulas are used in case the therapy is given for 7 or fewer days (Fig. 2).

Central Venous Catheters

If a peripheral vein is difficult to locate in the adult or the veins are not suitable for IV therapy, a catheter is inserted into the large subclavian vein and positioned in the superior vena cava or the right atrium. This type of catheter can be left in place for 6–8 weeks. The nurse assists the physician during the subclavian catheter insertion by providing the sterile catheter tray, draping the patient, opening sterile

Fig. 2: Intravenous cannula and its parts

TABLE 2: Size and color code of the cannula

Gauge	Color code	Ext. Dia. (nm)	Length (mm)	Flow rate (mL/min)
14G	Orange	2.1	45	240
16G	Gray	1.8	45	180
18G	Green	1.3	35/45	90
20G	Pink	1.1	32	60
22G	Blue	0.9	25	36
24G	Yellow	0.7	19	20
26G	Violet	0.6	19	13

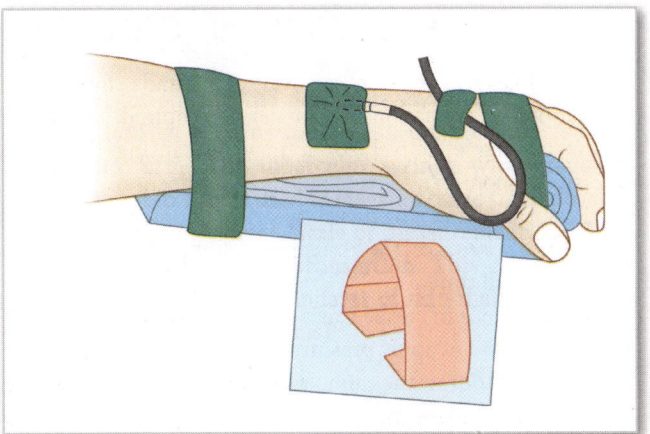

Fig. 3: Securing the intravenous cannula

packages, and preparing the IV administration set for use. If the patient needs a central line for more than 6–8 weeks, a long-term catheter such as a tunneled broviac, Hickman is inserted in the operating room.

Peripherally inserted central catheters (PICC) or midline catheters (ML), are often used in children or in adults who need peripheral IV therapy that requires placement where there is high blood flow. These catheters are long and are inserted in the larger basilic or cephalic vein of the upper arm. The ML catheters are ideally placed inside the subclavian vessel and the PICC may be advanced as far as superior vena cava.

Central venous catheters are used for the far patients who need long-term drug therapy, fluid therapy or chemotherapy. Remember not to take blood pressure on the arm of the patient of PICC of ML catheter in place. These catheters are periodically flushed with heparin to keep the lumen patent. Correct placement of subclavian catheters must be verified by radiographic studies before any fluid is infused through them.

Gauge Size Color Code

Injection port caps are color coded for instant identification of cannula gauge size (Table 2).

SECURING OF INTRAVENOUS CANNULA

- Dressing to peripheral intravenous (PIV) sites are the first line of defense against infections and must be kept secure, clean and dry.
- The type of secure dressing for the PIV cannula depends upon the child's age, condition of the skin, site of the IV, child's activity and/or mobility (Fig. 3).
- Consider placing a small piece of cotton wool ball or gauze underneath the hub of the cannula to reduce pressure.
- Cover the cannula site with sterile transparent or semipermeable occlusive dressing (e.g., Tegaderm, IV 3000) placed aseptically over the catheter.

- If desired, place sterile tape over the hub and wings of the device before placing the transparent dressing.
- IV board/splints are recommended to secure PIV cannula place in or adjacent to areas of flexion. This adequately immobilizes the joint and minimizes the risk of venous damage resulting from flexion.
  - While using splints, ensure these are positioned and strapped with the limb and digits in a neutral position to prevent restricting blood or nerve supply and pressure sores.
  - Inspect the splint at least daily and change if soiled by blood or fluid leakage.
- Cover with gauze or non-compression tubular bandage. Check for the following things:
  - While using non-compression tubular bandage (e.g., tubifast), ensure that there is a clear window where the cannula enters the skin so the site can be viewed
  - It is secure
  - The site is visible
  - The child can't injure himself/herself on the connections
  - The child can't remove or dislodge the cannula
  - That tapes are not too tight
- Change the dressing only if it becomes insecure or if there is blood or fluid leakage.

Changing Cannulas

Recannulation should be avoided if possible, as this causes the child and family further distress. There is no limit to the length of time that a cannula may remain in situ and with appropriate care, several days may be possible. Cannulas only need to be replaced if there is accidental dislodgement, occlusion, phlebitis and infection.

REMOVAL OF INTRAVENOUS CANNULA

The possible reasons for removal of cannula includes—infiltration, extravasations, no longer be required, no longer be functioning effectively or it may be causing the child excessive discomfort, signs of phlebitis or infection.

- Perform hand hygiene, wearing nonsterile gloves, carefully remove the dressing, holding the cannula in place at all times.
- Hold a piece of sterile gauze or cotton wool over the exit site but do not apply pressure.
- Slowly withdraw the cannula, maintaining a neutral angle with the child's skin.
- Cover site with cotton wool and tape or band-aid.
- Advise the child and family that the cotton wool and tape or band-aid should remain in situ for 24 hours.
- Document date and reason of removal.

COMPLICATIONS OF INTRAVENOUS THERAPY

Complications of IV therapy are potentially very serious. intravenous sites must be checked at least once an hour to prevent or catch and alleviate problems such as infiltration, phlebitis, blood stream infection and catheter embolus. Ask the patient about discomfort while inspecting and palpating the site time-to-time assess the flow of fluid at the patient's bedside (Table 3).

Infiltration

Infiltration is the most common problem. This occurs when fluid or medication leaks out of the vein into the tissue. There will often be edema around the site. The tissue will be cold. Skin appears pale. Flow gets reduced from the set rate when infiltration has occurred. In this condition, infiltration is discontinued and another site is initiated to continue the therapy.

Phlebitis

Phlebitis is caused due to irritation of the vessel by the needle, cannula, medications or additives in the IV solution. The typical signs of phlebitis are erythema, warmth, swelling, and tenderness. The IV must be discontinued and another site should be used for therapy. Warm compresses the inflamed site decreases discomfort.

Blood Stream Infection

Blood stream infection (septicemia) occurs if infections pathogens are introduced into the blood stream. This may occur due to break in sterile technique during cannula insertion or change of bag or tubing. Signs and symptoms are fever, chills, pain, headache, nausea, vomiting, and extreme fatigue. Blood cultures are ordered and accordingly antibiotics are started. The IV set is immediately discontinued.

TABLE 3: Complications of intravenous therapy and related interventions

Complications	Manifestations	Nursing care
Local		
Infiltration	Arm swollen, tender, cool to touch; Decrease in flow rate.	Remove IV catheter and restart IV in the other extremity.
Phlebitis	Vein gets hard with skin and red, swollen, tender, warm; blood return present; IV infusion may or may not be sluggish	Remove IV catheter, notify the physician apply warm soaks at the IV site.
Thrombophle-bitis	Site red, tender, warm; IV infusion sluggish	Never irrigate the IV catheter, remove the IV catheter, notify the physician, restart IV in opposite extremity.
IV site infection	Site hot, red, painful but not hard or swollen; IV infusion sluggish	Remove the IV catheter and inspect, place a tourniquet high on limb of IV site. Notify physician, obtain x-ray, prepare for surgery to remove pieces.
Systemic		
Infection	Fever, chills, general malaise	Change the infusion system, notify the physician, obtain cultures as ordered
Speed shock	Flushed face, severe headache, chest pain, irregular pulse, decreased BP, loss of consciousness, cardiac arrest	Stop the infusion, notify the physician, monitor vital signs frequently.
Circulatory overload	Increased BP, distended neck veins, rapid breathing, dyspnea, moist cough, crackles.	Elevate the head of the bed, keep warm, assess for edema, slow the infusion rate, notify the physician.
Air embolus	Sudden drop in BP, increase in pulse	Place on left side and lower head of the bed inspect IV infusion system for disconnection or leak, notify the physician.
Allergic reaction	Catheter—red streak along vein, pain at IV site Medication—site red, itching, rash	Remove IV catheter, restart IV using different type of IV catheter, notify the physician; discontinue the medication.

Catheter Embolus

Catheter embolus (piece of catheter obstructing blood flow) can occur if piece of the cannula breaks off and travels in the vein until it lodges. Air embolus can occur while changing bags. Speed shock occurs if fluids or medications is given by bolus administered too rapidly.

APPLICATION OF NURSING PROCESS

All nurses monitor IV therapy, add medications to IV solutions, calculate IV infusion rates, initiate IV therapy by inserting a cannula.

Assessment

A primary nursing responsibility is to check the patient's chart and verify the IV orders. The patient on IV infusion fluids must have the site assessed periodically, preferably hourly during the shift to ensure that the site is patent and that the solution is infusing correctly. The flow rate must be assessed to determine that the fluid is running at the prescribed rate. While giving IV medications the order must be carefully checked. Review the drug's action, possible side effects, correct dosage and nursing implications before preparing the drug. Assess for drug allergies before preparing the IV piggyback medication. Check for possible drug solutions incompatibilities. If incompatibilities exist; the IV line must be flushed with sterile saline before the other drug or solution is started and flushed again till the infusion or injection is finished. Assess for potential drug interactions in case more than one drug is being administered. Assess the existing IV site and cannula size before beginning the infusion of blood product through it. The site must be free of any signs of infection or inflammation. Blood products are not infused into the same IV line in which medications or other fluids are infused. Obtain baseline vital signs before starting the infusion of blood products.

Nursing Diagnosis

Common nursing diagnosis for patients who are undergoing various types of IV therapy might include:

- Fluid volume deficit related to inability to take fluids by mouth
- Risk for infection related to invasive procedure
- Altered nutrition less than body requirements, related to inability to take or use foods orally (total parenteral nutrition)
- Altered tissue perfusion related to loss of red blood cells/fluid volume

Planning

Any patient receiving IV fluids takes slightly more time to bathe, turn and he/she needs assistance in his/her daily activities. Allow time for the care of the patient's IV site, hanging of solutions, and needed assessments in the daily work schedule. The expected outcomes for the stated nursing diagnosis are:

- The patient's electrolyte values should be within normal limits within 24 hours
- No signs of dehydration are displayed
- The patient displays no signs of infection as evidenced by weight gain and protein levels are within normal limits
- The patient's nutritional status improves
- The patient's hemoglobin level should be within normal limits before discharge

CALCULATION OF FLOW RATES

To calculate the flow rate, it is important to know how many drops are contained in each milliliter as it passes through the drip chamber of the tubing because the size of drops varies for different types of administration sets. The standard set produces 10–20 drops/mL, the pediatric or micro drip chamber produces 50–60 drops/mL and the macro drip of the transfusion type sets give 10 drops/mL.

For the purposes of calculation 10 drop/mL is used for the macro drop, 15 drops/mL for the regular drop and 60 drops/mL for the micro drip chamber. The basic formula for calculating the flow rate is given below.

If the order reads 100 mL of D 500 over 10 hours

$$\frac{\text{amount of solution in mL} \times \text{no. of drop/mL}}{\text{time in minutes}} = \text{drop/minute}$$

Use a regular drop set (15 drops/mL)

$$\frac{100 \text{ mL} \times 15}{10 \times 60} = \frac{15000}{600} = 25 \text{ drops/mL}$$

While IV therapy is administered, the fluid enters the circulation immediately. An adult can adapt best to fluids at a steady rate of 20 to 60 regular drops/minute, i.e., 80–250 mL/hr. Larger amounts of fluids increase the work of the heart and the fluid overload could lead to congestive heart failure. The amount should infuse at an even rate so that equal amounts are given each hour. Keep the IV on time by regulating the drip rate. If IV fluids are infusing behind schedule, recalculate or reschedule the time in consultation with the physician (Table 4).

Factors that Influence the Rate of Flow

- **Size of needle:** Fluids flow less rapidly through a needle with a small bore than through a needle with a large bore.

TABLE 4: Troubleshooting intravenous flow

Check	Rationale
Height of infusion container	Patient may have changed position. The container should be at least 36 inches above the heart
System vent	Air vent may be absent or occluded, which will prevent the flow
Position of tubing	Tubing may be kinked, obstructing flow. Tubing may be hanging below the bed, interfering with the gravity flow
Position of the extremity where the site is located	Flexion of the extremity may have compressed the vein, slowing the flow
Attempt to aspirate blood from the cannula	A small clot may be obstructing the cannula. Aspiration may withdraw the clot
Position of the cannula within the vessel	Cannula may be lying against the vessel wall, obstructing flow. Slightly turning the cannula to reposition the tip may solve the problem

- **Height of the solution container:** The higher the container is held, the faster is the flow of fluid.
- **Viscosity of the fluid:** Packed red blood cells (RBCs) are more viscous and require a larger cannula. Table 4 indicates steps for attempting to get sluggish IV flow corrected.

Implementation

This phase of the nursing process includes all the tasks involved in caring for the patient receiving various types of IV therapy. The guideline for intravenous therapy are:

- **Keep the IV fluid sterile:** Make sure that everything coming in contact with the solution is sterile, including the cannula hub, all connecting points between the bag and drip chamber and between the tubing and the needle.
- **Protect the cannula site from contamination to avoid possible infection:** An airtight, transparent dressing is used over the cannula site.
- **Keep tubing free of air:** Clear tubing of air before connecting to the cannula by allowing the solution to run through. Does not allow the bag to run dry before changing the next one.
- **Hang fluids at the correct height:** Fluids flow through the tubing by the force of gravity. If there is negative pressure in the IV line, blood will flow back into the tubing. Keep the bag of fluid sufficiently above the level of the cannula site to maintain flow, but avoid having it too high because this significantly increases the effect of gravity.
- **Carefully regulate the rate of flow:** If the IV is behind the schedule, do not open the clamp and make the fluid run in

a large amount at one time to catch up. Rather, recalculate either the span of time for the infusion or the rate of drops per minute for the fluid to run at the ordered rate.

- Maintain intake and output of the patient receiving IV fluids or blood. Keep accurate intake and output records and compare intake and output over 24 hours.
- Assess the site frequently for signs of complications infiltration, swelling at the IV site, irritation of the vein, or formation of clot, stopping the flow, or systemic reaction should be identified quickly. Vital signs should be taken several times a day to detect early signs of infection or adverse reaction.
- **Observe closely for transfusion reactions:** Reactions to blood transfusion usually occur shortly after the start of transfusion (within 5–15 minutes) signs of reactions include hives, itching, facial flushing, chills back pain, apprehension and fever. If any of these occur stop the transfusion, start normal saline inform the physician for further orders.

Initiating Intravenous Therapy

Lot of preparation is necessary before initiating IV therapy. Equipment is gathered, the IV infusion is prepared, the most appropriate vessel is selected and the site prepared before venipuncture is performed.

- Selection of the IV site: Selection of a vein for IV use depends on several factors;
  - Accessibility of the vein
  - General condition of the vein
  - Type of fluid to be given
  - Duration of the IV infusion

The veins preferred for infusion and intermittent doses of medications are those distal to the antecubital area. The cephalic, basilic, and antebrachial veins of the lower arm and the veins of the back of the hand are the sites of choice for adult patients (Fig. 4). The most distal site is used first so that other sites are available, if therapy needs to be continued longer than 48–72 hours; a new site cannot be placed distal to an old site. The scalp veins are frequently used in infants because they are easily accessible. Veins of the foot are used only if no other site can be utilized.

Managing Intravenous Therapy

The nurse assigned to the patient is responsible for seeing to it that the IV infusion flows at the prescribed rate and that the solution is the one that was ordered. Movement of the patient can alter the rate. It is best to check the flow rate after the patient has been ambulating, returns from a test or a treatment, is settled after morning care, has been turned in bed, has been up to the bathroom, etc.

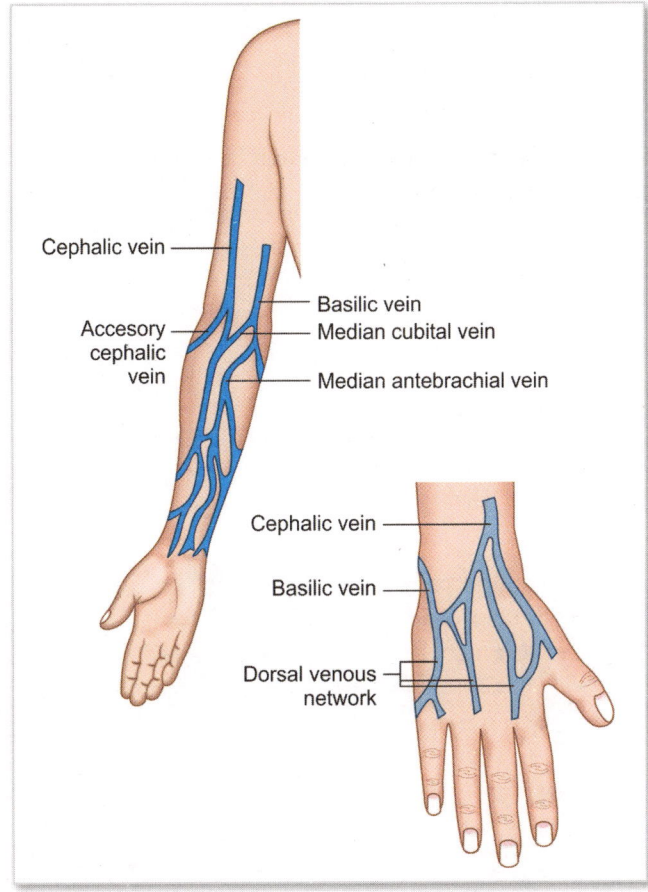

Fig. 4: Sites for insertion of intravenous cannula

Administering Intravenous Medications

Medications can be given by the IV route at one time or PRN doses, as multiple doses to be given at regularly scheduled times or by continuous infusion. Preparation of drugs to be used in IV requires dilution in 50–250 mL or more of fluid for certain drugs such as potassium chloride and antibiotics. In ICUs, drugs such as Lidocaine (Xylocaine) are given very slowly by bolus (a concentrated amount of medication at one time) and by infusion. If drug is given in bolus, the entire amount is injected over a short period into the vein to obtain immediate effects. Therefore, the nurse must be familiar with not only the drug's reaction and side effects but also the proper dose and time frames.

If a medication is administered too rapidly, speed shock may occur. In this the patient may lose consciousness, go into shock and cardiac arrest.

Various methods are used to administer IV medications, such as adding medications to the primary bag of fluids adding a secondary line or piggyback to the primary line, using controlled–volume burettes, or directly injecting the medication into the vein.

Some potent drugs and those causing irritation in concentrated strengths are diluted in 1000 mL of fluid. Drugs used in this way are potassium, insulin, sodium bicarbonate, calcium, magnesium sulphate, vitamin B complex, and vitamin C. Use strict aseptic technique while adding medication to IV fluids.

Medications that are given intermittently at timed intervals may be diluted in a small amount of fluid and administered by the piggyback method. Usually 50–150 mL of medication is added to a small bag of fluid if the patient is on PRN lock rather than on continuous IV infusion.

Another method of administering IV medications is to mix them in a small amount of solution in a controlled volume burette. Medications given by this method act to interrupt the primary infusion of fluids. Once the medicine is given the clamp is opened to restart the flow of primary solution.

Giving the medication directly into the vein over few minutes is termed giving a bolus, or IV push injection. The medication can be instilled via the injection port on the IV tubing, through a PRN lock or given into the vein.

Discontinuing an IV Infusion

If an infusion is to be discontinued, then the flow is stopped and the cannula is removed. Discontinuation is documented on the IV flow sheet.

The following guidelines are to be followed while managing intravenous therapy:

- **Keeping the IV solution running:** It is important to check every half an hour or so that fluid is running properly and note: the level of fluid remaining in the bag. If there is 50 mL left then a new bag may be added before the current solution is completely infused.
- **The IV flow:** The solution should drip into the chamber at regular intervals.
- The rate of the infusion to note. If it is too fast or too slow, it should be adjusted to the correct infusion rate per minute.
- **The needle site:** To check for signs of phlebitis.
- **Complaints from the patient:** There should not be any pain after the IV is started. There should not be any leaking at the site.

The solution container is hung from an IV stand. The tubing should be long enough to provide room for the patient to move about in bed, to turn over, or to carry out necessary activities.

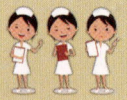

SKILL: STARTING THE INTRAVENOUS INFUSION

Before an IV cannula or needle is inserted, the solution to be infused is set up so that infusion can be started immediately. Maintain strict aseptic technique as IV site provides access for bacteria to enter the blood stream.

Articles Required

- Intravenous solution
- Intravenous administration set
- Scissors
- Intravenous stand
- Intravenous cannula
- Gloves
- Alcohol swabs
- Povidone iodine swabs
- Tape
- Transparent dressing
- Towels and protective covering
- Medication administration record
- Arm board or splint
- Kidney basin
- Paper bag.

Steps of Procedure

Review and carry out the standard steps as given in Appendix

Action/steps	Rationale
Assessment	
1. Inspect the patients hands and forearms, and select the site for venipuncture and choose the most distal site possible.	If repeated infusions are required, it is best to start the IV in the most distal vein and progress proximally with each successive site.
Planning	
2. Verify that the patient is ready for the procedure and gather all equipment.	Prepares the patient and prevents time loss.
Implementation	
3. Obtain the correct IV solution check the solution with the order.	Following the five rights of medicines administration applies to IV fluids.
4. Check the solution for clarity, leaks and particulate matter. Note the expiry date.	The solution should be free of sediments and must be in date.
5. Open the administration set, and position the roller clamp within the reach and regulate while watching the drops in the drip chamber. Close the roller clamp and remove the metal cap on the IV bottle and insert the spike, be careful, do not touch the spike or anything (keep it sterile).	If the roller camp is not closed, the fluid will run quickly through the tubing and out if the bag is inverted there will be break in aseptic technique the tubing or solution must be discarded.
6. Remove the air from the tubing slowly by opening the roller clamp after loosening the protector cap over the needle adapter to allow the air to escape, allow a small amount of fluid to escape from the tubing. Close the roller clamp and retighten the cap.	Air left in the tubing might cause an air embolism, although several milliliters of air must accumulate before serious damages could occur.
7. Place a time tape label on the IV container and mark it in gradations of the amount of fluid to be infused every 1–2 hours.	If time markings are indicated at different fluid levels, it is easy to see at glance the IV is flowing correctly according to the rate ordered.

Contd...

Action/steps	Rationale
8. Apply the tourniquet and check the site suitability. The tourniquet should be positioned on the mid-forearm, if the dorsum of hand is to be used. If the forearm area is to be used the tourniquet is placed on the upper arm or at least 4 – 6 inches above the site. Do not place the tourniquet so tight as to restrict arterial flow. Release the tourniquet	The venous flow must be restricted in the vein for it to distend enough to introduce the cannula. Releasing tourniquet promotes comfort.
9. Put the protective covering under the extremity and cleanse the site with povidone iodine, alcohol. Start at the center and work in circular motion outward for 2 inches. Allow area to dry. Wait for full 1 minute.	Microorganisms left on the skin may cause infection. A protective covering prevents bedding from being soiled.
10. Put on gloves, reapply the tourniquet and ask the patient to open and close the fist couple of times and hold it closed. Stabilize the skin below the IV site by placing thumb about 2 inches directly below the insertion site.	A tourniquet and opening and closing the fist distend the vein. Gloves are required in case the contact with blood is possible. For the needle to enter the vessel smoothly, the skin must be taut. This causes least discomfort to the patient.
11. Insert the IV needle into the vein by either method. By the **indirect method**, first insert the needle into the subcutaneous space directly parallel to the side of the vein, then move the tip of needle toward the vein. By the **direct method**, hold the needle with the bevel upright and at a 15–25 degrees angle to pierce the skin and then lower the needle until it is nearly parallel to the skin while piercing the vein. Enter the skin and vein in one quick, steady, forward thrust with the needle. An over the needle cannula should be placed all the way into the vein. Decreased resistance will be felt as the needle enters the vein. A pop may be felt. When the needle is in the vein, the blood return into the hub of the needle tubing. (Figs 5A and B)	The indirect method of cannula insertion has less chance of pushing the needle completely through the vein. The direct method is best in case the vein is large and stable.

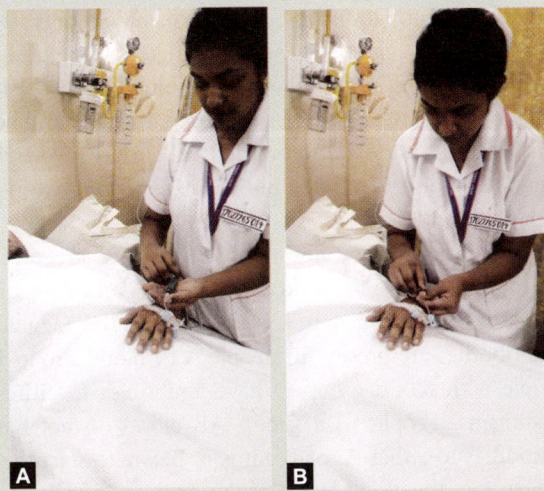

Figs 5A and B Administration of IV infusion

12. If it is certain that the catheter is in the vein, slide the catheter off the stylet into the vessel for its full length while keeping the stylet steady. Remove the stylet and advance the cannula. If needle is used, advance the needle to its full length into the vein. Remove the tourniquet and ask the patient to open the fist. If you go through the vein wall, remove the tourniquet, withdraw the needle and apply pressure.	Advancing the catheter or needle in case IV is not in the vein, causes pain and tissue damage. The stylet of the IV catheter should not be advanced after the catheter is positioned through the vein wall, only the cannula should be advanced into the vein. If IV catheter or needle goes through the vein, this site cannot be used as fluid leaks out of the vessel. Pressure need to be applied to prevent bleeding.

Contd...

Action/steps	Rationale
13. Remove the protective cap over the needle adapter on the IV tubing, attach the tubing to the catheter or needle hub, and open the clamp to begin the infusion slowly. Observe the site for swelling or leaking, indicating that the site is not patent.	Starting the solution flowing slowly establishes the patency of the IV before much fluid is infused. If the IV is not patent, little fluid infiltrates the tissue. The solution is stopped, and the cannula or needle is removed if the site is not patent.
14. If the site is patent, apply tape gently in a 'V' fashion across the hub of the catheter. Place a strip of ½ inch tape under the hub, sticky side up, crisscross the ends over the hub, and secure them to the skin. Sterile 2 × 2 gauze dressing may be applied. Loop the IV tubing on the extremity, and secure it again with tape. Immobilize the IV area with arm board.	Dressing protects the site from microorganisms. Taping the IV tubing prevents direct pull on the cannula, which could possibly dislodge if the patient moves around.
15. Regulate the solution flow according to the order by adjusting the roller clamp and counting the drops per minute.	The position of the arm, movement, and taping of the needle to stabilize it in the vein can alter the flow rate.
Evaluation	
16. Verify that the solution is running at the correct rate into the vein without pain and that the cannula is held securely in place.	Assures that the IV is patent and secure.
17. Clean up used supplies and make patient comfortable. Remove gloves and wash hands.	Prevents spread of microorganisms and helps patient's wellbeing.
Documentation	
18. It should include the site, the type of cannula inserted and the solution started. Record intake and output in the chart.	Documents the time of cannula insertion so that it can be changed at the appropriate time.

BLOOD TRANSFUSION

Intravenous fluids can be effective in restoring intravascular (blood) volume; however, they do not affect the oxygen carrying capacity of the blood. When red and white blood cells, platelets, or blood proteins are lost because of hemorrhage or disease, it may be necessary to replace these components to restore the ability of blood to transport oxygen and carbon dioxide, to fight infection, to clot, and to keep extracellular fluid within the intravascular compartment.

A blood transfusion is the introduction of whole blood or blood components into the venous circulation.

Blood Groups

Human body is commonly classified into four main groups (A B AB and O) (Table 5). The surface of an individual's red blood cells contains a member of proteins known as antigens that are unique for each person. Many blood antigens have been identified, but the antigen A, B and Rh are the most important in determining the blood group or type. Because antigens promote agglutination or clumping of blood cells, they are also known as agglutinogens. "A" antigen or agglutinogen is present on the RBC's of people with blood group A, the "B" antigen is present in people with blood group B, and both "A" and "B" antigen are found on the RBC surface in people with group AB blood. Neither A nor B antigen is present in people with O blood group.

Preformed antibodies to RBC antigens are present in the plasma; these antibodies are often called agglutinins. People with blood group A have B antibodies (agglutinins); A antibodies are present in people with blood group B; and people with blood group O have antibodies to either A or B antigens. People with group AB blood do not have any antibodies to either A or B antigen. Before to start the blood transfusion, the blood group of the donor and recipient must match to avoid an antigen antibody reaction and destruction (hemolysis) of RBCs.

Rhesus (Rh) Factor

The Rh factor antigen is present on the RBCs of approximately 85% of the people. Blood that contains the Rh factor is known as Rh positive (Rh+); and in which it is absent is Rh negative (Rh−). In contrast to the ABO blood groups, Rh blood does not naturally contain Rh antibodies. However, on exposure to blood containing Rh factor (e.g., an Rh− mother carrying a fetus with Rh+ blood, or transfusion of Rh+ blood into client

TABLE 5: The blood groups with their constituent agglutinogens and agglutinins

Blood type	RBC antigens (agglutinogens)	Plasma antibodies (agglutinins)
A	A	B
B	B	A
AB	A and B	–
O	–	A and B

who is Rh−), Rh antibodies develop. Subsequent exposures to Rh+ blood place the client at risk for an antigen – antibody reaction and hemolysis of RBC occurs.

Blood Typing and Cross Matching

To avoid transfusing incompatible red blood cells, both blood donor and recipient are typed and their blood cross-matched. Blood typing is done to determine the ABO blood group and Rh factor status. This test is also performed on pregnant women and neonates to assess for possible intrauterine exposure to incompatible blood type (particularly Rh factor incompatibilities).

Blood typing only determines the presence of the ABO and Rh antigens, cross matching is also necessary prior to transfusion to identify possible interactions of minor antigens with their corresponding antibodies. RBCs from the donor blood are mixed with serum from the recipient; a reagent (Coomb's serum) is added and the mixture is examined for visible agglutination. If no antibodies to the donated RBCs are present in the recipient's serum, agglutination does not occur and the risk of transfusion reaction is small.

Selection of Blood Donors

Screening of blood donors is rigorous. Criteria have been established to protect the donor from possible ill effects of donation and to protect the recipient from exposure to diseases transmitted through the blood. Criteria are:

- Blood donors are unpaid volunteers.
- Donor is free from disease. The blood must be tested for HIV (human immunodeficiency virus), hepatitis B and C virus (HBV and HCV) and syphilis.
- Donor with history of heart disease, cancer, severe asthma, bleeding disorders, convulsions, malaria or hepatitis, pregnancy, surgery, anemia, high or low blood pressure and certain drugs.
- Potential donors are questioned about their lifestyle and health history, including questions about diseases, past surgeries, tattoos, body piercing, travel, sex and drug use.
- Donors may give blood only if their blood count, Hb level, temperature, pulse, respiration, blood pressure, and weight are within normal limits.

Autologous Transfusion

This is a new concept and is growing in popularity. Autologous transfusion, also called auto transfusion, which eliminates the danger of transmitting cross-infection from donor to recipient and decreases the risk for complications from mismatched blood but requires advance planning. The blood must be donated 5 weeks before the surgery; which can be transfused later during surgery.

A patient's own blood can also be salvaged during surgery or collected from tubes and drains to allow for autologous transfusion.

Blood Components for Transfusion

Whole blood is rarely used unless blood loss is massive. With current technology, whole blood can be easily separated into its components, and patients receive only the blood product they need. For example, a patient may need red blood cells but not the blood plasma and its constituents. Red blood cells in concentrated form, called **packed red blood cells**, may be used in the following situations:

- Patient with anemia (reduction in RBCs or hemoglobin)
- Patient with cardiovascular failure, with a need to increase blood volume and red bed cells while avoiding circulatory overload.
- Patient with gastrointestinal (GI) bleeding, with a need to maintain adequate hemoglobin levels without increasing blood pressure, which would likely to more bleeding.

In other situations, only plasma is required, in case of low plasma protein or the blood clotting factors. **Fresh frozen plasma** is particularly useful in emergencies for immediate restoration of fluid because serum transfusion presents no compatibility problems and time need not be lost seeking donors and matching blood. It is also an excellent blood volume expander, for example, in a patient who is severely burned and losing plasma rapidly from burn areas. Components of plasma that are used therapeutically include human albumin (used for hypovolemic shock, albuminemia, liver failure), cryoprecipitates also contain fibrinogen used for bleeding due to hemophilia or disseminated intravascular coagulation (DIC), and gamma globulins the antibody containing part of plasma (used for gamma globulin deficiencies).

Platelet infusion is indicated for the treatment or prevention of bleeding associated with deficiencies in the number or function of patient's platelets. Platelet infusion is indicated in certain diseases such as Dengue fever in which the platelets count goes down.

Transfusion Reactions

Transfusion of ABO or Rh incompatible blood can result in hemolytic transfusion reactions with destruction of the transfused RBCs and subsequent risk of kidney damage or failures. Other forms of transfusion reaction may also occur, including febrile, allergic, circulatory overload and sepsis. Because the risk of an adverse reaction is high during blood transfusion, clients must be frequently and carefully assessed before and during transfusion. Many reactions become evident within 5–15 minutes of initiating the transfusion but they can develop any time during a transfusion. Clients should be closely monitored during the initial period of the transfusion. Stop the transfusion immediately, if signs of reaction develop.

Blood that has not been used within 30 minutes after its arrival from the blood bank must be returned, and blood that has been infusing for more than 4 hours must be discontinued to prevent the risk for bacterial contamination. Nurses are also responsible for monitoring the patient for adverse reactions to the blood transfusion. Table 6 describes the potential transfusion reactions.

Administering Blood

Special precautions are necessary while administering blood. Once a transfusion is ordered, obtain the blood from the blood bank just before starting the transfusion. Do not store the blood in the refrigerator in the nursing unit; lack of temperature control may damage the blood. Once blood

or blood product is removed from the refrigerator, there is limited amount of time to administer it (e.g., packed RBCs should not hang for more than 4 hours after being removed from the refrigerator). Blood is usually administered through 18–20–gauge intravenous needle. This size is necessary because of the viscosity of blood. The procedure for starting a blood transfusion is basically the same as for an IV infusion. If possible, select larger veins. A Y-type blood transfusion set with filter is used while administering blood. One arm of the administration set connects to the blood; normal saline (0.9% NaCl) is attached to the other arm of the Y-type set. Saline is used to prime the set and flush the needle before administering blood. It also provides a means to keep the vein open if a transfusion reaction occurs. No other IV solution should be administered with blood; they may cause the blood cells to clump or cause clotting.

TABLE 6: Transfusion reactions

Reaction: Cause	Clinical signs	Nursing Intervention*
Hemolytic reaction: Incompatibility between client's and donor's blood	Chills, fever, headache, backache, dyspnea, cyanosis, chest pain, tachycardia and hypotension	◆ Discontinue the transfusion immediately. **Note:** When the transfusion is discontinued, the blood tubing must be removed as well. Use *new* tubing for the normal saline infusion. ◆ Maintain vascular access with normal saline, or according to agency protocol. ◆ Notify the primary care provider immediately. ◆ Monitor vital signs. ◆ Monitor fluid intake and output. ◆ Send the remaining blood, bag, filter, tubing, a sample of the client's blood, and a urine sample to the laboratory.
Febrile reaction: Sensitivity of the client's blood to white blood cells, platelets, or plasma proteins	Fever, chills, warm, flushed skin, headache, anxiety and muscle pain	◆ Discontinue the transfusion immediately. ◆ Give antipyretics as ordered. ◆ Notify the primary care provider. ◆ Keep the vein open with a normal saline infusion.
Allergic reaction (mild): Sensitivity to infused plasma proteins	Flushing, itching, urticaria and bronchial wheezing	◆ Stop or slow the transfusion, depending on agency protocol. ◆ Notify the primary care provider. ◆ Administer medication (antihistamines) as ordered.
Allergic reaction (severe): antibody–antigen reaction	Dyspnea, chest pain, circulatory collapse and cardiac arrest	◆ Stop the transfusion. ◆ Keep the vein open with normal saline. ◆ Notify the primary care provider immediately. ◆ Monitor vital signs. Administer cardiopulmonary resuscitation, if needed. ◆ Administer medications and/or oxygen as ordered.
Circulatory overload: blood administered faster than the circulation can accommodate	Cough, dyspnea, crackles (rales, distended neck veins, tachycardia, hypertension	◆ Place the client upright, with feet dependent. ◆ Stop or slow the transfusion. ◆ Notify the primary care provider. ◆ Administer diuretics and oxygen as ordered.
Sepsis: contaminated blood administered	High fever, chills, vomiting, diarrhea, hypotension	◆ Stop the transfusion. ◆ Keep the vein open with a normal saline infusion. ◆ Notify the primary care provider. ◆ Administer IV fluids, antibiotics. ◆ Obtain a blood specimen from the client for culture. ◆ Sent the remaining blood and tubing to the laboratory.

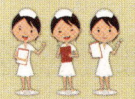

SKILL: ADMINISTRATION OF BLOOD PRODUCTS

Blood components are administered for a variety of reasons. There is no margin for error while administering blood products because adverse reactions can be considerable and life threatening. Most agencies require that two nurses verify the ordered blood component with the component supplied by blood bank and casualty match up the patient number with the blood component number. A signed consent is needed before a blood product administration begins.

Equipment and supplies:

- Blood transfusion set
- Ordered blood component
- Blood bank slip
- Normal saline (0.9% IV solution)
- Physician's order
- Alcohol swabs
- Gloves
- Tape
- Protective lining
- Waste receptacle
- Arm board/splint

Steps of Procedure

Review and carryout the standard steps as listed in Appendix

Action/steps	Rationale
Assessment	
1. See that the patient has a patent 18–20 gauge cannula or needle in place. Plasma products may be infused via 22 gauge needle.	A needle smaller than 19 gauge may break up red cells.
Planning	
2. Gather the equipment, verify that the patient is ready, and obtain the blood product from the blood bank.	Saves time; administration of the blood product must begin within 30 minutes of the time the product leaves the blood bank.
Implementation	
3. Verify the blood component with another nurse, and compare the donor number and the ABO group and Rh type on the request slip with the label and number on the blood component bag; check the bag for clots.	For safety, two nurses must verify the order and match the numbers on the blood component with those on the transfusion record slip. The blood component may not be transfused after the expiration date. If the unit contains clots, it should be returned to the blood bank.
4. Close all clamps on the Y administration set. Hang a normal saline container. Prime the filter and tubing with normal saline by opening the clamp below the drip chamber. Hang the blood component bag. For packed red cells, invert and lower the packed red cell bag. Open the clamp to the normal saline while keeping the roller clamp closed. Allow about 50 mL of saline to run into the packed red cells. Close the clamps.	A Y-set is always to be used for blood component infusion. Priming the filter and tubing with normal saline removes air and eases the way for blood flow. Combining a small amount of saline with packed red cells, decreases the viscosity and helps the blood infuse more easily. Care is taken to close clamps so that none of the blood product is accidentally lost.
5. Take the administration set to the patient's unit, identify the patient, comparing the full name and hospital identification number with the transfusion record information.	It is mandatory that all identifying information and numbers match exactly. If discrepancies occur, notify the blood bank. Transfusion does not begin until the discrepancy is resolved.
6. Put on gloves and face shield, and connect the administration set to the cannula. Start the normal saline to clear the cannula, and verify the patency of the site.	Gloves must be used when contact with blood is likely. The patency of the site must be verified before beginning the transfusion.
7. Obtain baseline vital signs. If the patient's temperature is over 100°F, consult the physician. Assess the patients physical status and look for signs and symptoms of transfusion reaction.	Baseline data are essential. It helps to determine later if a transfusion reaction is occurring.

Contd...

Action/steps	Rationale
8. Clamp off the saline, and open the clamp to the blood. Set the flow rate at 2 mL /minute for the first 15 minutes. Remain with the patient for at least the first 5 minutes. Reassess the patient and take vital signs at the end of 15 minutes. If there are no adverse reactions, the infusion rate may be increased to the calculated flow rate. Take vital signs at the end of 30 minutes and then every 30 minutes until the transfusion is complete. Blood must be infused within 4 hours of release from the blood bank.	Begins the transfusion. Adverse reactions occur most frequently during the first 5 minutes although delayed reaction can occur. The patient must be monitored throughout the transfusion for any signs of an adverse reaction. Average time is 2 hours per unit.
9. After the blood component has been infused, flush the line with normal saline and maintain at 50 mL/hr to keep vein patent, then convert to a PRN lock, or discontinue the IV as per order.	Previously hanging IV solution and tubing are considered contaminated and must be discarded.
Evaluation	
10. Monitor vital signs and assess for shortness of breath, rash, back pain, apprehension, fever, tachycardia, nausea and vomiting, and other signs of transfusion reaction.	Evaluates whether a reaction has occurred.
Documentation	
11. Document the infusion on the IV flow sheet. Add the amount infused to the IV intake record. Document cross match identification number with the donor type and Rh type, volume infused, date and time, any reaction, signs and symptoms any adverse reactions must be charted in the nurses notes.	Documents the transfusion and patient's response.

BIBLIOGRAPHY

1. *White L. Basic Nursing. Foundations of Nursing Skills and Concepts. Delmar Thomson Learning; 2002.*

2. *Carol A, McAthie LM. Fundamentals of Contemporary Nursing Practice. WD Saunder's Company.*

3. *Fuerst, Elinor V, Lewis, et al. Fundamentals of Nursing. Philadelphia PA: JB Lippincott Company; 1974*

4. *Taylor C, Lillis C, LeMone P, Lynn P. Fundamentals of Nursing, 6th edition. Lippincott Williams and Wilkins: Philadelphia. 2008.*

5. *McClain ME, Gragg SH. Scientific Principles in Nursing. C.V. Mosby Co, St. Louis; 1966.*

Advance Techniques

THORACENTESIS

Introduction

Excessive pleural fluid or air can accumulate in the pleural cavity as a result of injury or disease. This may alter the respiratory function.

Thoracentesis is performed for diagnostic or therapeutic purposes. The amount of fluid that is removed is usually about 20–30 mL, the specimen thus collected is examined in the laboratory for its color consistency, specific gravity, presence of abnormal cells and bacteria. When thoracentesis is done for therapeutic purpose a large amount of fluid is withdrawn to relieve the pressure symptoms in the chest caused by the accumulation of fluid in the pleural cavity.

Definition

Thoracentesis refers to the puncture done by needle through the chest wall into the pleural space for the purpose of removing pleural fluid (blood, serous fluid, pus, etc.) and air.

Related Anatomy and Physiology of Thorax, Lung and Pleura

The skeletal part of the thorax is the bony enclosure formed by the sternum, costal cartilages, ribs and the bodies of thoracic vertebrae.

Twelve pairs of ribs give structural support to the side of thoracic cavity. True ribs—the first seven pairs of ribs have a direct anterior attachment to sternum by a strip of hyaline cartilage called costal cartilage. False ribs–the remaining five pair of ribs are either indirectly or not attached with sternum costal cartilage called false ribs. The spaces in between the ribs are called intercostal space.

The lungs are cone-shaped, paired organs in the thoracic cavity. Left lung has two lobes—superior and inferior and right lung has three lobes—superior, middle and inferior.

Two layers of serous membrane enclose and protect each lung and called collectively as pleural membranes.

The superficial layer called the parietal pleura, lines the wall of thoracic cavity. The deep layer, and the visceral pleura cover the lungs themselves. The pleural cavity is filled with pleural fluid produced by pleural membrane. Pleural fluid has three functions:

1. It acts as a lubricant allowing the pleural membrane to slide each other during respiration.
2. It helps to hold the pleural membrane together.
3. During some disease condition there is increased amount of pleural fluid called pleural effusion.

Purposes of Thoracentesis

- Diagnostic
- Therapeutic

Diagnostic

To study the chemical, bacteriological and cellular composition which may reveal the presence of neoplastic cells effusions characterized by lymphocytosis carcinoma, etc.

Therapeutic

- To remove excessive pleural fluid, which could become infected and cause empyema.
- To relieve lung compression, pain and respiratory distress caused by the accumulation of fluid or air in the pleural space.
- To instill medication into the thoracic cavity.

Related Terms

- **Pneumothorax:** Air in the pleural cavity
- **Hemothorax:** Blood in the pleural cavity
- **Pyothorax:** Pus in the pleural cavity
- **Hemopneumothorax:** Presence of blood and air in the pleural cavity

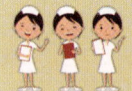 **SKILL: PERFORMING THORACENTESIS**

Equipment

- Spirit, Betadine, local anesthetic agent (1% lidocaine)
- Waterproof sheet with towel
- Sterile gloves, gown and mask
- Sterile collection bottle
- Kidney tray and paper bag
- Sterile tray containing:
  - Syringe with needle for local anesthesia
  - Aspiration needle
  - 20cc–30cc syringe with adapter three-way stopcock
  - Sterile bowls
  - Sterile cotton balls, gauze
  - Fenestrated towel (for maintaining sterile field)

Site of Thoracentesis

Physician uses a chest X-ray for the purpose of measuring the fluid level and the level at which the aspiration would be performed and may use the percussion method. The site of puncture is the region that is dullest to percussion. The site for thoracentesis is the area below the inferior angle of the scapula at the seventh intercostal space (Fig. 1).

Contd...

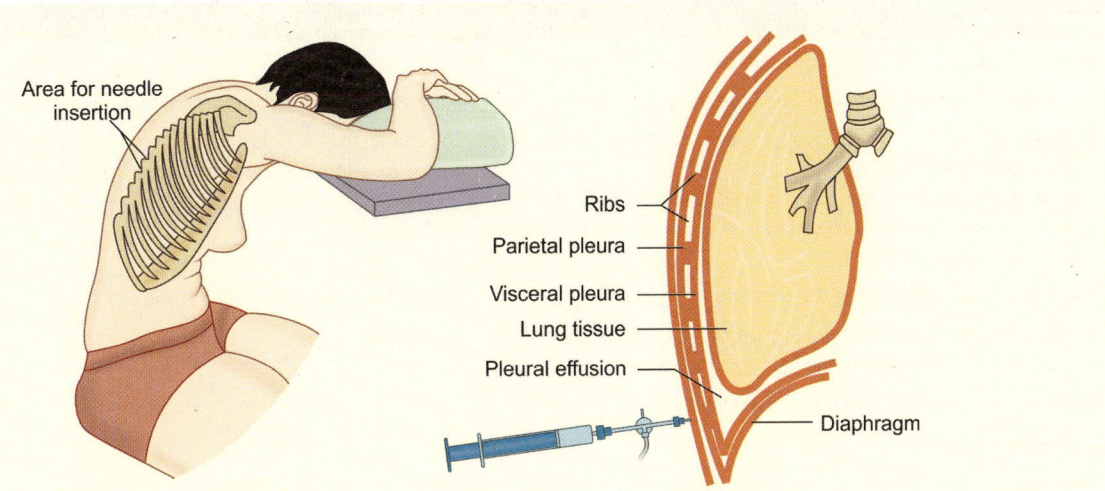

Fig. 1: Site for thoracentesis

Steps of Procedure

Review and follow the standard steps as given in Appendix

Action/steps	Rationale
Assessment	
1. Assess the client's ability to understand and follow instructions necessary to assume and maintain proper position	Helps to know what all information needs to be given and helps to accumulate the pleural fluid at the base of chest
Planning	
2. Obtain informed consent from the patient	For legal concerns
3. Assess vital signs and assess patient for allergy to local anesthetic	
4. Explain the procedure to the patient ▪ Importance of remaining immobile and refrain from coughing ▪ Explain where and when the procedure will be performed ▪ Have the patient empty the bladder and bowel	Helps patient's cooperation during the procedure
5. Position the patient ▪ Either sitting on the edge of bed with feet supported and arms on a padded bed-table ▪ Lying on the unaffected side with head of bed elevated 30°–45°, if unable to assume a sitting position (Fig. 2)	Helps for easy removal of fluid for the pleural space

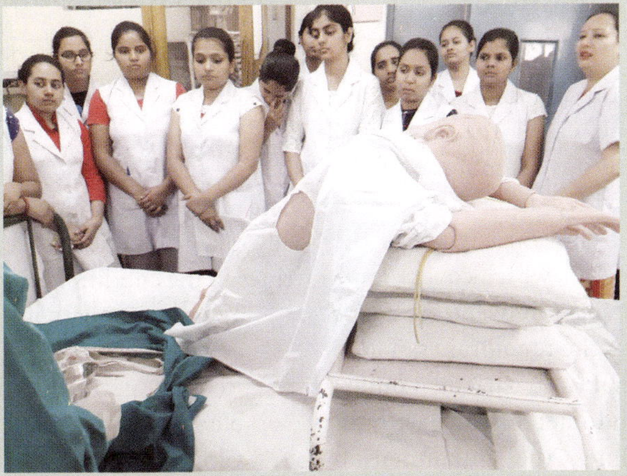

Fig. 2: Position the patient for thoracentesis

Contd...

Action/steps	Rationale
Implementation	
6. Expose the puncture site and clean the site with aseptic solution	For easy visibility and prevent infection
7. Give local anesthesia and assist physician to insert the needle in the intercostal space • A diagnostic thoracentesis requires 20–30 mL of fluid • A therapeutic thoracentesis can drain 1–2 liter at a time by using three-way stopcock	Local anesthesia helps to relieve pain as the needle is inserted to collect adequate amount of specimen required for tests
8. Observe vital signs during the procedure	Helps to monitor the patient properly
9. After the needle is withdrawn, pressure is applied over the puncture site and apply small, airtight sterile dressing	To prevent leakage and seal the area
10. Discard the used equipment and wash hands	Decreases transfer of microorganisms
Evaluation	
11. Determine how the patient tolerated and observe for coughing, decreased breath sounds, blood in sputum and rapid pulse rate	To report their occurrence immediately
Documentation	
12. Document the amount of fluid withdrawn and nature of fluid, its color and viscosity	Sample to be labeled and sent for laboratory evaluation

ABDOMINAL PARACENTESIS

Introduction

The peritoneal cavity is the largest serous membrane of the body. In certain diseases the peritoneal cavity may become distended by the accumulation of several liters of fluid in a condition called ascites.

Definition

Abdominal paracentesis is the removal of fluid from the peritoneal cavity through a small surgical incision or puncture made through the abdominal wall under sterile condition either to relieve pressure to drain the cavity or for diagnostic purpose.

Related Anatomy and Physiology of Peritoneal Cavity

♦ The body walls and organs of the abdominal cavity are lined with a serous membrane, called the peritoneal membrane. It is the largest serous membrane of the body. The peritoneum is divided into the parietal peritoneum, which covers the interior surface of the body wall and visceral peritoneum, which covers some of the organs in the cavity. The space between the layers is containing fluid secreted by the membranes. These membranes (visceral—internal and parietal—outer) allow the organs within the abdomen to move without producing friction. Sometimes the inflammation of the peritoneum by infectious microbes causes peritonitis.

Purpose of Paracentesis

♦ To make a diagnosis, to study chemical, bacteriological and cellular composition of the peritoneal fluid.
♦ To relieve pressure symptoms in ascitis
♦ To drain exudates
♦ To give treatment.

Sites for Abdominal Paracentesis

♦ A common site is the midway between the symphysis pubis and umbilicus on the midline.
♦ A point two-thirds along a line from the umbilicus to the anterior superior iliac spine.

This site is mainly selected to avoid injury to the urinary bladder and other abdominal organs.

Position for Abdominal Paracentesis

The patient is given Fowler's position and he/she is supported with back rest and pillows near the edge of the bed.

Physical Characteristics

The normal appearance of a sample of peritoneal fluid is usually straw-colored and clear. Abnormal appearances may give clues to the conditions or diseases present and may include:

♦ Yellow color with liver disease, milky from the lymphatic system and greenish from bile.
♦ Reddish peritoneal fluid may indicate the presence of blood.
♦ Cloudy peritoneal fluid may indicate the presence of microorganisms and with blood cells pointing to an infection.

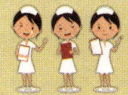

SKILL: PERFORMING ABDOMINAL PARACENTESIS

Equipment and Supplies

- Spirit, Betadine, local anesthetic agent 2% Lignocaine
- Waterproof sheet with towel
- Sterile gloves, gown and mask
- Kidney tray and paper bag
- Sterile tray containing:
  - Sponge-holding forceps
  - 5 mL syringe for local anesthesia

- 20 mL syringe for aspiration of fluid
- Three-way adapter and tubing
- Scalpel, trocar and cannula with rubber tubing
- Fenestrated towel (for maintaining sterile fluid)
- Cotton balls and sterile gauze
- Sterile specimen bottles
- Abdominal binder
- Pint measure
- Inch tape

Steps of Procedure

Review and follow the standard steps as given in Appendix

Action/steps	Rationale
Assessment	
1. Assess the client's ability to understand and follow instructions. Palpate client's bladder for distention and determine time for last voiding	To gain cooperation of the patient Ask the patient to empty bladder 5 minutes before the procedure to avoid injury to urinary bladder.
2. Measure abdominal girth in centimeters at the largest point of abdomen. Check weight and vital signs	To have the baseline observation
Planning	
3. Assess vital signs and keep patient warm and comfortable	To prevent peripheral vasoconstriction and monitor patient closely for signs of vascular collapse
4. Position the patient ▪ Give Fowler's position to the client	Comfortable for the patient and easy expansion of thoracic cavity
5. Change the clients garments and have gown during the procedure	Prevents interference with the procedure
Implementation	
6. Expose the area below the nipple to the pubic area	To minimize exposure of the client
7. Place the waterproof cover with towel	To protect the linen
8. Wash hands and open the sterile tray	To prevent cross-Infection
9. Assist the doctor in drawing local anesthesia and after infiltration with local anesthetic, the doctor will insert trocar and cannula halfway between umbilicus and anterior superior iliac spine after cleansing skin	To anesthetize the site of paracentesis and help in preventing local pain during procedure Cleaning with antiseptic prevent infection
10. Withdraw fluid slowly and in small quantity at a time. Apply many tailed abdominal blinder and tighten it from above downward as the fluid is drained	Sudden drop in intra-abdominal pressure may cause the client to go in hypovolemic shock
11. Attach the rubber tubing to the cannula after removal of trocar to drain the fluid into sterile pint measure and adjust the flow with screw clamp	To drain fluid and prevent cross infection
12. Monitor vital signs closely for vascular collapse, increased pulse rate, fall in blood pressure	Do not remove more than 1000 mL at a time
13. Collect specimen of peritoneal fluid	For diagnostic purpose
14. Seal the punctured area with sterile pressure dressing	To prevent infection and leakage
15. Return the equipment and make client comfortable. Continue to monitor vital signs every 15 minutes of 1st hour, every 30 minutes for 2 hours and then every 2 hours and then 4 hourly	Close monitoring is essential after removal of peritoneal fluid

Contd...

Action/steps	Rationale
16. Measure the abdominal girth and weight of the patient after the procedure	Reduction of abdominal girth and weight after procedure indicates effective fluid drain
Evaluation	
17. Determine how the patient tolerated and observe for complications such as injuries to bladder or bowel, peritonitis, etc.	To report their occurrence immediately to the physician
Documentation	
18. Document the amount of fluid withdrawn, its color and consistency. Record the vital signs	Sample collected to be labeled and sent to laboratory for evaluation

EPIDURAL PUNCTURE

Introduction

Continuous epidural analgesia is the most effective way of providing and maintaining labor analgesia. Over the past 20 years the technique has undergone a number of modifications that increased the safety efficacy and patient satisfaction. Epidural analgesia is administered into the epidural space through a catheter which is usually placed in the operating room and post anesthesia room unit of intensive care unit (ICU).

Definition

Epidural puncture is a form of local anesthesia and an effective therapy for the treatment of post-traumatic, chronic non-cancer and cancer pain. Epidural analgesia is short- or long-term, depending on the patient's condition and life expectancy. Short-term epidural analgesia is effective for pain after intrathoracic, abdominal, and orthopedic surgery. Useful in long-term therapy for pain non-responsive to oral or parental medications.

Related Anatomy and Physiology

The spinal cord lies within the spinal column, beginning at the foramen magnum and terminating about the level of the first lumber vertebra. Like the brain, the spinal cord is enclosed and protected by the meninges. The arachnoid and dura mater are separated by a potential space known as subdural space. Epidural puncture is done between the dura mater and subarachnoid mater.

Advantages

- Production of excellent analgesia
- Occurrence of minimal sedation
- Longer-lasting pain relief with fewer opioid doses
- Facilitation of early ambulation
- Avoidance of repeated injections

- No significant effect on sensation
- Little effect on blood pressure or heart rate
- Epidural is punctured either for epidural anesthesia or epidural analgesia

Purposes

To administer spinal anesthesia before surgery and to administer medications into the spinal canal.

Indications

- Administer anesthesia
- Diagnostic purpose radio contrast agent
- For treatment of chronic pain

Contraindications

- Anatomical abnormalities — spina bifida, scoliosis
- Previous spinal surgery
- Bleeding disorder

Position

Patient should be positioned either on his side in the fetal position (lateral decubitus) or seated on the edge of the bed, slightly bend forward with his feet dangling.

These positions open the spaces between the vertebrae and easy insertion of catheter in the epidural space.

Steps of Procedure

Preprocedural Steps

- Prepare the patient by introducing yourself and explaining
- Obtain informed consent
- Ensure the patient has an empty stomach
- Take the patient to a suitable site
- Institute monitoring
- Draw up any drugs that may be needed
- Obtain intravenous access

Intraprocedural Steps

- Position the patient, sitting or lateral with a flexed spine at the edge of the bed
- Use an aseptic technique that prepares the skin as for surgical procedure
- Provide local anesthetic infiltration
- Use a middle, paramedian or caudal approach
- Use an LP needle for cannulation—2 sizes with their stilet 22 g/24 g

Postprocedural Steps

- Monitor blood pressure, heart rate and respiration
- Review the patient for late onset complication

Aftercare of the Client

- As soon as the needle is withdrawn, seal the puncture site.
- Place the client comfortable on the bed in the supine position for 12–24 hours.
- If the client develops post-puncture headache, the following precautions should be taken:
  - Darken the room
  - Give plenty of oral fluids
  - Administer analgesics
  - Raise the foot end of the bed.
- Watch the client's color pulse, respiration, blood pressure and other signs of complications such as nausea, vomiting headache, etc.
- Record the procedure in nurses' records.

Nursing Care

- Monitor vital signs every 15 minutes for the first 2–3 hours and every hour for the first 24 hours as the client is at risk for respiratory depression, which may not manifest itself for several hours.
- Ensure the naloxone, a narcotic antagonist is immediately available to reverse respiratory depression.
- Monitor the effectiveness of the pain management.
- Monitor intake and output, intraspinal narcotic may block the micturition reflex, causing urinary retention and necessitating the insertion of Foley's catheter.
- Use sterile technique to care for the catheter.

LUMBAR PUNCTURE

Definition

Lumber puncture is a medical procedure, which involves withdrawing cerebrospinal fluid by the insertion of a hollow spinal needle with a stilet into the lumbar subarachnoid space.

Anatomy and Physiology

The spinal cord lies within the spinal column, beginning at the foramen magnum and terminating at the level of the first lumber vertebra. Like the brain, the spinal cord is enclosed and protected by meninges, that is, the dura mater, arachnoid mater and pia mater. The dura and arachnoid mater are separated by potential space known as subdural space. The arachnoid and pia mater are separated by the subarachnoid space, which contains the cerebrospinal fluid (CSF), the filum terminale and the cauda equins. To avoid damage to the spinal cord, the lumbar puncture is performed below the first lumbar vertebra where the cord terminates.

The cord serves as the main pathway for the ascending and descending fiber tracts that connect the peripheral and spinal nerves with brain. The peripheral nerves are attached to the spinal cord by 31 pair of spinal nerves.

Cerebrospinal fluid is formed primarily by filtration and secretion from networks of capillaries, called choroid plexus, locates in the ventricles of the brain. Eventually absorption takes place through the arachnoid villi, which are finger-like projections of the arachnoid mater that push into the dural venous sinuses.

Characteristics of CSF

Cerebrospinal fluid is clear, colorless and slightly alkaline with a specific gravity of 1005. In an adult, approximately 500 mL of CSF are produced and reabsorbed each day, with 120–150 mL present at one time.

Functions of CSF

- To act as a shock absorber
- To carry nutrients to the brain
- To remove metabolites from the brain
- To support and protect the brain and spinal cord
- To keep the brain and spinal cord moist.

Sampling and CSF Pressures

The amount of CSF withdrawn for sampling depends on the investigation required. In practice, approximately 5–10 mL.

Normal CSF pressure falls between a range of 60 and 180 mm of H_2O.

Normal Values of CSF Constituents

Test	Normal range in child	In adult
Color	Crystal clear	Crystal clear
Odor	Odorless	Odorless
CSF protein	5–40 mg/dL	15–45 mg/dL
CSF glucose	40–80 mg/dL	50–80 mg/dL
WBC	0–5 mm^3	0–7 mm^3

Physical Findings in Different Conditions (Abnormal Values)

Color/Appearance

Crystal clear	Normal
Turbid	Infection
Blood stained	Hemorrhage

Cell Count

0–5 cumm	Normal
Presence of RBC	Hemorrhage
Increased number of WBC (above 5 mm³)	Infection
Lymphocytes	Viral and tuberculosis infection
Increased polymorphonuclear leucocytes	Pyogenic infections

Sugar

50–80 mg/dL	Normal
Lower than normal level	Tubercular meningitis

Chloride

50–80 mg/dL	Normal
Lower than normal level	Bacterial infection

Protein

15–45 mg/dL	Normal
Increased than the normal level	Degenerative diseases and brain tumors

Diagnostic Tests Performed from CSF

- Culture and sensitivity:
    - Virology screening.
    - Serology for syphilis
- Protein: There is normally more albumin (80%) than globulin in CSF as albumins are smaller molecules, raised globulin levels are indicative of multiple sclerosis, neurosyphilis, degenerative cord or brain disease. However, raised levels of total protein can be indicative of meningitis, encephalitis, myelitis or the presence of a tumor.
- Cytology: Central nervous system tumors or secondary meningeal disease tend to shed cells into the CSF, where they float freely. Examination of these cells morphologically after lumbar puncture (LP) determines whether the tumor is benign or malignant.

Purposes

Diagnostic purposes and therapeutic purposes.

Indications

- To administer certain medications. For example, instillation of chemotherapy
- To administer spinal anesthesia
- To reduce intracranial pressure (ICP)
- To measure the pressure of CSF
- For diagnostic purpose
- To diagnose the brain tumors or other brain disorder, e.g., Pneumoencephalography, myelography

Contraindications

- Patients with papilledema or deteriorating neurological symptoms, where there is a chance of raised ICP.
- In the presence of local skin infection.
- Presence of frontal sinusitis, middle ear discharge, congenital heart diseases, or prosthetic heart valve may give rise to cerebral abscesses.
- Patients who are uncooperative or who are too drowsy to give a history.
- Patients who have severe degenerative spinal joint disease.
- Patients undergoing anticoagulant therapy or who have coagulopathies or thrombocytopenia.

Sites of Lumbar Puncture and Positioning of the Client

In Adults

- Usually between the 3rd and 4th lumbar vertebrae.
- The spinal needle is inserted in the midline between the spinous process of the vertebrae.

In Children and Infants

In children, the spinal cord extends up to the 3rd lumbar vertebra. So the site is lower than that, i.e., 4th and 5th lumbar vertebra (Fig. 3).

Positioning
Lying Down Position

- Patient is given side lying position (right or left) at the edge of the table or bed.
- One pillow under the patient's head.
- On side with knees drawn up to the chest and clasped by the hands. Fetal attitude or "C"-shaped position. Spine is fully flexed. Patient is asked to touch the chest with chin.
- Support patient in this position by holding him/her behind the knees and neck.

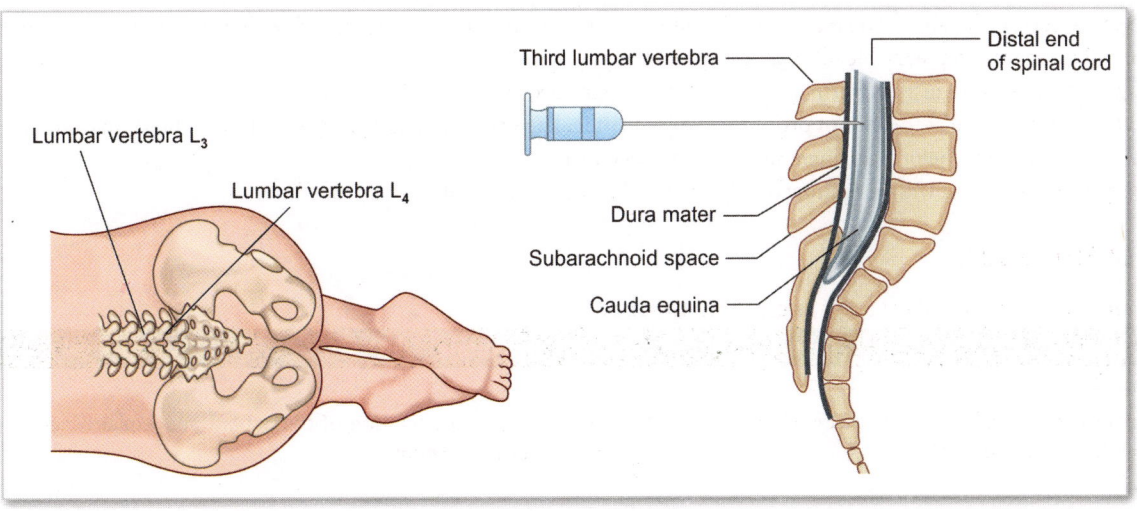

Fig. 3: Lumbar puncture: Position of client and insertion of the needle into the subarachnoid space are shown

Sitting Position

- Patient sits on a straight backed chair so that his/her back is facing the doctor.
- Patient folds arms on the back of the chair and rests head on them.

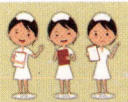 **SKILL: PERFORMING LUMBAR PUNCTURE**

A sterile tray containing the following articles
- Sponge-holding forceps
- Two bowls
- Cotton balls and gauze pieces
- Sterile drapes or fenestrated towel

Another tray containing the following articles
- Waterproof sheet with towel
- Inj. Xylocaine 2%
- Spirit, iodine (Betadine), tr. Benzoin
- Adhesive tape, scissors
- Disposable syringes 2 mL, 5 mL, and 10 mL
- Disposable lumbar puncture needles spinal needle 18, 22, 23, 24 gauge
- Disposable gloves, gown and mask
- Spirit swab in a container
- Specimen bottles
- Three-way stopcock, manometer
- Mackintosh and towel

General Instructions/Points to Remember

- Follow strict aseptic technique. Use sterile articles only.
- Give position as per doctor's preference (sitting or side lying).
- Use sharp and appropriate sized needles.
- The flow of cerebrospinal fluid (CSF) vary in different conditions. When intracranial pressure (ICP) is high, the fluid may spurt in jets. When the tension is low, the fluid may come out only on coughing and straining.
- The specimen should be sent to the laboratories immediately after the procedure.

- The specimen bottles should be numbered 1, 2 and 3 as the specimens are collected. The first specimen may contain a tinge of blood due to the capillary bleeding at the site of the puncture.
- Drugs to be injected must be warmed to the body temperature and it should be injected slowly.
- Seal the puncture site at the end of procedure to prevent leakage and the entry of infection into the spinal canal.
- Check the vital signs before, during and after the procedure.
- Give a supine position without pillow or slightly head down position after the procedure.

Steps of Procedure

Review and follow the standard steps as given in Appendix

Action/steps	Rationale
Assessment	
1. Assess the client's ability to understand and follow instructions, check for written consent	To gain cooperation of the patient and explain specific purpose of the procedure
Planning	
2. Explain the procedure to the patient. Ask the patient to empty the bladder	To reduce anxiety of the patient
3. Place the patient on the edge of the bed so that back is facing the doctor or in lateral position, at the edge of the bed with knees drawn up to abdomen, and chin tucking the chest (Fig. 4) Fig. 4: Position the patient for lumbar puncture	This position helps an easy entry to arachnoid space
Implementation	
4. Spread water proof sheet with towel	Protects bed linen from soiling
5. Wash your hands	Helps to control infection
6. Check vital signs	To obtain baseline data
• Assist the physician by opening and providing necessary items	
▪ Clean the puncture site area	To prevent infection
▪ Drape the area with fenestrated towel	To provide sterile field
▪ Assist in injecting local anesthetic	To reduce sensation of pain
▪ Locate L_3-L_4 space and insert the spinal needle 20–22 gauge usually 4–5 cm into the skin	To aid in accurate insertion of needle between L_3-L_4 space and avoid any spinal injury
▪ When needle is in place, remove stilet and attach a manometer with stopcock to the needle hub to read CSF pressure	To monitor CSF pressure (normal pressure 8–15 mm Hg)
▪ Disconnect manometer and collect approximately 2 or 3 mL of fluid in each labeled specimen container (1, 2)	To send for various investigations
▪ Administer contrast media for radiologic studies or anesthesia drugs for spinal anesthesia or chemotherapy drugs as per the requirement	For visualization of spinal cord or administer drugs
▪ Remove the spinal needle and apply pressure to the area and seal the site with Tr. Benzoin	Prevents post-lumbar puncture CSF leak
▪ Apply small dressing	To prevent infection

Contd...

Action/steps	Rationale
Evaluation	
7. After the procedure, assess for any discomfort, headache, and vital signs. Ask the client to remain in supine position for 12–24 hours	Supine position for 12–24 hours helps in preventing leakage of CSF and headache
Documentation	
8. Record the procedure on nurse's chart with date and time. Record the amount, characteristic of fluid withdrawn, any drug given, and whether specimen is sent to laboratory	Labeled specimen to be sent for laboratory evaluation

Complications

- Injury to the spinal cord and spinal nerves.
- Introduction of infection into spinal cavity which may lead to meningitis.
- Leakage of CSF through puncture site.
- Bleeding into the spinal canal
- Damage to the intervertebral discs.
- Pain radiating to the thighs, due to trauma of the spinal nerves.
- Rapid reduction in the intracranial pressure caused by the removal of CSF can cause **herniation of the brain structures** into the foramen magnum. This causes **pressure on the vital centers in the medulla** causing respiratory failure and sudden death.

BONE MARROW ASPIRATION

Definition

Bone marrow is the soft tissue inside bones that helps to form blood cells. It is found in the hollow part of most bones. Bone marrow aspiration is the removal of a small amount of this tissue in liquid form for examination.

Anatomy/Physiology

- Bone marrow is aspirated from:
  - The sternum
  - Iliac crest
  - Posterior superior iliac spine
  - Spine of the vertebrae
  - Tibia (in children)

Red marrow contains the myeloid tissue and the yellow marrow contains mainly the fatty tissue. Red marrow is found in the medullary cavities of all bones in the first 4 years of life. Between the years of 7 and 20 the red marrow recedes proximally from the extremities leaving the fatty marrow behind.

In adults, the red marrow is found in the ribs, clavicles, scapulae, sternum, vertebrae, skull, pelvis, and in the upper parts of femur and humerus.

Therefore, a site of puncture over these areas of bones facilitate the aspiration of the bone marrow. Certain areas are selected for the site of biopsy aspiration, because the bones are more superficial and there is less danger of injuring the vital organs lying underneath.

Purposes

- To diagnose the blood dyscrasias such as aplastic anemia, leukemia, thrombocytopenia, etc.
- To determine the number, size and shape of red cells, white cells and platelets as they evolve through their various developmental stages.
- To diagnose toxic states producing bone marrow depression or destruction.
- To diagnose metastatic neoplasms.
- To diagnose deficiency states of vitamin B6, folic acid, pyridoxine, etc.

Sites of Bone Marrow Aspiration/Biopsy, and Positioning of the Client

- **Sternal puncture:** The usual puncture site is either the manubrium sterni or the upper part of the body of the sternum. The client lies in the dorsal recumbent position (supine) with a pillow under the shoulders to raise the chest. The hands are kept at the sides of the body.
- **Iliac puncture:** This is a more common site. Since the site of biopsy is out of the sight of the client, therefore the client has less fear of the procedure. Also, this site is away from vital organs. The bone marrow biopsy is taken from the iliac crest 2 cm posterior and 2 cm interior to the anterior superior iliac spine. Alternatively, the posterior iliac spine is also used. For iliac puncture, the client should lie either on his side or abdomen, depends upon the site used.
- **Spinous process aspiration:** The spinous process of the lumbar vertebrae usually L3 or L4 is the puncture site. The client is placed in the lumbar puncture position.
- **Tibial puncture in children:** In children up to the age of 2 years the proximal end of tibia, just below the tibial condyles and medial to the tibial tuberosity is selected. In older children, the iliac sites are more appropriate as the tibial site is too thick for their age and the sternum is too thin.

Indications

- To diagnose hematological disorders
- To follow the course of disease and patient's response to treatment
- To diagnose disease conditions such as primary metastatic tumors, infectious diseases and certain granulomas.
- To isolate bacteria and other pathogens by culture.

Contraindications

- Coagulation defects.

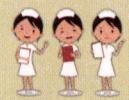

SKILL: PERFORMING BONE MARROW ASPIRATION

Articles Required

A sterile tray containing the following articles:

- Marrow puncture needle with obturator—1
- Aspiration syringe—1
- Sponge holding forceps—1
- Dissecting forceps—1
- Small bowls—2
- Sterile towels or fenestrated sheet
- Cotton swabs, gauze pieces, cotton pads, etc.
- Slides to make smears
- Glass syringes
- Scalpel blade and handle

Another tray containing the following articles:

- Spirit, iodine, tr. benzoin
- Lignocaine 2%
- Kidney tray and paper bag
- Mackintosh and towel
- Adhesive tapes, scissors

- Sterile containers with FAA solution (formalin, alcohol and acetic acid)
- Culture tubes
- Sterile gloves, gown, mask
- Disposable syringes and needles

General Instructions/Points to Remember

- Explain the procedure to the client/relative.
- Make sure that written consent is obtained.
- Shaving as a part preparation.
- All articles should be sterile and handled with aseptic technique.
- A sedation may be given to an apprehensive client and to children as per order.
- Place the patient in a correct position according to the site used.
- Remain with the client and reassure him/her.
- Monitor vital signs before, during and after the procedure.

Steps of Procedure

Review and follow the standard steps as given in Appendix

Action/steps	Rationale
Assessment	
1. Explain the procedure to the client	Reassurance helps in gaining patients cooperation and promotes relaxation
2. Place the screen	To provide privacy
Planning	
3. **Positioning of the client** Lying down position Patient is placed in the lateral recumbent position (right or left) at the edge of the table or bed with knees drawn up to the chest and clasped by the hands. Fetal attitude or "C" shaped position. Spine is fully flexed. Patient is asked to touch the chest with chin. One pillow may be placed under the patient's head	Iliac crest is visualized adequately. The pillow between the legs prevents the upper leg from rolling forward and separates the two bony prominence
4. **Supine position**	For sternal puncture
Spread the mackintosh and towel on the bed below the puncture site	To protect bed linen from soiling
5. Wash hands	It helps to control infection
6. Check vital signs	To obtain baseline data

Contd...

Action/steps	Rationale
Implementation	
7. Physician washes hands and wear sterile gown, mask and gloves	To prevent infection
8. Clean the site with Betadine and spirit and assist physician as he spreads the spinal sheet and drape	To prevent infection
9. The needle is advanced into the bone marrow and the required amount of bone marrow is withdrawn with syringe (0.2–0.5 mL)	To facilitate bone marrow aspiration
10. Once the physician removes the needle, apply pressure over puncture site for 5–10 minutes using sterile swab until the bleeding stops	To minimize bruising and hematoma formation. Prolonged pressure is required in case of thrombocytopenia (5–10 minutes)
11. Seal puncture site with tincture benzoin and apply small transparent firm dressing. Instruct the client not to wet the area for 24 hours	To provide an airtight seal over the puncture site and to prevent the entry of microorganisms
12. Make the patient comfortable. He/she may be mobile as desired depending on the level of sedation	Some patients may have this procedure performed in OPD so they may be asked to wait for 30 minutes to check bleeding
13. Send the specimen to laboratory immediately	Delay in sending the samples may cause changes in sample
Evaluation	
14. Determine how the patient tolerated the procedure.	If adverse effects occur such as bleeding from site inform the physician
15. Documentation <ul><li>Record the procedure on the nurse's chart and patient's flow sheet with date and time</li><li>Record the condition and reaction of the patient during or after the procedure</li><li>Record any drug given, name of the doctor who performed the procedure, any additional instructions given by the doctor.</li><li>Record whether the specimen is sent to laboratory or not, and give the details of tests</li><li>Make necessary entries in lab register also</li><li>Observe the puncture site for any leakage</li></ul>	Recording is an essential part of client care Early detection helps to prevent complications
16. Aftercare of the Articles <ul><li>Dispose all waste as per biomedical waste management protocol</li><li>Wash and clean all the reusable instruments. Send it for autoclave to the central sterile services department (CSSD)</li></ul>	To prevent cross-infection To make instruments ready for next use

Complications

- Bleeding
- Infection

Special Considerations

Aspirin containing analgesic should be avoided as it may cause bleeding.

INTRA-ARTERIAL ADMINISTRATION

Definition

It is the delivery of a cytotoxic drug to the tumor site by catheterization of the artery providing the blood supply to the affected organ. This allows a high concentration of drug to be delivered.

Indications

Intra-arterial chemotherapy has been used to treat a variety of **malignancies** at a number of different sites. These include:

- Head and neck lesions
- Liver metastases from colorectal cancer
- Sarcomas/melanomas of upper and lower limb
- Carcinoma of the stomach
- Carcinoma of the breast
- Carcinoma of the cervix

Advantages

The advantage of the route is that it facilitates the delivery to high concentrations of drug to the primary or secondary tumor mass.

A reduction in systemic circulating levels or drugs has been shown to occur in many circumstances resulting in a corresponding reduction in side effect to the patient, although this is difficult to predict.

The cytotoxic drugs used vary with the histology and site of the tumor. For example, actinomycin D, bleomycin, cisplatin, 5-fluorouracil, methotrexate, vincristine, etc.

Disadvantages

The main disadvantage of this route is that very high levels of drug in perfused organ may result in excessive tissue damage.

It also requires the insertion of an arterial device.

Methods

Two main methods are used for infusional chemotherapy; these are termed **external and internal arterial infusions**.

The external method involves radiographic placement of an arterial catheter and attachment to an external infusion pump for 3–7 days, during which the patient remains flat. Temporary catheter placement is used for short time therapies, i.e., from hours up to 5 days. Therapy can be given intermittently for several courses. This method is unsuitable for long-term use (6 months or longer) as it is uncomfortable, inconvenient and expensive, although a subcutaneous implanted port increases the patient's comfort and freedom.

Once the catheter is in place and secured, cytotoxic drugs may be administered by:

- Injection—using a syringe
- Small volume infusion—using a syringe pump
- Large volume infusion—using a volumetric pump

Internal or implantable methods involve the surgical placement of a totally implantable pump and appeared to have a lower complication rate than the external method. The catheter is inserted into an appropriate artery and attached to the pump, which is filled with chemotherapy. This approach is more frequently used for colorectal cancer which metastases to the liver.

All delivery systems must provide adequate pressure to combat arterial pressure, i.e., 300 mm Hg. The majority of infusion pumps meet this requirement. Patient education is important as the patient may have to maintain the implantable pump and be able to recognize any complications or malfunctions.

Procedure

- Insertion is an operative procedure so consent must be obtained.
- Explain the procedure and what is expected on return to the ward.
- Shaving as a part preparation
- Nil per os (NPO) status as per anesthetist's order

The catheter is inserted in OT or X-ray room, and its position is checked at that time.

The catheter is then secured and an occlusive dressing is applied.

Instruct the patient **not to touch** it as it may get dislodged. A three-or one-way stopcock is connected to the catheter and it is at this point where all manipulations take place. An extension line is attached with this to make the handling easy. The system consists of: catheter/tap/extension set/administration set and infusion device.

Nurses' Responsibilities

- Dressing must not be touched, but should be observed regularly for signs of bleeding.
- Follow strict aseptic technique.

- All connections must be locked to prevent exsanguination, air embolism or disconnection under pressure.
- The catheter must be clamped securely or switched off using the tape in situ before any equipment changes.
- A positive pressure greater than arterial pressure must be maintained at all times.
- If chemotherapy is not being infused, the flushing solution must be used to maintain patency. A syringe pump or infusion pump can be used for this. It should be delivered at the minimum rate sufficient to combat arterial pressure and maintain patency, approximately 3–5 mL per hour or 10 drops per minute, dependent on the device used. A nurse escort may be necessary for transfer of patient.
- Give proper instructions on the amount of mobility allowed. (Depends on the site of catheter).
- Assist the patient to maintain personal hygiene. Take measures to prevent pressure ulcers.
- Daily X-ray to check the position of the catheter.
- At the end of the treatment, patency of the arterial catheter should be maintained using an appropriate flushing solution until a decision has been made about removal.
- Amount of heparin to be used must be confirmed.
- Before removal, the tap may be switched off and the catheter is allowed to clot.
- The catheter is removed by a doctor and firm pressure is applied for at least 5 minutes or until the bleeding has stopped. A firm dressing is applied on the site.
- Monitoring vital signs throughout the period is important.

Complications

- Arterial occlusion and thrombosis
- Damage to the artery, arteriovenous fistula, aneurysm formation
- Chemical hepatitis and biliary sclerosis
- Exsanguination/air embolism

INTRAOSSEOUS ADMINISTRATION

Definition

Intraosseous infusion (IO) is the process of injecting directly into the bone marrow to provide a non-collapsible entry point into the systemic venous system. Technique is used in emergency situations to provide fluids and medication when intravenous access is not available or not feasible.

A comparison of intravenous (IV), intramuscular (IM), and intraosseous (IO) routes of administration concluded that **the intraosseous route is demonstrably superior to intramuscular** and comparable to intravenous administration (in delivering pediatric anesthetic drugs).

Needle is injected through the bone's hard cortex and into the soft marrow interior, which allows immediate access to the vascular system. An IO infusion can be used on adult or pediatric patients in case traditional methods of vascular access are difficult or impossible.

Sites

Often the anteromedial aspect of the upper tibia is used as it lies just under the skin and can easily be palpated and located.

The anterior aspect of the femur, the superior iliac crest and the head of the humerus are other sites that can be used.

Uses

This route of medication administration is an alternative one to the preferred intravascular route in case the latter cannot be established in a timely manner.

If intravascular access cannot be obtained intraosseous access is usually the next approach.

It can be maintained for 24–48 hours, after which another route of access should be obtained.

Although intravascular access is still the preferred method for medication delivery in the hospital area, advances in IO access for adults has caused many systems to re-think their preferred secondary access route. In Massachusetts, for example IO is now a preferred administration over endotracheal (ET) drug administration. In fact, the American Heart Association no longer recommends using the endotracheal tube for resuscitation drugs since the efficacy is unclear. Paramedics may perform intraosseous infusion in a cardiac arrest patient if no vein is clearly visible. The IO is becoming more and more common in **emergency medical services (EMS)** systems around the world.

Furthermore, any medication that can be introduced via IV can be introduced via IO. Because of this, adult IO systems (most of which use a mechanical or powered adjunct to place the catheter) have become more common across the united states in the pre-hospital setting. Intraosseous access has roughly the same absorption rate as IV access, and (Unlike ET administration) allows for fluid resuscitation as well as high-volume drugs such as sodium bicarbonate to be administered in the setting of a cardiac arrest in case IV access is unavailable. Endotracheal administration allows only specific drugs that have relatively low toxicity to tissue, and must be restricted to relatively low volumes to avoid drowning the patient.

Due to the rapid advances and adoption of superior access technology, IO access has now become the preferred method of establishing vascular access for patients in whom traditional access is difficult or impossible. This includes patients experiencing cardiac arrest, major trauma, airway compromise, severe dehydration, and/or hypoperfusion (shock). IO is also an alternative route for patients who typically have poor peripheral vasculature or challenging vascular access such as diabetics, renal patients, burn victims, IV drug users, obese patients, dehydrated patients, the very young or elderly patients, and other. Many EMS services and hospitals are now using IO as their first-line solution for vascular access in both adult and pediatric cardiac arrest victims, enabling administration of lifesaving drugs much earlier than previously possible with traditional peripheral IV placement.

INTRATHECAL INJECTIONS

Intrathecal ("Within a sheath") refers to something introduced into the anatomic space inside a sheath, most commonly the arachnoid membrane of the brain or spinal cord under which is the subarachnoid space.

For example, an intrathecal injection (often simply called "an intrathecal") is a route of administration for drugs via an injection into the spinal canal, more specifically into the subarachnoid space so that it reaches the CSF and is useful in spinal anesthesia, chemotherapy, or pain management applications.

This route is also used to introduce drugs that fight certain infections, particularly post-neurosurgical. The drug needs to be given this way to avoid the blood brain barrier. The same drug given orally must enter the blood stream and may not be able to pass out and into the brain. Drugs given intrathecal often have to be made up especially by a pharmacist technician because they cannot contain any preservative or other potentially harmful inactive ingredients that are sometimes found in standard injectable drug preparations.

An intrathecal pump is a medical device used to deliver medications directly into the space between the spinal cord and the protective sheath surrounding the spinal cord. Medications such as baclofen, or ziconotide may be delivered in this manner to minimize the side effects often associated with higher doses used in oral or intravenous delivery of these drugs. Preparation of patient and article are same as that of lumbar puncture.

BIBLIOGRAPHY

1. Altman G, Coxon V, Buchsel P. "Delmer Fundamental and Advanced Nursing Skills," Canada Delmer Thomas company; 2000. pp. 1322-9.

2. Smeltzer SC, Bare BG, Hinkle, et al. Brunner & Suddarth's Textbook of Medical-Surgical Nursing, 7th edition. Lippincott Williams & Wilkins. pp. 443-5.

3. Sr Nancy. "Stephanie's Principles and Practice of Nursing senior Nursing Procedure and Nursing administration", vol. 2, 4th edition. NR Brothers; 2006. pp. 365-73.

4. Berman AT, Snyder S, Kozier BJ, et al. Kozier and Erb's Fundamental of Nursing concept, process and practice, 8th edition. Delhi: Dorling Kindersely Pvt. Ltd; 2008. pp. 821-2, 824-5.

5. Bolander VB. Sorensen and Luckmann's Basic Nursing-A Physiologic Approach, 3rd edition. Saunders; 1994. pp. 719-720.

6. Taylor C, Lillis C, LeMone P, Lynn P. Fundamentals of Nursing, 6th edition. Lippincott Williams and Wilkins. Philadelphia: 2008. pp. 909- 10, 1190-1.

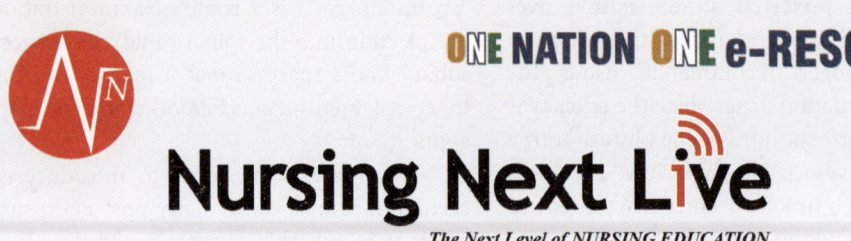
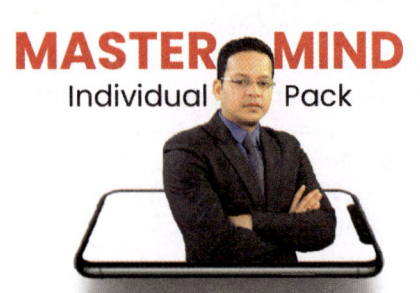 

Topical Applications: On Skin and Mucous Membranes

INTRODUCTION

Topical medications are administered directly to the skin and mucous membrane by painting or spreading it over an area, applying moist dressing or soaking body parts in a solution. They are applied to produce local effects, but certain topical preparations have systemic effects since they are absorbed through the skin mucous membrane.

Systemic effects will be more if skin is very thin, if the drug concentration is high or if skin contact is prolonged.

DEFINITION

It is the application of the medicine locally on the skin or mucous membranes in the form of lotion or ointment.

ADMINISTRATION VIA PERCUTANEOUS ROUTES

Percutaneous routes are those by which medicines are absorbed through the skin or mucous membranes. It includes:

• **Topical:** Applied to the skin
• **Instillation:** To the mucous membranes
• **Sublingual:** Under the tongue
• **Buccal:** In the cheek
• To the mucous membranes of eye, ear, nose and vagina
• **Inhalation:** Aerosolized liquids or gases

Advantages Over Systemic Administration

• Easy to administer
• Noninvasive

- Rapid onset of action
- Less side effects
- Bypasses the liver metabolism and acidic gastric environment.

Different forms of Percutaneous Medications

- Lotion
- Cream
- Ointment
- Gel
- Powder
- Paste
- Transdermal patch
- Nasal sprays
- Eye, ear and nasal drops
- Eye ointment
- Tablets

Skin Application

General Instructions

- The skin area should be thoroughly cleaned before the application of an ointment or lotion and should be checked for being intact.
- A lotion should be shaken well first, then applied on the skin and allowed to dry.
- The lotions have to be reapplied as necessary. Before the re-application, the lotion or ointment should be completely removed from the skin.

- The skin should be observed frequently after the application of the ointment or lotion for any skin irritation. Skin irritation should be reported immediately and the application should be discontinued.
- A thin coating is preferable to thick layer.
- The nurse may use a sterile/clean gloves depending upon the condition of the skin. The use of the gloves will prevent the cross-infection and the effect of medicine on herself.
- Take only sufficient amount of medicine for one application to the patient in order to prevent wastage.
- Look for the special instructions on the label.
- No ointment or lotion should be applied on any patient without doctor's prescription.

Different forms of Skin Applications

- **Ointments, lotion, paste and creams:** Smear lightly and evenly onto the skin's surface. Do not rub over the area.
- **Liniment:** Applied by rubbing it gently but firmly into the skin
- **Powder:** It is dusted lightly to cover the affected area with a thin layer.

Purposes

- To protect, soothen or soften surface areas
- To warm an affected area and also for muscle relaxation
- To relieve itching
- To check the growth of microorganisms.

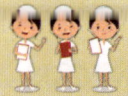 **SKILL: APPLICATION OF MEDICINE OF SKIN**

Articles Required

A tray containing:
- Gloves
- Cotton balls or gauze pieces
- Medicine (ointment, lotion) in appropriate container.
- Adhesive tape and dressing pad
- Kidney tray

Steps of Procedure

Review and follow the standard steps as given in Appendix

Action/steps	Rationale
Assessment	
1. Identify the patient and explain the procedure	Gains cooperation of patient
Planning	
2. Wash hand and put on gloves on dominant hand	Prevents spread of microorganisms and self protection
Implementation	
3. Expose only the area where lotion/ointment is to be applied	Prevents undue exposure

Contd...

Action/steps	Rationale
4. Clean the area with soap and water and pat dry it if required.	Previously applied medication remaining on the skin may reduce contact of medication with skin.
5. **Skin preparation** ■ **Powders:** Make sure that the skin surface is dry and sprinkle evenly over the area till a fine thin layer covers the skin. Cover the area with dressing if required.	Moisture can cause the powder to stick and cause uneven distribution.
■ **Lotion:** Shake the container and put a small amount of lotion on gauze dressing pad and apply it evenly in the direction of the hair growth	Shaking the container ensures proper mixing of medication.
■ **Cream, ointment and pastes:** Take a small amount of medicine in gloved hand, smear it evenly over skin using long strokes in the direction of the hair growth. Apply dressing if required.	Smearing medication evenly on the skin ensure uniform distribution.
■ **Aerosol spray:** Shake the container well to mix contents. Hold the container 15–30 cm away from the area and spray. Ensure that spray does not enter the eyes or nose.	Aerosol spray if enters in to eyes or nose can cause adverse effects.
■ **Transdermal patches:** Select clean dry area, which is free of hair. Take the patch, holding it without touching the adhesive edges and apply it firmly using palm of the hand and press it for 10 sec. Remove the patch at the appropriate time, folding it with the medicated side inside.	Hair growth in the area of a application can affect the absorption of medication. Applying the patch for longer than required can cause increased rate of absorption.
Evaluation	
6. Observe the area carefully for changes in the color, swelling, appearance of a rash or other observable signs.	
Documentation	
7. Recording of the procedure and care of the articles to be done at the end.	

Sublingual Administration

In this type of administration, tablets are placed beneath the tongue until they dissolve, e.g., nitroglycerine

Advantages

- The onset of action will be faster due to direct administration
- Bypasses liver metabolism
- Eases delivery for those who have trouble swallowing pills
- Bypasses gastrointestinal degradation from stomach acid

Buccal Administration

- Tablets are placed between the cheek and the gums.
- It is left there, until it dissolves.
- Drug is absorbed into the capillaries of the mucous membranes of the cheek which leads to rapid onset of action.

Nasal Instillation

- **Common forms:** Decongestant spray or drops.
- It is used to relieve symptoms of nasal congestion or cold and sinus infection.

- Avoid abuse of medication because of rebound effect, systemic effects.
- Saline drops are safer decongestants for children.

Contraindications

- Known allergies
- Hypertension
- Heart disease
- Diabetes mellitus
- Hyperthyroidism

Side Effects

- Transient hypertension
- Tachycardia
- Palpitation
- Headache

Assessment

Identification data of the patient, physician's order.

- History of the patient.
- Inspect the condition of the nose and sinuses using a penlight
- Explain the procedure to the client regarding positioning and sensations to expect
- Arrange supplies and medications at bedside

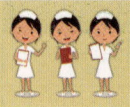

SKILL: ADMINISTRATION OF NASAL DROPS

Articles Required

- Prepared medication with clean dropper.
- Face towel
- Disposable gloves
- Penlight or torch
- Medicine card

Administration of Nasal Drops

- Instruct the client to clean or blow nose gently unless contraindicated.
- Assist the client to die in supine position
- **For posterior pharynx:** Tilt the head backward
- **For ethmoid or sphenoid sinus:** Tilt the head back over the edge of bed or place a small pillow under shoulder and tilt head back
- **For frontal and maxillary sinus:** Till head back over edge of bed or pillow with head turned toward side to be treated
- Support the client's head with non-dominant hand.
- Instruct the client to breathe through mouth.
- Hold dropper 1 cm above nares and instill prescribed number of drops toward midline of the ethmoid bone.
- Have the client remain in supine position for 5 minutes.

After Instillation

- Assist the client to a comfortable position
- After care of the articles.
- Observe for the onset of side effects 15–30 minutes after administration.
- Ask if client is able to breathe through nose after decongestant administration.
- Reinspect the condition of nasal passages between the instillations.

Unexpected Outcomes

- Wheezing or other signs of allergic reaction to the drug.
- Client is unable to breathe easily through nasal passages.
- Inflammation of nasal mucosa and discharge from the nares.
- Client complaints of sinus headache. Sinus remains congested.

Recording and Reporting

- Record name of the medicine, concentration, number of drops, nostril into which medicine was instilled and time of administration.
- Record client's response
- Report any unusual systemic side effects

BIBLIOGRAPHY

1. *Potter PA, Perry AG. Fundamentals of Nursing, 6th edition. New Delhi: Elsevier; 2008. pp. 855-863.*
2. *Sr. Nancy. "Stephanie's Principles and Practice of Nursing senior Nursing Procedure and Nursing administration", vol. 2, 4th edition. NR Brothers; 2006. pp. 153-236.*
3. *Annama J. Art of Nursing Procedures, 2nd edition. Elsevier. pp. 215-8.*
4. *Christensen BL, Kockrow EO. Foundations of Nursing, 3rd edition. Mosby; 1999. pp. 346-51.*
5. *www.wikipedia.org*

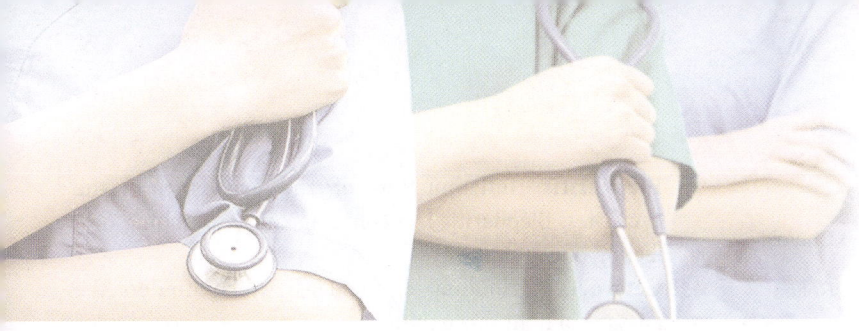

Treatments Related to Eye (Eye Care, Eye Irrigation, Instillation of Eye Drops)

Learning Objectives

After completing this chapter, you will be able to:

- Define terms used in eye conditions
- Enlist the purposes of procedures in eye conditions
- Explain the assessment of eye
- Demonstrate procedures used in eye conditions skillfully

Key Terms

- Astigmatism
- Blepharitis
- Cataract
- Conjunctivitis
- Diplopia
- Diabetic retinopathy
- Glaucoma
- Far-sightedness
- Myopia
- Retinal detachment
- Stye
- Uveitis
- Tonometry

Chapter Outline

- Introduction
- Related Anatomy and Physiology
- Terminologies of Various Eye Conditions
- Eye Treatments
- Examination of Eye
- How to Take Care of the Eyes?
- Eye Care
- Eye Irrigation
- Instillation of Eye Drops
- Eye Ointment Application

INTRODUCTION

Eye is one of the most precious gift possessed by the human beings. It is one of the five sensory organs, through which we perceive things. One-fourth of all the physical energy is used in seeing.

RELATED ANATOMY AND PHYSIOLOGY

The human eye is the organ that reacts to light and allows vision.

- The eyes are situated in the orbital cavity. The eye ball is nearly spherical in shape and one inch in diameter. The six extrinsic muscles move the eye ball in an orbit. Eyelids and eye lashes protect the eyes from the injury.

- The eye is a fused two-piece unit. The smaller frontal unit, transparent and more curved, called the cornea, is linked to the larger white unit called the sclera.
- The cornea and sclera are connected by a ring called the limbus. The iris is the colored, circular structure concentrically surrounding the center of the eye. The pupil appears to be black.
- The size of the pupil, which controls the amount of light entering the eye, is adjusted by the dilator and sphincter muscles of iris.
- The eye is made up of three coats, enclosing three transparent structures.
  - The outermost layer, known as the fibrous tunic, is composed of the cornea and sclera.

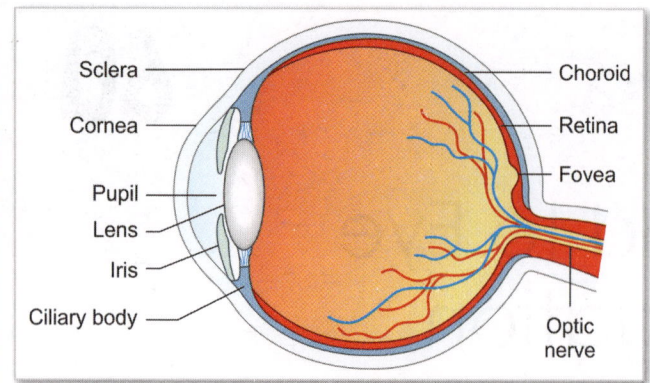

Fig. 1: Anatomy of eye

- The middle layer, known as the uvea, consists of the choroid, ciliary body, and iris.
- The innermost is the retina, which gets its circulation from the vessels of the choroid as well as the retinal vessels (Fig. 1).

- Within these coats are the aqueous humor, the vitreous body, and the flexible lens.
  - The aqueous humor is a clear fluid that is present in two areas: The anterior chamber between the cornea and the iris and the posterior chamber between the iris and the lens.
  - The lens is suspended to the ciliary body by the suspensory ligament made up of fine transparent fibers.
  - The vitreous body is a clear jelly that is much larger than the aqueous humor present behind the lens, and the rest is bordered by the sclera, suspensory ligament, and lens.
- They are connected via the pupil. The eyeball is covered with a sensitive mucous membrane called conjunctiva.
- Light enters the eye through the cornea, then the pupil and then through the lens controlled by ciliary muscles. Light falling on the light-sensitive cells of the retina is converted into electrical signals that are carried to the brain by the optic nerves.
- Rod and cone cells in the retina allow conscious light perception and vision including color differentiation and the perception of depth. The human eye can distinguish about 10 million colors.

TERMINOLOGIES OF VARIOUS EYE CONDITIONS

- **Age-related macular degeneration:** A loss of central vision of both eyes.
- **Astigmatism:** A defect that causes an inability to properly focus light on to the retina. Astigmatism causes blurry vision that can be corrected with glasses or contact lenses.

- **Blepharitis:** Inflammation of the eyelids near the eyelashes. Blepharitis is a common cause of itching or a feeling of grit in the eyes.
- **Cataract:** A clouding of the lens, which hinders the passage of light through the lens.
- **Conjunctivitis:** Also known as pink eye. Conjunctivitis is an infection or inflammation of the conjunctiva, the clear layer that covers the front of the eye. It is usually caused by allergies, a viral, or a bacterial infection.
- **Corneal abrasion:** A scratch on the clear part of the front of the eye. Pain, light, sensitivity, or a feeling of grit in the eye are the usual symptoms.
- **Diabetic retinopathy:** High blood sugar damages blood vessels in the eye. Eventually, weakened blood vessels may overgrow the retina or bleed, threatening the vision.
- **Diplopia (double vision):** Seeing double can be caused by many serious conditions. Diplopia requires immediate medical attention.
- **Glaucoma:** Increased pressure inside the eye slowly reduces vision. Peripheral vision is lost first, often going undetected for years.
- **Hyperopia (far-sightedness):** Inability to see near objects clearly. The eye is "too short" for the lens or certain eye muscles have weakened with age. It is also called as hypermetropia
- **Keratitis:** Inflammation or infection of the cornea. Keratitis typically occurs after germs enter a corneal abrasion.
- **Myopia (near-sightedness):** Inability to see clearly at a distance. The eye is "too long" for the lens, so light is not focused properly on the retina.
- **Retinal detachment:** The retina becomes loose from the back of the eye. Trauma and diabetes are common causes of this medical emergency.
- **Retinitis:** Inflammation or infection of retina. Retinitis may be long-term genetic condition or results from a viral infection.
- **Stye:** Bacteria infect the skin on the edge of the eyelid, creating a tender red bump.
- **Uveitis (iritis):** The colored part of the eye becomes inflamed or infected. An overactive immune system, bacteria or viruses can be responsible

EYE TREATMENTS

- **Contact lenses and glasses:** Glasses or contact lenses correct refractive errors such as near-sightedness, far-sightedness, and astigmatism.
- **Laser-assisted in situ keratomileusis (LASIK):** A doctor cuts a flap in the cornea with a tiny saw. A laser reshapes the cornea's surface, improving near-sightedness. It is used for correcting myopia, hyperopia and astigmatism.

- **Laser photocoagulation:** A doctor uses a laser to burn blood vessels in the retina that are leaking or growing abnormally. Laser photocoagulation is most often done for diabetic retinopathy.
- **Cataract surgery:** The cloudy cataract is removed from the lens and is replaced by a manmade lens.

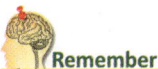
Remember

Common Abbreviations
- OD (oculus dexter) or RE: Right eye
- OS (oculus sinister) or LE: Left eye
- OU (oculus unitas): Both eye
- IOP: Intraocular pressure
- IOL: Intraocular lens
- EOL: Extraocular lens

EXAMINATION OF EYE

History

- **Demographic data**
  - Include age and gender. The incidences of cataract, dry eye, retinal detachment, glaucoma, etc. increases with age. Hereditary color vision deficits are common in men than women.
- **Current health**
  - Various disease conditions and treatments have potential negative impact on visual health. For example, diabetic retinopathy.
- **Symptoms analysis:**
  - Ask and see about the signs and symptoms of eye disorders. Most common include eye pain, burning, itching, photophobia, dryness, grittiness, edema and trauma.
- **Surgical history:**
  - Some eye surgeries such as that for glaucoma can precipitate other eye issues.
- **Past medical history:**
  - Focuses on systemic disorders commonly associated with ocular manifestations, e.g., diabetes mellitus, hypertension, and thyroid disorders.
- **Allergic manifestations:**
  - Note any allergies to eye medications or eye drops.
  - Has the client had an allergy to eye drops or other medication that have affected the eyes? Allergic manifestations include redness of the eye, etc. formation of terms, itching.
- **Medications:**
  - Include drugs which affect eyes. Ask about the use of over-the-counter eye drops like natural tears.
- **Dietary habits:**
  - Diet rich in fruits, vegetables, fish, and supplements of antioxidants. Vitamin C, E and beta-carotene have the potential to reduce visual problems.

- **Social history and lifestyle data:**
  - Significant to ocular health includes occupational hazards, leisure activities etc.
- **Family health history**
  - For glaucoma, myopia, hypermyopia

Physical Examination

External Eye

Eye Position

Assess position of the eyes for symmetry and alignment. Sunken or protusion of eyes are an abnormal findings (Exophthalmos: Bulging of eye caused by hyperthyroidism).

Eye Brows

Inspect the eye brows for symmetry, hair distribution, skin conditions and movements, the eye brows usually move up and down smoothly under control of the facial nerve. The skin may be dry and flaking (dandruff), which is abnormal.

Eyelids and Eyelashes

Examine eyelids and eyelashes for placement and symmetry. When open, the upper lids rest at the top of the iris and lower at the bottom so that the sclera is not visible above the iris. Sagging of the upper eyelids (ptosis), inversion of the eyelid (entropion), outward turning—(eversion) of the eyelid should be noted. Elevate the eye-brows to inspect the upper lids for lesions. Inspect the lower lids by asking to open the eyes, examine the skin of the eyelids and orbit by palpating for texture, firmness, mobility and integrity of the underlying tissues. Eyelashes should curl outside. Look for infections and stye.

Blink Responses

Blinking is an involuntary reflex that occurs bilaterally up to 20 times a minute. Rapid, infrequent or asymmetrical blinking is abnormal.

Eyeballs

Palpate the eyeballs for symmetry and firmness. Instruct the client to close the eyes and look down. Place the tip and index finger on the upper eyelids, over the sclera and palpate gently. Normally the eyeballs feel firm and symmetrical. If any abnormal findings occur, go for further examination.

Lacrimal Apparatus

Examine the lacrimal apparatus by retracting the upper lids and having the client look down so that part of the lacrimal gland can be visualized. Observe this area for swelling or tenderness.

Conjunctiva and Sclera

Inspect the conjunctiva and sclera for color changes, texture, vascularity, lesions, thickness, secretions and foreign bodies. The bulbar conjunctiva is colorless and transparent. Retract the lower eyelids to expose the conjunctiva without applying pressure to the eyeballs. You should gently push the lower lids down against the bony orbit while the client looks up. Healthy conjunctiva is pink to light red; paleness or bright red color is abnormal. After inspection, return the eyelid to its normal position by gently pulling the eye lashes forward while the client looks up.

Cornea

Inspect the cornea from an oblique angle while shining a penlight on the corneal surface. The iris is easily visible. Abnormalities include surface irregularities and cloudiness.

Iris and Pupil

The iris should light up with oblique lighting from the penlight and should have consistent color. Bulging or uneven coloring is abnormal. When light shines into the eyes, the iris constricts as the optic nerves are stimulated, causing the pupil to become smaller. Dim light causes iris to dilate.

Inspect the pupil for size, equality, shape and ability to react to light and accommodation. Pupils are normally black, round with smooth borders and are of the same size. Results of the pupil assessment are normally recorded as PERRLA (pupils equal, round, reactive to light and accommodation). Abnormal results include light intolerance (photophobia), irregular or unequal pupils or pupils that do not react to light or accommodation.

Visual Acuity

In cases of pain in eye, injury or visual loss, always check visual acuity before proceeding with the rest of the examination or putting medications in your patient's eyes.

- Position the patient 20 feet in front of the Snellen's eye chart (Fig. 2).
- Have the patient cover one eye at a time with a card
- Ask the patient to read progressively smaller letters until they can go no further.
- Visual acuity is recorded as smallest line of letters that can be read accurately with no more than two inaccurate readings (such as, 20/20 is considered normal)
- Repeat with the other eye
- Unexpected/unexplained loss of acuity is a sign of serious ocular pathology

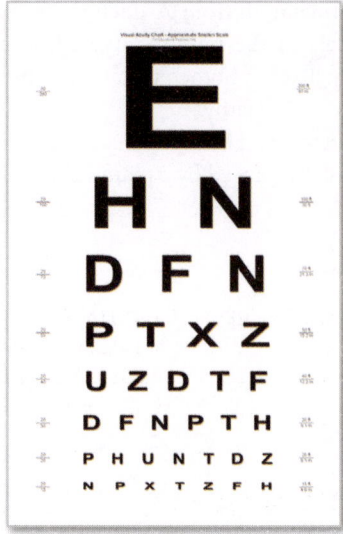

Fig. 2: Snellen's chart

- Use E-card or picture of familiar object if unable to read.
- The numerator is the distance from which the client is standing and denominator is the distance from which normal eye can read the chart. The larger the denominator poorer the visual acuity.

Testing Near Vision

Test near vision with a card or newsprint held 12–14 inches (30–36 cm) from the client's eye. Corrective lenses are worn if they are needed. The client with normal vision can read the material at that distance. Complaints of blurring or attempts by the client to move card either closer or further away signal abnormal near vision.

Extraocular Movements

Extraocular movements are assessed by assessing the cardinal fields of vision for coordination and alignment. Normally both eyes move together, are coordinated and are parallel. To assess range of motion (ROM) follow these three steps:

1. Ask the patient to sit or stand about 2 feet away, facing you by sitting or standing at eye level with patient.
2. Ask the patient to hold the head still and follow the movements of your forefinger or a pen light with the eyes
3. Keeping your finger or light 1 foot from the patient's face move it slowly through the cardinal positions up and down, left and right, diagonally up and down to the left and to the right.

Nystagmus is noted (involuntary rhythmical oscillation of eye by periodically stopping the movement of fingers).

Pupillary Reaction

Light

Dim the light. To test the direct response to light, bring the pen light in front then side to side directly over the center of pupil. The illuminated pupil should constrict briskly and evenly. Repeat this maneuver on the other eye. Both eyes should react to the same degree.

Accommodation

Test accommodation by holding the penlight 4–6 inches or 10–15 cm away from the client's nose. Instruct the client to look first at the penlight, then at the distant wall straight ahead and then back at the pen light. While the client gazes from near to far and back again, observe the pupil's response to changes in the distance. The pupils should dilate when the client look at the far point and should constrict when the client looks at the nearer object, then move the penlight towards the bridge of the nose, observing the pupils for convergence and constriction.

Examination of Internal Eye

Ophthalmoscopic Examination

Uses a strong light reflected into the interior of the eye through an instrument called ophthalmoscope (Fig. 3).

Tonometry

It is the measurement of tension or pressure. A tonometer is an instrument for measuring tension or pressure. In ophthalmoscopy, tonometry is the procedure professionals perform by the tonometer to determine the intraocular pressure (IOP) (the fluid pressure inside the eye). It is an important test in the evaluation of patients with glaucoma. Most tonometers are calibrated to measure pressure in mmHg. Pressure between 8 and 21 mm Hg is considered within normal range.

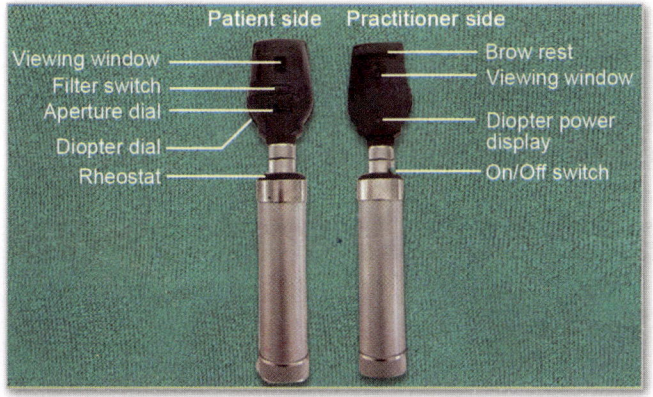

Fig. 3: Ophthalmoscope

Slit Lamp Examination

The slit lamp uses an instrument that provides a magnified, three dimensional views of the different parts of the eye. It is a special equipment that magnifies the cornea, sclera and anterior chamber.

- The patient sits with chin and forehead resting againt equipment support.
- The room is generally darkened, and the pupils are dilated.
- It helps to detect disorders of the anterior portion of the eye. Special lenses can be placed between slit lamp and the cornea (or directly on the cornea) to view deeper structures of the eye, such as the optic nerve, retina, and the area where fluid drains out the eye. A camera may be attached to the slit lamp to take photographs of different parts of the eye.

HOW TO TAKE CARE OF THE EYES?

- Have a regular annual eye checkup. This is helpful in preventing regularly eye problems and treat existing ones. If you are using contact lens, make sure to keep them properly clean. Have your reading glasses checked to provide the right vision for you.
- Eat a well-balanced diet of fresh fruits and vegetables. Eat food rich in vitamin A, E and C. Eat a lot of carrots, which is rich in beta carotene and include fish, which is high in omega fatty acids. Try a cup of broccoli since this is also good for the eyes.
- Take good care of your health and immune system. Avoid too much smoking and excessive drinking of alcohol as this can make your eyes look tired and droopy. Smoking has bad effects to blood circulating around the eye areas. If you have diabetes, have regular checkups because if neglected, this can severely affect the eyes. Try to keep your blood pressure and cholesterol at normal levels.
- Protect your eyes with sunglasses with high or at least 95% UV protection against the sun. Choose the kind of glasses which have wrap around frames to ensure full protection. Wear hats, caps and use umbrellas to further shade the eyes from heat and wind. Use protective glasses when engaging in strenuous sports and when working with heavy tools and machines.
- Make sure to always have clean hands before touching your eyes. Infection starts with dirty hands. Also try avoiding too much rubbing of the eyes. Keep hankies clean and use soft cotton fabrics to protect eyes.
- Remember to have a proper lighting when reading. In case of watching TV, make use of anti-glare screens. Avoid sitting too close. Do the same with the computers. Take time to briefly look away from the computer screen to relieve eye tension.

- Do some eye exercises like simple blinking to relieve eye stress. Blinking helps in lubricating the eyes. Try to close your eyes for about 15 minutes for them to be relaxed and to relieve eye strain. Have time to rest eyes as much as possible. Look at something green to relax the eyes.
- After some good amount of rest, wash your eyes with cold water to relax and to reduce eye strain. Use eye drops if prescribed by your doctor
- Take sufficient sleep
- Avoid reading while lying down
- Drink plenty of water
- Half an hour of meditation everyday helps keep the eyes healthy.
- Wash eyes frequently with tap water
- Wash hands after touching the infected eye
- Do not rub the eye, just pat it dry.

PROCEDURES RELATED TO EYE

- Eye care
- Eye irrigation
- Instillation of eye drops

Assessment

- Check the diagnosis of the patient
- Check the physician's order to see the specific precautions regarding the care of eyes, the patient's movement and positioning.
- Assess the general condition of patient and ability to follow the instructions
- Check the articles available in the patient's unit.

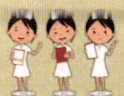

SKILL: PROVIDING EYE CARE TO THE PATIENT

Articles Required (Fig. 4)

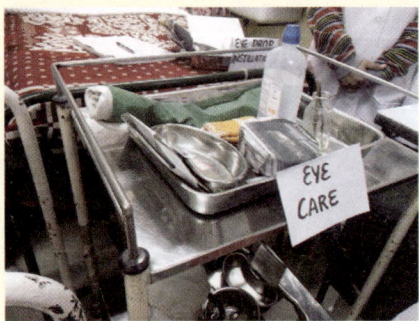

Fig. 4: Article tray for eye care

EYE CARE

Cleaning the eye using aseptic technique is called eye care.

Purposes

- To clean the eye
- To remove the irritating discharges from the eye
- To prevent the infection
- To prevent ophthalmia neonatorum in new born
- To prepare eye for any treatment e.g., eye instillation, eye irrigation

General Instructions

- Clean the eyes from inner to outer canthus
- Use a separate swab for each stroke
- Do not touch that part of cotton swab that will come directly in contact with the eyes
- Less infected eye should be cleaned or treated first before the infected one.

Articles	Rationale
A mackintosh and a towel	To protect the pillow and bed linen
A sterile bowl with sterile cotton swabs/boiled cool swabs	To clean the eyes
Sterile normal saline (if sterile swabs are used)	To clean the eyes

Contd...

Thumb forceps dipped in boiled cool water	To pick up the cotton swabs
A gauze piece in the bowl/towel	To dry the eyes
A kidney tray and a paper bag	To discard waste

Steps of Procedure

Review and follow the standard steps as given in Appendix

Action/steps	Rationale
Planning	
1. Explain the procedure to the patient	
2. Place the patient in the dorsal recumbent position slightly towards the infected side	Relaxed patient is more cooperative
3. Place the mackintosh and the towel under the head	To protect the bed linen
Implementation	
4. Wash hands	To prevent the cross-infection
5. If sterile swabs are used, pour sterile saline to wet the cotton swabs	For cleaning of eye discharge
6. Stand in front of the patient. Pick up the wet cotton swabs with the thump forceps, transfer it to hands and squeeze the excess of water without touching the part, which will come in direct contact with the eye. Squeeze in such a way so that water flows towards the hand and not the sterile swab. Clean the less infected eye first from inner canthus to the outer (one stroke with each swab) discard the used swabs in paper bag (Fig. 5).	To prevent the transmission of microorganisms to the lacrimal duct.

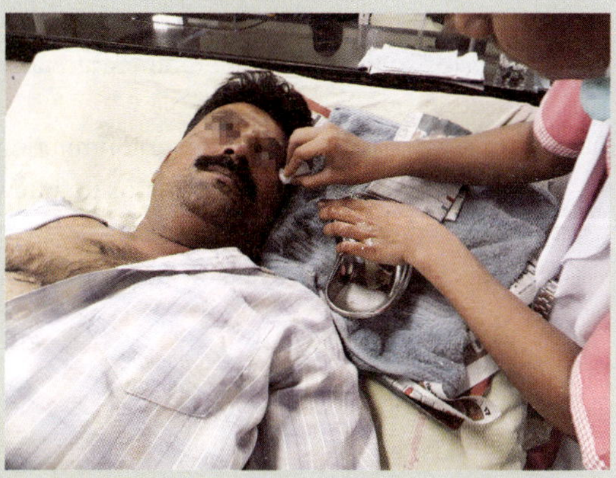

Fig. 5: Clean the eye from inner canthus to outer canthus

7. When the eye is clean, repeat the procedure for the other eye and make the patient comfortable	To prevent the infection
8. Record the procedure and the final condition of the eyes	Provides documentation for the nursing action
9. Wash and replace the articles in a proper place	To be able to use later

Evaluation

Check the patient's response to the treatment.

EYE IRRIGATION

Eye irrigation is washing the conjunctival sac by a stream of liquid.

Purposes

- ♦ To clean and remove secretions
- ♦ To relieve inflammation, congestion and pain
- ♦ To relieve foreign bodies
- ♦ To apply medication for an antiseptic effect
- ♦ For thermal effects
- ♦ To prepare for the eye surgery

Solutions Used

- Plain water
- Normal saline
- Boric acid (2%)
- Acriflavine (1%)
- Silver nitrate (1%)
- Mercurochrome (1%)

General Instructions

- Do the procedure in a sterile way.
- All the articles and the solutions that come in contact with eye during irrigation should be sterile.
- Wash hands thoroughly before and after procedure.
- It is best to treat each eye separately using separate equipment and solutions to prevent infection from one eye entering into the other.
- Place the head tilted to the affected side so that it allows drainage away from the unaffected side. Thus, potential contamination of the healthy eye is prevented.
- The nurse should take precautions to prevent infections being transmitted to herself and to others.
- Before irrigation starts, carefully clean the eyelids to remove any secretions or particles of dust adhering to the lashes, which would otherwise be carried to the conjunctival sac.
- Every movement of the nurse should be gentle.
- Never touch the eye with the irrigator.
- When both eyes are treated, treat the least infected eye first.
- Never direct forceful stream of solution into the eyes. If the solution is held very high, it will flow with great force,

which might injure the eye. The solutions are held to a height, which allows a steady flow of solution.

- The temperature of the solution varies according to the effects desired. Irrigations are usually given at body temperature. In inflammatory conditions, these may be prescribed as hot as the patient can tolerate. Test the temperature of the water at the inner surface of the wrist.
- The amount of solution varies according to the desired effect. When irrigations are intended to remove the chemicals, a large volume of solution is needed.
- Restrict the movement of the patient when he is likely to be non-cooperative.
- The eye irrigations should be carried out in good light.
- Direct the flow of the fluid from inner canthus to the outer canthus to prevent forcing the infection into the nasolacrimal duct.
- If any medicine is to be instilled, it should be done immediately after eye irrigation.

Assessment

- Check the name and identification data of the patient
- Check the diagnosis and purposes for irrigation
- Check the doctor's order for specific instruction regarding type of solution and the temperature at which it is to be used.
- Assess the patient's abilities and limitations
- Assess the patient's mental status to follow instructions
- Assess the need for any restraints
- Check the articles available in patient's unit

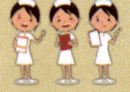 **SKILL: EYE IRRIGATION**

Articles Required (Fig. 6)

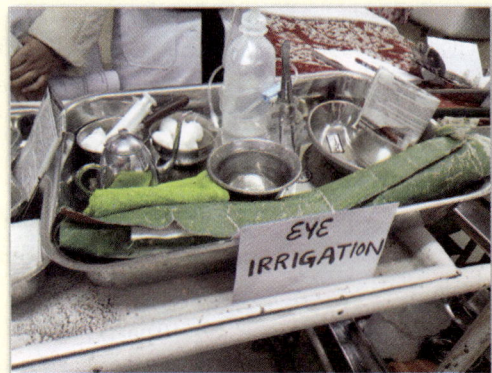

Fig. 6: Articles for eye irrigation

Contd...

Articles	Rationale
An eye dropper, a syringe or plastic bottle with prescribed solution and an intravenous (IV) set with attached tubing or a sterile irrigating can with tubing	To irrigate the eye
A bowl/jug with solution ordered (temperature varies according to the desired effect)	To irrigate the eye
Sterile wet swabs in a bowl	To clean eyes before procedure
Sterile cotton balls and a small towel	To dry the eyes after the procedure
Thumb forceps in boiled cold water	To handle sterile articles
A mackintosh and a towel	To protect bedding
A kidney tray and paper bag	To receive waste
An IV stand if needed	To adjust the height of the can/IV bottle as prescribed for the patient
Medication as ordered	

Steps of Procedure

Review and follow the standard steps as given in Appendix

Action/steps	Rationale
1. Explain the procedure to the patient and instruct him/her to tilt his head towards the side of the affected eye. The patient may sit or lie in supine position.	To win patient's confidence and co-operation
2. Place the mackintosh and towel under the head	To protect the linen from soiling
3. The kidney tray should be placed on the affected side of the face with convex side near the eye to receive the outflow	To prevent soiling of bedding and clothes.
4. Wash hands	To prevent transfer of microorganisms
5. Clean the eyelids and eye lashes from the inner canthus to the outer canthus using sterile wet swabs.	Any crust on the lids and lashes should be washed off before the procedure
6. Irrigate the eye using the irrigator: • Adjust the flow of liquid by adjusting the height of the irrigator • Test the temperature of the irrigating solution (98°–100°F) by pouring some fluid on the back of your hands and ask the client to close his/her eyes and pour a little solution on to his/her eyelids.	To prevent burns
7. Pull down the lower lid with the index finger. Instruct the client to look up. Avoid touching the eye with nozzle held 2 cm above	To prevent injury to sensitive cornea
8. Allow irrigating fluid to flow from inner canthus to outer canthus. Ask the patient to look up while irrigating.	To prevent infection to the nasolacrimal duct
9. Irrigate the eye till the desired effect is obtained	For proper cleaning of the eye
10. Repeat the procedure for the other side if needed, separate articles and solutions should be used	To avoid the spread of infection from one eye to the other.
11. Pat the eye and dry the face with a small towel/dry swab.	Provide comfort
12. Record the type and amount of fluid used as well as the effectiveness of the therapy	Provides documentation for nursing action
13. Discard the swabs. Wash and dismantle the articles	To keep the equipment ready for next use

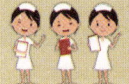

Evaluation

Check the patient's response to the treatment.

INSTILLATION OF EYE DROPS

Purposes

- To contract or dilate the pupil
- To combat infection and inflammation
- To relieve pain and discomfort.

General Instructions

- Check the physician's order
- Check the medication to be administered
- Medicines should not be cloudy or should not have any precipitate

- Only the desired dose should be administered
- Always start with the least affected eye

Assessment

- Assess the condition of external eye structure.
- Determine whether the patient has any known allergies to eye medication.
- Determine whether the client has any symptoms of visual alterations.
- Assess the client's level of consciousness and ability to follow directions.
- Assess the client's knowledge level regarding medication and desire to self-medication.
- Assess the client's ability to manipulate and hold dropper.

SKILL: INSTILLATION OF EYE DROPS

Articles Required (Fig. 7)

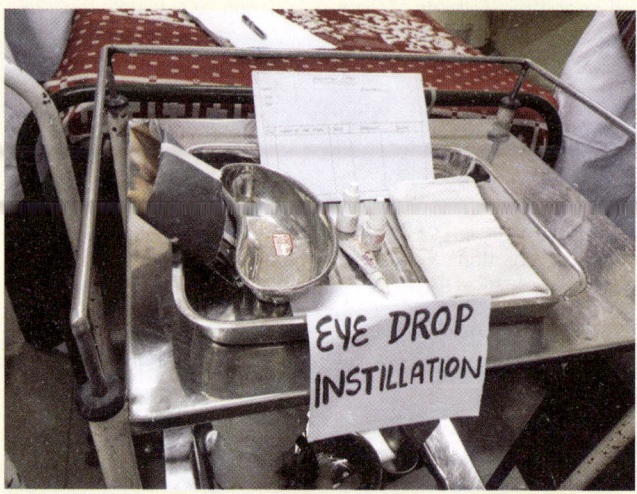

Fig. 7: Articles for eye drop instillation

Articles	Rationale
Medicine with a dropper	For accurate instillation of drops
A face towel/gauze pieces	To wipe off excess medication that escapes eye
A medication card	For correct administration of medicines
A kidney tray with paper bag	To discard used swabs

Contd...

Steps of Procedure

Review and follow the standard steps as given in Appendix

Action/steps	Rationale
Planning	
1. Check the patient's name and physician's prescription	For patient identification and ensure correct administration of medication
2. Explain the procedure to the patient	Relaxed patient is more cooperative
Implementation	
3. Wash hands	It reduces the transmission of microorganisms
4. Ask the patient to lie a supine position or sitting position with head slightly hyperextended and stand behind the patient	It provides easy access to the eyes for medication and instillation
5. If there is any discharge from eyes or crust is present, clean the eyes with boiled cooled swabs	It reduces pain
6. Ask the client to look up. Separate the lower lid of the eye by pressing it against the cheek bone	This exposes lower conjuctival sac and prevents pressure and trauma to eyeball
7. With dominant hand resting on client's forehead, hold a filled medication dropper approximately 1 or 2 cm above conjuctival sac and drop the prescribed number of drops into conjuctival sac/center of the lower eyelid.	Reduces the risk of injury to eyes and transfer of infection from dropper Enhances even distribution of drops across the eye
8. After instillation of drops, ask the client to close eyes. Gently move the eyeballs from side to side	Helps in distribution of medicine evenly
9. If excess medication is on eyelid, gently wipe it off from the inner to outer canthus with a towel or gauze. Make the patient comfortable.	Helps prevent trauma to eyes and promotes comfort
10. Observe response to medication	Helps to evaluate reaction to medication
11. Record the drug administered, its concentration, number of drops, time and eye in which drops are administered	Timely documentation prevents error.

Evaluation

Check the patients response to treatment.

EYE OINTMENT APPLICATION

Steps of Procedure

Action/steps	Rationale
1. Holding the applicator above lower lid margin, apply thin stream of ointment evenly along the inner edge of lower eyelid on conjunctiva from inner canthus to outer canthus.	Distributes medication evenly across eye and lid margin
2. Have the client close eyes and ask him to move the eyeballs in a circular motion	Further distributes the ointment

Evaluation

Check the patients response to treatment.

CONCLUSION

Eyes are the sensitive organs of the body. They need to be handled gently. The role of the nurse in the care of the patients receiving therapies of the eye is not only with administrating treatment but also to administer and rehabilitation of the client.

BIBLIOGRAPHY

1. Sr. Nancy. "Stephanie's Principles and Practice of Nursing senior Nursing Procedure and Nursing administration", vol. 2, 4th edition. NR Brothers; 2005. pp. 176-81.
2. Potter PA, Perry AG. Fundamentals of Nursing, 6th edition. New Delhi: Elsevier; 2008. pp. 859-62.
3. Taylor C. Fundamentals of Nursing, 5th edition. Lippincott Publications; 2006; pp. 761-4.
4. Mayer B. Nursing Procedures. Spring House Corporation; 3rd edition. 1999, pp. 679-82.
5. White L. Basic Nursing: Foundation of Skills and Concepts, 1st edition. Delmar/Thomson Learning; 2002; pp. 422-3.

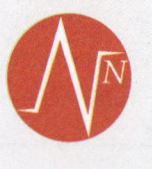
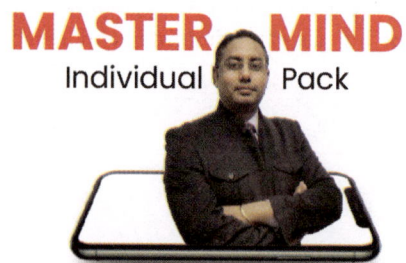

Treatments Related to ENT

INTRODUCTION

People are highly dependent on the sensory perceptions gained through the sense organs which are eye, ear, nose and throat. We not only receive important information about our surroundings through these sense organs of seeing, hearing, smelling and tasting, but move about safely and appreciate the beauty of nature and life.

ENT stands for Ear, Nose and Throat

Ear performs two main functions, hearing and maintaining the balance. They are delicate structures and need to be protected from any infection or injury that might affect hearing and balance.

Nose is the organ of smell. Normally, it has a variety of bacteria. Usually, they do not cause any harm. Many communicable diseases begin in the nose and the mouth.

Throat is the gateway to swallowing and breathing. It is important to keep it free and clean. Nurses play an important role in prevention, treatment and rehabilitation of patients with ear, nose and throat disorders.

ANATOMY AND PHYSIOLOGY OF EAR

Ear is the organ that detects sound. It not only receives sound, but also aids in balance and body positioning. The ear is part of the auditory system.

Structure of Ear

The ear is made up of three parts: the outer, middle and inner ear. All three parts of the ear are important for detecting sound by working together to move sound from the outer part through the middle and into the inner part of the ear. Ears also help to maintain balance.

The Outer Ear

The outer ear includes:
- Auricle (cartilage covered by skin placed on opposite sides of the head)
- Auditory canal (also called the ear canal)
- Eardrum outer layer (also called the tympanic membrane)

The outer part of the ear collects sound. Sound travels through the auricle and the auditory canal, a short tube that ends at the eardrum.

The Middle Ear

The middle ear includes:
- Eardrum
- Cavity (also called the tympanic cavity)
- Ossicles (3 tiny bones that are attached)
  - **Malleus (or hammer):** Long handle attached to the eardrum
  - **Incus (or anvil):** The bridge bone between the malleus and the stapes
  - **Stapes (or stirrup):** The foot plate; the smallest bone in the body

Sound entering the outer ear travels through the middle ear and causes the eardrum and ossicles in the middle ear to vibrate. As it travels, it amplifies (becomes louder) and changes from air to liquid.

The Inner Ear

The inner ear includes:
- **Oval window** that connects the middle ear with the inner ear
- **Semicircular ducts filled with fluid:** Attached to cochlea and nerves; send information on balance and head position to the brain
- **Cochlea:** Spiral-shaped organ of hearing; transforms sound into signals that get sent to the brain
- **Auditory tube** drains fluid from the middle ear into the throat behind the nose

Physiology of Hearing

Sound travels through the auricle and the auditory canal, a short tube that ends at the eardrum. Sound entering the outer ear travels through the middle ear and causes the eardrum and ossicles in the middle ear to vibrate. As it travels, it amplifies (get louder) and changes from air to liquid. When the stapes moves, it pushes the oval window, which then moves the cochlea. The cochlea takes the fluid vibration of sounds from the surrounding

semicircular ducts, translates them into signals sent to the brain by nerves like the vestibular nerve and cochlear nerve. The brain translates the information into recognizable sound patterns.

ANATOMY AND PHYSIOLOGY OF NOSE

The nose is the organ of smell located in the middle of the face. The internal part of the nose lies above the roof of the mouth. The nose consists of:
- **External meatus:** Triangular-shaped projection in the center of the face.
- **External nostrils:** Two chambers divided by the septum.
- **Septum:** Made up primarily of cartilages and bone and covered by mucous membranes. The cartilage also gives shape and support to the outer part of the nose.
- **Nasal passages:** Passages that are lined with mucous membranes and tiny hairs, (cilia) which help to filter the air.
- **Sinuses:** Four pairs of air-filled cavities, also lined with mucous membranes. The sinuses are cavities, or air-filled pockets, near the nasal passage. As in the nasal passage, the sinuses are lined with mucous membranes. There are four different types of sinuses:
  - **Ethmoid sinus:** This sinus is located inside the face, around the area of the bridge of the nose. It is present at birth, and continues to grow.
  - **Maxillary sinus:** This sinus is located inside the face, around the area of the cheeks. It is also present at birth, and continues to grow.
  - **Frontal sinus:** This sinus is located inside the face, in the area of the forehead. It does not develop until around 7 years of age.
  - **Sphenoid sinus:** This sinus is located deep in the face, behind the nose. It does not typically develops until adolescence.

Functions of the Nose

- **Respiration:** The nose is for breathing. Mouth breathing occurs when the nose is blocked.
- **Air conditioning:** The air inhaled through the nose is warmed, filtered and moistened before it reaches the lungs.
- **Protection:** Inhaled air is purified in the following ways:
  - Cilia removes smaller particles, which stick to the mucosa in the nose and are passed backwards into the pharynx by the ciliary's movements. The mucous, which reaches the pharynx is swallowed.
  - Lysozomes can kill the bacteria.
  - Sneezing throws out irritating particles or fumes from the nose.
- Olfaction is an important function of the nose and it has a protective value against approaching dangers.

ANATOMY AND PHYSIOLOGY OF THE THROAT (PHARYNX)

The pharynx is a funnel-shaped fibromuscular tube that forms the upper part of the digestive and respiratory tracts. It is lined by mucous membrane. It extends from the base of the skull to the level of the body of the sixth cervical vertebra. From above downwards, the nasal cavity, oral cavity, and laryngeal inlet open into the pharynx. The corresponding part of the pharynx is named as:

- **Nasopharynx:** Opening into the nasal cavity.
- **Oropharynx:** Opening into the oral cavity
- **Layngopharynx (Hypopharynx):** Opening into larynx

The lower end of the pharynx is continuous with the esophagus. This is the narrowest part of the gastro-intestinal tract and it is called cricopharynx which is situated behind the cricoid cartilage.

Size and Shape

It is about 10–15 cm long in adult. It is shaped like a funnel with the broad end at the top.

PROCEDURES RELATED TO EAR, NOES AND THROAT

EAR IRRIGATION

Ear irrigation is the washing of the external auditory canal with a stream of liquid.

Purposes

- To remove the ear wax
- To remove foreign bodies (except hygroscopic substances)
- To cleanse the ear in case of purulent discharge caused by middle ear infection
- For antiseptic effect
- To apply heat
- To evaluate vestibular functions

Assessment

- Check the name, bed number and other identification of the patient.
- Check the diagnosis and purpose of the ear irrigation.
- Check the doctor's order and the specific instructions regarding the type of the solutions used and the movement of the patient.
- Ascertain whether the impaction is due to a hygroscopic substance (attracts and absorbs moisture). In such case, the ear irrigation should not be carried out because the substance will absorb water, swell and will produce intense pain.
- Assess the patient's abilities and limitations.
- Assess the patient's mental status to follow instructions.
- Examine the ear for any perforation of the tympanic membrane by using an otoscope.
- Check the articles available in the patient's unit.
- If the patient is found to have impacted cerumen, instill 1–2 drops of mineral oil into the ear for 2–3 days before irrigation.

Solutions Used

- Boric Acid (2–4%)
- Sodium bicarbonate solution (1%)
- Normal saline
- Hydrogen peroxide (2%)
- Sterile water

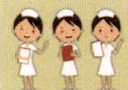 SKILL: EAR IRRIGATION

Articles Required (Fig. 1)

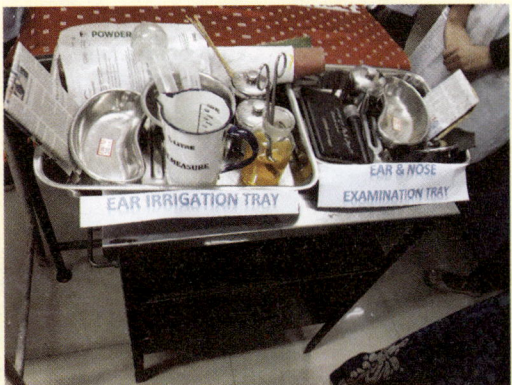

Fig. 1: Articles for ear irrigation

Contd...

Prescribed sterile irrigating solution (warmed to 37 degree centigrade) or at body temperature	To irrigate the ear
Irrigation set (container and irrigation bulb syringe)	To irrigate the ear
Waterproof pad/mackintosh and towel	To protect the bedding
Emesis basin/kidney tray and paper bag	To receive waste
Sterile cotton balls and cotton tipped applicators	To clean external auditory canal
Clean gloves	To protect the examiner
Spot light and head mirror	To visualize the tympanic membrane

Planning

- Explain the procedure to the patient.
- Unless contraindicated, make the patient to sit on the chair with a back support, leaning against the back of the chair. If the patient's condition does not permit for sitting position, have the patient lying on his back with the head turned slightly to the side to be irrigated.
- Place the mackintosh and towel under the head to protect the bedding and garments.
- Place the kidney tray under the ear to be irrigated. Ask the patient to adjust the position of the kidney tray against the neck to receive the return flow.
- Arrange to provide enough light for the procedure.
- Arrange the articles conveniently in the patient's unit.
- If the patient is a child or is non-cooperative, restraint the patient to prevent any interference in the procedure.

Steps of Procedure

Review and follow the standard steps as given in appendix

Action/steps	Rationale
1. Explain the procedure to the patient and inform him/her how he has to cooperate	It facilitates cooperation and provides reassurance
2. Bring the equipment to patient's bedside. Check the physician's order. Protect the patient and bed linen with a moisture proof pad.	Provides for an organized approach to the task
3. Wash hands	Prevent spread of microorganisms
4. Have the patient sit up or lie with the head tilted toward the side of the affected ear. Have the patient support the basin under the ear to receive the irrigating solution	Gravity causes the irrigating solution to flow from the ear to the basin.
5. Clean the pinna and meatus at the auditory canal as necessary with moistened cotton tipped applicators dipped in warm tap water or the irrigation solution	Materials lodged on the pinna and at the meatus may be washed into the ear
6. Ascertain whether impaction is due to foreign hygroscopic (attracts or absorbs moisture) body before proceeding.	If water contacts such a substance, it may cause it to swell and produce intense pain.
7. Fill the bulb syringe with warm solution, if an irrigating container is used, allow air to escape from the tubing (using 50 mL of fluid)	Air forced into the ear canal is noisy and therefore, unpleasant for the patient
8. Straighten the auditory canal by pulling the pinna up and back for an adult, upward and back for a child over 3 years, and down and back for an infant or child up to 3 years of age	Straightening the ear canal helps to allow the solution to reach all areas of the ear canal.
9. Direct a steady, slow stream of solution against the roof of the auditory canal, using only sufficient force to remove secretions holding tip 1 cm above the opening of ear canal. Do not occlude the auditory canal with the irrigating nozzle. Allow the solution to flow out unimpeded.	Directing solution at the roof the canal helps prevent injury to the tympanic membrane. Continuous in flow and outflow of the irrigating solution helps to prevent pressure in the canal.
10. When the irrigation is completed, place a cotton ball loosely in the auditory meatus and have the patient lie on the side of the affected ear on a towel or absorbent pad.	The cotton ball absorbs excess fluid and gravity allows the remaining solution in the canal to escape from the ear
11. Assess the drained fluid for foreign body, color and any discharge	To identify the foreign body or ear wax.

Contd...

After Care

♦ Discard the irrigated fluid and swabs. Clean and replace the reusable articles.

♦ Wash hands.

Documentation

♦ Record the irrigation: Check the appearance of the drainage and the patient's response.

Evaluation

Check the remove the cotton ball and assess drainage after 15 minutes. Canal is free of cerumen and foreign material.

INSTILLING MEDICATION INTO EAR

It is the process of the introduction of the medicine into the ear drop by drop for a localized effect.

Purposes

♦ To soften ear wax for removing it.

♦ To reduce localized inflammation and destroy infective organism in the external ear canal.

♦ To relieve pain

♦ To facilitate removal of foreign body

♦ To produce local anesthesia

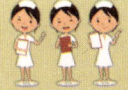 **SKILL: INSTILLATION OF MEDICINE INTO EAR**

Articles Required (Fig. 2)

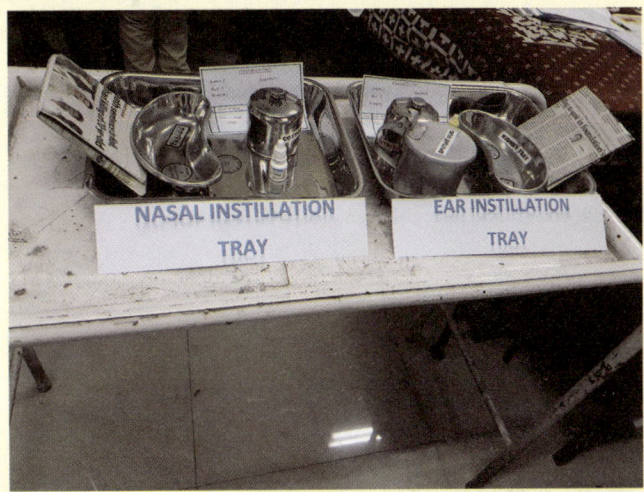

Fig. 2: Article tray for ear and nasal instillation

Clean gloves	For protection
Cotton tipped applicators	To wipe the cerumen and discharge
Medication bottle with dropper	To instill the drops
Cotton balls, cotton tipped applicator	To plug the ears and to clean the ear canal
Kidney tray	To discard the waste
Bowl with normal saline or Luke warm water	To instill the drops at room temperature

Steps of Procedure

Review and follow the standard steps as given in Appendix.

Contd...

Action/steps	Rationale
Assessment	
1. Assess for: ▪ Allergy to medication ▪ Redness/abrasion in the pinna/meatus ▪ Type and amount of discharge ▪ Complaints of discomfort ▪ Ability to cooperate during procedure ▪ Specific drug action and side effects ▪ Patient's knowledge about medication to be administered	Identifies contraindications for ear drop instillation
Planning	
2. Check medication order for name, dose time, amount and ear to be treated.	Reduces risk of medication errors
3. Identify patient and explain procedure, the purpose of medication and position to assume during and after instillation.	Reduces anxiety and promotes cooperation of patient.
4. Obtain assistance in case of children or infants to immobilize them	Prevents accidental injury due to sudden movement during the procedure.
Implementation	
5. Assist patient to a side lying position with ear being treated on the upper side	Positioning provides easy access for instillation of medication.
6. Wash hands	It reduces the transmission of microorganisms.
7. Clean meatus of ear canal, using cotton tipped applicators. Use normal saline, if necessary	Removes any discharge before instillation
8. Warm container in hand or by placing it for a short time in warm water	Promotes comfort of patient and prevents vertigo and nausea
9. Fill ear dropper partially with medication	
10. Straighten auditory canal. For an adult or child older than 3 years, pull pinna upward and backward and for children, downward and backwards	Straightening the canal can ensure solution to flow the entire length of the canal.
11. Instill correct number of drops along the side of ear canal by holding the dropper one centimeter (1/2 inch) above ear canal (Fig. 3)	Reduces trauma to tympanic membrane

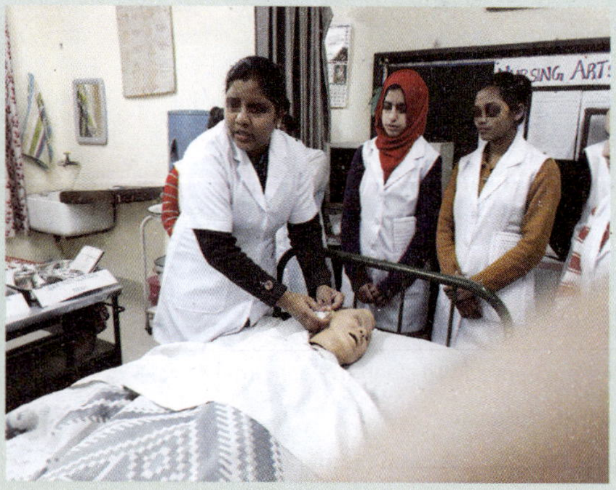

Fig. 3: Instillation of ear drops

Action/steps	Rationale
12. Press gently and firmly few times on the tragus area with fingers	Pressing on the tragus assists flow of medication into ear canal
13. Instruct the patient to remain in side-lying position for 5 minutes	Prevents drops from escaping and enables medication to reach all sides of canal.
14. Insert a small piece of cotton ball loosely at the meatus of auditory canal after 15–20 minutes	The cotton helps to retain medication and prevents leakage when patient is upright.

After Care

♦ Assess for patient's comfort, response and check for discharge/drainage from the ear.
♦ Replace medication and other articles.
♦ Wash hands.
♦ Document medication administration, name of the medication, number of drops administered and patient's response.

Evaluation

Check for patient's response and effectiveness of the treatment. Assess if patient can explain technique of instilling ear drops and demonstrates self administration of next dose.

NASAL INSTILLATION

The process of instilling the solution into the nose is called nasal instillation.

Purposes

♦ To shrink the swollen mucous membrane of nasal cavity
♦ To loosen the secretions and facilitate drainage
♦ To treat infections of the nasal cavity or sinuses
♦ To give local anesthesia.

General Instructions

♦ Caution the client to avoid the use of nasal decongestants for a prolonged period as it can lead to a rebound effect in which the nasal congestion worsens.
♦ The anterior nares should be clean and free from any discharge before instilling.
♦ The patient should be placed in proper position otherwise the drops will run down the throat and will be swallowed, thus making the procedure ineffective.
♦ Instruct the patient to remain in the same position after instilling of the drops to promote proper absorption of the medicine.
♦ Do not infect the dropper by touching the tip to the nose.

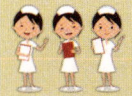 **SKILL: NASAL INSTILLATION**

Articles Required

Articles	Rationale
Medication with clean wrapper	For instilling the drop
A medication card	To ensure accurate nasal instillations
Small towel	To wipe the nose
Cotton tipped applicators (swab stick)	For cleaning

Steps of Procedure

Review and follow the standard steps as given in Appendix

Action/steps	Rationale
Assessment	
1. Check the physician's order for medication, name of the drug, concentration, number of drops and time of administration	To ensure safe and correct administration of drug.
Planning	
2. Explain the procedure to client to breathe through mouth until he/she is made up to sit up at the end of procedure	It helps to reduce the patient's anxiety. It reduces the chances of aspirating nasal drops into trachea and lungs.
3. Instruct the client to blow the nose gently unless contraindicated (e.g., risk of increased intracranial pressure or nose bleeds)	To clear the nasal passage of mucous and secretions that can block distribution of medication.

Contd...

Action/steps	Rationale
Implementation	
4. Wash hands	It reduces transmission of microorganisms
5. Assist the client to a supine position and place a pillow under the shoulders to fall over the edge of the pillow	It provides access to nasal passages
6. Hold the dropper 1 cm above the nares and instill the prescribed number of drops towards the midline of the ethmoid bone	It avoids contamination of the dropper. It also facilitates distribution of medication over the nasal mucosa
7. Instruct the client to remain in supine position for 5 minutes. Give him a towel. But caution should be taken not to blow nose for several minutes	It promotes maximum amount of medication to be absorbed
8. Discard any medication remaining in the dropper before returning the dropper to the bottle	To prevent contamination of medicine

After Care

- Assist the client to a comfortable position after the drug has been absorbed.
- Dispose off the soiled supplies in a proper container and wash hands.
- Document medication administration, name of the medication, number of drops administered and patient's response.

Evaluation

Check the patient's response and effectiveness of treatment.

PAINTING OF THROAT

Medication is applied to the throat locally by the way of spraying and painting.

Purposes

- To treat infections
- To relieve inflammation, pain and congestion
- To anesthetize the part.

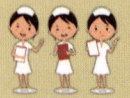

SKILL: PAINTING OF THROAT

Articles Required

Articles	Rationale
Spot light	To visualize the throat
Sterile/clean cotton applicators in a container	To apply medication
A tongue depressor	To visualize the throat
Kidney tray and paper bag	To receive the waste
Mackintosh and towel	To protect garments
Medication as ordered: Mandel's paint, tannic acid, glycerin, phenol glycerin.	

Steps of Procedure

Review and follow the standard steps as given in Appendix

Contd...

Action/steps	Rationale
Assessment	
1. Check for physician's order	To ensure safe and correct administration of drug.
2. Check the patients name and the indication for application	
3. Explain the procedure to the patient and make him/her sit on the chair and tilt his head backwards	To reduce the patient's anxiety
Implementation	
4. Place the mackintosh and towel around the neck	To prevent garments from soiling
5. Adjust the spotlights	To visualize the throat
6. Take the medication on the cotton applicators (squeeze off the excess medication)	To avoid dropping of the medication
7. Ask the patient to say "aaaa…" to open the mouth fully and place the tongue depressor over his tongue and apply slight pressure downwards	To visualize the back of the mouth
8. Paint the throat quickly (paint the tonsils and back of pharynx) using the circular movements. Allow the patient to breathe in between.	Taking too much time can cause throat irritation and choking

After Care

Record the procedure, date and time, type of medication and condition of patient. Dismantle the articles

Evaluation

Check the patient's response and effectiveness of treatment.

THROAT IRRIGATION

It is the process of flushing the throat with irrigating fluid

Purposes

♦ To clean the mouth and pharynx
♦ To relieve congestion
♦ To relieve dryness
♦ To relieve pain
♦ To combat infection
♦ To provide antiseptic effect

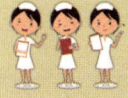 **SKILL: THROAT IRRIGATION**

Articles Required

A tray containing:
♦ **Irrigating solution:** Normal saline or warm water
♦ Gauze pieces
♦ Small towel
♦ Mackintosh
♦ Kidney tray
♦ Paper bag
♦ IV stand.

Steps of Procedure

♦ Check physician's order to obtain specific instructions
♦ Identify the patient and explain the procedure to patient
♦ Position the patient with his or her head bent slightly forward and tilted to one side.
♦ Cover his/her shoulder and neck with mackintosh and towel
♦ Hang the irrigating can up to 12 inches above patient's mouth
♦ Check the temperature of irrigation fluid as tolerated by the patient.
♦ Introduce the irrigating tip from the sides reaching behind the tongue avoiding the uvula.
♦ Rotate the tip to direct the fluid in all directions.
♦ When irrigation is complete, stop the procedure.
♦ Dry the mouth with towel.
♦ Remove the equipment and replace after washing.
♦ Wash hands after the procedure.
♦ Record the time of irrigation, kind and amount of solution used, nature of return flow and effect of treatment.

THROAT GARGLE

Gargle is letting hot salt solution roll in the throat for few seconds.

Purposes

- To relieve congestion
- To relax the throat muscles
- To reduce inflammation
- To relieve sore throat

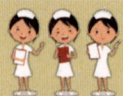

SKILL: THROAT GARGLE

Articles Required

- Two glasses of hot water
- One teaspoon of salt
- Half tea-spoon salt per glass of water

Procedure

- Explain procedure to the patient.
- Add half teaspoon of salt into glass of hot water as tolerated by patient.
- Stir the salt so that it is dissolved completely.
- Salt gargle can be done near the sink.
- Ask the patient to sip enough water and let it roll free in the throat for few seconds before spitting the water into the sink.
- Continue the procedure of throat-gargle until all the two glasses of salt solution are consumed.
- If sore throat is severe, it can be repeated every two hours.
- It is best done after meals.
- Do not take cold beverages until sore throat is healed.

BIBLIOGRAPHY

1. Annama J, Rekha R. Clinical Nursing Practice, 2nd edition, pp. 101-103, 296
2. The Trained Nurses Association of India. Fundamental of Nursing: Procedure Manual, 1st edition. TNAI Publication.
3. Tortora GJ, Grabowski SR. Principles of Anatomy and Physiology. John Wiley & Sons. pp. 355-9.

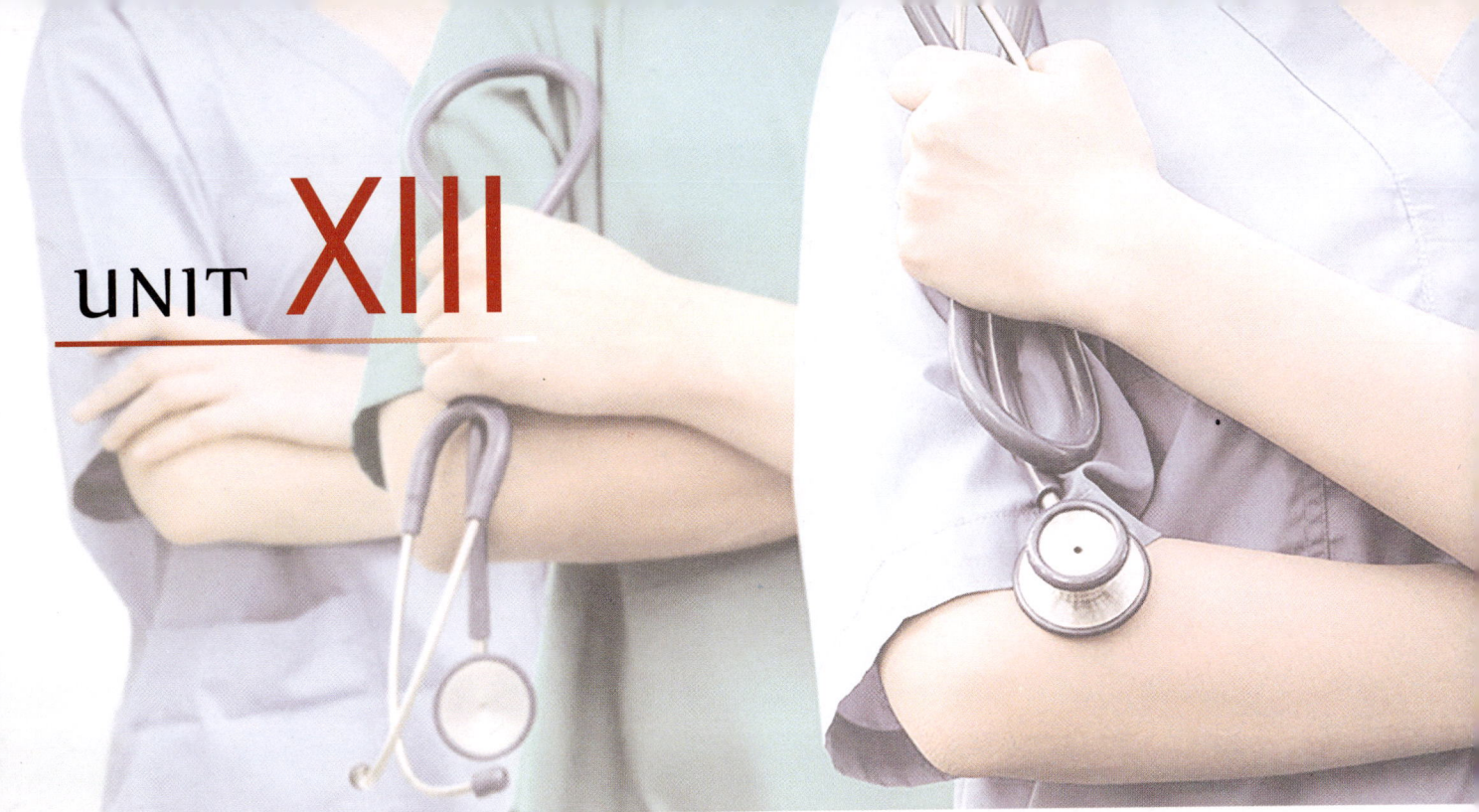

UNIT XIII

REHABILITATION

Unit Outline

Rehabilitation

Rehabilitation is a dynamic health related process that assists an ill or disabled individual to achieve the greatest possible level of physical, mental, spiritual, social and economic functioning. The rehabilitation process helps the person to achieve an acceptable quality of life with dignity, self-respect and independence. Rehabilitation programs are designed for individuals with physical, mental and emotional disabilities. During rehabilitation, the individual is assisted to adjust to the disability by learning how to use resources and to focus on existing abilities.

Rehabilitation is an integral part of nursing. Rehabilitation efforts should begin during the initial contact with the patient. Every major illness or injury carries with it the threat of disability. The emphasis of rehabilitation is to restore the patient to independence or to the pre-illness or pre-injury level of function in the shortest possible time. If this is not possible, the aims of rehabilitation are maximal independence and quality of life acceptable to the patient.

DEFINITIONS OF REHABILITATION

- Rehabilitation is a program designed to enable the individual who is physically disabled, chronically ill or convalescing to live and to work to the utmost of his capacity.
  —**Dr Howard Rusk**
- Rehabilitation means the restoration of one's physical, mental, social, vocational and economic capacity to the fullest extent to which one is capable.
- Rehabilitation is a creative procedure which includes the cooperative efforts of various medical specialists and their associates in other health fields to improve the mental, physical, social and vocational aptitudes of persons who are handicapped with the objective of prescribing their ability to live happily and productively on the same level and with the same opportunities as their neighbors.
  —**Frank Krusen**

- Rehabilitation is a treatment process designed to help physically handicapped individuals to make maximal use of residual capacities and to enable them to obtain optimal satisfaction and usefulness in terms of themselves, their families and their communities. —**Helen J Yesner**
- Rehabilitation is a creative process that allows maximal use of existing abilities. It is basically an optimistic process which concedes that despite continuing and even catastrophic disability a better way of life for the patient is possible.
- Rehabilitation is the process of maximizing an individual's abilities and resources to promote optimum growth and focusing on the individual's decision – making ability. This begins with preventive care in the initial stage of accident and/or illness. It continues through the restorative phase and it involves adaptation of new life.

AIMS OF REHABILITATION

To receive the greatest benefit from a rehabilitation program, it is imperative that the nurses perceive rehabilitation as a process that begins when a patient first suffers acute illness or injury. The elements of rehabilitation nursing need to be viewed as a part of basic nursing rather than as a specialty. Those who work at rehabilitation centers where patients are severely disabled, naturally have additional knowledge in this field of nursing.

Three aims of rehabilitation are considered in the care given by all members of the health. They are:

1. Prevent further impairment
2. Maintain existing abilities
3. Restore as much function as possible

Prevent Further Impairment

Prevention of further impairment must be considered throughout. Unfortunately preventive measures are never noticed unless they were not used. A pressure sore is visible but the lack of it is not. In case of an automobile accident, the driver is the first person to handle the patient. The way he moves and lifts the person from the site of accident into the ambulance prevent further injury. During the hospital stay the measures taken by nurses to prevent contractures, foot drop, pressure sores are the examples of preventing further impairment.

Maintain Existing Abilities

There is a need to emphasize regarding maintaining existing ability of non-injured parts. For example: Why should a person with fractured hip develop hypostatic pneumonia? Why should a young child develop a pressure sore from wearing a leg brace? Why should an amputee develop a hip flexion contracture?

Maintaining existing abilities actually entails preventing additional injury or deterioration of uninvolved parts. Nursing can make sure that no additional treatment or hospitalization is required because of a lack of knowledge in the part of those caring for the patient.

Restore as Much Function as Possible

The nurse works with the health team to help the patient to regain strength, to restore speech, to walk, to re-learn activities of daily living and to gain new ways to handle bowel and bladder problems. While prevention of further impairment and maintenance of existing ability continue throughout a patient's rehabilitation program, restoration plays role at this time it is the area of restoration that is often the responsibility of rehabilitation as a specialty.

The overall goal of restorative care is to assist the individual to regain maximal functional status, thereby enhancing the individual's quality of life. The restorative health care team supports the client's adaptation to or adjustment of the loss of function, maximization of the residual functional capacity and return of the client to the community.

TYPES OF REHABILITATION

There are different types of rehabilitation available for different types of disabilities. Some of them are as follows:

Neurological Rehabilitation

In this type of rehabilitation, patients suffering from stroke, neuromuscular disease, certain types of head trauma and spinal cord injury are treated. It aims at making the patient self-dependent and helps create a positive thinking in patient. The patient is treated so that he leads an improved life physically, emotionally and socially.

Cardiac Rehabilitation

The program is designed to help those people who have heart problem. Heart patients are educated to have a healthy life and reduce stress for the proper functioning of the heart. The main contents of the program include: educating people about the various risk factors that contribute to developing a heart disease. These risk factors include: high blood pressure, obesity, smoking, diabetes, drug abuse, drinking, lack of physical activity, etc. It also includes recovery programs from heart disease/surgery and educating people about improving their quality of life.

Physical Rehabilitation

This is designed for those people whose life style has changed after they have gone through a serious illness, surgery, accident or illness. Here the therapist introduces programs to improve the mobility and functioning of the injured body part of the patient. In this proper exercising program is designed to improve the functioning of body part. Massage, heat or cold therapy, balance and gait retraining, pain management and use of an artificial limb.

Vocational Rehabilitation

This program is designed to help those people who find it difficult to get employment or retain it after they have gone through certain situation that caused mental and physical disability in them. This program provides physiological and medical assessment for job placement, job training and on job training.

Speech Rehabilitation

Speech therapy can help treat a wide variety of issues involving language, communication, voice, swallowing and fluency. Common tactics used by speech therapist include language intervention activities, articulation therapy (demonstrating how to move tongue to create certain sounds), and feeding and swallowing therapy (tongue, lip and face exercises designed to strengthen the muscles of the mouth and throat). Conditions or illness that may require a speech therapist include:

- **Dyslexia:** Difficulty reading accurately and fluently
- **Dyspraxia:** Difficulty controlling muscle function for movement, coordination, language or speech
- **Aphasia:** A loss of ability to understand or express speech due to brain damage
- **Dysphagia:** Difficulty in swallowing
- **Articulation problems:** Difficulty in speaking clearly and making errors in sounds
- **Fluency problems:** Difficulty with flow of speech such as stuttering
- **Resonance or voice problems:** Difficulty with voice pitch, volume and quality

Occupational Therapy

It helps individuals who require assistance to participate in everyday activities, or "occupations". Occupations don't just refer to work or your job, but can also refer to self care practices, everyday tasks. The goal of occupational therapy is to help individuals participate in the things they want and need to do to live an independent and satisfying lifestyle. Occupational therapists help by making changes to things that hinder someone's ability to complete. Tasks such as eating, dressing, brushing one's teeth, and working. Modifications may include changing the way the task in approached changing the environment in which the task is completed or helping a person to develop skills necessary to complete certain tasks.

It may be needed by people of all ages such as children with disabilities—to develop their co-ordination needed to feed themselves, use a computer or improve their handwriting. Adults who have lost the ability to hold a fork due to an injury may need to regain grip strength and modify movements so that they can feed themselves independently.

REHABILITATION TEAM

Rehabilitation requires a team of professionals working together with patients and family. The team members represent a variety of disciplines with each health professional making a unique contribution. Each health professional assesses the patients needs within the discipline. Team members meet in group sessions at frequent intervals to collaborate, to evaluate progress, and to modify goals as needed to facilitate rehabilitation.

The rehabilitation team members promote independence, self respect and an acceptable quality of life. The patient is the key member of the rehabilitation team. Patient is the focus of the team effort and that one who determines the final outcomes of the process. The patient participates in goal setting in learning to function using remaining abilities, and in adjusting to living with disabilities.

The patient's family is incorporated into the team. Disability of one member of family affects other family members. By incorporating the family into the rehabilitation process, one can make the family adapt to the change in one of its members. The family provides ongoing support and participates in providing necessary ongoing care.

The rehabilitation nurse develops a therapeutic and supportive relationship with the patient and the family. The nurse during patient interactions, actively listens, encourages and shares the patient's strengths. The patient is praised for efforts to improve self-concept and self-care abilities. The nurse develops a plan of care designed to facilitate rehabilitation, to restore and maintain optimum health, and to prevent complication.

The nurse collaborates with and coordinates the services provided by all members of the health care team including the home health nurse who is responsible for directing the patients care after return to the home. The nurse assumes role of caregiver, teacher, counselor, patients advocate and consultant.

The rehabilitation team also may include: a physician, surgeon, psychiatrist, physical therapist, speech therapist, pathologist, psychologist, social worker, vocational counselor, prosthetist, respiratory therapist, and audiologist.

The team functions as a unit to assist the client to achieve the maximal possible level of functioning. Although the health care professionals work together as a team, members participate and contribute from the specific focus of their own respective disciplines. For example, for a client with self care deficit, the nurse assists the client with bathing, feeding, etc. While supervising and reinforcing the clients use of transfer techniques taught by the physical therapist and assistive devices provided by the occupational therapist.

Role of Nurse in Rehabilitation

The role of the rehabilitation nurse is similar to those of nurses in other settings. However, there are certain areas of priority and emphasis to which a rehabilitation nurse must address herself. Certain knowledge, skills and attitudes, while pertinent to many areas of nursing, are required in greater depth by the nurse who works with patients having chronic illness or in a rehabilitation program. First of all, the nurse needs a good understanding of the psychological effects of long–term illness in order to respond appropriately to patient needs during the various stages of adjustment to a disability. She needs to have thorough knowledge of anatomy, physiology and pathophysiology, especially of the nervous system, the musculoskeletal system and the urinary system. She needs to have knowledge about kinesiology the science of body movement.

The nurse needs to know how to plan ways in which the patient can achieve bowel and bladder control. She should be aware of the interrelatedness of psychosocial and economic problems. What radical changes are occurring to the family as a result of the disease? Is he the breadwinner who has been struck down by some accident or illness? Is she the housewife on whom the whole family, children depends? How do individual perceptions of the condition affect planning? In addition to specialized knowledge, the rehabilitation nurse needs to be expert in certain skills.

Change of position is essential for maintaining body alignment, to prevent skeletal deformities and to prevent pressure sores. Another necessary skill is the performance of transfer techniques like from bed to wheelchair and back to bed. Can the patient transfer independently or needs assistance?

Skills in performing range of motion exercises to clients who are disabled to prevent additional problems resulting from disease. These exercises vary with the age and condition of the patient.

The rehabilitation nurse needs to possess special attitudes as she has to deal with patients having long term problems. She must have patience and understanding in order to be sensitive to her patient and to adjust her actions accordingly. At certain times, the patient may need a lot of encouragement, at other times pressure is required. The nurse must encourage the patient and praise him not only for achievement but also for effort. This is very essential as the results may not be evident for weeks or even months.

Patients need time to perform their tasks. Practice is essential, this is true in learning new ways to eat, dress, walk and so forth. We want to allow the patient to take time to perform certain activities. This means allowing ourselves time to let patients do things for themselves. The helping role of the nurse in rehabilitation differs from that of in acute care the emphasis is not to help the patient but to help him to help himself. When a nurse first works with patient who have a disability or a chronic disease, she must be especially cognizant of the ultimate goal—patients must become independent in every way. While planning patient care, the rehabilitation nurse includes the objective data from the patients history and physical examination, careful observation of the patient, application of nursing knowledge and finally, patient participation. It helps the nurse to assess patient problems, more accurately and ultimately to assist him to a greater degree. The areas of concern include the physical, psychological, social and environmental spheres of the patients life.

The aim of rehabilitating nurse is to enhance patient care through the initiation of independent nursing measures. The use of footboards, turning schedules, positioning techniques, range of motion exercises, use of transfer belts, comfort measures are initiated by the nurse, not the physician. Her assessment of patient needs takes place over a 24-hour period and is more current than that of any other health professional, including the physician. Coordination is a key role of the nurse who cares for patients receiving care from a variety of health workers. In order to coordinate, the nurse must have open channels of communication between departments. Most of the rehabilitation centers find that interdisciplinary patient conferences provide an excellent avenue for sharing information.

A major role of the rehabilitation nurse is that of patient and family teaching. The patient usually has much to learn.

He may need to learn new ways of performing activation of daily living (ADL's) such as dressing, bathing, eating, toileting, the patient may need to learn to walk again, to use a wheel chair or a variety of other new living adaptation.

Rehabilitation services are required by more people than ever before, because of advances in technology that saves the lives of the seriously ill, injured and disabled. Increasing numbers of patients who are recovering from serious illness or injuries are returning to their homes and communities with ongoing needs of rehabilitation. Every patient regardless of age, socio-economic status, or diagnosis, has a right to rehabilitation services.

BIBLIOGRAPHY

1. *Handerson V. Textbook of the Principles and Practice of Nursing. The Macmillan Company.*
2. *Basavanthappa BT. Fundamentals of Nursing. Jaypee Publications.*

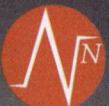
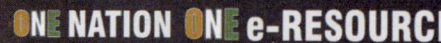

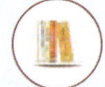

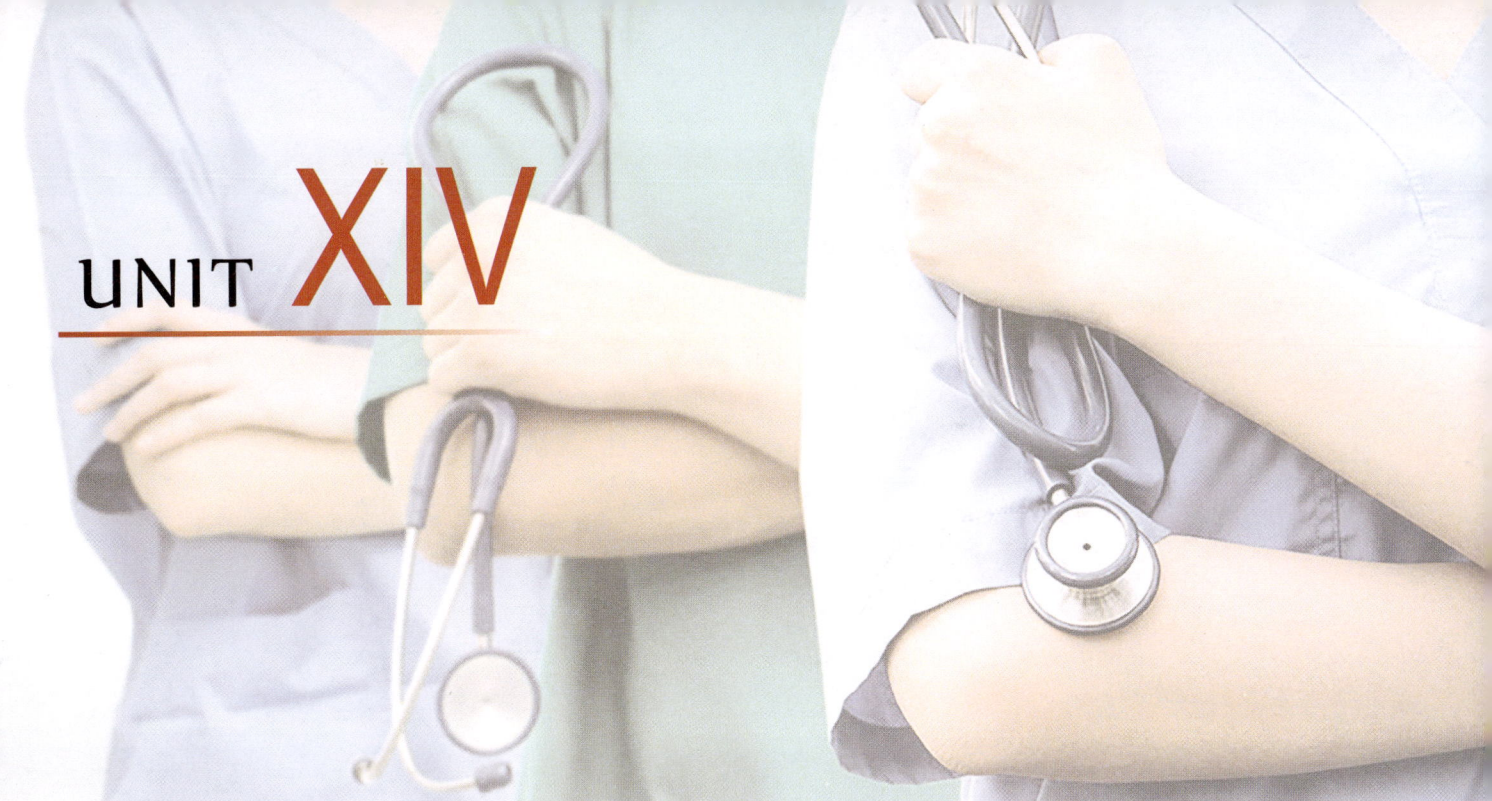

UNIT XIV

CARE OF TERMINALLY ILL PATIENT

Unit Outline

Care of Terminally Ill Patient

INTRODUCTION

Knowledge about terminal illness and principles of care is essential in supporting patients during decision making and in end-of-life closure in ways that recognize their unique responses to illness and that supports their values and goals.

DEFINITION

Terminal illness is a medical term used to describe a disease that cannot be cured or adequately treated and that is reasonably expected to result in the death of the patient within a short period of time.

IMPACT ON PATIENT

Many patients realize without being told that they are suffering from a terminal illness, they often pick up this knowledge from nonverbal communication by their families and by their health care professionals. Patients must be allowed to go through the stage of grieving process and to make decisions about their care; they must be supported in their decision making. Competent patients have the right to consent and refuse any and all indicated medical treatment, even life-sustaining treatment and should be made aware of this right.

IMPACT ON FAMILY

The family and significant others of terminally ill patients should be encouraged to participate in planning the patient's care. Health care personnel should be available to discuss the patient's condition with the family members and should support and care as the family begins the grieving process. The family may want to make arrangements with the patient for funeral or memorial services.

STAGES OF DYING ACCORDING TO KÜBLER–ROSS

- **Denial:** In denial and isolation stage, the patient denies that he or she will die, maybe repress what is discussed, and may isolate himself or herself from reality. Patient may think the doctor made a mistake in the diagnosis or may be his/her records got mixed with someone.
- **Anger:** In anger stage, patient expresses rage and hostility and adopts a why me attitude.
- **Bargaining:** In the bargaining stage, the patient tries to barter for more time, many patients put their own personal affairs in order, make wills and fulfill last wishes. "If I can just make it to my son's graduation, I will be satisfied, just let me live until then". It is important to meet these wishes, because bargaining helps people to move into later stages of dying.
- **Depression:** The patient goes through a period of grief before death, the grief is characterized by crying and not speaking much. "I just don't know how my wife will get along after I am gone".
- **Acceptance:** The patient feels tranquil. He or she has accepted death and is ready to die, have no regrets. "I have done everything I wanted to".

AIMS OF CARE OF TERMINALLY ILL PATIENT

- To improve the patient's and family's quality of life
- To provide prioritized care and symptom management
- To provide care of the multiple dimensions of the illness experience for both patients and families
- Promoting self-care and self-esteem
- Meeting client's needs
- Prepare for, and manage life closure and the dying process
- Coping with loss and grief during the illness and bereavement.

THREE ESSENTIAL COMPONENTS FOR CARE OF TERMINALLY ILL CLIENT

1. Team work and partnership
2. Assessing and to care for the needs
3. Psychosocial support

Team Work and Partnership

Care of patient during terminal illness by its very nature is a team effort, where members of diverse health care disciplines jointly plan, implement and evaluate care.

- **Physician:** The terminally ill patient comes in contact with many different doctors during their illness. It might be their general practitioner, a hospital physician, surgeon or oncologists.
- **Nurses:** Nurses working in acute settings such as medical, surgical or oncology section are a part of the multiprofessional team. Some also have specific post registration training in palliative care.
- **Physiotherapists, occupational therapists and speech therapists:**
- The usual roles of physiotherapists involve restoring musculoskeletal function, prevention of deformity and prevention of complications such as chest infections. They aim to maximize and maintain the patient's physical resources
- **Occupational therapists** often work closely with physiotherapists. Their main role is maximizing patient's safety, independent living potential. Occupational therapists perform detailed assessment of person's ability to carry out daily living tasks such as feeding, dressing and mobilizing, they provide adaptations and aids to enhance and maintain these skills.
- **Social worker:** The social worker's role is to help the patient, family and care givers to deal effectively, with the personal and social problems and impending death. They can provide the patient and family with advice on financial matters and benefits. Social workers are closely involved with counseling and bereavement support for families.
- **Dieticians:** The dietician's specialist knowledge and experience allows them to make a detailed assessment of patient's individual needs and what is best to advise them. They can provide not only individual meal choices but also supplements and according to the patient's taste.
- **Pharmacists:** The clinical pharmacist's role extends far beyond the provision of medicines. They are valuable source of information to patients, families and care givers.

Their detailed knowledge of pharmacology means they can advise on possible side effects or drug interactions and best combinations to avoid these.

- **Chaplains**: Chaplains are excellent talkers and are also trained to listen. Many patients experience a huge range of emotions and many people turn to religion during this period. This is a time when chaplain's help is invaluable. Once the patient has died the chaplain can usually be relied on to comfort and care for the bereaved family.

Assessing and to Care for the Needs

Physiological Needs

Pain

Assessment

In a nonresponsive client, agitation, restlessness, tense muscles moaning, frowning of face can be assessed for pain. Other measures are Wong Baker scale visual analogue scale (VAS) used for measuring pain.

Management

- Patient who have an established regimen of analgesics should continue to receive those medications as they approach the end of life.
- The route of administering the drugs should be considered.
- Assess the pain periodically and change the doses as required.
- In case of opioids, a regimen to combat constipation should be implemented.
- Patient controlled analgesia (PCA) pumps can provide the patient with a sense of independence and manage the pain at the same time.
- Provide distractions and verbal analgesia

Dyspnea

It is a subjective experience described as difficulty in breathing or as an uncomfortable awareness of breathing that accounts for a high proportion of the client's inability to carry out activities of daily living (ADL), and gravely affects the perceived quality of life. To manage dyspnea, patient may be given:

- Anti-anxiety agent, bronchodilators, corticosteroids
- Treat underlying pathology (cardiovascular disease or respiratory disease).
- Administer blood products and erythropoietin as prescribed
- Administer prescribed diuretics and monitor fluid balance
- Provide oxygen therapy
- Maintain high Fowler's position

- Ensure drainage of secretions, provide steam inhalation and chest physiotherapy
- Periodic suctioning is necessary
- Maintain adequate ventilation in the room
- Avoid overcrowding around the patient

Skin and Mucous Membrane

- Patient should be comfortably placed and their position should be frequently changed in the bed. The bedding should not be wrinkled
- Frequent skin care should be given with particular attention to the pressure points. Back massage is to be given
- Perineal care is to be given, to keep the patient clean and to prevent skin breakdown.
- Catheterization has to be done in an incontinent patient
- Protect the eyes from corneal ulceration with protective ointment
- Prevent drying of lips and skin breakdown
- Provide daily bath
- Assist in elimination and keep the area clean
- Assist the patient in mobilization
- Prevent fall and injury
- Maintain skin integrity especially in old patients
- Change the bed linen and clothes whenever soiled
- Assist in active and passive exercise.
- Keep the skin moist and clean

Nausea and Vomiting

- Provide small frequent meals
- Allow the patient to choose favorite foods and fluids
- Monitor the weight
- Provide Fowler's position and make the client to sit upright after food intake for at least 15 minutes
- Provide anti-emetics half hour before the meals
- Provide adequate fluid intake
- Provide IV fluids if oral intake is inadequate
- Explain the patient and the family that in chemotherapeutic drugs, nausea and vomiting are side effects
- Provide oral care after vomiting episodes
- Provide antacids

Altered Nutrition

- Maintain a strict input and output chart
- Provide meals as per the taste of the client
- Provide a pleasant environment while meals are served.
- Serve the foods as per the appropriate temperature
- Provide intravenous total (IV) fluids and parenteral nutrition (TPN) in case the patient is not tolerating orally
- Maintain adequate hydration
- Provide a well-balanced diet

- Do not force-feed the patient
- Provide-home-cooked food if allowed
- Prevent gas forming foods

Anorexia (Desire, Appetite)

- Offer small portions of food
- Cool foods may be better tolerated than hot foods
- Place nutritious foods at bedside (fruit juices, fruits, etc.)
- Schedule meals when family members are present to provide company and stimulation
- Avoid arguments at meal time
- Assist the patient to maintain a schedule of oral care. Rinse the mouth after each meal or snack. Use soft toothbrush, treat ulcers and lesions, and make sure that dentures fit well.
- Treat pain and other symptoms
- Allow the patient to refuse foods and fluids.

Cachexia

Cachexia is a complex syndrome associated with metabolic changes, fat and muscle wasting, loss of appetite and involuntary weight loss. The term is derived from Greek word *kakos* and *hexis* meaning poor condition.

Interventions

- Ensuring good mouth care
- Maintaining pleasant surroundings
- Encouraging small and frequent meals
- Providing active and passive exercises
- Periodic weight checking
- Nutritional supplements.

Bowel and Bladder Care

Constipation

- Provide small frequent meals and increased fluid intake
- Provide increased roughage in the diet
- Provide stool softeners
- Enema should be given as per prescription
- Encourage mobilization after meals
- Establish a schedule for elimination

Diarrhea

- Provide meticulous skin care during diarrhea to prevent skin breakdown
- Provide medications as prescribed to prevent diarrhea
- The food served should be properly cooked
- Proper hand-washing before meals should be ensured
- The hands of caregiver while feeding the patient should also be clean
- Provide IV fluid in case of severe diarrhea and dehydration

- Keep the anal area dry and clean
- Change the linen and clothes when wet and soiled

Bladder Care

- Maintain an intake and output chart
- Ensure adequate hydration
- Provide privacy
- Prescribe diuretics to be given
- Catheterize the patient, if urinary incontinence prolongs
- Provide for skin care after urination

Fatigue and Weakness

It is a distressing subjective experience that impedes functioning and impairs quality of life. Clients describe fatigue as tiredness, exhaustion, generalized weakness, and diminished energy, increased need to rest or sleep, diminished motivation, diminished capacity to pay attention or a disturbed mood.

Interventions

- **Planned activity:** Plan the activities maintaining the independence of the patient, throughout the day, so that the patient has time to take rest in between activities.
- **Energy conservation:** Prioritize the activities, discuss plan with patient and care givers. Provide calm and quiet environment and effective rest periods.
- **Emotional support:** Improve self-worth, social relationships and opportunity to share feelings.
- **Nutritional support:** Provide small frequent feeds according to the liking of the patient.
- Encourage mobilization.

Sleep Disturbances

Impaired sleep is a common often overlooked problem in clients with advanced illness. Many a times a disturbance in sleep is accepted as a part of being sick; however, it is important to recognize the importance of sleep. Sleep is associated with tissue restoration. Sleep deprivation alters immune function. Excessive sleepiness is also disabling, resulting in an inability to participate in treatment, comprehend information and share in social interactions.

Interventions

- Promote a regular fixed sleeping pattern
- Staying out of bed during the day
- Keeping active, mentally or physically during the day
- Avoid stimulants like coffee at night.
- Treat potential causes contributing to impaired sleep such as nausea and vomiting, itching and respiratory problems
- Minimizing night time disruptions
- A sedative or hypnotic can be given, as prescribed by the physician.

Psychological Needs

Delirium

Delirium—is one of the most common complications seen in clients with advanced illness. Characterized by concurrent disturbances of level of consciousness, attention, thinking, perception, memory, psychomotor behavior, emotion and the sleep wake cycle. It is often identified as a sudden and significant decline in previous level functioning and is conceptualized as a reversible process.

Intervention

- Haloperidol may reduce hallucinations and agitations
- Benzodiazepines reduce anxiety
- Treat the underlying cause such as hypoxia, dehydration, hypercalcemia, hyponatremia, sepsis, etc.
- Teach the family how to interact with the client
- Provide safety of the patient
- Spiritual intervention, music therapy, gentle massage and therapeutic touch may provide some relief
- Avoiding harsh lighting or very dim lighting.
- The presence of familiar faces and gentle reorientation and reassurance are also helpful.

Depression

The following symptoms are present: Depressive mood, weight loss or gain, insomnia or hypersomnia, agitation or motor retardation, fatigue or loss of energy, depreciation or guilt feelings and concentration difficulties. Sometimes, it goes unrecognized by clinicians because many of the clinical manifestations of depression, e.g., fatigue, anorexia or weight loss, can be attributed to the disease process itself.

Interventions

- Emotional and spiritual support
- Control of physical distressing symptoms
- Presence of relatives
- Provide space and time for family to experience sadness and to grieve
- Pharmacological intervention with psychostimulants, and tricyclic antidepressants.

Psychosocial Needs

Spiritual Needs

- Spiritual coping strategies enhance self-empowerment
- Assess the desire for spiritual counseling and support
- Obtain information regarding significant religious rituals, beliefs and practices

- Encourage their practice to the maximum extent possible
- Foster the insights.

Need of the Family Members

- Support the expression of feelings
- Encourage the telling of the story using open-ended questions or statements, e.g., tell me about your husband.
- Assist the mourner to find an outlet for his or her feelings by talking, attending a support group or writing letters that will not be mailed.
- Assess emotional affect and reinforce the normalcy of feelings.
- Assess coping skills and social support
- Assess signs of complicated grief and mourning and offer professional referral.

PALLIATIVE CARE

Palliative care means taking care of the whole person: body, mind and spirit and heart and soul. This mode of care looks at dying as something natural and personal. The goal of palliative care is to give patients the best quality of life they can have by the aggressive management of symptoms.

Palliative care, by definition of its derivative is to palliate, is a type of care that focuses on alleviation of a client's symptoms and not to cure.

Principles of Palliative Care

- Palliative care looks after the medical, emotional, social, and spiritual needs of the dying person,
- Palliative care supports the needs of the family members helping them with the responsibilities of care giving and even supporting them as they grieve.
- Palliative care involves a multidisciplinary team to look after the complete needs of the patient.

HOSPICE CARE

Hospice is a coordinated program of interdisciplinary services provided by professional caregivers and trained volunteers to patients with serious illness. In hospice setting, the patient and family together are a unit of care Hospice care can take place

- At home
- At a hospice center
- In a skilled nursing facility

A hospice care team typically includes: doctors. Nurses, home health aides, spiritual counselors, social worker, pharmacists and bereavement counselors.

DEATH

Definition

Death is defined as: "cessation of heart-lung function, or of whole brain function, or of higher brain function. "either irreversible cessation of circulatory and respiratory functions or irreversible cessation of all functions of the entire brain, including the brain stem."

Clinical Death

Clinical death is the medical term for cessation of blood circulation and breathing, the two necessary criteria to sustain life. This is called **cardiopulmonary arrest**, a period when a person's heartbeat and breathing stop, but can still be revived if early medical attention is given.

Biological Death

It occurs four–six minutes after clinical death. This is due to the fact that the heart is the main pumping machine of the body, and without the blood coming from the heart, the brain gradually ceases to function until it achieves irreversible damage.

Immediate Signs of Death

- The respiration becomes labored, irregular, rapid or very slow, noisy breathing (death rattle) sound of secretions moving in the airway.
- There is a weak thready pulse and falling blood pressure
- The heart rate decreases
- As the oxygen supply to the brain decreases, the patient may become restless
- Death rattle: A rattling sound heard in throat caused by secretions as the patient cannot cough longer
- The skin becomes pale and cool, there is peripheral cyanosis, the skin loses its turgor and has mottled appearance
- The extremities are cold to touch
- The sight gradually fails, the pupils fail to react to light, and sunken eyes are present
- Mental confusion arises
- Urinary output may decrease in amount and frequency
- There may be incontinence of urine and distension in bladder because of loss of sphincter control
- Difficulty talking or swallowing.

Changes in Body after Death

- **Rigor mortis:** Body becomes stiff within 4 hours after death as a result of decreased adenosine triphosphate (ATP) production. ATP keeps muscles soft and supple.
- **Algor mortis:** Temperature decreases by a few degrees each hour. The skin loses its elasticity and will tear easily.
- **Livor mortis:** Bluish color of death also known as hypostasis is the discoloration of the skin due to the pooling of blood in the dependent part of body following death.

Postmortem Care

Purposes

- To prepare the body for the morgue /discharge
- To prevent discoloration or deformity of the body.
- To provide death with dignity
- To prepare the body for burial/funeral

General Instructions

The procedure of care of dead must be according to the local policy of the hospital, which in turn is according to the state laws.

In general, nursing responsibilities include equally important duties:

- Immediate notification of the officials
- General consideration for other patients in the ward
- Preparation of the body for transfer to home/ morgue
- The nurse notifies the physician and the ward sister immediately if the patient has ceased breathing.
- It is the function of physician to declare death of the client
- When the death occurs following certain communicable diseases such as smallpox, the body requires special attention to prevent the spread of the disease.
- The personal care after death needs to be carried out within 2–4 hours of the person dying to preserve their appearance, condition and dignity.
- Pack personal property. Discuss the issue of soiled clothes sensitively with the family and ask whether they wish them to be disposed of or returned.
- **Organ donation:** Once brain death has been confirmed, the patient will remain connected to the ventilator while members of the medical team speak with the person's family about donation. If the family supports. The person will remain connected to the ventilator during this time

to keep blood and oxygen circulating to the organs, If it becomes clear that organs are no longer suitable for donation, donation of eye, heart, bone and skin tissues may still be possible.

- **The medicolegal case:** If death is caused by accident, suicide, homicide, etc. it should be brought to the notice of legal authorities and the body should not be handed over to the relatives without the permission of the legal authorities
- **Autopsy:** It is the examination of the body of a dead person. Autopsies are performed to determine the cause of death, for legal purposes, and for education and

research. If it is to be done, the doctor gets the consent from relatives.

- The concerned authority's signature should be obtained while handing over the body in the death proforma.
- The personal protective equipment should be worn while handling the body
- The waste management protocol must be followed
- Disinfection of the patient's room and the articles and equipment used should be done
- Sometimes the family members would want to be involved in the care that has to be dealt as per the institutional policy.

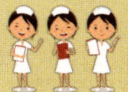

SKILL: POSTMORTEM CARE

Equipment Required

Articles	Rationale
Gloves, masks	To follow universal precautions
Bath basin	To take water for bath
Small bowl	To keep the sponge cloth
Soap with soap dish	To apply soap to the body
Face towels -2	One to apply soap and other to clean
Bath towel or sheet	To dry the skin
Nail filer, nail cutter	To smoothen and cut the nails
Comb and oil	To attend the hair
Laundry bag	To discard waste water
Gauze Pieces	To clean mouth
Mouth wash/potassium permanganate solution	To clean mouth
Bucket	To keep water
Cotton swabs	To clean the eyes
Cotton plugs	To plug the orifices
Bandages	To cover the eyes, if required, to tie the body
Cotton pads	To absorb the discharge
Large diaper	To prevent the soiling of clothes
Patients Clothes	To clothe the body
Blue, black and yellow bags	To segregate the waste
Identification tags	To put ID on the body
Ether	To remove the adhesive markings
Sheets/shroud	To cover and pack the body
Needle and thread	To tie the sheet
Syringe and scissors	To remove and cut the tubings, and remove air or water from endotracheal tube or Foleys catheter
Dressing pack, extra bandages	To clean the wound, if any

Contd...

Articles	Rationale
Plastic sheet, if required	To transport the body If the patient had infectious disease
Kidney tray and paper bag	To receive the waste
Stretcher	To transport the body

Review and carry out the standard steps as given in Appendix

Action/steps	Rationale
Assessment	
1. Verify the patients identification	Ensures that the patient is properly identified
2. Determine if the family wishes to assist with bathing or caring for the body, or if they wish to view the deceased after the nurse prepares the body	Involvement of family in care helps them to care for their loved one
3. Determine whether an autopsy will be done. Check for signed autopsy consent	Drainage or other tubes are not removed, if an autopsy is planned
Planning	
4. Collect equipment and prepare the working space by raising the bed to proper height	Promotes work efficiency and prevents back strain.
5. Maintain privacy by closing the door or drawing curtains	Protects privacy and dignity
Implementation	
6. Wash your hands and don gloves	Protects you from contact with body fluids
7. Position the patient in supine position with small pillow under head	Raising the head prevents pooling of blood, which might discolor the face
8. Replace the dentures if they are out of the mouth. Close the mouth. A small-rolled towel may be placed under the chin, if needed to keep the mouth closed.	Closing the eyes and mouth protects the eyes, keeps the face in the most natural position during rigor mortis that occurs after death
9. Remove all the valuables and hand over to the attendant according to agency policy	Return the personal property to the family.
10. Wash all areas of the body soiled with blood, feces, urine or drainage, place protective pads under rectum and between the legs to protect from drainage from rectum, vagina and urethra. Plug all body orifices such as ears, nose, mouth with cotton plugs.	After death, sphincter muscles relax, allowing leakage of stool, urine, or body fluid.
11. Comb the hair and arrange neatly	Combing the hair improves the appearance of the body
12. Remove all tubes (IVs, catheters, nasogastric) unless autopsy is planned	Properly deflating balloons before tube removal prevents tissue damage
13. Change any soiled dressings and remove adhesive marks with appropriate solvent	This improves appearance of the body
14. Dress the body in a clean gown/clothes, before the body is wrapped and ask family members to view the body.	Dressing the body preserves dignity.
15. After the family leaves, attach identifying tags usually on the big toe or ankle and the wrist.	Proper identification assures that the body will be transported to the right mortuary.
16. Place padded ties around the ankles; criss-cross the wrist over the abdomen and secure. You may place a gauze tie or chin strap under the jaw to keep the mouth closed.	Ankles and wrist are secured to prevent the arms and legs being hurt during transport.

Contd...

Action/steps	Rationale
17. Place the body on the shroud and check for placement of drainage pads. Fold the shroud according to agency procedure using the numerical order indicated (Fig. 1). Secure the shroud at the chest wrist and knees, and place in identification tag on the outside. 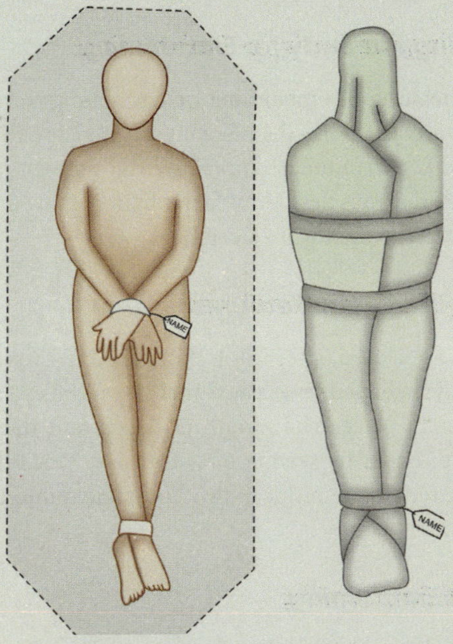	The shroud covers the body and prevents unnecessary exposure. The ID tag assures correct disposal of the body.

Fig. 1: Securing the should around the body

Action/steps	Rationale
18. Transfer the body to the structures or morgue cart. Secure the body properly and remove gloves and wash hands.	Transport to the morgue is done quickly, as it may be upsetting to other patients or visitors.
Evaluation	
19. Ask yourself, whether the procedure is carried out in respectful way? Was the family supported and did the diseased appear clean, peaceful and well cared for?	Determines if expected outcomes have been met.
Documentation	
20. Note the care provided in the chart and the time when the doctor pronounced death. Family assisted in washing and preparing the body for transport to morgue at time. Tags are attached to right toe, right ankle and outside of shroud	Documentation is a legal proof of nursing care provided

Note: If the patient died of a communicable disease the body may require special handling to prevent spread of disease. Requirements for such handing are usually specified in local laws and are contingent on the disease causing organisms, mode of transmission and other characteristics.

Caring for Other Patients

Other patients become aware of a death particularly, who have shared a room with dying patient. They may have grief reactions and should be supported by the nurse. Death of a patient may cause depression in other patients, so nurse needs to take care of these reactions.

AUTOPSY

Autopsy is defined as the medical procedure that consists of a thorough examination of a corpse to determine the cause and manner of death and to evaluate any disease or injury that may be present. It is an examination of the organs and tissues of a human body after death. Autopsy is usually performed by pathologist.

Purposes of Autopsy

Autopsy is done mainly for two reasons:
1. Legal purpose
2. Medical purpose

Legal Purpose

Under this, forensic autopsy is done. Forensic autopsy is done in case the deceased is having the clinical background.

Medical Purpose

It includes academic autopsy. It is done to find out the unknown cause of death.

Types of Autopsy

Internal Autopsy

In this, the dead body is dissected and the internal organs are examined. For this, consent form from next to kin or spouse is taken. It is commonly the physician's responsibility to obtain consent for autopsy. The nurse can assist by explaining reasons for autopsy. It is only done if it is required by law.

External Autopsy

This does not require any consent. This is the external examination of dead body.

Procedure

The body which is to undergo autopsy is first received in body bag. The body is then photographed from all angles to look for any external injury. After this, ultraviolet search is done to look for any minute abrasions, hairs, nails, etc. After this, radiography of the body is done to rule out any bone fracture. Then any external wound, if present, is examined. After that, the body is dissected. The actual part of internal dissection depends upon the cause of death. For example, if the cause of death is strangulation, then the neck is left intact and the dissection is done in V-shape down the neck.

After autopsy all the internal organs are replaced before handing over the body to the relatives.

EMBALMING

Embalming is the art and science of preserving human remains by treating them with chemicals to forestall decomposition. The intention is to keep them suitable for public display at a funeral, for religious reasons, or for medical and scientific purposes such as their use as "anatomical specimens".

Embalming Process

The first step in the embalming process is *surgical,* in which bodily fluids are removed and are replaced with formaldehyde-based chemical solutions. The second step is *cosmetic,* in which the body is prepared for viewing by styling the hair, applying make-up, and setting the facial features.

Preparing the Body for Embalming

Before the surgical embalming or cosmetic processes begin, the body is washed in a disinfectant solution and the limbs are massaged and manipulated to relieve rigor mortis (stiffness of the joints and muscles). Any facial hair is shaved off, unless the person who died wore facial hair.

Setting the Facial Features

The eyes are closed, after using skin glue and or plastic flesh-colored oval-shaped "eyes caps" that sit on the eye and secure the eyelid in place. The mouth is closed and the lower jaw is secured, either by sewing or with wires. Once the jaw has been secured, the mouth can be manipulated into the desired arrangement.

Arterial Embalming

For arterial embalming, the blood is removed from the body via the veins and replaced with an embalming solution via the arteries. The embalming solution is usually a combination of formaldehyde, glutaraldehyde, methanol, ethanol, phenol, and water, and may also contain dyes in order to stimulate a life-like skin tone.

Cavity Embalming

For cavity embalming, a small incision is made near the belly button and a sharp surgical instrument used for drainage, called a trocar, is inserted into the body cavity. Using the trocar, organs in the chest cavity and abdomen are punctured and drained of gas and fluid contents and then replaced with formaldehyde-based chemical mixture. The incision is closed and at this point the body is fully embalmed.

BIBLIOGRAPHY

1. *Bolander VB. Sorensen and Luckmann's Basic Nursing: A Psychological Approach. WB Saunders Company, Philadelphia, Pennsylvania; 1994. pp: 867-68.*

2. *Potter PA, Perry AG. Fundamentals of Nursing, 6th edition. Mosby Inc; 2008. pp. 1097-98.*

3. *Taylor C, Lillis C, LeMone P, Lynn P. Fundamentals of Nursing, 6th edition. Lippincott Williams and Wilkins. Philadelphia: 2008.*

4. *Taylor CR, Lillis C, LeMone P, et al. Fundamentals of Nursing – The Art and Science of Nursing Care, 5th edition. Lippincott Williams & Wilkins; 2004. pp. 1396-98.*

5. *Berman AT, Snyder S, Kozier BJ, et al. Kozier & Erb's. Fundamentals of Nursing: Concepts, Process and Practice, 8th edition. Pearson Education. pp. 982-1000.*

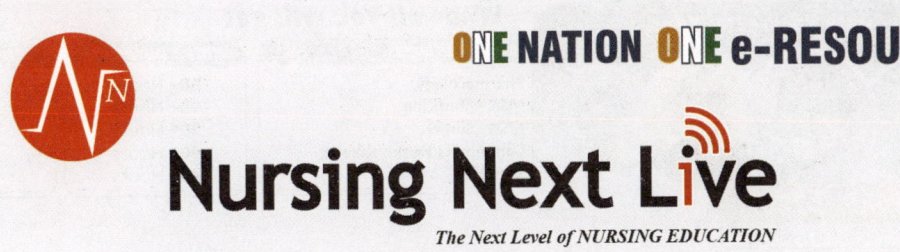
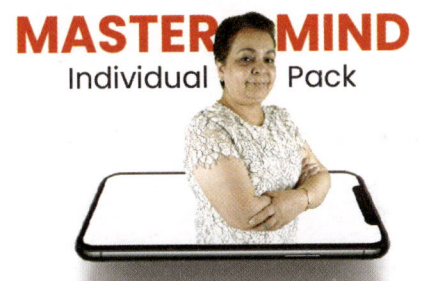
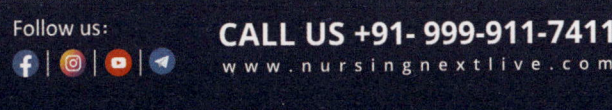

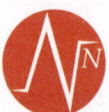
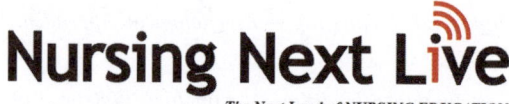
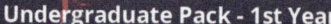
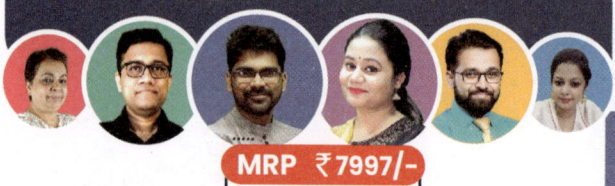
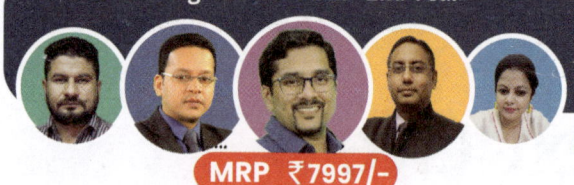
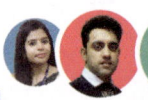 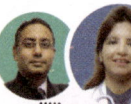

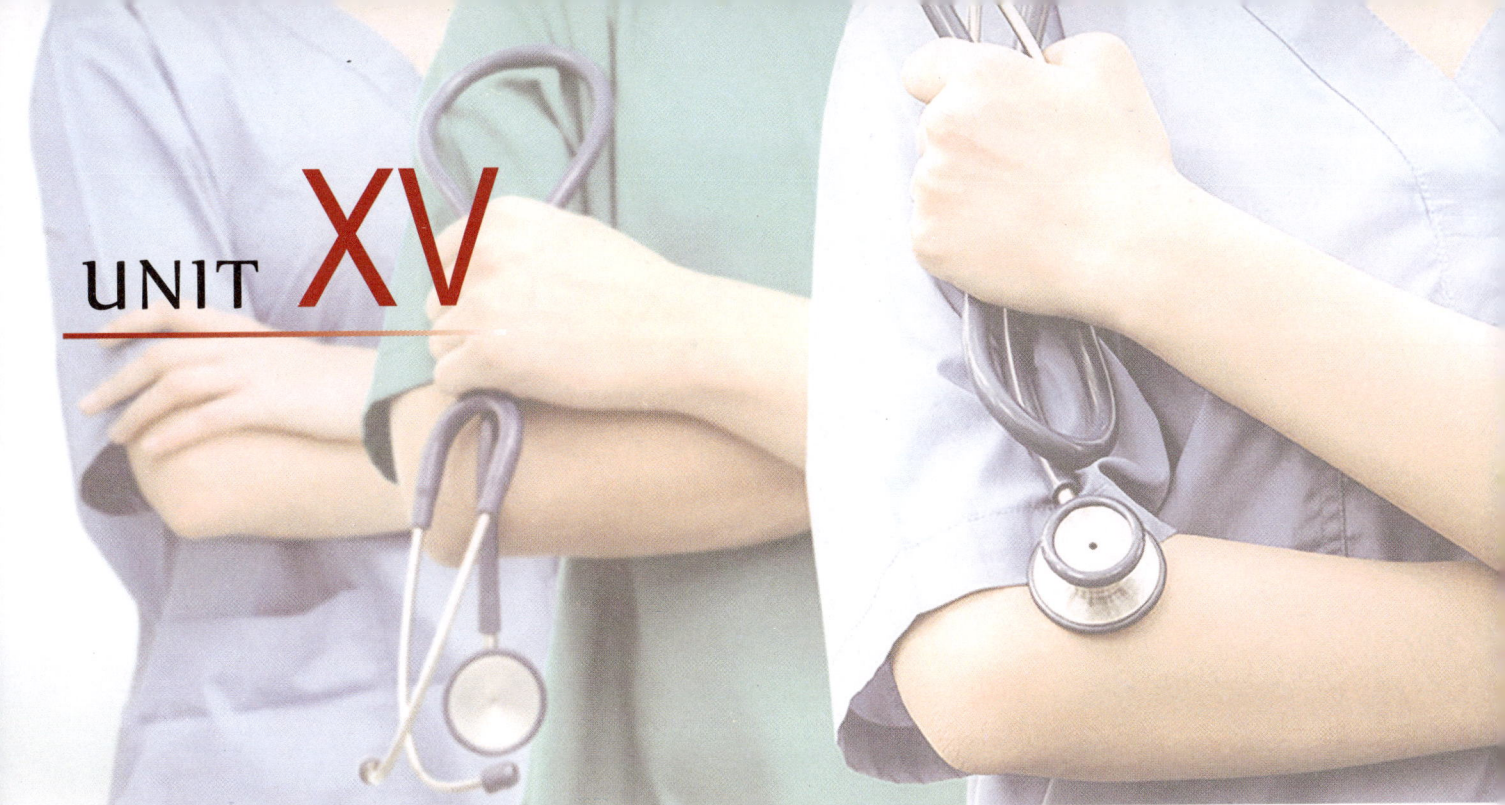

UNIT XV

FIRST AID NURSING

Unit Outline

Chapter 64 First Aid Nursing

First Aid Nursing

Learning Objectives

After completing this chapter, you will be able to:

- Identify the qualities of first aider
- Provide first aid in selected conditions given in the text

Key Terms

- Crepitus
- Ecchymosis
- Asphyxia
- Choking
- Precordial thump
- External cardiac compression
- Epistaxis
- Shock
- Poisoning

Chapter Outline

- Definition
- Objectives of First Aid
- Essential Qualities of a First Aider
- Principles of First Aid
- Fracture
- Heat Exhaustion
- Asphyxia
- Cardiopulmonary Resuscitation
- Bees and Wasp Bites
- Poisoning

An emergency is the unforeseen event which calls for prompt and quick action to save the life of a person or to prevent from further damage. At any moment, you or someone around you could experience an injury or illness. Using basic first aid, you may be able to stop a minor mishap from getting worse. In case of a serious medical emergency, you may even save a life.

DEFINITION

First aid is an immediate temporary assistance given to a person who is injured or suddenly becomes ill, using facilities or materials available at that time before regular medical help is imparted. First aid includes assessing the victim for life threatening condition, performing appropriate interventions to sustain life and keeping the person in the best possible physical and mental conditions until she/he can enter the emergency or casualty unit in the hospital

OBJECTIVES OF FIRST AID

The objectives of first aid are:

- To preserve life.
- To prevent further injury and deterioration of the condition.
- To prevent complications related to injury or illness or conditions.
- To make the victim as comfortable as possible to conserve the strength.
- To put the injured person under professional medical care at the earliest.

ESSENTIAL QUALITIES OF A FIRST AIDER

The following are the qualities, which a trained first aider, should possess:

- **Prompt and quick:** As soon as an accident or injury. takes place, the first aider should be prompt and quick, to render help to the victim, without delay.
- **Calm and controlled:** He should be a calm and controlled sort of person because he has to take immediate action, without any fuss or panic.
- **Wise and intelligent:** He should be intelligent and wise enough to decide the immediate treatment even before a complete diagnosis, especially in case of serious injuries and severe bleeding.
- **Resourceful:** He should be resourceful enough to make available his first aid material at once or get the required things on the spot, for giving immediate relief to the victim.
- **Sweet tempered and sympathetic:** The first aider should use sweet and encouraging words to lessen the victim's distress. He should keep the victim as comfortable as possible and should be able to allay the victim's fears with sympathy.
- **Skillful and tactful:** The first aider should be skillful and tactful to judge the symptom and history of the case without wasting any time. If need be, he should be able to master requisite support from the crowd.
- **Dexterous and clever:** Should be able to help the injured without causing and/or aggravating pain, and to use the appliances and/or procedure efficiently and effectively
- **Confidence and perseverance:** The first aider should have full faith in his skill to administer whatever assistance the situation demands, even if there is no response initially. He should have perseverance and should not give up. It may take time for the patient to respond to his handling.

Remember, an efficient and resourceful first aider maybe the link between the life and death.

PRINCIPLES OF FIRST AID

When any person comes across another seriously injured person, he should follow the following principles:

- Make sure that victim's airway is not blocked by the tongue, secretions or some foreign body–restore respiration.
- Make sure that the person is breathing. If not, administer artificial respiration–restore respiration.
- Make sure that the patient has a pulse, if no pulse is felt, administer cardiopulmonary resuscitation (CPR)–for restoration of circulation.
- Check for bleeding–take measures to control bleeding.

- Act fast if the victim is bleeding severely or if he has swallowed poison or if the heart or breathing has stopped, every second counts for his survival.
- Arrange without delay for shifting of the victim to hospital for medical attention, although most injured persons can be safely moved. It is very important, not to move a person with serious neck and/or back injuries unless taking proper measure to ensure him from further complications.
- Keep the victim/patient quiet and make him lie down. Turn the victim on his side to prevent choking if there is no danger about neck injury. Keep him warm with blanket.
- Have someone call for medical assistance while applying first aid. The persons who summons help should explain the nature of the emergency and ask what should be done if the arrival of ambulance is pending.
- Examining the victim gently, cut clothing of necessary length.
- Reassure the victim, try to remain calm yourself. Your calmness can allay the victim's fear and panic.
- Do not give fluids to an unconscious or semiconscious victim.
- Do not try to arouse an unconscious persons by slapping or shaking.
- Do not allow crowd to gather near the victim so that fresh air is allowed.
- Look for an emergency identification card for medical information related to victim.

Equipment for First AID—First Aid Kit

- Wound cleaner/antiseptic (100 mL)
- Swabs for cleaning wounds
- Cotton wool for padding
- Sterile gauze (minimum quantity 10)
- 1 pair of forceps (for splinters)
- 1 pair of scissors
- 1 set of safety pins
- 4 triangular bandages
- 4 roller bandages (75 mm)
- 4 roller bandages (100 mm)
- Crepe bandage
- 1 roll of elastic adhesive (25 mm × 3 m)
- 1 roll of non-allergenic adhesive strip (25 mm × 3 m)
- 1 packet of adhesive dressing strips (10)
- 4 first aid dressing (75 m × 100 mm)
- 4 first aid dressing (150 mm × 200 mm)
- 2 straight splints
- 2 pairs large and 2 pairs medium sized disposable latex gloves
- 2 CPR mouth pieces or similar devices
- Thermometer

- Bulb syringe
- Sterile eye dressings (at least 2 sterile dressings)

FRACTURE

Types of Fractures

- **Simple or closed fracture:** This is simply, a clean break or crack in a bone. The broken ends of the bone do no cut open the skin nor are visible outside.
- **Compound or open fracture:** This is accompanied by a wound, the skin is broken and the bone may be exposed to contamination from the skin surface.
- **Comminuted fracture:** The bone is broken into several small pieces, which surrounds the main break.
- **Impacted fracture:** Broken ends of the bone are driven or forcibly embedded into one another.
- **Depressed fracture:** Broken parts of the bone are driven inward, e.g., in cases of fracture of skull.
- **Greenstick fracture:** Bone is partially broken or bent, common in children due to incomplete calcification of bone.
- **Pathological fracture:** The pathological changes or carcinoma of the bone make the bone weak and brittle; it breaks spontaneously without or with little force common in old age.
- **Complicated fracture:** Along with the fracture there is associated injury to some internal structure like brain, spinal cord, liver, lungs, spleen, kidney, etc. (Fig. 1).

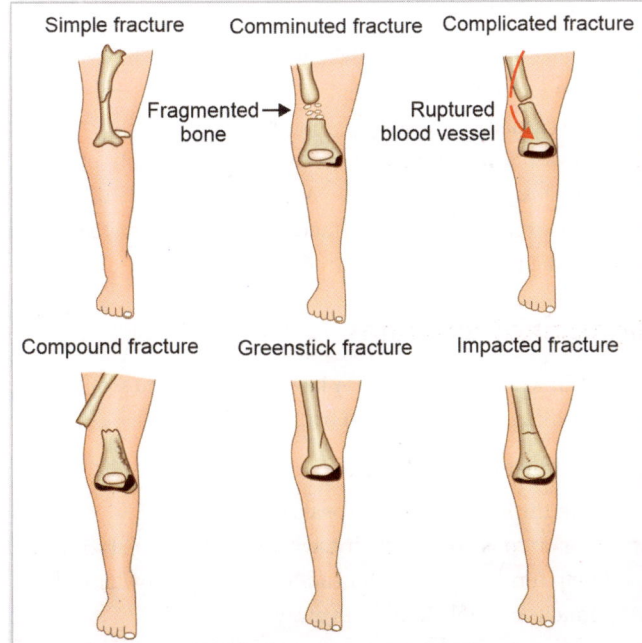

Fig. 1: Types of fractures

Signs and Symptoms of Fractures

- Pain and tenderness at the point of a fracture especially on movement.
- Deformity of the part: alteration in its shape, length.
- Irregularity of the bone often felt by passing of the hand over the skin, specially when it is near the skin.
- Limitation of loss of power or function of the part and unnatural mobility.
- **Crepitus:** A crackling sound is heard or a sensation of grating is felt when the ends of broken bone are moved against each other.
- **Ecchymosis:** Occurs when blood leaks from a broken capillary into surrounding tissue under the skin measuring 1 cm.

However, the presence of these signs vary with the site of fracture and the bone broken e.g., pain may be absent in simple fracture of small bones. Toes can be moved in case of fracture of tibia and fingers in case of Colle's fracture. Fracture of bones like fibula will hardly impair function of the leg if it is broken.

First Aid Measures for the Fractures

When bones are broken, a good rule to follow is "Do not permit motion of the broken ends or of the joints near the injury. This prevents pain and further damage".

- For closed or simple fracture, place the limb in as natural position as possible without causing discomfort to the victim. Handle very gently; avoid all unnecessary movements of the injured part.
- Since the danger of infection is very great in compound or open fractures, it is always better to get help from a doctor. In caring for the injury, clean the wound and apply dressing.
- If there is an excessive bleeding from open fracture, apply pressure dressing to control it. Transfer the patient to hospital.
- Never try to reduce the fracture, i.e., bringing bones to normal position (alignment).
- Before trying to move or carry a person with a broken bone, immobilize the broken ends with splints.
- Send the patient for medical aid as soon as possible.

Immobilization of the Fractured Part

The important thing to remember is immobilize the fracture site and the joints or both sides of fracture. This can be done by using bandages and using splints. The uninjured limb or body of the patient is used as splint. In case of upper limb fractures, the body is used as a splint; while in lower limb fractures, the other uninjured limb is used as a splint keeping the injured part steady and avoiding all unnecessary movements, bandaging should be done with broad bandages, towels or a big size cloth. Never apply bandage over the area of fracture. Apply knots on the sound side.

Splints must be long enough to extend beyond the joints above and below the fracture site. Wide splints are always better than narrow ones. Any firm material can be used—board, pole, metal rod, walking stick, a book or an umbrella or even thick magazines or thick folded newspaper. Use clothing or other soft material to pad splints to prevent skin injury. Fasten splints with bandages or cloth at maximum three sites: below joint below break, above joint above break and the level of break. The bandaging should be firm but not too tight to stop the circulation of blood in the area. Always place padding material like cotton, socks, handkerchief or small towel between the natural hollows like ankles and knees, if a splint is to be tied over them. After the fracture ends have been stabilized, do not waste time and arrange for quick transportation to a nearby hospital or doctor.

Slings are used for:

- Supporting an injured arm or wrist.
- Immobilizing fractures.
- Elevating to control external bleeding.

How to Apply an Upper Arm Sling

This sling is used for injuries to the upper arm, including the collarbone, shoulder or ribs.

- Position the arm across the body with the hand near the opposite shoulder.
- Place the triangular bandage under the arm with the apex at the elbow.
- Fold the lower half of the bandage over the arm.
- Twist the bandage firmly at the elbow and bring the twisted bandage around the back.
- Twist the bandage around the hand and over the uninjured shoulder and tie the ends together using a reef knot on opposite side of the injury and place a pad under the knot.
- Check the bandaged arm for circulation.

How to Apply a Lower Arm Sling

- This sling is used for injuries to the lower arm, including the wrist and hand.
- Place the arm across the chest and slightly raised.
- Place the triangular bandage between the arm and the body with the apex pointing towards the injured elbow.
- Bring the lower half of the bandage up and over the injured arm.
- Tie the ends together with a reef knot on the uninjured side and place a pad under the knot.
- Tie the tape or pin at the elbow.

- Check the injured arm for circulation.
- Ensure the arm is not sloping downwards as this will increase swelling and pressure.

How to Apply a Collar and Cuff Sling

This sling can be used for dislocated shoulder, fractured ribs, or a fracture of the upper arm.

- Make a clove hitch using a narrow fold bandage.
- Put the loops over the wrist of the injured arm.
- Gently elevate the injured arm against the casualty's chest.
- Tie the bandage ends together around the neck on the uninjured side, using a reef knot, place a pad under the knot.
- For extra support apply a broad bandage below the fracture site over the arm and around the body.

How to Fold a Triangular Bandage

Triangular bandages are used for slings, pads or bandaging:

- Fold the triangular bandage in half, and this makes a broad fold bandage.
- Fold the triangular bandage in half again and this is called a narrow fold bandage.

Facial Fractures

Common injuries to the face include a broken nose, cheekbone or jaw. The main danger is obstruction of the airway, either by swollen, displaced or lacerated tissue, by loose teeth or by blood and saliva. There may be damage to brain, skull or neck. There may be bleeding from the nose or mouth.

- **Cheekbone and nose fractures:** This may block the air passage in the nose. Apply a cold compress and transfer the casualty to hospital.
- **Lower jaw fractures:** Are usually the result of direct force, such as heavy blow. A blow on one side of the jaw can sometimes cause a fracture on the other side. A fall on the point of chin can fracture both sides.

Signs and Symptoms

- Pain which is increased by jaw movement and swallowing.
- Swelling, tenderness and bruising of mouth.

First aid measures to be taken:

- Ask the casualty not to speak.
- For a conscious casualty, who is not seriously injured, help him to sit up with head forward, to allow any blood, mucus and saliva to drain away.
- If the casualty vomits, support his jaw and head and gently clean his mouth.

- Ask the casualty to hold a soft pad firmly in place to support the jaw.
- If the patient is conscious, transfer to hospital with his face leaning forward and downward in sitting position. If the patient is unconscious, send the patient to hospital on a stretcher with the face place downwards.

Collar Bone Fracture

The two collar bones (clavicles) can be broken by indirect force such as fall on to the outstretched hand or impact at the shoulder.

Signs and Symptoms

- Pain and tenderness at the site of injury increased by movement.
- Casualty may support the arm at the elbow, and incline the head to the injured side.

First aid measures to be taken:

- Make the casualty sit down and place the arm on his injured side across his chest.
- Support the arm in an elevation sling.
- Secure the arm to his chest with the broad fold bandage over the sling.
- Send casualty to hospital in sitting position.

Upper Arm Fracture

The upper arm bone (Humerus) maybe fractured across its shaft by the direct blow, common among elderly. The casualty may walk around for sometime with this fracture and without seeking medical advice, because it is a stable injury.

Signs and Symptoms

- Pain which is increased by movement.
- Tenderness over the fracture site.
- Rapid swelling and bruising which develop slowly.

First aid measures to be taken:

- Make the casualty sit.
- Gently place the injured arm across his chest in the position that is most comfortable.
- Support the arm in arm sling, and secure the limb to his chest by placing soft padding between the arm and chest and tie a broad fold bandage around the chest over the sling.
- Transport the casualty to hospital in sitting position (Fig. 2A).

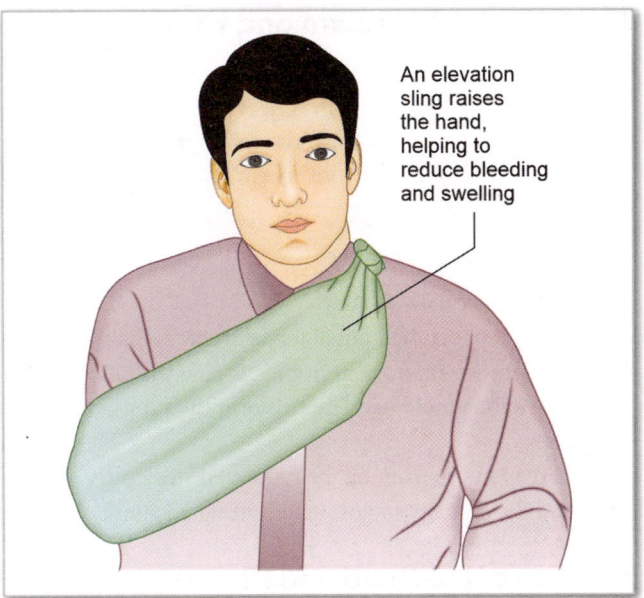

An elevation sling raises the hand, helping to reduce bleeding and swelling

Fig. 2A: First aid for fracture elbow

Elbow Fracture

Fracture at the elbow joint are common by a fall on to hand. A fracture to the hand of the radius is characterized by a stiff elbow that cannot be fully straightened.

Signs and Symptoms

- Pain increases by movement.
- Tenderness over the fracture site.
- Possible swelling and bruising.
- In case of stiff elbow which could be due to fracture of head of radius.

Initiate following measures for the elbow that cannot be bent:

- Lay the casualty down, and place the injured limb on the trunk.
- Do not attempt to forcibly bend or straighten elbow.
- Insert soft padding between the inured limb and the trunk.
- Do not attempt to forcibly bend or straighten elbow.
- Insert soft padding between the injured limb and the trunk.
- Bandage the injured limb to the trunk, first at the wrist and then above and below the elbow.
- Check the pulse at the wrist every 10 minutes.
- Treat as for the fracture of upper arm.
- Transfer the casualty to hospital.

Fracture of the Forearm and Wrist

The bones of the forearm (the radius and ulna) may be fractured across their shafts by a heavy blow. They are often associated with a wound. The most common fracture around the wrist is a Colle's fracture, occurs while falling on an outstretched hand.

First aid measures to be taken:

- Make the casualty sit down.
- Gently support the injured forearm across his chest.
- Support the arm in an arm sling. Secure the limb to chest using a broad fold bandage tied over the sling close to the elbow.
- Tie the knot in front on the uninjured side.
- Send the casualty to hospital in sitting position.

Fracture of the Hand and Fingers

The hand is made up of many small bones with movable joints, and any of which may be injured by direct or indirect force.

Multiple fractures affecting all of the hand are usually censed by crush injury, and there may be severe bleeding and swelling. The most common injury is the fracture of the knuckle between the little finger and the hand.

Dislocations and sprains may affect any of the fingers. The thumb is particularly prone to dislocation caused by a fall on to the hand.

First aid measures to be taken:

- Protect the injured hand by surrounding it in folds of soft padding.
- Gently support the affected arm in an elevation sling.
- If necessary secure the arm to the chest by applying a broad fold bandage over the sling.
- Tie the knot in front on the uninjured side.
- Send the casualty to hospital in sitting position.

Fracture of the Rib Cage

Rib fractures may be caused by direct force by a blow, fall on to chest or by indirect force produced by crush injury. If the fracture is complicated by a penetrating wound or a "flail chest" injury, breathing may be impaired.

Flail Chest Injuries

If multiple rib fractures isolate a portion of the chest wall, the portion will move out when casualty breathes in and the portion will move out when the person breathes out. This is opposite of the normal chest movement. This state of "Paradoxical breathing" produces severe respiratory difficulties.

Signs and Symptoms

- Sharp pain at the site of fracture.
- Pain on taking a deep breathe in order to reduce pain casualty may be having shallow breathing.
- Paradoxical breathing.
- An open wound over the fracture through which you might hear air being sucked into the chest cavity.

First Aid Measures

- In case of fractured rib, support the limb on the injured side in an arm sling and send casualty to the hospital.
- In case of open or multiple fractures, immediately cover and seal any wound on the chest wall.
- Have the casualty in a half–sitting position, with head and shoulders leaned and body inclined towards the injured side.
- Support the limb or the injured side in an elevation sling (Fig. 2B).
- Call for medical aid.
- If the casualty becomes unconscious or breathing becomes difficult, place him in the recovery position, uninjured side uppermost.

Fracture of Backbone/Spine

Injuries to the back include fractures of the bones of the spine, a displaced intervertebral disc, muscle strains and ligament sprains. The main danger with any back injury is the injury to spinal cord or nerves.

The spine is made up of a column of small bones, called vertebra. The spine supports the trunk and head, surrounds the spinal cord and protect it. The spinal column is supported

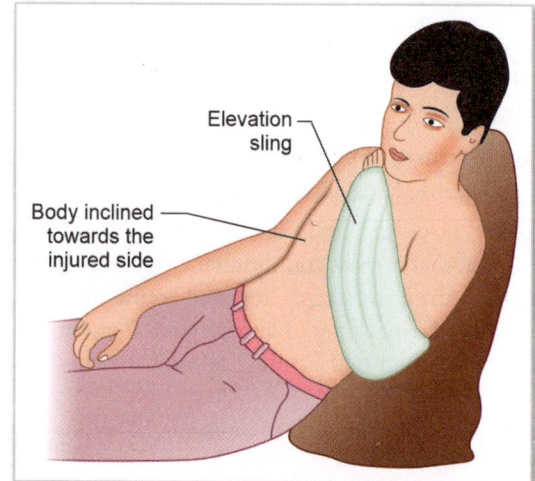

Elevation sling

Body inclined towards the injured side

Fig. 2B: Fracture rib cage

by many strong ligaments and the muscles of the trunk. The spinal cord is delicate and if damaged, loss of power or sensation can occur in parts of the body below the injured area, temporary damage can be caused if cord or peripheral nerves are pinched by displaced disc or bone fragments, permanent damage, will result if the cord is partially or completely severed. Fractures of the vertebrae can be caused by both direct and indirect force. The most vulnerable parts of the spine are the bones in the neck and in the lower back. Always, suspect spinal injury if the casualty complains of any disturbance of feeling or movement. The history of the injury is most important indicator.

Causes of Spinal Injury

* Falling from a height.
* Falling awkwardly while doing gymnastics.
* Diving into a shallow pool.
* Being thrown from a horse or from a motor bike.
* Sudden deceleration in a motor vehicle (a head on crash).
* A heavy object falling across the back.
* Injury to the head or face.

Signs and Symptoms in Spinal Injury

* **When only the spinal column is damaged:**
  * Pain in the neck or back at the level of injury.
  * Falling awkwardly while doing gymnastics.
  * Diving into a shallow pool.
  * Being thrown from a horse or from a motor bike.
  * Sudden deceleration in a motor vehicle (a head on crash).
  * A heavy object falling across the back.
  * Injury to the head or face.
* **When the spinal cord has also been damaged:**
  * Loss of control over limbs. Movement may be weak or absent.
  * Loss of sensation.
  * Abnormal sensations—burning or tingling.
  * The limbs may feel stiff, heavy, or clumsy.
  * Difficulty in breathing.

First Aid Measures (For Conscious Victim)

* Do not move the casualty from the position found unless there is danger.
* Reassure the casualty and tell not to move.
* Support the head in the neutral position by placing your hands over the ears.
* If neck injury is suspected, get helper to place rolled blankets/sheets ground the casualty's neck and shoulder.
* Remove the casualty in ambulance but continue to hold the head and neck till the collar is applied.

For Unconscious Victim

* Check breathing pulse and place the casualty in recovery position.
* Clear the airway by tilting the head and chin lift gently so that the head and neck remain in neutral position.
* Check breathing and pulse again if not present give artificial ventilation with chest compression till help arrives.
* If you have to turn the casualty on to her back to resuscitate, you should keep head, trunk and toes in a straight line, while you maintain support at the neck, ask helpers, (usually five) to gently straighten the casualty's limbs, and 'log roll' her over.
* Steady and support the casualty's head by placing your hands over his ears. Be prepared to maintain this support throughout, until help arrives.
* Ask your helper to straighten the casualty's legs and bring the arm nearest to him, elbow bent, palm uppermost, at right angles of the body.
* Your helper grasps the casualty's thigh, drawing up the knee; then bringing the other arm of casualty across the chart, grasps the far shoulder.
* As he pulls the casualty towards him, you control the neutral position of the head and neck.
* Do not pull the neck.
* Once the casualty is fully turned on to his side both you and, if possible, your helper should support the casualty in this position till help arrives.
* If injury is to the neck, a collar may be applied for further support.

Fracture of Pelvis

Injuries to the pelvis are usually caused by crushing, or by indirect force, such as might occur in a car crash. The impact of car dashboard on a knee can force the head of thigh bone through the hip socket. Pelvic injuries may be complicated by injury to internal tissues and organs, particularly the bladder and urinary passages, which the pelvis protects.

Signs and Symptoms

* Inability to walk or even stand.
* Pain and tenderness in the region of the hip, groin or back, increased when the casualty moves.
* Blood at the urinary orifice, especially in males. The casualty may not be able to pass urine.
* Signs of internal bleeding and shock.

First Aid Measures

* Help the casualty to lie on her back with her legs straight or if it is more comfortable, bend knees slightly and support them.

- Immobilize the legs by bandaging together; placing padding between bony points.
- Dial for ambulance, Treat the casualty for shock.
- Do not bandage the legs together, if this causes intolerable pain.

Fracture of Hip and Thigh

Fractures of the neck of the thigh bone (femur) at the hip joint are common in the elderly and more frequent in women, whose bones become more porous and brittle as they age. This can be a stable injury, the casualty may be able to walk around for some time before the fracture is discovered. The hip may also, more rarely, be dislocated.

It takes considerable force (such as on road accidents, or falls from heights) to fracture the shaft of the thigh bone. This is a serious injury because in most cases a large volume of blood is lost from the tissues. This may cause shock to develop.

Signs and Symptoms

- Pain at the site of the injury.
- Inability to walk.
- Signs of shock.
- Shortening of the thigh, a powerful muscle pull broken bone ends together.
- A turning outwards of the knee and foot.

First Aid Measures

- Lay the casualty down. Ask a helper to steady and support the limb by holding it above and below the injury.
- Gently straighten the lower leg and apply traction at the ankle, pulling steadily in the line of the limb.

- Call for an ambulance. If the ambulance arrives quickly, support the leg with your hands, until it arrives.
- Keep casualty warm. Treat for shock.
- If the ambulance is delayed, immobilize the limb by splinting it to the uninjured limb.
- Gently bring the casualty's sound limb alongside the injured one.
- Maintaining traction at the ankle, gently slide two bandages under the knees. Ease them into position above and below the fracture by sliding them backwards and forward. Position another bandage at the knees and one at the ankles.
- Insert padding between the thighs, knees and ankles, to prevent displacing the broken bone.
- Tie the bandages around his ankles and knees. Then tie the bandages below and above the fracture site.
- To transport the casualty over a distance, place a wooden leg splint, reaching from the armpit to the foot, against the injured side. Pad between the legs, and between the splint and body. Secure the splint with broad fold bandages, at the chest and pelvis, and then at the legs. Do not bandage directly over the fracture. During transport, keep the foot of the stretcher raised to minimize swelling and shock (Fig. 3).

Fracture of the Knee Joint

The knee is the joint between the thigh bone (femur) and shin bone (Tibia). It is a hinge joint which allows bending, straightening, and in the bent position, slight rotation. The knee joint is supported by strong muscles and ligaments and protected in front by a disc of bone, the knee cap (Patella). Any of these structures may be damaged by direct blows, violent twists and strains.

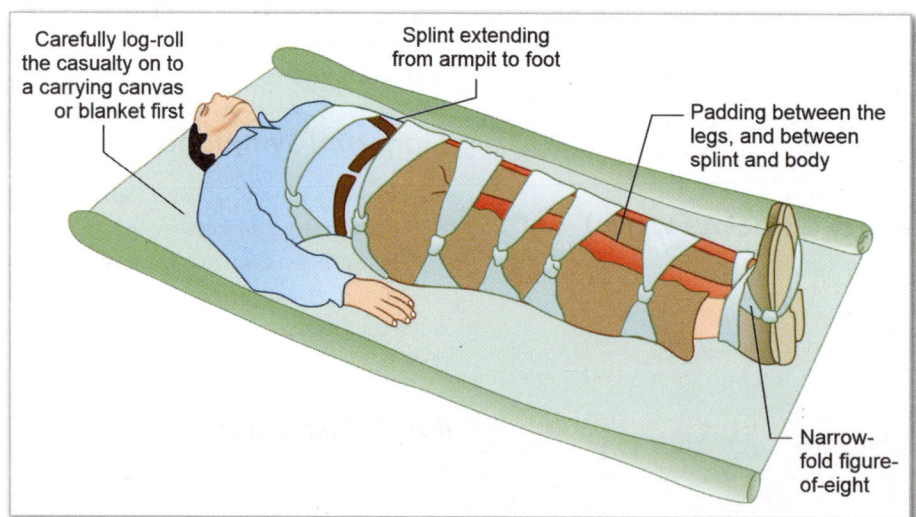

Carefully log-roll the casualty on to a carrying canvas or blanket first

Splint extending from armpit to foot

Padding between the legs, and between splint and body

Narrow-fold figure-of-eight

Fig. 3: Method of transporting the casualty over a distance

Signs and Symptoms

- History of a recent twist or blow to the knees.
- Pain, spreading from the injury to become deep seated in the joint.
- If the bent knee has 'locked, acute pain on attempting to straighten the leg.
- Rapid swelling of the knee joint.

First Aid Measures

- Help the casualty to lie down, supporting her leg and knee in the most comfortable position.
- Wrap soft padding around the joint, and bandage it carefully in place.
- Send the casualty to hospital, transporting as a stretcher case.
- Do not attempt to force the knee straight. Displaced cartilage or internal bleeding may make the joint impossible to straighten safely.
- Do not let the casualty walk.
- Do not give anything to eat or drink to casualty as the anesthetic may be needed.

Fracture of the Lower Leg

The shin bone (Tibia) of the lower leg usually requires a heavy blow to break e.g., from the bumper of a moving vehicle. The thinner splint bone (fibula) can be broken by the type of twisting injury that sprains the ankle. Because the load bearing shin bone remains intact, the casualty may be able to walk, and may be unaware that a fracture has occurred.

Signs and Symptoms

- Localized pain.
- Inability to walk.
- An open wound.

First Aid Measures

- Help the casualty to lie down.
- Straighten the leg using traction, pulling gently in the line of the shin.
- Call an ambulance, till then support the leg with your hands until it arrives.
- If there is delay in arrival of ambulance, splint the injured limb to the unaffected limb.
- Gently bring the unaffected limb alongside the injured one.
- Maintaining support at the ankle, gently slide bandages under the knees and ankles, one above and one below the fracture and at knees and ankles.
- Insert padding between the knees ankles and between the calves.

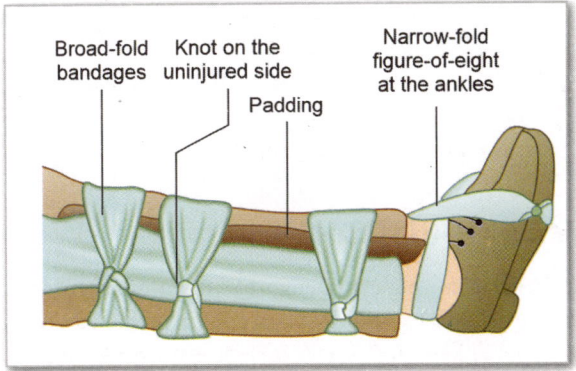

Fig. 4: First aid in fracture of the lower leg

- Tie the bandages around the ankles and knees, then above and below the fracture.
- Bandage firmly and avoid jerky move mats (Fig. 4).

First Aid Measures in Extremes of Heat

Individuals with certain health problems are at high risk such as cardiovascular disease, obesity, diabetes mellitus, malnutrition, alcoholism are more vulnerable to heat related problems. Farmers, athletes, infants and elderly are also at high risk.

There are three heat related problems which includes heat stroke, heat exhaustion and heat cramp.

Heat Stroke/Sun Stroke

Both these conditions are similar and can prove dangerous. Sunstroke is caused by too high temperature in atmosphere by the sun rays. While heat stroke may be caused by high temperatures in factories, furnaces, or high fever. In both conditions, the heat regulating mechanism of the body fails and body rapidly becomes dangerously overheated.

Signs and Symptoms

- Headache, dizziness and discomfort.
- Restlessness and confusion.
- Hot, flushed dry skin.
- Slow and rapid pulse.
- Rapid unconsciousness.
- The body temperature rises up to 104°F or more.

First Aid Measures

- Remove the patient to a dry and shady place, loosen collar and any tight clothes.
- Raise the head and sprinkle cool water on his body or wrap him in a thin wet sheet and fan him.
- Check temperature every 10 minutes.
- Do not allow the body temperature fall below 103°F.

- After this, wrap him in a dry sheet and keep fanning so that the temperature does not rise again.
- If the casualty is conscious, cool water mixed with salt and glucose can be given for drinking.
- Remove the casualty to hospital.

HEAT EXHAUSTION

It is caused by too high temperature in the atmosphere directly by the sun or due to hard work and confinement in a close, hot atmosphere like factories, etc. Excessive sweating with loss of body water and salts result in this condition.

Signs and Symptoms

- Headache, dizziness, nausea, vomiting, abdominal cramps and cramps in limbs.
- Pale face and cold sweat.
- Pulse is weak.
- Shallow breathing.
- Temperature is normal or slightly elevated.
- Sometimes there is unconsciousness.
- Person may be in shock.
- Loss of appetite.

First Aid Measures

- Remove the casualty to a cool place.
- Place him flat on his back.
- Give him plenty of fluids with added salt or fruit juice.

Heat Cramps

These are intermittent, painful contraction of skeletal muscles. These cramps often occur in individual who replace the fluid lost in sweat by drinking water, but do not replace sodium. The sodium depletion is believed to be responsible for the cramps. Heat cramps usually occur in muscle that have been involved in strenuous activity and most often of the legs. The cramps last a few minutes and disappear spontaneously. With heat cramps, the body temperature is normal and serum sodium may be normal or low.

The treatment is to replace sodium with electrolyte solution. In severe cases, intravenous salt solutions may be required.

Preventing Extreme Heat Condition

- Limiting the strenuous activities in the hot weather.
- Gradually exposing to hot weather to get acclimatized to extreme heat.

- Stay indoors and wear a minimum of clothing during heat waves.
- Wear clothes that are loose fitting, light in color, and covering the body properly when outdoors.
- Lose weight if obese.
- Use measures to improve ventilation and reduce heat by shades.
- Eating more salts but with increased amounts of fluids.

Extremes of Cold

Effects of excessive cold are common in persons who live or work in a climate where temperature falls below 32°F or are in high altitudes. Extent of the injury caused depends on the degree of the temperature and the period to which exposed to cold.

Frost Bite

During very cold weather, especially if there is also a strong wind, frost bite is liable to occur on nose, chin, ears, fingers, toes. After being painfully cold the affected parts become waxy white in appearance and feel quite numb. Whiteness and numbness are danger signals which must not be overlooked because prolonged freezing will do irreparable damage.

Signs and symptoms

- The exposed part becomes cold, painful and ultimately numb.
- Color first is red then becomes white, which may later lead to gangrene.
- The parts feel waxy and has no feeling while it is frozen.

First Aid Measures

- Remove all wet or tight clothing from the frost bitten area.
- Carry the casualty to a closed room without a fire and undress him carefully.
- Remove tight gloves, boots, socks, rings, etc.
- Do not rub – the frozen part with a snow.
- Cover the casualty with a dry sheet.
- Give him warm drinks.
- The hands and feet need to be wrapped in a blanket.
- Do not use hot water bottles or heat lamps.
- Do not allow the victim to walk, if the feet are affected.
- Do not allow the victim to smoke because the nicotine in tobacco may further constrict blood vessels.
- Send for the physician immediately.

Preventive Measures for Extreme Cold

- Plan activities carefully to minimize exposure.
- Dress for the weather. Protection is more important than fashion.
- Always let someone know where you are and when to expect you back.
- Apply protective cream to the face prior to exposure.
- Use hand protection. Mittens are generally more effective than gloves.
- Avoid alcohol and cigarettes.
- Avoid using excessive heat to cold freezing tissues.

ASPHYXIA

Asphyxia is a deficiency of oxygen in the blood and an increase of carbon-dioxide in blood and tissues. It occurs due to an interruption in the normal exchange of oxygen and carbon-dioxide between the lungs and atmospheric air. If this condition continues for some minutes, breathing and heart action stops and death occurs.

Causes of asphyxia are drowning, electric shock, foreign body in the air passages (choking), inhalation of smoke and poisonous gases, hanging and strangulation, etc.

Signs and Symptoms of Asphyxia

First Stage

- Rate of breathing increases.
- Breathing gets shorter.
- Neck veins become swollen.
- Face, lips, nails, fingers and toes turn blue.
- Pulse gets faster and feeble.

Second Stage

- Consciousness is lost totally or partially.
- Froth may appear at the mouth and nostrils.
- Fits may occur – If this occurs than place the casualty on his back. Support the nape of the neck on your palm and press the head backwards. This will extend the neck and open the airway. Check if breathing is restored, if not give mouth to mouth breathing.
- Keep the casualty covered.
- Call doctor and ambulance.

Drowning

- Water may enter the respiratory passage and cause asphyxia.
- Immediately put the victim in prone position (face down) and make sure that his air passage is not obstructed.
- Pull tongue forward and remove any foreign material.

- Raise the middle part of the body with your hands to cause water to drain out of the lungs.
- Remove wet clothing, keep body warm and continue artificial breathing until breathing comes back.
- Seek medical assistance.

Choking

Choking occurs due to blockage of the throat by foreign object. There is difficulty in speaking and breathing.

First Aid Measures (For Adult)

- Reassure the casualty, bent him forward so that his head is lower than the chest.
- Give up to five sharp blows to her back between the shoulder blades, with the palm of your hand.
- If back slaps fail, try abdominal thrust. The sudden pull up against the diaphragm compress the chest, and may expel the obstruction.
- For abdominal thrust:
  - Stand behind the victim.
  - Wrap your arms around the waist.
  - Make a first, clasp fist with free hand.
  - Press in with quick inward and upward thrust.
- If this does not free the blockage, try again four times, then alternate five back blows with five thrusts (Fig. 5).

First Aid Measures (For Child)

- Place the child over your knee, head down, slap him between the shoulder blades using less force then for an adult.
- If back blow fails, use the abdominal thrust only if you have been trained to do on a child–otherwise, begin resuscitation.

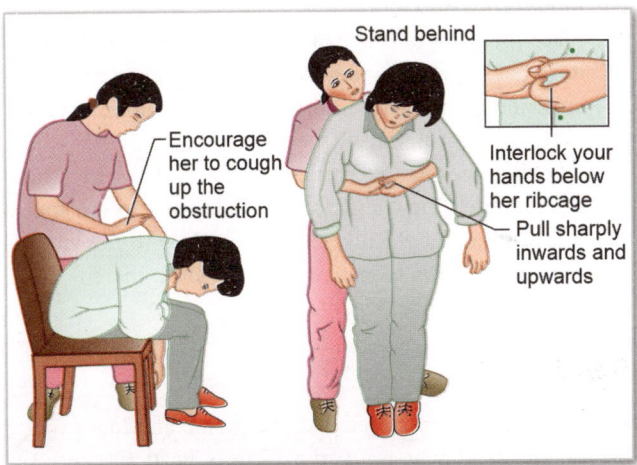

Fig. 5: Choking measures : Sharp blows on back and Abdominal thrust

First Aid Measures (For Baby)

- Lay the baby along your forearm.
- Slap the baby between the shoulder blades, using less force than for a child.
- If the baby becomes unconscious, begin resuscitation and do not use abdominal thrust.

Inhalation of Fumes and Gases

The inhalation of smoke, gases or toxic fumes can be dangerous. Two types of gases, carbon monoxide and carbon dioxide are common.

Carbon monoxide is lighter than air and is present in car–exhaust fumes, burning coal, coal mines, during fire, etc. Carbon dioxide is heavier than air and is found in coal mines, and sewerage.

First Aid Measures

- Before attempting to rescue a person, always open door and windows for proper ventilation.
- Pull out the casualty quickly while holding your breath.
- Crawl along the floor if the gas (CO) is lighter than air.
- Enter in upright position if poisonous gas is heavier than air, i.e., carbon dioxide.
- After bringing out the casualty in fresh air, if there is breathing difficulty, give artificial respiration.
- Send the casualty for medical assistance.

Artificial Respiration (Resuscitation Technique)

Step 1

- Open the airway, unless you suspect neck injury. Place the victim on his back.
- Wipe any foreign substance—solid or liquid—out of his mouth with the cloth.
- Place the palm of one hand on the forehead and tilt the head back, place the fingers of the other hand under the chin and lift to bring it forward. This position prevents obstruction of airway by the tongue (Fig. 6).
- Opening the airway may start the persons breathing again. Watch the chest rise and fall, listen to the sound of breathing by placing your cheek close to the victim's mouth and nose, to feel any exhaled air. It there is none, take step 2 at once (Fig. 7).

Step 2

- Pinch the nostril closed. Use the thumb and index finger of the hand that is on the victim's head to exert the necessary pressure and maintain proper tilt.

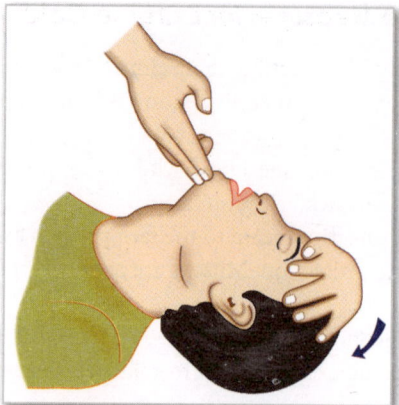

Fig. 6: Head tilt and Chin lift

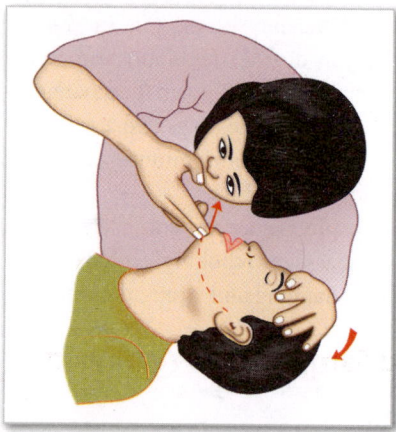

Fig. 7: Listen for breathing, watch chest, feel any exhaled air

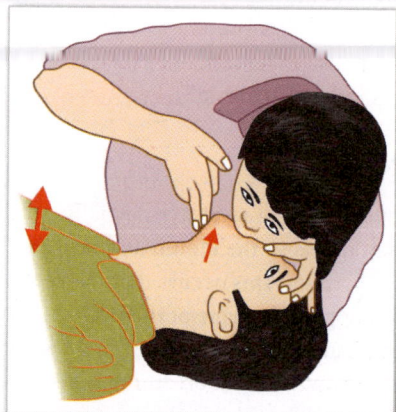

Fig. 8: Pinching nostrils and blowing into open mouth

- Place your mouth over the victim's mouth, and give two full breaths, each ventilation should cause the victim's chest to rise and fall.
- If this fails, suspect an obstruction of the airway (choking).
- When you are able to ventilate the victim quietly take step 3 (Fig. 8).

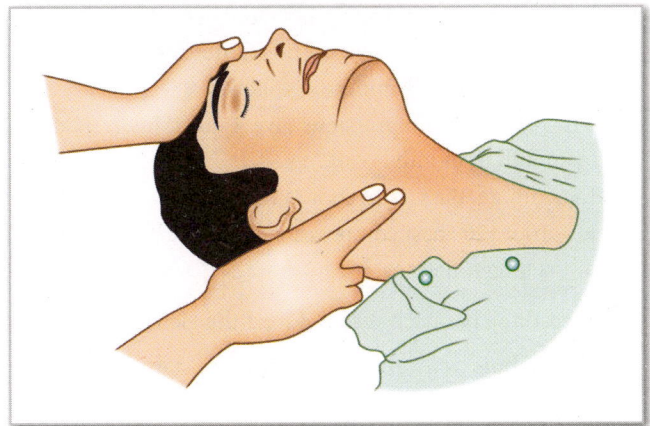

Fig. 9: Feeling carotid pulse

Step 3

♦ Feel the carotid pulse in the neck, if there is no pulse, give cardiopulmonary resuscitation (CPR). If there is pulse but still no breathing, begin step 4 (Fig. 9).

Step 4

♦ With victim's head tilted as in step 1, and his nose pinched shut, place your mouth over the victim's and blow hard.
♦ Remove your mouth and allow the victim to exhale and you take another deep breath.
♦ Watch for the rise and fall of the chest and listen for the sounds of inhaled air.
♦ Then blow again. Repeat the procedure, giving one vigorous breath every second until the victim starts to breathe spontaneously or help arrives.

CARDIOPULMONARY RESUSCITATION

Cardiopulmonary resuscitation (CPR) is a life-saving technique to be performed with skill and practice. When you come across a person with cardiac arrest, the quicker you start CPR, the better are the chances of survival.

Signs of Cardiopulmonary Arrest

♦ Immediate loss of consciousness.
♦ Absence of carotid pulse.
♦ Cessation of perceptible respirations.
♦ Dilation of pupils.

Resuscitation for Adults

When the victim appears unconscious, carry out the assessment as quickly as possible following these 4 steps:

♦ **Check for consciousness:** By shaking shoulders and asking him his name.
♦ **Open the air way (A):** By removing blockages and lifting chin.
♦ **Check for breathing (B):** By looking for chest movements. Listening for sounds of breathing and feeling for breath for 5 seconds.
♦ **Check for circulation (C):** By feeling for the carotid pulse for 5 seconds.

Airway

To clear the airway, remove obstructing substance from the mouth with finger.

♦ Use first finger as a hook to dislodge any material causing obstruction.
♦ Hyperextend the neck to open the airway.
♦ Place one hand under nape of neck.
♦ Place other hand on forehead and tilt head backward.
♦ Lift chin up gently without closing mouth.
♦ Check if breathing is restored.
♦ If not, start mouth to mouth breathing (Fig. 10).

Breathing

You are expected to act quickly and restore breathing by giving mouth-to-mouth resuscitation as follows:
♦ Pinch and compress nose to close nostrils.
♦ Take deep breaths.
♦ Place your mouth around victim's mouth, make an airtight seal.
♦ Quickly breathe into victim's mouth four times.
♦ Refill your lungs by inhaling deep.
♦ Watch victim's chest movements for rise and fall of chest
♦ Allow patient to exhale.

Circulation

You are expected to act quickly and restore circulation by pericardial thump and/or external cardiac compression.

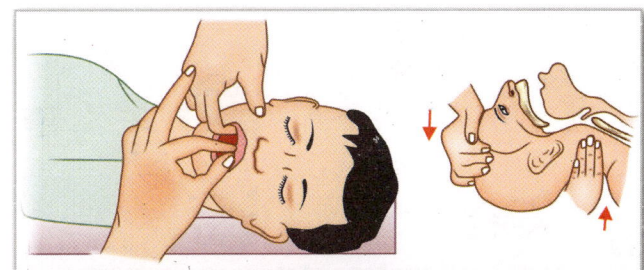

Fig. 10: Use of finger to remove obstructing material and hyperextending the neck

Precordial Thump

- Strike upper left chest forcibly in midsternum region with closed fist (except for patients with myocardial disease).
- This may result in resumption of normal heart beat, e.g., in electric shock cases.

External Cardiac Compression

This is also known as external cardiac massage, can be carried out by one or two individuals.

- Place victim on hard surface.
- Kneel at victim's side.
- Locate xiphoid process, measure 1–2 inch above xiphoid process.
- Place heel of one hand at this point on the sternum.
- Place the other hand on top of it.
- Interlock fingers to keep them off the victim's ribs.
- Keep elbows straight and lean forward.
- Make full use of your body weight when delivering downward compression (Figs 11A and B).
- Apply steady smooth pressure to depress victim's sternum 1½ to 2 inches.

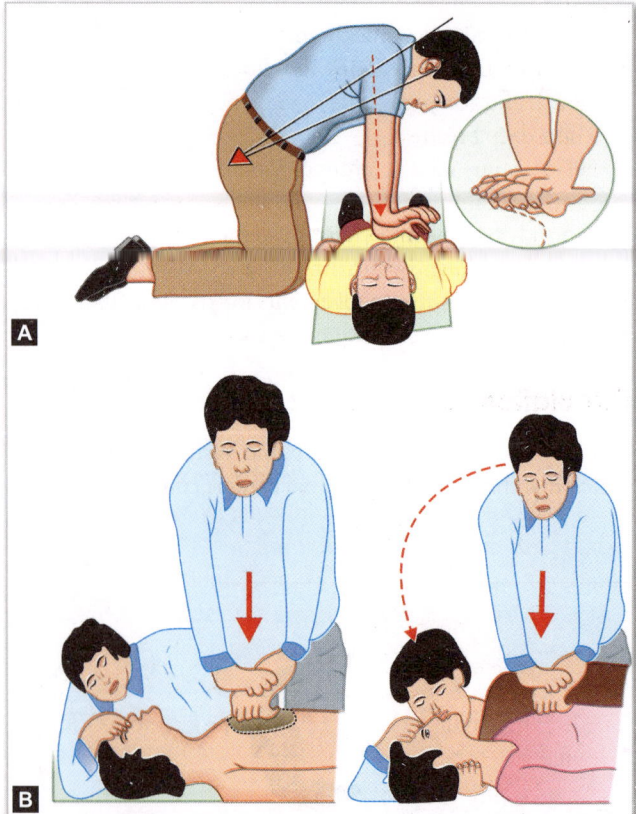

Figs 11A and B: A. Rescuers position for external compression; **B.** External cardiac compression

- Relax pressure completely but don't let your hand leave victim's chest so that correct position is not lost.
- Perform CPR for 1 minute as follows:
- After 30 chest compressions give 2 quick lung inflations by mouth to mouth breathing.
- In a minute, the victim should receive:
  - 100–120 chest compressions.
  - 8 lung inflations.

After breathing has been restored treat the victim as follows:

- To promote warmth and circulation, start rubbing the limbs upwards.
- Promote the warmth by giving blanket.
- If the victim can swallow, small quantities of tea or coffee can be given.
- The victim is rushed to hospital for further care. The CPR bridges the gap between the arrival of ambulance and casualty's collapse.

First Aid Measures in Wounds and Hemorrhage

Wound: A wound is an injury in which the skin is cut or penetrated. If wound is deep, severe bleeding may occur, depending on how they are caused e.g., by blunt force, sharp weapon or firearm. They are classified as:

- **Abrasion (scratches):** An abrasion is a superficial injury involving only the outer layers of the skin. It is caused by friction or pressure of some rough object. It bleeds very slightly.
- **Bruise (contusions):** A bruise is caused by blunt force, i.e., stick, stone or fist. There is infiltration of blood into the tissues following rupture of vessels, hence it appears red.
- **Lacerated wound:** These are wounds in which the skin and underlying tissues are torn as a result of application of blunt force. These wounds have irregular and torn edges and bleed less. They are usually caused by industrial accidents, falling on rough surfaces, pieces of shells and claws of animals.
- **Incised wound:** An incised wound is an injury caused by a weapon with a sharp cutting edge, e.g., knife, razor, etc. It leads to more bleeding.
- **Punctured wound:** Is an injury caused by a pointed weapon, when it is driven in through the skin. Such wounds are caused by needle, arrow, scissors, ice pick, etc. They have small openings but may be very deep.

Hemorrhage: Bleeding means the escape of blood from the blood vessels. It may be classified as external or internal hemorrhage.

External Hemorrhage

- **Arterial bleeding:** The blood, richly oxygenated is bright red and under pressure from the pumping heart, spurts from the wound in line with the heartbeat.
- **Venous bleeding:** Venous blood is dark red in color. It is under less pressure than arterial blood.
- **Capillary bleeding:** This type of bleeding characterized as oozing, occurs at the site of all wounds. Blood loss is generally negligible.

First Aid Management of Wounds

The main principles are control bleeding and prevent infection.

Control of Bleeding

- **Rest:** Make the casualty lie down still, so that amount of blood loss is less.
- **Elevation:** Elevate the wounded arm, or leg, above the level of the heart.
- **Direct pressure:** Apply firm pressure directly on the wound. Pressure is applied through a dressing which is bandaged firmly on the wound. The dressing should be thick and compressible to facilitate the application of even pressure over the whole wound area. It compresses all blood vessels leading into the wound and so lessens blood flow.
- **Indirect pressure:** If direct pressure is not possible to apply than indirect pressure may be applied to a "pressure point" where a main artery runs close to a bone. It must not be applied for longer than 10 minutes.
- For a wound of the scalp, compress the temporal artery (Fig. 12).
- For bleeding over lower face (below the eyes) apply pressure to the facial artery along the lower border of the mandible.
- For a neck wound, compress the wound site. Do not compress the carotid artery, as this could cause stroke.
- For a shoulder wound or hemorrhage of the upper arm compress the subclavian artery against the clavicle.
- For a wound of the lower part of the upper arm or of the elbow, press the brachial artery against the humerus.
- For foot wounds, compress the entire network of arteries in the ankle.
- For a wound of the lower arm, press the ulnar and radial arteries at the antecubital fossa.
- For thigh wounds, apply great pressure to the femoral artery against the femur.
- For wounds of the lower leg, apply pressure to the popliteal artery, behind the knee.

Immediately the victim should be shifted where facility to save victim are available.

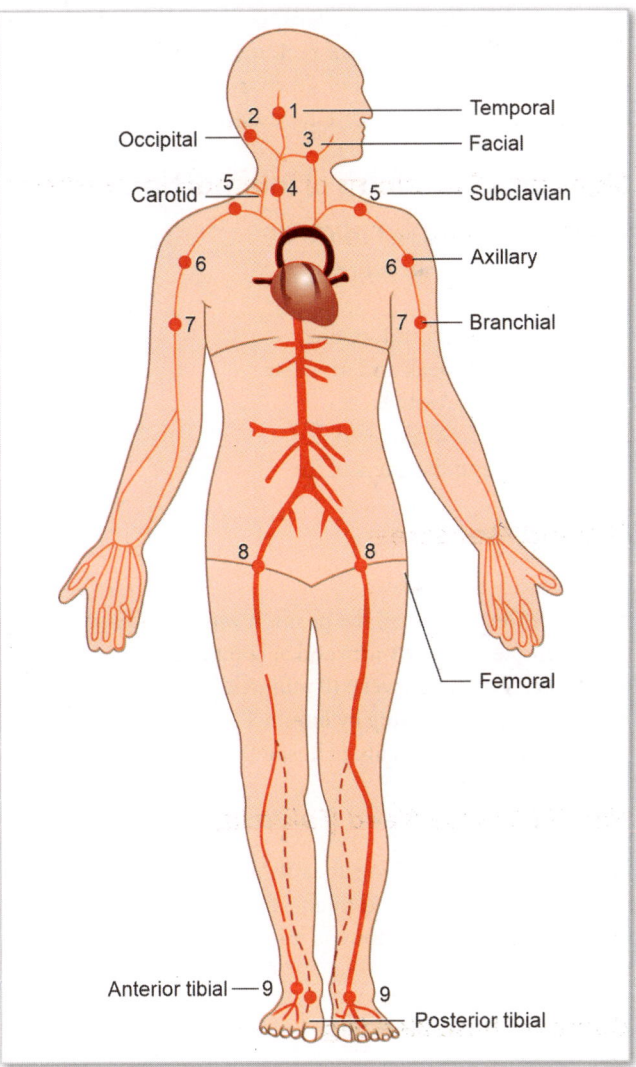

Fig. 12: Pressure points of artery

Prevention of Wound Infection

Before Applying the Dressing

- If possible, wash your hands carefully.
- To wash off the skin around the wound with soap and water.
- **While applying dressing:** Do not breathe, talk, cough or sneeze into or over the wound.
- Cover the wound as quickly as possible with a sterile or clean dressing.
- After bandaging, keep the injured part in a position of comfort.

Internal Hemorrhage

This is the bleeding within one of the cavities of the body, which is not visible, such as cerebral hemorrhage, or bleeding in peritoneal chest cavity. This is due to head injuries, accidents, falls or collapse of building. Initially there are no signs of internal bleeding but slowly a large amount of blood may be lost from the circulation, resulting into shock.

Signs and Symptoms of Internal Hemorrhage

- The skin is cold and clammy.
- Subnormal temperature.
- Eyes sunken.
- Breathing deep and sighing.
- Pulse rapid, weak and irregular.
- Low blood pressure.
- Victim feels thirsty, anxious.
- Fainting and dizziness occur.

First Aid Measures

- Reassure the casualty.
- Place the casualty in flat position with feet raised.
- Keep the casualty warm and at complete rest.
- Check vital signs every 10 minutes.
- Do not give anything by mouth.
- Transport the casualty to hospital as quickly as possible.

First Aid in Nose Bleed (Epistaxis)

Nose bleeds may be dangerous if blood loss is excessive. If nose bleed follows a head injury, the blood may appear thin and watery which is serious as it indicates that cerebrospinal fluid is present.

Causes of Nose Bleeding

- Picking out crusts and hair.
- Blowing the nose forcefully.
- High blood pressure.
- Bleeding disorders like leukemia.
- In summer due to excessive heat.
- Injury to the bones of the nose, skull.
- Common cold and other infections.

First Aid Measures

- Let the person sit up, with head slightly bent forwards.
- Press the nostrils together for several minutes and let him breathe through mouth.
- Apply a wet towel with ice over nose.
- Loosen clothing at neck.
- Do not let the person talk, cough, laugh, or blow the nose.
- Immediately take a narrow gauze and plug in nose for several hours and when bleeding has stopped, remove it carefully.
- Send the casualty for medical help.

Shock

Shock results from the failure of the cardiovascular system to provide sufficient blood circulation to all parts of the body.

Causes of Shock

- Severe loss of blood.
- Intense pain.
- Extensive trauma.
- Burns.
- Poisoning.
- Emotional stress or intense emotion.
- Extreme heat and cold.
- Electrical shock.
- Allergic reactions.
- A sudden or severe illness.

Types of Shock

- **Hypovolemic:** It is also known as hemorrhagic shock. It is caused by decrease in fluid volume form bleeding, prolonged vomiting, diarrhea or loss of blood during surgery or trauma.
- **Cardiogenic shock:** It results from poor heart pumping function and is caused by various cardiovascular abnormalities. The heart is not able to provide sufficient amount of blood to all parts of body.
- **Neurogenic shock:** It is caused by the failure of the nervous system to maintain a normal contraction of the blood vessels.
- **Septic shock:** It results from the severe infection.
- **Psychogenic shock:** It is caused by nervous system reactions to an emotional stimulus. The blood vessels dilate temporarily, decreasing blood flow to brain which result in syncope.
- **Anaphylactic shock:** It results from a sudden severe allergic body reaction to a foreign substance.

Signs and Symptoms

- Change in level of consciousness.
- Skin becomes pale, cold to touch, later cyanosis develops over lips and nail beds.
- Decrease in blood pressure.
- Pulse rate is increased but becomes weak and thready.
- Respiratory rate is increased, it may be shallow, labored or irregular.
- Urine output is decreased.
- Decreased oxygen to the tissues result in weakness and/or tremors of the arms and legs.
- Victim may complain of thirst, nausea, vomiting and dry mucous membranes may be present.

First Aid Measures

- Take measures to establish airway.
- Take steps to control bleeding if it is present.
- Take steps to reduce pain.
- Appropriate positioning of the victim in shock which is determined by the type and extent of injury.
  - The victim should lie flat with the head slightly lower than the rest of the body unless the victim has sustained head and chest injuries.
  - If victim is unconscious, position on the side to keep airway patent and encourage drainage.
  - If victim has difficulty in breathing, the head and shoulders should be elevated.
  - If neck or spinal injuries are suspected, not to move the victim to prevent further injury.
- Maintain the victim's body temperature by keeping him dry and warm.
- Take measures to relieve pain.
- Give emotional support and reassurance.
- Do not let crowd gather around the patient.
- Arrange for transportation.

Anaphylactic Shock

This is a severe body response to allergic substance or protein. Allergic substance on its introduction into the body causes sudden release of histamine into the blood stream and allows blood plasma to flow through capillary walls, thus decreasing blood flow to the heart, giving rise to circulatory failure. Its onset is sudden.

Causes of anaphylactic shock:

- Pollen
- Particular food, e.g., mushroom, milk, eggs, fish, etc.
- Wasp sting, bee sting.
- Drugs like penicillin, sulpha, iron, serum, etc.

Signs and Symptoms of Anaphylactic Shock

- Nausea, vomiting.
- Diarrhea.
- Anxiety.
- Widespread red, blotchy skin eruption, hives.
- Urticaria.
- Swelling of the face and neck.
- Rapid pulse.
- Wheezing and gasping for air.
- Itchy, red watery eyes.

First Aid Management

A person stands good chances of survival if he receives treatment within 20 minutes of its onset.

- The person urgently needs oxygen and a life-saving injection of adrenaline. There is no particular first–aid measure, except assisting in breathing and minimizing shock till the doctor arrives.
- Remove the allergen if possible and call for assistance.
- Keep the person cool and loosen any constrictive clothing.
- Reassure the person, stay with him until emergency aid arrives.
- Help the person for easy breathing by making him sit up and leaning forward a little.
- If the person stops breathing, administer CPR.

First Aid in Unconsciousness

Unconsciousness is the state in which a person is unable to respond to stimuli and appears to be asleep. Person may be unconscious for a few seconds as in fainting or for longer periods of time.

People who become unconscious don't respond to loud sounds or shaking. They may even stop breathing or their pulse may become faint. This calls for immediate emergency attention. The sooner the person receives emergency first aid, the better their outlook will be.

Causes of Unconsciousness

Unconsciousness can be brought on by a major illness or injury, or complications from drug use or alcohol misuse.

Common causes of unconsciousness include:

- A car accident
- Severe blood loss
- A blow to the chest or head
- A drug overdose
- Alcohol poisoning

A person may become temporarily unconscious, or faint, when sudden changes occur within the body. Common causes of temporary unconsciousness include:

- Cardiac arrest
- Low blood sugar
- Low blood pressure
- Syncope or loss of consciousness due to lack of blood flow to the brain (fainting)
- Neurologic syncope, or loss of consciousness caused by a seizure, stroke, or transient ischemic attacks (TIA)
- Dehydration
- Problems with heart rhythm
- Straining
- Hyperventilating

Note: Any sudden loss of consciousness is a medical emergency, bystanders should call for medical help immediately.

Symptoms that may indicate that unconsciousness is about to occur include:

- Sudden inability to respond
- Slurred speech
- A rapid heart rate
- Confusion
- Dizziness or lightheadedness

First Aid Measures

If person is breathing:

- Place him in recovery position, this will help to maintain a clear airway and decrease the risk of choking.
- For providing recovery position, follow the instructions listed below:
  - Kneel on the floor next to him
  - Take the arm that is closest to you and position it so that it is perpendicular to his body, forming a right angle. The head should be facing upward.
  - Take his other hand and position it so that the back of the hand is pressed against the cheek that is closest to you.
  - With your free hand, bend his knee that is farthest from you. His foot should be resting flat against the floor.
  - Help him get onto his side by pulling on the bent knee. After you roll him over, ensue that his top arm is still helping to support his head.
  - Tilt his head back and lift his chin. This helps open airway.
  - Make sure there is no obstruction in the airway.
  - Keep an eye on his condition, and remain with him until emergency personnel arrives.

If Person is not Breathing

Call for help immediately and begin CPR.

Other First Aid Measures

- Do not try to arouse an unconscious person. Let him lie quiet.
- Do not move the casualty unnecessarily, because of the possibility of spinal injury. Never attempt to make an unconscious person sit or stand.
- Do not let people gather around, give him fresh air.
- Loosen clothing at neck, chest and waist.
- Never give water to an unconscious person to drink, it might get into his windpipe.
- Apply specific treatment for the cause of unconsciousness.

Fainting

This occurs most frequently in healthy young people, especially during hot weather, and while standing for long

periods. People who are hungry, tired, emotionally upset, fearful may faint even though they are in good health. The cause is insufficient supply of blood to the brain.

Signs and Symptoms of Fainting

- The person feels giddy, looks pale and collapse on the ground
- Pulse is weak and slow
- Skin is cold and clammy
- Breathing becomes less deep

First Aid Measures

- Keep the victim lying flat, and raise the legs to improve the blood flow to the brain.
- Loosen tight clothing at neck.
- Do not let the crowd gather and let there be plenty of fresh air.
- Consciousness will return in one or two minutes.
- After he recovers consciousness, a cup of tea or coffee may be given.
- If the victim does not recover, medical help is advised.

Burns and its First Aid Measures

Burns are due to dry heat including friction, whereas scalds are due to wet heat. Burns and scalds are considered together as they produce the severe type of injury.

Causes of Burns and Scalds

- **Dry heat:** Fire, explosions, contact with hot object.
- **Moist heat:** Boiling water, steam, hot tea or coffee, oil.
- **Friction:** Contact with moving wheel, rope, wire.
- **Chemical:** Strong acids and alkalies.
- **Electrical:** Contact with live wire, electric pole.

The person who has sustained a major burn is critically ill. The body systems are threatened not only from physiologic and psychological effects of burn, but also from other physical trauma that may occur simultaneously. The extent of injury caused by burns and scalds depends on following factors:

- The duration of contact between the skin and the substance causing injury.
- The strength of the substance, this is particularly important when chemicals and electrical current are the cause of injury.

Characteristics of Burn Injuries

Severity of a burn injury is determined by following five factors:

1. Surface area of body burnt.
2. Depth of tissue damage.
3. Age of casualty.

4. Past medical history.

5. Part of body burnt.

Body Surface Area Burnt

A quick approximate estimate of the percentage of body surface area may be made using Rule of Nine. The rule of nine, is useful for adult patients only. The body is divided into areas, each of which represent 9% this system is based on anatomic regions, each representing approximately 9% of the TBSA (total burnt surface area) (Fig. 13).

Depth of Burn

- First degree or superficial partial thickness burn—involves total destruction of the epidermis. Healing usually occur within 7–10 days.
- Second degree or deep partial thickness burn— involves total destruction of the epidermis and major involvement of the upper dermal layers only. Lower dermal layers remain intact. Healing occurs within 14–21 days.
- Third degree of full thickness burn—involves total damage to the epidermis and major damage to both upper and lower dermal layers, subcutaneous tissue, muscle and bone may also be involved.

Age of Casualty

Persons younger than 2 years and older than 50 years have the highest incidence of morbidity and mortality. The severity of the burn increases with age.

Part of the Body Burnt

Burns of the face, eyes, ears, neck, hands or feet and genitals are major. Damage to the tracheobronchial tree through heat, and smoke inhalation is also a major problem.

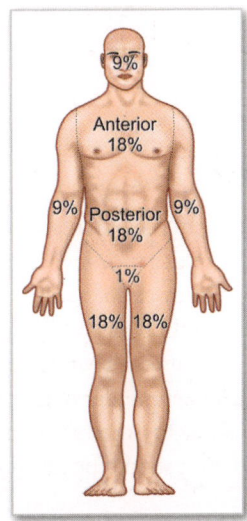

Fig. 13: Rule of Nine

Management of Burns

Goals of Burns Management

- Stopping the burning process.
- Reduce pain.
- Providing life support –oxygenation, fluids, etc.
- Preventing complications.
- Restoration of functions.
- For stopping the burning process do not allow the person to run about, as it increases the severity. Lay him flat on the ground, put any thick clothing which is available like blanket, carpet, shawl, etc. over the victim to extinguish flames. Do not try to remove the burning clothes.
- Immediately immerse the burnt area under cool running water or cool moistened towels can be applied. This reduces pain and decrease the effect of transmission through the tissues.
- Assess airway breathing and circulation.
- Blisters should not be touched.
- All articles like bangles, belt, boot should be removed.
- Cover the burnt area with clean sheet over which blanket can be placed to maintain heat and prevent hypothermia.
- Give warm fluids to drink if casualty can take it and restrict the movement.
- In case of extensive burns, person may go into shock, then the first aid for shock is given and victim rushed to a nearby hospital.
- **In acid burns:**
  - Cool area with stream of plain water.
  - Remove acid soaked clothing.
  - Bathe affected part with alkaline solution of 1 table spoon of baking soda and 1 L of water.
  - Cover with clean linen.
  - Give analgesics for pain.
- **In alkali burns:**
  - Flood burnt area with stream of plain water.
  - Remove alkali soaked clothing.
  - Bathe affected part with weak solution of vinegar and water in equal parts.
  - Cover with clean linen material only.
  - Give analgesics for pain.
- **In electrical burns:**
  - The passage of electrical current through the body may cause breathing problem and even heart to stop. A person while indoors may receive an electric shock, by touching a bare electric wire and the danger is greater if the floor or one's body is wet.
  - Outdoors one may be electrocuted by touching an electric wire or by flying a kite having a damp or metal string that touches an electric wire. Contact with high voltage current found in power lines and overhead high tension cables is usually fatal.

Severe burns always result. The power must be cut off before the casualty is approached.

Signs and Symptoms

- Burns—super facial or deep, depends on the strength of the electric current.
- Cardiac arrest.
- Sudden stoppage of breathing due to paralysis of muscles used in breathing.

First Aid Measures

- Free the victim from the circuit immediately.
- Remove the victim from contact with the wire by taking a dry wooden stick, dry towel.
- Stand on dry insulating material—wooden, rubber or plastic mat or thick pile of newspapers.
- Call the fire department for outdoors electrocution.
- Start artificial respiration and continue till natural breathing is restored.

Bites and Stings

Animal bites always require medical attention, because germs are harbored in the mouths of all animals. Bites from sharp, pointed teeth cause deep puncture wounds that carry germs to the tissues. They require prompt first aid followed by medical attention.

Snake Bite

Commonly two types of snakes Colubrine and Viper. Colubrine snakes are quite long and very poisonous. The common varieties are King cobra, Common krait and Striped krait. The vipers are found in the form of pit viper and Russell's viper. The snakes living in water are also poisonous.

Signs and Symptoms

- Cobra bite very quickly affects the nervous system Severe pain in the bitten area, uneasiness, giddiness and sometimes vomiting. Muscles get affected causing weakness of hands and legs, loss of sensation, watering of mouth, slow respiration and weak pulse rate. There is constriction of pupils of eye. If first aid is not given on time death occurs.
- Viper snake has effect on the blood vessels of the bitten area. The blood clotting process is disturbed due to the effect of viper snakes. There is excessive bleeding from the bitten area and the bitten area appears swollen. With the absorption of poison in the body there is uneasiness, giddiness, vomiting, weakness and slow pulse rate.

First Aid Measures

- Make the person lie down comfortably and reassure the casualty.
- Tie handkerchief or tourniquet at a distance away from the bitten area to avoid the venous blood flow towards the heart. Do not tie the tourniquet very tightly that the blood flow to the organ is inhibited. Put an inch long cut over the snake bitten area and start sucking/removing out the blood mixed liquid coming out from the wound. Send the casualty for medical help.

Scorpion Bite

Scorpion bite rarely leads to a serious condition but there is severe burning, intolerable increasing pain in the bitten area. Sometimes person complains of giddiness, vomiting and can become unconscious.

First Aid Measures

- Casualty should be made to lie comfortably and soothing cream should be applied.
- Pain should subside within an hour if it does not and the victim complains of feeling of unconsciousness call for medical help.

Dog Bite

Domestic dogs which are not immunized against rabies and which comes in contact with stray dogs/wild animals have a chance to contract the rabies virus and become rabid. Rabies virus is commonly found in dogs but can be carried by any animal like cats, rats, foxes, wolves, bats and monkeys. Saliva of infected animal can get injected into human being even by licking if there is a break in the skin.

Signs and Symptoms

- Headache, malaise, fever.
- Hydrophobia.
- Aerophobia.

First Aid Measures

- Thorough washing of the bitten area with soap and water for 5–10 minutes under running water.
- Dress the wound with clean sterile gauge and let wound bleed of suspected rabid dog.
- Victim should be immediately referred to doctor.
- The dog should be kept under observation for 10 days. If the dog remains healthy then there is no risk, but if the dog gets mad, then it should be killed.

BEES AND WASP BITES

Their sting causes local pain, itching and severe swelling because their sting has one type of poison which is little in quality. Some people are very sensitive to this poison they may have anaphylactic shock and may require immediate treatment in the hospital.

If the sting is visible, it can be taken out by slightly scrubbing the skin. So, that poison can come out easily. If swelling and pain is severe than keep wet bandage.

Foreign Bodies

Foreign Bodies in the Skin

Small foreign bodies (wood splinters, pieces of glass) usually cause minor puncture wounds with little or no bleeding. If a small portion of the object protrudes from the skin, it can be taken out. Foreign bodies may get deeply embedded in the skin, should not be removed by first aider. Doctor should be consulted.

Foreign Bodies in the Eye

Dust, sand particles, glass pieces, coal, insect may enter the eye. These particles usually are found under the eyelids or eyeball.

Signs and Symptoms

♦   Watering from the eyes.
♦   Pain, irritation in eye.
♦   Photophobia–Difficulty in opening eye in the light.
♦   Blurred vision or loss of vision in the affected eye.

First Aid Measures

♦   Do not allow the casualty to rub the eyes. Because by doing so it can cause further injury.
♦   Wash your hands before touching the eyes of victim.
♦   Do not try to take out foreign body by using means like matchstick, etc.
♦   Do not try to take out the embedded foreign body in eye. In such cases, immediately consult to doctor.
♦   If foreign body is visible, wet the corner of a soft handkerchief, and take out foreign body with the help of a pointed end.
♦   If foreign body is sticking on the inner portion of the lower eyelid, slide the lower eyelid under the upper one and open the eye. The foreign body sometimes comes out when the hairs of the upper eyelid get rubbed.
♦   If foreign body does not come out, close the eye put eye pad and person should be sent to hospital.

Foreign Body in the Ear

This usually occurs in children. They may insert buttons, peas inside the ear. Substances like seeds absorb moisture, swell up and obstruct the ear. Flies, mosquitoes or bed bugs can also enter the ear.

Signs and Symptoms

♦   Pain
♦   Infection
♦   Hearing loss

First Aid Measures

♦   Do not probe the ear with a tool such as a cotton swab or matchstick. There is a risk of pushing the object further in and damaging the ear.
♦   Remove the object if possible. If the object is clearly visible, and can be grasped easily with tweezers, gently remove it.
♦   Try using gravity. Tilt the head to the affected side to try to dislodge the object.
♦   Use oil for an insect. If the foreign object is an insect, tilt the person's head so that the ear with the insect is upward. Try to float the insect out by pouring mineral oil, olive oil or baby oil into the ear. The oil should be warm but not hot.
♦   Try washing the object out. Use a rubber bulb syringe and warm water to irrigate the object out of the canal.
♦   Do not pour water if any seed is suspected, to be obstructing the ear canal. It may swell up the seed and further block the ear canal.

Foreign Body in the Nose

Foreign bodies in nose like pieces of betel nut, grains or peas or other seeds, crayon, etc. may be put by children in nose while playing.

First Aid Measures

♦   Do not probe at the object with a cotton swab or other tool.
♦   Don't try to inhale the object by forcefully breathing in. Instead, breathe through your mouth until the object is removed.
♦   Blow out of your nose gently to try to free the object but don't blow hard or repeatedly. If only one nostril is affected, close the opposite nostril by applying gentle pressure and then blow out gently through the affected nostril.
♦   Gently remove the object if it is visible and you can easily grasp it with tweezers. Don't try to remove an object that is not visible or easily grasped.
♦   Call for emergency medical assistance if these methods fail.

Foreign Body in the Throat

A foreign body in the throat or upper part of the respiratory tract can cause choking and is a medical emergency that needs immediate attention. The foreign body may be pieces of food, small bones of fish, coins or artificial teeth.

First Aid Measures

- If the person is able to cough forcefully, the person should keep coughing. If the person is choking and cannot talk, cry or laugh forcefully, then the red cross recommends "five and five" approach is delivering first aid.
- Give 5 back blows. Stand to the side and just behind a choking adult. Place one arm across the person's chest for support. Bend the person over at the waist so that the upper body is parallel with the ground. Deliver five back blows between the person's shoulder blades with the heel of your hand.
- Give 5 abdominal thrusts. Perform five abdominal thrusts. Abdominal thrusts have been described in detail in first aid in asphyxia (also known as the Heimlich maneuver).
- Alternate between 5 blows and 5 thrusts until the blockage is dislodged.
- Call for help while you are performing first aid.

POISONING

Poisoning is a condition caused by introduction of harmful substances or chemicals into the body either by injection, inhalation or ingestion. A poison (or toxin) is a substance, which if taken into the body in sufficient quantity, can cause temporary or permanent damage. Once in the body, poisons may work their way into the blood stream. Signs and symptoms vary depending on the poison and the method of entry.

First Aid for Poisoning

If the poison is swallowed:
- **If the person is alert:** Do not induce vomiting (in case of acid or alkali). Immediately rinse the mouth. Keep the product or medicine container handy for sending to lab.

On the Skin

- Carefully remove contaminated clothing and wash exposed areas with copious amounts of water.

In the Eye

- Rinse eyes with a slow gentle stream of water for 10 to 15 minutes. Allow the stream of water to flow from the inner corner across the eye to the outer corner.

Inhaled

- Get the person to fresh air, without placing yourself at risk.
- Loosen any tight clothing at the neck.
- Avoid breathing fumes you may become a victim yourself.

When to Suspect Poisoning

Poisoning signs and symptoms can mimic other conditions, such as seizure, alcohol intoxication, stroke, insulin reaction.

Signs and Symptoms

- Burns or redness around the mouth and lips.
- Breath that smells like chemicals such as gasoline or paint thinner.
- Vomiting.
- Difficult breathing.
- Drowsiness.
- Confusion or other altered mental status.

If you suspect poisoning, be alert for cues such as empty pill bottles or packages, scattered pills, burns, stains and odor on a person or nearby objects.

When to Call for Help

Call for help immediately if the person is:
- Drowsy or unconscious.
- Having difficulty in breathing or has stopped breathing.
- Uncontrollably restless or agitated.
- Having seizures.
- Known to have taken medications or any other substance, intentionally or accidentally overdosed.
- Immediately send the casualty for medical assistance.

BIBLIOGRAPHY

1. *Keech. P. Practical Guide to First-aid.*
2. *Gupta. LC Manual of First-aid.*
3. *St. John Ambulance First-aid Book.*
4. *Practical First-aid by British Red Cross.*
5. *Linda Young L. Manual of First-aid and Emergency for Health Professionals.*

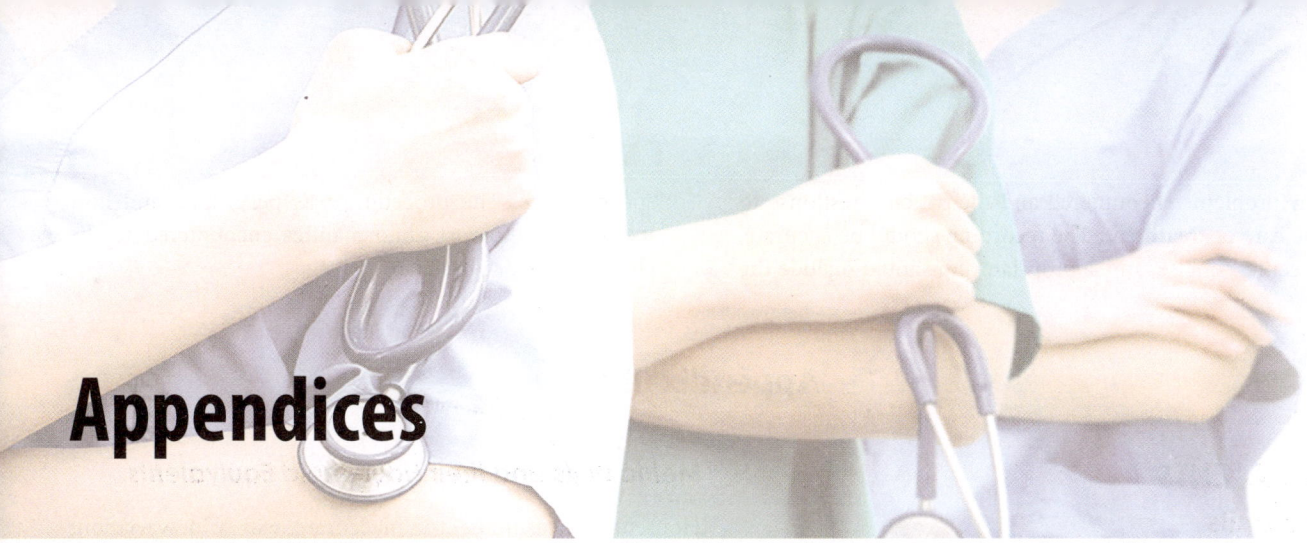

Appendices

STANDARD STEPS FOR ALL NURSING PROCEDURES

At the Beginning of the Procedure

- *STEP A: Check the order, collect the equipment and supplies, and wash your hands.*
  Verify the procedure to be done for the patient. Check the agency's policies and procedures manual for the accepted method of performing the procedure, process equipment and supply changes. Take all equipment and supplies to the patient's room.
- *STEP B: Identify and prepare the patient.*
  Greet the patient, introduce yourself, and check the patient's identification band. Explain what you are going to do in terms the patient can understand. Elicit questions and answer clearly. Provide necessary teaching related to the procedure to be performed.
- *STEP C: Provide privacy and perform safety precautions; arrange the supplies and equipment.*
  Close the door or curtains and drape the patient before beginning the procedure or discussing information, the person might want to keep confidential. Check equipment for proper function and for safety. Set up the equipment and supplies in an orderly, methodical fashion. Raise the bed to an appropriate working height. Raise the siderails before turning the patient and be certain that the wheels are locked. Wash your hands to prevent contaminating the patient with organisms from the chart, the nurses' station and the supply room.

During the Procedure

- *STEP D: Use standard precautions and aseptic technique as appropriate.*
  Protect yourself from blood and body fluids by wearing gloves. If there is a danger of splashing blood or body fluids, wear protective glasses or goggles and an impermeable cover gown or apron. Be very careful with sharp instruments and needles so as not to prick your skin.
- *STEP E: Perform the task according to protocol.*
  Mentally review the steps of the task beforehand. If you are uncertain how to do a task, ask your team leader, resource nurse, instructor, or charge nurse. Plan for efficiency of time and effort while delivering safe care.

At the End of the Procedure

- *STEP X: Remove gloves and other protective equipment.*
  After making certain the patient is clean and dry, dispose of used supplies, remove goggles and other protective equipment, and discard or store appropriately. To remove gloves without contaminating yourself, begin by pulling one glove off without touching your skin; hold the removed glove in the palm of the remaining gloved hand and then reach to the inside of the other glove and roll it down the hand. Dispose off the gloves in the trash. Wash your hands immediately.
- *STEP Y. Restore the unit. Collect the used equipment dispose off, clean, or store them in the proper places.*
  Make the person comfortable, tidy the bed and unit, place the call light and personal items within reach, and provide for safety by raising the side rails and lowering the bed. Remove used equipment. Soiled linens are to be placed in a soiled-linen hamper. Reuseable items are cleaned and returned to the storage or processing area (central supply). Document use of the equipment on the computer so no further changes will be made. Remove unsightly, odorous, or potentially infectious trash from the room. Inquire if anything else is needed. Wash your hands before leaving the room.
- *STEP Z. Record and report the procedure.*
  Document assessment findings and the details of the procedure performed, or care given, in the chart. Include

any problems encountered and the patient's response to the care or treatment. The recording should be accurate, specific, concise, and appropriate and should include the specific time. The procedure was performed and how it was done. Report abnormalities encountered to the charge nurse or physician

Appendix II

EQUIVALENTS

Metric Units

The metric system, developed by the French, uses the meter as the basic unit. The metric system is a decimal system, with prefixes that designate the various multiples or divisibles of 10. The most commonly used prefixes in medicine are:

Milli, which means one-thousandth (0.001)

Centi, which means one-hundredth (0.01)

Kilo, which means one thousand (1000)

These prefixes may be affixed to any of the three basic units of measurements, which are:

Meter (m), the unit of length

Gram (g). the unit of weight

Liter (L), the unit of volume

Therefore,

1 millimeter (mm) = 0.001 m

1 milligram (mg) = 0.001 g

1 milliliter (mL) = 0.001 L

1 kilometer (km) = 1000 m

1 kilogram (kg) = 1000 g

1 kiloliter (kL) = 1000 L

Length

The meter (a little longer than a yard) and the kilometer (about 0.6 mile) seldom are used in medicine or nursing. The commonly used measure of length is 1 centimeter (cm) = 0.01 m = about 0.4 inch.

Volume

The most frequently used measures of volume are the liter and the milliliter. Some useful equivalents to know are:

1000 milliliters (mL) = 1 liter (L)

1000 cubic centimeters = 1 liter (L)

Weight

The gram designates the weight of 1 mL of distilled water at 4°C. The most frequently used units of weight are:

1,000,000 micrograms (mcg) = 1 gram (g)

1000 micrograms (mcg) = 1 milligram (mg)

1000 milligrams (mg) = 1 gram (g) 1000 grams (g) = 1 kilogram (kg) = 2.2 pounds (lb)

Metric Units and their Household Equivalents

Household measurement is inaccurate, with wide variations in the size of teaspoons, teacups, and so forth. The generally accepted household measures are:

60 drops (gtt) = 1 teaspoon (tsp or t)

3 tsp = 1 tablespoon (Tbs or T)

12 Tbs = 1 teacup

16 Tbs = 1 glass (or a standard measuring cup)

Apothecary Units

In the apothecary system:

The unit of weight is the *grain*.

The unit of volume is the *minim*.

Of the many units of measure in the apothecary system, you should know the following units, abbreviations, and equivalents.

Weight

60 grains (gr) = 1 dram (dr or ʒ)

8 drams (dr or ʒ) = 1 ounce (oz or ʒ)

Volume

60 minims (min) = 1 fluid dram (fl dr or fʒ)

8 fl dr = 1 fluid ounce (fl oz or fʒ)

16 fl oz = 1 pint (pt)

2 pt, = 1 quart (qt)

4 qt = 1 gallon (gal)

In the apothecary system, when the symbol or abbreviation is used, the quantity is written in lowercase Roman numerals and follows the symbol. Arabic numerals are used, however in preference to large Roman numerals. For example

5gr = gr v

8 dr = ʒviii

Metric and household equivalents

Metric unit	Household unit
5 mL	1 tsp
15 mL	1 tbs
180 mL	1 full teacup
240 mL	1 full glass

The quantity one-half may be indicated by the symbol ss.

1 ½ , gr = gr iss

7 ½ gr = gr viiss

Other fractional parts are expressed as common fractions, for example. gr 1/250, gr 1/10.

When pint quart, and gallon are written, the quantity is expressed in Arabic numerals, (e.g., 11/2 pints or 71/2 quarts) 1.

Apothecary Units and Their Household Equivalents

1 drop = 1 minim (m i)

    1 tsp = 1 dr (ʒ i)

    1 Tbs = 1/2 oz (ʒ ss)

    2 Tbs = 1 oz (ʒ i)

    1 teacup = 6 oz (ʒ vi)

    1 glass or measuring cup = 8 oz (ʒ viii)

    2 measuring cups = 1 pt

TABLE 1: Most commonly used approximate equivalents

Metric	Apothecary	Household
0.06 g	Gr i gri	
0.06 mL	Min i	1 drop
1.0 g	Gr xv	
1.0 mL	Min xv	1/5 tsp
5 mL	(1 oz) ʒ i	1tsp
15 mL	(1/2 oz) ʒ ss	1tbs
30 mL	(1 ox) ʒ i	2tbs
500 mL	(16 oz) ʒ16	1 pt
1000 mL	(32 oz) ʒ32	1qt

*There are many discrepancies among these approximate equivalents. for example, 30 mL is the accepted equivalent for 1 oz (29 .57 mL is the exact equivalent). Such discrepancies are inevitable when two system are used whose equivalents are not exact If the discrepancies are within a 10% margin of error, they usually are acceptable in pharmacology.

Appendix III

MACHINERY, EQUIPMENT AND LINEN

Health care institution uses various items for diagnostic and therapeutic procedures. These items of different material like rubber, glass, plastic and enamel are common among most of the departments of hospital. A lot depends upon the care of these equipments to prevent cross-infection to the patients. Therefore, every professional nurse needs to have knowledges and practice for safe use of equipments and supplies for the care of an individual patient.

CARE AND MAINTENANCE OF EQUIPMENT

Rubber Items

Purposes

The purposes of care and maintenance of rubber items are as follows:

- To prevent spread of infection
- To clean the article and prepare for re-use
- To remove stains
- To preserve life of articles

Following are different types of rubber articles used in the hospital:

- Mackintosh (rubber protective)– Long and drawn
- Rubber tubes: Gavage, lavage, catheters, tubes. etc.
- Hot water bottle, ice caps, ice collars, air cushions
- Gloves
- Mouthpiece of ambu bag
- Pillows – air and water mattress
- Rubber bulb– asepto syringe and breast pump

General principles of care for rubber articles are as follows:

- Do not use hot water to clean or sunlight for drying.
- Do not keep near radiator–rubber articles get destroyed with heat
- Do not fold rubber sheets, instead roll them with paper of thin cloth lining after powdering them
- Do not stick pins, clamps on rubber tubes and catheters
- Store in wooden cupboards preferably
- Dry rubber goods in shade

Care of Rubber Articles after Use

Mackintosh

- Decontaminate by immersing in a tub of 0.5% chlorine/sodium hypochlorite solution
- Spread it on flat surface and pour water, and apply soap
- Repeat the above process on the other surface
- Rinse with water and dry it under shade
- When dry, powder it and roll it with paper lining in it

Rubber Tubes and Catheters

- Hold the tube upside down under running water
- Use swabsticks to remove any organic matter blocking the tip of the tube and eye of the catheter
- Ensure patency by seeing free flow of water

- Use soap and water to clean the tube and catheter
- Hang the tubes and catheters to dry in a cool/shaded place
- Powder the outer surface, coil the tube by securing the tip into the broader end
- Wrap individual tube and catheter using a thin piece of cloth and boil for 5 minutes or autoclave

Hot Water Bottle, Ice Caps, Ice Collars, Air Cushions

- Remove the outer cloth cover of each item after use
- Empty the contents, i.e. water from hot water bottle, ice cubes from ice cap and collar
- Deflate the air cushion: Clean the outside of the air cushion with soap and water, and decontaminate it.
- Hang the hot water bottle, ice cap upside down
- After the water is drained, wipe the outer surface with clean damp cloth
- Blow some air in these items and tighten the cap
- Check each item for leakage of air or water before storing it
- Store in a cool dry place

Gloves

- Gloves need to be decontaminated before removal by dipping them into disinfectant solution (0.5% chlorine) or just wash hands under running water if they are disposable gloves.
- Disposable gloves are sent for incineration
- Re-usable gloves are washed using soap and water first from outside surface and then the inside surface after reversing them
- Fill each glove with water to identify any tears or holes, if found leaking, discard them
- Hang the gloves to dry the inside surface and then the outside surface in shade
- Once dried, powder both the surfaces and pack them with paper or a cloth envelope by separating even number gloves of right and left hand
- Fold the upper end of the glove little before packing each glove. Label the size of glove on each envelope
- Pack in drum and send for autoclaving

Rubber Air/Water Mattress and Pillows

- Deflate the mattress, pillow, and remove the cloth cover. If soiled, decontaminate the cover with 0.5% chlorine solution and send it to laboratory.
- Clean the mattress and pillow using a piece of clean cloth and if soiled, decontaminate them with 0.5% sodium hypochlorite solution.
- Clean with soap and water on a flat surface.

- Dry under shade on a dry flat surface by exposing both surfaces to air.
- Inflate some air into mattress and pillow, and store.

Ambu Bag with Face Mask

- Wipe the bag and rubber part of the face mask using a piece of clean damp cloth
- Disinfect using a cotton ball soaked in pure Savlon or methylated spirit or 70% alcohol

Bulb Syringes

- Pinch the bulb creating a negative pressure and gently pull out the rubber bulb to separate it from the glass syringe
- Wipe it using a clean damp cloth
- Disinfect it using pure Savlon or spirit, if soiled
- Lightly powder the bulb using dusting powder and store in a cool dry place.

Sterilization of Rubber Articles

- **Autoclaving:** This is the best method. It is done at a lower temperature of 200°–250°F or 121°–123°C and pressure of 15–17 pounds per square inch, for 15 minutes
- **Boiling:** Wrap the rubber item in soft, thin cloth and boil it for 15–20 minutes. Hard rubber goods should not be boiled for more than 5 minutes and cooled fast to retain their shape
- Chemical sterilization can be used:
  - Savlon 100%: 30 minutes
  - Glutaraldehyde 2%: 10–20 minutes for disinfection and 10 hour for sterilization
  - Alcohol 50–70%: 20–30 minutes

Glass Items

Purposes

The following are the purposes of glass item:
- To prevent spread of infection
- To prepare for safe re-use
- To prevent damage to the item and to prolong its life

Different Glass Items are used in Hospitals
- Syringes
- Test tubes
- Funnel
- Ounce glass, drachm glass
- Undine: Used for irrigating eye
- Jars/bottles used for drainage and suction machines
- Slides
- Specimen bottles
- Connection tubes: Straight and y-shape
- Thermometer: Clinical, lotion

- Pipettes, glass rods, manometer column, dropper
- Intravenous fluid bottles

Care of Glass Articles

Cleaning, Disinfection and Sterilization of Glass Items in General

- Disinfect the item by immersing in 0.5% chlorine/sodium hypochlorite solution for 5 minutes in a plastic container covered with lid.
- Clean glass wares using mild soap.
- Use plastic brushes of an appropriate size to cleanse the tubes, jars and bottles.
- Rinse the glass items under cold running water, remove plunger from syringe and wash them separately. Keep plunger of each syringe beside it, to avoid mixing.
- Dry the item on a rack or appropriate stand by placing the item in an inverted position
- Remove any glass item with cracks
- Wrap the glass item in a piece of thin cloth before sending it for autoclaving or boiling
- Immerse glass item in 2% glutaraldehyde for 20–30 minutes.

Thermometers

- Remove the thermometer from antiseptic solution and wipe it dry from bulb to stem with a dry cotton ball before using
- After use clean the thermometer from stem to bulb using a wet soapy cotton ball in a circular movement
- Rinse the thermometer holding from the stem with bulb downward under running water
- Immerse the thermometer in a disinfectant solution as per hospital policy
- Dry and store in the container and cover the cap
- Use disposable sheath for electronic thermometers and wipe probe with 70% alcohol
- Lotion thermometer can be wiped, using a dry cotton swab before storing in a container

Enamel Items

Various enamel articles used in hospitals include trays, kidney trays, basins, bowls, funnel, jugs, pint measure, urinals, bed pans, enema cans, buckets, bath tubs, sputum mugs, knife dish, soap dish, etc.

General Principles of Care

- Handle gently because enamelware gets chipped off easily and becomes unsafe for care.
- Do not boil for long periods and rapidly cool them, as enamel cannot withstand heat

- Wash enamelware immediately when some antiseptic reagents are used in it

Cleaning, Disinfecting and Sterilizing the Enamelware

- Empty the contents from the used enamelware
- Immerse the enamelware in a chlorine solution of 0.5%
- Wash the enamelware with cold water and then hot soapy water, and rinse using water jet/stream
- Dry the item by keeping in an inverted position. Store separately. Keep in an inverted position in the appropriate cupboard/shelf
- Bedpans can also be kept in direct sunlight
- If needed, boil the item in a big water-filled container. Item should be completely dipped in water and, boil it for 10 minutes
- If needed, wrap it in a piece of cloth and send for autoclaving
- Terminal disinfection of client's bed-side items like basin, feeding cup, bowls, kidney tray with chlorine or phenol
- Clean, dry and store

Stainless Steel Items

These items includes items mentioned under enamel items and the additional items are:

- **Forceps:** Artery, thumb, mosquito, kockers, towel clips, cheatle forcep, sponge-holding, etc.
- **Different needles:** Needles used for intramuscular (IM), intravenous (IV), subcutaneous (SC), intradermal (ID) injections, biopsy needles, suture needles– curved, straight, needles for lumbar puncture, sternal puncture paracentesis, etc.
- **Different scopes:** Blades of laryngoscope, bron-choscope and proctoscope
- **Sharp instruments:** Surgical blades, different scissors, razors, etc.
- **Miscellaneous items:** Spatulas, tongue depressors, tracheal airway, tube clamps, tracheostomy tubes, mouth gag, dilators, etc.

Cleaning, Disinfection and Sterilization of Stainless Steel Items

- Always immerse the used instruments in 0.5% of chlorine solution for 5 minutes
- Wash the instrument in cold running water, paying special attention to the tips, toothed end and grooves of forceps
- Separate sharp instruments from other blunt and fine-tip instruments
- Put a hard rubber cap on fine-tip instrument. Sort out instruments of the same size and tie together

- Dry them thoroughly, wrap and make different packs, e.g., bowls, forceps etc. and prepare for autoclaving
- Hinged instruments such as artery clamp must be open for sterilization

Needles

- Decontaminate all needles and flush with 0.5% chlorine solution
- Discard the disposable injection needle with syringe either in a puncture-proof container or destroy the needle in needle destroyer
- Send the puncture-resistant container for incineration
- Send stainless steel needles for autoclaving, packed with syringes in mizor
- Remove cannula/stylet of centesis and biopsy needles
- Flush centesis, biopsy needles with 0.5% chlorine solution, wash with soapy water and rinse in running water
- Dry them, pack and send for autoclaving

Proctoscope

- Pull out obturator from the proctoscope
- Immerse both obturator and speculum in 0.5% chlorine solution for minimum 10 minutes
- Discard the chlorine solution and remove items
- Rinse in cold water and wash in soapy solution
- Boil for 10 minutes before storing
- Pack and send the proctoscope for autoclaving

Sharp Instruments

- Immerse the sharp instruments in 0.5% chlorine solution or in 2% glutaraldehyde for 20–30 minutes.
- Remove from the disinfectant solution, rinse in cold water, wipe dry using a dry piece of sterile cloth.
- Store in an appropriate container.

Laryngoscope

- Wipe off saliva from the blade of the laryngoscope, using a dry piece of clean gauze.
- Detach the blade and immerse in 2% glutaraldehyde solution for 20–30 minutes.
- Remove the blade from the solution, using cheatle forceps and dry it with a dry piece of sterile gauze.
- Re-attach the blade to the laryngoscope and store in the leather bag in resuscitation trolley.

Fiberoptics with Camera Items

Items consists of gastroscope, endoscope, bronchoscope, laparoscope, ventriculoscope, arthroscope, etc.

- All fiber optic scopes are expensive items and require careful handling

- Detach camera from the scope
- Wipe off the fiberoptic using a gauze soaked in 2% glutaraldehyde to disinfect
- Hang the scope or keep in container to avoid damage.

Items using Electric Current

Suction Machine

- Wear clean gloves before handling the jars
- Add the sodium hypochlorite solution in a sufficient amount to decontaminate the contents
- Disconnect the tubes, immerse fully in the sodium hypochlorite solution for 10 minutes
- Flush the tubings with soapy water and rinse with plain water
- Empty the contents of glass jars into sewage and flush with plain water
- Wash the jars with detergent and rinse thoroughly
- Keep jars inverted at a dry, safe place to remove water
- Dry and wrap the jars and tubing in fine cloth for autoclaving
- Ensure intact wiring of the electric cord with proper earthing
- Wipe the cord with piece of clean dry cloth daily
- Use oil, grease for wheels
- Change the jars and tubing, if client requires suction for more than 24 hours
- Periodically send the machine to workshop
- Attach fresh catheter to the tubings each time the machine is used
- Empty the jars daily, irrespective of the amount of secretion aspirated

Linen

Common linen items used in hospital are:

- Bed sheets, draw sheets, counterpanes, packsheets
- Cloth covers for pillow, mattress, blanket, IV fluid bottle, hot water bottle, ice collar, air cushion, inhaler cover, sandbag cover
- Pillows, blankets and mattresses
- Bath blankets
- Curtains
- Towels: face, bath, hand, dressing, treatment, anesthesia, doctors towel
- Wrappers for tray, dressing sets, bowls, syringes,
- Patients clothes– jacket gown, shirt, pyjama, leggings
- Staff clothes, shirt, pyjama, caps, head tie
- Binders
- Restraints–elbow, jacket, cribnet and mittens
- Wringers
- Guard, spinal sheets
- Diet napkin, tray covers
- Dusters

Cleaning and Disinfection of Linen

- Send the dirty linen to laundry for washing and ironing
- Dust the mattress regularly of any food particles using a piece of clean damp cloth
- Protect the mattress with mackintosh from potential areas of soiling like the middle part
- Use small rubber/plastic mackintosh over top linen during therapeutic procedures
- Remove fresh stains, using an appropriate solvent
- Routinely inspect and send torn linen for repair in time to prevent further damage
- Send instructions on time to keep extra linen at hand
- Fold and keep different linen sorted out in cupboards with proper labels
- Check your inventory periodically and keep a proper record
- Never put used linen on the floor. Use laundry bags.
- Prepare a record of linen sent for laundry
- Neatly store laundered linen in the cupboard.

Note:

- Contaminated linen need to be soaked in a big plastic bucket/drum with chlorine 0.5% solution minimum for 10 minutes for decontamination
- Rinse in cold water to prepare for autoclaving
- Dry in the sun
- Send for autoclaving and store neatly in appropriate cupboards

Removal of Stains from the Linen

- **Tea, cocoa, coffee:** Spread the cloth over a hole and pour boiling water from a reasonable height. Rub lemon, boric powder over the stain and put for sunning. Wash with soap and water. Milk and sodium carbonate can also be used to remove stains and then the cloth can be washed with soap and water
- **Vegetable stains:** Apply salt over the stain and pour hot water from a height or else apply ammonia (NH_3) or Hydrogen peroxide (H_2O_2) solution.
- **Gentian violet stain:** Soak the stained area in a bowl/mug with raw milk for several hours then wash as usual
- **Ink stain:** Wet the stain area with cold water, sprinkle salt and rub lemon juice or apply NH_3 and wash as usual
- **Medicine stain:** Apply alcohol/spirit and wash
- **Iron stain:** Rub the stain with lemon juice and salt or pour kerosene. Wash with soap and water and dry in sun
- **Grease and oil:** Soak the stained area in a mug filled with kerosene oil, rub it lightly, wash with soap and water and dry in the sun. Thereafter, put a blotting paper over the cleaned area of stain and iron it

- **Paint and varnish:** Same as grease and oil, turpentine can also be used to soak, in addition to kerosene oil
- **Perspiration:** Put a few drops of ammonia, over the stained area and wash as usual

Blankets

- Woollen blankets should be dusted in an open area and spread in sunlight for sunning both sides for 15–20 minutes each to prevent frequent washing and to disinfect, using ultra-violet rays of sun
- Soak soiled blankets in cold water and dry in the sun before sending to the laundry
- Store blankets in cupboards with naphthalene balls to protect them from moths

Mattresses and Pillows

- Clean and wipe any fluid contamination with chlorine bleach, disinfect before putting in the sun.
- Place mattresses and pillows on a dry, flat, clean surface for sunning both sides for 15–20 minutes each to disinfect surfaces.
- Do not fold the mattress at acute angles to prevent formation of folds.
- Store with cover on it by placing on the beds or a long flat surface, piled one over another in linen store to prolong life of the item. Do not store in the patient treatment area.
- Place anti-moth balls in the cupboard or in between the piles wrapped in thin perforated cloth to protect from moths and mites and to prolong the life.

Furniture

Types of Furniture

- **Wooden:** Tables, chairs, cupboards, shock blocks, stools, patients attendant bed/ settings, sofa, cardiac tables, benches, stands for drying articles
- **Metal (Iron/steel):** Tables, chairs, cupboard, beds, trolleys (dressing, patient transfer stretcher), treatment tables, lockers, foot stools, wheelchair, IV stand, bed cradle, backrest, screens, wheel commode, monitor stand, cradles in nursery, patients diet trolley, ward diet trolleys, bed keys, cylinder key, bed rolling, etc.

Cleaning and Disinfection of Furniture

- Wipe the dust on furniture, using a piece of dry soft cloth daily followed by damp dusting.
- Wipe any water or chemical from the polished surface of furniture to avoid stains and damage to the polished surface.

- Disinfect iron, steel, plastic furniture and incubators using 2% glutaraldehyde, 2% savlon every day after discharge or death of the patient. Trolleys, lockers, IV stands should be disinfected daily.
- **Patient beds and lockers:** To be cleaned and disinfected daily.
- Use insecticides pure or in dilution as per the manufacture's instructions to spray in crevices/grooves of wooden, iron, stainless steel furniture items like tables, lockers, cupboards, etc.
- Use oil/grease for wheels of chairs, trolleys, beds.
- Do not over load the shelves of cupboards.
- Protect wooden furniture from fire.
- Ensure timely repair of handles, wheels, railings.
- Keep an inventory of the furniture in the stock register and indent books.
- Put proper labels in different cupboards for the items contained in them.
- Periodically clean and damp dust the cupboards by emptying them and changing paper linings in them.

Every organization big or small need variety of materials for patient care. Materials are the major cost factor in an organization. It is one of the very important functions of the management. In health care institutions about 40% of budgetary allocation is on procurement and management of stores.

NURSES ACTIVITIES IN EQUIPMENT AND SUPPLY MANAGEMENT

Managing supplies and equipment involves much more than keeping the storage area neat. Managing a hospitals nursing department includes managing the supplies and equipment needed for patient care and treatment. The head nurse/nurse manager is responsible for proper management of equipment and supplies required for patient care.

Following are the key activities of nurse managers

- **Procurement:** It involves several steps:
  - Requirements must be established
  - Send requisitions of the supplies and equipment through proper channels
  - Place indent by specifying a detailed description of equipment, specifications including whether the requirement is fresh or additional or replacement.
- **Receiving:** When the indent items arrive in work place. They must be properly received, inspected and counted.
- **Storing:** The supplies and equipments are stored in appropriate place and in a correct way. Group-wise and alphabetical arrangement helps in identification and retrieval. Monitor expiry date.

Issuing, Distribution and Maintaining Inventory

Nurses managers must make sure that their nurses have the supplies they need. She distributes the supplies in the morning for the use to the operational level nurses. She also ensures that adequate supplies are there for evening and night staff.

She maintains the current inventory of equipment and inspects and properly issues for use. She is responsible for accountability of supplies and equipment.

Repairing and Disposal

Equipment found damaged must be sent for repair. The nurse manager should ensure the quality of equipment keeping in mind the safety of the patient. She showed conduct routine checking of equipment, label, isolate or remove facility equipment to prevent injury.

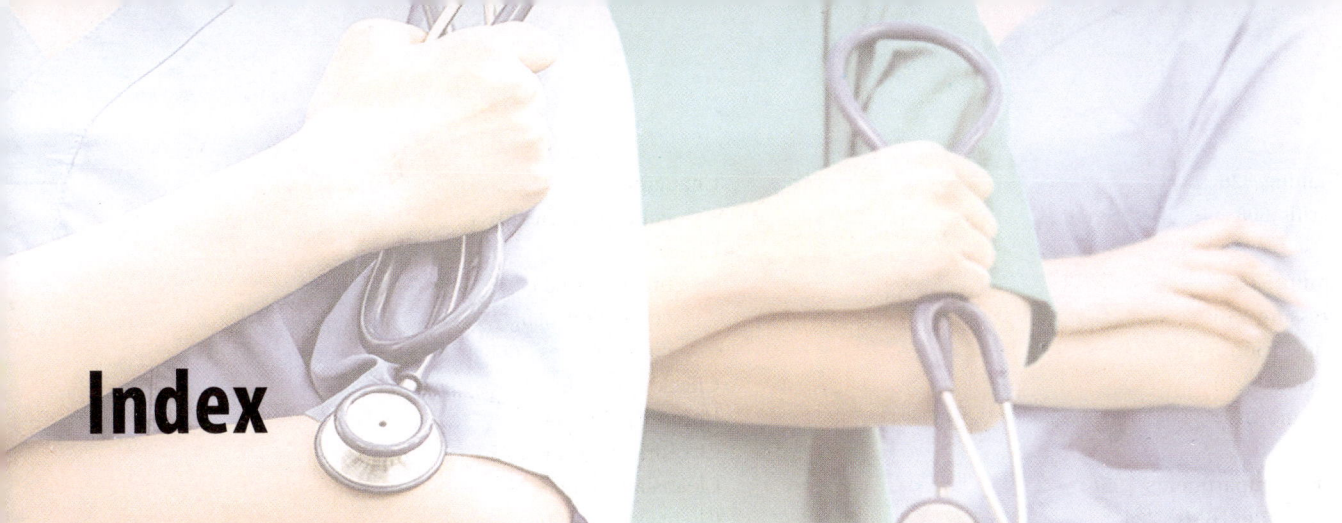

Index

Refer 'f' for figure and 't' for table respectively

C

W

Z

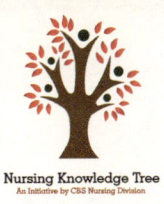

Nursing Knowledge Tree
An Initiative by CBS Nursing Division

Nursing Books Catalogue 2021-22

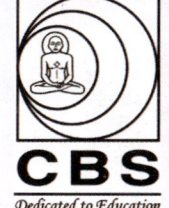

CBS
Dedicated to Education

Books for All

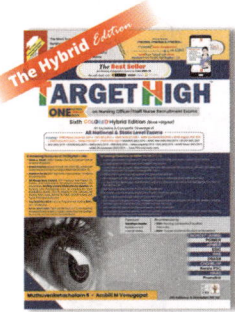

Target High
Muthuvenkatachalam S et al.
978-93-90619-55-9
6/e, 2022
MRP: ₹1499/-

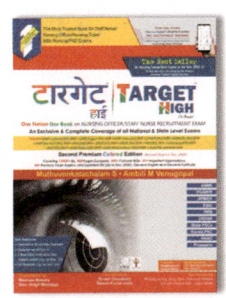

Target High (In Hindi)
Muthuvenkatachalam S et al.
978-81-94025-65-8
2/e, 2020
MRP: ₹1299/-

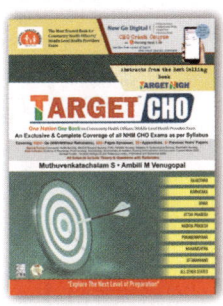

Target CHO
Muthuvenkatachalam S et al.
978-81-940256-0-3
1/e, 2020
MRP: ₹495/-

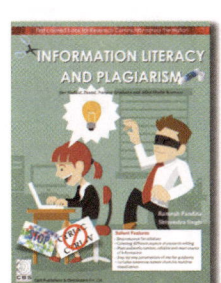

Information Literacy and Plagiarism
for Medical, Dental, Nursing Graduates
and Allied Health Sciences
Ramesh Pandita et al.
978-93-86827-13-5
1/e, 2018
MRP: ₹370/-

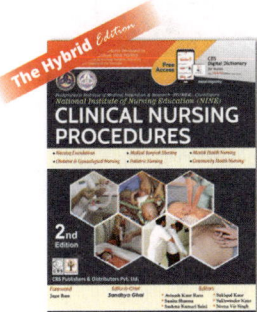

PGI NINE
Clinical Nursing Procedures
Sandhya Ghai
978-93-89261-97-4
2/e, 2020
MRP: ₹1295/-

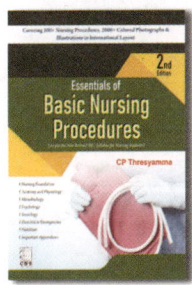

Essentials of
Basic Nursing Procedures
CP Thresyamma
978-81-94523-47-5
2/e, 2020
MRP: ₹795/-

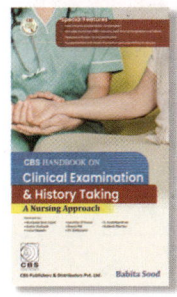

CBS Nursing Drug Guide
2020-2021
Yogesh Gulati et al.
978-93-88178-53-2
1/e, 2020
MRP: ₹1050/-

CBS Handbook on
Clinical Examination & History Taking
A Nursing Approach
Babita Sood
978-81-948693-9-9
1/e, 2021
MRP: ₹350/-

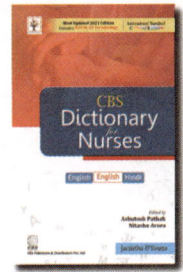

CBS Dictionary for Nurses
Jacintha D'Souza
978-93-90619-06-1
1/e, 2021
MRP: ₹595/-

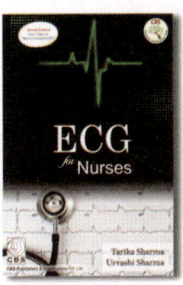

ECG for Nurses
Tarika Sharma et al.
978-93-89261-88-2
1/e, 2019
MRP: ₹350/-

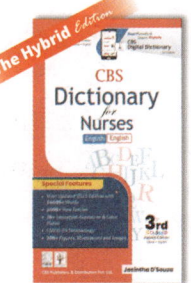

CBS Dictionary for Nurses
Jacintha D'Souza
978-93-90619-29-0
3/e, 2022
MRP: ₹450/-

 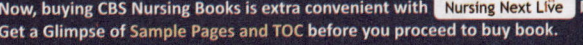

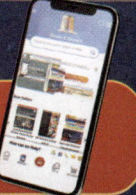

Community Health Nursing

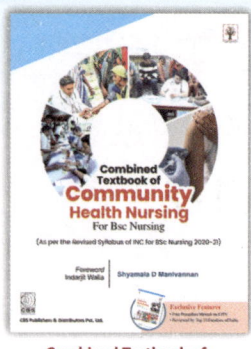

Combined Textbook of Community Health Nursing
For BSc Nursing
Shyamala D Manivannan
978-93-90619-37-5
1/e, 2022
TBA

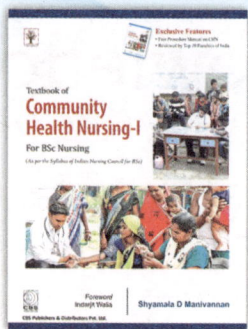

Textbook of Community Health Nursing-I
For BSc Nursing
Shyamala D Manivannan
978-81-23927-01-5
1/e, 2018
MRP: ₹750/-

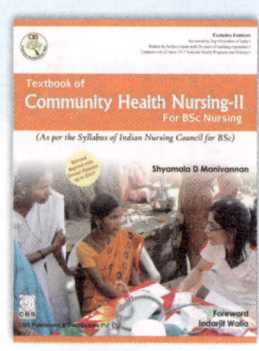

Textbook of Community Health Nursing-II
For BSc Nursing
Shyamala D Manivannan
978-93-86827-22-7
1/e, 2018
MRP: ₹450/-

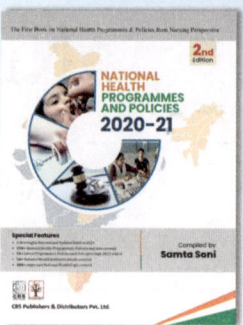

National Health Programmes & Policies 2020-21
Samta Soni
978-93-90619-13-9
2/e, 2022
MRP: ₹695/-

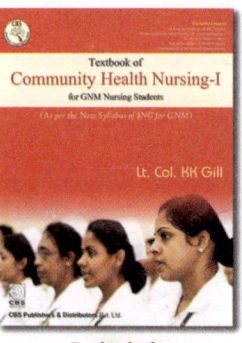

Textbook of Community Health Nursing-I
For GNM Nursing Students
Lt. Col. KK Gill
978-93-86827-17-3
1/e, 2018
MRP: ₹550/-

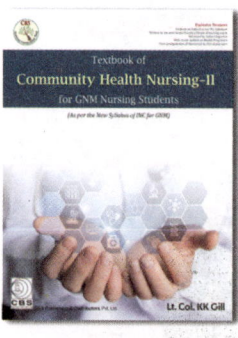

Textbook of Community Health Nursing-II
for GNM Nursing Students
Lt. Col. KK Gill
978-93-88178-57-0
1/e, 2019
MRP: ₹525/-

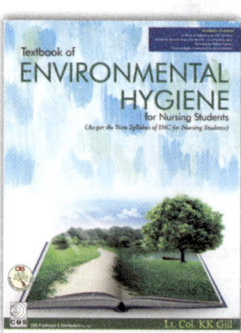

Textbook of Environmental Hygiene
for Nursing Students
Lt. Col. KK Gill
978-93-88178-56-3
1/e, 2018-19
MRP: ₹225/-

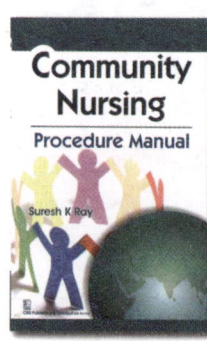

Community Nursing Procedure Manual
Suresh K Ray
978-81-23929-35-4
1/e, 2017
MRP: ₹265/-

Procedure Manual for Community Health Nursing
N Gowri et al.
978-81-948693-6-8
1/e, 2021
MRP: ₹195/-

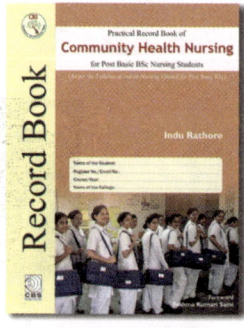

Practical Record Book of Community Health Nursing-I
for BSc Nursing 2nd Year Students
M Vijaya Santhi
978-81-23926-84-1
1/e, 2016
MRP: ₹450/-

Practical Record Book of Community Health Nursing-II
for BSc Nursing 4th Year Students
M Vijaya Santhi
978-93-88108-77-5
1/e, 2018-19
MRP: ₹575/-

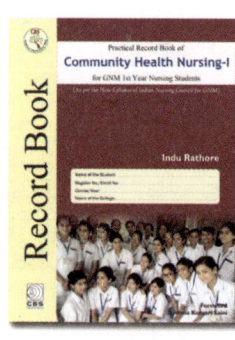

Practical Record Book of Community Health Nursing
for Post Basic BSc Nursing Students
Indu Rathore
978-93-86827-06-7
1/e, 2017
MRP: ₹475/-

Practical Record Book of Community Health Nursing-I
for GNM 1st Year Nursing Students
Indu Rathore
978-93-86827-07-4
1/e, 2018-19
MRP: ₹350/-

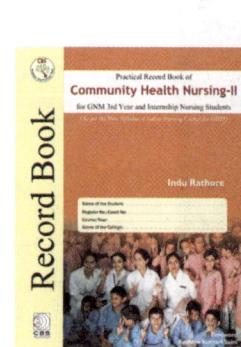

Practical Record Book of Community Health Nursing-II
for GNM 3rd Year and Internship Nursing Students
Indu Rathore
978-93-86827-30-2
1/e, 2018-19
MRP: ₹395/-

Buy online :
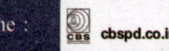 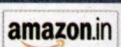 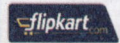 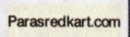 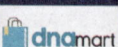

Nursing Foundation

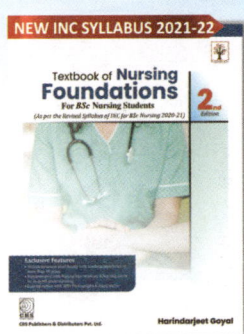

NEW INC SYLLABUS 2021-22

**Textbook of
Nursing Foundations
for BSc Nursing Students**
Harindarjeet Goyal
978-93-90619-12-2
2/e, 2022
MRP: ₹950/-

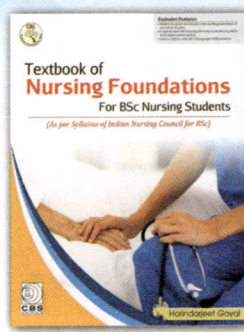

**Textbook of
Nursing Foundations
for BSc Nursing Students**
Harindarjeet Goyal
978-93-88108-94-2
1/e, 2020
MRP: ₹950/-

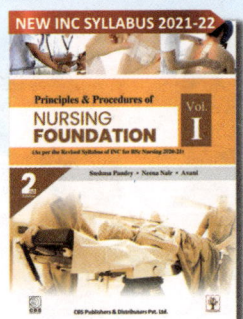

NEW INC SYLLABUS 2021-22

**Principles & Procedures of
Nursing Foundation Vol-I
for BSc Nursing**
Sushma Pandey et al.
978-93-90619-57-3
2/e, 2022
TBA

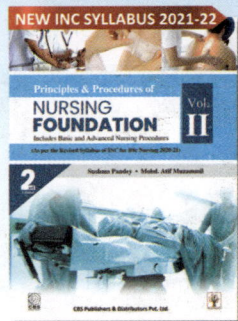

NEW INC SYLLABUS 2021-22

**Principles & Procedures of
Nursing Foundation Vol-II
for BSc Nursing**
Sushma Pandey et al.
978-93-90619-19-1
2/e, 2022
TBA

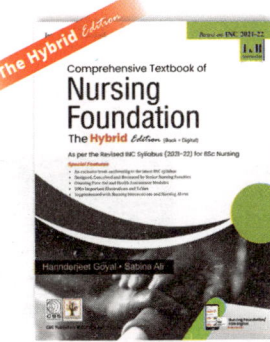

**Textbook of
Nursing Foundations
for GNM Nursing Students**
Harindarjeet Goyal
978-93-90619-70-2
1/e, 2022
MRP: ₹850/-

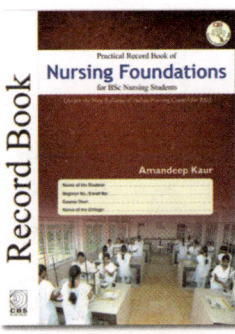

**Practical Record Book of
Nursing Foundations
for BSc Nursing Students**
Amandeep Kaur
978-93-88108-96-6
1/e, 2018-19
MRP: ₹425/-

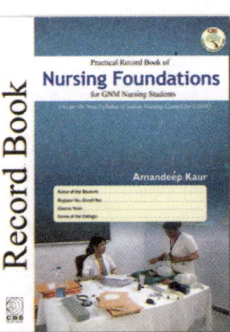

**Practical Record Book of
Nursing Foundations
for GNM Nursing Students**
Amandeep Kaur
978-93-88178-50-1
1/e, 2018-19
MRP: ₹350/-

Medical Surgical Nursing

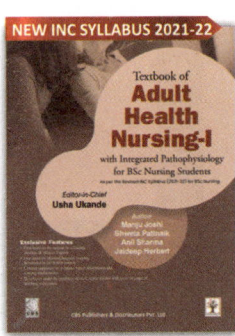

NEW INC SYLLABUS 2021-22

**Textbook of
Adult Health Nursing-I
with Integrated Pathophysiology
for BSc Nursing Students**
Usha Ukande
978-93-90619-20-7
1/e, 2022
TBA

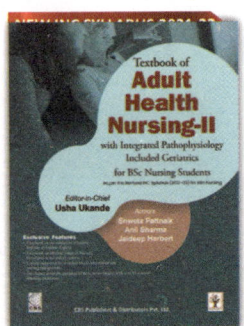

NEW INC SYLLABUS 2021-22

**Textbook of
Adult Health Nursing-II
with Integrated Pathophysiology
Included Geriatrics for BSc Nursing Students**
Usha Ukande
978-93-90619-86-3
1/e, 2022
TBA

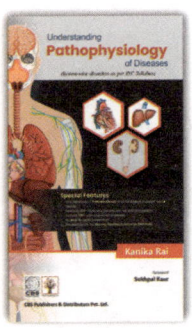

**Understanding
Pathophysiology of Diseases**
Kanika Rai
978-93-90619-11-5
1/e, 2022
MRP: ₹395/-

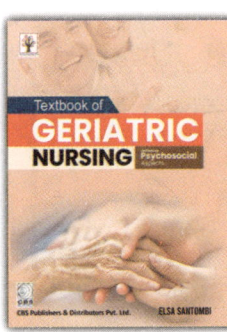

**Textbook of
Geriatric Nursing
Including Psychosocial Aspects**
Elsa Santombi
978-93-90619-79-5
1/e, 2022
TBA

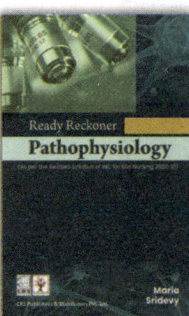

**Ready Reckoner
Pathophysiology
for Nurses**
Maria et al.
978-93-90619-05-4
1/e, 2022
TBA

CBS

MSN/Pharmacology/Pathology

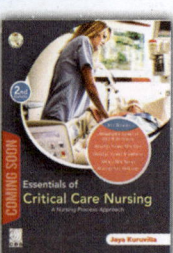

Essentials of
Critical Care Nursing
A Nursing Process Approach
Jaya Kuruvilla
978-93-90619-61-0
2/e, 2022

TBA

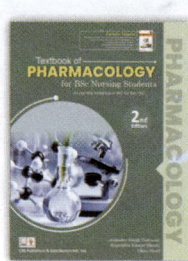

Textbook of
Pharmacology
For BSc Nursing Students
Joginder Singh Pathania et al.
978-93-90619-27-6
2/e, 2022

MRP: ₹650/-

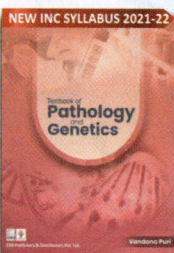

Textbook of
Pathology and Genetics
Vandana Puri
978-93-90619-87-0
1/e, 2022

TBA

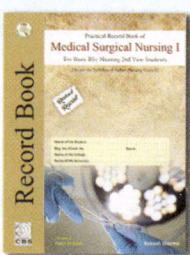

Practical Record Book of
Medical Surgical Nursing I
for Basic BSc Nursing 2nd Year Students
Rakesh Sharma
978-81-23928-00-5
1/e, 2018-19

MRP: ₹550/-

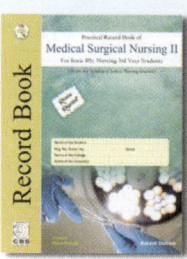

Practical Record Book of
Medical Surgical Nursing II
for Basic BSc Nursing 3nd Year Students
Rakesh Sharma
978-81-23928-01-2
1/e, 2018-19

MRP: ₹475/-

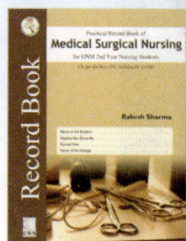

Practical Record Book of
Medical Surgical Nursing
for GNM 2nd Year Nursing Stude
Rakesh Sharma
978-93-86827-04-3
1/e, 2017

MRP: ₹475/-

Child Health Nursing & Pediatric Nursing

Exclusive Marketing & Distribution Rights

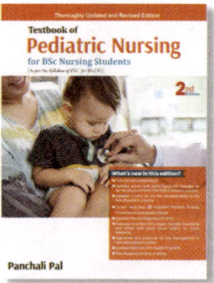

Textbook of
Pediatric Nursing
for BSc Nursing Students
Panchali Pal
978-81-948693-2-0
2/e, 2021

MRP: ₹795/-

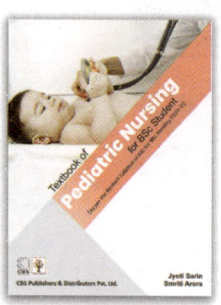

Textbook of
Pediatric Nursing
for BSc Nursing Students
Jyoti Sarin et al.
978-93-90619-78-8
1/e, 2022

TBA

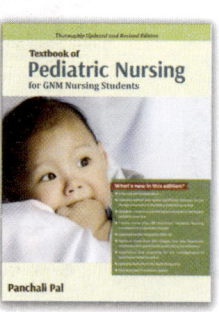

Textbook of
Pediatric Nursing
for GNM Nursing Students
Panchali Pal
978-93-90619-71-9
1/e, 2022

TBA

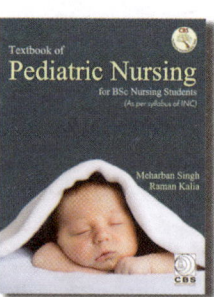

Textbook of
Pediatric Nursing
for BSc Nursing Students
Meharban Singh et al.
978-93-88108-72-0
1/e, 2018

MRP: ₹725/-

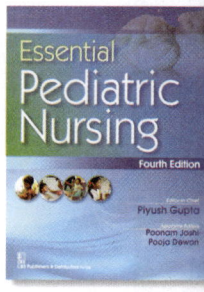

Essential
Pediatric Nursing
Piyush Gupta
978-93-86217-87-5
4/e, 2017

MRP: ₹750/-

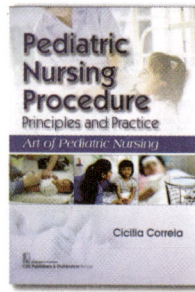

Procedure Manual for
Pediatric Nursing
Niyati Das
978-93-88108-86-7
1/e, 2018

MRP: ₹325/-

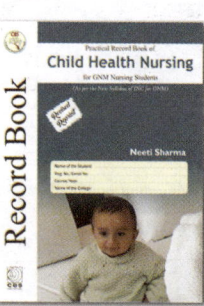

Pediatric Nursing Procedure
Principles and Practice
Cicilia Correia
978-93-86310-74-3
1/e, 2017

MRP: ₹450/-

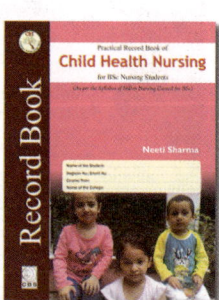

Practial Record Book of
Child Health Nursing
for GNM Nursing Students
Neeti Sharma
978-93-86827-53-1
1/e, 2017

MRP: ₹325/-

Practial Record Book of
Child Health Nursing
for BSc Nursing Students
Neeti Sharma
978-93-86827-05-0
1/e, 2017

MRP: ₹310/-

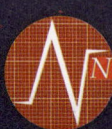

Read, Review & Buy

Now, buying CBS Nursing Books is extra convenient with Nursing Next Live Mobile App.
Get a Glimpse of Sample Pages and TOC before you proceed to buy book.

Download the App from
Google Playstore or scan
here to download

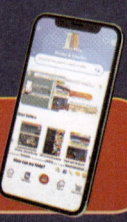

Mental Health Nursing & Psychiatric Nursing

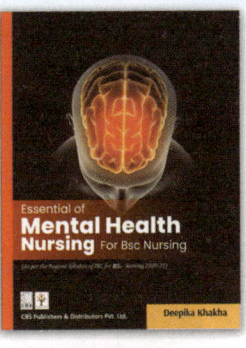

Essential of Mental Health Nursing
for BSc Nursing
Deepika Khakha
978-93-90619-73-3
1/e, 2022

TBA

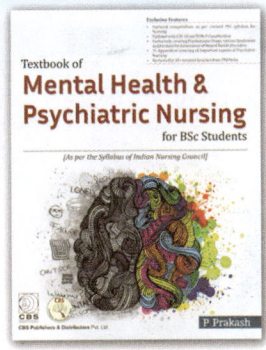

Textbook of Mental Health & Psychiatric Nursing
P Prakash
978-93-89261-91-2
1/e, 2019

MRP: ₹625/-

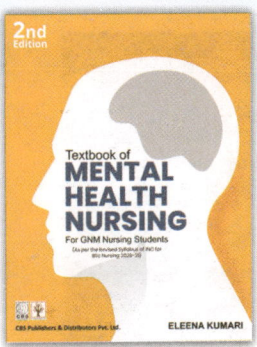

Textbook of Mental Health Nursing
for GNM Nursing Students
Eleena Kumari
978-93-90619-72-6
2/e, 2022

MRP: ₹395/-

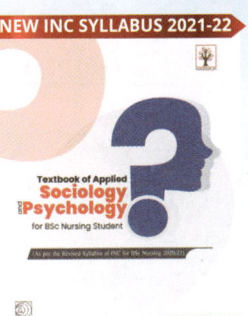

Textbook of Applied Sociology and Psychology
for BSc Nursing Students
P Prakash
978-93-90619-54-2
1/e, 2022

MRP: ₹395/-

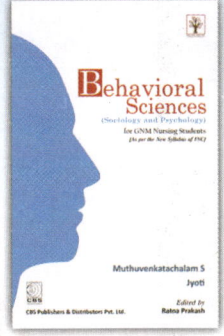

Behavioral Sciences
(Sociology and Psychology)
Muthuvenkatachalam S et al.
978-93-90619-04-7
1/e , 2021

MRP: ₹350/-

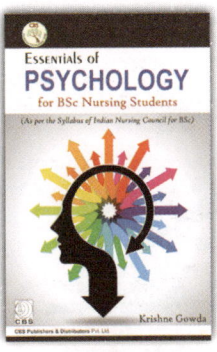

Essentials of Psychology
for BSc Nursing Students
Krishne Gowda
978-81-23927-11-4
1/e, 2017

MRP: ₹340/-

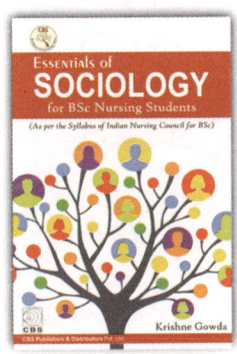

Essentials of Sociology
for BSc Nursing Students
Krishne Gowda
978-93-86217-51-6
1/e, 2017

MRP: ₹395/-

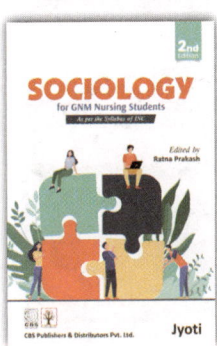

Sociology
for GNM Nursing Students
Jyoti
978-81-948693-1-3
2/e, 2022

MRP: ₹210/-

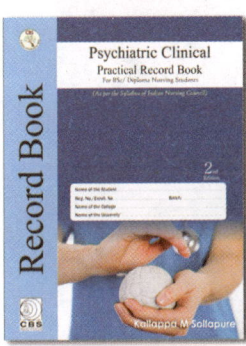

Psychiatric Clinical Practical Record Book
for BSc/Diploma Nursing Students
Kallappa M Sollapure
978-93-88108-81-2
2/e, 2018-19

MRP: ₹395/-

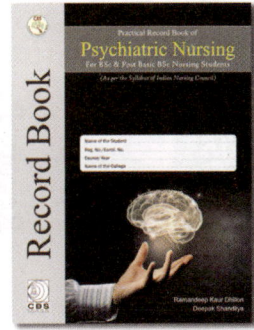

Practial Record Book of Psychiatric Nursing
for BSc & Post Basic BSc Nursing Students
Ramandeep Kaur Dhillon
978-93-88108-80-5
1/e, 2019

MRP: ₹415/-

Midwifery, Obstetrical & Gynecological Nursing

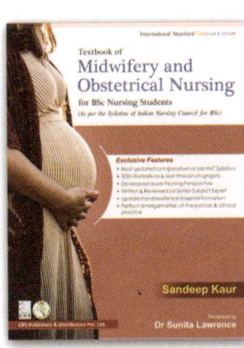

Textbook of Midwifery & Obstetrical Nursing
for BSc Nursing Students
Sandeep Kaur
978-93-89261-90-5
1/e, 2020

MRP: ₹995/-

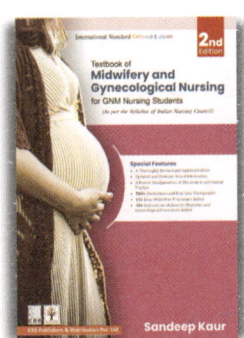

Textbook of Midwifery & Gynecological Nursing
for GNM Nursing Students
Sandeep Kaur
978-93-90619-18-4
2/e, 2022

MRP: ₹895/-

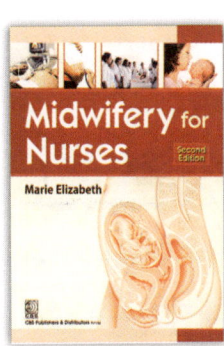

Textbook of Midwifery for Nurses
Marie Elizabeth
978-81-23922-14-0
2/e, 2018

MRP: ₹650/-

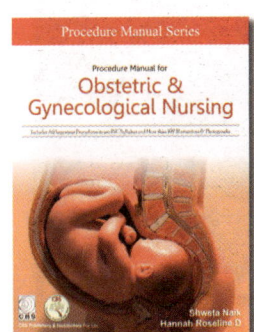

Procedure Manual for Obstetric & Gynecological Nursing
Sheweta Naik et al.
978-93-88178-60-0
1/e, 2018-19

MRP: ₹235/-

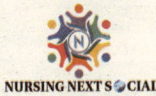

Midwifery, Obstetrical & Gynecological Nursing

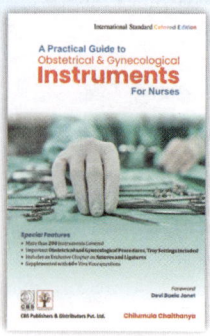

A Practical Guide to Obstetric & Gynecological Instruments for Nurses
Chilumula Chaithanya
978-93-90619-03-0
1/e, 2022

MRP: ₹250/-

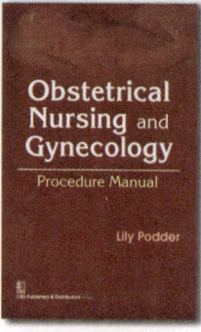

Obstetrical Nursing and Gynecology Procedure Manual
Lily Podder
978-81-23925-81-3
1/e, 2017

MRP: ₹265/-

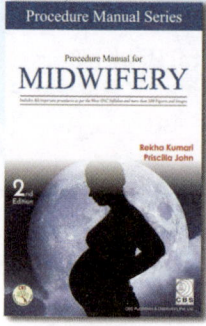

Procedure Manual for Midwifery
Rekha Kumari et al.
978-93-89261-94-3
2/e, 2019

MRP: ₹225/-

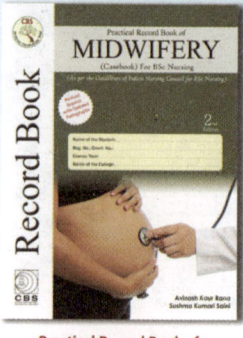

Practical Record Book of Midwifery (Casebook) For BSc Nursing
Avinash Kaur Rana et al.
978-93-88178-65-5
2/e (R/R), 2018-19

MRP: ₹675/-

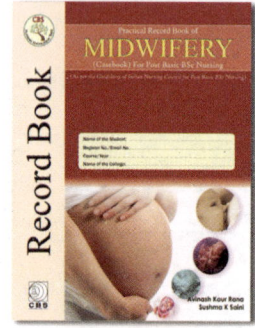

Practical Record Book of Midwifery (Casebook) for Post Basic BSc Nursing
Avinash Kaur Rana et al.
978-81-23927-07-7
1/e, 2016

MRP: ₹375/-

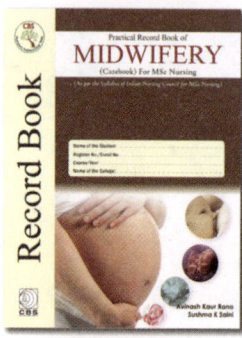

Practical Record Book of Midwifery (Casebook) for MSc Nursing
Avinash Kaur Rana et al.
978-93-86217-97-4
1/e, 2017

MRP: ₹625/-

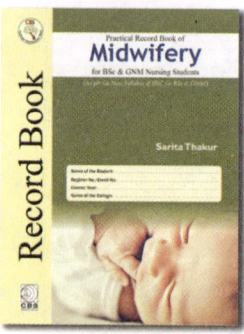

Practical Record Book of Midwifery for BSc & GNM Nursing Students
Sarita Thakur
978-93-86827-33-3
1/e, 2017

MRP: ₹415/-

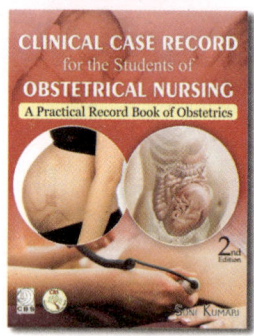

Clinical Case Record for the Students of Obstetrical Nursing
A Practical Record Book of Obstetrics
Soni Kumari
978-93-88178-51-8
2/e, 2018

MRP: ₹475/-

Nursing Research/Biostatistics

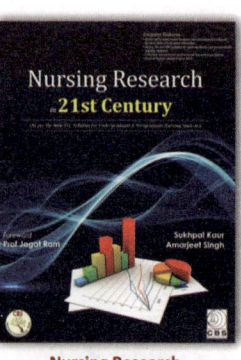

Nursing Research in 21st Century
Sukhpal Kaur et al.
978-93-89261-89-9
1/e, 2020

MRP: ₹725/-

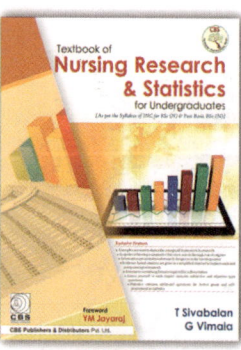

Textbook of Nursing Research & Statistics for Undergraduates
T Sivabalan et al.
978-93-88178-61-7
1/e, 2018

MRP: ₹525/-

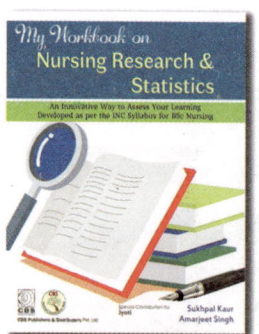

My Workbook on Nursing Research & Statistics
Sukhpal Kaur et al.
978-93-88108-75-1
1/e, 2019

MRP: ₹150/-

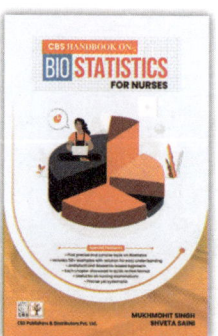

CBS Handbook on Biostatistics for Nurses
Mukhmohit Singh et al.
978-93-90619-10-8
1/e, 2022

MRP: ₹195/-

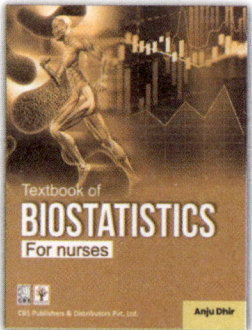

Textbook of Biostatistics for Nurses
Anju Dhir
978-93-90619-47-4
1/e, 2022

TBA

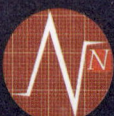

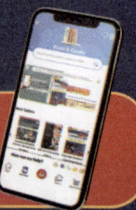

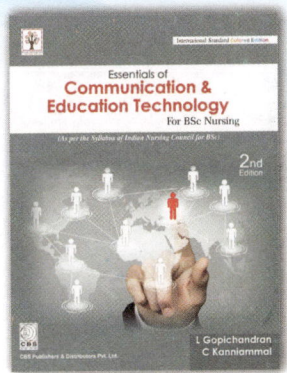

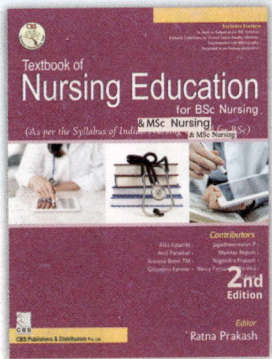

Essentials of
Communication & Education Technology
for BSc Nursing
L Gopichandran et al.
978-93-88178-58-7
2/e, 2019

MRP: ₹495/-

Textbook of
Nursing Education
for BSc & MSc Nursing
Ratna Prakash
978-93-86827-34-0
1/e, 2018

MRP: ₹450/-

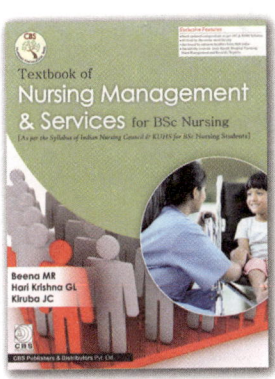

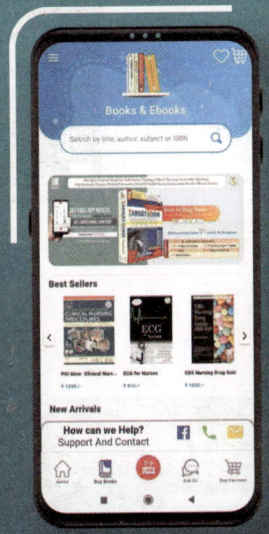

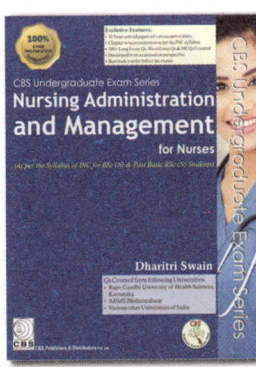

Textbook of
Nursing Management & Services
for BSc Nursing
Beena MR et al.
978-93-88178-62-4
1/e, 2019

MRP: ₹625/-

Textbook of Nursing
Management & Leadership
Johny Joseph Kutty
978-93-90619-40-5
1/e, 2022

MRP: MRPV

CBS Undergraduate Exam Series
Nursing Administration
and Management for Nurses
Dharitri Swain
978-93-86827-42-5
1/e, 2018

MRP: ₹350/-

Read, Review & Buy

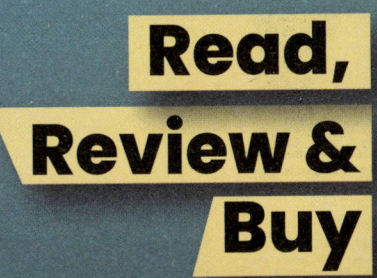

Now, buying CBS Nursing Books is extra convenient with Nursing Next Live Mobile App.

Get a Glimpse of **Sample Pages and TOC** before you proceed to buy books.

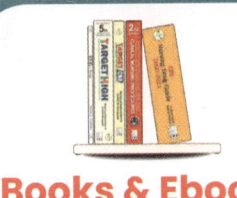

Books & Ebooks
Section is Live Now

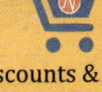

Best Discounts & Special Offers on all the Books.

Microbiology

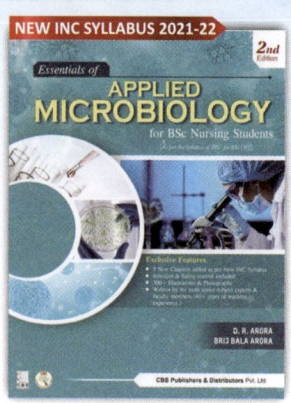
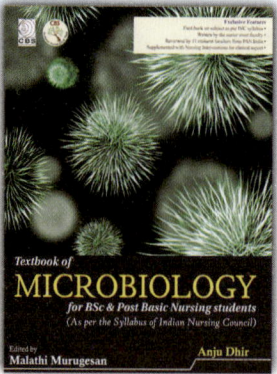
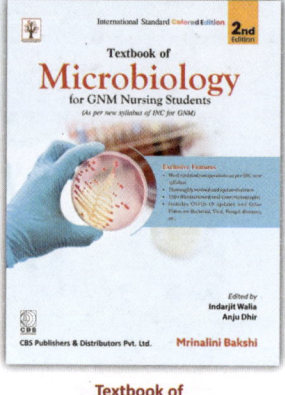
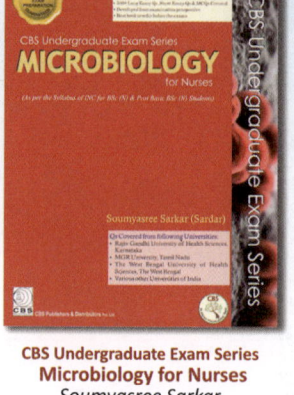

**Essentials of
Applied Microbiology
for BSc Nursing Students**
D.R. Arora et al.
978-81-945234-4-4
2/e, 2020

MRP: ₹575/-

**Textbook of
Microbiology
for BSc & Post Basic Nursing Students**
Anju Dhir
978-93-88108-82-9
1/e, 2018

MRP: ₹725/-

**Textbook of
Microbiology
for GNM Nursing Students**
Mrinalini Bakshi
978-93-90619-12-2
2/e, 2021

MRP: ₹225/-

**CBS Undergraduate Exam Series
Microbiology for Nurses**
Soumyasree Sarkar
978-93-86310-49-1
1/e, 2017

MRP: ₹275/-

English/First Aid/Computer

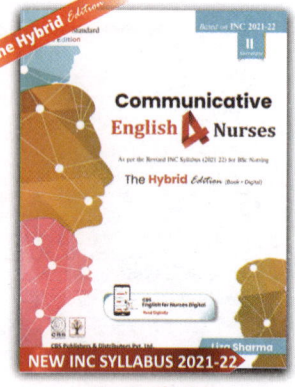
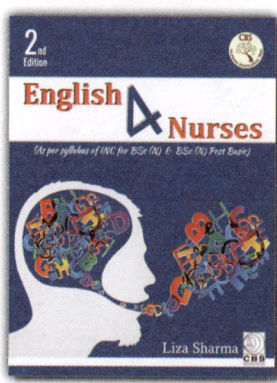
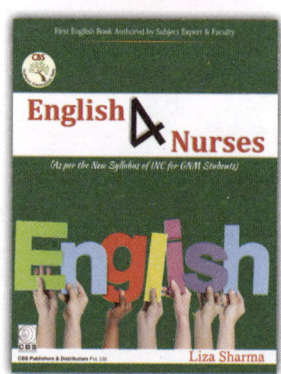
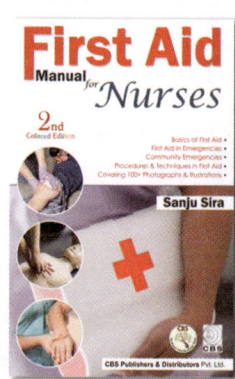

**Communicative
English 4 Nurses
for BSc Nursing Students**
Liza Sharma
978-93-90619-26-9
1/e, 2022

TBA

English 4 Nurses (BSc)
Liza Sharma
978-93-89261-95-0
2/e, 2019

MRP: ₹415/-

English 4 Nurses (GNM)
Liza Sharma
978-93-86827-09-8
1/e, 2017

MRP: ₹350/-

First Aid Manual for Nurses
Sanju Sira
978-93-88178-55-6
2/e, 2019

MRP: ₹310/-

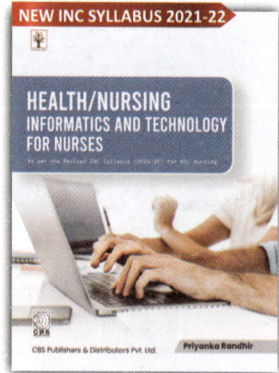
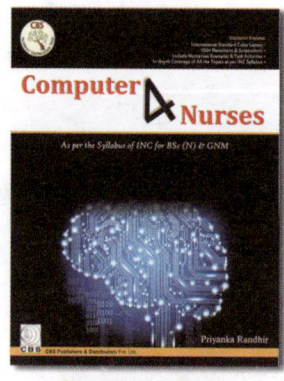

**Health/Nursing Informatics and
Technology for Nurses**
Priyanka Randhir
978-93-90619-21-4
1/e, 2022

TBA

Computer 4 Nurses
Priyanka Randhir
978-93-86310-48-4
1/e, 2017

MRP: ₹370/-

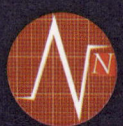
Read, Review & Buy
Now, buying CBS Nursing Books is extra convenient with Nursing Next Live Mobile App.
Get a Glimpse of Sample Pages and TOC before you proceed to buy book.

Download the App from Google Playstore or scan here to download
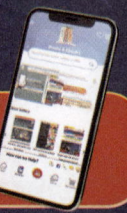

Anatomy & Physiology/Biochemistry & Nutrition

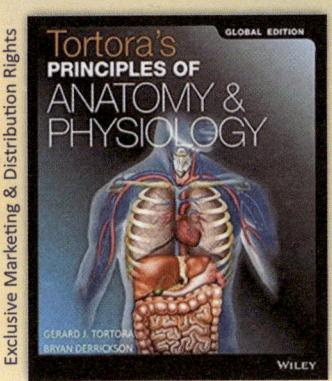

Tortora's Principles of
Anatomy & Physiology
Gerard J. Tortora
978-81-26567-61-4
GLOBAL Edition, 2017

MRP: ₹3495/-

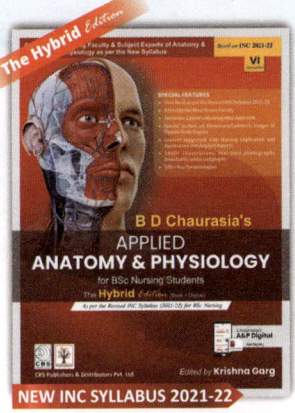

NEW INC SYLLABUS 2021-22

BD Chaurasia's
Applied Anatomy and Physiology
for BSc Nursing Students
Krishna Garg
978-93-90619-65-8
1/e, 2022

TBA

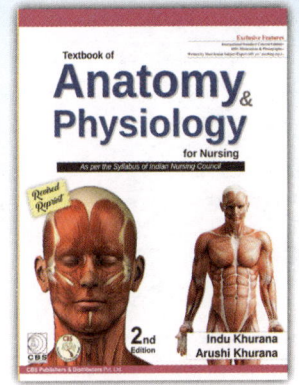

Textbook of
Anatomy & Physiology for Nursing
Indu Khurana et al.
978-93-86827-12-8
2/e, 2018

MRP: ₹995/-

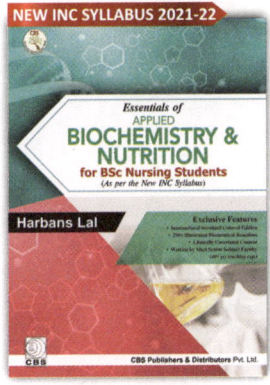

Essentials of APPLIED
Biochemistry & Nutrition
for BSc Nursing Students
Harbans Lal
978-93-90619-41-2
1/e, 2022

MRP: ₹450/-

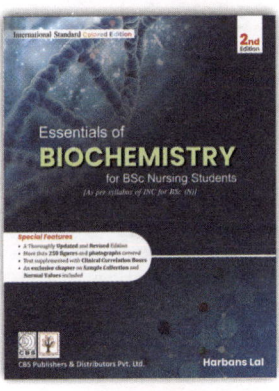

Essentials of
Biochemistry
for BSc Nursing Students
Harbans Lal
978-81-948693-3-7
2/e, 2022

MRP: ₹450/-

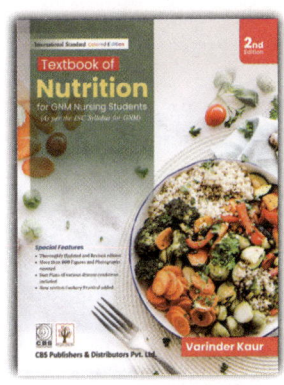

Textbook of
Nutrition
for GNM Nursing Students
Varinder Kaur
978-93-90619-02-3
2/e, 2022

MRP: ₹295/-

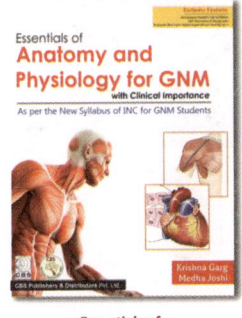

Essentials of
Anatomy & Physiology for GNM
with Clinical Importance
Krishna Garg et al.
978-93-86827-11-1
1/e, 2018

MRP: ₹475/-

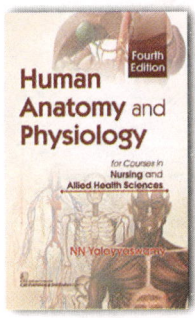

Human Anatomy and Physiology
for Nurses
N.N. Yalayyaswamy
978-93-87085-16-9
4/e, 2018

MRP: ₹395/-

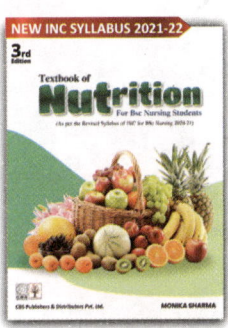

Textbook of
Nutrition
for BSc Nursing Students
Monika Sharma
978-93-90619-02-3
3/e, 2022

MRP: ₹370/-

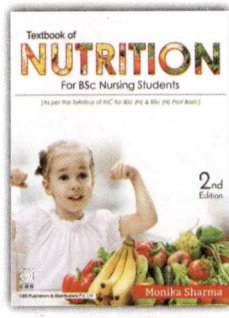

Textbook of Nutrition
for BSc Nursing Students
Monika Sharma
978-93-89261-92-9
2/e, 2019

MRP: ₹370/-

CBS

Nursing Knowledge Tree

NURSING NEXT SOCIAL

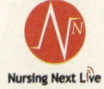
Nursing Next Live

Others

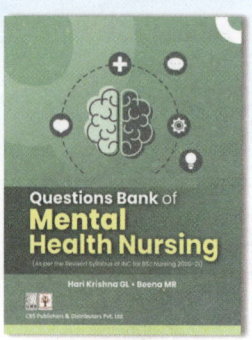

Questions Bank of
Mental Health Nursing
Hari Krishna GL et al.
978-93-90619-46-7
1/e, 2022

TBA

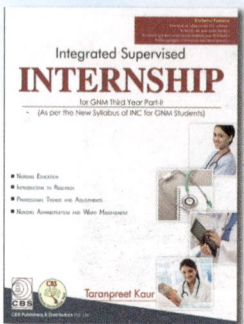

Integrated Supervised
Internship
for GNM Third Year Part-II
Taranpreet Kaur
978-93-88108-89-8
1/e, 2018

MRP: ₹415/-

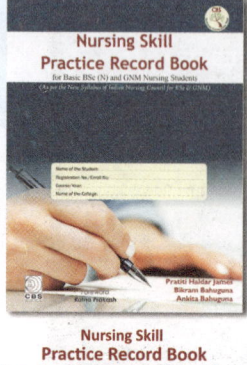

Nursing Skill
Practice Record Book
for Basic BSc (N) and GNM Nursing Students
Pratiti Haldar James et al.
978-93-86827-38-8
1/e, 2018-19

MRP: ₹310/-

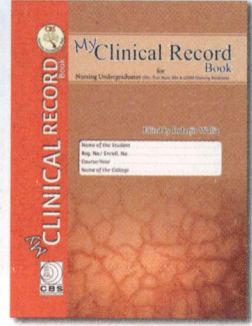

***My* Clinical Record Book**
for Nursing Undergraduates
(BSc, Post Basic BSc & GNM Nursing Students)
Indarjit Walia
978-81-23927-04-6
1/e, 2017-18

MRP: ₹325/-

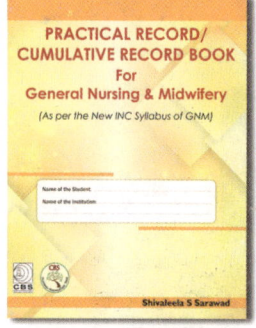

Practical Record/Cumulative Record Book
for General Nursing & Midwifery
Shivaleela S Sarawad
978-93-86827-03-6
1/e, 2018

MRP: ₹225/-

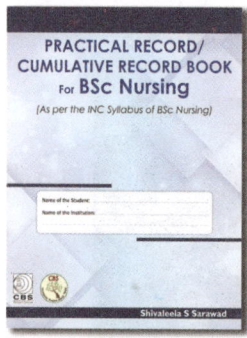

Practical Record/Cumulative Record Book
for BSc Nursing
Shivaleela S Sarawad
978-93-86827-01-2
1/e, 2017

MRP: ₹210/-

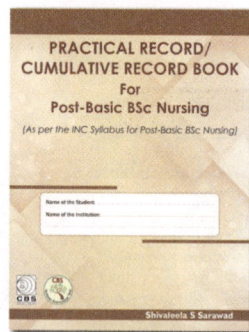

Practical Record/Cumulative Record Book
for Post-Basic BSc Nursing
Shivaleela S Sarawad
978-93-86827-02-9
1/e, 2018

MRP: ₹225/-

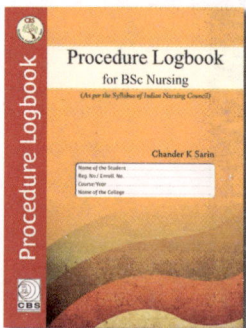

Procedure Logbook
for BSc Nursing
Chander K Sarin
978-93-86310-46-0
1/e, 2017

MRP: ₹210/-

Read, Review & Buy

Now, buying CBS Nursing Books is extra convenient with **Nursing Next Live** Mobile App.

Get a Glimpse of **Sample Pages and TOC** before you proceed to buy books.

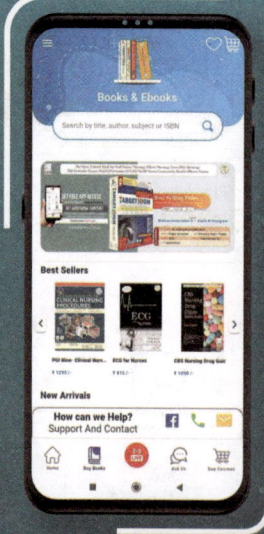

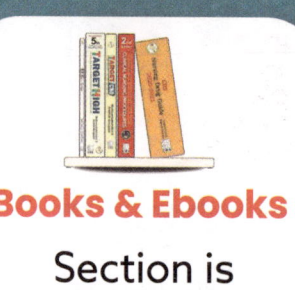

Books & Ebooks

Section is **Live** Now

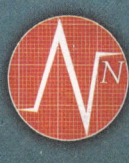

Best Discounts & Special Offers on all the Books.

KUHS Series (Kerala University of Health Sciences)

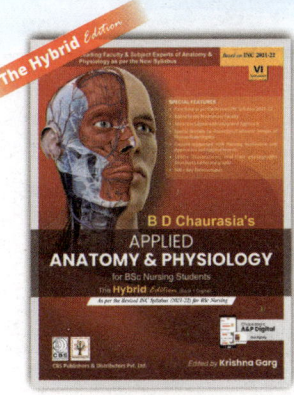

BD Chaurasia's
Applied Anatomy and Physiology
for BSc Nursing Students
Krishna Garg
978-93-90619-65-8
1/e, 2022

TBA

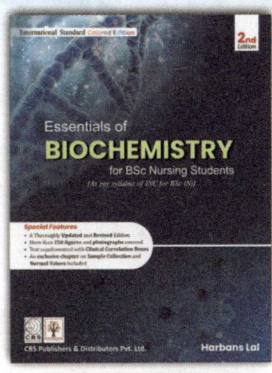

Essentials of Biochemistry
for BSc Nursing Students (As per KUHS)
Harbans Lal
978-81-948693-3-7
2/e, 2022

MRP: ₹450/-

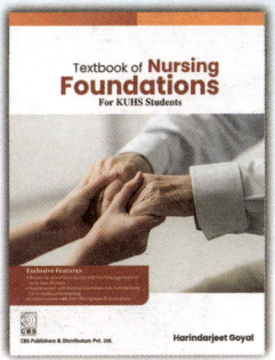

Textbook of
Nursing Foundations
for BSc Nursing (As per KUHS)
Harindarjeet Goyal
978-93-90619-38-2
1/e, 2022

MRP: ₹950/-

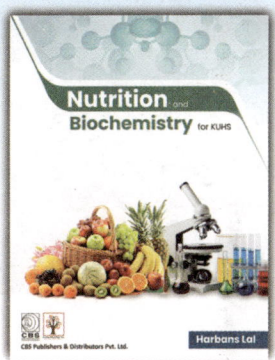

Textbook of
Nutrition & Biochemistry
for BSc Nursing (As per KUHS)
Harbans Lal
978-93-90619-32-0
1/e, 2022

MRP: ₹450/-

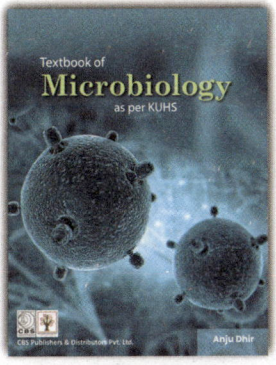

Textbook of
Microbiology
for BSc Nursing (As per KUHS)
Anju Dhir
978-93-90619-49-8
1/e, 2022

MRP: ₹725/-

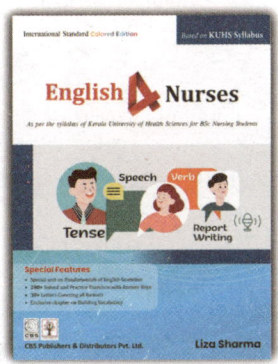

English 4 Nurses
for BSc Nursing (As per KUHS)
Liza Sharma
978-93-90619-33-7
1/e, 2022

MRP: ₹495/-

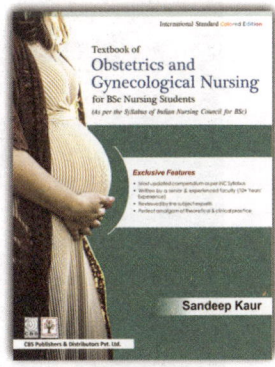

Textbook of
Obstetrics & Gynecological Nursing
for BSc Nursing (As per KUHS)
Sandeep Kaur
978-93-90619-48-1
1/e, 2022

MRP: ₹895/-

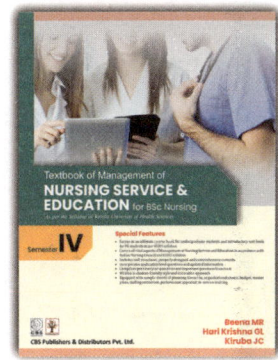

Textbook of
Nursing Management
for BSc Nursing (As per KUHS)
Hari Krishna GL et al.
978-93-90619-39-9
1/e, 2022

MRP: ₹695/-

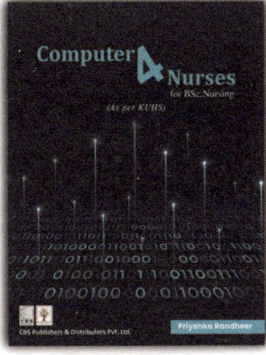

Computer 4 Nurses
for BSc Nursing (As per KUHS)
Priyanka Randheer
978-93-90619-62-7
1/e, 2022

MRP: ₹370/-

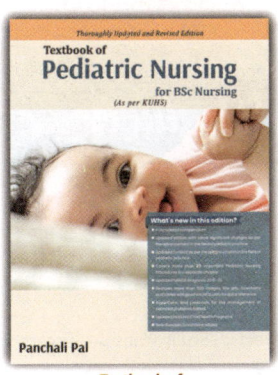

Textbook of
Pediatric Nursing
for BSc Nursing (As per KUHS)
Panchali Pal
978-93-90619-80-1
1/e, 2022

MRP: ₹795/-

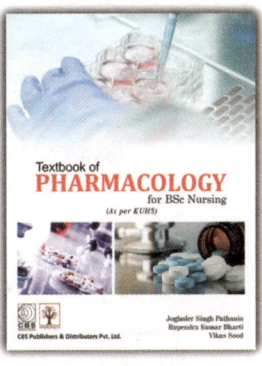

Textbook of
Pharmacology
for BSc Nursing (As per KUHS)
Joginder Singh Pathania et al.
978-93-90619-28-3
1/e, 2022

MRP: ₹650/-

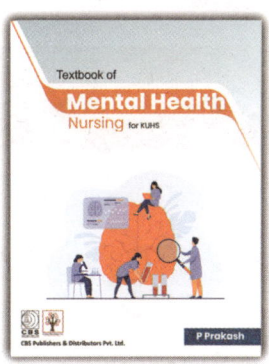

Textbook of
Mental Health Nursing
for BSc Nursing (As per KUHS)
P Prakash
978-93-90619-81-8
1/e, 2022

MRP: ₹625/-

Nursing Knowledge Tree

NURSING NEXT SOCIAL

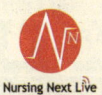
Nursing Next Live

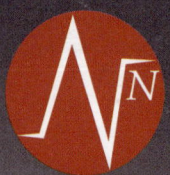
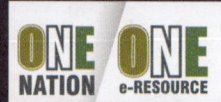
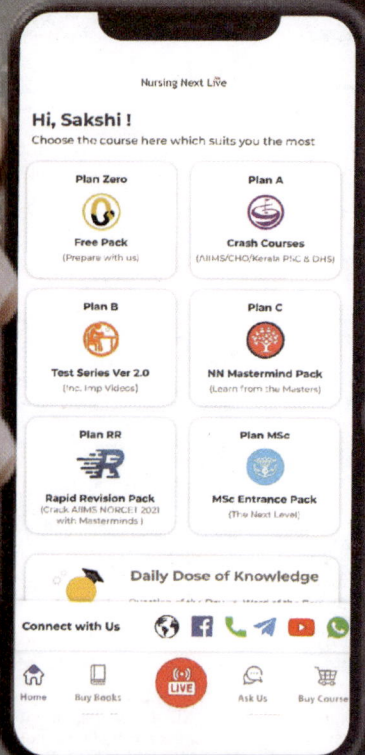

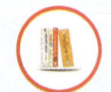

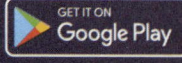
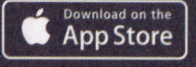